Synopsis of
PATHOLOGY

Synopsis of PATHOLOGY

(William Arnold Douglas)

W. A. D. ANDERSON, M.A., M.D., F.A.C.P., F.C.A.P., F.R.C.P.A. (Hon.)

Professor Emeritus of Pathology and formerly
Chairman, Department of Pathology,
University of Miami School of Medicine, Miami, Florida

THOMAS M. SCOTTI, A.B., M.D.

Adjunct Professor, Department of Pathology,
University of North Carolina School of Medicine,
Chapel Hill, North Carolina; formerly Professor of Pathology,
University of Miami School of Medicine, Miami, Florida

TENTH EDITION

With 506 illustrations

The C. V. Mosby Company

ST. LOUIS • TORONTO • LONDON   1980

TENTH EDITION

The C. V. Mosby Company
11830 Westline Industrial Drive, St. Louis, Missouri 63141

Library of Congress Cataloging in Publication Data

Anderson, William Arnold Douglas, 1910-
  Synopsis of pathology.

  Bibliography: p.
  Includes index.
  1. Pathology. I. Scotti, Thomas M., 1917-
joint author. II. Title. [DNLM: 1. Pathology.
QZ4 A552s]
RB111.A5 1980   616.07   80-13985
ISBN 0-8016-0231-9

C/VH/VH 9 8 7 6 5 4 3 2   01/B/008

To

Our wives and children

Preface

Synopsis of Pathology has been in print since 1942, when the first edition appeared. The favorable reception of the book during these years is truly gratifying. We are pleased also that the translation of previous editions into several languages has permitted wider distribution and usage. The comments and helpful criticisms that have been received from students, pathologists, and others are greatly valued and have furnished us with useful ideas for some of the changes in the revisions.

In the present edition we have not departed from our original purpose of presenting a concise but comprehensive view of pathology. The basic plan and structure of the text remain essentially the same, although for this revision all chapters received attention and required some changes. Several sections were rewritten, and some subjects were enlarged as seemed advisable because of relative importance, current interest, or recent new information. A major consideration has been to up-date the book as much as was feasible. Several diseases and syndromes that have been recognized recently were added to the text. It is our hope that the user of this book will be aware of the constantly expanding and changing knowledge of disease but will understand as well the basic foundation of knowledge on which the advances are built.

This presentation is designed to be useful to medical students, to other students studying general pathology, to clinicians and resident physicians who must maintain familiarity with fundamental sciences of medical practice, and to others in the medical and paramedical fields who need basic knowledge of disease processes.

We wish to thank those who have submitted comments, suggestions, or criticisms and to express our gratitude to the publishers for their continued interest and cooperation and for their helpfulness throughout all phases of this revision.

W. A. D. Anderson
Thomas M. Scotti

Contents

Synopsis of
PATHOLOGY

1

Cell injury and genetic disorders

The basic concepts concerning cells are as follows:

1 Cells are the fundamental morphologic and functional units of the body.
2 All tissues are composed of cells and products of cells.
3 All cells are derived from preexisting cells—i.e., *omnis cellula e cellula* (aphorism of Rudolph Virchow, 1859).

Developments in cell biology have advanced at a rapid rate in recent years, largely because of the progress that has been made in instrumental analysis (including electron microscopy and x-ray diffraction techniques) and the integration of cytology with other fields of biologic research (e.g., genetics, physiology, and biochemistry). As a result, new fields of study have come into being: *submicroscopic morphology* (ultrastructure), *molecular biology, cytogenetics, cell physiology,* and *cytochemistry*.

STRUCTURE AND FUNCTION OF CELLS

Cells vary in size and shape, but they have a number of characteristics in common (Fig. 1-1). Each cell consists of a mass of *cytoplasm* and a *nucleus*. Surrounding the cell is a very thin *plasma membrane (plasmalemma)*, composed chiefly of lipids and protein, through which the exchange of materials takes place between the cell and its environment. The limiting membrane may be simple and smooth, or it may be a complex structure adapted to spe-

cial functions of cells. For example, the numerous minute folds (microvilli) in the plasma membrane of epithelial cells in the intestine, renal tubules, and bile canaliculi increase the effective absorptive or secretory surface. Permeability of the cell membrane, one of its major functions, includes not only the process of diffusion or "passive transport" (in relation to water and certain solutes) but also the mechanism of "active transport" (as in the exchange of ions), which involves energy originating in the cell's own metabolism. Some substances are brought into the cell by *pinocytosis* (Gr. *pinein,* to drink). In this process, the plasma membrane encircles fluid droplets in the environment (e.g., solutions of protein, glucose, hormones). It then invaginates into the cell and becomes pinched off, so that the fluids can be incorporated into the cytoplasm. For the induction of pinocytosis, certain substances other than water must be present in the environment—viz., certain amino acids, proteins, and salts. Carbohydrates and nucleic acid do not induce the process. Pinocytosis is somewhat like *phagocytosis* (Gr. *phagein,* to eat), a process whereby solid particles are ingested by a cell (p. 61).

There exists on the external surface of the plasma membrane of almost all cells a thin layer of carbohydrate-rich material ("surface coat," "cell coat," or "glycocalyx") that probably is derived from the cell it coats. This surface material may have immunologic or filtration properties or may help in the mainte-

1

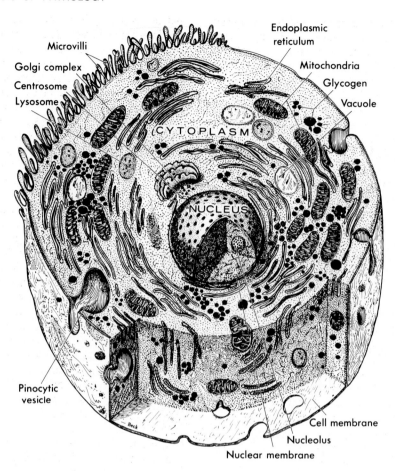

Microvilli

Golgi complex

Centrosome

Lysosome

Endoplasmic
reticulum

Mitochondria

Glycogen

Vacuole

CYTOPLASM

NUCLEUS

Pinocytic
vesicle

Cell membrane

Nucleolus

Nuclear membrane

Fig. 1-1. Diagram of a typical cell based on electron microscopic appearances. (From Anthony, C. P., and Kolthoff, N. J.: Textbook of anatomy and physiology, ed. 9, St. Louis, 1975, The C. V. Mosby Co.)

nance of the microenvironment of the cell. It is not known to what extent it acts as an "intercellular cement," although it has been suggested that it may play some role in maintaining cohesion of cells in tissues. Certain structural modifications appear in plasma membranes, particularly in epithelial cells, which apparently serve to hold cells together. On the lateral surfaces of some cells, there are membranous folds that permit interdigitation of adjacent cells. Specialized areas or zones,

referred to as *junctional complexes,* are present along lateral cellular surfaces in many types of epithelium, appearing usually in the following order in an apical-basal direction: *tight junction (zonula occludens), intermediate junction (zonula adherens),* and *desmosome (macula adherens).* At the *tight junction* the membranes of adjacent cells are closely apposed and possibly fused along their outer aspects, so that the intercellular space is obliterated. At the *intermediate junction* there is a distinct intercellular space, and the cytoplasm adjacent to the inner layer of the cell membrane contains a dense accumulation of filaments arranged parallel to this zone. At the *desmosome,* characterized as a plaquelike or buttonlike area, there is also an intercellular space, but this space contains an electron dense material. In this area the cell membrane appears thickened as fine cytoplasmic filaments *(tonofilaments)* converge on the cell membrane.

The plasma membrane connects with a membranous cytoplasmic network of tubules and vesicles, the *endoplasmic reticulum,* that courses throughout the cytoplasm to the nuclear membrane. Some of the cytoplasmic membranes are rough or granular *(ergastoplasm)* because of the attachment of dense granules to their outer surface. These granules, known as *ribosomes,* are present also in the cytoplasmic matrix outside the membrane system. They are composed of protein and ribonucleic acid (RNA) and serve as the centers for the synthesis of proteins (including enzymes, the accelerators of chemical reactions within the cell). The cytoplasmic ribosomes tend to form aggregates, referred to as *polyribosomes* or simply *polysomes.* The ribosomes are responsible for the basophilic properties of cytoplasm. The rest of the endoplasmic reticulum is of the smooth-surfaced variety without a granular component.

The *Golgi apparatus (complex)* is generally considered to be a part of the agranular endoplasmic reticulum, although some investigators regard it as a separate membranous structure. It apparently is involved in the secretory activities of a cell, probably serving as a site where the products of secretion elaborated elsewhere in the cell are concentrated into granules or droplets prior to their liberation from the cell. The Golgi apparatus in developing spermatids participates in the formation of the *acrosome.*

Lysosomes are varying-sized, single membrane–enveloped intracytoplasmic bodies that contain hydrolytic enzymes and have a high content of acid phosphatase. Lysosomes are most numerous in phagocytes (macrophages and neutrophils), liver cells, and cells of the proximal convoluted tubules of the kidney, but they are also seen in all-other cells, except erythrocytes. The lysosomal enzymes are involved in the intracellular digestion of material derived from outside the cell (by means of endocytosis) or of parts of a living cell's own cytoplasm *(cellular autophagy)* and in the digestion of a cell after its death *(autolysis).* It is also possible that certain cells may release lysosomal enzymes to produce lytic effects on surrounding structures, as in the removal of bone by osteoclasts.

Lysosomes are classified as primary or secondary. In *primary lysosomes* (also called *storage vacuoles),* which are newly formed, the digestive enzymes are in an inactive state. The enzymes are first formed in the granular endoplasmic reticulum and then pass to the Golgi complex, where they are packaged into the primary lysosomes, after which the latter are released to the cytoplasmic matrix. Digestive vacuoles and autophagic vacuoles are *secondary lysosomes,* which are formed by fusion of primary lysosomes with other membrane-enveloped bodies. For example, during phagocytosis an endocytic vesicle containing ingested material (i.e., a *phagosome)* is fused with a primary lysosome, resulting in a *digestive vacuole* or *phagolysosome,* in which degradation of the ingested material occurs. A primary lysosome may also fuse with an intracytoplasmic, membrane-enveloped body containing one or more organelles of the cell itself, forming an *autophagic vacuole (autolysosome* or *cytolysosome).* This process is referred to as *cellular autophagy,* a type of intracellular digestion (sometimes referred to as "focal autolysis") in which a focus of cytoplasmic degradation occurs during the normal course of organelle turnover or as a result of cellular injury. After enzymatic action in a secondary lysosome, the material that is not returned to the cytoplasm for further use by the cell remains in an incompletely digested form and appears as membrane-enveloped debris known as a *residual body.* The latter may fuse with the plasma membrane and be discharged from the cell, a process that is essentially the reverse of the endocytic processes, pinocytosis and phagocytosis, i.e., *exocytosis*. Membrane-bound *peroxisomes* or *microbodies,* which are observed in renal and hepatic cells and contain catalase and oxidases, bear some similarity to lysosomes. The exact role of peroxisomes has not been determined, although it has been suggested that participation in lipid and carbohydrate metabolism may be one of their functions.

There are genetic disorders in which a deficiency of certain lysosomal enzymes results in an overloading of the lysosomes by material that cannot be hydrolyzed because of the enzyme defect *(lysosomal storage diseases)*. Some of these disorders are discussed elsewhere in this book, including *Pompe's, Tay-Sachs, Gaucher's,* and *Niemann-Pick diseases* and *Hunter's* and *Hurler's syndromes.* Another genetic disorder is characterized by giant lysosomes in phagocytes, as in the *Chédiak-Higashi syndrome,* which is also discussed later.

Mitochondria are granular, rodlike, or filamentous cytoplasmic organelles. Each mitochondrion is limited by a double (outer and inner) membrane. The inner membrane forms a series of complex infoldings (crests or cristae) that project into the mitochondrial cavity and are responsible for the characteristic striated appearance of the organelles. The inner cavity contains a granular matrix. The mitochondria are the main "power plants" of the cell that supply the energy for it metabolic functions, the generation of energy being provided by the various intramitochondrial enzyme systems. The mitochondria are one of the major sources of adenosine triphosphate (ATP) in the cell. The mitochondrial membrane seems to be selectively permeable, so that the mitochondria swell or shrink as a result of chemical or osmotic changes in the cytoplasmic medium. Various *mitochondrial inclusions* may occur in cells that have been injured. Enlarged mitochondria *(megamitochondria)* with crystalline or paracrystalline inclusions have been described in liver cells in persons with or without hepatic diseases.

Microtubules and *microfilaments* are cytoplasmic organelles that are composed of protein molecules and participate in different cellular processes. They apparently are involved in the maintenance of cell shape and cell movement and possibly in the transport of material within the cytoplasm. In a sense, they serve as the cellular cytoskeleton. Microtubules play a role in the motility of cilia and make up the mitotic spindle in dividing cells. Colchicine inhibits cell division by disrupting microtubule function. *Neurotubules* are the microtubules in cell bodies and axons of neurons. Microfilaments in voluntary and cardiac muscle are identified as *actin* and *myosin,* and in other cells they resemble actin. In certain cells, they form the *terminal web* beneath the plasma membrane. Bundles of microfilaments converge in the desmosomes as *tonofilaments.* Some investigators have suggested that a defect in formation of microtubules and microfilaments in leukocytes impairs the chemotactic response of these cells in inflammation (p. 63).

The *centrosome,* within which are two small granules called the *centrioles,* usually occupies the geometric center of the cell near the nucleus and is in close relationship to the Golgi complex. During cell division, two pairs of centrioles and surrounding astral rays appear. The pairs separate and become situated at the poles of the mitotic spindle. After mitosis, each daughter cell receives two centrioles.

The *cytoplasmic matrix,* or *cytosol,* in which are embedded the various organelles previously mentioned, is a clear homogeneous substance with colloidal properties, such as those related to sol-gel transformations, viscosity changes, ameboid movements, spindle formation, and cell cleavage. In certain specialized cells, the cytoplasmic matrix is the site of differentiation of fibrillar structures (e.g., keratin fibers, myofibrils, and neurotubules). Much of the cytoplasmic matrix consists of water that contains electrolytes, soluble proteins and enzymes, lipids, carbohydrates, and soluble (transfer) RNA. Visible particles in the cytoplasm, other than the organelles, are called *inclusions* and comprise such structures as secretion granules, stored substances (lipids, glycogen), and various pigments.

The *nucleus* is the most conspicuous structure in a cell. It is present in all cells, although it disappears in the late stages of development of the human erythrocyte. Its size and shape vary in different cells. Generally, it is spherical or ovoid, but it may be indented or lobulated. Usually a single nucleus is present, but a few cells are binucleated (e.g., some plasma cells) or multinucleated (e.g., osteoclasts). The position of the nucleus in the cell is variable, being centrally or eccentrically located. As a rule, its position is constant for a given type of cell.

The nucleus serves as the control and regulating center of most of the cell's activities and plays a fundamental role in cell division and heredity. The nucleus of a living cell is not clearly visible microscopically unless phase contrast microscopy is used, by which technique only the nuclear membrane and one or two nucleoli are observed in the interphase (nondividing) stage. The details of nuclear structure are best seen in fixed cells by means of routine staining procedures, by histochemical techniques, and especially by electron microscopy (Fig. 1-2). The basic constituents are a *nuclear envelope,* filaments and granules of *chromatin* (considered to be the interphase form of chromosomes), one or more *nucleoli,* and the *nucleoplasm,* or *nuclear sap.* The latter, like the cytoplasm, is of a colloidal nature, being composed of water, electrolytes, protein (including enzymes), lipids, and carbohydrates. The nuclear envelope is a double membrane system that encloses a perinuclear space. Polyribosomes are attached to the outer membrane, whereas chromatin is closely associated with the inner membrane. At various sites, the outer and inner membranes blend together to form nuclear pores, which contain nonmembranous granular and filamentous material *(pore complex).* Ringlike material that lies on the outer and inner margins of a pore is known as the *annulus.* The nuclear pores may be one means by which certain material may be transferred from the nucleoplasm to the cytoplasm. The most important chemical constituent in the nucleus is nucleic acid, of which there are two types: deoxyribonucleic acid (DNA) and ribonucleic acid (RNA). DNA is the more abundant, being present mainly in the chromatin. RNA is concentrated mostly in the nucleolus in the form of loosely bound, ribosomelike granules and also is found in small amounts in the chromatin. DNA, the essential component of genetic material, controls or directs protein synthesis within a cell, whereas RNA is concerned with the actual synthesis of protein.

In a high percentage of cells in females, a prominent mass of chromatin is found next to the nuclear membrane in interphase nuclei. This structure, known as the *X chromatin* or *Barr body,* is present in persons with two or more X chromosomes. In fact, more than one Barr body may be present (the number of bodies is usually one less than the number of X chromosomes). The term *sex chromatin* was previously used as a synonym for the Barr body before a sex chromatin mass was identified in the cells of males. The sex chromatin observed in a high proportion of males is referred to as the *Y chromatin* or *Y body.* It is smaller than the Barr body and requires a special fluorescent method for identification; thus, it is sometimes called the *fluorescent* (or *F) body.* It occurs as a single body in XY males, but there may be 2 Y bodies in XYY and XXYY males.

CELLULAR INJURY

Various techniques of investigating cells, such as electron microscopy, ultracentrifugation, and cytochemistry, have increased our knowledge of the changes occurring in cells as a result of injury, which may be caused by many types of agents, including ischemia or hypoxia, hyperoxia, chemicals and drugs, radiant energy, heat, cold, nutritional disturbances, bacteria and their products, and immune complexes. The injury may be *nonlethal,* resulting in reversible cellular changes (e.g., degenerations), or *lethal,* with the outcome being death of the cell.

In some nonlethal injuries, the *cells may*

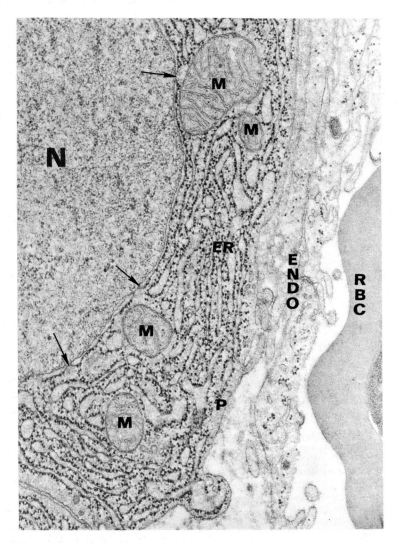

Fig. 1-2. Electron micrograph of pancreatic acinar cell showing nucleus, cytoplasmic organelles, and adjacent capillary. Nucleus, *N,* is surrounded by double-layered nuclear envelope with pores (arrows). Endoplasmic reticulum, *ER,* is of rough type (with attachment of ribosomes). Mitochondria, *M,* vary in size and show characteristic internal membranes (cristae). Next to edge of cell, *P,* are capillary endothelium, *ENDO,* and a red blood cell, *RBC,* in capillary lumen. (×52,500; courtesy Dr. D. R. Anderson.)

appear normal morphologically by the existing methods of examination, as in certain biochemical disturbances or genetic mutations, or there may be only minimal ultrastructural changes, such as an *increase in the number of autophagic vacuoles,* which is evidence of ac-

celerated focal cytoplasmic degradation. In other nonlethal injuries there may be more obvious changes that are characteristic of the reversible *retrograde cellular processes* or *degenerations,* the details of which are described in Chapter 2. Alterations in specific components (organelles) of the cell may readily be seen in the early stages of development of these pathologic processes. It is generally believed that damage begins in the endoplasmic reticulum and/or the mitochondria. Among the early ultrastructural and biochemical alterations that may occur are the following:

1 Loss of granules in the mitochondrial matrix, followed by swelling of the mitochondria and clearness of their matrix
2 Vesicular distention of the endoplasmic reticulum, which in some instances may result in formation of large cytoplasmic vesicles
3 Depletion of RNA granules with loss of cell basophilia
4 Decrease in cytoplasmic glycogen
5 Reduction of enzymes such as adenosine triphosphatase (ATPase) and succinodehydrogenase
6 Appearance of lipid droplets in vesicles of the endoplasmic reticulum and in the cytoplasmic matrix
7 Also, in certain nonlethal injuries, intracytoplasmic, multilaminated, whorled membranous structures (''whorls,'' ''myelin figures,'' or ''myeloid bodies'') as well as an increased number of autophagic vacuoles

As a result of the damage to the mitochondria and the endoplasmic reticulum and the subsequent changes in the enzymatic reactions within them, certain functional derangements may occur in the cell, including alterations in the ''active transport'' mechanism and cell membrane permeability (with changes in water and electrolyte content) and disturbances in the metabolism of protein, fat, and carbohydrate. Thus may be explained, at least in part, such pathologic processes as *cellular (cloudy) swelling, hydropic degeneration, hyaline degeneration,* and *fatty metamorphosis.*

When cells in a living body are exposed to lethal injury, the damage is such that it results in death of the cells. After cell death, certain intracellular and extracellular enzymes cause nuclear and cytoplasmic changes that are visible under the light microscope. These structural alterations, which represent the histologic criteria of the process known as *necrosis,* are evident mainly in the nucleus (i.e., pyknosis, karyorrhexis, and karyolysis), but cytoplasmic changes such as coagulation of proteins, cytolysis, and contraction of cells may also be seen. In a normal piece of tissue that has been killed instantly by immersion in a fixative, the cell structure may remain apparently unaltered because of the sudden cessation of all enzymatic activity. Necrosis, which is a form of acute death of cells in the living body, is commonly differentiated from the process *necrobiosis.* The latter refers to the slow gradual death of cells that occurs as part of the constant turnover of cells in certain tissues (e.g., skin) after the cells have passed through a period of ''senescence.''

In contrast to the degenerative cellular changes, from which the cells may recover, the structural alterations in cells following lethal injury are irreversible. Formerly, it was believed that rupture of lysosomes with release of their destructive enzymes was responsible for death of a cell. However, now it is apparent that the lysosomal membranes are intact at the time when irreversible changes have already occurred, but there may be some leakage of lysosomal enzymes because of increased permeability of their membranes. Rupture of lysosomes occurs late in the process of necrosis. Although recognition of necrotic cells under the light microscope is based chiefly on the prominent nuclear changes, submicroscopic morphologic alterations may be demonstrated in cytoplasmic organelles (particularly mitochondria and ergastoplasm) even before modifications in the nucleus become evident. The ultrastructural changes in lethal injury may at first be similar to those described previously as early manifestations of cell injury, including the presence of ''myelin figures'' and an increased number of autophagic vacuoles, some of which may be gigantic. Subsequently, the following may be seen:

1 Severe swelling of mitochondria, disappearance or disruption of cristae, formation of dense particles in matrix occasionally calcium deposits

2 Vesiculation, distortion, and fragmentation of mitochondrial membranes
3 Breakdown of endoplasmic reticulum, loss and dissociation of polysomes
4 Alteration of plasma membrane
5 Distortion of microvilli, disruption of cell junctions
6 Clumping of nuclear chromatin, disruption and dissolution of nucleolus, irregularity of nuclear membrane
7 Formation of intranuclear and intracytoplasmic blebs and vacuoles
8 Rupture and contraction of cell

THE CELL IN GENETICS

Nuclear DNA is responsible for transmission of hereditary characteristics. The genetic information that is transmitted from generation to generation is coded in the DNA of the *genes,* the hereditary units of the chromosomes. The sequence of purine and pyrimidine bases in the DNA molecule forms the genetic code. Prior to cell division, DNA is able to replicate itself accurately so as to ensure the integrity of the genetic information during its transmission to future cells or generations. The DNA, through its genetic code, determines the biochemical processes of the cell by it control of protein synthesis. It dictates the specific sequence in which amino acids are incorporated into the polypeptides that combine to form structural proteins and enzymes. This information is transcribed to ''messenger'' RNA (formed in the nucleus upon a template or cast of DNA) and is carried by the RNA to the site of protein synthesis in the cytoplasm, the ribosomes.

The usually stable genetic and structural organization of chromosomes may be altered spontaneously, without apparent cause, or may be affected by injurious agents (e.g., ionizing radiation, chemicals, infections), resulting in two types of chromosomal changes: (1) a change at the molecular level in the genetic material, occurring at definite points in the chromosome and usually involving individual gene loci without detectable microscopic alterations of the chromosomes (so-called *point mutation,* or *gene mutation*), and (2) micro-scopically recognizable *chromosomal aberrations,* consisting of abnormalities of number or structure. The study of the microscopic appearance of chromosomes and their behavior during cell division is referred to as *cytogenetics.* The genetic makeup of an individual is called the *genotype,* and the expression of the genetic constitution (physical, physiologic, and biochemical traits) is called the *phenotype.*

Point mutation. In point mutation there is a loss or change of function of a gene, caused by a defect in the DNA, that may lead to formation of an abnormal enzyme or other type of protein or be responsible for lack of production of certain enzymes. Examples of diseases characterized by such biochemical genetic disturbances are the *hemoglobinopathies* (e.g., sickle cell disease), in which abnormal hemoglobins are produced by mutations in the genes controlling the formation of the globin portion of the hemoglobin molecule, and *inborn errors of metabolism,* in which deficiency of a specific enzyme is evident (e.g., alkaptonuria, phenylketonuria, glycogen storage diseases, galactosemia, cystinuria, homocystinuria, Wilson's hepatolenticular degeneration, and many others).

Chromosomal aberrations. Chromosomal aberrations characterized by alterations in number or structure of chromosomes are known to occur in association with a variety of disorders. Before reference is made to some of the abnormalities, however, it should be recalled that normally each sex cell, or gamete, contributes 23 chromosomes to the fertilized ovum—22 autosomes and a Y or an X chromosome; the sperm contributes either a Y or an X chromosome and the ovum only an X chromosome. Each cell of a normal person, except for the gametes, contains 46 chromosomes—22 pairs of homologous autosomes and a pair of sex chromosomes (XX in females, XY in males).

Chromosomal aberrations affect both autosomal and sex chromosomes. The frequency of chromosomal abnormalities among unselected infants born alive is about 0.5%. In a recent survey, chromosomal abnormalities were noted in 5.6% of unselected infants dying in the perinatal period. The frequency was 13% among infants with malformations (stillbirths and neonatal) and 2.5% among infants dying from other causes. In studies of spontaneous abortions during the early phases of pregnancy, chromosomal abnormalities are found usually in about 35% of the fetuses. In the surviving patients with alterations of chromosomes, structural anomalies and abnormal function of many organs are frequently associated. Mental retardation commonly occurs in clinical disorders associated with chromosomal abnormalities, especially in those with autosomal anomalies. In general, autosomal defects are associated with more severe physical and mental disturbances than sex chromosome abnormalities.

Chromosome analysis. Chromosomes are usually studied in cells that are grown in tissue cultures, either leukocytes obtained from the blood (Fig. 1-3) or cells derived from a small specimen of living tissue. Even amniotic fluid cells obtained from pregnant women by amniocentesis have been studied successfully for detection of genetic disorders in the fetus. The dividing cells are treated with colchicine, which halts them at the metaphase; then a hypotonic salt solution is added to cause swelling of the nuclei and separation of the chromatids, with the centromeres left intact. After the cells are fixed, placed on slides, stained and examined microscopically, a photograph is made and enlarged. Each chromosome is cut out of the picture, arranged in pairs, and classified into seven groups (A through G) on the basis of size of chromosomes and position of the centromere, and each pair of autosomal chromosomes is numbered in the order of decreasing size. The X chromosome (resembling those of the C6-C12 group, especially chromosome 6) and the Y chromosome (similar to the G21-G22 chromosomes) are not numbered. This systematic arrangement of the photographs of the chromosomes is referred to as the *karyotype* (Fig. 1-4). (The word *idiogram* is sometimes used synonymously, but strictly used, this term applies to a diagrammatic representation of a karyotype.)

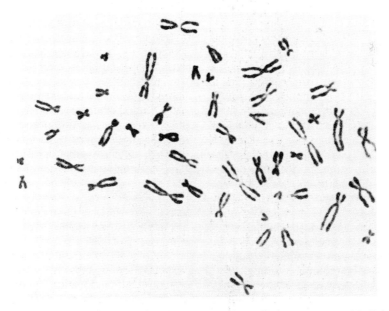

Fig. 1-3. Metaphase of cultured, normal, blood leukocyte from female subject with diploid number of chromosomes (2n = 46). (From Sandberg, A. A.: CA **15**:2-13, 1965.)

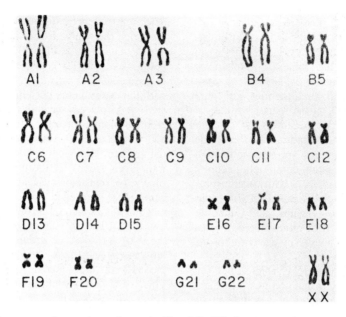

Fig. 1-4. Karyotype of metaphase shown in Fig. 1-3. B5 chromosomes are somewhat shorter, relative to B4 chromosomes, than usual. (From Sandberg, A. A.: CA **15**:2-13, 1965.)

A standardized system for describing the karyotype was proposed at a conference in Chicago in 1966 and modified at another conference in Paris in 1971. A supplement to the Paris conference was issued in 1975. By means of symbols, the total number of chromosomes, the sex chromosome complement, and the description of the anomaly are noted. A plus or minus sign placed before a chromosome letter or number indicates additional or missing whole chromosomes. A plus or minus sign placed after a symbol designating the short or long arm expresses increase or decrease in length of the arm, the letter "p" representing the short arm and "q" the long arm. For example, 47,XY,+G is a male karyotype with 47 chromosomes, including an additional G-group chromosome; 45,XY,−21 is a male karyotype with 45 chromosomes and missing one chromosome number 21; 48,XXY,+G is a karyotype with 48 chromosomes, including XXY sex chromosomes and an additional G-group chromosome; 47,XY,+14p+ is a male karyotype with 47

chromosomes, including an additional number 14 chromosome with an increase in length of its short arm; and 46,XX,18q− is a female karyotype with 46 chromosomes and a number 18 chromosome lacking part or all of its long arm. Translocation is indicated by the letter "t" followed by parentheses, which include the chromosomes involved. The letter "i" placed after the chromosome arm involved indicates an isochromosome. An "r" placed after a chromosome indicates a ring chromosome. Other symbols are used to express the remaining types of chromosomal anomalies.

In the preparation of karyotypes by the conventional means, it is sometimes difficult to distinguish between chromosome pairs in the various groups. The use of autoradiography has permitted distinctions in some but not all groups. New chromosome staining techniques, such as quinacrine fluorescent and Giemsa methods, demonstrate structural details (e.g., banded regions on chromosomes) that are characteristic for each chromosome.

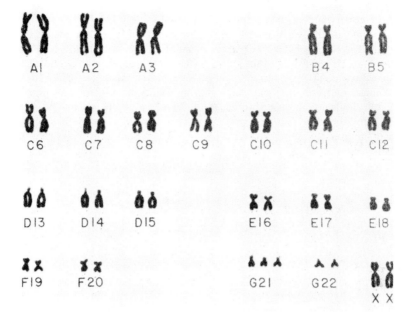

Fig. 1-5. Karyotype from female patient with mongolism (Down's syndrome). Note trisomy (extra chromosome) in Group G21. (From Sandberg, A. A.: CA **15:**2-13, 1965.)

These methods not only permit easier identification of chromosomes but also increase the information that may be obtained by study of individual chromosomes.

Some investigators have successfully used certain "direct" fixation methods of studying freshly aspirated bone marrow that do not require in vitro cell culture, particularly in patients with leukemia. Others have used automated computer systems to analyze chromosomes.

Alterations in number. An abnormal number of chromosomes may result from *nondisjunction* in meiosis—a failure of the usual separation of two chromosomes of a pair, so that one daughter cell receives both and the other daughter cell receives neither chromosome of the pair. A gamete with an extra chromosome (24 chromosomes) fertilizing a normal gamete (23 chromosomes) results in a trisomic zygote. Such an abnormality is seen in *mongolism* (Down's syndrome), in which there is a *trisomy* of one of the autosomal chromosomes, number 21 (Fig. 1-5), with the result that

there is a total of 47 chromosomes in that individual. Trisomies may involve other autosomal chromosomes, e.g., the E and D groups. They may also be noted in certain abnormalities of the sex chromosomes, as in *Klinefelter's syndrome* (47,XXY), in the *triple X syndrome* (47,XXX), and in males with an extra Y (the *XYY syndrome*). When only one chromosome is present instead of the usual pair, the abnormality is referred to as a *monosomy.* For example, in the monosomic state known as *Turner's syndrome,* only one sex chromosome, an X, exists. Monosomes with only a Y chromosome are not known to occur. In some sex chromosomal aberrations, the individual may have more than one extra chromosome, as in variants of *Klinefelter's syndrome* (48,XXXY or XXYY, etc.) and in some multi-X females (48,XXXX). Another type of chromosomal abnormality that may occur is *mosaicism,* i.e., the presence in the same individual of cells that differ in their chromosomal constitution. This defect apparently arises during mitosis after fertilization, perhaps as a result of nondisjunction or complete loss of a chromosome in the early stages of growth of the zygote.

DOWN'S SYNDROME. Characteristic features of Down's syndrome include hypotonia, mental retardation, a flat occiput, oblique palpebral fissures, epicanthic folds, flat nasal bridge, speckled irises, protruding tongue, short broad hands with curved little fingers, characteristic dermal pattern of palms, fingers, and soles, and associated cardiovascular anomalies and other congenital abnormalities. Mongoloids have a greater susceptibility to infections and an increased incidence of leukemia compared with nonmongoloids of the same age group. The incidence of Down's syndrome tends to increase in relation to maternal age at the time of birth. Although, as already noted, this syndrome is usually associated with a trisomy 21 karyotype, in a few patients the extra chromosomal material is not arranged as a separate chromosome but is attached to another chromosome, usually number 15 (so-called translocation Down's syndrome). This type of mongolism apparently is not related to maternal age. It may be familial but frequently arises de novo. Patients with translocation Down's syndrome have 46 chromosomes, including the translocation chromosome, and clinical features similar to those with the usual trisomy 21. In another small group of mongoloids, chromosomal analysis reveals cells of two different genotypes (mosaicism) in the same patient, i.e., 47 chromosomes with trisomy 21 in some cells and a normal number of chromosomes (46) in other cells. In these patients, the clinical features may differ from those of the usual Down's syndrome. For example, external mongoloid features may be present, but the patient may have a normal mentality.

TRISOMY E AND D. Other congenital abnormalities with trisomy of autosomal chromosomes have been described (e.g., trisomy of a chromosome of the E group, most likely number 18, and trisomy of one of the D group of chromosomes). External and internal abnormalities are seen characteristically in the E and D trisomies, and death usually occurs early in life. The E(18) trisomy (Fig. 1-6), for example, is characterized by a prominent occiput, micrognathia, low-set eyes and ears (the latter often malformed), flexion of fingers with overlapping (the index on the third finger and the fifth on the fourth finger), cardiovascular defects, mental deficiency, and death usually by 6 months of age. The D(13 to 15) trisomy is characterized by small, wide-set eyes, cleft palate and lip, polydactyly, retroflexed thumbs (trigger thumbs), microcephaly, capillary hemangiomas, and cardiovascular anomalies, along with other abnormalities.

Sex chromosome abnormalities. A patient with *Klinefelter's syndrome* (seminiferous tubule dysgenesis) is usually a tall phenotypic male who is eunuchoid with small testes, frequently gynecomastia, and sometimes mental retardation. The cells usually have a Barr body (X chromatin) in the nucleus and 47 chromosomes, including 22 pairs of autosomes and two X and one Y sex chromosomes. Some have 48 or 49 chromosomes with a sex chromosome composition of XXXY, XXYY, XXXXY, or XXXYY. Even mosaicism has been identified. For example, some cells may contain XY chromosomes while others contain XXY chromosomes (expressed as XY/XXY). Another mosaic type may be XY/XXXY. The degree of mental retardation appears to be related to the number of X chromosomes in patients with this syndrome.

A patient with *Turner's syndrome* (ovarian dysgenesis) is usually a phenotypic female with amenorrhea, hypoplastic ovaries or absence of ovarian tissue, which is replaced by fibrous tissue, and other physical abnormalities. The chromosomal number is usually 45, one less than normal, with 22 pairs of autosomes and a single X sex chromosome, expressed as XO. The nuclei of the cells are usually negative for Barr bodies (X chromatin). Mosaicism also may be noted (e.g., XO/XY, XO/XX, XO/XXX, or XO/XX/XXX).

Phenotypic females with XXX chromosomes and 22 pairs of autosomes, a total of 47 chromosomes, have been described (*triple X syndrome* or *superfemales*). Usually, two

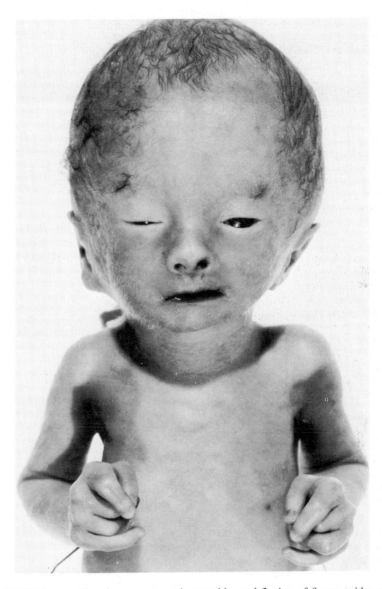

Fig. 1-6. E(18) trisomy. Note low-set ears, micrognathia, and flexion of fingers with overlapping (index on third finger and fifth on fourth finger).

sex chromatin masses can be demonstrated in many of the nuclei of the patients' cells. There may be no striking clinical features except menstrual irregularities and sometimes mental retardation. A few instances of females with 48 chromosomes, including XXXX chromo-somes, have been reported. There have been several reports of males with 47 chromo-somes, including an extra Y chromosome (i.e., an XYY chromosomal complement), who tend to be tall and show behavioral ab-normalities. Although it is generally believed that a correlation exists between XYY and criminal or antisocial impulses, some investigators urge caution in accepting the interpretation that there is a specific association of XYY with criminal behavior.

Aberrations in structure. Certain genetic disorders are characterized by structural aberrations of the chromosomes:

deletion a loss of a portion of a chromosome (when both terminal portions are lost, the broken ends may unite to form a *ring chromosome*)

duplication the presence of an extra piece of a chromosome

inversion the fragmentation of a chromosome, followed by a rejoining of the fragments in such a way that they are inverted or reversed with respect to the rest of the chromosome

translocation the transfer of a portion of one chromosome to a nonhomologous chromosome

isochromosomes abnormal chromosomes resulting from division of the centromere perpendicularly to the long axis of a chromosome rather than parallel to it

An example of deletion involving the short arm of a chromosome of the B group (number 5) is observed in the *cri du chat syndrome,* so called because the affected infant's cry resembles the meowing of a cat. Microcephaly, mental retardation, hypertelorism, prominent epicanthal folds, and low-set ears commonly occur in these patients. The catlike cry and prominent epicanthal folds disappear with aging. Other deletion syndromes associated with microcephaly, mental retardation, hypertelorism, and a variety of malformations have been described, involving chromosomes number 4 (short arm) and number 18 (short or long arm) and one of the D group, 13 to 15, forming a ring chromosome. The Philadelphia chromosome (Ph[1]) observed in the leukocytes of patients with chronic granulocytic leukemia, an abbreviated 21 autosome with its long arms substantially shortened, is another example of deletion (Fig. 1-7). Recently, it has been shown that the material from this chromosome may be translocated to another chromosome, usually one of the number 9 chromosomes. In

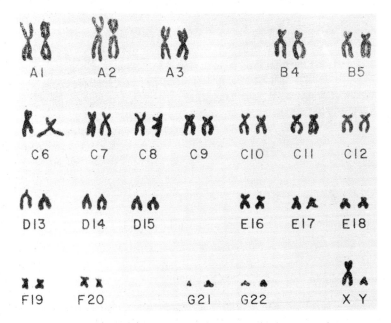

Fig. 1-7. Karyotype from patient with chronic myelocytic (granulocytic) leukemia. Note abbreviated G21 chromosome with long arms substantially shortened—Philadelphia (Ph[1]) chromosome. (From Sandberg, A. A.: CA **15:**2-13, 1965.)

the forms of acute leukemia, aneuploidy (an abnormal number of chromosomes) has been demonstrated in bone marrow cells, particularly when prepared by the "direct" fixation technique. Chromosomal abnormalities, such as breakage with translocation or deletions, including an anomaly similar to the Philadelphia chromosome of leukemia, have been observed in patients who have been using LSD (lysergic acid diethylamide), but in the published reports, there is no general agreement among investigators that LSD or other hallucinogens cause chromosomal damage. Chromosomal aberrations have been detected in cells of neoplasms (p. 264) other than leukemia, as well as in cells of tissues exposed to ionizing radiation.

There are a number of recent reports concerning the association of a familial form of mental retardation in males with a *fragile X* (or *marker X*) *chromosome*. The defect in the chromosome is a fragile site that predisposes to an increased breakage frequency. In some studies, the abnormality has been described as a secondary constriction near the end of the long arms of the X chromosome, presenting the appearance of large satellites.

Recent improvements in cell culture techniques have permitted not only the identification of chromosomal anomalies but also the diagnosis of inborn errors of metabolism and the detection of heterozygous carriers of these disorders. The detection of enzymes in cells cultured from amniotic fluid obtained by amniocentesis has been helpful in establishing the prenatal diagnosis of certain familial metabolic disorders.

INHERITANCE PATTERNS

Inherited disorders resulting from mutant genes are known as *autosomal* or *sex-linked,* depending on whether the affected genes are in the autosomes or in the sex chromosomes. A *dominant* disease is one that is clinically manifest in an individual who has only one mutant gene (a *heterozygous* state). A person with two abnormal dominant genes (a *homozygous* state) would be phenotypically similar to the heterozygote. However, since diseases

related to dominant genes are so uncommon, it is extremely unlikely in practice to encounter such a homozygous individual, because the latter can result only from mating of two affected persons. A *recessive* disease is one that is apparent only in a *homozygous* subject. It is not evident in a heterozygote, but the latter is a carrier of the condition.

The patterns of hereditary transmission are classified according to the classic mendelian categories. A variety of patterns of inheritance have been observed—some simple, others complex. Those readily recognized are the simple patterns produced by rare genes at a single locus that include *autosomal dominant, autosomal recessive, sex-linked dominant,* and *sex-linked recessive*. In almost all of the sex-linked disorders, the mutant gene is on the X chromosome, and this is the entity referred to when the term *sex-linked* is used without qualification. Well-substantiated examples of Y-linked traits are rare, occurring only in males.

Although the concepts of dominance and recessiveness are being presented here according to the simple hereditary patterns, it should be emphasized that some genes are neither strictly dominant nor strictly recessive. Genes may be *codominant* if both alleles of a pair are fully expressed in the heterozygote. In one form of hereditary transmission, a harmful gene occurring alone in an individual (heterozygote) may produce a mild effect, but when two of the genes occur in the same person (homozygote), a greater degree of the abnormality may appear. This is referred to as *intermediate inheritance,* since the heterozygote is not identical to either the normal or the affected homozygote but is intermediate between the two. As an example, patients who are heterozygous for an abnormal hemoglobin may have sickling of the red blood cells but are asymptomatic (sickle cell trait), whereas those who are homozygous develop severe effects, including hemolytic anemia (e.g., sickle cell anemia). It is to be noted, however, that some individuals may refer to the inheritance of this condition differently—that is, as codominant (because the gene for normal hemoglobin and the gene for sickle cell hemoglobin are both present in the heterozygote), as dominant (because the phenotypic feature, sickling of red blood cells, is expressed in the heterozygote), or as recessive (because the phenotypic feature, sickle cell anemia, is expressed only in the homozygote).

In the autosomal forms of inheritance, dominant or recessive, males and females tend to be equally affected. An *autosomal dominant* disorder is transmitted directly from affected person to affected person, appearing in every generation, as a rule, without skips or breaks in continuity. About half of the children of an affected parent will be affected. An *autosomal recessive* disease characteristically appears in siblings whose parents, offspring, and other relatives are usually phenotypically normal. The parents of an affected child are generally both heterozygous carriers. On the average, one out of four children of two heterozygous parents is affected (homozygous). An increase in the occurrence of the recessive condition occurs in consanguineous marriages because of the great proportion of carriers marrying other carriers.

In sex-linked (i.e., X-linked) disorders, whether dominant or recessive, the abnormality is expressed in all males who possess the mutant gene on the X chromosome, since it is not paired with any gene on the essentially genetically inert Y chromosome. Males are neither heterozygous nor homozygous with reference to the X-linked gene but are known as *hemizygous.* Females, on the other hand, are heterozygous or homozygous for a mutant gene since they have two X chromosomes, and the abnormal trait may be manifested as recessive or dominant. The vast majority of X-linked diseases in man are inherited as recessive, whereas only a few X-linked dominant disorders are known.

In *X-linked dominant* states (when mating occurs between an affected and a normal person), the affected (hemizygous) male transmits the disorder to all daughters, not to sons, whereas the affected heterozygous female transmits it to half the offspring, male or female, and the homozygous female transmits it to all her children. In *X-linked recessive* disorders, the mutant gene is expressed by all males who possess it, but females must be homozygous for expression of the abnormality. A heterozygous female appears normal but is a carrier of the mutant gene. An affected father (mating with a normal mother) does not transmit the disease directly to his sons—and the disease appears only in males after the mating of a carrier female and a normal male. It is rare to see serious sex-linked recessive disorders (e.g., hemophilia) in females, because mating of an affected male and a carrier female, which would be necessary, is an uncommon occurrence.

SOME MENDELIAN INHERITED DISORDERS

Some examples of diseases inherited according to the four mendelian patterns are the following:

Autosomal dominant

Familial intestinal polyposis—neoplasia (pp. 272 and 566)

Huntington's chorea—cerebral disease, pathogenesis undetermined (p. 752)

Marfan's syndrome—deficiency in formation of elastic fibers (discussed below)

Milroy's disease—congenital lymphedema resulting from abnormal development of lymphatic vessels (p. 98)

Osteogenesis imperfecta—defect in collagen synthesis and formation of osteoid in bones (p. 701)

Recklinghausen's neurofibromatosis—neoplasia (pp. 266 and 743)

Autosomal recessive

Alkaptonuria—disturbance in phenylalanine-tyrosine metabolism with homogentisic acid oxidase deficiency (p. 46)

Cystic fibrosis—disturbance in secretion of exocrine glands (discussed below)

Galactosemia—inability to metabolize galactose because of galactose-1-phosphate uridyl transferase deficiency (discussed below)

Phenylketonuria (PKU)—phenylalanine hydroxylase deficiency (discussed below)

Tay-Sachs disease (amaurotic family idiocy)—lipid (ganglioside) storage disease with hexosaminidase A deficiency (pp. 493 and 748); other inherited lipid storage diseases (lipidoses)

include *Gaucher's disease* or cerebroside lipidosis (p. 493) and *Niemann-Pick disease* or
phosphatide lipidosis (p. 493)
Wilson's disease—inborn error of copper metabolism associated with defective synthesis of
ceruloplasmin (pp. 451 and 751)

X-linked recessive
*Glucose-6-phosphate dehydrogenase (G6PD) de-
ficiency*—the basis for hemolytic anemia that is
induced by certain drugs or associated with
favism (p. 20)
Hemophilia A—deficiency of antihemophilic
globulin (factor VIII) (p. 510)
Lesch-Nyhan syndrome—hypoxanthine-guanine
phosphoribosyltransferase deficiency (p. 40)
Muscular dystrophy (Duchenne type)—so-called
pseudohypertrophic muscular dystrophy, pathogenesis undetermined (p. 751)

X-linked dominant
*Vitamin D–resistant⁻ (hypophosphatemic) rick-
ets*—impairment of reabsorption of phosphate
with resulting hyperphosphaturia, hypophosphatemia, rickets, or osteomalacia

Marfan's syndrome. The basic defect in
this syndrome is a deficiency in the formation
of elastic fibers. Many organs and tissues are
involved. The articular capsules, ligaments,
skeleton, and large arteries are especially affected. Patients with this disorder are characteristically tall with elongation of the extremities. The fingers are long and spiderlike
(arachnodactyly). In the aorta the defect may
be associated with the development of a dissecting aneurysm (p. 290).

Galactosemia. Patients with this disorder
are unable to convert galactose to glucose because of a lack of the enzyme galactose-1-phos-
phate uridyl transferase. The resulting elevation of galactose in the blood (galactosemia)
may be associated with serious physical and
mental disturbances. The liver is particularly
affected, showing hepatomegaly resulting
from fatty metamorphosis, which is followed
by cirrhosis. Jaundice occurs, and in addition,
morphologic changes are observed in the brain
and eyes (e.g., cataracts).

Phenylketonuria (PKU). This is an inborn
error of metabolism caused by a deficiency of
phenylalanine hydroxylase, the enzyme that
converts phenylalanine to tyrosine. This dis-

order is characterized by an elevation of serum
phenylalanine and often is associated with cerebral and mental retardation. Abnormal metabolites of phenylalanine, e.g., phenylpyru-
vic acid and orthohydroxyphenylacetic acid,
are excreted in the urine. The changes in the
brain are nonspecific and include areas of demyelination in the white matter. The pathogenesis of the cerebral damage and mental retardation is not clearly understood. It has been
attributed to the elevated levels of phenylalanine in the serum, although some investigators
have suggested that an increase in serum glutamine concentration may be responsible.
Whatever the cause, it has been shown that
mental retardation may be prevented by feeding the infant a low phenylalanine diet, thus
lowering the level of this amino acid in the
serum. However, some patients with elevated
phenylalanine levels do not develop mental
retardation.

Cystic fibrosis. Cystic fibrosis is a familial,
autosomal recessive genetic disease of children, adolescents, and young adults in which
there is abnormality of secretion by exocrine
glands. Formerly, the disease had been known
as *pancreatic cystic fibrosis* or *fibrocystic disease of the pancreas* because of the prominent
anatomic changes in the pancreas and associated enzyme deficiencies. Later, the disease
was termed *mucoviscidosis*, since many of the
glands affected produce a thick viscid mucus.
This term is appropriate only in part, for it has
since been observed that an abnormality of
sweat (i.e., an increase in sodium and chloride) is consistently present also. The sweat
test for detection of this abnormality is presently the most reliable of any general method
for the diagnosis of this disorder. As yet, the
pathogenetic mechanism for the disturbance in
secretion by the exocrine glands in the various
organs is not known, although dysfunction of
the autonomic nervous system control of the
exocrine glands has been considered.

Cystic fibrosis is the most prevalent inherited disease among white children, the highest
frequency being observed in persons of mid-
European heritage. The incidence in the United
States is variously estimated as one in 1,500

to one in 3,700 live births, according to reports since 1960, and the disease is comparatively rare in blacks and Orientals. Mild or incomplete forms that are difficult to recognize probably exist. Characteristic sweat electrolyte patterns may be present in asymptomatic relatives of known patients.

The pancreas and lungs are most seriously involved and, less commonly, the liver and salivary glands. In the pancreas, amorphous inspissated eosinophilic material obstructs ducts, which show prominent dilatation. There is progressive atrophy of the parenchyma and gradual replacement by fibrosis, with infiltration by some lymphocytes and other mononuclear cells. Fatty replacement of atrophic parenchyma as well as fibrosis may occur. Ultrastructural changes in the atrophic acinar cells include dilatation of ergastoplasm, decrease in zymogen granules, spherulation of mitochondria, and atrophy of microvilli. The islets of Langerhans remain intact, although there are some reports of an increased incidence of diabetes mellitus. The pancreas may show little gross change except to be firmer and thinner than normal

In about 10% of cases, there is "meconium ileus" at birth, an intestinal obstruction caused by abnormal inspissated meconium, which possibly results from deficiency of pancreatic secretion before birth. The obstruction is usually in the distal part of the small intestine, and proximally the dilated ileum is filled with a large amount of tenacious viscid meconium.

With pancreatic involvement and deficiency of the pancreatic enzymes trypsin, amylase, and lipase, food is poorly digested and absorbed. Fatty foods particularly are poorly digested, and steatorrhea is commonly present. Malnutrition, including deficiency of vitamins A, D, and K, may be a prominent feature.

Pulmonary involvement is present in almost all cases at some time during the course of the disease and is the important factor in most deaths. The paranasal sinuses also are consistently involved, and nasal polyposis is sometimes present. A respiratory infection with increased mucus production may initiate pulmonary disturbance. Inspissated abnormal bronchial secretions cause obstruction, leading to secondary infection, emphysema or atelectasis, bronchial damage, and bronchiectasis. Squamous metaplasia of bronchial linings, in which vitamin A deficiency may be a factor, complicates the problem of the removal of secretions. Mucous glands of the trachea, bronchi, and bronchioles become distended with inspissated material similar to that in pancreatic acini and ducts. Recurrent resistant bronchopneumonia and lung abscesses are common results and often appear to be caused by *Staphylococcus aureus* or *Pseudomonas* species. Pulmonary hypertension and cor pulmonale develop in some patients.

The liver may show a focal fibrosis in portal areas, with amorphous eosinophilic material plugging bile ductules. There is usually some bile duct proliferation and inflammatory reaction in the areas of fibrosis. The hepatic changes vary greatly in their severity and extensiveness. A few cases may progress to widespread and severe biliary cirrhosis with portal hypertension and enlargement of the spleen.

Submaxillary glands have increased secretion and show a similar mucinous obstruction. They are consistently enlarged by the age of 6 years. On the other hand, the parotid gland produces largely a serous secretion and usually does not show obstruction of ducts. Sweat glands show a consistent abnormality of sweat electrolytes, and sodium and chloride are increased two to four times above normal. Various sweat tests (e.g., pilocarpine iontophoresis sweat tests) have been devised that are important diagnostically and as simplified screening procedures. Handprints on filter paper or agar plates impregnated with silver chromate have been used as a simplified screening test. Abnormally high losses of sodium chloride in the sweat during hot weather may lead to massive salt depletion in these patients, which may be followed by peripheral vascular collapse, hyperpyrexia, coma, and death.

Changes in the reproductive system have been described in the postpubertal male—

viz., azoospermia associated with absence of vasa deferentia and small fibrotic epididymides.

Of interest is the observation that fibroblasts, obtained by culturing skin biopsies of patients with cystic fibrosis, stain metachromatically and that parents and relatives frequently show a similar change in their fibroblasts. The possibility of detecting heterozygotes for cystic fibrosis by this means has been suggested. It should be noted, however, that metachromasia in cultured fibroblasts has been demonstrated in other genetic disorders in which intracellular mucopolysaccharides may appear, e.g., Hurler's syndrome, Marfan's syndrome, late infantile amaurotic idiocy, and certain lipid-storage diseases. It is sometimes seen in fibroblasts of healthy individuals.

A serum factor (a protein or protein complex) has been identified in cystic fibrosis patients and heterozygotes that inhibits ciliary activity in explants of rabbit tracheal epithelium and oyster gill cilia. This factor has also been identified in culture media of fibroblasts derived from cystic fibrosis patients and is produced by cells cultured from amniotic fluid of a fetus with the cystic fibrosis gene. Some studies have suggested that there may be an inhibiting factor in the sweat of cystic fibrosis patients that interferes with reabsorption of sodium and chloride in the ducts of sweat glands, resulting in the elevated concentration of the electrolytes in sweat.

Localized malformations. In addition to the preceding as well as other related inherited disorders, it has been shown that some of the localized congenital malformations (i.e., limited to specific anatomic sites) may be caused by single mutant genes. These can be considered *inborn errors of morphogenesis* (e.g., postaxial polydactyly, type B, an extra digit that hangs from the ulnar side of the fifth finger; aniridia, congenital absence of part or all of the iris of the eye; split hand-foot deformity; absent radius; brachydactyly). It must be noted, however, that several malformations may be caused by either a single mutant gene or other conditions. Thus, the malformations caused by mendelian inheritance must be dif-

ferentiated from those resulting from multifactorial inheritance (involving both genetic and environmental factors), teratogenic agents (such as radiation; viruses, e.g., rubella; and drugs, e.g., thalidomide), and chromosomal abnormalities and from those that occur as sporadic, nonhereditary malformations.

• • •

Chromosomal aberrations generally do not show the familial tendencies seen in the truly inherited disorders related to mutant genes. In many of the chromosomal anomalies, transmission to the next generation is not possible because of their tendency to produce severe abnormalities and sterility. There is some evidence that about one third of *spontaneous abortions* may be caused by chromosomal aberrations. In several family studies, one chromosomal disorder, mongolism, was observed to have been transmitted through subsequent generations, thus designated familial mongolism.

In addition to the diseases that are the direct result of mutant genes or chromosomal aberrations, there are certain disorders, such as hypertension, atherosclerosis, and some of the congenital malformations, that probably result from the interaction of genetic and environmental factors. It is difficult to assess the exact role that heredity plays in these diseases, but it usually is regarded as a predisposing factor. It is to be noted that the term *congenital,* meaning born with, is not synonymous with the term *hereditary*. A congenital disease may or may not be hereditary. Also, although many hereditary diseases are congenital, in the sense that manifestations are present at birth, in some of them the clinical features do not appear until later in life. A *familial disease* is one that tends to run in families or affects two or more siblings in a particular family, and it may be either genetic in origin or caused by environmental factors.

In certain hereditary disorders, clinical manifestation of the genetic defect may not be apparent unless some environmental influence supervenes. For example, persons with a deficiency in the activity of the enzyme glucose-

6-phosphate dehydrogenase (G6PD) in the erythrocytes may show no ill effects, and the affected red blood cells may not be associated with any decrease in life span unless the patient is exposed to certain chemical or other toxic agents. Drugs such as the antimalarial compound primaquine result in increased destruction of the genetically defective red blood cells, causing hemolytic anemia *(primaquine sensitivity)*. Some patients who develop hemolytic anemia as a result of sensitivity to the fava bean or its pollen *(favism)* are known to have G6PD deficiency of the erythrocytes.

REFERENCES

Ashworth, C. T., et al.: Arch. Pathol. **75:**212-225, 1963 (hepatic cell degeneration).

Baker, D., et al.: J.A.M.A. **214:**869-878, 1970 (chromosomal errors and antisocial behavior).

Barnett, D. R., et al.: Tex. Rep. Biol. Med. **31:**691-696, 1973 (ciliary inhibitor in cystic fibrosis).

Bourne, G. H., editor: Cytology and cell physiology, ed. 3, New York, 1964, Academic Press, Inc.

Carr, D. H.: In Harris, H., and Hirschhorn, K., editors: Advances in human genetics, New York, 1971, Plenum Press, pp. 201-257 (chromosomes and abortion).

Cheville, N. F.: Cell pathology, Ames, Iowa, 1976, The Iowa State University Press.

Cloutier, M. M., and Mangos, J. A.: J. Fla. Med. Assoc. **65:**259-263, 1978 (cystic fibrosis).

Danes, B. S., and Bearn, A. G.: J. Exp. Med. **129:**775-793, 1969 (cell culture in cystic fibrosis).

DeRobertis, E. D. P., et al.: Cell biology, ed. 6, Philadelphia, 1975, W. B. Saunders Co.

Desforges, J. F.: N. Engl. J. Med. **294:**1438-1440, 1976 (G6PD deficiency).

di Sant'Agnese, P. A., and Davis, P. B.: N. Engl. J. Med. **295:**481-485, 534-541, 597-607, 1976 (cystic fibrosis).

Dorrance, D., et al.: J.A.M.A. **212:**1488-1491, 1970 (hallucinogens and chromosomes).

Egozcue, J., et al.: J.A.M.A. **204:**214-218, 1968 (chromosome damage in LSD users).

Erbe, R. W.: N. Engl. J. Med. **294:**381-383, 480-482, 1976 (principles of medical genetics).

Farquhar, M. G., and Palade, G. E.: J. Cell Biol. **17:**375-412, 1963 (junctional complexes).

Franke, W. W.: Int. Rev. Cytol. (Suppl.)**4:**71-236, 1974 (nuclear envelope).

Freeman, J. A.: Cellular fine structure, New York, 1964, McGraw-Hill Book Co.

Gerald, P. S..: N. Engl. J. Med. **294:**706-708, 1976 (sex chromosome disorders).

Gottlieb, S. K.: J.A.M.A. **209:**1063-1066, 1969 (chromosomal abnormalities in malignant neoplasms).

Hansen, R. G.: J.A.M.A. **208:**2077-2082, 1969 (hereditary galactosemia).

Harvey, J., et al.: J. Med. Genet. **14:**46-50, 1977 (familial mental retardation and X chromosome abnormality).

Hecht, F., et al.: N. Engl. J. Med. **285:**1482-1484, 1971 (cytogenetics).

Hirschhorn, K.: J.A.M.A. **224:**597-604, 1973 (human genetics).

Holmes, L. B.: N. Engl. J. Med. **291:**763-773, 1974 (inborn errors of morphogenesis).

Holmes, L. B.: N. Engl. J. Med. **295:**204-207, 1976 (congenital malformations).

Irwin, S., and Egozcue, J.: Science **157:**313-314, 1967 (chromosome abnormalities in LSD-25 users).

Ito, S.: Fed. Proc. **28:**12-25, 1969 (glycocalyx).

King, D. W., editor: Ultrastructure aspects of disease, New York, 1966, Hoeber Medical Division, Harper & Row, Publishers, Inc.

Kolodny, E. H.: N. Engl. J. Med. **294:**1217-1220, 1976 (lysosomal storage diseases).

Landing, B. H., et al.: Arch. Pathol. **88:**569-580, 1969 (epididymis and vas deferen in cystic fibrosis).

Lubs, H. A.: Am. J. Hum. Genet. **21:**231-244, 1979 (marker X chromosome and mental retardation).

Machin, G. A.: Lancet **1:**549-551, 1974 (chromosome abnormality and perinatal death).

Mandel, E. N., et al.: Am. J. Med. Sci. **274:**61-67, 1977 (intramitochondrial crystalline inclusions).

Matalon, R., and Dorfman, A.: Lancet **2:**838-841, 1969 (acid mucopolysaccharides in cultured human fibroblasts).

McCombs, M. L.: Tex. Rep. Biol. Med. **31:**615-629, 1973 (cystic fibrosis—a review).

McKean, C. M., and Peterson, N. A.: N. Engl. J. Med. **283:**1364-1367, 1970 (glutamine in phenylketonuria).

McKusick, V. A.: Mendelian inheritance in man, ed. 4, Baltimore, 1975, The Johns Hopkins University Press.

Miller, J. Q.: Neurology **23:**1141-1146, 1973 (chromosome deletions).

Miller, O. J., and Breg, W. R.: N. Engl. J. Med. **294:**596-598, 1976 (autosomal chromosome disorders).

Milunsky, A.: N. Engl. J. Med. **295:**377-380, 1976 (prenatal diagnosis of genetic disorders).

Nadler, H. L.: Birth defects **7**(5):5-9, 1971 (amniocentesis and detection of genetic disorders).

Nora, J. J., and Fraser, F. C.: Medical genetics, Philadelphia, 1974, Lea & Febiger.

Paris Conference (1971): Standardization in human cytogenetics, Birth Defects: Orig. Art. Series **8**(7), 1972.

Paris Conference (1971), Supplement (1975): Standardization in human cytogenetics, Birth Defects: Orig. Art. Series **11**(9), 1975.

Perry, T. L.: N. Engl. J. Med. **282:**761-766, 1970 (glutamine in phenylketonuria).

Porta, E. A., et al.: Am. J. Clin. Pathol. **42:**451-465, 1964 (electron microscopy in cystic fibrosis).

Pyeritz, R. E., and McKusick, V. A.: N. Engl. J. Med. **300:**772-777, 1979 (Marfan syndrome).

Rambourg, A., and Leblond, C. P.: J. Cell Biol. **32:**27-53, 1967 (surface coat on cells).

Ross, L. M.: Clin. Symp. **25**(4):4-35, 1973 (the cell).

2

Retrograde cellular changes and infiltrations

Among the fundamental results of injury to tissues are the *retrograde cellular changes,* e., atrophy, degeneration, and necrosis. A ide variety of injurious agents, including acterial and chemical poisons, immune complexes, trauma, radiant energy, heat, ischnia, and nutritional disturbances, cause such ffects. Retrograde cellular changes may or ay not be accompanied by an inflammatory action, depending on the degree of damage the cells and the rate at which cells die and t free toxic decomposition products. Closely lated to the retrograde cellular changes are filtrations or depositions—the abnormal accmulation of substances in tissues (within or tween cells)—e.g., adiposity (adipose tis- e infiltration) and deposition of amyloid, ur- s, calcium, or pigments. The degenerative anges, as well as the infiltrations or deposi- ns, are often looked on as disturbances of tabolism of various substances (e.g., pro- n, fat, carbohydrate, mineral, or pigment).

TROPHY

Atrophy is an acquired decrease in the size organs (or cells) that were once of normal portions. This is to be distinguished from tain congenital abnormalities: *agenesia* or enesis, which denotes complete absence of organ or tissue; *aplasia,* which indicates ost complete failure of development; and

hypoplasia, which is a failure of full development.

Atrophy of an organ or tissue may be caused by a reduction in size or in number of component cells, or in both. When atrophy affects cells, the organ or tissue is usually. but not necessarily, reduced in size. Frequently the atrophied cells are replaced by connective tissue or fat, which helps to maintain the size of the organ. In certain atrophic parenchymal cells, an accumulation of a granular yellowish brown pigment (lipofuscin) occurs, as in the heart, which causes a brown appearance of the organ on gross examination (brown atrophy). Function is disturbed by atrophy if the reserve capacity of the organ is encroached on.

The general cause of atrophy is inadequate nutrition of the cells, which, in turn, results from a variety of causes. The disturbed cellular nutrition leads to a negative balance between the metabolic processes, anabolism and catabolism, resulting in a progressive breakdown of cellular constituents and decrease in cell mass. If the causative agent is removed, restoration of equilibrium between these processes with recovery of the cell may occur. Persistence of the disturbed equilibrium causes slow death of cells, thus accounting for the reduction in number of cells. In certain organs, a normal, or *physiologic, atrophy* occurs at certain periods of life, as in the thymus

Sandberg, A. A.: The chromosomes in human cancer and leukemia, New York, 1980, Elsevier North-Hoiland, Inc.

Sandberg, A. A., et al.: Cancer Res. **21:**678-689, 1961 (chromosomes in leukemia).

Sergovich, F., et al.: N. Engl. J. Med. **280:**851-855, 1969 (chromosome aberrations in newborn infants).

Smuckler, E. A., and Arcasoy, M.: Int. Rev. Exp. Pathol. **7:**305-418, 1969 (changes in endoplasmic reticulum).

Spock, A. H., et al.: Pediatr. Res. **1:**173-177, 1967 (abnormal serum factor in cystic fibrosis).

Telfer, M. A., et al.: Science **159:**1249-1250, 1968 (chromosomal aberrations in male criminals).

Thompson, J. S., and Thompson, M. W.: (medicine, ed. 2, Philadelphia, 1973, W. B Co.

Tjio, J.-H., et al,: J.A.M.A. **210:**849-856, and chromosomes).

Trump, B. F., et al.: Hum. Pathol. **4:**89-109 lular changes in human disease).

Turpin, R., and Lejeune, J.: Human afflictior mosomal aberrations, Oxford, 1969, Pergan

Weiner, S., et al.: Lancet **1:**150, 1968 (XYY

Witkin, H. A., et al.: Science **183:**547-554, of XYY and XXY men).

Yunis, J. J., editor: Human chromosome r ed. 2, New York, 1974, Academic Press, at puberty and in the breasts and uterus after menopause.

Whether the atrophy that occurs in many organs and tissues in advanced age *(senile atrophy)* is physiologic or pathologic is a debatable point. During this period, endocrine changes bring about the atrophy of some tissues (e.g., the breasts). Lymphoid tissues, elastic tissues (as in the skin and blood vessels), bones (osteoporosis), and the nervous system all participate prominently. The possibility that ischemia resulting from arteriosclerosis contributes to atrophy in some of the tissues must be considered. *Pathologic atrophy* may be either general or local.

General atrophy

A major cause of general atrophy, involving widespread tissues and organs of the body, is starvation or inanition. The atrophy of starvation results from the using up of stored carbohydrate, fat, and eventually protein. It may be caused by lesions of the digestive tract such as an obstructing tumor of the esophagus, by loss of appetite without organic cause (anorexia nervosa), or by lack of essential foodstuffs. The central nervous system, bones, and muscles that are in active use participate less in the atrophy than do other tissues of the body. The basis for the generalized wasting (cachexia) of advanced cancer is not always certain, but in some instances it is a nutritive disturbance related to an inadequate food intake. Senile atrophy is a form of general atrophy, which, to a certain extent, may be physiologic, but the atrophy of some of the tissues or organs may, at least in part, be caused by pathologic influences (e.g., circulatory insufficiency brought about by arteriosclerosis).

Local atrophy

Local atrophy may be caused by disuse of a part, by ischemia, by pressure, by loss of endocrine stimulation, or by unknown causes.

Disuse atrophy. Forced inactivity of muscle soon results in decrease in size, the atrophy being particularly great when there is loss of motor nerve supply. It is not certain whether the interruption of the nerve supply leads to an absence of a "trophic" (nutritional) influence. Glandular organs forced to inactivity by occlusion of their ducts soon show atrophy of their functional cells. In the case of the pancreas, occlusion of the duct results in atrophy of the acinar tissue, whereas the endocrine islet tissue, the secretion of which goes directly into the bloodstream, remains relatively unaffected (Fig. 2-1).

Ischemic atrophy. A slow, progressive narrowing of the arteries (as in atherosclerosis), in the absence of an adequate collateral circulation, may result in atrophy of an organ or tissue. A similar effect may be produced by pressure upon a vessel by an extrinsic tumor or other mass.

Pressure atrophy. Pressure atrophy is commonly the result of prolonged or continuous pressure upon a local area or group of cells. Pressure apparently affects cells by interfering with blood flow and tissue fluid circulation thus preventing proper nutriment from reaching and being absorbed by the cells. Pressure exerted by a growing tumor causes such atrophy of the adjacent nontumor tissue. Amyloid deposited within tissue spaces brings about atrophy of the adjacent cells. The constant pulsating pressure of an aneurysm causes atrophy of any tissue, even bone, on which it impinges. Obstruction of a ureter with distention of the pelvis of the kidney (hydronephrosis) eventually leads to severe atrophy of renal tissue.

Endocrine atrophy. Endocrine atrophy occurs in organs that depend for their functional activity on endocrine stimulation, and it results whenever such stimulation decreases or ceases. Cessation of pituitary activity results in atrophic changes in the thyroid gland, adrenal glands, ovaries, and other organs that are influenced by pituitary hormones (Simmonds' disease, p. 579). Long-term administration of adrenal steroids may suppress the release of adrenocorticotropic hormone (ACTH) from the pituitary gland and lead to adrenal cortical atrophy. Prolonged hyperfunction of an endocrine gland (e.g., thyroid, islets of pancreas) may be followed by atrophy of the gland *(exhaustion atrophy)*.

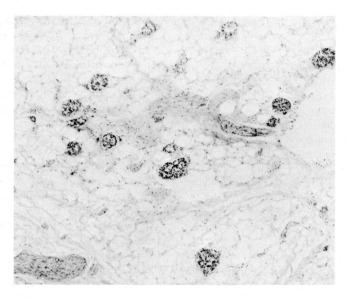

Fig. 2-1. Pancreas with severe acinar atrophy and fatty replacement following duct obstruction. Only islets remain.

Idiopathic atrophy. Idiopathic atrophy is a rare type of atrophy in which the cause has not yet been identified. Some investigators have attributed it to an unknown toxic influence—thus, it is sometimes called "toxic atrophy." Some cases of Addison's disease (p. 609) have as their basis an idiopathic bilateral atrophy of the adrenal cortices. However, it has not been proved that this disease is not the result of adrenal cortical necrosis. The presence of circulating antibodies against adrenal tissue in some patients with Addison's disease has suggested the possible role of autoimmunity.

DEGENERATIONS AND CERTAIN INFILTRATIONS

A form of cellular injury is *degeneration,* characterized by a disturbance of intracellular metabolism, a swelling of the cell, and an accumulation in the cytoplasm of substances that normally are invisible, absent, or present only in small amounts. The degeneration is named—according to the morphologic change or the nature of the abnormally accumulated material—cellular swelling (cloudy swelling), hydropic, vacuolar, fatty, or hyaline degeneration. These degenerative changes vary in severity and usually are reversible. However, severe degenerations may proceed to death of the cells.

Cellular swelling. Most acute infections and toxic conditions are accompanied by some degree of cellular swelling. It is the mildest and most common type of degeneration and is easily reversible. It is best seen in the liver and kidneys and sometimes in the heart. Other terms used for this form of degeneration are parenchymatous degeneration and cloudy swelling, the latter being descriptive of the gross appearance. The affected organ is swollen, so that the capsule is tense and the cut surface bulges. The tissue appears more opaque (cloudy) than normal, pale, and soft. Microscopically, the affected cells are swollen and have a granular cytoplasm, the granules being of a protein nature. Changes in the mitochondria contribute to the granular appearance. The ultrastructural and cytochemical alterations include certain of the changes already described under cellular injury in Chapter 1—viz., swelling of the mitochondria, vesicular distention of the endoplasmic reticulum, depletion of RNA granules, and reduction in cytoplasmic glycogen.

The swelling of the cell mainly results from an increased water content of the cytoplasm, although increase in the water content of the organ as a whole may not be demonstrable. It has been postulated that the energy function of the damaged mitochondria is disturbed, leading to a diminished output of ATP. The decrease in ATP impairs cellular membrane permeability and the "active transport" mechanism of the cell, which normally maintain a low concentration of intracellular sodium. The result is an increase in sodium ion within the cell, followed by an increased water content. Generally, the nucleus is unaffected in cloudy swelling, but in one investigation a decrease in DNA of the nucleus was detected. As noted previously, the RNA of the cell also may be diminished after injury to the cell. The parenchymal cells of the liver and convoluted tubular cells of the kidney show the change most severely. It is to be noted that postmortem autolysis may produce changes in certain tissues that simulate those of cellular swelling.

Hydropic degeneration. In cellular swelling, there is some imbibition of water into the cell, but in hydropic degeneration this is of greater degree. Hydropic degeneration is a more severe form of cellular injury than cellular swelling, but it, too, is reversible. The cell is swollen, and its cytoplasm is pale and vacuolated or reticulated. The clear vacuoles may be small and multiple, or they may be confluent, producing larger vacuoles or a single large vacuole replacing much of the cytoplasm and displacing the nucleus. When larger vacuoles appear, the term "vacuolar degeneration" often is used. The latter is a characteristic lesion affecting the renal tubular epithelium in dioxane and diethylene glycol poisoning and also in potassium deficiency (p. 355). Electron microscopically, the cytoplasmic vacuoles in hydropic degeneration are seen to be caused by vesicular distention of the endoplasmic reticulum that is more prominent than in cellular swelling.

Fatty metamorphosis. Another common form of retrograde cellular change is that characterized by an abnormal accumulation of lipid *in parenchymal cells* of an organ in which lipid normally is not demonstrable histologically. This disturbance has been designated by various terms, such as fatty metamorphosis (fatty change), fatty degeneration, steatosis, and parenchymal fatty infiltration or deposition. The most widely used term, however, is *fatty metamorphosis (fatty change)*. This process is to be differentiated from interstitial fatty infiltration, or adiposity, a condition characterized by the abnormal accumulation of adipose tissue in the stroma of parenchymatous organs (i.e., *between* parenchymal cells). Fatty metamorphosis is a disturbance of fat metabolism but is often preceded by cellular swelling or hydropic degeneration. Fatty change, although a more serious disturbance than the latter degenerative lesions, is generally reversible, but when severe it may result in death of cells (necrosis). Functional impairment of affected organs sometimes occurs when the process is extensive. In preparations of ordinary paraffin sections, the intracellular lipid is dissolved out, so that it appears as small or large vacuoles in the cytoplasm. Special staining procedures are available for demonstration of the lipid (e.g., scarlet red or Sudan III used on frozen sections, or osmic acid stain).

Fatty metamorphosis is seen most frequently in the liver, kidneys, and heart. The gross appearance of the affected organ depends on the amount of fatty change. Little or no alteration is observed when there is only a slight degree of involvement.

The severely involved *liver* is enlarged, yellow, and decreased in consistency, the margins are rounded, the cut surface is greasy and bulges, and the lobular markings are obscured when the change is diffuse but may be accentuated if the lipid is limited to a particular zone of the hepatic lobules (e.g., centrilobular regions). Microscopically, the vacuoles in the cytoplasm of the hepatic cells may be tiny and numerous or may be large, sometimes replacing the cell and pushing aside the nucleus (Figs. 2-2 and 2-3). In some areas there may be rupture of the membranes of adjacent cells

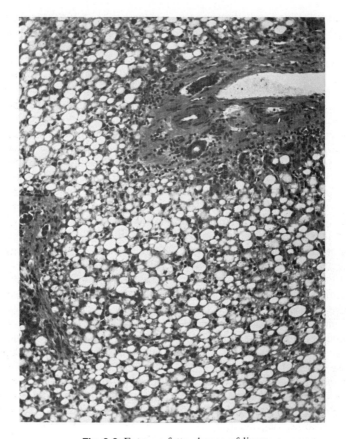

Fig. 2-2. Extreme fatty change of liver.

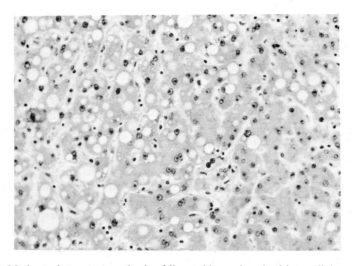

Fig. 2-3. Moderate fatty metamorphosis of liver with varying-sized intracellular vacuoles.

with confluence of large vacuoles, producing so-called lipid cysts. It is said that these lipid cysts may rupture into sinusoids and release the lipid into the venous circulation as fat emboli.

The fatty *kidney* may be normal in size or slightly enlarged, and the cut surfaces are pale grayish brown or yellowish brown and soft or friable. Microscopically, small vacuoles are found mainly in the epithelial cells of the convoluted tubules, particularly the proximal.

In the *heart,* fatty change affects the myocardium and may be patchy or diffuse. In patchy involvement, such as occurs in severe anemias, the change is best seen in the subendocardial region of the ventricles as irregular yellow streaks or lines alternating with lines of unaffected muscle, producing the so-called tigroid, tabby cat, or thrush breast appearance. In diffuse fatty change, usually caused by severe infections or toxic states, the entire myocardium is pale yellow or yellowish brown, soft, and flabby when the condition is severe, but lesser degrees are detected only upon histologic examination. Microscopically, a fine vacuolization is observed within the sarcoplasm of myocardial fibers in ordinary paraffin sections (Fig. 2-4). The minute droplets are often less distinct than the small or large vacuoles usually seen in liver or renal tubular cells.

The *causes* of fatty metamorphosis in both clinical and experimental situations include a variety of noxious agents, such as toxins of infectious diseases, phosphorus, carbon tetrachloride, chloroform, ethionine, puromycin, orotic acid, and ethanol, and also anoxia resulting from circulatory insufficiency or severe anemias. A deficiency of lipotropic substances (e.g., choline and methionine) also can induce fatty change, particularly in the liver. This state may be brought about by an inadequate diet, as in starvation or chronic alcoholism. In fatty livers said to be caused by excessive amounts of lipids brought to the cells, as in overfeeding, a relative deficiency of lipotropic substances may play a role. Certain studies suggest that alcohol (ethanol) itself may cause fatty change in the liver, probably by an increased uptake of plasma fat by the liver and

a decreased hepatic oxidation of fatty acids. That alcohol also directly interferes with release of lipids from hepatic cells has not been proved. A deficiency of intracellular carbohydrate, such as occurs in diabetes mellitus or starvation, is another cause of fatty change in the liver. Apparently, decreased liver glycogen leads to an increased oxidation of fat in hepatic cells, with a resultant increase of mobilization of lipid from the fat depots.

In the various instances of fatty metamorphosis, the predominant lipid that accumulates intracellularly is triglyceride. Thus, the factors in the *pathogenesis* of fatty change are those mechanisms that produce an excess of triglyceride within cells. Most of the information concerning these mechanisms has been derived mainly from investigations of fatty change in the liver rather than in the heart, kidneys, or other organs. These studies have shown that the various causative agents or conditions previously mentioned may bring about triglyceride accumulation in a cell by the following mechanisms, singly or in combination:

1 There may be an *increased synthesis of triglyceride.* Since triglyceride normally is formed from fatty acids, some of which are utilized also in phospholipid and cholesterol ester synthesis, an increased triglyceride synthesis would be related to an elevated concentration of fatty acids in the liver. The rise in hepatic fatty acids may occur as a result of (1) increased uptake of plasma fat by liver cells (increased mobilization from fat depots or excess dietary fats), (2) increased hepatic synthesis of fatty acids (from acetate), (3) decreased hepatic oxidation of fatty acids, or (4) impairment in the esterification of fatty acids to esters other than triglyceride.

2 There may be a *decrease in the release or secretion of triglyceride from the cell.* Normally, after synthesis in the endoplasmic reticulum of the liver cell, triglyceride is coupled with protein, cholesterol, cholesterol ester, and phospholipid to become lipoprotein, the form in which it is secreted from the cell. Interference with protein synthesis, such as may occur following administration of carbon tetrachloride, phosphorus, ethionine, or

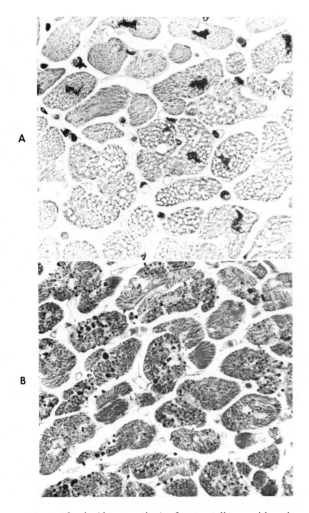

Fig. 2-4. A, Fatty metamorphosis (degeneration) of myocardium, with rather uniform, fine vacuolization in myocardial fibers. **B,** Fatty metamorphosis (degeneration) of myocardium in phosphorus poisoning. Black droplets in myocardial fibers are globules of fat (osmic acid stain). Note occasional fat globules in interstitial tissue, which appear to have been expelled from fibers. (From Scotti, T. M.: Heart. In Anderson, W. A. D., editor: Pathology, ed. 7, St. Louis, 1977, The C. V. Mosby Co.)

puromycin, blocks lipoprotein synthesis and thus prevents release of hepatic triglyceride. The impairment may be in the phospholipid moiety of the lipoprotein, as may happen in fatty livers caused by choline deficiency. In orotic acid–induced fatty livers, the defect appears not to involve the synthesis of the protein or the lipid moieties but a later event in the metabolism of lipoprotein, either the coupling of lipid with protein or the release of the formed lipoprotein from the liver cell. Ultrastructural changes have been identified in the endoplasmic reticulum to support some of the foregoing concepts.

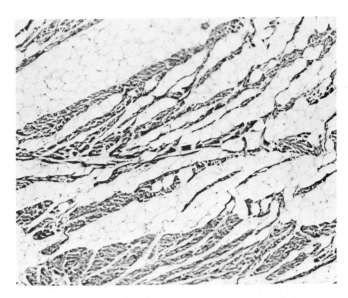

Fig. 2-5. Marked interstitial fatty infiltration of myocardium with atrophy of muscle fibers.

Adiposity (interstitial fatty infiltration). In adiposity, which is commonly associated with generalized obesity, there is an abnormal or excessive accumulation of adipose tissue (adult fat cells) between parenchymal cells of an organ. The increase in adult fat cells is believed to result from the transformation of interstitial connective tissue cells after the deposition of lipid within them. The heart and pancreas are the two organs principally affected.

In the heart, the adipose tissue appears between myocardial fibers and frequently is continuous with the overlying epicardial fat, which usually is increased in amount. Atrophy of muscle fibers may occur (Fig. 2-5). Only rarely will myocardial adiposity produce clinical manifestations. In the pancreas, there is an accumulation of adipose tissue in the interlobular septa that may also affect the interacinar stroma within the lobules. Usually, fatty infiltration of the pancreas produces no functional disturbance of the acinar tissue or islets. Areas of necrosis or atrophy in an organ or tissue may be replaced by adipose tissue (so-called fatty replacement; Fig. 2-1).

Hyaline degeneration and extracellular hy- **alins.** The term *hyaline* is a descriptive adjective used to qualify any translucent, homogeneous, structureless material that stains with eosin. There are a variety of intracellular or extracellular hyaline substances (or *hyalins*), which are mainly of a protein nature. To speak of a substance as a hyalin does not disclose its specific chemical nature nor its localization. Certain types of hyalin, such as amyloid, have distinctive characteristics or staining reactions and hence are separable from the general group.

After injury to certain cells, a hyaline change of varying degree may take place in the cytoplasm; this is termed **hyaline degeneration.** However, not all intracellular hyaline changes, even though commonly termed "hyaline degeneration," represent a true degenerative process. Examples of intracellular hyaline change are the following:

1 *Hyaline droplets in renal tubular epithelium,* particularly in proximal convoluted tubules, appear as numerous, closely grouped, eosinophilic structures within the cytoplasm (Fig. 2-6). Some investigators have considered them to be cytoplasmic alterations resulting from renal

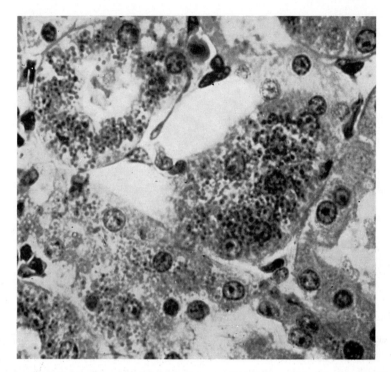

Fig. 2-6. Hyaline droplets in epithelial cells lining renal tubules. (From Anderson, W. A. D.: Degenerative changes and disturbances of metabolism. In Anderson, W. A. D., editor: Pathology, ed. 6, St. Louis, 1971, The C. V. Mosby Co.)

tubular cell injury (thus the formerly used term "hyaline droplet degeneration"). However, the prevalent opinion is that the hyaline droplets represent excessive protein that has passed through injured and abnormally permeable glomeruli and been reabsorbed into tubular cells.

2 *Mallory bodies* are hyaline masses within degenerating liver cells in active nutritional ("alcoholic") cirrhosis.

3 *Councilman bodies* are hyaline masses in liver cells in yellow fever.

4 *Acidophilic bodies* are hyaline rounded masses in liver cells in viral hepatitis, in primary cancer of the liver, and in other hepatic lesions.

5 *Crooke's hyaline change* occurs in basophils of the pituitary gland in Cushing's disease.

6 *Russell bodies* in plasma cells are rounded hyaline masses that contain gamma globulin formed apparently in response to antigenic stimuli, thus not a true degenerative process.

7 *Zenker's (waxy) degeneration* is a hyaline change in voluntary muscle that was originally described by Zenker in cases of typhoid fever but is also seen in other severe infections. The alteration is not caused by the localization of the infection in the muscle but rather by the toxins or excess accumulation of lactic acid. The lesion is best seen in the rectus abdominis and diaphragmatic muscles. The involved muscle is very pale and friable, so that rupture of the fibers and small hemorrhages are frequent. Microscopically, the affected fibers are swollen, they lose their

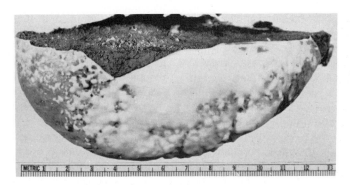

Fig. 2-7. Hyalinization of splenic capsule.

striations, and they have a hyaline appearance. When advanced, the lesion progresses to necrosis.

Of the three types of hepatocellular hyaline change mentioned, the Mallory body is the most distinctive. It is a protein complex consisting of hyaline clumps about the nucleus. The origin of Mallory bodies has not been definitely established, although in ultrastructural studies it has been determined that they are fibrillar or filamentous in nature. Various investigators have suggested that they are derived either from organelles (mitochondria, rough endoplasmic reticulum, or microfilaments) or from the cytosol (as a result of fragmentation and unfolding of certain cytoplasmic proteins). The Councilman body of yellow fever is a condensation of the cytoplasm, affecting first a part of the cell and later the entire cell, after which the latter becomes contracted and distorted, since by that time death of the cell already has occurred. Councilman bodies do not contain virus particles and thus are not to be confused with true viral inclusions. The acidophilic body is somewhat like a Councilman body, consisting of condensed cytoplasm. When a cell is totally involved, it may become reduced in size and separated from neighboring cells and may be found free in tissue spaces or even in the sinusoids.

Extracellular hyalins include connective tissue hyalin, fibrinoid, vascular hyalin, and amyloid. Amyloid will be discussed in the next section.

Hyaline change in connective tissue is common, occurring in old scars, in thickened serosae (e.g., pleura) after chronic inflammation, in a thickened capsule of the spleen (Fig. 2-7), in the intima of arteries (atherosclerosis), in the stroma of tumors (e.g., leiomyomas), and in other sites. The change actually is a physical alteration of the collagen fibers, which become fused to form a homogeneous, acellular area, but the collagen retains its usual staining quality. This change is sometimes referred to as "hyaline degeneration" of connective tissue, but it is better called "hyalinization."

Fibrinoid represents altered collagen that appears homogeneous and stains deeply eosinophilic so that it resembles fibrin. Fibrinoid change (often called "fibrinoid degeneration" or "fibrinoid necrosis") is a characteristic lesion that may occur in connective tissue diseases associated with hypersensitivity (e.g., polyarteritis nodosa, rheumatic fever, and systemic lupus erythematosus). It also is present in the arteriolar walls in malignant hypertension. Studies have shown that fibrinoid consists of a mixture of substances including fragments of collagen, acid mucopolysaccharide, fibrin, and, in certain situations, also gamma globulin.

Vascular hyalin occurs in the walls of arterioles in the hyaline form of arteriolosclerosis.

Despite several thorough electron microscopic studies of vascular hyalin, the origin of this substance is still not settled. Some investigators believe that the hyaline deposits are derived from plasma proteins that filter through the endothelium and are deposited predominantly within intimal spaces. When the deposits are larger, they infiltrate the adjacent elastic tissue and smooth muscle of the media. Others claim that the hyalin is essentially an excessive elaboration of endothelial and smooth muscle cell basement membrane material, followed by atrophy and disappearance of smooth muscle.

It should be mentioned that certain substances of a different nature may have a hyaline appearance, e.g., protein casts in the lumen of renal tubules, colloid in thyroid acini, clumped masses of fibrin, inspissated secretions in glandular ducts, and thrombi in small blood vessels as in thrombotic thrombocytopenic purpura.

Amyloid deposition (amyloidosis). Amyloid is a hyaline material characterized by deposition intercellularly, rather than in cells, and by specific staining reactions with iodine, methyl violet, Congo red, silver, and thioflavine-T. Amyloid stains orange-red (light microscopy) and shows a green birefringence (polarization microscopy) when stained with Congo red. The green birefringence may appear in hematoxylin- and eosin-stained sections but does so with less frequency and less intensity than in Congo red–stained sections. It stains purple-red with methyl or crystal violet (metachromatic stain), mahogany brown with iodine, and dark brown to black with silver stains. Thioflavine-T causes a yellow fluorescence of amyloid in ultraviolet light. The Congo red test (to determine amount of absorption of the dye from the serum after its injection into the circulation) is seldom used today for the diagnosis of amyloidosis. More usual diagnostic tests include biopsy of the rectal mucosa or of the gingiva and needle biopsy of organs (e.g., liver or kidney).

Nature and pathogenesis. Originally, amyloid ("starchlike") was so named because its gross deposits in tissues or organs were stained blue by the application of iodine followed by dilute sulfuric acid. The exact chemical composition of amyloid is unknown, but it appears to be essentially a proteinous substance, although a polysaccharide component has been identified. Some investigators have suggested that it is a glycoprotein in which a mucopolysaccharide is attached to a globulin. However, it has been demonstrated in certain studies that mucopolysaccharide is not a significant part of the amyloid itself but that it represents the ground substance in which amyloid is deposited.

Electron microscopically, amyloid is seen to be made up primarily of characteristic fibrils (Fig. 2-8), which are considered to be the components responsible for the Congo red staining and green polarization color by which the deposits are identified histologically. The fibrils are shown by x-ray crystallographic analysis to be composed of protein consisting of polypeptide chains arranged in an antiparallel β-pleated sheet conformation.

The origin of amyloid has been a mystery for a long time, but in some cases an immunologic mechanism is probably responsible for its appearance in tissues. Experimentally, it has been produced in animals by various antigenic stimuli, such as repeated injections of bacteria and of the protein casein. Horses hyperimmunized for production of diphtheria antitoxin may develop amyloidosis. In man, some of the conditions in which amyloid is found are characterized by hyperglobulinemia. Observations such as the preceding have led to the theory that amyloid results from an antigen-antibody reaction and that it represents the tissue localization of a circulating abnormal protein complex. Another hypothesis, which is supported by electron microscopic, fluorescent antibody, and autoradiographic evidence, states that a wide variety of immunologic stimuli may stimulate reticuloendothelial and possibly other cells to produce amyloid fibrils locally. Among the other cells incriminated in the production of amyloid are fibroblasts, endothelial cells, and plasma cells.

Recently, immunoglobulin proteins have been shown to be a source of amyloid fibrils

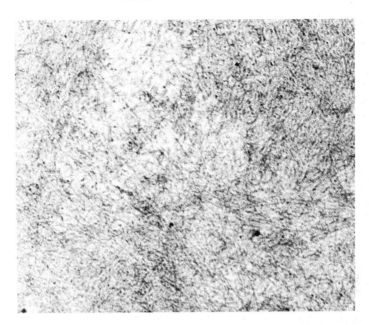

Fig. 2-8. Electron microscopic appearance of meshwork of amyloid fibrils in mesangial area of renal glomerulus. (×47,500; courtesy Dr. V. Pardo.)

in many cases of human amyloidosis. Osserman and co-workers have emphasized the relationship of amyloidosis to a plasma cell dyscrasia in which there is a decreased synthesis of complete immunoglobulin molecules, resulting in the formation of an excess of low molecular weight fragments of the Bence Jones (light chain) type. Glenner and associates have presented physicochemical and immunochemical evidence that the major component of amyloid fibrils is an immunoglobulin light polypeptide chain and/or its amino-terminal fragment. One of the mechanisms suggested for the production of amyloid is the following: light polypeptide chains or their fragments formed by immunocompetent cells are taken up by cells of the macrophage system and enter the lysosomes, where they are degraded to insoluble fibril aggregates, which are subsequently deposited extracellularly as amyloid fibrils. However, in addition to this mechanism, the possibility has been considered that a physicochemical change in circulating immunoglobulin protein precursors could produce fibrils from a whole polypeptide chain

in the absence of proteolysis. The evidence presented by Osserman and co-workers that amyloid-related Bence Jones proteins have a greater binding affinity for certain normal tissue components than nonamyloid-related Bence Jones proteins suggests a physicochemical characteristic residing in the amyloid-related light chains.

The amyloid fibrils of immunoglobulin origin appear to be more frequently, but not exclusively, associated with plasma cell dyscrasias or with "primary" (idiopathic) amyloidosis. Another major protein, which is of nonimmunoglobulin origin, has been obtained from amyloid fibrils derived predominantly from patients with amyloidosis that is associated with predisposing diseases ("secondary" amyloidosis). This protein was first identified by Benditt and Eriksen in amyloid associated with chronic inflammatory diseases and was designated by them as "protein A." Others subsequently demonstrated this protein in secondary amyloidosis associated with chronic infections, rheumatoid arthritis, and Hodgkin's disease and in one type of familial amyloidosis (familial Mediterranean fever). Franklin and co-workers termed the protein "acid soluble fraction" (ASF), and Glenner and associates referred to it as "amyloid of unknown origin" (AUO). Recently, it has been designated "AA protein." It is of interest that in some studies of amyloid fibrils with this protein as the major component, some light chain–related material was also demonstrated.

Classification. Amyloidosis and incidental deposits of amyloid may be classified as follows:

A Systemic amyloidosis
  1 Secondary amyloidosis (usually secondary to chronic infections or other chronic inflammations, but also to Hodgkin's disease and other neoplasms)
  2 Primary amyloidosis (not associated with other diseases)
  3 Amyloidosis associated with multiple myeloma and other plasma cell dyscrasias
  4 Hereditary forms of amyloidosis
B Localized (or organ-limited) primary amyloidosis (not associated with another disease process)
C Incidental localized amyloid deposits (associated with another process, e.g., in tumors of certain endocrine glands and in pancreatic islets in association with diabetes mellitus)

Secondary amyloidosis is a systemic form of amyloidosis that is associated with chronic tissue-destructive infections (e.g., tuberculosis, leprosy, and syphilis), with other chronic inflamations (e.g., rheumatoid arthritis, regional enteritis, and chronic ulcerative colitis), and sometimes with certain malignant neoplasms (e.g., Hodgkin's disease). The organs most frequently involved in the secondary form are the spleen, kidneys, liver, and adrenal glands. Blood vessel walls tend to be affected first and most prominently in these organs. The earliest amyloid deposits are characteristically subendothelial, along reticulin fibers ("perireticulin amyloidosis"), in contrast to the deposition in primary or similar forms of amyloidosis, in which deposits are along collagen fibers ("pericollagen amyloidosis").

The amyloid *spleen* is enlarged, firm, and of rubbery or elastic consistency. On the cut surface, the amyloid areas have a characteristic pale translucent appearance. The involvement may be focal or diffuse. In the *focal form* (sago spleen), the deposition is in arteriolar walls and extends into surrounding lymph follicles (Figs. 2-9 and 2-10). The involved foci are prominently pale and translucent against the red background of the remainder of the spleen. In the *diffuse form* (lardaceous spleen) there is widespread deposition between the fibrous reticulum of the spleen, the follicles tending to be spared.

Amyloid disease of the *kidney* (Fig. 2-11) is occasionally severe enough to disturb renal function and give a picture of renal disease. With glomerular involvement, the nephrotic syndrome may occur. Amyloid is deposited chiefly in glomeruli and blood vessel walls. In the glomeruli, as noted by electron microscopy, the amyloid fibrils are deposited in the mesangium and between the basement membrane and the endothelial lining of the capillaries (Fig. 2-8). Later, in some instances, amyloid may appear in the membrane and on the epithelial side. The capillaries are narrowed and finally obliterated, so that the glomerulus becomes functionless and secondary changes develop in the tubules. Amyloid also may be deposited in the basement membrane of some of the tubules, and in the peritubular stroma, as well as in the walls of some blood vessels.

Considerable amyloid deposition in the *liver* causes it to be enlarged, firm, and unusually translucent. Deposition tends to occur first in the midzonal region of the liver lobule, appearing in the space between the sinus endothelium and the liver cells. In the liver, as elsewhere, the deposition of amyloid tends to cause pressure atrophy of the parenchymatous cells.

Primary systemic amyloidosis is not associated with known predisposing diseases. Deposition of amyloid is seen especially in mesenchymal tissues, such as the tongue, gastrointestinal tract, heart, blood vessels, lungs, adipose tissue, carpal ligaments, skin, and gums. The liver, kidneys, spleen, and adrenal glands are affected less frequently, although in occasional instances one or more of these organs may be prominently involved.

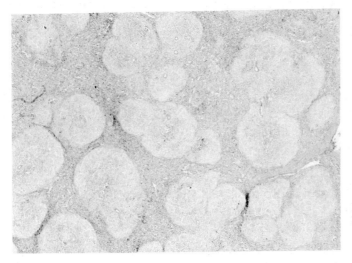

Fig. 2-9. Focal form of amyloidosis of spleen (sago spleen) involving lymphoid follicles. Note confluence of nodules.

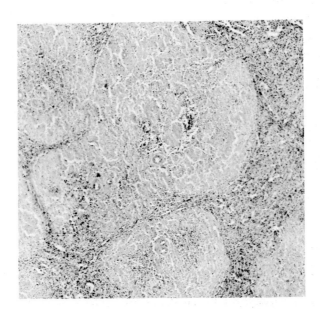

Fig. 2-10. Amyloidosis of spleen. High-power view of section shown in Fig. 2-9 to show involvement of arterioles and adjacent follicle with atrophy of follicle cells.

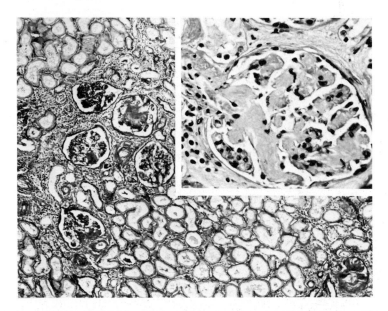

Fig. 2-11. Amyloidosis of kidney in a patient with severe long-standing infection of bone (osteomyelitis) occurring after trauma. Amyloid deposits obliterate normal structure of glomeruli. *Inset,* Higher magnification of glomerulus shows amyloid deposited along the course of capillaries. There is a reduction in the number of nuclei and patency of capillary lumina. (From Scarpelli, D. G., and Chiga, M.: Cell injury and errors of metabolism. In Anderson, W. A. D., and Kissane, J. M., editors: Pathology, ed. 7, St. Louis, 1977, The C. V. Mosby Co.)

Amyloid may be deposited in irregular masses or in the form of "rings" in fatty tissue. The amyloid in the primary systemic form tends to stain atypically, for which reason it is sometimes referred to as "atypical amyloid" or "paramyloid."

Multiple myeloma may be complicated by amyloidosis that is similar to primary systemic amyloidosis in its tissue distribution and variable staining reaction.

Several *hereditary forms* of amyloidosis have been described. One of these is associated with familial Mediterranean fever, an autosomal recessive disorder in which renal involvement is the most prominent lesion. Other organs are affected as in the usual secondary form, except that deposits of amyloid in the liver are not striking. Another hereditary form is the neuropathic type, transmitted by an autosomal dominant gene, with amyloid deposition as in the classic primary systemic form but with prominent involvement of the peripheral nerves and sympathetic ganglia. An autosomal, probably dominant, hereditary amyloidosis with myocardiopathy and progressive cardiac insufficiency also has been reported.

Primary localized amyloidosis is characterized by deposition of amyloid confined to an organ system and thus is also called " organ-limited" amyloidosis. As with the primary systemic form, there is no known predisposing or associated disease that is responsible for the formation of amyloid. Primary amyloidosis restricted to the heart has been reported in elderly patients. Localized amyloidosis, sometimes forming nodular or tumorlike masses of amyloid, may occur in other sites, including the respiratory tract, tongue, pharynx, and urinary tract. Infiltration of lymphocytes and plasma cells may be associated with the amyloid deposits.

Incidental localized amyloid deposits may

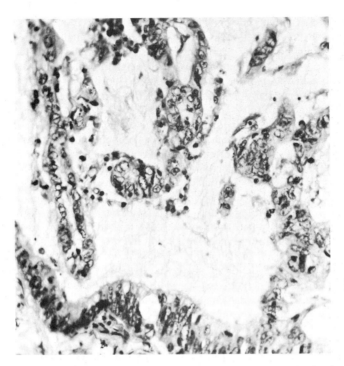

Fig. 2-12. Abundant mucin (pale reticulated substance) in lumen of neoplastic glands, produced by cancer cells (adenocarcinoma of colon).

be seen in certain neoplasms, e.g., medullary carcinoma of the thyroid gland and islet cell tumor of the pancreas. They may also be found in the pancreatic islets in association with diabetes mellitus and/or advanced age.

Various classifications of amyloidosis have been suggested in addition to the preceding one. Isobe and Osserman have proposed a classification that is based on the predominant clinical patterns of amyloid distribution. These patterns are:

Pattern I: Involvement chiefly of the tongue, heart, gastointestinal tract, skeletal and smooth muscles, carpal ligaments, nerves, and skin

Pattern II: Involvement chiefly of the liver, spleen, kidneys, and adrenal glands

Mixed pattern I and II: Amyloid in both pattern I and pattern II sites

Localized: Involvement of a single tissue or organ exclusively

It can be seen that the distribution in pattern I is that occurring in the "primary" type and in multiple myeloma, and the distribution in pattern II is that observed in the "secondary" type and in familial Mediterranean fever.

Mucinous degeneration. Mucin is a clear, structureless material that stains lightly with basic dyes (hematoxylin). In certain epithelial tumors, such as intestinal carcinoma (Fig. 2-12), and in some catarrhal inflammations of mucous membranes, an excess is secreted by the epithelial cells. A somewhat similar (mucoid or myxomatous) material may be formed by connective tissue (normally in the umbilical cord) and is found in the subcutaneous tissue in thyroid deficiency (myxedema) and in the connective tissue tumors called myxomas.

Actually, the designation "mucinous degeneration," which is commonly used for these epithelial and connective tissue disturbances, does not seem to be appropriate. The alteration appears to be one of overproduction of mucin, although secondary adverse effects may be produced in cells surrounded by the abundant material. What is probably a true retrograde cellular change is so-called *basophilic (mucinous) degeneration* of myocardial fibers, characterized by the appearance of a blue intrasarcoplasmic substance in sections stained with hematoxylin-eosin. Because of its histochemical reactions, it has been designated variously as an acid mucopolysaccharide, a mucoprotein, or a glycoprotein. However, its mucinous nature has been questioned recently. The suggestion has been made, based on histochemical and electron microscopic studies, that the basophilic substance may be a complex glucose polymer related to an abnormal glycogen. The cause of basophilic degeneration of the myocardium is not certain, but it may be a form of ischemia. A similar change has been described in voluntary skeletal muscle in myxedema.

Disturbances of purine metabolism. Uric acid, which is derived mainly from nucleoproteins of food and body tissues, is important under pathologic conditions in the formation of uric acid calculi and so-called uric acid infarcts of the kidneys and in gout.

Gout, a disturbance of purine metabolism, is characterized by an acute or chronic arthritis with deposition of crystalline urates in articular cartilages, synovial membranes and fluid, and ligaments about joints. They also occur in bursae and tendon sheaths, in cartilages of the ears, in eyelids, in subcutaneous tissues about joints, in heart valves, and in the interstitial tissue and tubules of the medullae of the kidneys. The deposits form small masses (tophi), which may be visible or palpable clinically, particularly in tissues about the joints. Microscopically, tophi consist of masses of needle-like crystals or amorphous granules of urates surrounded by a foreign body reaction (lymphocytes, plasma cells, macrophages, giant cells, and fibrous tissue) (Figs. 2-13 and 2-14).

The classic and usual form of gout is a hereditary disorder, commonly referred to as *primary gout.* The vast majority of patients are men. Only about 5% are women. The pattern of inheritance is not definite but probably is autosomal dominant with variable penetrance or multifactorial type rather than sex-linked. The hyperuricemia in these patients is explained on the basis of (1) an overproduction of uric acid, perhaps as a result of an enzymatic defect, (2) a deficient renal excretion of uric acid, presumably resulting from impaired distal tubular secretion, or (3) a combination of both mechanisms. In some patients, symptoms of a nonhereditary form of gout may occur as a result of various diseases or disturbances that produce hyperuricemia *(secondary* or *symptomatic gout),* e.g., (1) myeloproliferative disorders, such as polycythemia vera, chronic granulocytic leukemia, and myeloid metaplasia, in which there is an accelerated turnover of nucleic acids with overproduction of purines, including uric acid, (2) following administration of certain drugs that impair the excretion of uric acid, (3) chronic renal diseases resulting in decreased excretion of uric acid, and (4) various other conditions, such as hyperparathyroidism, sarcoidosis, and psoriasis, in which the mechanism is not clear.

The mechanism whereby urate crystals induce gouty inflammation and tissue damage apparently is related to release of lysosomal enzymes after ingestion of the crystals by phagocytes. It has been thought that the sharp crystals cause mechanical rupture of lysosomes, but there is evidence that hydrogen bonding between crystals and lysosomal membranes may be responsible for the rupture of membranes. This theory does not exclude the role of kinins or other vasoactive agents in the early phase of inflammation.

Sometimes, urate deposits occur in the kidneys of nongouty subjects as a clinically insignificant finding, particularly in newborn infants. The deposits appear prominently in the renal pyramids as wedge-shaped areas made up of yellowish gray streaks of crystalline material. The uric acid and urates are within the lumina of collecting tubules and normally are excreted without damage to the kidney. These lesions are called *uric acid infarcts,* although there are no features of a true infarct and there is no associated inflammatory reaction.

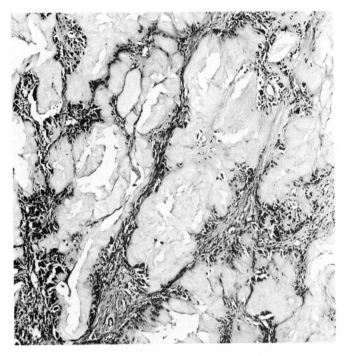

Fig. 2-13. Tophus of gout. Urate deposits are surrounded by bands of fibrous tissue infiltrated by mononuclear cells and giant cells (see Fig. 2-14).

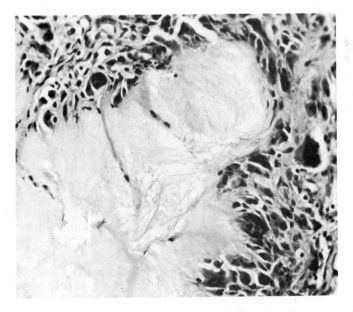

Fig. 2-14. High-power view of section shown in Fig. 2-13 to show fine crystals of urates and surrounding cells (lymphocytes, histiocytes, and giant cells) and fibrous tissue.

A hyperuricemic syndrome occurs in children (the so-called *Lesch-Nyhan syndrome*) that is characterized by self-destructive behavior (chewing one's own lips and fingers) and is associated with mental retardation, cerebral palsy, and athetosis. Deficiency of the enzyme hypoxanthine-guanine phosphoribosyltransferase is regarded as the basic defect, which in some families has been inherited apparently as a sex-linked recessive trait.

Disturbances of glycogen distribution. Glucose is not identifiable histologically in tissues, but glycogen can be demonstrated by Best's carmine stain after fixation in alcohol or Carnoy's fluid or by periodic acid–Schiff (PAS) stain. The normal liver of a well-nourished individual contains abundant glycogen in the cytoplasm of the hepatic cells. In ordinary sections, this gives the hepatic cells a foamy or finely reticulated appearance. Postmortem tissues may show a little of this appearance but may show a greater change if only a short time has elapsed between food intake and death. Glycogen is normally quite abundant in various other tissues such as skin, muscle, heart, and parathyroid glands. Histochemical methods have indicated that potassium and glycogen are closely related in the heart and liver and that the potassium appears to invest the glycogen droplets intimately. Excess glycogen within cells is usually regarded as a form of "infiltration," but some consider it a "degeneration." Glycogen may be increased in areas of inflammatory reaction around dead tissues.

Diabetes mellitus that is inadequately controlled by insulin shows depletion of the normal store of glycogen in the liver and skin. In the presence of glycosuria, excess glycogen content may be demonstrable in renal tubules, particularly in the cells lining the terminal straight segment of proximal convoluted tubules and contiguous portion of Henle's loops. The glycogen content of hepatic cell nuclei is often increased in diabetes (p. 471).

Various forms of *glycogen storage disease* have been reported. They are characterized by an inborn error of glycogen metabolism resulting from deficiency or absence of certain enzymes and an abnormal accumulation of glycogen in various tissues. Among these is the classic form, Type I or *von Gierke's disease,* which is usually manifested in infancy and affects particularly the liver and kidneys. It is associated with an enzyme defect of glucose-6-phosphatase. Type II is the cardiac form (called *Pompe's disease*), which is associated with a deficiency of lysosomal enzyme, α-1,4-glycosidase. It is part of a generalized glycogenosis in which the major manifestation is in the heart. The sarcoplasm of practically all the myocardial fibers is replaced by glycogen, so that the fibers appear as hollow cylinders surrounded by a thin rim of sarcoplasm (Fig. 2-15.) The heart is enlarged. Pompe's disease is usually fatal during the first year of life. Another glycogenic disorder of the heart consists of congenital tumorlike nodules of myocardial fibers distended with glycogen, so-called rhabdomyomas, the cause of which is obscure.

NECROSIS

The most serious effect of injury is death, which may be of the body as a whole (somatic death) or of localized areas of tissue or cells. Cell or tissue death within the living body is termed *necrosis* and is recognizable by the changes that the dead tissues and cells undergo after their death. As mentioned previously (p. 7), the earliest change in necrotic cells seen by light microscopy appears to be in the nucleus. Most investigators, however, have identified ultrastructural alterations in the cytoplasmic membranes and particulate systems and disturbances in their functions before any nuclear changes, although in certain experimental models of cell injury, clumping of nuclear chromatin has been observed almost as early as some of the cytoplasmic alterations. Whether or not the release of enzymes from the lysosomes is responsible for initiating the cellular changes leading to cell death is not settled, but it is generally accepted that these, as well as extracellular enzymes, act upon the cells after their death to produce the morphologic effects that are characteristic of necrosis.

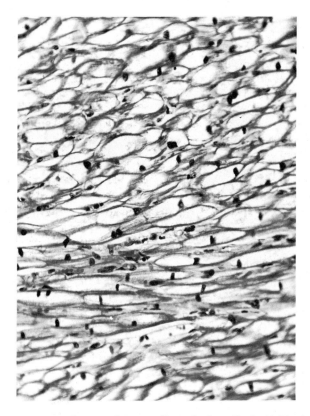

Fig. 2-15. Glycogen storage disease of myocardium. In formalin-fixed histologic preparations stained with hematoxylin-eosin, muscle fibers appear as clear spaces surrounded by a thin rim of sarcoplasm.

Necrosis may be caused by almost any type of severe injury. Macroscopic areas of dead tissue tend to be opaque, i.e., the normal translucency of most living tissues is lost, and a whitish or yellowish color is assumed. However, gross appearance of necrotic tissue may differ, varying with the type of tissue affected and the causative agent, so that several types are described.

Microscopic recognition of necrosis is aided by nuclear changes in necrotic cells. The nucleus may shrink and stain more intensely basophilic (pyknosis), or it may fragment (karyorrhexis). More commonly, the nucleus simply loses its ability to stain differentially with basic dyes (karyolysis), for it gradually fades and eventually becomes indistinguishable. Necrotic tissue tends to stain diffusely with red acid dyes such as eosin, with lack of any blue or hematoxylin-staining material. Any calcium that precipitates in the necrotic material stains with hematoxylin, thus appearing as bluish masses.

Coagulation necrosis. Coagulation necrosis is commonly produced by the cutting off of blood supply (i.e., in infarction) (Fig. 2-16) but may also be caused by other means, e.g., by certain poisons (phenol, formaldehyde, and mercuric chloride). It is characterized by a protoplasmic coagulative process. In such

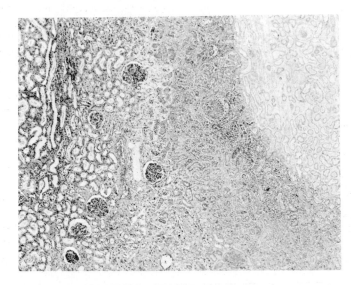

Fig. 2-16. Coagulation necrosis in infarct of kidney on right. Outlines of tubules and glomeruli are evident, although individual cells are indistinct. Necrotic tissue at junction of normal tissue (on left) and infarct appears darker because of leukocytic infiltration.

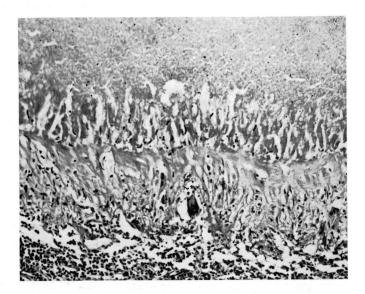

Fig. 2-17. Caseous necrosis in tuberculosis. Necrotic tissue in upper part lacks both structural outlines and discernible individual cells and their nuclei.

necrosis, general architectural features may be preserved for a considerable period, although cellular detail is lost.

Caseous necrosis. Caseous necrosis is so called because of a cheesy macroscopic appearance. It is particularly characteristic of the necrotic tissue resulting from tuberculous infection (Fig. 2-17), although it is seen in other lesions (e.g., tularemia and certain fungal infections). Microscopically, the architectural outline of the necrotic tissue is completely lost.

Gummatous necrosis. Gummatous necrosis results from syphilis and presents features of both caseous and coagulation necrosis microscopically, but in the gross form it has a more rubbery consistency. The individual inflammatory lesion of syphilis containing this type of necrosis is called a *gumma*.

Liquefactive necrosis. In liquefactive necrosis, the dead area softens and eventually liquefies. It is especially characteristic of necrosis in the central nervous system. It may follow other types of necrosis in other tissues, and the term may be applied to the liquefaction of pus in abscesses.

Fat necrosis. Fat necrosis is most commonly the result of pancreatic disease, which allows release of enzymes that act upon fat *(enzymatic fat necrosis)*. The traditional concept is that lipase and possibly other enzymes from the pancreas permeate the fat, causing hydrolysis of the neutral fat, and the free fatty acids that are split off in this process combine with calcium and other cations in the tissue fluid. An alternative theory is that the membrane of the fat cell is damaged by pancreatic enzymes (amylase, lecithinase, or both) and then lipase and possibly other enzymes are freed from the cytoplasm and cell membrane complexes that cause self-digestion of the cell fat.

The fat of the pancreas, omentum, or other intra-abdominal tissues shows whitish opaque nodules of very characteristic appearance. A zone of congestion and leukocytes surrounds the necrotic area. Eventually, calcium tends to be deposited in the necrotic tissue. In rare instances of acute pancreatitis, foci of enzymatic fat necrosis may occur outside the abdominal cavity (e.g., subcutaneous tissue). Fat necrosis also may occur in the breast and other subcutaneous areas as a result of trauma *(traumatic fat necrosis)*. With necrosis of the fat cells, there is release of neutral fat into tissues, followed by its change into fatty acids or soaps, probably more slowly than in enzymatic fat necrosis. An inflammatory reaction occurs, often of foreign body type with formation of giant cells, and a tumorlike mass may result.

Gangrene. In the strict sense, the term *gangrene* refers to necrotic tissue in which there is putrefaction resulting from invasion by saprophytic bacteria (e.g., moist gangrene). By usage, however, the term also is applied to massive areas of necrosis, even without invasion by saprophytes (e.g., dry gangrene).

Dry gangrene (or mummification) is a term usually applied to ischemic necrosis of a portion of an extremity, i.e., an infarction of the extremity. The tissue becomes dried out, greenish yellow, and finally dark brown or black. Inflammatory reaction in the adjacent living tissue causes a sharp line of demarcation separating healthy and dead tissues. In *moist gangrene,* which may be found in almost any part of the body, saprophytic organisms invade the dead tissue through wounds or from the respiratory or intestinal tract, causing putrefactive changes. *Gas gangrene* occurs when the invading saprophytes are of the gas-forming group (e.g., *Clostridium perfringens*).

Senile gangrene is a necrosis in an extremity in older persons resulting from interference with blood supply by arteriosclerosis, frequently with thrombosis. It is often a dry type but may be moist and putrefactive. *Diabetic gangrene* (Fig. 2-18) is similar and also caused by arteriosclerosis, but it is likely to occur at an earlier age. Gangrenous extremities resulting from interference with blood supply also may be caused by Raynaud's disease (vascular spasm), ergot poisoning (vascular spasm), and thromboangiitis obliterans (thrombosis).

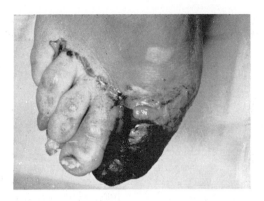

Fig. 2-18. Diabetic gangrene of great toe (53-year-old white woman). (From Gore, I.: Blood and lymphatic vessels. In Anderson, W. A. D., editor: Pathology, ed. 6, St. Louis, 1971, The C. V. Mosby Co.)

POSTMORTEM CHANGES

Somatic death, or death of the body as a whole, is followed by some early changes with which some familiarity is necessary.

Rigor mortis. Rigor mortis is a stiffening of muscles resulting from a chemical change in which there is precipitation of protein. At first it involves involuntary muscles, then usually begins in voluntary muscles in about 2 to 4 hours after death, and becomes complete in approximately 12 hours. Rigor gradually disappears in 24 to 48 hours but may persist up to 4 days. Since time of appearance and degree of rigor mortis are affected by a number of conditions, it is unreliable as an indicator of the exact time of death.

Livor mortis. Livor mortis is the reddish discoloration of dependent portions of the body resulting from the gravitational sinking of blood. Internal organs, such as the lungs, as well as the skin are affected. Hemolysis of red cells occurs with varying rapidity after death, and hemoglobin may lightly stain the aortic lining or serous surfaces. Hemoglobin staining may be hastened in death from infections, particularly if caused by hemolytic organisms.

Algor mortis. Algor mortis (cooling of the body) occurs gradually until the temperature of the environment is reached. The rate of cooling varies with factors such as environmental temperature, clothing of the body, and state of nutrition.

Postmortem clots. Postmortem clots are described in a subsequent section (p. 111) and compared with antemortem clots, or thrombi.

Autolysis. Postmortem autolysis is the self-digestion or breakdown of tissues caused by ferments released in the body after death. In some tissues, such as the mucosa of the stomach or gallbladder, autolytic changes are rapid, and good microscopic preparations of such tissues may be difficult to obtain after death. In general, the highly differentiated tissues (e.g., the ganglion cells in the nervous system and glandular epithelium) undergo more rapid autolysis than do supporting or connective tissue structures. Early autolysis results in loss of cellular detail in staining and may cause some confusion in differentiating it from such degenerative processes as cellular (cloudy) swelling. In postmortem autolysis, there is no inflammatory cell response, in contrast to that which may be seen in relation to necrotic tissue.

Putrefaction. Putrefaction in the dead body follows entrance of saprophytes, usually from the intestinal tract. It results in production of gases and a greenish discoloration of tissues. Gas-producing saprophytes may cause a foamy or spongy appearance of organs, particularly the liver.

CALCIFICATION

Calcium salts are normally deposited only in bone and teeth, but pathologic calcification is frequent in soft tissues and as concretions (calculi) in excretory or secretory passages. The calcium deposits contain calcium phosphate, calcium carbonate, and variable amounts of other salts, the composition being similar to that in normal bone. Frequent sites of pathologic calcification are blood vessel walls and kidneys, but some tissues contain calcium deposits with such regularity that the calcification may be a normal event (e.g., pineal gland in adults). Pathologic calcification is commonly classified as *dystrophic* and *metastatic*.

Dystrophic calcification. Dystrophic calcification is the deposition of calcium salts in dead or degenerating tissue. This is the most frequent type of pathologic calcification, occurring in areas of tuberculous necrosis, in blood vessels in arteriosclerosis, in areas of fatty degeneration and necrosis, in degenerating thyroid tissue, in degenerating tumors, etc. A retained ectopic fetus may become calcified (lithopedion). Dystrophic calcification is not dependent on an increase in the calcium content of the blood but appears to be influenced by a local relative alkalinity of the damaged tissue. Another suggestion is that an abnormal amount of phosphatase accumulating in necrotic tissue may favor the deposition of calcium salts. In areas of fat necrosis, calcium combines with released fatty acids (p. 43).

Metastatic calcification. Metastatic calcification is a precipitation of calcium salts resulting from a disturbance in calcium and phosphorus metabolism and is associated with an excess of calcium in the circulating blood. It occurs particularly as a result of hyperparathyroidism (p. 600) but also is seen in hypervitaminosis D (pp. 237 and 361) and in some conditions associated with destructive bone lesions, particularly tumors. The calcification occurs in previously undamaged tissues, especially in the kidneys, lungs, gastric mucosa, and media of blood vessels. In addition, any degenerating or necrotic tissue that may be present in the body also tends to become infiltrated by the excess calcium circulating in the blood, the factor of dystrophic calcification thus being present in some circumstances.

Calcinosis. Calcinosis is a disorder of unknown cause characterized by calcification, particularly in or under the skin. Circumscribed and generalized forms occur, the latter often having calcium deposits in tendons, fasciae, muscles, and nerves. Progressive systemic sclerosis (scleroderma) may have an associated calcinosis.

Pathologic ossification. In extraosseous sites, pathologic ossification is characterized by the formation of bone structures, such as lamellae, lacunae, and sometimes marrow. Such abnormal bone formation, which usually is preceded by calcification, is produced by osteoblasts arising from transformed fibroblasts in the area. The process occurs in a variety of tissues (e.g., arteries, cardiac valves, organizing hematomas, pleural scars) and even in an injured eye with chronic inflammation. *Myositis ossificans* is a pathologic calcification and ossification that may occur in a localized form after trauma to a muscle, or it may progress to involve tendons, fasciae, and ligaments also.

PIGMENTATION

In a number of conditions, colored materials are deposited in the skin or internal tissues. Although considered here together, they have nothing in common except the pigment deposition. There are two classes of pigmentation: (1) *endogenous,* in which the colored substance is produced within the body, and (2) *exogenous,* in which the pigment is introduced into the body by way of the intestinal tract, skin, or lungs.

Endogenous pigmentation

There are three types of pigments produced within the body: *melanins, those related to hemoglobin,* and *lipochromes.*

Melanin. Melanin, an insoluble polymer of high molecular weight, forms the normal coloring matter of the skin and of the uveal tract and retina of the eye. It is produced in the skin by melanoblasts (melanocytes) situated in the basal layers of the epidermis. These specialized cells may be distinguished, even though they contain no pigment at the time, by the dopa reaction (p. 694.) The precursor is tyrosine, which by a series of oxidations under the influence of the enzyme tyrosinase forms melanin. Pigment-carrying cells are present in the subepithelial tissues. The amount of melanin in the skin is increased by exposure to sunlight. Skin pigmentation is increased in Addison's disease (p. 609), and pigmented spots are common in association with multiple neurofibromatosis. Patchy areas lacking pigment also occur, and there may be a congenital absence of melanin pigment *(albinism)* resulting from a genetically transmitted lack of tyrosinase.

Partial albinism is a rare congenital defect with permanent absence of melanin pigment in various areas of the body (e.g., white forelock and spotting of the skin, a simple dominant condition, or albinism of the eye alone, a sex-linked recessive disorder). The also rare *total albinism,* involving skin, eyes, and hair, is transmitted as a simple autosomal recessive trait. *Vitiligo* is an acquired depigmentation of areas of the skin, in which the size and distribution of the lesions may alter.

Benign pigmented nevi and malignant melanomas are tumors composed of melanocytes. The amount of pigment found in such tumors shows extreme variation. Melanomas commonly arise from the skin or eye.

A melanocyte-stimulating hormone is produced by the pituitary gland. This hormone appears to be mainly responsible for the increased melanin pigmentation of the skin in Addison's disease and in pregnancy. Hydrocortisone from the adrenal cortex inhibits the release of the melanocyte-stimulating hormone, and adrenal medullary hormones appear to interfere with the action of the melanocyte-stimulating hormone on the melanocytes. Pigmentation may follow the administration of estrogens or corticotropin but not of cortisone.

Ochronosis is a rare type of pigmentation by a melanin in which cartilage is affected. Discoloration of the cartilage of the ear and nose may be visible through the skin. Ocular and renal tubular pigmentation also may be present. Most cases result from an inborn error of metabolism evidenced by *alkaptonuria.* This metabolic disorder is a genetic (autosomal recessive) defect of phenylalanine and tyrosine intermediary metabolism, resulting in abnormal accumulation of homogentisic acid, which tends to localize selectively in cartilage and is excreted in the urine. The basic defect is a lack of the enzyme homogentisic acid oxidase, which normally metabolizes homogentisic acid. Oxidation of homogentisic acid in the presence of alkali produces the dark urine (alkaptonuria), which is the main evidence of the disease in early life. Ocular pigmentation, with brownish blue spots on the sclera or on margins of the cornea, is a common finding. In later years, a degenerative arthritis of severe degree may develop and is the main clinical disturbance. The spine, knees, shoulders, and hips are affected most frequently.

Melanosis coli is a black discoloration of the mucosa of the large intestine, occurring in chronically constipated persons. The pigment resembles but is not a true melanin (p. 560).

Hemoglobin-related pigments. Hemoglobin, the pigment of red blood cells, is a combination of a pigment complex, *heme,* plus a protein, *globin.* The heme fraction consists of iron and protoporphyrin III. Several types of pigments are related to hemoglobin: hemosiderin, bilirubin (hematoidin), hematin, and the porphyrins.

Hemosiderin. Hemosiderin appears microscopically as golden brown, varying-sized, refractive crystals and granules of pigment. It may be formed locally when hemoglobin breaks down in tissues (e.g., as the result of hemorrhage) or systemically when there is excessive destruction of erythrocytes in the circulation. In these instances, the pigment is formed from hemoglobin within phagocytic cells, and the time for its production may be as short as 1 day. Hemosiderin deposition in various tissues also may occur as a result of excessive absorption of iron (e.g., in hemochromatosis). Hemosiderin has no exact chemical composition but contains loosely bound iron, which gives a Prussian blue reaction (a blue color with potassium ferrocyanide and hydrochloric acid). The iron is present mainly in the ferric form.

The normal continuous breakdown of red blood cells in the reticuloendothelial system results in some hemosiderin deposition in the liver and spleen. Pathologic excess of hemosiderin deposit (hemosiderosis) occurs in these organs and elsewhere whenever there is excessive breakdown of blood. Such occurs systemically in hemolytic anemias (e.g., thalassemia and sickle cell anemia) or after numerous blood transfusions and locally in areas of hemorrhage or in passive congestion of an organ, in which stagnation in capillaries results in increased blood destruction. In the spleen, hemosiderin pigment is found in phagocytic cells of the pulp and sinuses. In the liver, the pigment is found both in the phagocytic Kupffer cells of the sinusoids and in the liver cells. In the kidney, tubular lining cells as well as interstitial tissue and endothelial cells may contain pigment. In the lung, hemosiderin pigment is often abundant in large mononuclear phagocytic cells in alveoli when there is chronic congestion. These pigmented alveolar macrophages often are called "heart failure cells" because of their association with circulatory failure. Cardiac failure is the most common cause of pulmonary hemosiderosis, but idiopathic forms also occur, usually in association with repeated pulmonary hemorrhages. A related syndrome (Goodpasture's disease) is characterized by pulmonary hemorrhage and glomerulonephritis.

Iron storage disorders, characterized by excessive iron deposition in parenchymal cells and/or reticuloendothelial cells, are brought about by an increased absorption of iron from the gastrointestinal tract or by parenteral injection or by both. The excess iron originating from the intestine is deposited predominantly in the parenchymal cells of the liver and other organs; that which is introduced parenterally (e.g., by blood transfusions) is distributed mainly in reticuloendothelial cells, although some may be deposited subsequently in parenchymal cells. When cirrhosis of the liver and frequently when anatomic and functional changes in other organs are present also, the iron storage disease is designated *hemochromatosis,* either primary or secondary.

Primary, or *idiopathic, hemochromatosis* is a rare disturbance of iron-pigment metabolism, occurring almost exclusively in middle-aged and older men (80% between 40 and 60 years of age). A familial occurrence has been reported by some authors. In its classic form, it is characterized clinically by cirrhosis of the liver, diabetes mellitus, and skin pigmentation ("bronzed diabetes"), but the diabetes or the skin pigmentation is sometimes absent. Splenomegaly often accompanies the hepatic cirrhosis (portal hypertension), and ascites may be present in late stages. Endocrine disturbances are sometimes present, and cardiac complications may occur late in the disease. Primary carcinoma of the liver is a terminal complication in about 7% of the patients.

This form of hemochromatosis is due to an excessive absorption of iron from a usually normal diet. The nature of the absorptive defect in the intestine has not been clearly defined, but it is believed to have a genetic basis. Some reports have suggested that there is an increased avidity of the tissues for iron, but this mechanism is not generally accepted. The relative infrequency of the disease in women is attributed to the losses of iron during menstruation and childbearing. In some studies, relatives of patients with primary hemochromatosis have been found to have higher serum iron levels and plasma transferrin saturation than control subjects. In patients with this disease, the serum iron level is high, the plasma transferrin is saturated, and the total amount of iron in the body is increased from a normal of 4 to 5 g to 25 to 50 g. Most of the iron deposited in the tissues is in the form of hemosiderin. The liver contains the most iron, with increased amounts also in the pancreas, thyroid gland, pituitary gland, adrenal glands, salivary glands, and myocardium. There is little increase of iron in the spleen and bone marrow, the excess iron being predominantly in epithelial or parenchymatous cells rather than in the reticuloendothelial system. The excess iron may be mobilized from the body by repeated phlebotomy. There has been some controversy as to whether cell damage and fibrosis of organs are caused by the iron or simply occur concurrently.

The liver is enlarged and shows a portal type of cirrhosis with irregular hepatic nodules separated by thick fibrous bands. Hemosiderin is demonstrable predominantly in liver cells (not always distributed uniformly throughout) but is also present in the connective tissue, Kupffer cells, and epithelial cells of bile ducts (Figs. 2-19 and 2-20). The pancreas is enlarged, hard, and pigmented, with variable degrees of fibrosis. Hemosiderin is present in the cells of the acini, ducts, and islets as well as in connective tissue cells. Pigmentation in the skin is often caused by an increase of melanin, but in about 50% of the cases there is also demonstrable hemosiderin in the dermis of the skin, particularly about sweat glands. The heart almost always has an increased iron content with hemosiderin in muscle fibers. An excess of a yellowish fatty pigment, lipofuscin (hemofuscin), may be present in the heart, in walls of blood vessels and connective tissues of the involved organs, and in the smooth muscle of the intestinal tract.

It should be noted that some investigators have questioned the genetic nature of this disease and even have challenged the view that there is such an entity as primary or idiopathic hemochromatosis. They believe it is, instead, a "dietary hemochromatosis" resulting from two factors—viz., ingestion of excess iron in the diet and conditions, such as alcoholism and malnutrition, that lead to cirrhosis of the liver. According to this concept, the disease is regarded as a variant of nutritional cirrhosis of the liver, in which the associated conditions (malnutrition, alcoholism, anemia, etc.) enhance the absorption of iron, and the hepatic cirrhosis and fibrosis in other organs are independent of the iron deposits in the tissues.

Those who maintain that there is a primary form of the disease agree that an intake of excess iron and diseases or conditions promoting enhanced iron absorption may produce in some patients a pattern of iron overload similar to that of *primary hemochromatosis*. Such instances they classify in the group of disorders referred to as *secondary hemochromatosis*. Examples of "secondary hemochromatosis" of dietary origin are:

1 Patients with portal cirrhosis of the liver (often with a history of alcoholism or malnutrition)
2 Alcoholics imbibing wines and other beverages having a high iron content
3 Bantu subjects of South Africa who ingest excess iron in foods and alcoholic beverages prepared in iron pots (particularly if there is also nutritional deficiency)
4 Patients with refractory anemias in whom ineffective erythropoiesis may be a stimulus to increased iron absorption
5 Persons receiving prolonged oral iron therapy for anemia not secondary to iron deficiency

Transfusional hemosiderosis is an excessive iron storage in tissues as a result of multiple transfusions, usually given for the treatment of refractory anemia. It occurs in young adults of both sexes. The excess iron is deposited first and predominantly in the spleen and reticuloendothelial system. The skin, liver, and pancreas all may show hemosiderin deposits, but great degrees of fibrosis of the liver and pancreas are not usually present. When fibrosis and functional derangement of these organs exist, the condition is regarded as another example of secondary hemochromatosis *(transfusional hemochromatosis)*.

Recently, an association between primary hemochromatosis and certain HLA antigens (mainly A3) has been demonstrated by some investigators. As a result of their findings, they believe that there now exists a genetic marker of the disease by which idiopathic hemochromatosis may be differentiated from secondary iron overload, such as occurs in alcoholic liver disease.

Bilirubin and hematoidin. Bile pigment is formed from the breakdown of hemoglobin by reticuloendothelial cells, particularly in the

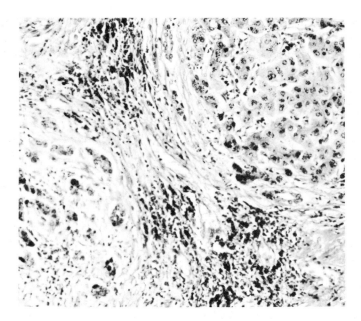

Fig. 2-19. Hemochromatosis of liver. Hemosiderin granules are present in liver cells, Kupffer cells, bile duct epithelium, and fibrous bands that separate nodules of liver cells. (Hematoxylin-eosin.)

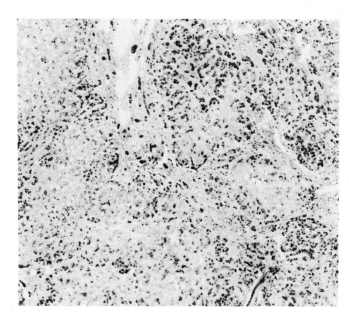

Fig. 2-20. Hemochromatosis of liver. Hemosiderin granules stand out prominently—Prussian blue reaction. (Iron stain.)

spleen, liver, and bone marrow. Excessive bilirubin in the circulation causes the yellowish pigmentation known as jaundice, or icterus (p. 458).

Hematoidin is a pigment closely related to or identical with bilirubin and is formed in tissues from hemoglobin. Like that of hemosiderin, its formation is intracellular, but several days are required to produce hematoidin. It is formed mainly in tissues in which good oxygen supply is lacking. Hence, it is often found where there is breakdown of blood in dead or dying tissues, as in infarcts, and usually appears extracellularly. Hematoidin may be seen as amorphous yellow granules or sheaves of crystals, which are frequently burr shaped. It does not give the Prussian blue reaction for free iron, since it is iron free, but it does give the Gmelin reaction for bile.

Hematin and malarial pigment. Hematin, which may be formed by the action of acids or alkalies on hemoglobin, is not a normal breakdown product of hemoglobin or a precursor of hemosiderin and bile pigments. However, there is a possibility of its formation in some cases of intravascular hemolysis or hemoglobinemia. In such cases, it rapidly combines with blood proteins to form methemalbumin. In the tissues, hematin appears as minute, rather uniform-sized rhomboid, dark brown pigment granules. Sometimes it is mistaken for hemosiderin, but its iron is firmly bound so that it fails to give a Prussian blue reaction as does hemosiderin.

In massive hemoglobinurias such as may result from transfusion reactions, casts of hematin pigment may be formed in renal tubules by the action of an acid urine and are a contributing factor in the resulting renal failure.

Malarial pigment is a closely related (hematin) compound formed by action of the malarial parasite on the hemoglobin in the red blood cell. Massive deposits of this brown pigment, which fails to stain for iron, are formed in reticuloendothelial cells of the spleen and liver (p. 208). In malignant pernicious malaria, the pigment is especially seen in red blood cells within capillaries and other small vessels of many organs, particularly the brain.

Formalin pigment, a hematin, is formed in tissues containing much blood when they are exposed to prolonged fixation in formalin, especially if it is acidified.

Porphyrins. Porphyrins are pigments that are normally found in minute amounts in the urine. In a rare inborn metabolic disturbance, *congenital (erythropoietic) porphyria,* large amounts of porphyrins are found in the urine, which is colored Burgundy red. Individuals having this disease are abnormally sensitive to light. This erythropoietic porphyria appears in infancy or childhood, transmitted as an autosomal recessive characteristic. It appears to be caused by an abnormal (increased) porphyrin formation in the bone marrow. Splenomegaly is commonly present. *Hepatic porphyria,* apparently an autosomal dominant disorder, occurs in adults, with high concentrations of porphyrins and porphyrin precursors in the liver. It may occur in an intermittent acute or a chronic cutaneous form. *Acquired porphyrinuria* occurs as a result of various conditions (e.g., lead poisoning and other chemical intoxications, hemolytic anemia, pernicious anemia, liver diseases, and carcinoma).

Lipochrome pigments. Lipoid pigments are found in small amounts in various places in the body. Some of these are probably related to carotene, a vegetable pigment ingested with food. The yellowish pigment of the corpus luteum is a lipochrome. Certain lipochromes are said to be the result of wear and tear of tissues. Brown atrophy of the heart is a senile condition in which lipochrome pigments are visible at the nuclear poles of heart muscle fibers. The heart has a brownish discoloration and is small as a result of atrophy of the muscle fibers.

Exogenous pigmentation

Colored materials may gain entrance to the body by inspiration, ingestion, and inoculation into the skin. Pigmentation of the lung by inspired substances such as carbon forms an important group of pulmonary conditions known as the pneumoconioses (p. 427).

Silver poisoning (argyria). Silver poisoning may cause a permanent pigmentation of the skin. Excessive administration of a silver compound over a long period results in deposition of pigment in the upper layers of the corium, immediately under the epithelium, and around sweat and sebaceous glands. The skin acquires an unpleasant, permanent, ashen gray hue. In severe cases, pigment is present in the kidney and liver as well. The pigment, an insoluble albuminate of silver, appears to be deposited between the connective tissue cells of the skin and in the basement membranes in the liver and kidneys.

Lead poisoning (plumbism). Lead poisoning may cause pigmentation of the oral mucosa. A line of deep blue pigmentation develops at the junction of teeth and gums because of the formation of lead sulfide.

Carotenemia. Carotenemia is a pale yellowish discoloration of the skin resulting from excessive ingestion of plant pigments, such as the carotene found in carrots. No deleterious effects are known.

Tattoos. Tattoos are pigments introduced into the skin by a needle or other sharp instrument for decorative purposes. The pigment may be seen as small granules held in the corium by macrophages. Infections, such as serum hepatitis, may be introduced at the time of tattooing as a result of unclean habits of the operator.

REFERENCES

Albukerk, J., et al.: Arch. Pathol. **93:**510-517, 1972 (Mallory bodies).

Baruch, E., et al.: Exp. Cell Res. **29:**50-53, 1963 (Councilman bodies).

Bearcroft, W. G. C.: J. Pathol. Bacteriol. **80:**19-31, 1960 (yellow fever in monkeys).

Benditt, E. P., and Eriksen, N.: Am. J. Pathol. **65:**231-249, 1971 (chemical classes of amyloid substances).

Biava, C.: Lab. Invest. **13:**301-320, 1964 (alcoholic hyalin).

Biava, C. G., et al.: Am. J. Pathol. **44:**349-363, 1964 (renal hyaline arteriolosclerosis—electron microscope study).

Bordin, G. M.: Am. J. Clin. Pathol. **66:**1029-1030, 1976. (green birefringence of amyloid).

Boss, G. R., and Seegmiller, J. E.: N. Engl. J. Med. **300:**1459-1468, 1979 (hyperuricemia and gout).

Brewer, D. B., and Eguren, L. M.: J. Pathol. Bacteriol. **83:**107-116, 1962 (hyaline droplet degeneration).

Brown, S. B.: Semin. Hematol. **3:**314-339, 1966 (clinical aspects of iron metabolism.)

Charlton, R. W., and Bothwell, T. H.: Progr. Hematol. **5:**298-323, 1966 (hemochromatosis).

Child, P. L., and Ruiz, A.: Arch. Pathol. **85:**45-50, 1968 (acidophilic bodies).

Cohen, A. S.: Int. Rev. Exp. Pathol. **4:**159-243, 1965 (constitution and genesis of amyloid).

Cohen, A. S.: Lab. Invest. **15:**66-83, 1966 (amyloid fibrils).

Cooper, J. A., and Moran, T. J.: Arch. Pathol. **64:**46-53, 1957 (ochronosis).

Cooper, J. H.: Am. J. Clin. Pathol. **66:**1028-1029, 1976 (green birefringence of amyloid).

Franklin, E. C., and Rosenthal, C. J.: Fed. Proc. **33:**758, 1974 (chemical heterogeneity of human amyloid).

Glenner, G. G., and Page, D. L.: Int. Rev. Exp. Pathol. **15:**1-92, 1976 (amyloid, amyloidosis, and amyloidogenesis).

Glenner, G. G., and Terry, W. D.: Annu. Rev. Med. **25:**131-135, 1974 (characterization of amyloid).

Glenner, G. G., et al.: Semin. Hematol. **10:**65-86, 1973 (amyloidosis: its nature and pathogenesis).

Haust, M. D., et al.: Am. J. Pathol. **40:**185-197, 1962 (cardiac colloid).

Heller, H., et al.: J. Pathol. Bacteriol. **88:**15-34, 1964 (amyloidosis).

Isobe, T., and Osserman, E. F.: N. Engl. J. Med. **290:**473-477, 1974 (patterns of amyloidosis and immunoglobin abnormalities).

Kazuhiro, O., et al.:. Lab. Invest. **33:**193-199, 1975 (Mallory bodies).

Kennedy, J. S.: Pathol. Bacteriol. **83:**165-181, 1962 (amyloidosis).

Kennedy, J. S.: Lab. Invest. **15:**84-97, 1966 (amyloidosis).

Klion, F. M., and Schaffner, F.: Am. J. Pathol. **48:**755-767, 1966 (Councilman-like bodies).

Kosek, J. C., and Angell, W.: Arch. Pathol. **89:**491-499, 1970 (basophilic myocardial degeneration).

Levin, M., et al.: J. Clin. Invest. **51:**2773-2776, 1972 (nonimmunoglobulin component of amyloid fibrils).

Lichtenstein, L., et al.: Am. J. Pathol. **32:**871-895, 1956 (gout).

Lombardi, B.: Lab. Invest. **15:**1-20, 1966 (pathogenesis of fatty liver).

MacDonald, R. A.: Arch. Intern. Med. **107:**606-616, 1961 (idiopathic hemochromatosis).

MacDonald, R. A.: Progr. Hematol. **5:**324-353, 1969 (hemochromatosis).

Mandema, E., Ruinen, L., Scholten, J. H., and Cohen, A. S., editors: Amyloidosis, Amsterdam, 1968, Excerpta Medica Foundation.

McGee, W. G., and Ashworth, C. T.: Am. J. Pathol. **43:**273-299, 1963 (fine structure of hypertensive arteriopathy).

Med. World News **12:**21, May 7, 1972 (amyloidosis—light chains).

Novikoff, A. B., et al.: Lab. Invest. **15:**27-49, 1966 (liver cell changes induced by orotic acid).

Olcott, C. T.: Am. J. Pathol. **24:**813-833, 1948 (argyria).

Osserman, E. F.: In Beeson, P. B., McDermott, W., and Wyngaarden, J. B., editors: Cecil textbook of medicine, ed. 15, Philadelphia, 1979, W. B. Saunders Co., pp. 1863-1865 (amyloidosis).

Panabokké, R. J.: J. Pathol. Bacteriol. **75:**319-331, 1958 (fat necrosis).

Roheim P. S., et al.: Lab. Invest. **15:**21-26, 1966 (orotic acid–induced fatty liver).

Rosai, J., and Lascano, E. F.: Am. J. Pathol. **61:**99-116, 1970 (basophilic degeneration of myocardium).

Simon, M., et al.: N. Engl. J. Med. **297:**1017-1021, 1977 (idiophathic hemochromatosis and HLA typing).

Sinniah, R.: Arch. Intern. Med. **124:**455-460, 1969 (hemochromatosis).

Smuckler, E. A., et al.: J. Exp. Med. **116:**55-72, 1962 (ultrastructural changes induced by carbon tetrachloride).

Soergel, K. H., and Sommers, S. C.: Am. J. Med. **32:**499-511, 1962 (pulmonary hemosiderosis).

Stetton, D., Jr., and Stetten, M. R.: Physiol. Rev. **40:**505-537, 1960 (glycogen).

Sweetman, L., and Nyhan, W. L.: Nature (Lond.) **215:**859-860, 1967 (genetic disease of purine metabolism).

Talbott, J. H.: Gout, ed. 3, New York, 1967, Grune &. Stratton, Inc.

Tedeschi, C. G.: In Renold, A. E., and Cahill, G. F., Jr., editors: Handbook of physiology, Sect. 5, Baltimore, 1965, The Williams & Wilkins Co., pp. 141-168 (pathologic anatomy of adipose tissue).

Teilum, G.: Am. J. Pathol. **24:**389-407, 1948 (paramyloidosis).

Teilum, G.: Ann. Rheum, Dis. **11:**119-135, 1952 (amyloidosis).

Teilum, G.: Lab. Invest. **15:**98-110, 1966 (amyloidosis).

Trump, B. F., et al.: Lab. Invest. **14:**343-371, 1965 (necrosis).

Uys, C. J., et al.: S. Afr. J. Lab. Clin. Med. **6:**1-11, 1960 (siderosis of liver).

Van Campen, D.: Fed. Proc. **33:**100-105, 1974 (regulation of iron absorption).

Wagner, B. M., and Siew, S.: In Sommers, S. C., editor: Pathology annual, vol. 2, New York, 1967, Appleton-Century-Crofts (significance of extracellular hyaline substances)

Weissmann, G.: Hosp. Pract. **6:**43-52, July 1971 (molecular basis of acute gout).

Wolman, M., editor: Pigments in pathology, New York, 1969, Academic Press, Inc.

Zucker-Franklin, D., and Franklin, E. C.: Am. J. Pathol. **59:**23-41, 1970 (intracellular localization of amyloid).

3

Inflammation and repair

INFLAMMATION

Inflammation is a local reactive change in tissues following injury or irritation. Wright defines inflammation as "the process by means of which cells and exudate accumulate in irritated tissues and tend to protect them from further injury."* It is a progressive reaction in living tissues, accompanied or followed by the process of repair or healing. The agents causing the injury, and hence leading to inflammation, may be of a microbial, immunologic, physical, chemical, or traumatic nature. The irritant apparently induces direct injury of cells, whose resulting altered metabolism liberates materials that initiate the inflammatory process. Inflammation is the most common and fundamental pathologic reaction and, in general, is protective, tending to localize or dispose of the injurious agent and to set the stage for repair.

In the local area, there are vascular (microcirculatory) effects, disturbances of fluid exchange, and emigration of the white blood cells (leukocytes) from the blood into the tissues. The accumulation of fluid and cells is referred to as an exudate. The cells of the local area show some effect of the injury, which may vary from mild degenerative changes to massive death and destruction. These alternative changes in tissue are essential in the initiation of the vascular, exudative, and reparative changes that follow. The mechanism of the inflammatory reaction may be understood best by reviewing the events of a typical acute inflammation (Fig. 3-1).

Vascular reactions in acute inflammation

After a local acute injury, there sometimes occurs a momentary or transitory contraction of vessels and hence local anemia. This evanescent constriction is rapidly replaced by hyperemia of the part, resulting from dilatation of arterioles, capillaries, and venules. The increased rate of flow also is transitory and gives way to a slowing of the current in the dilated vessels, progressing to capillary and venular stagnation and stasis. The stasis probably results, in part, from the loss of fluid from the vessels, which leads to an increase in concentration of red blood cells (hemoconcentration) and increased blood viscosity, and possibly from swelling and irregularity of the endothelial lining of the vessels.

The increased passage of fluid through the vessel walls is caused by elevation of capillary pressure and increased vascular permeability. Formerly, the concept was that the increased vascular permeability associated with inflammation occurred only in the capillaries. However, evidence from various investigations, mainly by electron microscopy, suggests that venules (20 to 30 μ in diameter) contribute substantially to the fluid of the exudate. Indeed, these studies show that the venules may

---

*From Wright, G. P.: An introduction to pathology, ed. 3, London, 1958, Longman Group Ltd.

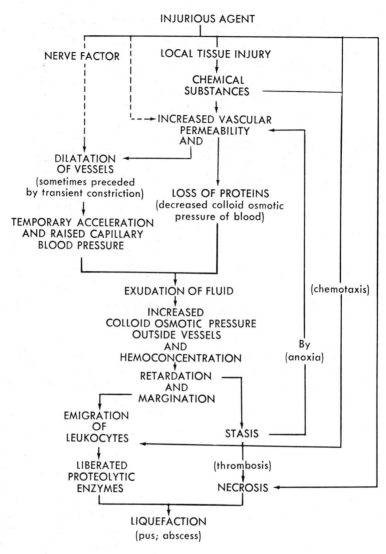

Fig. 3-1. Mechanism of acute inflammation.

be the most permeable segment of the micro-circulation. Further, it has been demonstrated that increased permeability, under the influence of vasoactive substances, may be caused not only by the intensification of the physiologic mechanisms of fluid exudation but also by the appearance of intercellular gaps in the endothelium through which even the larger molecules of the plasma (e.g., protein) and cells could pass.

Observations in various types of experimental injury have shown that the pattern of increased vascular permeability varies, depending on the type of injury, the species of experimental animal, and the intensity of the injury, the last factor being the most impor-

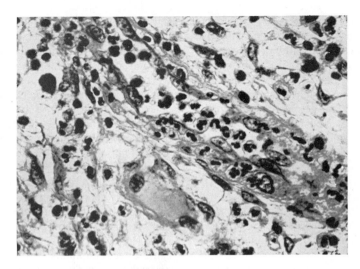

Fig. 3-2. Emigration of leukocytes in nasal polyp. Vessel in center contains a number of granulocytes. Others are seen in wall of vessel, apparently in process of emigrating. (×640; from Wilhelm, D. L.: Inflammation and healing. In Anderson, W. A. D., and Kissane, J. M., editors: Pathology, ed. 7, St. Louis, 1977, The C. V. Mosby Co.)

tant. With a mild or short-lived injury there is a transient, *immediate* increased permeability response, appearing rapidly and reaching its peak within a few minutes. Normal permeability is restored in about 15 to 30 minutes. Leakage occurs in the venules where intercellular gaps can be demonstrated in the endothelium. A slightly more severe injury causes a *delayed* response, in which there is a comparatively late onset of increased permeability preceded by a period of low permeability; this effect lasts for hours. Frequently, there is a *biphasic* response characterized by a transient immediate phase of increased vascular permeability, followed by a delayed type of response. In the delayed response, leakage occurs in the capillaries as well as in the venules, and intercellular endothelial gaps are demonstrated, although there also may be evidence of endothelial damage, particularly in the capillaries. After a strong stimulus, a *sustained* permeability response occurs, also referred to as an "early" or "immediate sustained" response. There is a rapid onset of increased vascular permeability, reaching a peak within minutes and persisting for hours. The affected vessels include venules, capillaries, and even arterioles. In this pattern of response, endothelial damage with disruption of endothelial cells is prominent.

Another phenomenon that occurs in the affected vessels is a change in the distribution of the leukocytes. Partly because of the slowing circulation, the leukocytes move from the central part of the bloodstream, where they are normally concentrated, and line up along and adhere to the endothelium (*margination* and *pavementing* of leukocytes), mainly in venules. They pass through the vessel wall into the tissue spaces by ameboid motion (*emigration* of leukocytes—Fig. 3-2).

The essential causes of the vascular reactions in acute inflammation have not been clearly established, but several factors have been suggested on the basis of experimental evidence. It is believed that vascular dilatation is brought about by certain chemical substances (mediators) liberated or formed at the site of injury, such as histamine released from damaged cells, although neurogenic influences (e.g., local axon reflexes) may play a less important role in the development of this response. Among the better known chemical mediators that are likely to be responsible for increased vascular permeability are histamine, 5-hydroxytryptamine (serotonin), polypeptides (such as "leukotaxine," bradykinin, and kallidin), and proteases (such as plasmin, kallikrein, and "globulin permeability factor"). The proteases act as mediators mainly because of their ability to produce polypeptides. Experimentally, it has been shown that the amines, particularly histamine, are important in the immediate type of permeability response. The polypeptides and their related proteases can act rapidly too. Whether any of these mediators also are involved in the delayed permeability response has not been definitely established.

Other agents that have been considered as possible mediators include slow reactive substance of anaphylaxis (SRS-A), nucleosides and nucleotides released from injured tissue, various products (such as enzymes and peptides) set free from neutrophils, lactic acid produced by anaerobic glycolysis or possibly produced by leukocytes in the exudate, lysolecithin, and certain bacteria or bacterial toxins. Lysolecithin is a cytolytic agent that may be released locally in tissues through the action of complement. It has been found to cause leakage from capillaries as well as venules, which is characteristic of the delayed type of increased vascular permeability. Such an action has not been demonstrated by the better known chemical mediators. The delayed permeability response also has been observed in some experimentally induced bacterial infections and following the application of the α-toxin of *Clostridium perfringens,* a lecithinase.

In certain immunologic reactions, an antigen-antibody complex is the likely cause of increased vascular permeability. In such instances, one mechanism may be fixation of antibody ("reagin") to mast cells and release of histamine from the cells after attachment of antigen to the antibody on the cells. Another mechanism may be the generation of certain vasoactive peptides, such as anaphylatoxin, from components of complement (e.g., C3 or

C5), which apparently cause the release of histamine from cells. A permeability factor has been obtained from lymph node cells, termed "lymph node permeability factor" (LNPF), which differs from the better known chemical mediators and is said to be particlarly active in delayed hypersensitivity reactions. Certain substances, known as prostaglandins, have been shown to cause increased vascular permeability, but their role in inflammation is not clearly established.

Although the etiologic stimulus of acute inflammation generally produces increased vascular permeability through the action of chemical mediators, the possibility should be considered that, if severe enough, it may cause direct endothelial injury followed by increased permeability. This appears to be the mechanism in the immediate sustained permeability response and possibly, in part, in some instances of the delayed type of response. Another consideration is that the stasis of blood that occurs in the microcirculation during the inflammatory process may cause a local anoxic effect on endothelium, thus contributing to the vascular leakage. The stasis of blood may play another role in inflammation, i.e., with or without accompanying microthrombi it may cause a critical level of microcirculatory insufficiency and consequent extravascular tissue damage (necrosis), which, in some instances, may be more than that produced by the etiologic agent itself.

The exudate

The accumulation of an exudate of fluid and cells in the area of injury is dependent on the vascular effects. The fluid part of the exudate is largely plasma from the blood and, when abundant, may be referred to as inflammatory edema. The fluid coagulates with the precipitation of a network of fibrin. The inflamed area tends to be walled off, and the injurious agent is localized by the fibrinous material. When immunity is present, localization of bacterial irritants is aided also by agglutinins, the invading organisms adhering to each other and to the tissues. The early fixation of a bacterial irritant in the area allows time in which leukocytes can assemble for phagocytosis. Neutrophils migrate through the vessel walls by ameboid motion, apparently by dissecting into and passing through the cellular junctions of inflamed endothelium, and then they pass through the basement membrane, possibly by enzyme action. After this, the membrane apparently is re-formed, perhaps by secretion of the cells of the vessel wall. Other leukocytes also pass through the gaps between the endothelial cells.

The cellular movement is aided in some cases by attraction to the site of injury by a chemical stimulus, a process referred to as *chemotaxis*. Some of the permeability factors (e.g., "leukotaxine," "globulin permeability factor," bradykinin, and serotonin) apparently exert only a slight chemotactic influence. Bacteria and products of tissue breakdown act as more powerful chemotactic agents, intensifying the emigration of leukocytes from blood vessels and directing them toward the injurious agent, leading them to the actual contact with the foreign particle, which makes phagocytosis possible. Adenine compounds released by the breakdown of nucleoproteins in injured tissue appear to promote chemotaxis and also to stimulate leukocyte formation in the bone marrow. It is possible that products of tissue breakdown participate indirectly by combining with or activating a factor in the serum, such as a component of complement, making it chemotactic. Three complement-derived chemotactic factors have been identified (viz., C3a, C5a, and C5,6,7 complex). These factors may be induced by sequential interaction of the complement system, as by an immune complex. C3a and C5a also may be generated by the direct action on C3 and C5 of an enzyme that is extrinsic to the complement system. The lymph node permeability factor, mentioned previously as a mediator of increased vascular permeability, also causes emigration of leukocytes. Viruses apparently do not attract leukocytes. The inflammatory cell response is probably evoked by products of cells damaged by viruses rather than by the viruses themselves.

The mechanism of the directional movement has been thought to depend on changes in surface tension, but McCutcheon has presented reasons for considering it to be caused by a directional orientation of colloidal changes within the cell. Chemotaxis is a directional reaction superimposed on ameboid motion. The rate of motion probably is not influenced. Toxic degenerative changes of leukocytes may interfere with chemotaxis and with rate of motion. Negative chemotaxis is a repelling of leukocytes by certain substances (e.g., silicic acid). Neutrophils move faster than other cells and thus usually are the first to emigrate. Monocytes are slower in chemotactic motion, and lymphocytes have little or no chemotactic activity. Positive chemotaxis is of great value in placing leukocytes in position to phagocytize bacteria and to form a wall about bacteria to prevent their spread.

In infections with pyogenic organisms, bacterial toxins and enzymes are probably largely responsible for the dissolution of tissues and destruction of leukocytes, which result in a purulent exudate and abscess formation. Proteolytic enzymes released from dead neutrophils lyse dead tissue, cells, and fibrin, contributing much to the formation of pus. In fact, it is by this means that suppuration occurs in nonbacterial lesions (e.g., after turpentine injection).

The fluid of an exudate usually has a specific gravity of 1.020 or higher, due mainly to an abundant content of serum proteins (1 to 6 g/100 ml). Ordinary edema fluid (a transudate) has a distinctly lower specific gravity. Antibodies of the blood are brought into the tissues with the exudate.

In inflammatory processes, there is frequently an increase in the number of circulating leukocytes (leukocytosis). Leukocytosis is a factor that aids in quickly bringing great numbers of phagocytic cells to the area of injury. The leukocytosis results from stimulation of the bone marrow by products released or formed in the area of inflammation (e.g., substances from disintegrating neutrophils or tissue cell breakdown and globulins and polypeptides from the exudate). Bacterial proteins also stimulate leukocytosis. In acute inflammations, particularly those caused by pyogenic bacteria, the neutrophils predominate in the blood (neutrophilia), and in some infections the ratio of immature (band) forms of neutrophils to mature (segmented) forms in the circulation is increased (''Shift to left''). The reversal to a normal ratio occurs as the infection is brought under control. Certain infectious diseases, however, are characterized by a decreased number of circulating neutrophils (neutropenia), e.g., typhoid fever, brucellosis, and various viral infections. In bacterial diseases ordinarily accompanied by neutrophilia, the presence of neutropenia is an unfavorable sign, since it implies an overwhelming infection with disturbance of the bone marrow function. Fever is also an accompaniment of many inflammations and is caused by toxic products from bacteria or other microorganisms (exogenous pyrogens) or by protein substances derived from leukocytes, mainly neutrophils, and possibly from damaged tissue (endogenous pyrogens).

Corticoids, such as hydrocortisone, appear to inhibit the development of an inflammatory reaction but without impeding necrosis as a result of the injurious agent.

Cells of inflammation

Cells in an inflammatory exudate may include various types of leukocytes, red blood cells, and giant cells.

Neutrophils. Neutrophilic leukocytes are the important cells of most acute inflammations. They migrate through the vessel walls and proceed by their ameboid activity to the site of injury, influenced by chemotaxis. Their function is phagocytosis of bacteria and tissue fragments, under the stimulus of substances of antibody or complementlike nature (opsonins) and other factors in the surrounding medium. They disintegrate and release proteolytic ferments, which digest necrotic tissue, fibrin, and other structures, producing liquefaction of the area. They also liberate enzymes and other substances that act as mediators of vascular permeability, stimulate leukocytosis, and cause fever (pyrogens).

The neutrophils tend to increase progressively until the irritant is overcome, provided the bone marrow is capable of increased production. Neutrophils are recognized by their segmented or lobulated nucleus. Faintly stained fine granules are present in their cytoplasm.

Lymphocytes. Lymphocytes are not present in significant numbers in acute inflammatory reactions except in lymph nodes and in the nervous system. However, they are numerous and important in many subacute and chronic inflammations. They are most important in immunologic reactions.

Lymphocytes are rounded cells, each with a relatively large dark nucleus and very scanty cytoplasm. It has been demonstrated that lymphoblasts, when studied in tissue culture, have a characteristic type of locomotion and shape that enables their differentiation from other cells, which often are morphologically similar (e.g., myeloblasts and monocytes). Lymphocytes are rarely phagocytic, but it has been maintained by Maximow and others that lymphocytes may be transformed into large mononuclear cells (macrophages) that have an active phagocytic function. It is generally believed that lymphocytes, unlike neutrophils and macrophages, pass through the venular endothelium not by way of the intercellular junctions but by invaginating the endothelial cells on the luminal side and traversing their cytoplasm. However, a recent study presents evidence that lymphocytes cross the vascular wall by insinuating themselves between endothelial cells.

Lymphocytes play an essential role in antibody production and in cell-mediated immune responses (e.g., delayed hypersensitivity, graft rejection, cellular immunity). For the immunologic properties of lymphocytes, see Chapter 4. Adrenal cortical activity appears to exert some control over lymphocytes and antibody production. Administration of cortisone causes lysis of lymphocytes but apparently before the cells are sensitized to antigen. It also has been suggested that the lymphocyte has a function in protein synthesis, acting as a carrier of reserve nucleoprotein, which some investigators believe may be utilized by other cells in the area of inflammation (e.g., by fibroblasts, thus enhancing fibrous tissue proliferation and repair). In studies of immune inflammatory responses, three types of substances have been derived from lymphocytes that may contribute to the tissue destruction in these states: lysosomal enzymes, a cytotoxic factor (possibly a phospholipid), and "lymphotoxin," which appears to be a heat-labile protein. The role of the lymph node permeability factor, derived from lymphocytes, was discussed previously (p. 56). Other substances liberated by sensitized lymphocytes as a result of an antigenic stimulus are referred to on p. 87.

Plasma cells. Plasma cells may be present in small numbers in acute and subacute inflammations but are particularly characteristic of chronic inflammation. Plasma cells are slightly larger than lymphocytes and have a basophilic cytoplasm that contains RNA and an eccentric nucleus in which the chromatin is collected in small masses around the periphery to give it a cartwheel or clock-face appearance. They are rarely seen in the circulating blood.

The plasma cell elaborates protein substances that accumulate in the ergastoplasm and under certain conditions may become condensed into acidophilic intracellular hyaline bodies (Russell bodies). Experimentally, these bodies may be produced by antigenic stimulus, and antibody may be a component of such bodies. Plasma cells are involved in the production of antibodies and other globulins (see Chapter 4). Plasma cell hyperplasia occurs during immunization. Antibodies are demonstrable in plasma cells by fluorescent microscopy and autoradiography. Gamma globulins and specific antibodies have been demonstrated in tissue extracts composed largely of plasma cells. In cases of agammaglobulinemia, there is as lack of plasma cells, and plasmacytomas may be accompanied by hyperglobulinemia. Plasma cells generally are not regarded as being phagocytic, although occasional phagocytosis by these cells has been reported. For example, phagocytosis of spirochetes and red blood cells has been demonstrated. Iron has been identified in plasma cells in diseases characterized by iron overload, but it is not certain whether this resulted from phagocytosis or from some other mechanism. A recent electron microscopic study offered evidence for incorporation of iron into the plasma cells by pinocytosis, although direct transfer of iron to the cells by macrophages was not excluded.

Eosinophils. Eosinophils have large reddish granules in their cytoplasm, and lobulation of the nucleus is less marked than in the neutrophilic polymorphonuclear leukocytes. Eosinophils once were believed to contain histamine, but more recently investigators have reported histamine-neutralizing substances in them. They are numerous in allergic inflammations, e.g., in the nose, sinuses, and bronchi (asthma). It is not certain, however, whether their presence in these lesions is directly related to antihistaminic activity. It has been proposed that they release substances that antagonize serotonin and bradykinin as well as histamine. Eosinophils also appear as a reaction to certain parasites, especially worms. Subacute and chronic inflammations in the uterus, fallopian tubes, and intestinal tract (especially the appendix) often show numerous eosinophils. In some pathologic conditions there may be an increased number of eosinophils in the blood (eosinophilia). The degree of eosinophilia may be marked in association with certain parasitic diseases, allergic disorders, Hodgkin's disease, and other neoplasms. In addition, a marked eosinophilia of unknown cause (idiopathic eosinophilia) may occur in the so-called hypereosinophilic syndrome. This syndrome also includes an increase of eosinophils in the bone marrow and an infiltration of eosinophils in various organs, such as the heart, lungs, nervous system, and skin, frequently with severe dysfunction of the affected organs.

Eosinophils are capable of phagocytosis. Since they frequently appear in hypersensitivity reactions, perhaps their role is to phagocytize antigen-antibody complexes, which apparently are able to attract eosinophils. Complement derived factors C3a and C5a as well as ECF-A (eosinophil chemotactic factor of anaphylaxis) also are capable of attracting eosinophils.

Circulating eosinophils decrease in number under conditions of stress because of increased pituitary–adrenal cortical activity. A decrease of circulating eosinophils following the administration of ACTH of the pituitary gland is an indication of adrenal cortical response to the stimulating hormone.

Basophils and mast cells. Basophils are present normally in small numbers in the blood (0.5%). Their cytoplasm contains granules that have a strong affinity for basic dyes and may alter the color of such dyes (metachromasia). The metachromasia appears to be caused by heparin content. The basophil also contains histamine, and most of the histamine in the bloodstream is carried by the basophils. Heparin is an anticoagulant and may be significant in fat transport and clearing in the bloodstream. Because of its histamine content, the basophil has a role in allergy, particularly in the histamine shock of anaphylaxis.

Mast cells, which also contain basophilic, metachromatic cytoplasmic granules, are found in connective tissues and sometimes appear particularly numerous in perivascular connective tissues. They have many similarities to the basophils of the blood. Mast cells have been shown to contain histamine, heparin, and 5-hydroxytryptamine. It is likely that the histamine involved in the acute inflammatory process in tissues is largely derived from mast cells. It has been suggested that a function of mast cells is to store and release mucopolysaccharides for connective tissues. Mast cells may be present in increased numbers in some chronic or healing inflammations. The skin lesions of *urticaria pigmentosa* are characterized by large numbers of mast cells.

Macrophages. Macrophages are large phagocytic cells described under a variety of names—monocytes, histiocytes, large mononuclear cells, polyblasts, endothelial cells, clasmatocytes, etc. At the site of inflammation, most of the macrophages are derived from blood monocytes, the major source of which may be the bone marrow. Some of the macrophages, however, may arise locally from the cells of the reticuloendothelial system, both those lining certain vascular spaces (sinusoids of liver, spleen, and lymph nodes) and those that are intimately mingled with fibroblasts in nearly all tissues. They also arise from alveolar cells of the lungs. The corresponding cells in the nervous system are the microglial cells.

Macrophages are large rounded or oval cells with an oval or indented nucleus and abundant relatively dense cytoplasm devoid of specific granules. They are highly important in both acute and chronic inflammatory reactions. In acute inflammations, they appear later than the neutrophilic leukocytes but persist after the latter have broken down. Some studies suggest that they may start to emigrate from the vessels at about the same time as neutrophils but appear later in the exudate because of their slower movement. Macrophages are highly phagocytic, ingesting bacteria, foreign material, and degenerating leukocytes, red cells, and tissue cells. They contain nucleases, proteinases, and carbohydrases and are rich in lipases. Thus, they act as scavengers and prepare the way for repair. They are the predominant and characteristic cells in certain inflammatory processes, e.g., in typhoid fever and tuberculosis, being transformed in the latter into "epithelioid" cells by the waxy material of the tubercle bacillus. It has been suggested that in delayed hypersensitivity states, lysosomal enzymes and a distinctive cytotoxin are released from macrophages, which may contribute to the tissue damage that usually accompanies these states.

Acquired resistance to certain infections depends, in part, on the presence of numerous macrophages in the tissues. The important role that they play in antimicrobial cellular immunity and in the induction of immune responses (e.g., antibody production) is discussed in Chapter 4. Their participation in cell-mediated cytotoxicity to tumor cells is discussed on p. 253.

Erythrocytes. Red blood cells appear in the exudate by passage through the excessively permeable vessel walls in the area of inflammation (diapedesis). In other cases, there are small hemorrhages due to rupture of injured vessel walls, so that red cells are more abundant in the exudate. An exudate of hemorrhagic character is present in reactions to certain organisms, such as those of anthrax.

Giant cells. Multinucleated cells of giant size are generally found in the presence of materials that resist absorption (e.g., foreign bodies and bone) and are a particular feature of certain inflammatory processes, e.g., tuberculosis and foreign body reactions. They appear to be formed by fusion of monocytes around some insoluble material, although nuclear division without cytoplasmic division probably occurs also. The Langhans' giant cell of tuberculosis usually has peripheral nuclei, and foreign body giant cells have diffuse or central nuclei, but they are probably essentially the same.

Other types of giant cells may occur in various situations, some of which are of a noninflammatory nature, e.g., megakaryocytes of the bone marrow, osteoclasts at the site of bone resorption or in giant cell tumors, tumor giant cells (as in osteogenic sarcoma), Sternberg-Reed giant cells in Hodgkin's disease, multinucleated Aschoff cells in rheumatic carditis, muscle giant cells at the site of repair of skeletal muscle, fusion giant cells in lymphoid tissue in measles (Warthin-Finkeldey cells), syncytial giant cells of placental chorionic villi, and epidermal giant cells in viral vesicles of skin (as in chickenpox).

Phagocytosis

Phagocytosis is the process of ingestion of foreign material or particulate matter. Its importance in the inflammatory reaction and as a defense of the body was first stressed by Metchnikoff. The neutrophilic leukocytes (Fig. 3-3) and the large mononuclear cells or macrophages are the important phagocytic

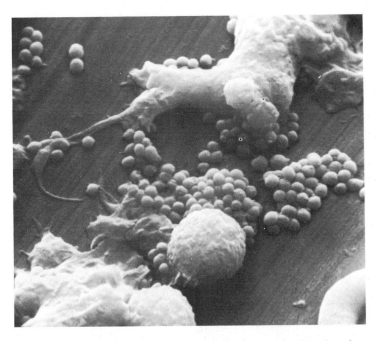

Fig. 3-3. Three-dimensional view of phagocytosis in vitro as seen by scanning electron microscopy. Neutrophil at top, with pseudopod at center left, is beginning to engulf several staphylococci. Two spherical cells with convoluted surfaces (center bottom) are lymphocytes. Part of erythrocyte may be seen in lower right-hand corner. Part of another neutrophil appears in lower left-hand corner. (Original magnification, ×5,000; from Klainer, A. S., and Perkins, R. L.: Hosp. Pract. **6:** 88-91, 95-97, 1971.)

cells, although a number of other cells exhibit lesser degrees of phagocytic power. Macrophages occur as monocytes in the blood, as wandering cells in all organs, and as cells lining the sinusoids of the liver, spleen, and lymph nodes. Giant cells, formed from macrophages, frequently show evidence of phagocytosis (Fig. 3-4).

The actual mechanism of ingestion was thought to be simply a passive, physical process dependent on surface tension changes. However, while surface tension may be a factor in phagocytosis, this process is now believed to be mainly an active one related to changes in metabolism of the phagocyte. It is apparent that phagocytosis requires expenditure of energy, since it is accompanied by an increase in oxygen consumption, glucose utilization, and lactic acid production and by an increased phospholipid turnover. The phagocytosis of bacteria is influenced by the nature of their surfaces and is aided by substances present in tissue fluids, such as opsonins and bivalent (e.g., calcium) ions. In some instances, phagocytosis of bacteria can occur in the absence of opsonizing antibody. This is done by the process of "surface phagocytosis"—i.e., the bacteria are trapped by leukocytes against surfaces provided by adjacent leukocytes, tissue cells (e.g., alveolar wall), fibrin strands, etc. and then ingested. The more highly virulent bacteria tend to resist phagocytosis.

During phagocytosis, the cytoplasm of the leukocyte extends out as pseudopods (Fig. 3-3) that encircle the particle to be ingested and then fuse to form an intracytoplasmic vacuole enclosed by pinched-off plasma membrane. This *phagocytic vacuole (phagosome)* fuses with lysosomes. The latter empty their contents into the vacuole, which now is referred to as a *digestive vacuole* or *phagolysosome*. Degranulation of leukocytes follows discharge of lysosomal contents into phagocytic vacuoles. The engulfed bacteria, tissue and cell fragments, foreign particles, etc. tend to be digested by the lysosomal contents, which include hydrolytic enzymes and nonenzymatic bactericidal substances such as phagocytin. Not all bacteria are killed by phagocytosis.

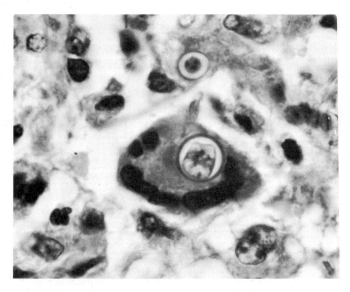

Fig. 3-4. Phagocytosis of pathogenic fungus *Blastomyces dermatitidis* by giant cell in human lung. Another organism may be seen above.

Some continue to live and even multiply within the phagocytes. This is true of the organisms of histoplasmosis, kala-azar, and leprosy. Tubercle bacilli also have considerable resistance to intracellular digestion. The inability of the macrophages to digest these microorganisms may be caused by failure of lysosomal fusion with phagosomes containing the organisms.

Phagocytic disorders. Various clinical syndromes characterized by impairment of the microbicidal function of phagocytes have been described; they may result from defective chemotaxis, phagocytosis, or intracellular microbicidal action or from a combination of these defects. The phagocytic defect may be caused by extrinsic or intrinsic factors and may or may not be characterized by morphologic abnormalities of the leukocytes. Some examples of the phagocytic disorders are listed below. In addition, a severe reduction of phagocytes, particularly of neutrophils (neutropenia), may result in a decreased resistance to infection, so that examples of this disorder are also included below even though defects in individual leukocytes may not exist.

A *Defective chemotaxis* caused by
  1 An inhibitor substance in the patient's serum
  2 A deficiency or abnormality of the complement factors
  3 Intrinsic phagocyte dysfunction, as in
    a Severe bacterial infections
    b Certain systemic diseases (e.g., diabetes mellitus)
    c Chédiak-Higashi syndrome (see below)
B *Defective phagocytosis* caused by
  1 Deficiency in opsonization resulting from
    a Deficiency of antibody (e.g., hypogammaglobulinemia)
    b Deficiency of complement factor
    c Specific lack of opsonin for certain microorganisms (e.g., for pneumococci in sickle cell disease)
  2 Defective lysosomal degranulation (disturbance in discharge of lysosomal contents into phagosomes), as in
    a Drug therapy (e.g., colchicine, corticosteroids)
    b Chédiak-Higashi syndrome (see below)
C *Defective intracellular microbicidal action* caused by

  1 Certain drugs (e.g., hydrocortisone)
  2 An inherent cellular defect, as in the genetic disorder known as "chronic granulomatous disease of childhood" (p. 123)
D *Reduction in number of phagocytic cells* caused by a defective production and/or excessive destruction of phagocytes, as in
  1 Congenital neutropenias
  2 Neutropenias caused by severe infections, chemicals, or drugs
  3 Autoantibodies against leukocytic antigens
  4 Bone marrow failure resulting from sepsis, leukemia, etc.

In the *Chédiak-Higashi syndrome,* an autosomal recessive condition, the leukocytes are characterized by a morphologic abnormality, i.e., abnormal giant lysosomal granules. There is an impairment of fusion of the abnormal granules with phagosomes as well as a delay or absence of release of the lysosomal enzymes into the phagosomes. The defective leukocytes also show impaired chemotaxis. An abnormality in formation of microtubules in the leukocytes has been considered to be responsible for this functional disturbance.

Signs of acute inflammation

The classic clinical signs of an acute inflammation on the surface of the body, where it can be seen and felt, are redness, swelling, heat, pain, and disturbance of function. The redness results from the vascular dilatation and congestion. The swelling is due to the edema (exudation) and congestion in the area. The inflamed area feels hot in comparison with surrounding areas because the dilated vessels bring a large amount of warm blood to the area. The heat is only that of the interior of the body. Pain is due to the swelling and tension on tissues caused by the exudate, with pressure on nerves. The accumulation of chemical substances (e.g., the kinins) or of hydrogen ions in the area may contribute to the pain by their action on the nerve endings. The cells and tissues involved by inflammation have their normal function disturbed.

Types of inflammation

Inflammation may be classified according to the following.

1 Duration and severity, as acute, subacute, and chronic
2 Predominant nature of the exudate and associated tissue change, as serous, fibrinous, hemorrhagic, catarrhal, purulent, phlegmonous, necrotizing, ulcerative, pseudomembranous, gangrenous, and granulomatous
3 Causative agent, as tuberculous, syphilitic, staphylococcic, foreign body type, and allergic

These classifications can often be combined. The ending ''itis'' added to the name of an organ or tissue indicates an inflammatory process (e.g., appendicitis—inflammation of the appendix; hepatitis—inflammation of the liver; dermatitis—inflammation of the skin). The various constituents of exudates often occur in combination, so that the reaction may be termed serofibrinous, fibrinopurulent, seromucinous, mucopurulent, etc. The inflammatory reactions induced by specific pathogenic organisms are described in Chapters 6 to 10.

In some inflammatory processes, proliferation (i.e., multiplication of cells) may be more prominent than exudation. Proliferation is not great in most acute inflammations caused by bacteria, except in the lymph nodules in typhoid fever, in which there is early multiplication of mononuclear cells, but many viral infections stimulate proliferation in their early stages. In subacute inflammations proliferation is usually evident, and in chronic inflammation it is often predominant. Proliferation of mononuclear cells (e.g., lymphocytes and macrophages), as well as connective tissue cells, is evident in nonspecific chronic inflammations, in chronic granulomatous inflammations (e.g., tuberculosis and foreign body reactions), and in delayed hypersensitivity reactions (e.g., at site of allograft rejection).

Pathologists frequently use the terms ''specific'' and ''nonspecific'' inflammation. A specific inflammation is one characterized by a well-recognized histologic appearance that is highly suggestive or diagnostic of a disease (e.g., the granulomatous lesions of tuberculosis and syphilis or the pathognomonic Aschoff body of rheumatic carditis). A nonspe-

cific inflammation does not conform to any distinctive pattern.

Acute inflammation. The acute inflammations are those that have a rapid course, the lesions clinically exhibiting the classic signs of heat, redness, swelling, and pain, or they are associated with severe or sharp constitutional reactions, such as fever, malaise, and leukocytosis.

Pathologically, the prominent features are vascular changes and exudation of fluid and leukocytes, particularly neutrophils. Although macrophages may be present, especially in the later phases of the acute process, other mononuclear cells, such as lymphocytes, appear infrequently or not at all. Connective tissue proliferation is not a feature. There are exceptional instances in which acute inflammations are characterized by mononuclear cell infiltration and not neutrophils (e.g., typhoid fever).

An acute inflammation may subside or proceed to subacute or chronic phases.

Subacute inflammation. Subacute inflammation is considered a transitional phase between acute and chronic stages. The exudative changes of acute inflammation may be still present to some degree while the proliferative changes characteristic of a chronic process have begun. Eosinophils are commonly present in association with macrophages, lymphocytes, and perhaps some neutrophils.

The use of the term subacute probably has little value except for those cases that cannot clearly be classed as either acute or chronic.

Chronic inflammation. Chronic inflammation is a process that is prolonged, and proliferation (especially of connective tissues) forms a prominent feature. It may occur as a late stage of a more acute process, or it may be essentially chronic (characterized by proliferative activity) from the beginning. The latter is likely to be the case with organisms of low virulence whose pathogenicity tends to be nearly balanced by the resistance of the body.

The predominant cells in chronic inflammation are lymphocytes, plasma cells, and macrophages, although a few polymorphonuclear leukocytes may be present. The proliferative activity, leading to the production of abundant scar tissue, may in itself be distinctly harmful. This is the case in chronic glomerulonephritis, in which the progressive glomerular scarring eventually results in functional failure of the kidneys.

Serous inflammation. Serous exudates, in which there is outpouring of abundant fluid in the inflammatory reaction, occur particularly in acute inflammations of serous cavities. The fluid contains a larger amount of protein and tends to have a higher specific gravity than a transudate. However, the specific gravity of fluids in serous cavities is not always an accurate guide to their nature. If fibrin precipitates from the fluid and appears on the inflamed surfaces, the exudate is termed serofibrinous. Reactions in other areas, such as some early acute inflammations of the skin, also may have an exudate of a predominantly serous nature.

Fibrinous inflammation. An abundance of fibrin in an exudate frequently is seen in inflammations of serous surfaces such as the pericardium, e.g., acute bacterial, rheumatic, uremic, tuberculous, or viral fibrinous pericarditis or that associated with myocardial infarction or invading neoplasms. Fibrin also is seen in the reaction to diphtheria bacilli, in which it entangles cells and necrotic material to form a false membrane on the surface. Fibrin formation decreases permeability of tissues and contributes to localization in acute inflammatory processes.

Hemorrhagic inflammation. Exudates containing so large a proportion of red blood cells as to have a grossly bloody appearance are usually caused by highly virulent organisms that damage small blood vessels. The reactions in severe cases of smallpox, anthrax, and meningococcal and hemolytic streptococcal infections are often hemorrhagic.

Catarrhal inflammation. Catarrhal inflammation is a superficial and usually mild inflammation of mucous surfaces, in which mucinous material forms a prominent part of the exudate. It is seen commonly in inflammations of the upper respiratory tract (Fig. 3-5) and large intestine.

Purulent (suppurative) inflammation. Pu-rulent inflammations are those in which there is production of pus, which is a creamy, semifluid opaque substance containing mainly liquefied necrotic material and many neutrophilic leukocytes (pus cells), both intact and disintegrated. A suppurative reaction results from a number of injurious agents, mainly bacteria but also some chemicals such as turpentine. Bacteria that commonly result in abundant pus production (pyogenic organisms) include staphylococci, gonococci, and pyocyaneus bacilli. Suppurative inflammation may be (1) on a surface, (2) localized in the tissues (abscess), or (3) diffusely spreading through tissue spaces (phlegmon or cellulitis).

An *abscess* is a localized area of pus accumulation within a tissue. It is found in an acute inflammation in which there is circum-

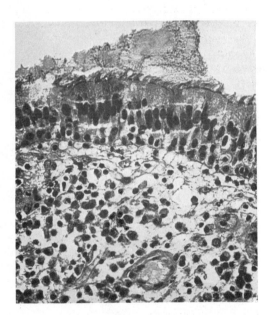

Fig. 3-5. Catarrhal inflammation in nasal polyp. Tissue is edematous and infiltrated with leukocytes. Observe mucous secretion beyond ciliated epithelial cells at top. (×350; from Wilhelm, D. L.: Inflammation and healing. In Anderson, W. A. D., and Kissane, J. M., editors: Pathology, ed. 7, St. Louis, 1977, The C. V. Mosby Co.)

scribed destruction of tissue and a collection of many neutrophils, which undergo disintegration (Figs. 3-6 and 3-7). Thus, a cavity is formed that contains the pus. Abscesses are fluctuant swellings because of their semifluid consistency. Healing is facilitated by drainage and removal of the purulent material. Otherwise, a relatively slow process of absorption is necessary. Abscesses may become walled off by fibrous tissue or may spread and extend, with the bacteria gaining entrance into the bloodstream (pyemia) and forming new (metastatic) abscesses in distant tissues.

Boils or *furuncles* are small abscesses of the skin. A *carbuncle* is a more extensive or spreading abscess of the skin that tends to discharge at several points. When an abscess discharges on a free surface, the tract along which it drains is a *sinus*. If the abscess discharges onto two body surfaces (e.g., skin and peritoneal cavity), the tract communicating with the two surfaces is a *fistula*.

Most, but not all, acute inflammations in which neutrophils predominate in the exudate are purulent, i.e., produce pus. A common example in which pus production does not usually occur is pneumococcal (lobar) pneumonia (p. 405), although leukocytes are abundant in the alveolar exudate.

Cellulitis. Cellulitis is an inflammation char-

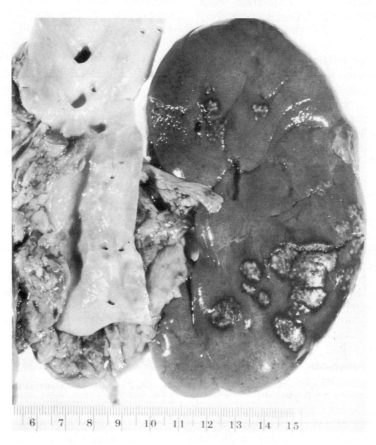

Fig. 3-6. Multiple recent abscesses of kidney, surrounded by reddish hyperemic or hemorrhagic zone.

acterized by a diffuse spread through tissue spaces and along tissue planes and frequently is of a suppurative nature. In contrast to an abscess, which is a localized lesion, cellulitis tends to be unlimited. Erysipelas, caused by β-hemolytic streptococci, is a form of cellulitis (p. 124). The terms *cellulitis* and *phlegmon (phlegmonous inflammation)* are commonly used synonymously, but some authors prefer to restrict the term phlegmon to the suppurative form of cellulitis (Fig. 3-8).

Pseudomembranous inflammation. Inflammations on mucous surfaces caused by a powerful necrotizing agent, such as diphtheria toxin or certain irritant gases, are characterized by formation of a false membrane. The surface pseudomembrane is composed of necrotic epithelium, coagulated plasma, and fibrin (p. 127).

Ulcer. An ulcer is a loss of substance from a surface (skin or mucous membrane) with in-flammation of adjacent tissue. Necrotic tissue discharged from the surface, leaving the ulcer, is termed a slough.

Granulomatous inflammation. Granulomatous inflammation is, in almost all instances, a form of chronic inflammation, with a distinctive histologic appearance. It is characterized by focal accumulation of mononuclear cells, chiefly macrophages (histiocytes). Admixed with the histiocytes are usually lymphocytes, sometimes plasma cells, and giant cells. Frequently there is a proliferation of fibrous tissue. In certain granulomatous inflammations, the macrophages become transformed to "epithelial-like" cells as a result of ingestion of certain substances and become known as "epithelioid cells."

Granulomatous lesions (granulomas) may occur as a result of certain microorganisms, in which case they are known as *infectious granulomas*. The lesion of tuberculosis, the "tuber-

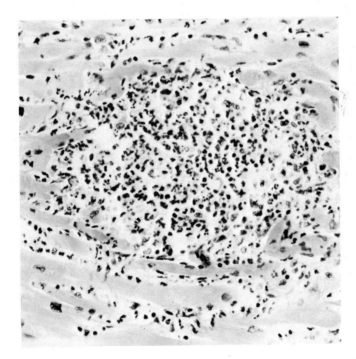

Fig. 3-7. Abscess of myocardium. Local accumulation of neutrophils in area in which necrotic muscle fibers have been digested (liquefaction necrosis).

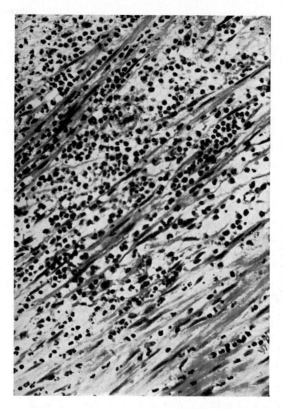

Fig. 3-8. Phlegmon of appendix. Fibers of muscularis are separated by exudate in which many polymorphonuclear leukocytes are recognizable. Lesion is not circumscribed. (×270; from Wilhelm, D. L.: Inflammation and healing. In Anderson, W. A. D., and Kissane, J. M., editors: Pathology, ed. 7, St. Louis, 1977, The C. V. Mosby Co.)

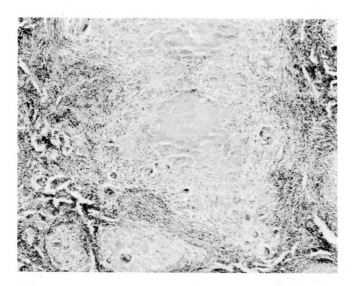

Fig. 3-9. Granulomatous inflammation in tuberculosis of lung (low power). Multiple nodules of histiocytes (epithelioid cells) with giant cells (details in Fig. 3-10). Confluence of nodules with foci of caseation necrosis may be seen in center and at top.

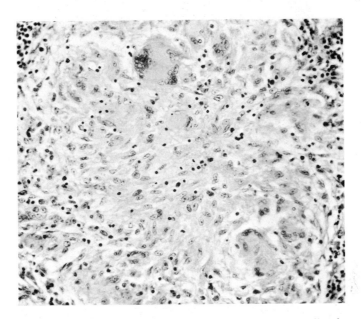

Fig. 3-10. High-power view of section illustrated in Fig. 3-9 to show details of granulomatous inflammation. Nodule consists of a collection of epithelioid cells with several Langhans' giant cells and lymphocytes, particularly in the periphery.

cle,'' is characteristic of this type, being composed of epithelioid cells, lymphocytes, and Langhans' giant cells (Figs. 3-9 and 3-10). Other infections, such as syphilis, leprosy, and certain fungal infections, produce similar lesions (''tuberculoid granulomas''). Sarcoidosis, a disease of unknown cause, also produces this type of reaction. Another form of chronic granulomatous inflammation is the *foreign body reaction*. Foreign materials, such as surgical sutures, cholesterol crystals, ingrowing hairs (as in pilonidal sinuses), and talcum powder, which are too large to be ingested by phagocytes, become surrounded by macrophages that fuse to form multinucleated giant cells (Fig. 3-11). Also included in the reaction are lymphocytes and proliferating fibroblasts. Granulomas also occur in diseases of immunologic origin (e.g., *allergic granulomas* in certain hypersensitivity states and *Aschoff bodies* in rheumatic carditis).

Allergic inflammation (hypersensitivity). Although the immune system is capable of protecting an individual, e.g., by production of antibodies against microbial agents, there are times when an immune response may induce a harmful reaction in the tissues. This type of reaction is seen in the various hypersensitivity states (e.g., anaphylaxis, Arthus reaction, serum sickness, and delayed hypersensitivity). These are discussed in Chapter 4.

The type of inflammation varies in the allergic responses. In certain of the immediate-type hypersensitivities, the inflammatory reaction may be nonspecific with granulocytes, including eosinophils, being prominent. Necrosis with fibrinoid change (e.g., in vascular walls) may be evident. In the delayed type of hypersensitivity, the mononuclear cells—lymphocytes and macrophages—predominate. In some allergic diseases, granulomatous inflammation is observed (e.g., necrotizing granulomas in Wegener's granulomatosis). Fibrinoid necrosis (p. 31) is frequently seen in hypersensitivity lesions, although it is not limited to these lesions. It commonly occurs in the so-

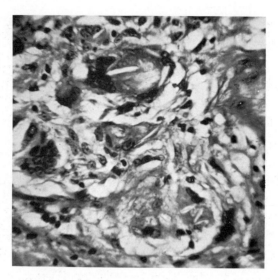

Fig. 3-11. Foreign body reaction with crystalline material in giant cells.

called collagen diseases, which are of a probable autoimmune nature, and frequently involves small vessels and the interstitial connective tissues.

REPAIR OR HEALING

Repair or healing of an injured tissue (e.g., an area of inflammation or a wound) may be brought about by one or more of three processes:

1 *Resolution* (or restoration of the involved part to a normal state) may occur when the injury is slight and there is degeneration of parenchymal cells without necrosis, as in certain inflammations. After subsidence of the inflammatory response and recovery of the degenerated cells, the area is restored to normal.

2 *Healing by granulation tissue or scar formation* may take place if resolution is delayed or if the injury is severe enough to produce destruction of tissue.

3 There may be replacement of destroyed or lost cells by proliferating cells of similar type from adjacent living cells *(regeneration).*

It is to be noted that the terms "healing" and "repair" are used synonymously here.

Some authors restrict the term "repair" to healing of an area by formation of scar tissue, using the term "healing" as a generic one, referring to any means by which tissue is restored after injury.

Repair by scar formation

A connective tissue reaction is a fundamental part of the response of the body to injury when tissue destruction occurs. Whether this reparative process is considered as part of inflammation or as a separate process is immaterial. Proliferative and reparative activity tends to follow the vascular and exudative phenomena of inflammation and often proceeds coincidentally. The final healed state is achieved by development of a connective tissue scar and by regeneration of cells. The degree of each and the balance between scarring and regeneration depend primarily on the nature and the extent of the destroyed tissue.

Repair by scar formation is a common type of healing. It begins as a proliferation of young connective tissue cells (fibroblasts) and multiplication of small blood vessels by mitotic division of connective tissue and endothelial cells, respectively. The elongated fibroblasts and buds of endothelial cells grow into

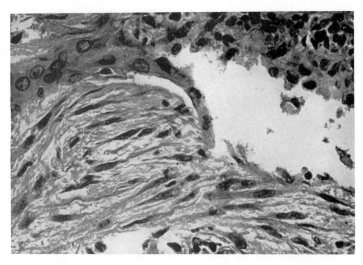

Fig. 3-12. Scar, early stage. Connective tissue cells lie parallel and are bipolar, provided with processes, and separated by extracellular collagen fibers. (×370; from Anderson, W. A. D., and McCutcheon, M.: Inflammation. In Anderson, W. A. D., editor: Pathology, ed. 5, St. Louis, 1966, The C. V. Mosby Co.)

and permeate the exudate, producing a highly vascularized, reddish granular mass termed *granulation tissue*. The granulation tissue replaces the exudate and fills any gaps in the tissue. This loose and highly vascularized young connective tissue is very resistant to infection. The replacement of necrotic material, exudate, or a thrombus by granulation tissue is referred to as *organization*. Infiltrating the granulation tissue are leukocytes, particularly macrophages, which assist in the repair process by removing necrotic tissue, cellular debris, and fibrin. Another role of the macrophages may be to promote fibroblastic proliferation in some way. There is a gradual laying down of collagen by the proliferating fibroblasts (Fig. 3-12), and eventually a dense fibrous scar is formed (Fig. 3-13).

A large abscess cavity or a tuberculous cavity from which the contents have been discharged may not be filled by granulation tissue. Rather, a fibrous wall may form around it. If, however, the cavity can be collapsed so that the walls are in contact, healing may be completed.

In the healing of a surface wound or ulcer, in addition to filling of the defect by granulation tissue, there is proliferation of epithelial cells at the edge, the cells gradually growing from the periphery to cover the surface gap. When the area to be covered is too large, the epithelial cells may be unable to complete the covering process. If any skin appendages (e.g., hair follicles) persist in the depths of a wound, they may contribute proliferating epithelium to help cover the defect. Skin grafting may be used to supply other foci of epithelial cells from which extension can occur.

When organization is complete and the defect has been filled by granulation tissue, the capillaries decrease in size and number and largely disappear. The connective tissue shrinks, becomes condensed, develops more collagenous fibers, and acquires the appearance of adult connective tissue. The scar (cicatrix) thus produced is transformed slowly from a soft red area to a pale or white, shrunken, firm fibrous tissue. Shrinkage or contracture may produce deformities of internal organs or disability if the scar is situated over a joint.

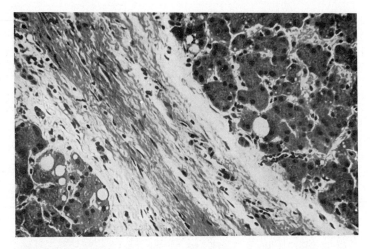

Fig. 3-13. Scar, late stage, in cirrhotic liver. Scar composed largely of collagen fibers with scanty elongated nuclei of connective tissue cells. (×180; from Anderson, W. A. D., and Mc-Cutcheon, M.: Inflammation. In Anderson, W. A. D., editor: Pathology, ed. 5, St. Louis, 1966, The C. V. Mosby Co.)

Adhesions of serous surfaces, as between visceral and parietal layers of peritoneum, pleura, or pericardium, frequently result from the organization of fibrinous exudates on apposing surfaces. In the pericardium, the effect may be to obliterate the sac and throw an added functional burden on the heart. Adhesions as a result of arthritis may limit the movement of a joint.

Healing of skin wounds. The healing of a clean uninfected incised wound, in which there is little destruction of tissue and where the edges of the wound are held in apposition, occurs with a minimum of granulation and scar tissue and is referred to as "primary union," or "healing by first intention." In such an instance, a coagulum of extravasated blood fills and seals the defect. Neutrophils and macrophages appear in the area because of the accompanying acute inflammation in the margins of the incised tissue and remove the necrotic tissue and erythrocytes. The fibrin network in the coagulum serves as a scaffolding along which proliferating fibroblasts extend, followed by newly formed blood vessels. Subsequently, collagen formation occurs. The migrating and proliferating epithelium from the

wound margins advances beneath the fibrin clot and eventually covers the defect. In the earlier stages of healing, the epithelium extends down into the wound along the sides of the incision, but as healing in the dermis occurs, the epithelial ingrowths regress and the surface epithelium completes its regeneration. Tensile strength, which is related to collagen formation and is the factor that combats dehiscence of a surgical wound, increases progressively from the fourth to the fourteenth or fifteenth day of the healing process, at which time it is nearly normal. Maximum tensile strength, however, generally occurs later.

In larger wounds with much loss of tissue or in wounds complicated by infection, the healing process is more delayed ("secondary union" or "healing by second intention"), and greater scarring results. Although the healing process in these circumstances is essentially similar to that in "primary union," some differences are that more tissue and other debris must be removed, the infection must be overcome, and the growth of granulation tissue filling the defect is more abundant. The granulation tissue must be built up slowly from the bottom and sides of the wound, and epithelium grows over the granulation tissue. In extensive, full-thickness wounds, it appears that a bed of granulation tissue is necessary before the defect undergoes epithelialization.

The nature and efficiency of the healing process may be influenced by various factors. The state of nutrition is of importance. Vitamin C is essential for proper collagen formation, and in severe deficiency of this vitamin, wounds fail to heal properly and are easily disrupted. Proper healing of bone is promoted by a sufficiency of vitamins C and D. An adequate protein diet also may be important, for some experiments have indicated that wound healing is delayed when plasma proteins are sufficiently reduced. Local factors that delay healing of a wound include excessive trauma of tissue during surgery, poor blood supply to the area, hematoma (collection of blood) in and about the wound, and infection.

Foreign substances vary widely in the type of tissue response that they elicit. Certain metal alloys used to hold fractured bone fragments in position elicit only little tissue response and do not delay healing. Similarly, certain suture materials, such as silk, cotton, and some synthetic fibers, produce relatively little inflammatory response in tissues as compared with other materials, such as catgut. Sulfonamides applied to wounds cause some reaction in tissues but apparently not sufficient to retard healing seriously. Experimentally, administration of cortisone or ACTH appears to depress formation of granulation tissue and delay wound healing.

Regeneration

Regeneration is the replacement of lost or destroyed tissue by newly formed similar tissue, which is accomplished by proliferation of the adjacent living specialized cells. Physiologic regeneration is the reproduction of tissue lost by the normal wear of life, e. g., of surface epithelium and red blood cells. Regeneration also acts to replace tissues destroyed by disease. Capacity for regeneration decreases as age increases and also is affected by the state of nutrition of the individual. The most important factor, however, is the type of tissue destroyed. The more highly specialized the tissue, the less its capacity for regeneration. Thus, connective tissue regenerates most readily, whereas ganglion cells of the central nervous system have no ability to regenerate. The power of the various tissues to regenerate may be outlined as follows:

blood-forming tissues regenerate readily

bone regenerates readily from periosteum or endosteum, with preliminary formation of uncalcified osteoid tissue

cartilage regenerates to some extent from perichondrium

connective tissue regenerates very readily

glandular epithelium individual cells regenerate, but specialized structures are not so readily formed; e.g., in the kidney, tubular epithelial cells regenerate easily, but whole tubular or glomerular structures are not replaced after their destruction

liver shows marked capacity for regeneration, provided its blood supply and connective tissue framework are intact

myocardium achieves practially no regeneration, except possibly in infancy

neuroglial tissue regenerates quite readily

neurons of central nervous system have no power of regeneration

peripheral nerve fibers regenerate easily if injured ends are in apposition

striated voluntary muscle has limited capacity for replacement after destruction of limited size

surface epithelium has marked capacity for regeneration, but in skin, associated structures such as hair follicles and sweat glands do not regenerate if completely destroyed

When tissues without the ability to regenerate are destroyed, repair is by connective tissue, or, in the central nervous system, by neuroglial cells. Even in tissues with good regenerative ability, such as the liver, the repair of extensive destruction is partly by connective tissue.

Biochemical changes associated with regeneration are similar, to a large extent, regardless of the tissues involved. Following the initial trauma, there is a regressive phase characterized by proteolysis, increase in sulfhydryl groups and lactic acid, and decrease in RNA concentration. In the subsequent progressive phase of growth and differentiation, there is augmented synthetic activity with increase in RNA and DNA concentrations and reversal to preexisting pH.

Several theories have been proposed concerning the pathogenetic mechanisms of regeneration. One is that there are organ-specific hormones released from tissue that stimulate proliferation of the same type of tissue. Another is that systemic hormones promote growth. This may be so in regeneration of endocrine tissues, which is possibly influenced by pituitary tropic hormones, or in the process of erythropoiesis induced by the hormone erythropoietin, which is believed to be released mainly by the kidney. A third concept is that certain intracellular inhibitory humoral factors (e.g., chalones), which normally prevent proliferation, disappear from the cells or are reduced in concentration because of uptake of water by the cells when tissue is damaged, allowing regeneration. A fourth hypothesis, not related to a humoral factor, is based on the concept of a regulatory mechanism between cytoplasmic and nuclear structures. Differentiation of cytoplasmic structures, such as the endoplasmic reticulum, restrains DNA synthesis. Thus, after damage of the cytoplasm, loss of the restraining influence occurs, followed by increase in DNA synthesis and cell division.

REFERENCES

Abramson, N., et al.: N. Engl. J. Med. **283:**248-250, 1970 (phagocytic plasma cells).

Adams, D. O.: Am. J. Pathol. **84:**163-192, 1976 (the granulomatous inflammatory response—a review).

Azar, H. A., et al.: Arch. Pathol. **90:**143-150, 1970 (phagocytosis of spirochetes by plasma cells).

Benditt, E. P.: Gastroenterology **40:**338-343, 1961 (mechanisms).

Curran, R. S.: In Crawford, T., editor: Modern trends in pathology, vol. 2, London, 1967, Butterworth & Co. (Publishers) Ltd., pp. 40-101 (recent developments in field of inflammation and repair).

Dannenberg, A. M.: N. Engl. J. Med. **293:**489-493, 1975 (macrophages in inflammation).

Douglas, S. D.: Blood **35:**851-866, 1970 (disorders of phagocytic function).

Dvorak, A. M., and Dvorak, H. F.: Arch. Pathol. Lab. Med. **103:**551-557, 1979 (the basophil).

Editorial: Lancet **1:**438-440, 1974 (disorders of neutrophil function).

Fisher, E. R.: J.A.M.A. **173:**171-173, 1960 (tissue mast cells).

Fisher, E. R.: In Sommers, S. C., editor: Pathology annual, vol. 4, New York, 1969, Appleton-Century-Crofts, p. 89 (repair by regeneration).

Florey, H. W., editor: General pathology, ed. 4, Philadephia, 1970, W. B. Saunders Co.

Forscher, B., and Houck, J. C., editors: Immunology of inflammation, Amsterdam, 1971, Excerpta Medica Foundation.

Goetzel, E. J., et al.: Arch. Pathol. **99:**1-4, 1975 (eosinophils in immediate hypersensitivity).

Hardy, W. R., and Anderson, R. E.: Ann. Intern. Med. **68:**1220-1229, 1968 (hypereosinophilic syndromes).

Jensen, J. A.: Microcirculation, perfusion, and transplantation of organs, New York, 1970, Academic Press, Inc., p. 191 (immunoresponse and vascular permeability).

Kaliner, M. A.: N. Engl. J. Med. **301:**498-499, 1979 (mast cells).

Karcioglu, G. L., and Hardison, J. E.: Arch. Intern. Med. **138:**97-100, 1978 (iron-containing plasma cells).

Kellermeyer, R. W., and Graham, R. C., Jr.: N. Engl. J. Med. **279:**754-759, 802-807, 859-866, 1968 (kinins—physiologic and pathologic roles).

Leibovich, S. J., and Ross, R.: Am. J. Pathol. **78:**71-100, 1975 (role of macrophage in wound repair).

Marchesi, V. T.: Q. J. Exp. Physiol. **46:**115-118, 1961 (emigration of leukocytes).

McCutcheon, M.: Arch. Pathol. **34:**167-181, 1942 (chemotaxis).

McGovern, V. J.: J. Pathol. Bacteriol. **73:**99-106, 1957 (inflammation).

McKinn, R. M. H.: Tissue repair, New York, 1969, Academic Press, Inc.

Menkin, V.: Biochemical mechanisms in inflammation, ed. 2, Springfield, Ill., 1956, Charles C Thomas, Publisher.

Movat, H. Z.: Am. J. Med. Sci. **236:**373-382, 1958 (fibrinoid).

Movat, H. Z., editor: Inflammation, immunity and hypersensitivity, ed. 2, New York, 1979, Harper & Row, Publishers, Inc.

Oliver, J. M.: Am. J. Pathol. **85:**395-418, 1976 (microtubules in Chédiak-Higashi syndrome).

Parrillo, J. E., et al.: Ann. Intern. Med. **89:**167-172, 1978 (hypereosinophilic syndrome).

Pearsall, N. N., and Weiser, R. S.: The macrophage, Philadelphia, 1970, Lea & Febiger.

Rausch, P. G., et al.: N. Engl. J. Med. **298:**693-698, 1978 (study of granules in Chédiak-Higashi leukocytes).

Rebuck, J. W., editor: The lymphocyte and lymphocytic tissue, New York, 1960, Hoeber Medical Division, Harper & Row, Publishers, Inc.

Ryan, G. B., and Majno, G.: Am. J. Pathol. **86:**183-276, 1977 (review of acute inflammation).

Schlegel, R. J.: J.A.M.A. **231:**615-617, 1975 (chronic granulomatous disease).

Schoefl, G. I.: J. Exp. Med. **136:**568-588, 1972 (migration of lymphocytes across vascular endothelium).

Shanmugathasa, M.: Arch. Pathol. Lab. Med. **103:**577-582, 1979 (plasma cells with iron inclusions).

Spector, W. G., editor: Ann. N.Y. Acad. Sci. **116:**747-1084, 1964 (acute inflammatory response [symposium]).

Spector, W. G., and Willoughby, D. A.: The pharmacology of inflammation, London, 1968, The English Universities Press Ltd.

Stossel, T. P.: N. Engl. J. Med **290:**717-723, 774-780, 833-839, 1974 (phagocytosis).

Thomas, L., Uhr, J. W., and Grant, L., editors: International symposium on injury, inflammation and immunity, Baltimore, 1964, The Williams & Wilkins Co.

Ward, P. A.: Am. J. Pathol. **77:**519-538, 1974 (review of leukotaxis and leukotactic disorders).

Weiss, L.: The cells and tissues of the immune system, Englewood Cliffs, N.J., 1972, Prentice-Hall, Inc.

Zweifach, B. W., Grant, L., and McCluskey, R. T., editors: The inflammatory process, ed. 2, New York, 1973, Academic Press, Inc.

4

Immunologic disorders

Under certain circumstances, the immune response in an individual is a protective mechanism *(protective immunity)*. This type of response may occur after a clinical or subclinical infection, in which instance it is specific in that the individual exhibits a resistance to the particular microorganism with which he has had previous contact. Protective immunity also may be conferred by immunization procedures. For example, inoculation of a relatively harmless antigen, such as an attenuated or killed bacterium or virus, will stimulate the production of specific antibodies against the microorganism. This protection, whether conferred naturally by previous exposure to an infection or artificially by the administration of an antigen, is known as "active immunity," since the individual produces his own antibodies through activation of the immune system as a result of antigenic stimulation. This differs from "passive immunity" in which protection, usually transient, is acquired by administration of preformed antibodies from another individual of the same or different species.

The protective effect of antibodies results from their ability to inhibit or destroy infectious agents, neutralize their toxins, and enhance phagocytosis by opsonizing or agglutinating microorganisms. Resistance to infections caused by bacteria, fungi, and viruses that can survive and multiply in macrophages is not mediated by humoral antibodies but by a cell-mediated mechanism, *antimicrobial cellular immunity*. Lymphocytes sensitized by the microbial antigen are able to "activate" macrophages, which means that the latter develop an increased ability to destroy microorganisms and contain an increased amount of lysosomal enzymes (p. 87). It should be noted that whereas the induction of this cellular activation is immunologically specific (i.e., it is mediated by a response to a specific microbial antigen), the expression is nonspecific in that the microbicidal activity of the macrophages is effective against a variety of microorganisms.

Protective immunity is not the only expression of an immune response. In an individual who has been sensitized by previous contact with an antigen, a second exposure to that antigen may result in a harmful reaction, commonly referred to as *allergy* or *hypersensitivity*. On the basis of experimental studies, hypersensitivity has been divided into two types: (1) *immediate hypersensitivity,* in which the reaction develops rapidly after administration of antigen, and (2) *delayed hypersensitivity,* in which the response occurs after 24 to 48 hours. However, investigations have shown that a more fundamental difference exists between these two responses than their time of appearance. The "immediate" reaction is humoral-mediated and is associated with specific circulating antibodies, whereas in "delayed" hypersensitivity the reaction is mediated by sensitized cells (lymphocytes) and is not dependent on the usual serum antibodies. Therefore, it is now common to refer to these basic responses as *humoral-mediated (antibody-dependent) hypersensitivity* and *cell-mediated (cellular) hypersensitivity*.

CHARACTERISTICS OF AN IMMUNE RESPONSE

Three essential features of an immune reaction are antigenic specificity, recognition of "nonself," and immunologic memory.

Antigenic specificity

The essence of any immune response is the capacity to recognize an antigen. An antigen may be *complete* or *incomplete*. A complete antigen is a macromolecule that is capable of inducing an immune response and of reacting specifically with the products (antibody or sensitized cells) of that response. Complete antigens usually consist of proteins, but other substances such as the polysaccharides may also act as complete antigens. An incomplete antigen *(hapten)* is a chemically active substance of low molecular weight (e.g., dinitrophenol) that is unable to induce an immune response by itself but can become immunogenic by combining with larger molecules, usually a protein (called a "carrier"). However, once the specific antibody has been produced, the hapten will combine with it, even though the hapten is not coupled with the protein carrier.

The reaction of an antigen is very specific, i.e., a particular antigen will react only with antibodies induced by its own kind or by a related kind of antigen. Only certain limited parts of antigen molecules determine immunologic specificity. These structural units are known as the antigenic determinant groups or sites. When cross-reactions occur between antigens and their antibodies, they probably occur because of the similarity of the antigenic determinant groups.

Recognition of "nonself"

Generally, the immune system discriminates between "self" and "nonself." In a normal individual, it responds to foreign proteins (recognition of nonself) but usually does not react against the host's own tissue antigens (self). Under certain circumstances, however,

an immune response is directed against self-antigens (see autoimmunity, p. 87).

Nonreactivity of the host to antigens is known as *immunologic tolerance*. This state is induced by previous antigenic exposure and is specific for a given antigen. It has been suggested that natural tolerance to one's own tissue antigens *(self-tolerance)* is acquired during fetal life. One view is that newly formed antigens come in contact with the immune system at a time when it is immunologically immature and specifically suppress any future responses to the antigens after immunologic maturity is attained. The responsive cells are either eliminated or inactivated. However, it has been shown that specific sensitization of lymphocytes to self-cells can be established in vitro and that this sensitization is inhibited by normal serum of the same animal. Such evidence as this has led to the suggestion that cells that can respond to self-antigens are present in a normal individual but that some factor exists in the serum that blocks the response against self. Some investigators have proposed that the effect of the responding cells is inhibited by a regulatory mechanism involving autoantibodies combined with autoantigens without fixation of complement ("blocking" antigen-antibody complexes). That harmless autoantibodies can occur is shown by the demonstration of autoantibodies of different types in some healthy subjects with no evidence of clinical disease.

Immunologic tolerance to a foreign antigen may be induced by injecting the antigen into fetal or newborn animals. When exposed to the same antigen in adult life, the treated animals do not develop an immune response. Apparently, it is more difficult to establish tolerance in the adult animal, but if the animal is subjected to immunosuppressive therapy at about the time an antigen is administered, tolerance to that antigen develops more readily. A state of *immunologic paralysis* (a form of tolerance) may be brought about by exposing the immune system to massive doses of antigen. Immunologic tolerance to a foreign antigen has been attributed to a decrease in or a suppression of responding cells induced directly by the antigen during previous exposure to it. More recently, however, it has been suggested that it is caused by inhibition of activity of the immunocompetent cells by "blocking" antigen-antibody complexes.

Immunologic memory

Immunologic memory results from the host's first contact with an antigen (i.e., during the primary response). After the second contact with the antigen, a more rapid immune reaction and a higher titer of antibody occur than in the primary response. This secondary (anamnestic) response is believed to be due to the presence of certain "memory" cells induced by the first antigenic stimulus. These are antigen-reactive cells, which respond to the challenging dose of antigen in an accelerated manner.

ANTIBODIES (IMMUNOGLOBULINS)

Antibodies are modified serum proteins that consist of various molecular forms known as *immunoglobulins*. Most of the antibodies are associated with the gamma globulin fraction of the serum.

Classes of immunoglobulins

Five major classes of immunoglobulins (Ig) are recognized: IgG, IgA, IgM, IgD, and IgE. The basic structure of each class of immunoglobulin consists of two heavy (H) and two light (L) polypeptide chains linked by disulfide bonds. The H-chain structure is different for each class of immunoglobulin. The L chains are antigenically divided into two main groups, kappa (κ) and lambda (λ). Both types occur in all classes of immunoglobulins, but a given molecule contains only one type of L chain.

The immunoglobulin molecules may be separated into subunits or fragments by enzymatic digestion. For example, the enzyme papain will cleave the IgG molecule into three fragments. Two of these are identical, each termed Fab ("fragment, antigen-binding") because of its binding affinity for antigen. The third fragment, referred to as Fc ("fragment,

crystallizable") because it spontaneously crystallizes at 4° C, does not combine with antigen but is responsible for the biologic properties of the immunoglobulin (i.e., complement fixation, placental transfer, etc.).

IgG is the most abundant immunoglobulin throughout the intravascular and extravascular body fluids and contains most of the antibacterial, antiviral, and antitoxic antibodies. It is effective in precipitation, complement fixation, and toxin neutralization serologic reactions. In man, IgG makes up about 80% of the total antibody in the serum. It is also named 7S,γG, the 7S indicating its Svedberg sedimentation coefficient and the γ referring to its electrophoretic migration into the gamma globulin region. Since IgG has the ability to cross the placenta during the latter part of pregnancy, it affords protection (passive immunity) to the newborn infant in the first few weeks of life, during which time the infant's own immune system is unable to provide an adequate defense.

IgA antibodies (7S or 11S,γA) are present chiefly in the external secretions (e.g., saliva, lacrimal and nasal fluids, and intestinal and bronchial secretions) and serve as part of the first line of defense against microorganisms. Transepithelial passage of IgA is facilitated by a protein component ("transport piece"), which is combined with it. IgA antibodies are present in low concentration in the serum and extravascular fluids, representing only 5% to 10% of serum gamma globulins. They do not fix complement nor do they cross the placenta.

IgM (19S,γM), also referred to as "macroglobulin" because of its high molecular weight, is present mainly in the blood, representing 5% to 10% of the total immunoglobulins in the serum of adults. It is the first immunoglobulin to be formed during fetal life and usually is the first to appear in an immunologic response. It is very effective in fixing complement and participating in agglutination and cytotoxic or cytolytic reactions. Anti-A and anti-B isohemagglutinins, antibodies to typhoid "O" antigen, and the rheumatoid factor are among antibodies in the IgM class. IgM usually does not cross the placenta.

IgD (γD) and IgE (γE) are present in very low concentrations in blood and extravascular fluids. They do not fix complement nor do they cross the placenta. Antibody activity is rarely demonstrated in the IgD class. IgE is a reaginic antibody *(reagin)* that becomes fixed to the surface of target cells (e.g., mast cells), thus sensitizing them. Subsequent contact with antigen leads to degranulation of the mast cells with release of vasoactive substances. This type of response is characteristic of anaphylaxis (p. 84).

Formation of antibodies

Immunoglobulins are produced in the lymphoid tissues by the progeny of B lymphocytes (p. 80). The plasma cell is the principal cell that synthesizes and secrets antibodies. There is evidence that antigens are first taken up by macrophages within the lymphoid organs. These macrophages do not synthesize antibodies, but they somehow participate in the induction of antibody formation. They are able to carry antigen to antigen-reactive cells, but before the antigen is released it probably is modified or "processed" within macrophages. It has been suggested that antigen is degraded by hydrolytic enzymes contained in these cells, so that nonessential parts are removed, leaving the critical portion, which has the antigenic determinant sites. Some investigators believe that the preserved portion becomes attached to RNA within the macrophage, forming an RNA-antigen complex, or that the macrophage reacts to the antigen by synthesizing and liberating a messenger-type RNA that is free of antigen. One of the functions of the macrophages may be that they prevent immunologic paralysis or tolerance by taking up excess antigen (since there is more than is needed for an immune response), thus permitting only a small amount to reach the antigen-reactive cells.

The mechanism by which antibodies are produced is debatable. According to one theory, an antigen in some way instructs the responding cell to make antibodies against that antigen. Some proponents of this theory claim that the antigen enters the cell and serves as a template for the de novo synthesis of the antibody. Others assume that the RNA-antigen complex formed in macrophages transfers information to the antibody-producing cell for synthesis of immunoglobulin of the IgG class and that the macrophagic messenger RNA devoid of antigen is a selective stimulant for IgM production. Many immunologists, however, hold the view, as expressed by Burnet, that the pattern of antibody released by an immunologically competent cell is determined by genetic processes in the ancestral line of the cell and that transfer of genetic material from another cell plays no role. It is not certain how an immunologically reactive cell recognizes antigen, but it appears that antibodies or antibodylike molecules on the surfaces of reactive cells (receptor sites) participate in this process. Antigen combines with these receptor sites and stimulates the cells to proliferate and form antibody-producing cells.

Complement

The complement system is a complex series of serum proteins consisting of nine functioning components (C1 through C9) and a number of subcomponents (i.e., C1q, C1r, C1s, C2a, C2b, C3a, C3b, C4a, C4b, C5a, and C5b). Activation of the complement system is usually set in motion by the binding of C1 to the Fc portion of an antibody after the latter has formed an antibody-antigen complex *(classic pathway of complement activation)*. This is followed by activation of C4, C2, and C3 in that order and then sequential activation of C5 through C9. Complement activation is involved in cytolysis and a variety of tissue reactions in many diseases.

An *alternative pathway of complement activation* exists that does not require antibody-antigen activation. This pathway involves activation of components C3 to C9 without previous activation of C1, C4, and C2. Complement activation is brought about by properdin and related serum proteins (the properdin system) following initial activation of the properdin system by bacterial polysaccharides, endotoxin, or IgA.

CELLULAR ASPECTS OF AN IMMUNE RESPONSE

The ability of the host to react to immunologic stimuli is based principally on the presence of certain cells in the lymphoid tissues. During early fetal life, hematopoietic tissue is first noted in the yolk sac as blood islands, which contain multipotential hematopoietic cells *(stem cells)* that give rise to all forms of blood cells, including the lymphocytes destined to participate in immune reactions. Subsequently, the liver and other tissues show evidence of hematopoiesis. It is not until the latter half of gestation that blood-forming tissue appears in the bone marrow. Postnatally, while the extramedullary hematopoietic foci recede, the bone marrow becomes the definitive hematopoietic organ and is the principal source of stem cells.

T and B lymphocytes

Two lymphocyte populations are derived from the stem cells, one that is dependent on the thymus *(T lymphocytes)* and another that is independent of the thymus and is analogous to the lymphocytes derived from the *bursa of Fabricius* in birds *(B lymphocytes)*. The cells of both populations undergo proliferation and morphologic changes upon stimulation by appropriate antigens. They eventually become the effector cells of an immune response, i.e., sensitized lymphocytes (T cell system) and antibody-producing plasma cells (B cell system). In addition, during the proliferative phase, memory cells (morphologically lymphocytes), which can respond to a subsequent antigenic stimulus with a secondary-type response, are also produced.

The stem cells released from the bone marrow to the thymus are processed in some way, proliferate, and develop into lymphocytes. Many lymphocytes die within the thymus, but those that persist acquire a characteristic antigen, θ (theta) antigen, and are rendered immunologically competent (immunocompetent T cells). Then they are released by the thymus and circulate through the blood and lymphatics. T cells account for most of the circulating lymphocytes, making up 80% to 90% of nucleated cells in the thoracic duct (in contrast to only about 5% for B cells). The life span of the immunocompetent T cells is said to be months or years, generally longer than the B cells (days or weeks). The T cells are found in the deep, perinodular cortical areas of the lymph nodes and the periarterial lymphatic sheaths of the spleen—the so-called thymic-dependent areas. T cells are stimulated by the mitogen phytohemagglutinin to undergo transformation to blast cells, whereas B cells are not. The T cells play a key role in cell-mediated reactions but do not produce any appreciable amounts of antibody, if any, in response to an antigenic stimulus.

The B cells are found in the cortical lymphoid follicles and medullary cords of the lymph nodes and in the splenic lymphoid follicles. Antibody is produced and released in significant quantities by cells of the B series, predominantly plasma cells. B lymphocytes and plasma cells have patches of immunoglobulin on the cell membranes but do not have theta antigen. Characteristic receptors for the C3 complement component have also been identified on the surface of B cells. It is probable that most of the B cells do not recirculate as the T cells do. In birds, the bursa of Fabricius (a lymphoepithelial organ on the posterior cloacal wall) controls the development of the B cell line and the production of antibody. The bursa does not exist in man, and it is not certain how the B cells are made immunocompetent after they are released by the bone marrow. It has been suggested that they may be processed by gut-associated lymphoid tissue (e.g., Peyer's patches, appendix, tonsil), which may be the equivalent of the bursa of Fabricius.

In addition to the aforementioned specific characteristics ("markers") that distinguish T and B cells (e.g., the θ antigen on the surface of T cells and the immunoglobulins and C3 complement component on the B cells), the means by which these cells bind sheep red blood cells (SRBCs) also serves to differentiate them. Human T cells incubated with normal, nonsensitized SRBCs bind the SRBCs in a characteristic morphologic pattern, i.e., the grouping of SRBCs about a lymphocyte in the form of a rosette, referred to as the *E (erythrocyte) rosette*. On the other hand, human B cells do not form rosettes with untreated normal SRBCs but do so with SRBCs coated with antibody and complement, so-called *EAC (erythrocyte-amboceptor-complement) rosettes*. Ox red blood cells, which do not bind spontaneously to human lymphocytes, may be used to form rosettes with B cells, after being coated with antibody and complement, in order to avoid confusion with T cell rosettes.

There are certain lymphocytes that do not have the characteristic markers of T or B cells. These cells, which have been referred to as "null cells," "K cells," "nil cells," or "negative immunoglobulin lymphocytes," apparently are involved in antibody-dependent cytotoxicity.

Role of the thymus

The immunologic function of the thymus, a lymphoepithelial organ, has been suggested by various observations. For example, thymectomy in mice at birth is followed by (1) decrease in circulating lymphocytes, (2) reduction of lymphocytes in the thymic-dependent areas of the lymph nodes and spleen, (3) impairment of graft rejection, related to decreased capacity to react by delayed hypersensitivity, (4) depression in humoral antibody response to certain antigens, and (5) apparent lowering of resistance to infection, associated with wasting of the animals.

Another pertinent observation is that decreased immunologic responsiveness caused by x-radiation of adult mice may be alleviated by injection of bone marrow cells if the mice were not previously thymectomized. On the other hand, x-irradiated adult mice that have been thymectomized are not benefited by the inoculation of bone marrow cells, suggesting that the thymus induces the primitive bone marrow cells to differentiate and become immunologically competent.

The prevalent view is that the thymic influence, which results in the production of immunocompetent T cells, is hormonal in nature. Certain hormonelike substances derived from the thymus have been shown to be related to maturation of T cells. For example, "thymosin" accelerates development of T cell function in newborn mice and partially restores cell-mediated immunity in thymectomized newborn mice, and "thymin," recently designated "thymopoietin," has been shown to induce T cell (not B cell) differentiation in vitro. Lymphopoietic differentiating effect may occur in vivo chiefly within the thymus, but there is evidence that the thymus also has an effect on cells in the peripheral lymphoid organs. It has been shown that lymphoid tissues and immunologic capacity in thymectomized neonatal mice can be restored in some instances by thymic tissue contained in a millepore chamber implanted intraperitoneally, the pores in the chamber being small enough to prevent passage of cells through them but not particles of large molecular size. The source of the humoral factors in the thymus is probably the epithelial component.

Cellular interactions

Although the presence of lymphocytes and various types of interactions between these cells are necessary for the induction and development of an immune response, the macrophage also makes a significant contribution. The available evidence suggests that the macrophage may play an important role in the induction of immune responses by interacting with antigen and lymphocytes. Macrophages themselves do not synthesize antibody. However, they seem to provide an effective system for presentation of antigen to immunologically competent (antigen-reactive) B cells, which subsequently divide and differentiate into antibody-secreting plasma cells. As pointed out below, interaction between T and B cells may be required for activation of B cells and formation of antibody, but it is also possible that soluble factors released from macrophages may assist in the activation of B cells.

It has been noted that in animals certain antigens are taken up first by phagocytic macrophages, which line the medullary sinuses of lymph nodes draining the injection site, a process known as "antigen trapping." Later, these antigens appear in the cortical lymphoid follicles of the nodes, where the antigens become absorbed to the surfaces of dendritic processes of reticular cells (nonphagocytic macrophages). Very likely, the antigen within phagocytic macrophages is processed in some way before it is carried to the immunologically competent cells (p. 79). Although some question has been raised as to whether processing of antigen is essential for induction of an immune response, in experimental studies some investigators found that this macrophagic activity was necessary for production of antibodies. In addition to modifying the antigen, the macrophages serve to transmit the antigen to the immunocompetent cells. The significance of antigen adhering to the dendritic macrophages in lymphoid follicles (germinal centers) is not clear. However, it is possible that this may be a means of facilitating antibody production, since the dendritic processes with the attached antigen can bring the latter into more intimate contact with reactive lymphocytes.

Antigen trapping and processing probably also play a role in antigen recognition by immunocompetent T cells during the inductive phase of delayed hypersensitivity. It has been suggested that macrophages enzymatically degrade antigens to produce small fragments that have the ability to invoke delayed hypersensitivity in preference to antibody production. In this type of response the recognition of antigen by T cells, which circulate, actually may occur at a site distant from the lymphoid organs (e.g., in the skin), after which the cells return to the lymphoid tissue where they proliferate, forming more sensitized cells. However, it is possible that some antigen also may be brought by macrophages to antigen-reactive cells in the lymphoid tissues.

Another type of interaction occurs between the B and T cells in certain antibody responses. For some antigens, B cells require the *cooperation of T lymphocytes* before antibody can be produced. However, there are a few antigens, such as pneumococcal polysaccharide, for which such cooperation is not necessary. The nature of this cell interaction is not understood, but it is probable that both T

and B cells must carry specific receptors for the particular antigen in order to have effective cooperation. The possibility has been considered that a humoral substance secreted by stimulated T lymphocytes enhances the antibody response of B cells.

In addition to the T-B lymphocyte collaboration in antibody production, there may be cooperation between different kinds of T cells. In the cell-mediated immune responses (delayed-type hypersensitivity reaction, graft rejection, antitumor cellular immunity), the effector T lymphocytes have the capacity of specifically damaging or destroying tissue without antibody synthesis (thus sometimes called "killer" cells). Some investigators have postulated that a population of T cells is produced that "helps" another population of T lymphocytes to divide and differentiate into effector ("killer") cells. The immunologic basis of this T-T cell collaboration is not known.

There is some evidence that T cells may be able to exert an inhibitory (suppressor) as well as a cooperative function in antibody formation. This function may serve as a feedback control mechanism that limits the formation of certain antibodies. These two functions of the T cell are opposed but balanced in a normal individual.

PRIMARY IMMUNOLOGIC DEFICIENCIES

The essential feature of primary immunologic deficiency disorders is failure to manifest an efficient humoral or cell-mediated response because of a developmental abnormality of the immune system. In most instances, a definite hereditary pattern is evident. The basic defect involves either the T cell or B cell system or both the T and B cell systems, so that some of the disorders are characterized by deficiency in antibody production, others by depression of cell-mediated immune responses, and others by both types of deficiency. Patients with immunologic deficiencies show an increased susceptibility to infections, particularly the pyogenic types. Individuals with impaired cellular immunity are more susceptible to certain mycotic and viral infections than those with deficiencies in immunoglobulins (agammaglobulinemia or hypogammaglobulinemia). Increased susceptibility to infections also may be related to primary phagocytic cell defects, which are discussed on p. 63. The following are just a few examples of primary immunodeficiencies.

X-linked agammaglobulinemia (Bruton's disease). This form of agammaglobulinemia is a sex-linked recessive disorder (manifested in males) that is characterized by (1) deficiency of all immunoglobulins, (2) lack of follicles (germinal centers) and plasma cells in lymphoid tissues, (3) deficient antibody response to all antigens, (4) susceptibility to serious infections, and (5) a normal thymus and ability to develop cell-mediated immune responses. The essential defect is in the B cell system.

Thymic aplasia (DiGeorge's syndrome). This condition is a congenital abnormality characterized by (1) absent or vestigial thymus and parathyroid glands resulting from a failure of development of the third and fourth pharyngeal pouches, (2) depletion of lymphocytes in thymic-dependent areas of the lymphoid tissues, (3) depression of cell-mediated immune responses, (4) susceptibility to infections, especially certain viral and fungal infections, (5) usually normal serum immunoglobulin levels, but with possible deficiency of some humoral responses, and (6) tetany in the neonatal period caused by parathyroid insufficiency. The basic defect involves the T cell system.

Immunodeficiency with ataxia telangiectasia. An autosomal recessive disorder, this immunodeficiency is characterized by (1) an embryonic-type thymus, which is small and lacks cortical and medullary organization and usually lacks Hassall's corpuscles, (2) depletion of lymphocytes in thymic-dependent areas of lymphoid tissues, (3) presence or absence of plasma cells, (4) depression of cell-mediated responses, (5) deficiency of IgA, low or normal IgG serum level, and usually normal IgM level, (6) deficient antibody response to some antigens, and (7) certain clinical manifestations, including progressive cerebellar ataxia, telangiectasia (particularly ocular and cutaneous), and recurrent infections. The defect involves the T cell system and usually the B cell system also.

Severe combined immunodeficiency disease. This disorder may be inherited either as an autosomal recessive form *(Swiss-type lymphocytopenic agammaglobulinemia)* or as an X-linked form *(X-linked lymphocytopenic agammaglobulinemia)*. The disorder is characterized by (1) depression of all major immunoglobulin classes, (2) deficiency of lymphocytes in the circulation and the tissues, (3) absence of plasma cells, (4) a hypoplastic thymus lacking lymphocytes and Hassall's corpuscles, (5) depressed humoral and cell-mediated immune responses, and (6) susceptibility to serious infections. The patient usually dies during infancy. The immunodeficiency involves both the T and B cell systems. It has been suggested that the basic defect lies in the stem cells, which fail to differentiate into T and B cells, although some investigators claim that the defect is at the thymic and bursa equivalent level and that normal stem cells are unable to differentiate in these defective sites.

SECONDARY IMMUNOLOGIC DEFICIENCIES

The secondary immunodeficiencies are acquired disorders that are associated with a variety of diseases, nonneoplastic or neoplastic, or are induced iatrogenically. Depression of humoral immune responses occurs in hypercatabolic states, such as protein-losing enteropathies and the nephrotic syndrome, in which serum proteins are decreased (hypogammaglobulinemia). Patients with lymphosarcoma or chronic lymphocytic leukemia have decreased levels of serum immunoglobulins and poor antibody response to antigens. In multiple myeloma, a neoplasm of plasma cells, there is a decrease in the level of normal immunoglobulins accompanied by an impairment of antibody production, despite the fact that the serum level of myeloma proteins is high.

In Hodgkin's disease a deficiency of cell-mediated responses occurs as evidenced by a reduced capacity for rejection of grafts and a depression of antimicrobial cellular immunity.

Patients with Hodgkin's disease are susceptible to viral and fungal infections. In some instances, antibody responses may be impaired. In patients with sarcoidosis, there is a depression in cell-mediated hypersensitivity response, although there is no impairment of antimicrobial cellular immunity. These patients, therefore, are not prone to fungal or viral infections as are those with Hodgkin's disease. Cell-mediated responses are diminished in lepromatous leprosy, as noted by depressed skin reactivity to tuberculin and prolonged survival of skin allografts. Depressed reaction of peripheral blood lymphocytes to phytohemagglutinin stimulation also occurs. Humoral-mediated immunity appears to be unaffected. Studies have shown that in patients with lepromatous leprosy, the T lymphocytes in the blood are decreased whereas the B lymphocytes are increased. Decreased cell-mediated immune responses have been observed in patients with alcoholic cirrhosis of the liver, probably resulting from a T cell defect.

Certain viral infections, e.g., infectious mononucleosis, may be associated with a suppression of cell-mediated responses. This is believed to be the result of an immunologic mechanism stimulated by the viral antigen rather than the result of injury to lymphocytes by the viral infection. The administration of certain agents, such as x-rays, gamma rays, corticosteroids, antimetabolites, alkylating agents, and antilymphocyte serum, causes a suppression of immune responses.

HYPERSENSITIVITY

As pointed out previously, an immune response may cause a harmful reaction in the host, referred to as *allergy* or *hypersensitivity*. Often, hypersensitivity reactions are classified into two groups on the basis of the time that elapses between the administration of an antigen and the appearance of the response, namely, "immediate" and "delayed" hypersensitivity. In accordance with this classification, *anaphylaxis* is a good example of an immediate response, since its manifestations occur promptly after the second exposure to an antigen. However, there are other conditions that also are commonly referred to as immediate hypersensitivity reactions in which the manifestations appear within hours instead of minutes. These sometimes are termed "intermediate" reactions (e.g., the *Arthus phenomenon*). An example of "delayed" hypersensitivity (i.e., occurring after a day or two) is the well-known tuberculin reaction, which is a local reaction to proteins of the tubercle bacillus after intradermal injection of tuberculin in a sensitized host.

A more fundamental differentiation of the types of hypersensitivity is based on the immunologic mechanism by which a reaction is brought about. Thus, the response may be mediated by humoral factors, i.e., serum immunoglobulins, as in immediate hypersensitivity, or it may be mediated by cells (lymphocytes) sensitized to antigen, as in delayed hypersensitivity. Generally, the types of inflammatory cell response differ in the immediate and delayed-type reactions. Usually, polymorphonuclear leukocytes (neutrophils and/or eosinophils) predominate in the former, and mononuclear cells (lymphocytes and macrophages) are characteristically present in the latter. The types of hypersensitivity reactions may be classified as follows:

Humoral (antibody-dependent) type
Reagin-mediated (e.g., anaphylaxis)
Immune complex–mediated (e.g., Arthus phenomenon and serum sickness)
Cell-mediated (cellular) type
Mediated by sensitized T cells (e.g., delayed hypersensitivity as in tuberculin reaction and contact dermatitis)

Anaphylaxis. Anaphylaxis is the typical example of hypersensitivity of the immediate type, the manifestations occurring in a previously sensitized host immediately or within minutes after exposure to the antigen. An antigen-antibody reaction causes formation or release of chemical mediators, such as histamine, bradykinin, serotonin, and "slow-reacting substance of anaphylaxis" (SRS-A), that are responsible for the various clinical effects (e.g., bronchospasm, pulmonary and laryngeal edema, visceral congestion, and shock). The antibody that sensitizes the cells (mast cells) from which vasoactive amines are released is principally immunoglobulin E (IgE), a *reagin*. Release of the vasoactive substances is triggered after the attachment of antigen to antibody on the surface of the cells.

Arthus phenomenon. The Arthus reaction is another humoral-mediated hypersensitivity that is grouped with the hypersensitivities of the immediate type, although the changes are not apparent grossly until several hours after administration of the antigen. The lesion is a local inflammation with necrosis, which is observed several hours after injection of antigen into the skin of an animal previously sensitized to the same antigenic protein.

Tissue injury is initiated by insoluble *antigen-antibody complexes* (precipitates), which are deposited in blood vessel walls and can be demonstrated by immunofluorescence and electron microscopy. The complexes activate the complement system, causing enhanced vascular permeability, chemotaxis, and enhanced phagocytosis. During phagocytosis of the complexes, the neutrophils of the exudate release lysosomal enzymes that cause vascular necrosis. The antibodies involved in this reac-

tion are principally of the IgG type. Figs. 4-1 and 4-2 show the lesion.

Serum sickness. Also an immune complex–mediated disorder, serum sickness is induced not only by administration of foreign serum or serum proteins (e.g., tetanus antitoxin or rabies antiserum) but also by various drugs, particularly antimicrobial agents. Features of the disease are fever, lymphadenopathy, splenomegaly, erythematous and urticarial skin lesions, and arthralgia. Often, the clinical manifestations appear days or weeks after exposure to the antigen (viz., in patients not previously sensitized to the antigen). During the time before onset of clinical features in these patients, antibodies are being produced, which then form complexes with the antigen. In individuals previously sensitized, the effects appear more rapidly, since antibodies already are present.

In a sense, serum sickness is a systemic form of the Arthus reaction. Necrotizing vasculitis with fibrinoid change, thrombosis, perivascular inflammation, and tissue damage occur in various organs, and immune complexes are demonstrated beneath the endothelium and within the basement membranes of

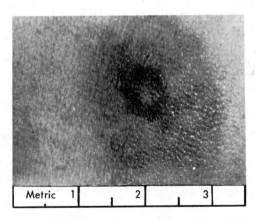

Fig. 4-1. Appearance of Arthus reaction 24 hours after injection of 0.2 ml of 1% solution of bovine serum albumin (BSA) intradermally into a rabbit sensitized to BSA. Central pale area represents necrosis. About this is a zone of hemorrhage surrounded by a wider zone of hyperemia and edema. (From Hopps, H. C.: Hypersensitivity diseases. In Anderson, W. A. D., editor: Pathology, ed. 6, St. Louis, 1971, The C. V. Mosby Co.)

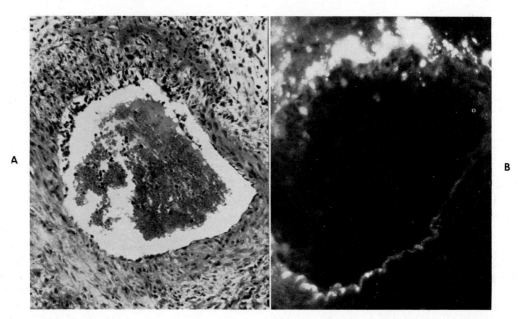

Fig. 4-2. Arthus reaction in rabbit. Antigen, bovine serum albumin (BSA), was injected intradermally, and biopsy of the lesion was performed 5 hours later. Photomicrographs of different sections from same block of tissue were stained, respectively, by hematoxylin-eosin, **A**, and fluorescent, anti-BSA, rabbit serum, **B**. Observe fibrinoid necrosis within wall of artery and associated granulocytic infiltration. Specific fluorescence indicates presence of BSA at site of fibrinoid necrosis. (Rabbit gamma globulin was also demonstrable at this site, indicating presence of antigen-antibody complex.) (**A** and **B**, approximately ×300; courtesy Dr. Charles G. Cochrane.) (From Hopps, H. C.: Hypersensitivity diseases. In Anderson, W. A. D., editor: Pathology, ed. 6, St. Louis, 1971, The C. V. Mosby Co.)

vessels. A form of immune complex glomerulonephritis may be seen in some patients (p. 336). Also, features suggestive of an anaphylactic reaction may be seen, e.g., the wheal and erythema of skin lesions and sometimes edema in certain tissues apparently result from humoral-mediated vasoactive amines.

Other diseases in which lesions are induced by immune complexes include poststreptococcal glomerulonephritis, polyarteritis nodosa, and systemic lupus erythematosus.

Delayed (cellular) hypersensitivity. Unlike the other immune reactions just discussed, delayed (cellular) hypersensitivity is not dependent on circulating antibodies but on sensitized cells, viz., T lymphocytes. It can be transferred from a sensitized to a normal host by living immunocompetent cells but not by serum. The transfer can also be accomplished by injecting an extract of lymphocytes from a sensitized individual into a nonsensitized subject, suggesting that some biologic substance ("transfer factor") exists in the lymphoid cells that is responsible for transfer of cellular hypersensitivity. Mononuclear cells (lymphocytes and macrophages) are characteristic of the cellular reaction in delayed hypersensitivity lesions. This is in contrast to the usual inflammatory response in immediate hypersensitivity reactions consisting of neutrophils and sometimes eosinophils. Neutrophils, however, may be present in delayed hypersensitivity, particularly early in the reaction. In the inflammatory site, parenchymal and vascular damage of varying degree is evident, with necrosis occurring in the more severe reactions.

The typical examples of delayed reaction are the tuberculin-type hypersensitivity and contact dermatitis. The tissue reactions that occur in certain infectious diseases, the rejection of allografts, and autoimmune diseases show characteristics of delayed hypersensitivity.

The mechanism by which the sensitized T lymphocytes induce the inflammatory response and tissue damage at the site of reaction is not clearly understood. It has been proposed that certain biologically active substances, sometimes referred to collectively as the "lymphokines," which are liberated by the sensitized lymphocytes as a result of the antigenic stimulus. may play an important role. Among these substances, named according to their function, are: *transfer factor, lymphocyte-stimulating factor, macrophage-chemotactic factor, macrophage-activating factor, macrophage-inhibiting factor, lymphocyte* (or *lymph node*) *permeability factor, cytotoxic factor,* and *interferon.*

Theoretically, the following events may occur. At first, there are only a relatively few sensitized lymphocytes in the reaction site, but their number is increased by the transfer factor, which sensitizes neutral lymphocytes, and by the lymphocyte-stimulating factor, which induces proliferation of the cells. Macrophages are attracted to the area, in part by the macrophage-chemotactic factor and possibly also by other factors liberated at the inflammatory site. These macrophages are then "activated" by the macrophage-activating factor, i.e., they become more actively phagocytic, have increased microbicidal properties, and exhibit a greatly increased formation of lysosomal enzymes. The migration of the macrophages is believed to be restrained by the macrophage-inhibiting factor, which serves to localize the cells. The lymphocyte permeability factor increases vascular permeability, enhancing the accumulation of inflammatory cells in the area.

The role that the T cells play in bringing about death of tissue cells in the reaction site is not certain. In vitro studies have shown that (1) sensitized lymphocytes can exert a direct cytotoxic effect on target cells (those bearing the antigen), following close contact with the target cells, and (2) "innocent bystander" cells may be killed as a result of cytotoxic factors released by sensitized lymphocytes reacting with antigen in solution. Possibly both mechanisms occur in vivo. In addition to the role of lymphocytes, certain cytotoxins and lysosomal enzymes released from activated macrophages may be responsible in part for the necrosis.

Interferon is a factor that inhibits viruses (p. 161). It does not inactivate the viruses directly but acts upon cells, inducing the cellular gene to produce a protein that inhibits viral multiplication. It probably protects cells involved in an immune response from destruction by viruses. Perhaps, in individuals who do not have the ability to generate an adequate cell-mediated immune response, a lack of interferon production may be one reason why their defense against viral infections tends to be inadequate. It has been shown that interferon has other effects on cells, e.g., it inhibits cell division (both tumor and normal cells), enhances phagocytic activity of macrophages, and causes alterations of the surface of cells. Recent studies have led to the hypothesis that interferon may possibly suppress certain aspects of the immune response and may perform an immunoregulatory function during the normal immune response. This may be the mechanism responsible for the transient depression of cell-mediated immune reactions that may occur during viral infections.

AUTOIMMUNE DISEASES

Normally, there are mechanisms in the body that prevent the immune system from reacting against self, but when the mechanisms break down, autoantibodies and autosensitized T lymphocytes may be produced, which can react against the individual's own tissues *(autoimmunity)*. Various hypotheses have been proposed to explain how autoimmunity may be developed, among which are the following:

1 Normally, certain tissues and proteins do not come in contact with immunocompetent cells (i.e., they are sequestered), but as a result of injury or disease, they may

be exposed to the circulation or may be infiltrated by immunocompetent cells, so that an immune response may develop.

2 Mutation of a gene occurs in cells of the immune system that normally are tolerant to self-antigens, and as a result the altered cells react against tissue that previously was tolerated.

3 Tissue antigen is altered by injury or disease or as a result of a somatic mutation, so that the host recognizes it as "foreign."

4 A foreign antigen (e.g., bacteria) in the body may stimulate antibodies against certain tissue antigens as well as against itself ("cross-reactive" antibodies).

5 T lymphocytes normally are unresponsive to self-antigens because of antigenic exposure in fetal life or the "blocking" effect of antigen-antibody complexes (see self-tolerance, p. 77). Also, B cells do not produce autoantibodies because of the inability of T cells to cooperate with them. Under certain circumstances the need for antigen-specific stimulation of the T cells may be overcome by some other mechanism, e.g., nonspecific stimulation by adjuvants or viruses, so that the T cells can cooperate with B cells in autoimmune responses.

6 The specific feedback control on synthesis of autoantibodies by B cells through the inhibitory (suppressor) function of T cells, which occurs normally, may be relaxed, particularly in aging individuals, thus contributing to development of autoimmunity.

Diseases that result from the reaction between self-antigens and autoantibodies or autosensitized T lymphocytes are referred to as *autoimmune diseases*. Examples of autoimmune diseases are Hashimoto's disease of the thyroid gland, autoimmune hemolytic anemia, allergic encephalomyelitis, some forms of aspermatogenesis, and uveitis. Rheumatic fever, some types of glomerulonephritis, and rheumatoid arthritis, as well as some other connective tissue diseases, are likely the result of autoimmunity. Not all diseases associated with autoantibodies are autoimmune diseases. In some instances the antibodies are apparently harmless and play no role in the pathogenesis of the disease. For example, in myocardial infarction, autoantibodies against heart tissue may occur as a result of damage to the myocardium.

Only a few of the autoimmune disorders will be considered here to illustrate some of the immunologic features of this group of diseases. Often the reactions that are encountered bear a similarity to the humoral and cell-mediated hypersensitivity responses discussed previously. These examples and other diseases of autoimmune nature are described in greater detail in other chapters.

Hashimoto's disease. Hashimoto's disease is a form of thyroiditis characterized by an enlarged thyroid gland infiltrated by lymphocytes, often with lymphoid follicles containing germinal centers (p. 592). The initial insult that induces the disease is not known. Deficiency in thyroid function may occur, and serum specific antibodies against thyroid antigens have been identified, including antithyroglobulin and antibodies against portions of thyroid epithelial cells, colloid, and cell nuclei. It is uncertain whether any of the antibodies are responsible for the thyroid damage. There is some evidence that the thyroiditis may be induced by sensitized lymphocytes that accumulate in the gland. In patients with the disease, skin reactions of delayed hypersensitivity may result from intradermal injection of thyroid extracts. Experimentally, rabbits receiving homologous thyroid gland extracts develop certain antibodies against thyroid antigens and histologic changes in the thyroid gland that closely resemble those seen in Hashimoto's disease in man. Transfer of experimental thyroiditis may be accomplished by lymphocytes, but it is difficult to transfer by serum.

Hematologic disorders. Various hematologic disorders, such as some forms of hemolytic anemia and thrombocytopenia, are attributed to the presence of autoantibodies against red blood cells or platelets or to the attachment of immune complexes to the cell surfaces fol-

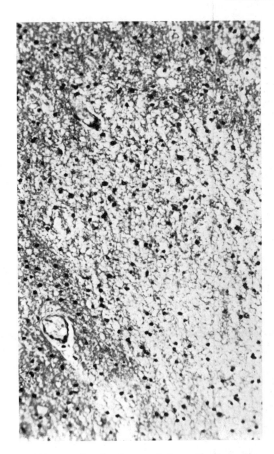

Fig. 4-3. Measles encephalitis showing focal area of demyelination of type often seen in postinfection encephalomyelitis. (From Pinkerton, H.: Rickettsial, chlamydial, and viral diseases. In Anderson, W. A. D., and Kissane, J. M., editors: Pathology, ed. 7, St. Louis, 1977, The C. V. Mosby Co.)

lowed by destruction of the cells. Autoimmunity may play a role in pernicious anemia (p. 497). Antibodies to intrinsic factor and to parietal cells of the stomach, lymphocytic infiltration, and atrophy are seen in the gastric mucosa.

Allergic encephalomyelitis (Fig. 4-3). *Postinfectious encephalomyelitis* may occur following infections with measles, mumps, and chickenpox, and *postvaccinal encephalomyelitis* may occur after immunization with rabies or smallpox vaccines. In both of these conditions the disease process is the same and may

be referred to as *allergic (autoimmune) encephalomyelitis.* Perivascular infiltration by lymphocytes, macrophages, and plasma cells is observed in the central nervous system, but the prominent feature is demyelination about the vessels (p. 166). The loss of myelin is probably caused by the activity of specifically sensitized lymphocytes as noted in delayed hypersensitivity reactions. The disease is believed to be related to an autoimmune response to brain tissue antigen.

Experimental allergic encephalomyelitis is produced by injecting animal brain tissue mixed with Freund's adjuvant into other animals of the same species. It has been shown that the experimental disease may be transferred passively by sensitized lymphocytes but not by serum. Some investigators have suggested that multiple (disseminated) sclerosis, a demyelinating disease of the central nervous system (p. 749), may be of an autoimmune nature.

Rheumatic fever. Acute rheumatic fever (p. 305) occurs after infection by members of the group A β-hemolytic streptococci. Elevated serum titers of antistreptolysin and other antibodies against other streptococcal enzymes and toxins are found in patients with this disease. The heart lesions with characteristic fibrinoid change and inflammatory reaction, including the pathognomonic Aschoff bodies, are the most striking feature, although many other tissues throughout the body are affected also. Antibodies against heart tissue have been demonstrated. A cross-reacting antigen mechanism is considered to be responsible for the autoimmunity in rheumatic fever. In support of this view, fluorescent antibody studies have shown that antibody against group A streptococcus cell membrane will bind to cardiac tissues, including myocardial fibers and sarcolemma.

Systemic lupus erythematosus. Systemic lupus erythematosus involves many tissues in the body (p. 686). Several features of the disease suggest that it is an autoimmune disorder. An LE factor, which is an antibody of the IgG type that reacts with nuclear DNA, has been identified. This factor converts nuclei of normal leukocytes in vitro to homogeneous rounded masses (LE bodies), which are engulfed by phagocytes, usually neutrophils, forming LE cells (p. 686). In addition to anti-DNA antibodies, autoantibodies against other nuclear and cytoplasmic constituents have been demonstrated. Hematoxylin bodies, which are analogous to the LE bodies described above, are present in various tissues. In the kidney lesion (p. 349), deposits of immunoglobulin, mainly IgG, and complement are demonstrated in the glomerular mesangium and basement membrane by immunofluorescence microscopy.

IMMUNOLOGIC ASPECTS OF TUMORS

The relationship between the immune system and neoplastic disease is discussed in Chapter 12, where the immune response to tumors (p. 253) and the immunologic factors in the etiology of tumors (p. 264) are considered. As a result of the recent advances that have led to a better understanding of the nature and function of the immune system, much research is being devoted to the immunologic control of cancer. Among the methods being tried is the administration of BCG, the attenuated tuberculosis vaccine, and other bacterial cell extracts, as nonspecific stimulants of T lymphocytes, in order to activate the immune system to react against malignant neoplasms. Reports of beneficial antitumor effects of BCG in some patients with leukemia and malignant melanoma have appeared, but further studies are necessary to determine the value and limitations of BCG for the treatment of cancer. Immunotherapy has been attempted also by the passive transfer of immunocompetent cells and the administration of the transfer factor in the hope of improving the patient's cell-mediated response against cancer cells.

In a previous section it was noted that certain specific characteristics ("markers") of T and B cells, including their rosette-forming ability, serve to distinguish these cells (p. 80). Immunologic techniques for studying these markers on B and T cells are being applied to the study of lymphocytes in leukemia and malignant lymphomas in an attempt to develop a more functional classification of the neoplastic conditions. Furthermore, the evaluation of the rosette-forming ability of T cells is being used to determine the immune status of patients with malignant tumors as well as other diseases associated with decreased cellular immunodeficiencies.

The impairment of immune responses in patients with leukemia, malignant lymphomas including Hodgkin's disease, and multiple myeloma (a form of plasma cell dyscrasia) was discussed earlier. The details of these neoplastic processes are discussed elsewhere (Chapter 17 and p. 718). The relationship of amyloidosis to plasma cell dyscrasia and to immunoglobulin light chains is discussed on p. 33.

TRANSPLANTATION

Transplantation (grafting) is not only a procedure for studying the reaction of a host to foreign cells or tissues but also a useful procedure employed in the surgical repair or replacement of diseased tissues or organs. Unfortunately, however, because of immune responses in the host a transplant may not be successful unless it involves grafting of tissue from one site to another in the same individual or between persons who are genetically identical.

Types of transplants

Transplants (grafts) and the usual response to them by a normal recipient are as follows.

An *autograft (autogeneic graft)* is a tissue of one site engrafted to another site in the same individual. Such a graft is usually accepted and survives, causing a minimum of inflammatory reaction.

A *syngraft (syngeneic graft)* is a graft between two genetically identical members of a species (e.g., monozygous twins or members of inbred strains) that is accepted by the recipient. This was formerly called an isograft (isogeneic graft). Syngrafts actually behave biologically like autografts.

An *allograft (allogeneic graft)* is a transplant between two genetically different members of the same species. It excites an inflammatory reaction in the recipient's tissue, characterized by proliferations of cells (especially lymphocytes). The graft undergoes necrosis and is rejected. This immunologic mechanism is referred to as the *allograft* (formerly "homograft") *reaction.*

A *xenograft (xenogeneic graft),* formerly known as heterograft (heterologous graft), is a tissue transplanted between members of different species, which induces more intense reaction and is more rapidly rejected than an allograft.

The immune response to a graft may be suppressed by several means, including localized irradiation, the administration of certain drugs and steroid hormones, and the use of antilymphocyte serum (ALS). Other approaches to prolonging survival of transplanted organs and tissues that are being investigated include induction of tolerance to foreign antigens by pretreatment with transfusions of blood from a potential living donor of an organ, thoracic duct drainage of lymphatic fluid to reduce the body's antagonism toward poorly matched grafts, and use of total lymphoid irradiation or of the fungal peptide cyclosporin A to induce immunosuppression. An unfortunate complication of immunosuppressive therapy is an increased susceptibility of the individual to infectious diseases. A serious consequence of transplantation that has been demonstrated in experimental animals and may occasionally occur in human beings is the *graft-vs.-host reaction,* i.e., a graft that contains immunologically competent cells can recognize the antigens of the host's tissues and react against them.

Mechanisms of rejection

The immunologic response of the host to a graft may be mediated by sensitized lymphocytes or by antibodies. The cell-mediated mechanism is usually thought to play a more important role than the humoral mechanism, although the latter, by means of cytotoxic antibodies or formation of immune complexes, may be effective under certain circumstances, especially in the hyperacute or acute rejection reactions.

Antigens are associated with the surface membranes of tissue cells. They are specific for each individual of a species and are the ones that induce an immune response when tissues are transplanted to another individual. The specificity of these antigens, known as *histocompatibility antigens,* is under genetic control. When these antigens are identical in donor and recipient the transplantation is usually successful. If they are dissimilar, there is the possibility that the transplant may be unsuccessful since the immunocompetent cells of the recipient can recognize the antigens and react against them. Histocompatibility antigens are present on all nucleated cells, including leukocytes. In man, the major histocompatibility antigens, designated *HLA (human leu-*

kocyte) antigens, were first demonstrated on the surface of white blood cells. In attempts to select a compatible donor for transplantation, certain tests for typing the antigenic profile of the tissues of donor and recipient are performed using principally blood lymphocytes. In addition, red blood cell antigens are typed to confirm blood group, particularly ABO, compatibility between donor and recipient.

Patterns of rejection reactions

Kidney transplantation has been the most successful form of organ transplant in man. Transplantation of other organs, including the heart and liver, has been attempted with less success. Most information concerning rejection has been derived from experiences with renal transplants. Therefore, the pertinent changes observed in human renal allograft rejections will be summarized to illustrate the rejection patterns, which are referred to as *hyperacute, acute,* and *chronic.*

In *hyperacute rejection,* within minutes or hours after transplantation, neutrophils appear along the endothelial surface of venules and capillaries. This is followed by endothelial damage, clumping of platelets, thrombosis, and cortical necrosis. The reaction apparently is associated with preformed antibodies in the serum.

In *acute rejection* occurring within the first 2 weeks, the prominent feature is interstitial infiltration by immature mononuclear cells, which synthesize proteins but seldom contain immunoglobulins. In later rejections of the acute type, these cells are mature (lymphocytes and plasma cells), and immunoglobulin (IgG) is demonstrable in some of them. Other changes that may be seen in acute rejections, particularly after about 2 weeks, are interstitial edema and hemorrhage, clumping of platelets and/or fibrin on endothelial surfaces (including the glomerular capillaries), venous thrombosis, necrotizing vasculitis, tubular necrosis, and presence of immune complexes in the walls of vessels and glomerular capillaries. Apparently, both cellular and humoral immune responses are involved in acute rejection.

The later *chronic rejection* is characterized by interstitial fibrosis and infiltration by mature mononuclear cells, tubular atrophy, obliterative vascular lesions, thickening of glomerular capillary walls, and deposition of fibrin on endothelial surfaces. The principal mechanism in this type of rejection is cell-mediated. Immune complexes may be demonstrated in capillary walls, particularly in the glomeruli. The obliterative vascular lesions consist of arterial intimal thickening with disruption of elastic lamellae and narrowing of the lumen. The intimal thickening, in part, may be caused by organization of fibrin deposits and healing of previous necrotizing vasculitis.

HLA antigens in various diseases

As noted previously, cell surface antigens that determine the rejection or survival of transplanted tissues *(histocompatibility antigens)* are under genetic control. Involved in this control is a closely linked group of genes known as the *major histocompatibility complex* (MHC). The importance of the MHC lies not only in its role in transplantation immunology but also in its control of other biologic processes or factors, such as immune responses to a variety of antigens, cell-to-cell interactions, and some components of the complement system. In man, the MHC has been designated the *HLA gene complex.* It is located on the short arm of chromosome 6 and is composed of four major genetic loci (A, B, C, D). Three of the loci (A, B, and C) code for antigens that are serologically determined. The D locus codes for antigens that are identified by specific lymphocytic interactions (e.g., mixed lymphocyte culture reaction).

In recent years, a statistical association of various diseases with particular HLA antigens has been observed, which has led to the suggestion that susceptibility to disease may be under the genetic control of the HLA complex. A similar association, although not as strong, had previously been shown to exist between particular blood groups of the ABO red cell antigen system and certain diseases, e.g., between blood group O and duodenal ulcer and between blood group A and gastric carcinoma. Many of the diseases associated with the HLA system are of uncertain or unknown cause and include disorders of an infectious, autoimmune, or neoplastic nature. Not infrequently, familial occurrence of the disease is evident.

One of the strongest histocompatibility associations is that of the antigen HLA-B27 with ankylosing spondylitis. In the United States, B27 is found in about 90% of white patients with this disease as compared with about 8% of normal whites. Individuals with Reiter's syndrome, psoriatic spondylitis, or other diseases associated with spondylitis resembling ankylosing spondylitis also have a greatly increased prevalence of B27. It is of interest, however, that the frequency of B27 is only about 50% to 60% in American black patients with ankylosing spondylitis and about 4% in normal blacks, although this disease is rare in the black population.

A number of diseases appear to be associated with HLA-B8, but the associations are not as strong as the disease associations with B27. A significantly high percentage of patients with gluten-sensitive enteropathy, dermatitis herpetiformis (particularly when associated with enteropathy), myasthenia gravis, Grave's disease, chronic active hepatitis, or insulin-dependent diabetes mellitus have antigen B8. An increased incidence of Bw15 as well as B8 has been observed in patients with insulin-dependent diabetes. A strong association has also been demonstrated between insulin-dependent diabetes and antigens in the D locus (Dw3 and Dw4). No HLA associations have been noted in insulin-independent diabetes, suggesting that it may be a different entity than the insulin-dependent variety.

Other diseases that have been reported to be associated with HLA antigens (shown in parentheses) include psoriasis without arthritis (both B13 and Bw17), pemphigus (B13), various immune deficiency disorders (A1), and certain congenital cardiac defects (A2). Some studies have shown HLA associations with certain neoplastic states, e.g., Hodgkin's disease, in which various antigens have been reported, including B5, B18, and A1. Of interest is the discovery that HLA antigen frequency and disease association may differ in different geographic areas and in different races. For example, HLA-B8 is associated with Grave's disease in white patients, but in Japanese patients with this disease, HLA-Bw35 is associated.

REFERENCES

Ainsberg, A. C., and Block, K. J.: J.A.M.A. **287**:272-276, 1972 (immunoglobulins on surface of neoplastic lymphocytes).

Allison, A. C., et al.: Lancet **2**:135-140, 1971 (cooperation and controlling functions of T cells in autoimmunity).

Askonas, B. A., and Jaroškova, L.: Antigen in macrophages and antibody induction. In van Furth, R., editor: Mononuclear phagocytes, Oxford, 1970, Blackwell Scientific Publications Ltd., pp. 595-612.

Bach, F. H., and van Rood, J. J.: N. Engl. J. Med. **295**:806-813, 827-878, 927-936, 1976 (major histocompatibility complex—genetics and biology).

Bankhurst, A. D., et al.: Lancet **1**:226-230, 1973 (lymphocytes binding thyroglobulin in healthy people—relevance to self-tolerance).

Baron, S., and Johnson, H. M.: The Sciences **18**(4):18-19, 29, April 1978 (interferon regulation in immunity?)

Barrett, J. T.: Textbook of immunology, ed. 3, St. Louis, 1978, The C. V. Mosby Co.

Bast, R. C., Jr., et al.: N. Engl. J. Med. **290**:1413-1420, 1458-1469, 1974 (BCG and cancer).

Berenyi, M. R., et al.: J.A.M.A. **232**:44-46, 1975 (T-rosettes in alcoholic cirrhosis of the liver).

Burnet, M.: Auto-immunity and auto-immune disease, Philadelphia, 1972, F. A. Davis Co.

Calderon, J., and Unanue, E. R.: J. Immunol. **112**:1804-1814, 1974 (antigen and macrophages).

Check, W. A.: J.A.M.A. (Medical News) **242**:2265-2269, 1979 (new approaches to induction of immunosuppression).

Cohen, S.: Am. J. Pathol. **88**:501-528, 1977 (cell-mediated immunity).

Cooper, M. D., et al.: N. Engl. J. Med. **288**:966-967, 1973 (classification of primary immune deficiencies).

Cosenza, H., and Nordin, A. A.: J. Immunol. **104**:976-983, 1970 (immunoglobulin classes of antibody-forming cells).

Craddock, C. G., et al.: N. Engl. J. Med. **285**:324-331, 378-384, 1971 (lymphocytes and immune response).

Danilevicius, Z.: J.A.M.A. **231**:965-966, 1975 (HLA antigens—genetic markers of many diseases).

David, J. R.: The role of macrophages in delayed hypersensitivity reactions. In van Furth, R., editor: Mononuclear phagocytes, Oxford, 1970, Blackwell Scientific Publications, Ltd., pp. 486-494.

David, J. R.: N. Engl. J. Med. **288:**143-149, 1973 (lymphocyte mediators and cellular hypersensitivity).

Dwyer, J. M., et al.: N. Engl. J. Med. **288:**1036-1039, 1973 (T:B lymphocyte ratio in lepromatous leprosy).

Editorial: Lancet **1:**1490-1491, 1973 (lymphokines).

Editorial: Lancet **2:**949-950, 1973 (lymphocytes reactive to autoantigens).

Editorial: Lancet **2:**79-81, 1973 (transfer factor).

Fishman, M., and Adler, F. L.: Heterogeneity of macrophage functions in relation to the immune response. In van Furth, R., editor: Mononuclear phagocytes, Oxford, 1970, Blackwell Scientific Publications Ltd., pp. 581-594.

Friedman, H., editor: Ann. N.Y. Acad. Sci. **249:**1-547, 1975 (thymus factors in immunity—a conference).

Friedman, H.: Fed. Proc. **37:**102-104, 1978 (macrophages in immunity).

Fudenberg, H. H., et al.: N. Engl. J. Med. **283:**656-657, 1970 (classification of primary deficiences—WHO recommendation).

Fudenberg, H. H., et al.: N. Engl. J. Med. **292:**475-476, 1975 (T-rosette forming cells, cellular immunity, and cancer).

Fudenberg, H. H., Stites, D. P., Caldwell, J. L., and Wells, J. V., editors: Basic and clinical immunology, Los Altos, Calif., 1976, Lange Medical Publications.

Gajl-Peczalska, K. J., et al.: N. Engl. J. Med. **288:**1033-1035, 1973 (B lymphocytes in lepromatous leprosy).

Gell, P. G. H., Coombs, R. R. A., and Lachmann, P. J.: Clinical aspects of immunology, ed. 3, Oxford, 1975, Blackwell Scientific Publications Ltd.

Gill, T. J. III, Cramer, D. V., and Kunz, H. W.: Am. J. Pathol. **90:**735-778 (major histocompatibility complex—a review).

Goldstein, G.: Nature **247:**11-14, 1974 (thymin: a polypeptide hormone of the thymus).

Good, R. A.: J.A.M.A. **287:**305-306, 1972 (lymphocyte surface markers).

Graber, P.: Lancet **1:**1320-1322, 1974 ("self" and "nonself" in immunology).

Gresser, I.: Cell. Immunol. **34:**406-515, 1977 (biologic effects of interferon).

Gross, R. L., et al.: N. Engl. J. Med. **292:**439-443, 1975 (rosette formation in lung carcinoma).

Henney, C. S.: J.A.M.A. **291:**1357-1358, 1974 (killer T cells).

Jaffe, E. S., et al.: N. Engl. J. Med. **290:**813-819, 1974 (nodular lymphoma—origin from B lymphocytes).

Kantor, F. S.: N. Engl. J. Med. **292:**629-634, 1975 (infection, anergy, and cell-mediated immunity).

Kelly, J. F., and Patterson, R.: J.A.M.A. **227:**1431-1436, 1974 (anaphylaxis).

Kemple, K., and Bluestone, R.: Med. Clin. North Am. **61:**331-345, 1977 (histocompatibility complex and rheumatic diseases).

Lindquist, R. R., et al.: Am. J. Pathol. **53:**851-881, 1968 (human renal allografts).

Marx, J. L.: Science **187:**1183-1185, 1217, 1975 (thymic hormones—inducers of T cell maturation).

McCluskey, R. T., and Cohen, S., editors: Mechanisms of cell mediated immunity, New York, 1974, John Wiley & Sons, Inc.

McDevitt, H. O., and Bodmer, W. F.: Lancet **1:**1269-1275, 1974 (HLA, immune response genes, and disease).

Miller, J.F.A.P.: N. Engl. J. Med. **290:**1255-1256, 1974 (endocrine function of the thymus).

Mills, D. M., et al.: J.A.M.A. **231:**268-270, 1975 (HLA antigens in ankylosing spondylitis).

Mitchell, D. N., and Scadding, J. G.: Am. Rev. Respir. Dis. **110:**774-802, 1974 (sarcoidosis).

Nakao, Y., et al.: Arch. Intern. Med. **138:**567-570, 1978 (HLA antigens in thyroid diseases).

Neel, J. V.: N. Engl. J. Med. **297:**1062-1063, 1977 (genetics of juvenile onset diabetes).

Nerup, J., et al.: Lancet **2:**864-866, 1974 (HLA antigens and diabetes mellitus).

Nossal, G. J. V.: The biological basis of histocompatibility and its implication for development and tissue grafting. In Motulsky, A. G., and Lenz, W., editors: Birth defects, New York, 1974, American Elsevier Publishing Co., Inc., pp. 105-113.

Pearsall, N. N., and Weiser, R. S.: The macrophage, Philadelphia, 1970, Lea & Febiger.

Pearson, M. N., and Raffel, S.: J. Exp. Med. **133:**494-505, 1971 (macrophage-digested antigen and delayed hypersensitivity).

Pincus, W. B.: Ann. allergy **28:**93-97, 1970 (tissue injury and delayed-type hypersensitivity).

Pyke, K. W., et al.: N. Engl. J. Med. **293:**424-426, 1975 (severe combined immunodeficiency disease).

Roit, I.: Essential immunology, ed. 3, London, 1977, Blackwell Scientific Publications Ltd.

Russell, P. S., and Cosimi, A. B.: N. Engl. J. Med. **301:**470-479, 1979 (progress in tissue and organ transplantation).

Russell, P. S., and Winn, H. J.: N. Engl. J. Med. **282:**896-906, 1970 (transplantation).

Samter, M., editor: Immunological diseases, ed. 3, Boston, 1978, Little, Brown & Co.

Schaller, J. G., and Omenn, G. S.: J. Pediatr. **88:**913-925, 1976 (histocompatibility system and human disease).

Scope Monograph on Immunology, ed. 2, Kalamazoo, Mich., 1972, The Upjohn Company.

Seligmann, M.: J.A.M.A. **290:**1483-1484, 1974 (B cell and T cell markers in lymphoid proliferations).

Sell, S.: Immunology, immunopathology, and immunity, ed. 2, New York, 1975, Harper & Row, Publishers, Inc.

Sell, S.: Am. J. Pathol. **90:**211-280, 1978 (immunopathology—a teaching monograph).

Sjögren, H. O., et al.: Proc. Natl. Acad. Sci. U.S.A. **68:**1372-1375, 1971 (antigen-antibody complexes blocking antitumor lymphocyte reactivity).

Stiller, C. R., et al.: Ann. Intern. Med. **82:**405-410, 1975 (autoimmunity—present concepts).

Taylor, H. E.: Pathology of organ transplantation in man.

In Sommers, S. C., editor: Pathology annual, vol, 7, New York, 1972, Appleton-Century-Crofts.

Thaler, M. S., Klausner, R. D., and Cohen, H. J.: Medical immunology, Philadelphia, 1977, J. B. Lippincott Co.

Unanue, E. R.: Am. J. Pathol. **83:**395-418, 1976 (secretory function of mononuclear phagocytes—a review).

Waldron, J. A., et al.: J. Immunol. **112:**746-755, 1974 (antigen handling by macrophages).

Weiss, L.: The cells and tissues of the immune system, Englewood Cliffs, N.J., 1972, Prentice-Hall, Inc.

Wright, P. W., et al.: Proc. Natl. Acad. Sci. U.S.A. **70:**2539-2543, 1973 ("blocking" antigen-antibody complexes in allograft tolerance).

5

Disturbances of body water and electrolytes and of circulation of blood

For the maintenance of health, there must be a proper distribution and normal balance of fluids and their electrolytes throughout the body—viz., in the intravascular, interstitial-lymph, and intracellular compartments. For the continuance of a state of equilibrium, it is necessary that there be a normal circulation of blood and lymph and a constant, dynamic exchange of fluids and electrolytes among the body compartments through their intervening permeable membranes. When disturbances arise, they are either (1) abnormalities of body water (including electrolytes) and/or disturbances in the volume of circulating blood (i.e., edema, dehydration, electrolyte deficits and excesses, hyperemia, hemorrhage, and shock) or (2) disorders interfering with the circulation of blood (e.g., thrombosis and embolism) and their consequences (i.e. ischemia and infarction).

Disturbances of body water and electrolytes

EDEMA

Edema is an excess of fluid within tissue spaces and/or serous cavities, either localized or generalized. An excessive accumulation of fluid in the pleural, pericardial, and peritoneal cavities is known as *hydrothorax, hydroperi-*cardium, and *hydroperitoneum (ascites),* respectively. *Anasarca (dropsy)* is a generalized edema that is evident particularly in the subcutaneous tissues and in the body cavities. Subcutaneous edema causes swelling of the part, and the overlying tissue is usually tense. When severe, it "pits on pressure," i.e., digital pressure displaces fluid from the tissue and leaves a dent, which slowly fills in as fluid flows back into the area after release of pressure *(pitting edema).* Edema fluid of noninflammatory origin is commonly referrred to as a *transudate,* having less protein content and a lower specific gravity than an inflammatory *exudate* (p. 57).

Generally, an edematous organ is heavier and larger than normal and may be boggy, and the capsule or covering serous surface may be stretched and glistening. The cut surface exudes fluid, which, in the case of the lung, may be frothy since it is contained within alveoli, where it is mixed with air. Microscopically, the fluid may be very pale and barely stained, or it may appear as an acidophilic material, the density of which varies in direct proportion to the amount of protein it contains.

Factors that govern the interchange between intravascular fluid (blood plasma) and interstitial fluid and that serve to maintain normal volumes in these compartments are as follows:

1 Hydrostatic pressure of the blood, tending to force fluid through capillary walls

2 Colloid osmotic pressure of plasma proteins, which tends to hold fluid in the vessels and to draw it from tissues into the blood
3 Permeability of vascular endothelium
4 Extravascular tissue factors (hydrostatic pressure and osmotic pressure), which normally are so low that they do not counteract the action of the same type of forces in the vessels
5 Normal concentration of sodium in intravascular and interstitial fluids
6 Free flow of lymph in the lymphatic vessels, which normally serve as a route for return of some of the extravascular fluid and its protein to the blood

Disturbances in any of these factors may lead to edema. Although edema may result from any one of the mechanisms discussed in the following paragraphs, frequently several factors are operative at the same time in a particular disorder.

Increased hydrostatic pressure in capillaries. Normally, the hydrostatic pressure in the arterial end of capillaries is such that the reverse force exerted by plasma proteins is overcome and fluid flows into intercellular spaces, whereas the pressure in the venous end of capillaries is low and the fluid that has not been carried away by lymphatics is drawn from tissue spaces into the blood. This balance of hydrostatic pressure is upset by passive or venous congestion, which results in increased intracapillary hydrostatic pressure. The generalized venous congestion of heart failure is the most common cause; hence, cardiac failure is commonly associated with widespread edema *(cardiac edema)*. However, in cardiac failure, sodium retention also influences the development of edema. Localized venous congestion also may cause edema, e.g., edema of the lower extremities resulting from thrombosis of the iliac veins or from pressure on these veins by a tumor or a pregnant uterus and ascites associated with portal congestion in cirrhosis of the liver. It is to be noted that additional factors are operative in the development of ascites in hepatic cirrhosis, e.g., hypoproteinemia, renal retention of sodium and water, and increased production of lymph in the liver because of intrahepatic passive congestion. The lymph exudes from the surface of the liver. Along with the ascites, edema may occur elsewhere in the body because of the low plasma proteins and sodium and water retention.

Decreased plasma proteins. The osmotic pressure of any body fluid is dependent on the concentration of its active chemical constituents, including the electrolytes. The nondiffusible colloids, particularly the proteins, which are more abundant in the blood plasma than in the interstitial tissue, make up a relatively small part of the total osmotic pressure of the blood, but they represent the effective part *(colloid osmotic pressure)* that promotes the exchange of water between the intravascular and interstitial compartments.

Edema is caused by a lowering of the colloid osmotic pressure of blood, which results when there is a decrease in plasma proteins (hypoproteinemia), particularly in the albumin fraction, since the osmotic attraction of plasma depends largely on the albumin content. Edema tends to appear when the plasma albumin is reduced to a level below 2.5 g/100 ml. A common cause of hypoproteinemic edema is renal disease associated with prominent loss of protein in the urine, e.g., in the nephrotic syndrome *(renal,* or *nephrotic, edema)*. Hypoproteinemic edema also may be caused by the failure of sufficient formation of serum albumin, as in undernourishment from famine *(nutritional edema)* or in *hepatic disease* (e.g., cirrhosis). However, it has been shown that hypoproteinemia is not always present in starvation, so that perhaps other factors, such as sodium and water retention, may play a role. Also, in renal and liver diseases, retention of sodium and water, as well as other factors, contributes to the edema.

Increased vascular permeability. Vascular endothelium acts as a semipermeable membrane in that, normally, water, crystalloids, and dissolved gases pass through it freely but only a very small amount of protein is permitted to pass through. Agents that are injurious to the endothelium increase its permeability to protein colloids. Diffusion of proteins, which occurs apparently through the walls of the venules as well as the capillaries, lowers the plasma osmotic pressure and increases the interstitial fluid osmotic pressure, both factors favoring the development of edema.

Systemic edema resulting from increased endothelial permeability occurs in a variety of conditions, including *severe infections, anaphylactic reactions, poisonings* with drugs and chemicals, and *anoxia,* such as may occur in secondary shock. The generalized edema in *acute glomerulonephritis* may be caused by increased vascular permeability, although retention of sodium and water and hypoalbuminemia may be significant causative factors also. Local edema resulting from increased endothelial permeability is seen in the inflammatory reaction *(inflammatory edema)* and in *angioneurotic edema,* the latter being allergic or neurogenic in origin.

Tissue factors. Normally, the tissue fluid colloid osmotic pressure is so small that it is insignificant in opposing the osmotic pressure of the plasma. However, in clinical states associated with increased vascular permeability or when there is lymphatic obstruction, the protein concentration of the interstitial fluid increases, which assists the production of edema. An *increased sodium concentration* of tissue fluid occurring in those states characterized by renal retention of this ion contributes to edema. The relatively low hydrostatic pressure of the interstitial fluid in certain areas of the body (e.g., in the subcutaneous tissues of the eyelids and external genitalia) enhances the edema caused by other factors.

Lymphatic obstruction. Lymphedema is the term applied to an increase of interstitial fluid resulting from interference with the flow of lymph from an area of the body. This may be caused by surgical removal of the axillary lymph nodes, as in radical mastectomy for cancer of the breast. Lymphatic obstruction may be caused by infiltrating cells of a malignant neoplasm, by extrinsic pressure of tumors, by inflammatory fibrosis, or by parasites (as in filariasis). An enlargement of the scrotum or an extremity resulting from lym-

phedema and associated fibrosis is often referred to as *elephantiasis.* Congenital lymphedema is caused by abnormal development of the lymphatic vessels, which causes defective lymph drainage (e.g., *Milroy's disease*).

Sodium and water retention. Retention of sodium occurs when its excretion in the urine is less than the intake. The excess sodium results in a retention of water. With progressive retention of sodium and water, there is expansion of the extracellular fluid volume, both intravascularly and interstitially, with resultant edema. At first, the retention of sodium produces an increased concentration of this ion in the extracellular fluids, so that *hypertonicity* exists. In response to this state, water is retained until normal concentration of sodium *(isotonicity)* is reached. As a rule, the amounts of sodium and water retained are proportionate, so that the serum in edematous patients contains a normal concentration of sodium *(normonatremic edema).* In some patients, a greater amount of water is retained, so that there is a low concentration of sodium *(hypotonicity)* in the plasma and interstitial fluid *(hyponatremic edema),* despite an excess of total body sodium.

The retention of these substances occurs in a variety of edematous states, as in *congestive heart failure, hepatic cirrhosis,* the *nephrotic syndrome,* and *acute glomerulonephritis.* This mechanism of edema production may be secondary in these conditions, although some investigators believe that it is primary in cardiac failure, resulting from decreased cardiac output and renal blood flow (forward failure) or from an increase in circulating aldosterone.

The retention of sodium may be caused by intrinsic renal mechanisms or extrarenal hormonal or neural influences, e.g., reduction in glomerular filtration, enhanced tubular reabsorption, and increased filtration factor in the kidneys and increased secretion of aldosterone or decreased rate of inactivation of aldosterone by the liver. A factor causing or contributing to retention of water is increased secretion of antidiuretic hormone (ADH). The stimulus for aldosterone secretion may be a reduction in the volume of extracellular fluid, particularly the intravascular phase, sodium deprivation, positive potassium balance, or formation of angiotensin. The renin-angiotensin mechanism, set in motion by ineffective perfusion of the kidneys due to reduction of intravascular volume or decreased blood flow, is apparently a major influence leading to aldosterone secretion in edematous states. A contributing factor may be an increased activity of the sympathetic nervous system in response to the intravascular deficit, causing renal arteriolar constriction and renin release. ACTH may play a part in aldosterone secretion.

DEHYDRATION

Dehydration is a disturbance of water balance in which body water is below the normal level, but there is also an accompanying abnormality of the electrolytes. Dehydration may be the result of water or sodium depletion, but usually both types of depletion exist in a given case, although one or the other may predominate.

Water depletion (primary dehydration). Pure water depletion, or primary dehydration, occurs as a result of restriction of intake of water, as in a patient who has a severe physical or mental illness and cannot or refuses to drink or in a person in the desert or at sea without fresh water. The increased sodium concentration (hypertonicity) that occurs in the extracellular fluids draws water from the cells (intracellular dehydration), which results in thirst. It also stimulates the release of ADH, leading to oliguria. In addition to thirst and oliguria, decreased salivary flow, dryness of the mouth, weakness, and, subsequently, mental disturbances are characteristic features. Death occurs in 7 to 10 days, as a rule, after complete water deprivation.

Sodium depletion (secondary dehydration). Sodium depletion, or secondary dehydration, is caused by loss of electrolyte-containing fluids from the body, which occurs commonly by means of vomiting, diarrhea, pancreatic and biliary fistulas, and continuous aspiration through intubation. It also may result from excessive perspiration when only water is taken as a replacement or from loss of sodium in the urine in certain conditions such as Addison's disease, diabetic acidosis, cerebral salt-wasting syndrome, and some instances of chronic renal disease. Lack of sodium in the diet does not cause sodium depletion in a healthy subject as a rule, because the kidney can conserve this ion effectively.

As a result of sodium depletion, the extracellular fluid becomes hypotonic, inhibiting the release of ADH, so that the kidneys excrete water in an attempt to maintain normal extracellular sodium concentration. The result is a decrease in the volumes of the plasma and interstitial fluid, but because the extracellular fluids are hypotonic in relation to the intracellular fluid, water flows into the cells. Nausea, vomiting, cramps, lassitude, headache, and loss of weight are common symptoms. Alterations of serum potassium and chloride and a disturbance of acid-base balance also may appear. The lowered blood volume may result in decreased cardiac output, low blood pressure, a tendency to orthostatic fainting, and decreased glomerular filtration with subsequent nitrogen retention. When there is a great reduction in the volume of extracellular fluid, shock may develop.

ELECTROLYTE DISTURBANCES

The electrolytes play a significant role in the maintenance of osmotic pressure and of normal balance and distribution of the body fluids and also are concerned with the preservation of acid-base balance and normal neuromuscular irritability.

In the extracellular fluids, the electrolytes that are highest in concentration are sodium and chloride ions, next are bicarbonate ions, and in comparatively low concentrations are potassium, magnesium, phosphate, and sulfate ions. The blood plasma and interstitial fluid have a similar chemical composition, except for the presence of a larger amount of protein in the former, which is responsible for adjustments of the concentration of diffusible ions in order to preserve the total cation-anion equivalence (Gibbs-Donnan equilibrium). The intracellular water, in contrast, has a high concentration of potassium and a low concentration of sodium and chloride. It contains more phosphate, sulfate, magnesium, and protein but less bicarbonate than the extracellular fluids.

Hyponatremia and hypernatremia. A *decreased sodium concentration* in the plasma *(hyponatremia)* may be brought about by sodium depletion (depletional hyponatremia) or by retention of water over and above the retention of sodium (dilutional hyponatremia). Sodium depletion was discussed above. Dilutional hyponatremia occurs in such states as overhydration (water intoxication), congestive heart failure and cirrhosis of the liver with impaired water diuresis, and other entities thought to be caused by an excess secretion of ADH. Usually, hyponatremia, especially when severe, results in various clinical manifestations. Instances of "asymptomatic hyponatremia" have been described in patients with the salt-wasting or salt-losing syndromes associated with cerebral or pulmonary disease (e.g., tuberculosis and bronchogenic carcinoma) or without evidence of other disease (idiopathic).

An *increased sodium concentration* in the blood *(hypernatremia)* occurs when there is either an output of water in excess of sodium or a severe restriction of water with dehydration (see water depletion above). It may occur in patients with cerebral lesions (e.g., encephalomalacia, hemorrhage, lacerations, malignant tumors, and meningitis), which probably interfere with production of ADH, causing an acute diabetes insipidus that is not compensated by adequate water intake. In primary aldosteronism, hypernatremia develops while potassium concentration is decreased. Acute salt poisoning has been reported in infants who were inadvertently given a formula containing salt instead of sugar. Alterations in the central nervous system may be produced by hypernatremia. There is a relationship between excess sodium and hypertension.

Hypopotassemia and hyperpotassemia. *Hypopotassemia (hypokalemia)* is caused by inadequate intake (as in starvation) or by excessive loss of potassium from the body (as in vomiting, diarrhea, diuresis, adrenal cortical hyperactivity, administration of adrenocortical hormones, and surgical trauma). In familial periodic paralysis, there is hypokalemia without an increased excretion of potassium. It is probable that in this disease the potassium is shifted into the muscle cells.

The effects of hypokalemia include foci of necrosis and leukocytic infiltration in the myocardium, electrocardiographic changes, fatty degeneration and necrosis of renal tubular epithelium, vacuolar nephropathy, and metabolic alkalosis.

Hyperpotassemia (hyperkalemia) does not occur as commonly as hypopotassemia. It may be seen in patients who receive excessive administrations of potassium parenterally or orally, in acute renal failure and in chronic renal disease with inability to excrete potassium, and in adrenal insufficiency with resultant retention of potassium. It also may be caused by a shift of cell potassium to the extracellular fluids as a result of injury to cells by noxious agents (e.g., anoxia in late stages of secondary shock) or in destruction of cells (e.g., extensive hemolysis of red blood cells).

The effects of hyperkalemia include paresthesias, flaccid paralysis, listlessness, mental confusion, decline in blood pressure, and certain electrocardiographic changes.

Hypochloremia and hyperchloremia. A decreased concentration of chloride in the plasma *(hypochloremia)* occurs in vomiting, adrenal insufficiency, acute infections, and renal failure. *Hyperchloremia* may be seen in patients receiving parenteral administrations of hypertonic sodium chloride solutions and in those suffering from water depletion. Alterations in acid-base balance may result from changes in chloride concentration: hypochloremia is counterbalanced by increased bicarbonate concentration, causing metabolic alkalosis, and hyperchloremia is associated with decreased bicarbonate concentration and metabolic acidosis.

Hypomagnesemia and hypermagnesemia. The concentration of magnesium in the plasma is decreased *(hypomagnesemia)* in chronic alcoholism, prolonged diuresis in congestive heart failure, rehydration therapy for dehydration in diabetic acidosis, and starvation. It causes muscular twitching, choreiform movements, convulsions, and coma. *Hypermagnesemia* is seen in severe dehydration, untreated diabetic acidosis, renal failure, or excess administration of magnesium. Clinical features include muscle relaxation, lethargy, coma, and respiratory failure.

Disturbances in volume of circulating blood

HYPEREMIA (CONGESTION)

An increased volume of blood within dilated blood vessels in an organ or a part of the body is referred to as *hyperemia*, or *conges-*

tion. It may be rapid in onset (*acute* congestion) or may occur gradually and be prolonged (*chronic* congestion).

Active hyperemia. Active hyperemia is the result of increased arterial blood to a part, is usually acute, and is characterized by dilatation of arterioles and capillaries. It occurs during functional activity of any tissue (e.g., exercised muscle) and as a result of emotion or heat (flushing of skin). It also occurs in the early stages in inflammation. Usually, the only change in active hyperemia is a deep pink or red appearance of the affected tissue *(erythema)*. In the case of acute inflammation, the additional factor of endothelial damage causes edema.

Passive hyperemia. Passive hyperemia is brought about by diminished venous blood flow from an area and is characterized by di-

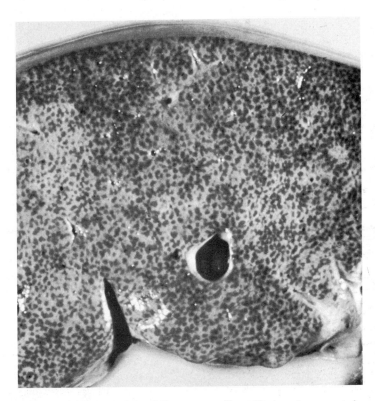

Fig. 5-1. Chronic passive congestion of liver, cut surface. Dark red, congested centrilobular zones contrast with paler adjacent liver tissue to cause "nutmeg" appearance.

latation of the veins and capillaries. It may be acute but often is prolonged, resulting in chronic passive congestion.

Hypostatic congestion is a form of passive hyperemia that involves the dependent portion of an organ and is caused by gravitation of the blood in a relaxed vascular system. *Local venous congestion* is caused by interference with the venous outflow from an organ or a part of the body, as in venous thrombosis, extrinsic pressure on a vein by a tumor or other masses, and constriction by ligatures, tight bandages, scar tissue, hernia, volvulus, etc. The severity of the congestion depends on the adequacy of the collateral circulation. *Systemic venous congestion* is observed in congestive heart failure, affects organs and tissues throughout the body, and is commonly associated with dyspnea, cyanosis, and edema.

In certain organs, chronic passive congestion produces characteristic changes. The *liver* is enlarged and its cut surface has a mottled appearance, resembling the cut surface of a nutmeg *(nutmeg liver;* Fig. 5-1). The mottling is caused by redness of the central part of the liver lobules around the central veins, contrasted with grayish peripheral portions of the lobules. Because of the anoxia of continued congestion, the liver cells in the centrilobular zones undergo fatty metamorphosis and/or atrophy. In more severe congestion, necrosis of the cells occurs.

The congested *spleen* is enlarged and has a tense capsule and a dark red, firm cut surface. The sinuses are engorged with blood. In long-standing cases, the trabeculae and walls of the sinusoids undergo fibrosis and the malpighian corpuscles are atrophic. Iron deposits are likely to occur in passive congestion caused by portal hypertension. They occur in areas of hemorrhage and are followed by fibrosis (siderofibrotic nodules or Gandy-Gamna nodules).

Chronic passive congestion of the *lung* results in pulmonary edema and extravasation of red blood cells from the distended venules and capillaries into alveolar spaces (Figs. 5-2 and 5-3). The hemoglobin of the red cells breaks down, forming hemosiderin, which is present within macrophages. The hemosiderin-laden macrophages are sometimes referred to as "heart failure cells" because of their frequent association with congestive heart failure. In long-standing cases, fibrosis of the edematous alveolar walls develops, and this, together with the brownish pigmentation of hemosiderin, produces a gross appearance of the lung called "brown induration" (p. 419).

HEMORRHAGE

Hemorrhage denotes escape of blood from the cardiovascular system, usually the result of *rupture* of a vessel or the heart. Extravasation of erythrocytes because of their passage through apparently unruptured venular and capillary walls is known as *hemorrhage by diapedesis*. When a vessel is severed, hemostatic mechanisms are set into motion in an attempt to control the hemorrhage. Vasoconstriction and retraction of the severed vessel at the site of injury produce a temporary mechanical barrier to the escape of blood. Of greater importance and more lasting benefit is the formation of a hemostatic plug (clot), which tends to occlude the defect. This consists at first of adherence of platelets to the rim of the severed vessel, followed by aggregation of platelets and formation of a coagulum of fibrin in which platelets, leukocytes, and red blood cells are enmeshed. A vasoconstrictor substance (e.g., serotonin) is probably released from the platelets, which may contribute to the vasoconstriction. The mechanisms in the formation of the hemostatic plug are basically similar to those involved in the formation of intravascular clots or thrombi (pp. 107-108).

Types. Hemorrhage may be classified as follows:

1 *Capillary, venous, arterial,* or *cardiac* (depending on its origin)
2 *External* or *internal* (in relation to the body)
3 *Traumatic* (when incident to various wounds) or *spontaneous* (when it occurs in the absence of obvious trauma)
4 According to type of lesion, e.g., *petechiae* (minute hemorrhagic spots, usually of capillary origin), *ecchymoses* (larger, blotchy areas of extravasated blood),

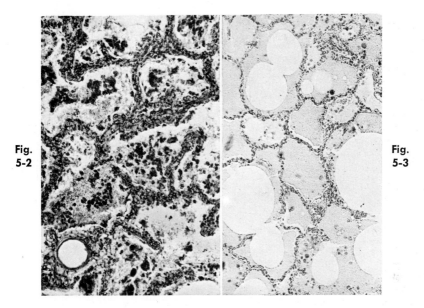

Fig. 5-2. Chronic congestion of lung. Alveolar walls are thickened. Alveoli contain pigment-laden macrophages and protein. (From Millard, M.: Lung, pleura, and mediastinum. In Anderson, W. A. D., and Kissane, J. M., editors: Pathology, ed. 7, St. Louis, 1977, The C. V. Mosby Co.)
Fig. 5-3. Pulmonary edema. (From Millard, M.: Lung, pleura, and mediastinum. In Anderson, W. A. D., and Kissane, J. M., editors: Pathology, ed. 7, St. Louis, 1977, The C. V. Mosby Co.)

purpura (characterized by spontaneous hemorrhages, varying in size from petechiae to ecchymoses throughout various tissues of the body), *hematoma* (localized collection of blood, forming tumorlike swelling in the tissue), *apoplexy* (copious effusion of blood in an organ, as in the brain)

Hemorrhages may be designated according to their location, e.g., *epistaxis* (bleeding from the nose), *hemoptysis* (expectoration of blood from hemorrhage in the lungs or elsewhere in the respiratory tract), *hematemesis* (vomiting of blood), *melena* (presence of dark, decomposed blood in the stools), *hemothorax, hemopericardium,* and *hemoperitoneum* (hemorrhage in the pleural, pericardial, and peritoneal cavities, respectively), and *hematuria* (blood in the urine).

Etiology. *Local hemorrhages* may be caused by trauma (as in abrasions, lacera-

tions, contusions, fractures, and penetrating injuries) or may occur in the absence of trauma (i.e., spontaneously) as a result of rupture of diseased vessels or the heart (e.g., atherosclerosis, cystic medial degeneration, inflammations, and congenital defects of arteries, which cause weakening of arterial walls, often with aneurysmal formation; erosions and ulcerations of the gastrointestinal tract, producing discontinuity of vascular walls; neoplastic invasion of vessels; and infarct of the myocardium). Hypertension (high blood pressure) may be a factor in the development of local hemorrhage, particularly if there is underlying disease of the arteries (e.g., in cerebral atherosclerosis).

Systemic hemorrhages are seen in a group of disorders characterized by a *hemorrhagic diathesis* (i.e., a hemorrhagic tendency) (Fig. 5-4), in which multiple tissues and organs are involved, often simultaneously (p. 508).

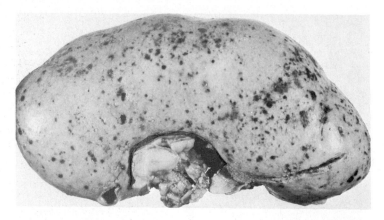

Fig. 5-4. Hemorrhages, chiefly petechial, on surface of kidney of leukemic patient with hemorrhagic diathesis.

These disorders are caused by defects of the coagulation mechanism, by defects of the vascular walls, or by both, and include such entities as hemophilia, hypoprothrombinemia, hypofibrinogenemia, the various purpuras associated with platelet deficiencies, hereditary hemorrhagic telangiectasia, vitamin C deficiency, Schönlein-Henoch ("anaphylactoid") purpura, and purpuras associated with endothelial damage caused by anoxia, chemicals, snake venom, fulminating infections, etc.

Effects. The effects of hemorrhage may be local or systemic. The *local effects* may be of a mechanical nature and will depend on the size and the location of the hemorrhage, e.g., subdural hematoma with pressure on the brain, pericardial hemorrhage causing interference with filling of the cardiac chambers *(cardiac tamponade),* and hemorrhage in the larynx, causing swelling of tissues and narrowing of the lumen, resulting in asphyxiation. If the hemorrhage is slight, it may be completely resorbed, leaving little or no trace behind, or it may undergo fibrosis (organization). Discoloration may occur at the site because of breakdown of erythrocytes and formation of hemoglobin-derived pigments.

Systemic effects of hemorrhage depend on the rapidity of bleeding (acute or chronic) and the amount of blood loss. Acute hemorrhage may be massive enough to cause shock and death. A transient anemia may result from acute blood loss, which may be followed by response of the bone marrow to produce erythrocytes. Chronic blood loss leads to an iron-deficiency anemia of the hypochromic type.

Certain *compensatory mechanisms* may be activated as a result of a sudden loss of a considerable amount of blood:

1 Lowered blood pressure affects the pressoreceptors, altering impulses to the cardiac and vasomotor centers and resulting in increased cardiac rate, peripheral vasoconstriction, and increased secretion of catecholamines (the latter contributing to the vasoconstriction).

2 Lack of oxygen in the circulation (a) activates the chemoreceptors and (b) increases renal secretion of a vasoexcitor material (VEM) or renin (which is important in the formation of angiotensin), and both a and b contribute to peripheral vasoconstriction.

3 Under the influence of epinephrine the spleen contracts and discharges blood into the circulation.

4 Sympathetic reflexes also may produce constriction of systemic veins (capacitance vessels), which normally serve as a reservoir from which blood is pumped by the heart. The venoconstriction causes a decrease in the capacity of veins, an increase in venous pressure, and an improvement in venous return to the heart.

5 Reduction of intravascular volume may stimulate release of ADH and aldosterone (release of the latter being contributed to by angiotensin). These hormones, as well as the reduced renal blood flow and glomerular filtration rate that follow arteriolar vasoconstriction in the kidneys, participate in the restoration of intravascular fluid volume.

Thus, these compensatory mechanisms assist in the recovery of plasma volume and blood pressure and divert the blood from the less vital to the vital organs (viz., heart and brain).

SHOCK

Shock is a circulatory disturbance characterized by an acute reduction of blood flow and an inadequate perfusion of the tissues. The effective blood flow is reduced rapidly as a consequence of a decreased cardiac output, brought about by a deficiency of venous return to the heart or primary impairment of cardiac function. A transient form, so-called primary shock, results from a neurogenic vasodilatation with pooling of blood in the peripheral microcirculation, particularly in the splanchnic area, which causes a sudden reduction of venous return to the heart and diversion of blood from the brain, leading to prostration and unconsciousness. This condition occurs immediately after trauma or may result from pain due to various causes or from emotional reactions (e.g., fear, grief, and emotion associated with the sight of blood or a wound).

The more serious, and sometimes fatal, disorder is *true shock,* often referred to as "secondary shock," which tends toward progressive circulatory failure with resultant damage to the body tissues. This is the form usually meant when the term "shock" is used without qualification and the one that is to be discussed. Among the usual clinical manifestations are weakness, cold moist skin, collapse of superficial veins, shallow respirations, rapid weak pulse, low blood pressure, and

oliguria. The skin may be warm in instances of shock due to severe infections.

Etiology. The causes of shock include many forms of injury and disease, e.g., trauma, hemorrhage, burns, surgical operations, bacterial infections, drug toxicity, ionizing radiation, intestinal obstruction, perforated viscera, dehydration, and cardiac insufficiency (as in myocardial infarction).

Types. The types of shock are generally classified on the basis of the principal cause, e.g., traumatic shock, hemorrhagic shock, surgical shock, septic (or endotoxin) shock, and cardiac or cardiogenic shock.

Pathogenesis. Concerning the pathogenesis of shock, the essential feature is the *reduction of blood flow with reduced delivery of oxygen to the tissues (anoxia) to the point where metabolic needs are no longer met.* The various clinical states mentioned previously induce this basic disturbance by means of one or more of the following factors (so-called *initiating factors of shock):*

I Factors causing acute deficiency of venous return because of a reduction of the *effective* circulating blood volume:
   A Diminution of actual blood volume resulting from:
      1 Local loss of blood and/or plasma at site of wound, burn, or operation
      2 Loss of fluid by vomiting, diarrhea, adrenal insufficiency, etc., as in dehydration
      3 Escape of fluid into interstitial compartment due to generalized increased vascular permeability
   B Vasodilatation in peripheral vascular bed, resulting in withdrawal of blood from general circulation into widened vessels (peripheral pooling of blood) without loss of actual blood volume and producing, in effect, reduction of circulating blood volume
   C Vasoconstriction or thrombosis in peripheral vascular bed, impeding flow of blood, or postcapillary vasoconstriction resulting in pooling and stasis of blood in capillary beds (as suggested in endotoxin shock)
II Factors causing decreased cardiac output primarily (cardiogenic shock) because of a sudden impairment of cardiac function, such as:
   A Deficiency in filling (e.g., cardiac tamponade)

B Deficiency in emptying (e.g., myocardial insufficiency, as in myocardial infarction, or mechanical obstructions, as in massive pulmonary embolism, ball valve thrombus, etc.)

Any of the foregoing factors, singly or in combination, initiate shock by setting in motion the same fundamental hemodynamic mechanism: *reduction of effective circulating blood volume ⟶ decreased venous return to heart ⟶ decreased cardiac output ⟶ reduced blood flow ⟶ reduced delivery of oxygen to tissues (anoxia).* If the anoxic state of the tissues is permitted to continue, it aggravates the circulatory deficiency and introduces a self-perpetuating feature into the mechanism, causing it to progress to a vicious cycle. In many instances of shock, the initial manifestation of this cyclic mechanism is the reduction of effective circulating blood volume (caused by group I factors), whereas in others, it is the decreased cardiac output (caused by group II factors).

In most of the clinical forms of shock, the initiating factors are readily apparent. However, in the type of septic shock caused by powerful endotoxins of gram-negative organisms ("endotoxin shock"), the initiating events are not so well understood as in other forms of shock. On the basis of experimental work, there is evidence that vasoconstriction in the microcirculation or thrombosis in these minute vessels may be the initiating factor by impeding the venous return to the heart. Some investigators have emphasized that the major site of vasoconstriction is in the postcapillary venules, thus leading to pooling and stasis of blood in the capillaries with possible escape of fluid into the interstitial tissues. Certain hemodynamic studies in cases of clinical septic shock, however, suggest that in some patients, peripheral vasodilatation may be the initiating factor, perhaps caused by circulating polypeptides (plasma kinins) activated by endotoxins, possibly through release of proteolytic enzymes from cells injured by the toxins.

When shock is associated with actual loss of blood volume, it is termed *hypovolemic.*

Shock that is not accompanied by actual loss of blood, as in vasodilatation with peripheral pooling of blood or in cardiac shock, is known as *normovolemic.*

Compensatory mechanisms occur early in shock in an attempt to prevent deterioration of the circulation. These mechanisms, which develop in response to reduced blood flow (hypotension), diminished blood volume, or anoxia, include:

1 Widespread peripheral vasoconstriction, most prominently in the splanchnic region
2 Cardioacceleration
3 Constriction of systemic veins
4 Retention of salt and water

These phenomena assist in the recovery of blood pressure and plasma volume and divert the blood from the less vital organs to the heart and brain. The participation of pressoreceptors, chemoreceptors, catecholamines, humoral factors (e.g., renin and vasoexcitor material) from hypoxic kidneys, and the secretion of aldosterone and ADH is similar to that already discussed in relation to acute hemorrhage (p. 104). Although peripheral vasoconstriction aids in maintaining systemic blood pressure, it may, if prolonged, accentuate the anoxic effects upon the tissues, particularly in the splanchnic region. The persistent vasoconstriction may lead to ischemic necrosis of certain organs (e.g., liver and intestines) and ultimately to paralysis of vascular muscle (vasodilatation) and decreased venous return to the heart. Thus, a state of *irreversibility,* or decompensation, in shock ensues by the establishment of a "vicious cycle."

A number of other mechanisms have been suggested as being responsible for irreversibility in shock as follows:

1 Ischemic myocardium causes decreased cardiac output, thus perpetuating the vicious cycle.
2 Cerebral ischemia results in depression of the vasomotor center with consequent vasodilatation and pooling of blood in the peripheral circulation, reducing the venous return to the heart and lessening the cardiac output.
3 As a result of the hypoxic state, a vasodilator material (VDM) is released from the

liver, spleen, and skeletal muscle and, unable to be inactivated by the hypoxic liver, causes terminal vessels to be refractory to epinephrine, resulting in vasodilatation.

4 A product of bacterial activity (e.g., endotoxin) derived from the intestinal flora is absorbed in the circulation, and since the antibacterial defense mechanism of the reticuloendothelial system of the liver and spleen is impaired by anoxia (especially as a result of persistent vasoconstriction), an endotoxemia results, which accentuates the vasoconstriction that was originally induced as a compensatory mechanism. The endotoxins elicit this effect by stimulating sympathetic activity. It is within the realm of speculation that endotoxins may produce the opposite effect in some patients (viz., microcirculatory vasodilatation) by means of their activation of vasoactive plasma kinins.

5 Hemorrhagic lesions in the intestines, caused by persistent vasoconstriction or by thrombosis in minute vessels, lead to loss of blood and serum into the intestinal lumen and a reduced circulating blood volume. This mechanism is much more characteristic of shock induced experimentally in dogs than of naturally occurring shock in man.

6 Decreased venous return may result from multiple thrombi in the microcirculation. The tendency to thrombosis is the result of several possible factors, including stasis and sludging of blood, anaerobic metabolism with excess of lactic acid in the blood that neutralizes the normally present heparin, increased coagulability of the blood because of the release of a clot-promoting factor caused by the catecholamines in the circulation, and endothelial damage resulting from anoxia or noxious products released from damaged tissue.

7 The hypoxic state causes damage to capillaries and venules, leading to vasodilatation and/or increased vascular permeability with escape of fluid to the interstitial spaces, both resulting in a decreased return of venous blood to the heart.

Morphologic changes. The morphologic changes in shock include (1) capillovenous hyperemia, (2) petechiae in serous cavities, (3)

edema, at least in certain organs such as the lungs, (4) congested gastrointestinal mucosa, with petechiae and acute ulcers, especially in the stomach, (5) degenerative changes in the kidneys, liver, heart, and adrenal glands, (6) foci of necrosis in the lymph nodes, spleen, pancreas, and liver, and (7) the characteristic lesion in the kidneys known as "hemoglobinuric nephrosis" or "lower nephron nephrosis" (p. 352).

Multiple thrombi, particularly in minute vessels, may be found in various organs. The blood is likely to be hypercoagulable in earlier stages of shock, but later it is characterized by hypocoagulability and fibrinolysis. A respiratory complication of intravascular coagulation in shock has been described (so-called shock lung or acute pulmonary failure) that is characterized by pulmonary congestion, hemorrhage, atelectasis, edema, and microcirculatory thrombi or emboli.

Circulatory disturbances of obstructive nature

THROMBOSIS

A *thrombus* is a mass formed from the constituents of the blood within the vessels or the heart during life. The process of its formation is known as *thrombosis*. The typical thrombus is initiated by clumping of the platelets and is further developed by coagulation of the blood (fibrin formation) (Fig. 5-5). A thrombus consisting entirely of erythrocytes or of platelets is not as common. Sometimes referred to as an "antemortem clot," a thrombus is to be differentiated from a clot that forms extravascularly in an area of hemorrhage and from a clot occurring within the vessels after death (postmortem clot).

Formation and structure of a thrombus. The initial event in thrombosis appears to be the adherence of platelets to the inner wall of a vessel or the heart. As seen by electron microscopy, the platelets at first are loosely aggregated (agglutinated), retaining their normal structure. With the deposition of more plate-

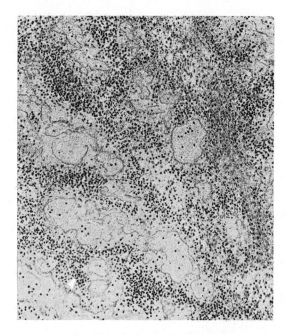

Fig. 5-5. Recent thrombus, with lamellae of platelets (pale areas) cut across at different angles. Other blood elements, particularly fibrin and leukocytes, are present between layers of platelets. (From Scotti, T. M.: Disturbances of body water and electrolytes and of circulation of blood. In Anderson, W. A. D., editor: Pathology, ed. 6, St. Louis, 1971, The C. V. Mosby Co.)

lets, the aggregates become closely packed and some platelets lose their granules. Leukocytes tend to adhere to the degranulated platelets. The agglutinated platelets form a small mound on the endothelial surface, referred to as the *primary platelet thrombus*. Disintegration of some of the platelets causes liberation of a substance that is used in the generation of plasma thromboplastin, which initiates the clotting mechanism: thromboplastin converts prothrombin to thrombin, which in turn reacts with fibrinogen to form fibrin. Tissue thromboplastin from an injured vessel wall may contribute to the process. As the thrombus develops, the platelets project from the vessel wall in the form of lamellae, bent in the direction of blood flow, and these in turn branch out as secondary lamellae, giving rise to a corallike mass. The bands of platelets, outlined by leukocytes and interlaid with fibrin, erythro-

cytes, and other leukocytes, are known as the *lines of Zahn,* which appear grossly as wavy, pale gray-white striae.

The characteristic structure of the thrombus depends on the velocity of blood flow. When the mass grows sufficiently large to obstruct the flow of blood, a homogeneous, dark red coagulum, lacking the lamellar arrangement of platelets, forms upon the coralline thrombus and is sometimes referred to as the "tail." The propagated part of the thrombus, occurring in a relatively stagnant column of blood proximally (toward the heart) in a vein, is at first unattached to the vessel wall. If it proceeds to the next tributary of the vein, a new platelet thrombus may form at the site of contact with flowing blood, followed by the events previously outlined. With repetition of this process, an elongated propagated thrombus ultimately exhibits small, pale masses of platelets alternating with longer red zones of coagulum. Propagation may occur to some extent on the other side of the thrombus as well.

Etiology. Three factors predispose to the formation of a thrombus: changes in the vessel wall, changes in blood flow (e.g., slowing, stasis, and eddying of the current), and changes in the blood constituents. An alteration of the lining endothelium is perhaps the most important factor causing thrombosis. This is operative in a wide variety of conditions, e.g., atherosclerosis of the aorta or its branches, inflammation of the wall of arteries (as in polyarteritis nodosa, thromboangiitis obliterans), of veins (thrombophlebitis), or of heart valves, physical or chemical injury of a vessel, and ischemic injury of the heart wall (as in myocardial infarction).

Experimental evidence suggests that the injured vessel wall may release certain substances, such as adenosine diphosphate (ADP), that facilitate platelet aggregation. A mechanism in the initiation of a thrombus may be the adherence of platelets to exposed subendothelial tissue (e.g., collagen) rather than to endothelium itself. It is postulated that the platelet-collagen interaction induces platelets to release ADP, which causes them to adhere to each other. It is also possible that ADP released from damaged red blood cells in the area may contribute to platelet aggregation.

The importance of changes in the blood flow is indicated by the frequency of thrombosis in the veins, where slowness and stasis are more likely to occur than in the arteries. Thrombi occur frequently in the veins of the lower extremities in bedridden patients, especially in those with heart disease, which is attended by slowing of the peripheral circulation, and in those in the postoperative period. Thrombosis is common in varicose veins, in which stasis and eddying of the blood are present. Eddying of the bloodstream promotes thrombus formation in an aortic aneurysm. There is evidence that stasis of the blood produces alterations of the endothelium and that this may be the means by which stasis predisposes to thrombosis.

Changes in the blood constituents favoring thrombosis include increase in number and adhesiveness of platelets (as in the postoperative and puerperal states, accidental trauma, cancer, and certain peripheral vascular diseases), increased viscosity of blood (as in polycythemia), release of thromboplastinlike substance (as in visceral carcinoma), and increase in fibrinogen and other clotting factors of the blood (as in pregnancy and possibly in users of oral contraceptives). An increased secretion of catecholamines into the circulation (such as may occur in hemorrhagic shock) may be a factor causing hypercoagulability of the blood and may predispose to thrombosis. One of the effects of the catecholamines may be release of ADP from platelets, thus causing platelet aggregation.

Thrombosis occurring in a vein in the absence of inflammation may be termed phlebothrombosis. The sudden, spontaneous appearance of thrombosis in a large vein or the recurrent formation of venous thrombi in widely scattered areas of the body ("migratory phlebothrombosis"), occurring in association with visceral cancer, is sometimes referred to as *Trousseau's syndrome*.

Types and fate of thrombi. Thrombi form anywhere within the heart or blood vessels but most frequently in veins and particularly in those of the lower extremities. A thrombus that completely obstructs the lumen of a vessel is referred to as occlusive, and one that extends along a vessel from the primary occlusive part is a *propagating* thrombus. A nonocclusive thrombus adherent to the vessel or cardiac wall is known as *mural* (Fig. 5-6) or *parietal*. When the latter occurs in the heart, it may be *pedunculated* or may appear as a rounded mass, which may become dislodged and move about freely in the chamber (a ball thrombus). Thrombi occurring on the valves of the heart as a result of underlying damage (infectious or noninfectious) are known as *vegetations*. Widespread thrombosis in the microcirculation is referred to as *disseminated intravascular coagulation (DIC)* (p. 510).

Thrombi are referred to as *recent* or *old* depending on their age, as *septic* or *bland* depending on whether or not they are infected,

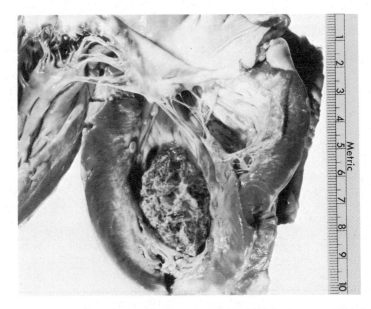

Fig. 5-6. Mural thrombus in left ventricle of heart, overlying organized myocardial infarct. (From Scotti, T. M.: Disturbances of body water and electrolytes and of circulation of blood. In Anderson, W. A. D., editor: Pathology, ed. 6, St. Louis, 1971, The C. V. Mosby Co.)

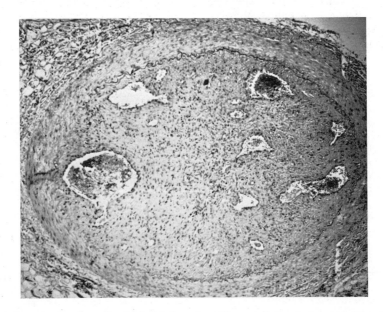

Fig. 5-7. Organized and canalized arterial thrombus. Wavy dark line is internal elastic lamina.

and as *hyaline* when the elements of the thrombus are so altered as to produce a homogeneous mass.

Various changes occur in thrombi. There may be a *softening* in the center of a large sterile thrombus caused by proteolytic enzymes released from disintegrating leukocytes or in an infected (septic) thrombus that is invaded by pyogenic organisms. The latter may give rise to septic emboli and abscesses in distant organs. *Dissolution* and removal of a small thrombus by fibrinolysis may occur. *Healing* of a thrombus is accomplished by the process of organization, proceeding from the periphery toward the center. Some degree of circulation may be reestablished through an occlusive thrombus by contraction of the mass and by formation of newly formed vascular channels *(canalization)* within it (Fig. 5-7). *Calcification* occurs in some organizing thrombi, especially in small veins *(phleboliths)*. There may be *detachment* of a whole thrombus or parts of it before it undergoes organization, forming emboli that are transported elsewhere.

Effects of thrombi. The local effects of thrombosis result from the interference of the circulation in an organ or part of the body. The effects depend on the size and type of a thrombus, the degree of vascular occlusion, the kind of vessel involved, the degree of collateral circulation, and the organ affected. Thrombotic occlusion of a vein may lead to stasis of blood, edema, and even necrosis in the area drained by the vessel. Occlusive arterial thrombi may cause localized ischemic necrosis *(infarct)* in an organ or *gangrene* of an extremity. If collateral circulation is adequate, little or no change may result from the vascular obstruction. A pedunculated or ball thrombus in the left atrium of the heart may suddenly occlude the mitral orifice and cause dyspnea, cyanosis, syncope, and even death. Detached masses of thrombi, set free in the circulation, result in *embolism* with its serious consequences (see below).

DIC may be a factor contributing to the initiation of some forms of shock (p. 105) or to the irreversibility in shock (p. 107). In certain conditions it may induce a hemorrhagic tendency due to the reduction of fibrinogen, platelets, and other coagulation factors that occurs during the formation of the microvascular thrombi throughout the body (p. 510).

Postmortem intravascular clot. It is important to distinguish between a thrombus and an intravascular postmortem clot at autopsy. A thrombus tends to be dry, friable, and mottled gray-white and red, is adherent to the lining endothelium, exhibits lines of Zahn, and sometimes produces distention of the affected vessel. A postmortem clot is moist, elastic, homogeneous, and without lines of Zahn, is not adherent to the lining endothelium, forms a cast of the vessel and its branches or tributaries, and is deep red throughout ("currant jelly" clot) when clotting occurs rapidly after death, or is layered with a lower deep red part consisting of settled erythrocytes and an uppermost gray-yellow plasma layer ("chicken fat" clot) when clotting occurs slowly.

EMBOLISM

Embolism is a partial or complete obstruction of some part of the vascular system by any mass carried there in the circulation. The transported material is an *embolus*.

Emboli are classified as *solid* (detached thrombi, fragments of tissue, clumps of tumor cells, etc.), *liquid* (fat globules), or *gaseous* (air). They may be *bland* or *septic*. They are also designated according to their location—*venous, arterial,* or *lymphatic*. A *paradoxical embolus* is one that arises in the venous circulation but enters the arterial side, or vice versa, usually through an arteriovenous communication such as a patent foramen ovale or some other septal defect in the heart. An embolus that travels against the flow of blood is a *retrograde* embolus.

The *effects* of emboli, as with thrombi, may be caused by the obstruction of the circulation in an organ or a part of the body, so that infarcts or gangrene may occur. Septic emboli may produce foci of inflammation, abscesses, and "mycotic" aneurysms at the sites of blockage. Dissemination of a malignant neoplasm occurs, locally or systemically, by means of tumor emboli in the bloodstream or in the lymphatics. Sudden death may result from emboli in the pulmonary or the coronary arterial vessels.

Thromboembolism. The most frequent type of embolus is a detached thrombus or portion thereof that arises in the venous or arterial circulation. The *arterial* emboli arise usually from mural thrombi in the heart (left ventricle or atrium), from vegetations on the aortic or mitral valves, and occasionally from thrombi on atheromatous plaques or in aneurysms of the aorta. They produce occlusions most frequently in the spleen, kidneys, brain, and lower extremities, often with resultant infarcts in the organs and gangrene in the limbs. Septic emboli (as from vegetations of bacterial endocarditis) may cause abscesses or arteritis with

formation of "mycotic" aneurysms. Coronary arterial embolism occurs in rare instances. *Venous* emboli originate most commonly from thrombi in veins of the lower extremities, less frequently from thrombi in the pelvic veins or in the right side of the heart, and rarely from thrombi in veins of the upper extremities. The most significant complication of venous embolism is the obstruction of the pulmonary arterial circulation.

The effects of *pulmonary embolism* include sudden or delayed death, infarction, and hemorrhage. Death is usually related to a large embolus in one or both main pulmonary arteries, sometimes in the form of a "saddle embolus" overriding the bifurcation of the vessel (Fig. 5-8), or it may be found in the right ventricle

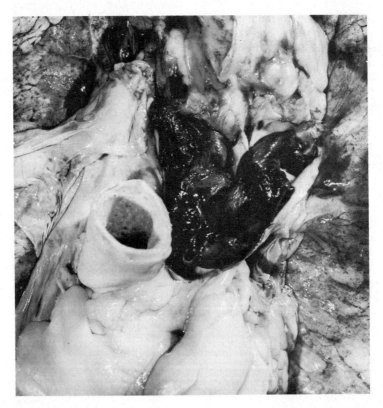

Fig. 5-8. Pulmonary embolism. Large detached mass from thrombus in leg vein is impacted in pulmonary artery and extends into both main branches—saddle embolus. (From Scotti, T. M.: Disturbances of body water and electrolytes and of circulation of blood. In Anderson, W. A. D., editor: Pathology, ed. 6, St. Louis, 1971, The C. V. Mosby Co.)

obstructing the outflow tract. Sudden death is attributed to one or several of the following mechanisms: asphyxia; acute cor pulmonale; diminished cardiac output with arterial hypotension, coronary insufficiency and myocardial failure, cerebral anoxemia, or shock; pulmonocoronary reflex causing widespread pulmonary and coronary vascular spasm, a reflex eventuating in peripheral circulatory failure, and a reflex producing cardiac standstill. *Chronic cor pulmonale* may result from widespread organized pulmonary emboli in the smaller vessels after recurrent thromboembolism.

Fat embolism. The presence of *fat globules* in the circulation with impaction of the minute vessels in various organs is termed *fat embolism*. This entity occurs most commonly as a result of trauma to bones, particularly after fractures of the long bones. Fat embolism also may be caused by contusion or laceration of adipose tissue, and in the absence of trauma it may occur in association with extensive cutaneous burns, inflammation in fatty marrow or adipose tissue, fatty livers, and decompression sickness. Fat emboli also may arise from extrinsic fat or oil introduced into the body for therapeutic or other purposes. The minute emboli in the pulmonary circulation do not produce infarcts of the lungs but may cause congestion, edema, and focal hemorrhages. Respiratory symptoms may occur with extensive involvement.

Systemic fat embolism is characterized by the presence of fat globules in the greater circulation as well as the pulmonary, so that emboli are disseminated to the brain, kidneys (Figs. 5-9 and 5-10), heart, and other organs. Death may result from cerebral involvement. Microinfarcts and focal hemorrhages may be observed in the brain.

The major theory regarding the source of fat

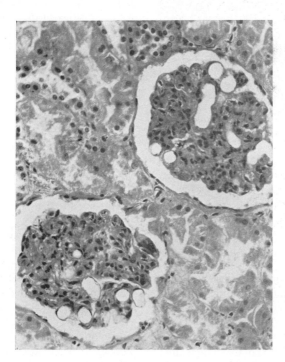

Fig. 5-9. Fat embolism in kidney. Clear, prominent vacuoles in glomerular capillaries are fat emboli (dissolved out in preparation of section). (From Scotti, T. M.: Disturbances of body water and electrolytes and of circulation of blood. In Anderson, W. A. D., editor: Pathology, ed. 6, St. Louis, 1971, The C. V. Mosby Co.)

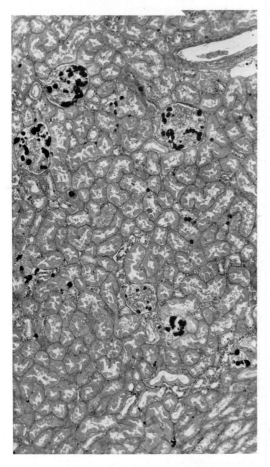

Fig. 5-10. Fat embolism in kidney. Glomerular capillaries and interstitial vessels contain fat globules (stained with osmic acid). (From Scotti, T. M.: Disturbances of body water and electrolytes and of circulation of blood. In Anderson, W. A. D., editor: Pathology, ed. 6, St. Louis, 1971, The C. V. Mosby Co.)

emboli, which is plausible in those instances associated with mechanical trauma, is that they arise from injured fat or bone marrow or other fat depots. The globules enter the venous circulation through ruptured blood vessels and are carried to the lungs and from there may pass to the systemic circulation by way of the pulmonary capillaries or arteriovenous shunts. On the other hand, some investigators are of the opinion that fat emboli are derived from aggregations of plasma lipids due to a disturbance in the natural emulsification of fat resulting from a biochemical event that is initiated by various forms of stress, whether the latter is of a traumatic or nontraumatic nature. In some patients, embolic fat is assumed to originate from hepatic cells affected by fatty metamorphosis, even in the absence of trauma.

Amniotic fluid embolism. Amniotic fluid embolism may be a cause of severe or fatal shock coming on during or soon after labor. Although the incidence is low, it is an important cause of obstetric death. The pulmonary vessels contain the components of amniotic fluid—epithelial squames, vernix caseosa, and sometimes mucus and lanugo hairs—admixed with leukocytes (Fig. 5-11). Pulmonary edema may be present. It is not always clear how the amniotic fluid enters the circulation from the uterus, although in some instances it is probably accomplished through tears or surgical incisions in the myometrium or endocervix. Amniotic fluid emboli have been found in vessels of organs other than the lungs (e.g., heart, kidneys, brain, liver, spleen, and pancreas).

Death may result from mechanical blockage of the pulmonary circulation, superimposed reflex vascular spasms, or "anaphylactoid" reaction. In some patients, DIC may appear as a result of thromboplastin entering the circulation along with amniotic fluid. This may result in a deficiency of fibrin, followed by a reduction of other coagulation factors and platelets, so that a hemorrhagic tendency develops.

Air embolism. *Venous air embolism* may occur as a complication of surgical operations, particularly of the chest and neck, during which air may be sucked into opened veins. Air also may be introduced into veins by various diagnostic or therapeutic procedures (e.g., during peritoneoscopy and induction of pneumoperitoneum). Venous embolism also is known to occur after the accidental injection of air, by means of a syringe, into endometrial veins during attempted abortion.

Death may result from pulmonary embo-

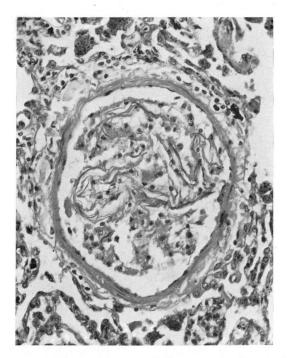

Fig. 5-11. Amniotic fluid embolism. Clump of squames and granular debris admixed with leukocytes in pulmonary vessel. (Courtesy Dr. R. J. Poppiti; from Scotti, T. M.: Disturbances of body water and electrolytes and of circulation of blood. In Anderson, W. A. D., editor: Pathology, ed. 6, St. Louis, 1971, The C. V. Mosby Co.)

lism, and in such cases frothy blood is usually found in the right side of the heart at autopsy. In fatal venous air embolism induced in animals, fibrin clots have been found in association with the air emboli in the distal branches of the pulmonary arteries. The intravascular coagulation was attributed to platelet damage caused by the whipping action of the heart on the air bubbles.

Arterial air embolism may result from the introduction of air into a pulmonary vein during thoracic operations or induction of pneumothorax. Since the air enters the systemic circulation, air bubbles may be found in the coronary or cerebral arteries. In such instances, smaller amounts may produce death than in the case of venous air embolism.

Decompression sickness. When divers or workers in caissons descend to levels of high pressure, the amount of gases held in solution

in the blood and tissues increases. If the pressure is rapidly reduced during ascent to normal pressure, the gases (particularly nitrogen) come out of solution as bubbles in the blood and tissues, causing a variety of symptoms, depending on their location *(caisson disease* or *diver's palsy)*. The same effect may be produced in aviators who ascend from normal atmospheric pressure to low atmospheric pressures of high altitudes.

Fat emboli are sometimes found in association with the gas emboli. The fat globules are presumed to be derived from fat-containing tissue cells that are ruptured upon release of the gases or from aggregations of plasma lipids.

Other types of embolism. In *bone marrow embolism,* fragments of marrow *(adipose tissue* and marrow cells) enter the venous circulation after bone fractures or as a result of sternal puncture, closed chest cardiac massage, or bone marrow infarction (as in hemoglobin C and S disease). Sometimes, fat embolism (liquid *globules* of fat) is associated with bone marrow embolism. *Atheromatous embolism* may result when fragments of eroded atheromatous plaques enter the arterial circulation (Fig. 5-12).

Emboli of other tissues may sometimes appear, e.g., *placental fragments, cerebral* or *hepatic tissues,* and *clumps of tumor cells*

(Fig. 5-13). *Bacteria, parasites,* and certain *foreign bodies* entering the circulation (e.g., needles, shrapnel, bullets, polyethylene catheters) are other forms of emboli.

ISCHEMIA

Ischemia refers to the diminution or the obliteration of the blood supply to a localized area of the body. As a result, the affected part is deprived of vital nutritional substances, particularly oxygen, while certain potentially in-

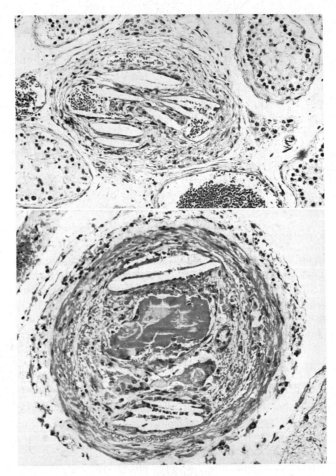

Fig. 5-12. Atheromatous emboli in arteries of testis (top) and meninges (bottom). Slitlike spaces are areas from which lipid (cholesterol) crystals have been dissolved in preparation of sections. (From Winter, W. J.: Arch. Pathol. **64:**137-142, 1957.)

jurious metabolic products accumulate in the area. The term ischemia generally is used in reference to interference with arterial blood flow to a part, but it should be noted that venous obstruction also may cause local tissue damage because of stagnant anoxia and lack of removal of metabolites.

Causes of ischemia include thrombosis, embolism, arteriosclerosis, polyarteritis nodosa, thromboangiitis obliterans, vasospasm (as in Raynaud's disease, hypothermia, ergotism), outside pressure on a vessel by tumors or other masses, and constriction by a ligature or volvulus. The extent of damage depends on (1) the rapidity of development of ischemia (gradual or sudden,) (2) the degree of occlusion (partial or complete), (3) the vulnerability of the organ or tissue involved, and (4) the degree of sufficiency of the collateral circulation.

Among the changes associated with gradual incomplete ischemia are degenerations, atrophy, and fibrosis and/or adipose tissue replacement (gliosis in the central nervous system). The change associated with sudden, complete ischemia is usually necrosis (infarct or gangrene), unless, as in the case of acute myocardial ischemia, sudden death ensues. In instances in which the collateral circulation is good, an occlusion of a vessel may not be associated with visible effect.

INFARCTION

An *infarct* is a localized area of necrosis resulting from some form of circulatory insufficiency. The process whereby this lesion is developed is known as *infarction*. Causes of infarcts are those just noted in the discussion of ischemia, particularly thrombosis and embolism. Arterial obstructions produce infarcts more frequently than do venous obstructions.

Infarcts are most common in the spleen, kidneys, lungs, intestines, heart, and brain. Cardiac infarcts usually are the result of coronary arterial atherosclerosis with or without thrombosis rather than embolism and are an important cause of disability and death (p. 320). Intestinal infarcts involve a segment of the bowel, are associated with paralytic intestinal obstruction, and, unless surgical relief is prompt, result in death from peritonitis or shock (p. 557).

In the lung, because of its abundant circulation, infarction tends to follow pulmonary embolism only when there is already some interference with the circulation, such as chronic passive congestion. The liver likewise has an abundant circulation, and in this organ infarction is rare.

In the spleen, kidneys, and lungs, an infarct forms a slightly raised pyramidal mass of dead tissue, with its base at the periphery of

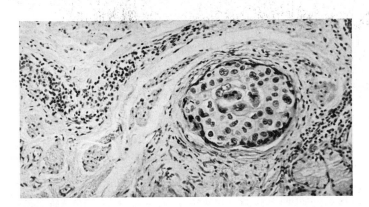

Fig. 5-13. Tumor embolism. Cells of squamous carcinoma occupying lumen of blood vessel.

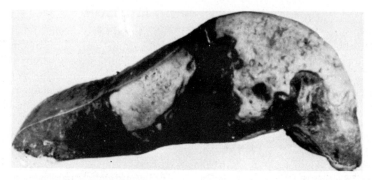

Fig. 5-14. Multiple infarcts of spleen due to emboli from bacterial endocarditis. (From Scotti, T. M.: Disturbances of body water and electrolytes and of circulation of blood. In Anderson, W. A. D., editor: Pathology, ed. 6, St. Louis, 1971, The C. V. Mosby Co.)

the organ and its apex toward the point of arterial obstruction (Fig. 5-14). In the myocardium, the pattern of an infarct is more irregular. Shortly after the vascular obstruction, the area becomes red and congested as a result of dilatation of the vessels and flowing of blood into the part from adjacent vessels. Hemorrhage occurs as a result of ischemic damage to vessel walls and is particularly severe in infarcts of the lungs and spleen. The area becomes swollen and edematous. In some cases, the amount of redness, congestion, and hemorrhage is slight. Degenerative changes appear, and necrosis is evident within 48 hours (sometimes as early as 12 to 24 hours), first affecting the parenchymatous tissue, but eventually the less sensitive supporting connective tissue is affected as well.

The tissue around certain infarcts responds to breakdown products of the necrotic tissue by an inflammatory reaction (hyperemia and infiltration of neutrophils and, if the area is covered by a serous layer, a fibrinous exudate may occur on the surface). The necrosis is of the coagulative type, except in the brain, where it is liquefactive. The infarct is gradually decolorized, as erythrocytes are lysed and removed from the area, and appears pale or yellow-white (*pale* or *white* infarct). Hematoidin and hemosiderin may be seen microscopically in some infarcts. However, in organs composed of soft, loose tissue (e.g., lungs

and intestines), and especially in organs with a double blood supply (e.g., lungs), infarcts tend to remain hemorrhagic *(red infarcts)*.

Healing of an infarct is accomplished by removal of dead tissue and replacement of fibrous tissue (organization), so that an older infarct shrinks beneath the surface of an organ and appears as a pale, depressed area.

REFERENCES

Brinkhous, K. M., et al., editors: The platelet, Baltimore, 1971, The Williams & Wilkins Co.

Chien, S., and Gregersen, M. I.: In Mountcastle, V. B., editor: Medical physiology, St. Louis, 1968, The C. V. Mosby Co., pp. 262-283 (hemorrhage and shock).

Collins, R. D.: Illustrated manual of fluid and electrolyte disorders, Philadelphia, 1976, J. B. Lippincott Co.

Edelman, I. S., and Leibman, J.: Am. J. Med. **27**:256-277, 1959 (body water and electrolytes).

Elton, N. W., et al.: Am. J. Clin. Pathol. **39**:252-264, 1963 (acute salt poisoning in infants).

Fine, J.: J.A.M.A. **188**:427-432, 1964 (septic shock).

French, J. E.: In Crawford, T., editor: Modern trends in pathology, vol. 2, New York, 1967, Appleton-Century-Crofts, pp. 208-237 (electron microscopy of thrombus formation).

Goodman, J. R., et al.: Am. J. Pathol. **52**:391-400, 1968 (pulmonary microembolism in shock).

Hardaway, R. M., et al.: J.A.M.A. **199**:779-790, 1967 (pulmonary microthrombi in shock).

Hartviet, F., et al.: Br. J. Exp. Pathol. **49**:81-86, 1968 (venous air embolism).

Jacobson, E. D.: N. Engl. J. Med. **278**:834-839, 1968 (physiologic approach to shock).

Jorgensen, L., et al.: Lab. Invest. **17**:616-644, 1967 (ADP and platelet aggregation).

Liban, E., and Raz, S.: Am. J. Clin. Pathol. **51:**477-486, 1969 (amniotic fluid embolism).

Liljedahl, S. O., and Westermark, L.: Acta Anaesthesiol. Scand. **11:**177-194, 1967 (fat embolism).

Marcus, A. J.: N. Engl. J. Med. **280:**1213-1220, 1278-1284, 1330-1335, 1969 (platelet function).

Mason, R. G., and Saba, H. I.: Am. J. Pathol. **92:**773-812, 1978 (normal and abnormal hemostasis—a review).

Maxwell, M. H., and Kleeman, C. R., editors: Clinical disorders of fluid and electrolyte metabolism, ed. 3, New York, 1980, McGraw-Hill Book Co.

Mills, L. C., and Moyer, J. H.: Shock and hypotension; pathogenesis and treatment, New York, 1965, Grune & Stratton, Inc.

Moser, K. M., and Stein, M., editors: Pulmonary thromboembolism, Chicago, 1973, Year Book Medical Publishers, Inc.

Mustard, J. F., et al.: Am. J. Med. Sci. **248:**469-496, 1964 (review of thrombosis)

Nicolaides, A. N., editor: Thromboembolism; etiology, advances in prevention and treatment, Baltimore, 1975, University Park Press.

Sevitt, S.: J. Pathol. **111:**1-11, 1973 (vascularization of deep-vein thrombi).

Sherry, S., Brinkhous, K. M., Genton, E., and Stengle, J. M., editors: Thrombosis, Washington, 1969, National Academy of Sciences.

Thal, A. P., and Sardesai, V. M.: Am. J. Surg. **110:**308-312, 1965 (shock and circulating polypeptides).

Thomas, D. P.: Clin. Haematol. **1:**267-282, 1972 (platelets in venous thrombosis).

Weisberg, H. F.: Water, electrolyte, and acid-base balance, ed. 2, Baltimore, 1962, The Williams & Wilkins Co.

6

Bacterial infections

Infectious diseases are caused by a variety of microorganisms, including bacteria. Pathogenic bacteria have the ability not only to establish and reproduce themselves within the host but also to elaborate certain metabolic products, including toxins, which participate in the development of the disease. *Transmission* of the organisms is by direct contact with infected animals or human beings or by means of contaminated food, water, milk, or other substances that may harbor the infectious agents (i.e., fomites). A characteristic of these diseases is a *period of incubation,* i.e., the interval between invasion by organisms and the clinical manifestations, which may vary from a few minutes or hours to weeks or months, or even longer. The microorganisms enter the body through various routes *(portals of entry),* i.e., the skin and the mucous membranes, the respiratory tract, the alimentary tract, and the genitourinary tract.

The *course of an infection* depends on (1) the organism, its nature, virulence, invasiveness, specificity, portal of entry into the body, and number (dose) and on (2) the resistance of the host to the organism and its growth and spread. The resistance is influenced not only by such factors as age, nutritional status, racial factors, and presence of other diseases that may predispose to infections but also by certain defensive factors in the host. For example, the organisms may be prevented from invading the tissues by maintenance of intact skin and mucous membranes,

the presence of lysozyme in secretions such as the tears, and the ciliary action of respiratory epithelium. Also important in defense of the host at the epithelial surface is the presence of mucosal (e.g., intestinal) antibodies. Their source is not the systemic immunoglobulins. The mucosal antibodies probably prevent adherence of microorganisms to the epithelial surface and thus prevent their invasion. They also appear to protect against the effects of bacterial toxins. When the microorganisms overcome the local defense mechanisms and invasion occurs, phagocytic cells of the reticuloendothelial system and the mobile phagocytes play an important defensive role by removing and destroying the organisms. Also, serum antibodies formed by immunocompetent cells in the host tend to inhibit or destroy the bacteria or neutralize their toxins.

Individuals with hypogammaglobulinemia or agammaglobulinemia have lessened resistance to infections. Such persons, children or adults, have recurrent infections, diminished or absent circulating gamma globulin (although other blood proteins may be normal in amount), inability to form circulating antibodies in response to administered antigens or infecting organisms, and absence of the normal blood-group isoagglutinins. Lymphoid tissue in nodes, the spleen, or elsewhere may show absence of germinal centers and of plasma cells. Decreased resistance to infections is evident also in patients with phagocytic cell defects (p. 63) and in those with impaired cell

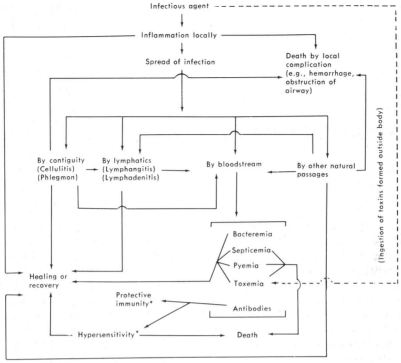

Fig. 6-1. Effects of infection.

*In certain infections, protective immunity and hypersensitivity
are mediated by lymphocytes sensitized to microbial antigens.

immunity (p. 82), the latter being more susceptible to viral and mycotic infections than patients with immunoglobulin deficiencies.

The various *effects of infection,* local and systemic, are summarized in Fig. 6-1. The local effect is inflammation, which may be represented by one or more types (acute, chronic, nonspecific, purulent, necrotizing, ulcerative, granulomatous, etc.), depending on the organism. The term *nonspecific* is often used when the inflammatory reaction does not conform to any distinctive histologic pattern. Spread of an infection may be by contiguity (cellulitis or phlegmon), by the lymphatics (lymphangitis and lymphadenitis), by other natural passages (bronchi and ureters), by the bloodstream (bacteremia, septicemia, pyemia, and toxemia), or by a combination of these

means. A significant effect is the production of antibodies. The antibodies may be beneficial to the body in that they tend to destroy or immobilize the invading organisms or neutralize their toxins (protective immunity), or they may sensitize the tissues of the host, resulting in a hypersensitivity state. In certain infections, hypersensitivity is mediated by sensitized cells (delayed hypersensitivity), as in tuberculosis, tularemia, brucellosis, and some mycotic and viral diseases. Hypersensitivity is important in these infectious diseases because of its influence on the character of the lesions and the progress of the disease. The intense tissue reactions usually associated with this state may be detrimental to the host and even severe enough to cause the death of the patient. An unsettled question is whether hypersensitivity reactions ever enhance protective immunity by serving as a defense mechanism against infection.

Bacteremia, the circulation of organisms in the bloodstream without clinical evidence of their presence, is probably frequent, is usually transient, and, in most cases, leads to no distant injury or new focus of infection. However, under certain circumstances it may lead to isolated infections, such as osteomyelitis and bacterial endocarditis. The term *septicemia* is applied when the bacteria and their toxins in the circulation are associated with clinical manifestations such as chills, fever, and petechial hemorrhages of skin. Pathologic changes associated with septicemia include the following:

1 Degenerative changes in parenchymatous organs
2 Foci of necrosis and reticuloendothelial hyperplasia in lymph nodes, spleen, liver, and bone marrow
3 Acute splenitis
4 Congestion and hemorrhages (e.g., in skin, serosae, and adrenal glands) and generalized edema
5 Thrombi in the small vessels of the microcirculation
6 Hemolysis of erythrocytes with slight jaundice or more severe hemolytic anemia in some instances
7 Acute inflammation in various organs (e.g., bacterial endocarditis, meningitis)

The term *pyemia* is used for that type of septicemia (septicopyemia) in which pyogenic organisms are spread by the blood and result in multiple abscesses in distant areas. *Toxemia* is the effect on the tissues of circulating bacterial toxins, whether or not the bacterial organisms are also circulating in the blood. Toxemia is of prime importance as the effect of certain organisms, e.g., in diphtheria, tetanus, and botulism. However, unlike diphtheria and tetanus, in which the toxins are derived from organisms within tissues of the host, the toxins of botulism are usually formed outside the body and ingested, causing a pure toxemia without invasion of the host's tissues by the organisms (p. 130). In severe infections with toxemia, shock may develop.

The various chemotherapeutic and antibiotic agents so effective in a wide range of infections apparently act by influencing or inhibiting growth of organisms rather than by augmenting natural defense mechanisms.

STAPHYLOCOCCAL INFECTION

Staphylococci are pus-producing organisms of the family Micrococcaceae that grow in grapelike or irregular clusters and are gram-positive and aerobic but facultatively anaerobic. The main pathogenic types are the golden *Staphylococcus aureus* and the white *Staphylococcus epidermidis*. In cultures, a hemolysin is produced that, by laking of red cells, produces a clear zone around colonies on blood agar plates. Staphylococci produce several potent toxins and enzymes, e.g., necrotoxin, leukocidin, hemolysins, enterotoxin, hyaluronidase, and coagulase. The toxin causing necrosis of the skin in dermal infections may act by direct injury to cells or by production of prolonged ischemia as a result of its vasoconstrictive effect. There has been an increase of staphylococcal infections in recent years because of the appearance of strains of staphylococci that are resistant to antimicrobial agents.

Wherever a foothold is gained in the body, staphylococci tend to produce a localized abscess. The skin is most commonly affected, with the production of furuncles (boils) and carbuncles. Staphylococci are commonly present on healthy skin, and although most are saprophytic, some forms are pathogenic. Predisposing factors of lowered resistance or abrasions allow these organisms to enter tissues and produce lesions.

Furuncle. Furuncles usually start about hair follicles, with production of a small localized but painful abscess. The abscess ruptures and discharges its pus on the surface, and healing follows. The inflammation may extend and burrow in the subepithelial tissues, and a number of discrete areas of necrosis form in the skin, from which pus is discharged.

Carbuncle. A more extensive lesion than the furuncle, the carbuncle is particularly dangerous on the upper lip or upper half of the face, where thrombophlebitic extension may lead to cavernous sinus and meningeal involvement.

Staphylococcal pyemia. Staphylococcal septicopyemia may occur by extension from any localized focus. This is an extremely dangerous condition with a mortality (without antibiotic therapy) of about 80%. It results in multiple pyemic abscesses in the kidneys, heart (Fig. 6-2), lungs, joints, etc. In some cases, the original focus may be difficult to identify because it has healed or is hidden among the multiple lesions.

Suppurative nephritis. When caused by staphylococci, suppurative nephritis may appear as a focal disease resulting from pyemia ("pyemic kidney") or as a suppurative pyelonephritis.

Staphylococcal endocarditis. Staphylococcal endocarditis is one form of acute bacterial endocarditis (p. 310) and has large, soft vegetations.

Staphylococcal pneumonia. Staphylococcal pneumonia represents 5% or less of bacterial pneumonias. It may be a primary infection, but more often it occurs when resistance is depressed, as by epidemic influenza. It also occurs as a complication of pertussis, measles, mucoviscidosis, leukemia, and various chronic debilitating diseases. It is often rapidly fatal, with an alveolar exudate of hemorrhagic and edematous character, although abscess formation occurs if life continues for more than 3 or 4 days.

Osteomyelitis. Osteomyelitis is commonly a localized staphylococcal infection in bone (p. 708). The organisms reach the bone by the bloodstream from some primary, and often inconspicuous, focus. The localization in a certain site may be determined by some particular stress or injury to the bone.

Food poisoning. Food poisoning is sometimes caused by growth of staphylococci in contaminated food. The manifestations are the result of ingestion of enterotoxin elaborated by the organisms in the food and not by a true infection of the intestinal tract.

Chronic granulomatous disease of childhood. Bacteria of low virulence, including certain strains of staphylococci as well as other organisms (e.g., *Aerobacter* and *Serratia*),

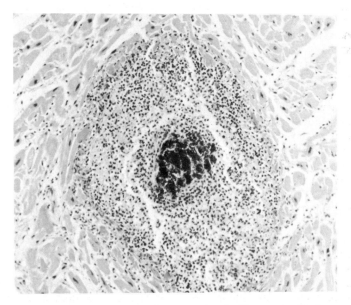

Fig. 6-2. Staphylococcal abscess of myocardium associated with pyemia. Dark mass in center of abscess is clump of staphylococci.

are sometimes associated with an uncommon, frequently fatal syndrome characterized by chronic suppurative and granulomatous (tuberculoid) lesions of the lymph nodes, lungs, liver, bones, and skin. The basic defect in this syndrome is the inability of phagocytes to kill or digest the microorganisms after phagocytosis. When first described, the syndrome was noted only in males as an X-linked recessive disorder. It has since been observed to occur in females, in whom the inheritance has been postulated to be autosomal recessive. It has been suggested that an enzyme deficiency in the phagocytes, which may be different in the two forms of the disease, causes an abnormal intracellular metabolism with decreased production of bactericidal hydrogen peroxide, thus preventing intracellular killing of the bacteria.

STREPTOCOCCAL INFECTION

Streptococci are gram-positive spherical organisms that grow in chains. They are widely distributed and very common bacteria that are associated with a diversity of lesions, including tonsillitis, otitis media, cellulitis, appendicitis, wound infections, puerperal infections, bronchopneumonia, endocarditis, erysipelas, scarlet fever, and certain abscesses.

The hemolytic streptococci, although pyogenic, tend to produce a diffuse and spreading type of inflammation rather than the circumscribed abscesses so characteristic of staphylococci. In addition to their pyogenicity and invasiveness, the hemolytic streptococci may produce an erythrogenic or rash-producing exotoxin. Other streptococcal toxins and enzymes include (1) the hemolysins, streptolysin O and streptolysin S, the former producing antibodies that can be demonstrated in the serum, (2) streptokinase, which activates plasminogen to form the enzyme plasmin (fibrinolysin), which dissolves fibrin, (3) hyaluronidase, (4) proteinase, and (5) a leukocytotoxic enzyme.

The nonsuppurative inflammatory diseases, rheumatic fever and acute diffuse glomerulonephritis, are considered to be complications of infections caused by group A β-hemolytic streptococci, not as infective lesions resulting from invasion by organisms but as poststreptococcal hypersensitivity diseases. It has been observed that acute glomerulonephritis, not rheumatic fever, may follow streptococcal infections of the skin. On the other hand, either rheumatic fever or acute glomerulonephritis may be preceded by streptococcal pharyngitis, with or without scarlet fever.

Wound infection. Invasion of streptococci through any wound of the skin, even a small cut or abrasion, may result in a dangerous infection. The organisms may spread rapidly in subcutaneous tissues, producing a cellulitis, with diffuse suppuration in later stages. Spread is often along the lymphatics, with the formation of reddish streaks (lymphangitis). When reached, the lymphatic glands also become swollen and tender (lymphadenitis). The more virulent infections reach the bloodstream and produce general septicemia. This may be associated with severe symptoms—chills, a high fever, and a rapidly developing hemolytic anemia. Focal pyogenic lesions are not so common with streptococcal septicemia as with staphylococcal pyemia, although the lungs, joints, or heart valves may be affected. Toxic degenerative changes (cloudy swelling and fatty degeneration) are severe in the heart, liver, and kidneys, and the spleen is enlarged and soft and is purplish red on the cut surface (acute splenitis).

Puerperal endometritis and myometritis are particularly dangerous forms of streptococcal wound infection. The raw surfaces of the postpartum uterus facilitate invasion, and rapid spread may occur by infection of lymphatics and blood vessels.

Erysipelas. Erysipelas is a spreading streptococcal infection of the skin. The organisms enter through some minute wound or abrasion. Spread occurs by the lymphatics, which are especially involved. The lesion appears as an elevated reddened area of skin with an irregular advancing margin. The inflammatory reaction in the corium is characterized by neutrophils, lymphocytes, and mononuclear wandering cells. Suppuration is unusual unless deeper parts of the skin and subcutaneous tissues are invaded.

Scarlet fever (scarlatina). Scarlet fever is

caused by a strain of hemolytic streptococci in which production of an erythrogenic or rash-producing exotoxin is a prominent character-istic. The infection is usually local with sore throat accompanied by fever and a widespread skin rash. It sometimes is complicated by glo-merulonephritis or otitis media.

The organism produces a potent exotoxin, which by injection into the skin may be used to demonstrate susceptibility or immunity to the toxin (the Dick test). In susceptible per-sons, a bright red swollen area develops in about 24 hours. If the serum from a scarlet fe-ver convalescent is injected into the skin of a patient suffering from the disease, the rash is blanched in that area because of local neutral-ization of the toxin (Schültz-Charlton phenom-enon).

An inflammatory lesion of the throat is con-stantly present. Occasionally, invasion by the streptococci produces suppurative lesions, but most of the distant manifestations are due to toxin production. The skin rash shows marked vascular dilatation, and in late stages the le-sion is infiltrated by leukocytes. A generalized lymphoid hyperplasia and some degree of acute splenic enlargement are usually present. Cloudy swelling of the heart, liver, and kid-neys accompanies the infection.

Acute glomerulonephritis is a possible com-plication that may develop during convales-cence. The damage is believed to be caused not by the direct effects of the streptococci on the kidneys but appears to be a manifestation of an immunologic reaction.

Streptococcal sore throat. The hemolytic streptococcus is a common cause of sore throat (nasopharyngitis), which sometimes occurs in epidemic form. Direct spread from one person to another is common, but milk-borne epi-demics also have occurred. Possible compli-cations and sequelae include peritonsillar ab-scess, cellulitis (Ludwig's angina), otitis media, sinusitis, septicemia, rheumatic fe-ver, and glomerulonephritis.

Streptococcal bronchopneumonia. The streptococcus is particularly important as a cause of bronchopneumonia complicating other infections, such as epidemic influenza (p. 167).

Streptococcal endocarditis. The hemolytic streptococcus is one of the organisms that may cause acute ulcerative valvular endocarditis. The α-hemolytic streptococcus (*Streptococcus viridans*) is a common cause of the more pro-longed subacute bacterial endocarditis (p. 310).

PNEUMOCOCCAL INFECTION

The principal disease caused by the pneu-mococcus is lobar pneumonia (p. 405). Less commonly, it is the etiologic agent in perito-nitis (in children), endocarditis, and menin-gitis.

MENINGOCOCCAL INFECTION

The meningococci (*Neisseria intracellularis* or *meningitidis*) are gram-negative organisms that are pathogenic for man only. Meningitis is the common manifestation of meningococcal infection, although lesions may also occur in other sites. Meningococcal strains A, B, and C have been the most common cause of epi-demic meningococcal disease, and of these, the group C organisms have been the most fre-quent cause in recent years. Other serogroups of meningococci exist.

The organisms probably enter the body from the nasopharynx, where the local infection may be so mild that the patient is not aware of it. The bacteria invade the bloodstream and lo-calize in the meninges, skin, and sometimes joints, heart, and other tissues. Before locali-zation of the organisms in the tissues, the bac-teria in the blood may be unaccompanied by symptoms or signs (bacteremia), but in some cases generalized clinical manifestations (e.g., fever, chills, malaise) without signs of local inflammation may appear (septicemia).

The meningeal infection produces a purulent exudate, and often there is also some involve-ment of brain tissue (p.759). The septicemic stage presents skin involvement with reddish petechial lesions of the skin that are caused by thrombotic involvement of the capillaries. Septicemia without meningeal involvement is not uncommon. Occasionally, the septicemia is fulminant and overwhelming and may lead to rapid death with peripheral circulatory fail-ure (shock). In some of these cases, there is hemorrhage into the adrenal glands in addition to cutaneous hemorrhages (Waterhouse-Friderichsen syndrome, p. 609). It is to be noted that the Waterhouse-Friderichsen syndrome may be caused by organisms other than the meningococci (e.g., *Haemophilus influenzae*, hemolytic streptococci, and pneumococci).

GONOCOCCAL INFECTION

The gonococcus, described by Neisser in 1879, is a gram-negative pyogenic organism *(Neisseria gonorrhoeae)* characteristically seen in diplococcal form within the cytoplasm of neutrophils. Gonorrhea is a disease of venereal nature, the primary acute infection involving the urethra in the male and the urethra, cervix, and Bartholin's glands in the female. In the acute stage, the inflammation is characterized by congestion, swelling, and a profuse purulent exudate.

Although in many cases the condition rapidly subsides and may completely clear up, there is often spread or development of chronicity. In the male, spread occurs to the posterior urethra, with involvement of the prostate gland, seminal vesicles, and epididymis (p. 378). Spread by the bloodstream may lead to joint involvement (arthritis). Healing may cause damage by fibrosis, which in a joint causes decreased mobility. Fibrosis in the epididymis may result in sterility, and in the urethra it produces stricture and interference with urination. In the female, spread from the cervix results in salpingitis following a transient and mild endometritis (p. 637). Peritonitis of the upper part of the abdomen (perihepatitis) is an occasional complication in young women. In healing, it may lead to thin (''violin string'') adhesions between the liver and abdominal wall. Proctitis, an uncommon lesion, is more prevalent in females than in males. The anorectal region may be involved in women by rectal intercourse or by direct spread from the infectious vaginal discharge, and in men, by rectal intercourse or less likely by rupture of a prostatic or pelvic abscess.

Gonococcal endocarditis may result from spread of the organism via the bloodstream. It is an acute destructive valvular involvement, with very large and friable vegetations. This is an infrequent complication of gonorrhea today.

Gonococcal nonvenereal infection in infancy particularly involves the conjunctiva and vagina. In newborn infants, an acute conjunctivitis may arise from organisms acquired in passage through the birth canal. It produces severe injury of the cornea and blindness, but its occurrence is prevented in most cases by a routine prophylactic instillation of silver solution or penicillin into the conjunctival sac.

Vulvovaginitis caused by the gonococcus occurs in female infants, whereas the more cornified adult vaginal mucosa resists the infection. It is usually due to contact with materials contaminated by gonorrheal pus. The infection usually is mild and complications are uncommon.

PSEUDOMONAS INFECTION

Infections due to *Pseudomonas aeruginosa (Bacillus pyocyaneus)* are usually local and mild. Superficial skin wounds and the lower urinary tract are the most frequent sites. Otitis media or externa and infections of the nasal fossa also may occur. The lesions caused by *Pseudomonas aeruginosa* are characterized by the presence of a blue-green purulent exudate and often by necrosis. More serious lesions include corneal ulcer, pneumonia, pyelonephritis, endocarditis, and meningitis. Necrotic, ulcerative skin lesions (ecthyma gangrenosum) may accompany *Pseudomonas* sepsis. Septicemia is a serious complication that may result in shock and death. *Pseudomonas aeruginosa* infections are particularly prevalent in debilitated patients and in those receiving prolonged antibiotic therapy, which suppresses other bacteria, allowing the resistant *Pseudomonas* organisms to flourish.

Melioidosis is an infectious disease of the tropics caused by *Pseudomonas pseudomallei*. Although it is not commonly seen in the United Staets, the disease occurs in countries (e.g., in Southeast Asia) in which American troops have been stationed and able to contract it. Melioidosis commonly appears as an acute respiratory disease, varying from a mild bronchitis to an overwhelming fatal pneumonia. An acute fulminating form is characterized by severe diarrhea, overwhelming pneumonia, septicemia, and death. A chronic localized form has been described that involves the lungs, lymph nodes, skin, or bone. Suppurative inflammation with abcess formation is common in the acute disease, and tuberculoid granulomas, sometimes with necrosis (suppurative or caseous), are characteristic of the chronic lesions. Chronic cavitary pulmonary lesions, mimicking tuberculosis, have been described.

DIPHTHERIA

Diphtheria is a disease in which the organism forms a characteristic local lesion on the mucosa of the pharynx or upper respiratory passages. Widespread effects are produced by formation of a powerful exotoxin (toxemia) rather than by invasion or by spread of the organisms through the bloodstream. The function of the exotoxin is to inhibit the inflammatory reaction of the tissues, thus enabling the bacteria to become established. If the inflammatory response is inadequate, the bacteria proliferate rapidly, and the toxin produced soon overwhelms the defense mechanism. *Corynebacterium diphtheriae* may be identified in cultures by swabs obtained from involved mucosa and spread on Löffler's medium, The diphtheria virulence test is a method of determining whether a strain of *Corynebacterium diphtheriae* is capable of forming significant quantities of the exotoxin. Diphtheria is most common in children between 2 and 10 years of age, which is the period of greatest susceptibility.

Immunity to diphtheria depends on immunity to the toxin due to the possession of a requisite amount of antitoxin. In the Schick test to determine immunity, a minute amount of toxin is injected intracutaneously. If antitoxin (immunity) is present, no reaction occurs. A positive local reaction of congestion and inflammation, reaching a peak in about 4 days, indicates lack of immunity. Evanescent passive immunity is produced by injection of antitoxin contained in the serum from immunized horses. More lasting (active) immunity results from injection of modified toxin or toxoid.

The local lesion of diphtheria on the mucosa of the pharynx, larynx, trachea, or elsewhere is characterized by formation of a false membrane. This is composed of necrotic surface tissue welded together by fibrin and infiltrated by leukocytes. The term *diphtheritic membrane* frequently is used for such a pseudomembranous layer on a mucosal surface, whether it is caused by *Corynebacterium diphtheriae,* or other bacteria, or by injurious chemicals such as strong acids, alkalies, or heavy metal salts. Marked cervical lymphadenitis with prominent enlargement of the nodes (bull neck) may occur in severe forms of diphtheria.

In the pharynx, the diphtheritic membrane is closely adherent, but in the trachea and bronchi, it is more easily detached and often coughed up in large fragments. The chief danger of the membrane is obstruction of respiratory passages, and asphyxiation is one of the major causes of death in diphtheria. The mechanical obstruction due to the membrane is enhanced by local inflammatory swelling and edema and by laryngeal spasm. Occasionally, the diphtheria organism attacks other mucous membranes, such as those of the nose, conjunctiva, or vagina. Other primary sites of infection may be the umbilical cord *(diphtheria neonatorum),* the genital tract (e.g., in circumcision), and traumatic wounds or burns.

The more distant effects of diphtheria are also serious, and death frequently is due to circulatory failure. This is contributed to by relaxation of blood vessels from loss of vasomotor control as well as by toxic degenerative changes in the myocardium. Myocarditis has been reported in 70% of fatal cases of diphtheria. It may be a late manifestation after apparent improvement. The heart is enlarged, dilated, flabby, and pale. There is a primary toxic degeneration of myocardial fibers that elicits an inflammatory response and culminates in scarring. Bronchopneumonia, due to streptococci or other organisms, is a common complication. Degenerative changes occur in the liver, adrenal glands, and kidneys. In some cases, the kidneys show, in addition, an acute interstitial nephritis (p. 356). Nerve paralyses are common and are due to degenerative changes in nerve fibers. The muscles of the palate and the eyes are most frequently paralyzed.

PERTUSSIS (WHOOPING COUGH)

Whooping cough, caused by *Bordetella pertussis,* is an important infection of early childhood. The major changes occur in the air passages and lungs. Tracheitis, bronchitis, and bronchiolitis with excessive production of thick mucus are the most prominent findings. Emphysema is usually present. Secondary bronchopneumonia is a common complication. The blood count in this disease is rather characteristic. There is leukocytosis, but unlike most acute infections, there is not a neutrophilia but a lymphocytosis (i.e., an increase in the number of circulating lymphocytes).

INTESTINAL INFECTIONS

The intestinal infections are considered in Chapter 20—typhoid fever, p. 543; paratyphoid fever, p. 545; bacillary dysentery, p. 545; cholera, p. 547. Food poisoning caused by infection (botulism, staphylococcal and *Salmonella* infections) is discussed on pp. 130, 123, and 545.

TETANUS

In tetanus, as in diphtheria, there is production of a powerful exotoxin with distant and far-reaching effects, although growth of the bacteria remains localized, with little or no invasion. The organism, *Clostridium tetani,* is anaerobic, rod-shaped, and gram-positive and forms characteristic terminal spores. The spores are very resistant and are common in dust and soil that has been contaminated by excreta. Infection occurs particularly in deep penetrating wounds that are soiled by such dirt and in which growth is promoted by anaerobic conditions and by the presence of injured or dead tissues. The disease also has been known to result from infected burns, ompha-

litis *(tetanus neonatorum),* surgical procedures (contaminated sutures, dressings, and plaster casts), and endometritis (puerperal sepsis or attempted abortions). The incubation period varies from 3 or 4 days to several months. The more severe and serious cases have shorter incubation periods.

The tetanus toxin has a direct effect upon the central nervous system. Whether it is carried there by the bloodstream or by nerve fibers is a matter of debate. Hyperexcitability of the nervous system results, giving rise to muscle spasms and convulsions. The spasms often begin in the masseter muscles; hence, the term *lockjaw.* No specific anatomic changes are usually recognizable in the nervous system or elsewhere by ordinary methods of examination, although chromatolysis of cells of motor nuclei and perivascular demyelination have been described in patients living 3 days or more.

GAS GANGRENE

Gas gangrene is an infection by one or more pathogenic anaerobes of the saccharolytic group of the genus *Clostridium,* i.e., *Clostridium perfringens (welchii), Clostridium novyi (oedematiens), Clostridium septicum, Clostridium histolyticum, Clostridium bifermentans,* and *Clostridium fallax.* Frequently more than one of these species are present in the individual lesions. *Clostridium perfringens* is the most common species recovered from the lesions (80%), followed by *Clostridium novyi* (40%), and *Clostridium septicum* (20%). These organisms, being anaerobic, thrive best in dead tissue and where oxygen tension is low. Hence, this infection is particularly likely to complicate wounds in which there is destruction of tissues, pyogenic infection, absence of free drainage, and some interference with circulation (ischemia). The condition develops in a few hours up to a few days after infection of the wound or dead tissue.

A limb in which the circulation has been cut off may have very massive involvement. In other cases of wound infection, there is an active, spreading involvement of muscle. Gas production makes the tissue crepitant, and bubbles of gas may appear when the tissue is pressed upon. Muscle particularly is involved, the dead muscle appearing brown and opaque. The necrosis appears to be a direct action on the muscle fiber of alpha toxin (lecithinase) in *Clostridium perfringens* infections. This toxin destroys cell membranes and alters vascular permeability. Other toxins and enzymes produced by the organisms enhance their effect (e.g., hyaluronidase, collagenase, leukocidin, deoxyribonuclease, fibrinolysin, and he-

molytic toxins). Later, the skin and other tissues become affected and appear yellowish, greenish, or black and putrefactive. The pigmentation is the result of breakdown of red blood cells in the lesion.

Associated with the necrosis are congestion and edema, a relatively sparse leukocytic infiltration, hemorrhages, and thrombosis of minute vessels. In severe cases, systemic reactions include fever, tachycardia, nausea, vomiting, prostration, and shock. Anemia

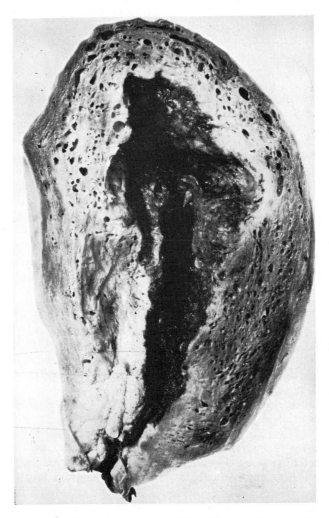

Fig. 6-3. Puerperal endometritis and myometritis *(Clostridium perfringens)*. Note sponginess of myometrium, caused by gas formation.

caused by hemolysis may develop rapidly. In terminal stages, there may be wide dissemination of the organisms. However, in most cases where such widespread involvement of tissues is found at autopsy, the spread has occurred post-mortem. Various internal organs, such as the liver, are found to be spongy and full of gas.

Puerperal infection with *Clostridium perfringens* or related organisms occasionally occurs, the anaerobes gaining a foothold in the necrotic material inevitably left in the uterus after delivery of the child. The wall of the uterus becomes involved (Fig. 6-3), and terminally there may be extensive spread throughout the body.

BOTULISM

The term botulism (L. *botulus*, sausage) came into use because in early times the disease was associated with the ingestion of poorly cooked sausage. Botulism is a form of *toxemia* without actual infection and results from ingestion of food in which *Clostridium botulinum* has grown and produced toxin. In man, the disease is usually caused by toxins, A, B, or E rather than C, D, of F. The effect is chiefly upon the nervous system. The toxin probably interferes with release or production of acetylcholine at synapses and neuromuscular junctions, resulting in muscle paralyses that usually are first manifested as visual disturbances (incoordination of eye muscles, diplopia) and difficulty in swallowing. These may be followed by paralysis of neck muscles and, eventually, of respiratory muscles. Death usually results from respiratory failure or cardiac arrest. At autopsy the pathologic findings are generally nonspecific, but usually hyperemia, minute hemorrhages, and thrombosis of small vessels are evident in the brainstem and meninges.

Recently, botulism has been observed in infants, particularly those between 4 and 26 weeks of age, and is characterized initially by lethargy, weakness, feeding difficulty, and constipation and eventually by respiratory insufficiency. Infant botulism is of particular interest, since the evidence suggests that ingestion of preformed toxin is not the cause of the disease; rather, ingested organisms produce the toxin in the intestinal tract.

ANTHRAX

Anthrax is a septicemic bacterial infection caused by a large, square-ended, gram-positive, encapsulated bacillus *(Bacillus anthracis)* that readily forms highly resistant spores. The disease is enzootic in certain regions among sheep, cattle, and other herbivorous animals. Human infection is mainly among persons who handle the hides or hair of infected animals, and hence the disease is most common among tanners, butchers, brush and hair workers, and woolsorters. In animals infection is by way of the gastrointestinal tract, but in man this is uncommon.

Anthrax in man is commonly an infection of the skin *(malignant pustule)* or of the lungs *(woolsorters' disease)*. The skin lesion is characterized by an acute inflammatory reaction with congestion, abundant edema, hemorrhage, relatively few neutrophils, and infarct-like necrosis of the tissue and is usually accompanied by local acute lymphadenitis. In the respiratory form of the disease a hemorrhagic bronchopneumonia occurs. Septicemic manifestations tend to be more severe in the respiratory form.

PLAGUE

Plague is an acute, highly fatal, infectious disease caused by *Yersinia pestis (Pasteurella pestis),* a gram-negative coccobacillus. It is primarily a disease of rats and other rodents and is transmitted to man by fleas. Cases have occurred in the western United States, where endemic foci of sylvatic plague exist among California ground squirrels. India and China are important endemic centers of plague.

The disease has been classified into bubonic, septicemic, and pneumonic forms, according to whether the lymphatic system, blood, or lungs are involved primarily.

In the bubonic form, following a fleabite or contact with infected material, spread occurs to lymph nodes, usually without development of a lesion at the site of entry, although a small lesion (vesicle, pustule, or ulcer) may appear. The involved lymph nodes (buboes) are necrotic and enlarged by intense congestion and hemorrhagic edema. Areas of suppuration may be associated with the acute necrotizing hemorrhagic inflammation. The tissues surrounding the lymph nodes are involved in the reaction. Septicemic spread may follow, with involvement of many tissues, including the lungs (secondary pneumonic plague). There is a pronounced destructive effect on blood vessels, and marked congestion of all organs and extensive hemorrhagic extravasations are usual. Primary pneumonic plague spreads from person to person by droplets of infected sputum. Bronchioles and alveoli are distended by a hemorrhagic exudate containing little fibrin and many organisms. Necrosis of pulmonary tissue is conspicuous in areas. Primary septicemic plague is probably acquired through mucous membranes of the mouth, throat, and conjunctiva. Localizing lesions are not clinically apparent.

OTHER YERSINIAE

Yersinia pseudotuberculosis and *Y. enterocolitica,* believed to be transmitted to man by means of food contaminated with excreta of infected animals (birds, rodents), may cause acute enterocolitis, mesenteric lymphadenitis with necrosis *(pseudotuberculosis),* and septicemia. The septicemic form resembles typhoid fever and frequently occurs in patients with other serious diseases. Acute mesenteric lymphadenitis, which tends to occur in children, may mimic acute appendicitis.

TULAREMIA

Tularemia is an infectious disease caused by *Francisella tularensis* (formerly *Pasteurella tularensis* or *Bacterium tularensis).* It is characterized by necrosis, with subacute and chronic granulomatous lesions in the lymph nodes, liver (Fig. 6-4), spleen, and lungs. Wild rabbits form a reservoir of the disease, and most human cases result from the handling of infected rabbits. The condition also occurs in ground squirrels, wild rats, and mice. The organisms are transferred among animals by

the wood tick. Although most human infections are caused by the handling of infected carcasses, transfer also may be by the bites of ticks and deerflies. Transmission by ingestion of contaminated food or water is possible.

The clinical types of the disease are as follows:

1 Ulceroglandular, in which a primary lesion forms at the site of inoculation in the skin and is followed by enlargement of regional lymph nodes
2 Oculoglandular, wherein the primary involvement is in the conjunctiva and is followed by lymph node enlargement
3 Typhoid type, in which septicemic manifestations occur while the primary point of inoculation and the lymph node enlargement are not obvious
4 Intestinal form, caused by the ingestion of organisms in contaminated food or water
5 Primary pneumonic form, caused by inhalation of material from cultures or contaminated particles

Septicemia may occur in any of the forms of the disease in addition to the typhoid type. Most cases are of the ulceroglandular type. Specific agglutinins, useful in diagnosis, develop during the second week of the infection. The disease has a mortality of about 4%. A nonfatal attack confers lasting immunity.

In tularemia, there are two effects in human tissues: (1) a necrotizing effect caused by the organism, producing areas of suppuration or caseous necrosis, and (2) a tissue reaction in which monocytes and epithelioid cells predominate. These granulomatous lesions, with or without caseous centers, resemble those of tuberculosis. In early lesions, the necrosis tends to predominate, whereas in old lesions the cellular reaction and fibrosis are more prominent.

The characteristic lesions of focal caseous necrosis and mononuclear cell reaction are found in the lymph nodes draining the primary lesions and also commonly in the spleen (70%), liver (55%), and lung (70%). The pulmonary involvement, which may be primary or, more often, secondary to one of the other forms of the disease, is a nodular or confluent

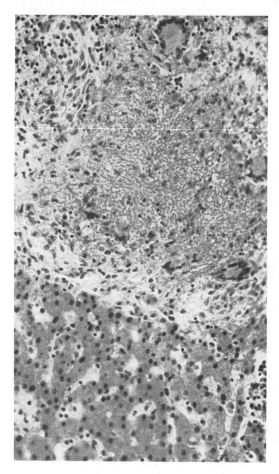

Fig. 6-4. Tularemia. Granulomatous reaction in liver very closely simulates tuberculosis. (From Hopps, H. C.: Bacterial diseases. In Anderson, W. A. D., editor: Pathology, ed. 6, St. Louis, 1971, The C. V. Mosby Co.)

pneumonia with mononuclear cell exudate and a tendency to caseous necrosis of the exudate and the alveolar walls. In fatal cases, the necrotizing factor in tularemic lesions is particularly prominent, whereas in specimens from nonfatal cases, the epithelioid cell reaction is more striking and there may be multinucleated giant cells of Langhans' type. The organisms are found in the lesions of lower animals but are scarce and usually not demonstrable in human lesions.

UNDULANT FEVER (BRUCELLOSIS)

Undulant fever has become recognized within recent years as a frequent and widespread infectious disease. The *Brucella* organisms causing the disease are of three strains: *Brucella abortus,* the bovine strain from cattle; *Brucella suis,* the porcine strain from swine; and *Brucella melitensis,* the caprine strain from goats. The term *undulant* fever refers to the intermittent febrile periods, which are a common manifestation.

The organisms enter the body through abrasions of the skin and mucous membranes after direct contact with tissues or body fluids of infected animals. Less frequently, they enter through the ingestion of contaminated milk or milk products. Positive diagnosis depends largely on laboratory procedures. The mortality is low, and the lesions found post-mortem have varied from slight reticuloendothelial hyperplasia to granulomatous lesions of the spleen and lymph nodes resembling tuberculosis or sarcoidosis, since the granulomas are usually of the noncaseating type. However, in the more chronic forms of the disease, suppuration and caseation occasionally occur, particularly in *Brucella suis* infections. Endocarditis, meningitis, and arthritis caused by *Brucella abortus* have been reported.

LEGIONNAIRES' DISEASE

A recently recognized disease, characterized by pneumonia, is caused by a gram-negative, rodlike bacterium that has been named *Legionella pneumophila*. The details of this disease will be described later in the section dealing with pneumonias (p. 417).

MYCOPLASMA

Organisms of the genus *Mycoplasma,* or pleuropneumonialike organisms (PPLO), are very small pleomorphic bodies that have no rigid cell wall, such as bacteria do, but they are bounded by a plasma membrane. Their size is quite variable. Although generally they are reported to be 125 to 250 mμ, smaller forms (80 to 100 mμ) and larger forms (400 to

BACTERIAL INFECTIONS **133**

1,000 mμ) have been identified. The mycoplasmas are classifed somewhere between the
large viruses and the bacteria, but they are
distinguished from the rickettsiae. Many instances of what was formerly called "primary
atypical pneumonia" or "viral pneumonia"
have been shown to be caused by *Mycoplasma
pneumoniae* (Eaton's agent). The organism is
probably transmitted by infected respiratory
secretions. An increase in titers of cold agglutinins in the serum is a feature of this disease.
The more specific complement fixation, indirect hemagglutination, and fluorescent antibody tests are more useful diagnostic procedures. Tracheal organ cultures and electron
microscopy have been found to be useful tools
for the study of *Mycoplasma pneumoniae* disease. *Mycoplasma hominis* type 1 has produced exudative pharyngitis in human volunteers under experimental conditions. Its
relationship, and that of other *Mycoplasma* organisms, to naturally occurring pharyngitis is
under investigation. Infections of the genitourinary tract, particularly urethritis and infections of the female genital system, and *Reiter's syndrome* (arthritis, nongonococcal
urethritis, and conjunctivitis) have been attributed to mycoplasmas by some investigators,
including the T-strain mycoplasma *(Urea-
plasma urealyticum)*. Although these organisms have been found in such infections, a
causative relationship has not been definitely
established. Other organisms have also been
identified in nongonococcal urinary tract infections, e.g., chlamydiae.

REFERENCES

Amies, C. R.: J. Pathol. Bacteriol. **67**:25-41, 1954 (diphtheria).
Anderson, D. R., and Barile, M. F.: J. Bacteriol. **90**:180-192, 1965 (structure of *Mycoplasma*).
Anderson, D. R., and Manaker, R. A.: J. Natl. Cancer Inst. **36**:139-154, 1966 (structure of *Mycoplasma*).
Anderson, D. R., et al.: J. Bacteriol. **90**:1387-1404, 1965 (structure of *Mycoplasma*).
Christie, A. B.: Infectious diseases; epidemiology and clinical practice, ed. 2, Edinburgh, 1974, Churchill Livingstone.
Cohen, L. S., et al.: N. Engl. J. Med. **266**:367-372, 1962 (staphylococcal infections).
Collier, A. M., and Clyde, W. A., Jr.: Am. Rev. Res-
pir. Dis. **110**:765-773, 1974 (*Mycoplasma pneumoniae* in experimental and natural disease).
Davis, B. D., et al.: Microbiology, ed. 2, New York, 1973, Harper & Row, Publishers, Inc.
Dobie, R. A., and Tobey, D. N.: J.A.M.A. **242**:2197-2201, 1979 (diphtheria—clinical features).
Dubos, R. J., and Hirsch, J. G.: Bacterial and mycotic infections in man, ed. 4, Philadelphia, 1965, J. B. Lippincott Co.
Feldman, R. A., and Koehler, R. E.: J.A.M.A. **226**:189, 1973 (editorial—tularemia).
Finland, M.: N. Engl. J. Med. **299**:770-771, 1978 (antibiotic-resistant bacteria).
Francis, E., and Callender, G. R.: Arch. Pathol. **3**:577-607, 1927 (tularemia).
Freundt, E. A.: Pathol. Microbiol. **40**:155-187, 1974 (*Mycoplasma* infections).
Good, R. A., et al.: Semin. Hematol. **5**:215-254, 1968 (fatal, chronic, granulomatous disease of childhood).
Hoeprich, P., editor: Infectious diseases; a modern treatise of infectious processes, ed. 2, New York, 1977, Harper & Row, Publishers, Inc.
Holmes, B., et al.: N. Engl. J. Med. **283**:217-221, 1970 (chronic granulomatous disease in females).
Hussey, H. H.: J.A.M.A. **227**:194, 1974 (mycoplasmas in arthritis and urethritis).
Jannini, P. B., et al.: J.A.M.A. **230**:558-561, 1974 (*Pseudomonas* pneumonia).
Jao, R. L., et al.: Arch. Intern. Med. **117**:520-526, 1966 (*Mycoplasma* in respiratory infections).
Jawetz, E., Melnick, J. L., and Adelberg, E. A.: Review of microbiology, ed. 12, Los Altos, Calif., 1976, Lange Medical Publications.
Johnston, R. B., Jr., and Baehner, R. L.: Blood **35**:350-355, 1970 (chronic granulomatous disease).
Kilpatrick, Z. M.: N. Engl. J. Med. **287**:967-969, 1972 (gonorrheal proctitis).
Klock, L. E., et al.: J.A.M.A. **226**:149-152, 1973 (tularemia epidemic).
McCormack, W. M., et al.: Lancet **1**:1182-1185, 1977 (gonococcal infection in women).
Merson, M. H., et al.: J.A.M.A. **229**:1305-1308, 1974 (botulism in the United States).
Mudd, S., editor: Infectious agents and host reactions, Philadelphia, 1970, W. B. Saunders Co.
Mufson, M. A., et al.: J.A.M.A. **192**:1146-1152, 1965 (*Mycoplasma* in pharyngitis).
Murray, H. W., et al.: Am. J. Med. **58**:229-242, 1975 (*Mycoplasma pneumoniae* infections).
Nelson, K. E.: J.A.M.A. **241**:503-504, 1979 (botulism).
Pickett, J., et al.: N. Engl. J. Med. **295**:770-772, 1976 (infant botulism).
Piggott, J. A., and Hochholzer, L.: Arch. Pathol **90**:101-111, 1970 (medioidosis).
Rodriguez, W. J., et al.: J.A.M.A. **242**:1978-1980, 1979 (*Yersinia enterocolitica* enteritis in children).
Simberkoff, M. S.: J.A.M.A. **236**:2522-2524, 1976 (mycoplasmemia in adult males).
Smilack, J. D.: Ann. Intern. Med. **81**:740-743, 1974 (meningococcal infection).

Spink, W. W.: Lancet **2:**161-164, 1964 (brucellosis).

Top, F. H., Sr. and Wehrle, P. F., editors: Communicable and infectious diseases, ed. 8, St. Louis, 1976, The C. V. Mosby Co.

Walker, W. A., and Isselbacher, K. J.: N. Engl. J. Med. **297:**767-773, 1977 (intestinal antibodies).

Weinstein, L.: N. Engl. J. Med. **289:**1293-1296, 1973 (tetanus).

Weinstein, L., and Barza, M. A.: N. Engl. J. Med. **289:**1129-1131, 1973 (gas gangrene).

7

Tuberculosis, leprosy, and sarcoidosis

Tuberculosis

Tuberculosis is still a serious disease and a major cause of death in certain parts of the world, although in other areas, such as the United States, the mortality is steadily declining. In 1900 there were 200 deaths per 100,000 population in the United States, but in 1972 the death rate was estimated to be only 2.1 per 100,000. The high mortality that was associated with infancy and early adult life years ago has been greatly reduced. Today, most of the deaths occur in elderly persons.

The prevalence of tuberculosis also has decreased over the past 50 years, but not at the same rate as the mortality. Despite the decline in the prevalence and mortality of the disease, particularly as a result of better socioeconomic conditions, earlier and more efficient diagnosis, and improvement in therapy, tuberculosis is still a significant health hazard in the United States. Over 40,000 new active cases are reported each year, and well over 300,000 active and inactive cases of tuberculosis are under medical supervision.

The causative organism, *Mycobacterium tuberculosis,* stimulates a specific granulomatous tissue reaction characterized by caseous necrosis, pale mononuclear "epithelioid" cells, and giant cells with multiple peripheral nuclei. Human and bovine strains of the organism are important. Most pulmonary tuberculosis is caused by the human strain, but in

countries in which bovine tuberculosis is common, the bovine strain is quite commonly found in intestinal, bone, and joint tuberculosis in children. Infection with the latter type is spread by milk from infected cows and has become rare in certain countries, such as the United States, because of pasteurization of milk, and eradication of tuberculosis in cattle. Infection with the human strain takes place by means of inhalation directly into the lungs of organisms contained in droplets or dust. In most cases, resistance is sufficient to overcome infection with a small dose of organisms. After this early infection, there is an enhanced sensitivity or allergy to products of the organism, as manifested by a reaction to a tuberculin skin test. The lung is the organ most frequently affected, but the lymph nodes, intestine, kidney, brain, meninges, spleen, and liver also are commonly involved. Spread in the body occurs by direct extension, the lymphatics, the bloodstream, and natural passages such as bronchi.

TUBERCLE BACILLUS

The tubercle bacillus, discovered by Koch in 1882, belongs to the group of mycobacteria. This group of acid-fast bacilli also includes the bacillus of leprosy and certain anonymous or atypical mycobacteria. Human and bovine strains of the tubercle bacillus commonly infect man, but human infection with the avian strain is very rare. The human strain is virulent in man and the guinea pig but much less pathogenic for rabbits. The bovine strain, in addition to infecting cattle, is virulent for the rabbit, guinea pig, and man. The human and bovine strains, although distinguishable by cultural methods, are best differentiated by studying their relative virulence for rabbits.

The tubercle bacillus is a slender rod with a somewhat beaded or granular appearance. It can be stained in smears or tissues by the Ziehl-Neelsen method, which consists of staining by hot basic fuchsin and decolorization by acid. The organisms, being acid fast, retain the dye and are colored red. When the organisms are scanty, a concentration method, using antiformin, may be useful. When the organisms are small in number, staining methods may fail, but inoculation of infected material into a guinea pig will reveal their presence, for this animal will develop characteristic tuberculous lesions within 6 weeks.

Tubercle bacilli do not have exotoxins or endotoxins to account for their effects. However, certain chemical fractions have been isolated from them that, upon injection, cause reproduction of the cellular reactions of tuberculosis. These chemical fractions include lipids, polysaccharides, and proteins. One of the lipids, a phosphatide, is taken up by phagocytic mononuclear cells and converts them into epithelioid cells and derivative giant cells, the characteristic cells of tuberculous lesions. Certain waxes, higher hydroxy acids, are responsible for the acid fastness of the bacilli and, upon injection, induce the formation of multinucleated giant cells. The polysaccharides have a chemotactic effect on neutrophils, causing an accumulation of these cells at the site of injection. The proteins induce a neutrophilic and macrophagic response and stimulate the monocytes to form epithelioid cells and giant cells. Sensitization of the tissues is attributed to this protein fraction.

ROUTES OF INFECTION

The routes of infection of tuberculosis are as follows:

1 Direct infection of the lung by inhalation

of organisms contained in droplets or dust particles is the most important method of infection in man.

2 Infection through the alimentary tract occurs in bovine bacillus infection by the ingestion of contaminated milk. The organisms enter through the mucosa and the lymphoid tissues of the tonsils or pharynx to involve cervical lymph nodes or through the intestine to reach mesenteric lymph nodes. No lesion may be left at the point of entry. In the United States, primary infection by the alimentary tract is rare.

3 Infection through the skin is rare, but it may occur in surgeons and pathologists who handle infected tissues. It usually results in a local lesion rather than in generalized infection.

4 Congenital infection may occur when there are placental lesions, but this is rare and unimportant.

TISSUE REACTIONS

The typical lesion in tuberculosis is a chronic granulomatous inflammation with formation of localized nodules known as tubercles, which consist of aggregates of mononuclear (epithelioid) cells, giant cells, and a border of lymphocytes (Fig. 7-1). Caseation necrosis frequently is present in the centers of the tubercles (Fig. 7-2).

When tubercle bacilli are injected into tissues, there is a prompt outpouring of polymorphonuclear leukocytes. Very rapidly, however, the reaction becomes mononuclear. These cells are phagocytic macrophages, which rapidly engulf the organisms and degenerated neutrophils. The fatty material thus engulfed becomes dispersed in fine particles throughout the cell, giving it a distinctive appearance with resemblance to an epithelial cell. These transformed macrophages are called epithelioid cells. They have large, oval, pale nuclei and abundant pale, eosin-staining cytoplasm and are bound together by irregular branching processes. Cell boundaries are often indistinct, and the appearance is that of a syncytium. Near the central part of the cluster of epithelioid cells there may be one or

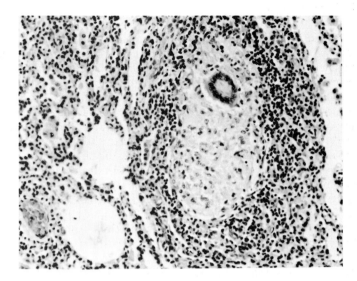

Fig. 7-1. Tubercle in pulmonary tuberculosis, consisting of collection of epithelioid cells, Langhans' giant cell, and lymphocytic infiltration about nodule.

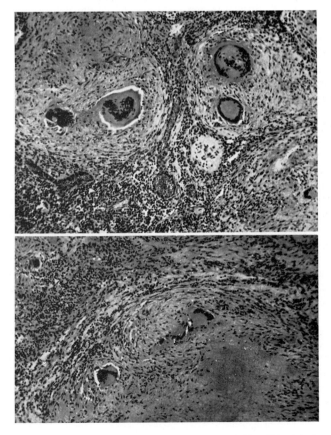

Fig. 7-2. Tuberculosis of lymph node. Note caseation, epithelioid cells, and characteristic multinucleated giant cells.

more giant cells. These are formed by fusion of epithelioid cells or possibly by amitotic division of nuclei without cellular division. The nuclei usually form a ring about the periphery or cluster at one or more poles of the giant cell (Langhans' giant cell), but occasionally they are scattered uniformly throughout the cytoplasm, resembling a foreign body giant cell.

Caseous necrosis develops in the center of the tubercle at about the end of the second week after injection of the tubercle bacilli. The necrosis is probably the result of acquired hypersensitivity to the tuberculoproteins, which can develop in about 10 to 14 days after inoculation of the organisms in a previously uninfected animal. There is a possibility that avascularity of the tubercle contributes to the necrosis. No blood vessels are present within the tubercle itself. The necrotic material is granular and cheesy in its gross appearance, and usually no residual histologic evidence of tissue structure can be seen in it. Lymphocytes border the periphery of the epithelioid cluster and, as the lesion ages, fibrosis develops around the tubercle.

The several elements that compose the tubercle vary quantitatively. When dosage and virulence of the organisms are low and resistance is high, epithelioid cells are predominant, giant cells may be scarce, and there is little or no necrosis. This type of lesion is often termed a "hard tubercle." On the other hand, when the dosage and virulence are high in comparison with resistance, necrosis may predominate and epithelioid cells may be relatively scarce. This lesion is termed a "soft tubercle."

The smallest tubercles are of microscopic size, but their enlargement or fusion produces visible lesions. The smallest of these, about the size of a millet seed, are little grayish areas, 1 or 2 mm in diameter, with or without a minute yellowish point of necrosis in their centers, called "miliary tubercles."

The aforementioned reactions are essentially productive, but in certain situations tuberculous inflammation may be exudative. On serous surfaces such as the peritoneum and in tuberculous pneumonia and tuberculous meningitis, there may be a serofibrinous exudate in addition to tubercle formation. Rare cases of nonreactive (acute caseating) tuberculosis occur and are characterized by necrosis and many organisms but minimal reaction in surrounding tissue. Cortisone administration may cause a similar failure of tissue response.

If the tubercle is very small, healing may result in its disappearance or replacement by a fibrous scar. A considerable amount of caseous material may not be absorbed but becomes calcified by the deposition of calcium salts. This tendency to calcification is comparable to calcium deposition in any devitalized tissues in the body (dystrophic calcification) and possibly depends on a localized increased alkalinity of the necrotic material. Although calcified tuberculous lesions ordinarily are considered healed, it is sometimes possible to demonstrate living tubercle bacilli in them. Under certain circumstances, the necrotic material of tubercles can be disposed of by natural passages, e.g., a tubercle in the lung may rupture into a bronchus and the caseous mass be transferred by bronchial passages, leaving a cavity. As a result, progression of the disease may occur throughout the lung, or the infective material may be coughed up and inhaled into the opposite lung or be swallowed into the gastrointestinal tract.

Chemotherapeutic agents may have an effect on the progress of tuberculosis and also may produce a change in the tissue reactions and microscopic appearance. *Streptomycin* promotes healing of surface lesions and liquefaction of the content of tuberculous cavities. In such lesions, the tubercle bacilli may be demonstrable by staining, although they may not grow on culture media or produce disease upon injection into susceptible animals. *Isoniazid* treatment may result in the presence of numerous multinucleated giant cells of foreign body type and of atypical appearance and location. The contents of cavities and caseous nodules tend to become liquefied, with a marked polymorphonuclear leukocytic reaction.

RESISTANCE AND HYPERSENSITIVITY

As with any other infection, the development and course of tuberculosis are dependent on the virulence, dosage, and portal of entry of the organisms. Also important, however, are the variable factors in the host: (1) native and acquired resistance and (2) hypersensitivity.

Differences in native resistance are both racial and individual. Blacks and American Indians are more susceptible than whites, although certain environmental factors probably contribute to the decreased resistance. There is evidence that heredity or genetic factors play a role in individual resistance. Significant environmental factors that tend to decrease native resistance include malnutrition, physical and psychologic stress, fatigue, and certain diseases (e.g., diabetes mellitus and alcoholism). There is a high incidence of tuberculosis in patients with silicosis, but the reason for this is not clear—whether it is related to decreased pulmonary resistance brought about by the injurious effects of silica or to enhancement of growth and virulence of the organisms resulting from a synergism between the silica and tubercle bacilli. Other factors, such as overcrowding and slum conditions, are favorable for exposure to infection.

Age and sex appear to influence susceptibility. Whereas infants, young adults, and elderly persons are susceptible to the disease, children in the age group of 5 to 14 years are more resistant. Today, it appears that tuberculosis in the United States is becoming a disease of older persons, particularly men. Resistance in males and females is similar until puberty, but during the reproductive period the disease is more serious in females. From about 40 years of age on, the mortality is greater in men and increases progressively with advancing age.

The problem of acquired resistance (immunity) and hypersensitivity is a complex one. A certain degree of protective immunity results from a previous infection, but it does not appear to be related to specific circulating antibodies. Although antibodies have been demonstrated in the sera of tuberculous patients, these have not been found to be protective against the bacilli. This acquired immunity appears to be a cellular phenomenon, whereby macrophages proliferate and inhibit further growth of tubercle bacilli. Hypersensitivity to bacterial products also occurs as a result of infection with tubercle bacilli, and it is characterized by an accelerated and intense inflammatory reaction, with tissue destruction and caseous necrosis. Although hypersensitivity develops shortly after the first infection by tubercle bacilli, the reaction tends to be more severe in a host who has previously been infected. However, at the same time that this vehement tissue reaction is taking place, there is an apparent attempt to localize the infection, which is a feature of protective immunity. When this immunity factor is dominant, the proliferative (macrophagic and fibroblastic) response is prominent, and there is a tendency toward healing of the lesions. The hypersensitivity reaction is especially severe in a host with low resistance who is infected by a large dose of virulent organisms. It has been suggested that acquired immunity and hypersensitivity in tuberculosis are different manifestations of the same mechanism, both being mediated by T cells sensitized to the bacterial antigen, although some investigators have expressed the opinion that the two processes are independent, at least partially.

MILIARY TUBERCULOSIS AND SINGLE ORGAN DISEASE

Miliary tuberculosis is the result of widespread dissemination of large numbers of tubercle bacilli by the bloodstream. When the dissemination is massive, myriads of tiny miliary tubercles develop in the lungs, spleen, liver, kidneys, meninges, and other organs. The tubercles are seen as grayish nodules, 1 or 2 mm in diameter, fairly uniform in size, studding the outer and cut surfaces of affected organs. The patient exhibits fever and intense intoxication, and death usually results in a few weeks. Less massive discharge of bacilli into the circulation may give rise to subacute and chronic forms of miliary tuberculosis.

The spread of such large numbers of tubercle bacilli by the blood may be the result of tuberculous infection of a vessel wall from an adjacent lesion (as in the lung or mediastinal lymph node), followed by rupture of an intimal tuberculous lesion into the lumen. Occasionally, a lesion of the thoracic duct similarly causes massive vascular spread. Miliary dissemination commonly may be from an extrapulmonary lesion into the draining lymphatic system and, in turn, into the venous system.

Organisms spread in small numbers by the bloodstream may cause a few clinically silent tuberculous lesions, particularly in the spleen, liver, or kidney. Many such lesions heal and are seen as rounded, grayish white, fibrous or calcified nodules a few millimeters in diameter. Sometimes, a few bacilli in the circulation may result in progressive disease in only a single tissue or organ, accounting for the extrapulmonary clinical form known as "single organ," "isolated organ," or "local metastatic" tuberculosis, as in bone, kidney, adrenal gland, fallopian tube, or epididymis. This type of disease may be clinically manifest while the initial (e.g., pulmonary) lesion from which it arose is still active or, frequently, does not become apparent until years after the initial lesion has healed. Prior to the days of effective chemotherapy, these localized extrapulmonary lesions were treated principally by surgery and often were referred to as "surgical tuberculosis."

PULMONARY TUBERCULOSIS

The first infection with tubercle bacilli is referred to as *primary tuberculosis*. Although the primary lesion in man may occur in the tonsils, intestine, or skin, the usual site is in the lungs. *Reinfection tuberculosis* is the type that one sees in an individual who has had infection in the past. It is not settled, however, whether the "reinfection" is exogenous or endogenous (i.e., reactivation of a latent tuberculous focus).

Primary tuberculosis. The primary type of pulmonary tuberculosis, particularly as it ap-

pears in infants and children, is characterized by the development of a small peripheral or subpleural tubercle (sometimes multiple). Although the lesion may develop in any portion of any lobe, it is found most frequently in the lower or middle part of the lung, rarely at the apex.

This tuberculous lesion was minutely studied by Ghon and is frequently termed the *Ghon tubercle*. It develops to a size of 1 to 3 cm, and spread from it occurs by the lymphatics to the mediastinal lymph nodes, which become greatly enlarged and caseous (Fig. 7-3). The combination of the peripheral lung lesion and enlargement of the tracheobronchial lymph nodes is characteristic, and the two lesions together are called the *primary* (or *Ghon*) *complex*. Progression by direct extension or by bronchial, lymphatic, or bloodstream dissemination may occur, but in most cases there is healing by resolution, fibrosis, or calcification. Careful search frequently reveals healed remnants of primary tuberculous infection in adult lungs.

In the few patients who develop progressive disease, direct extension of the pulmonary lesion and bronchial dissemination to other parts of the lung occur. Involvement of the bronchi, with subsequent rupture of lesions into the lumen, results either from the pulmonary lesion itself or from an adjacent caseous lymph node. Small and large areas of tuberculous bronchopneumonia are scattered throughout the lung. When a significant degree of immunity exists, the lesions are likely to be of a proliferative nature. In a poorly resistant patient, however, especially when a large number of bacilli have been disseminated and tissue hypersensitivity has developed, an extensive pneumonia with exudation and severe caseation necrosis may be produced ("caseous pneumonia"). Cavitation, which occasionally occurs in the progressive lesions, is not so striking a feature as it is in reinfection tuberculosis. Other possible complications of bronchial spread may result from the coughing up of infected material and from initiation of lesions in the opposite lung, larynx, and intestines.

Lymphohematogenous spread may lead to

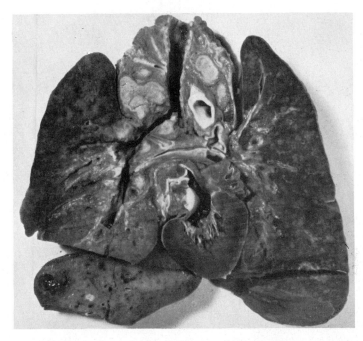

Fig. 7-3. Primary tuberculosis. Large caseous masses in mediastinal lymph nodes.

generalized miliary tuberculosis or to local-ized, progressive disease in a single site (i.e., single, or isolated, organ tuberculosis).

The pattern of primary pulmonary tubercu-losis just described has been referred to com-monly as "childhood type." Although it is true that this is the usual manifestation of the dis-ease in children and infants, it also may ap-pear in adolescents and adults not previously infected, particularly in black adults and oth-ers with lowered resistance to tuberculous in-fection. However, many white adults, in whom there is no evidence of previous infec-tion, do not develop the "childhood" type of tuberculosis. Instead, the apparent first infec-tion in these adults produces anatomic features that resemble more closely the "reinfection" type of tuberculosis.

Reinfection tuberculosis. Reinfection tu-berculosis, also referred to as "adult," "post-primary," or "secondary" type, is the type most commonly seen in adults, although it may appear in adolescents. The patient has had

a previous infection, which might have been detected by a positive tuberculin skin test but which otherwise usually remained clinically unnoticed. The interval between the primary infection and reinfection tuberculosis is vari-able, often many years. A debated problem is whether reinfection tuberculosis represents a fresh infection from without or a lighting up or reinvasion from a partially healed earlier le-sion in which tubercle bacilli have remained viable. There is no doubt that both types can and do occur, and it is generally considered that exogenous reinfection is the more frequent process in older adults, whereas endogenous reactivation is the more common mechanism in younger patients.

In adult pulmonary tuberculosis, there is a very constant localization of lesions in the up-per part of the lung (apical region). The reason for this has never been adequately explained.

A localized pneumonic focus consisting of exudative and proliferative features, usually with some caseation, develops in the subapi-

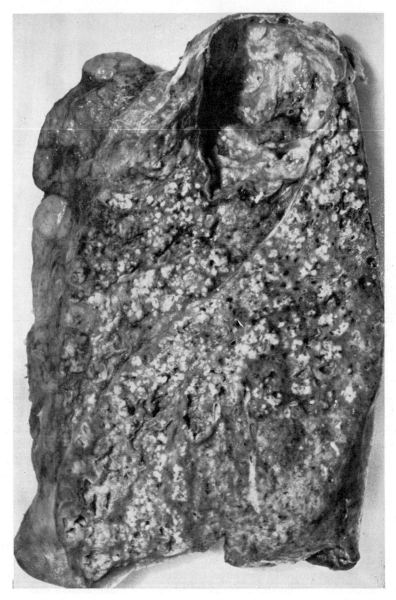

Fig. 7-4. Pulmonary tuberculosis. Note large cavity at apex and metastasis throughout rest of lung.

cal portion of the lung. If the infection is overcome, healing occurs with fibrosis, leaving a depressed fibrous scar at or near the apex. The scar is often blackened by coal dust pigment and occasionally is ossified. Such scars are very commonly found at autopsy. It is to be noted that other diseases also may produce apical scars (e.g., localized silicotic lesions and histoplasmosis). The regional lymph nodes usually are normal or involved only slightly in

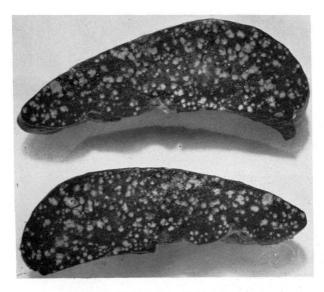

Fig. 7-5. Miliary tuberculosis of spleen.

the healed cases of reinfection tuberculosis.

If the lesion progresses, the tubercles coalesce to form a nodular expanding mass with more extensive caseation necrosis. Healing and fibrosis about the margins result in a fibrocaseous lesion that, in some cases, is well walled off and may be stationary. If healing is less complete, irregular extensions into the adjacent lung tissue occur. When a bronchial wall becomes involved in such extension, the caseous material is discharged and coughed up, leaving a cavity in the lung (Fig. 7-4). Such cavities may be as large as 4 or 5 cm and may have thickened fibrocaseous walls and rough irregular linings. Severe hemorrhage may occur into a cavity, but hemorrhage is usually slight or entirely lacking as a result of the narrowing of the lumen of involved vessels by intimal thickening (endarteritis obliterans) and thrombosis. The thickened vessels are sometimes seen as firm cords traversing the cavity.

Spread to uninvolved portions of the lung from the active apical lesion may occur as a result of bronchial dissemination of the organisms (Fig. 7-4). Isolated tuberculous nodules may appear, and, in places, the tubercles coalesce, replacing large areas of parenchyma. Some of the foci undergo caseation necrosis and are surrounded by fibrous tissue (fibrocaseous tuberculosis). Multiple cavities are likely to form in the involved areas. In addition to the role they play in cavitation, the bronchi may be involved by mucosal tuberculous lesions (endobronchial tuberculosis), strictures, and dilatation (bronchiectasis). Patches of pulmonary collapse usually are present. Fibrosis of the lung may be severe enough in some cases to produce pulmonary hypertension and cor pulmonale. With progressive disease of the lungs, the pleura is commonly affected (pleural effusions, fibrinous pleuritis, tuberculous empyema, or fibrosis with partial or complete obliteration of the pleural cavity). Foci of tuberculosis, with little or no caseation necrosis, may be present in the regional lymph nodes. Lesions in the opposite lung, the larynx, or the intestines may result from bronchial spread of the infection.

Hematogenous dissemination may lead to miliary tuberculosis in many organs, including the lungs (Figs. 7-5 and 7-6), or to localized progressive disease in a single tissue or organ (isolated organ tuberculosis).

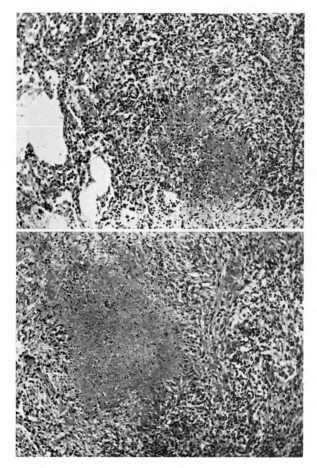

Fig. 7-6. Miliary tubercles in lung. Note focal areas of caseous necrosis, about which there is relatively little epithelioid cell formation.

When a large number of bacilli are spread by way of the bronchi, in the presence of a high degree of hypersensitivity and relatively low resistance, a caseous tuberculous pneumonia develops and progresses rapidly to a fatal ending (galloping consumption). With such an event, the involved portions of the lung are grayish white or yellowish white, consolidated, and airless. Microscopically, there is a massive caseation, the alveoli being filled with necrotic material. There is some protein-containing exudate, and few epithelioid or giant cells are formed.

Healing of tuberculous cavities of the lung is most commonly by inspissated caseous contents filling the lumen and becoming surrounded by contracted scar tissue. The bronchi entering the area become narrowed and finally have their lumina occluded. Rarely, there may be healing by scar tissue with no caseous remnants remaining, or there may be "open healing," the cavity remaining open and in communication with bronchi, the fibrous wall tending to develop an epithelial lining. There is evidence that streptomycin therapy promotes regression and healing of tuberculous lesions,

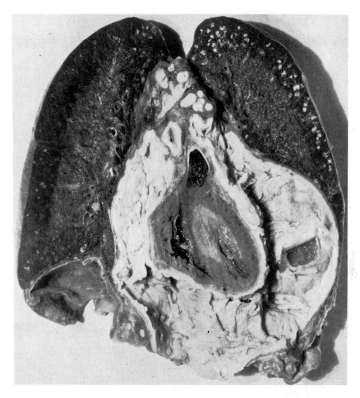

Fig. 7-7. Tuberculous pericarditis. Note tremendous thickening of pericardium, caseation of mediastinal lymph nodes, and tubercles in lungs.

particularly those that are recent and predominantly exudative.

EXTRAPULMONARY TUBERCULOSIS

Tuberculous pericarditis. Tuberculous involvement in the pericardium is usually an extension from the lungs or mediastinal lymph nodes. It is characterized by extreme thickening of visceral and parietal layers because of the tuberculous lesions, frequently with much caseation necrosis (Fig. 7-7), and because of organizing fibrinous exudate (p. 303).

Intestinal tuberculosis. Intestinal tuberculosis usually is a complication of pulmonary tuberculosis resulting from the swallowing of infected sputum. Only rarely does it occur in this country as a primary disease caused by the ingestion of bacilli in milk from infected cows. It begins in lymphoid tissue of the ileum or cecum and results in ulcers whose long axes run transversely (Fig. 7-8 and p. 547).

Tuberculous peritonitis. Peritoneal tuberculosis may be localized around an infected mesenteric node, fallopian tube, or other visceral lesion. A general form also occurs in which both visceral and parietal peritoneum become studded with tiny tubercles. There may be abundant peritoneal exudate (wet form) or a fibrinous exudate causing marked adhesions of viscera (dry or plastic form) (p. 572).

Tuberculosis of larynx. The larynx most often becomes infected by sputum from pulmonary lesions. Ulceration is usual, and there may be considerable destruction or fibrosis.

Tuberculosis of kidney. The kidney is usu-

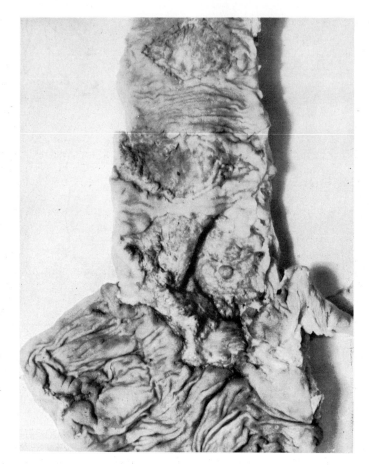

Fig. 7-8. Tuberculous enteritis, terminal ileum. Note oval ulcers that tend to encircle bowel.

ally involved in generalized miliary tuberculosis. Hematogenous spread of tubercle bacilli also causes isolated organ tuberculosis, resulting in a chronic ulcerative type of tuberculous pyonephrosis (p. 360).

Tuberculosis of ureter and bladder. Tuberculosis of the ureter and bladder is usually secondary to involvement of the kidney. In the bladder, it is most prominent around ureteral openings. Cystitis often gives the first evidence of renal infection.

Tuberculosis of male genitalia. Tuberculosis of the male genital organs occurs most often by hematogenous spread. The epididymis, seminal vesicles, and prostate gland are infected often, but the testis is less commonly affected, with involvement usually secondary to the lesion in the epididymis. Another possible source of infection of the prostate is infected urine from a tuberculous kidney, and the prostate disease, in turn, may extend to the seminal vesicles and epididymis.

Tuberculosis of female genitalia. Of the female genitalia, the fallopian tubes are most commonly involved, and from them the infection may spread to the endometrium or to the peritoneal cavity (p. 638). Infection of the tubes is by way of the bloodstream.

Tuberculous meningitis. Except when occurring as part of a miliary tuberculosis, meningeal infection is usually a spread from a caseous focus in the brain substance or choroid plexus. An abundant translucent exudate covers basal portions of the brain. The exudate is less noticeable over the convexities of the brain. Minute tubercles may be seen along the course of blood vessels and are frequently obvious on the margins of the Sylvian fissure. In the nervous tissue itself, localized tumorlike tuberculous lesions (tuberculomas) may develop to considerable size (p. 761).

Tuberculosis of bones and joints. Children are particularly susceptible to tuberculosis of the bones and joints, which is sometimes caused by bovine infection. Spongy bone especially is attacked. Tuberculosis of the vertebral bodies (Pott's disease) may cause deformities such as kyphosis (p. 710).

Tuberculosis of skin. There are several types of tuberculous skin lesions, of which *lupus vulgaris* is most common. *Tuberculides* are skin lesions that histologically resemble tuberculosis but in which the organisms are rarely demonstrable.

ATYPICAL MYCOBACTERIOSIS

In recent years, there has been a growing awareness of a group of mycobacteria that resemble but differ from *Mycobacterium tuberculosis* in several respects and are known as the "atypical," "anonymous," or "unclassified" mycobacteria. Many of these organisms produce colonial pigmentation, and all of them are nonpathogenic for guinea pigs. They include Group I, photochromogens (e.g., *Mycobacterium kansasii,* "yellow bacillus"); Group II, scotochromogens (e.g., *Mycobacterium scrofulaceum,* "orange bacillus"); Group III, nonphotochromogens .(e.g., "Battey bacillus"); and Group IV, rapid growers (e.g., *Mycobacterium fortuitum*).

The disease caused in man by these organisms (atypical mycobacteriosis) may be localized or disseminated. The mode of transmission of the infection is not known, and evidence of man-to-man transmission is lacking. The localized form is most common in the lungs, particularly in middle-aged persons, and in the cervical lymph nodes of children.

Rarely, the bones and joints may be affected. Athough any of the atypical mycobacteria may be identified with pulmonary disease, one of the photochromogens or the nonphotochromogens is usually the responsible agent. Most of the cases of cervical lymphadenopathy attributed to atypical mycobacteria (in the United States) are caused by the scotochromogens. The microscopic appearance of the local disease is similar to that of tuberculosis. Although there are certain differences, it is generally believed that it is impossible to make a positive differential histopathologic diagnosis between the two. The pulmonary disease simulates tuberculosis clinically and radiologically.

Disseminated atypical mycobacteriosis is rare and fatal, usually occurring in young children debilitated by other diseases or receiving steroid therapy. Lesions occur most frequently in the lymph nodes, reticuloendothelial system, and bones, being characterized by varying degrees of noncaseous necrosis, hypertrophy and hyperplasia of the reticuloendothelial cells, and numerous acid-fast bacilli within and outside histiocytes. Granulomas and caseous necrosis are rarely seen.

Mycobacterium balnei (Mycobacterium marinum) and *Mycobacterium ulcerans,* which are also atypical mycobacteria, cause tuberculoid lesions of the skin without visceral involvement. *Mycobacterium balnei (Mycobacterium marinum)* has been incriminated as a cause of swimming pool granuloma.

Leprosy (Hansen's disease)

The leprosy bacillus *(Mycobacterium leprae),* like the tubercle bacillus, is an acid-fast organism. It does not grow on artificial culture media, but it is able to grow in certain animal tissues. Recently, a disseminated infection resembling lepromatous leprosy has been produced in the nine-banded armadillo following inoculation with leprosy bacilli. The low body temperature of this animal is probably the reason that the bacilli grow well in its tissues.

In man, prolonged contact with an infected person appears to be necessary for transmission of the microorganisms. They may enter the body through the skin or the nasal or oral mucous membrane, but spread by airborne droplets *via* the respiratory tract is also possible. Leprosy most commonly affects the skin, nasal mucosa, and peripheral nerves, although lesions also may be found in the liver, spleen, lymph nodes, testes, and elsewhere. Duration of life with the disease is often 20 years or more, and secondary amyloidosis is common. Renal insufficiency from amyloidosis is a frequent cause of death. Secondary bacterial infections may complicate the disease and cause death. Only the two principal types of leprosy *(lepromatous* and *tuberculoid)* are considered here. The others are the "indeterminate" and "borderline" types.

In the *lepromatous* type, the more progressive form, the skin is most commonly involved, with irregular nodules or elevations and more diffuse infiltrating lesions affecting the face, hands, feet, and, less commonly, the trunk. The resultant thickening and wrinkling of the skin produces a characteristic "leonine facies" (Fig. 7-9). Sections from these nodules show an atrophy and flattening of the epidermis and characteristic changes in the corium. In the latter situation, there occurs a peculiar granulomatous reaction characterized by histiocytes (lepra cells), some of which contain abundant intracytoplasmic lipid. In ordinary sections, the lipid in the cells is dissolved out, and the cells exhibit a pale, vacuolated, and foamy cytoplasm (Virchow's cells). The histiocytes vary in size, occasionally are multinucleated, and contain clusters of the causative bacilli within them (Fig. 7-10). The lepra bacillus multiplies within these cells. Globular masses of the bacteria, within or outside cells, are known as *globi*. Because organisms are abundant in lesions of the skin and nasal mucosa, lepromatous leprosy is the more infectious type. An abundant network of loose connective tissue and blood vessels is present in the lesions.

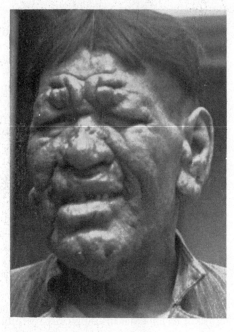

Fig. 7-9. Nodular (lepromatous) leprosy.

In the *tuberculoid* type, the histologic picture closely simulates that of tuberculosis. Noncaseating granulomas are characteristically seen, and organisms are difficult to find or are not demonstrable. Maculopapular lesions of the skin occur, but the considerable nodular thickening is absent.

Peripheral nerve lesions occur in both types of leprosy but are especially prominent in the tuberculoid type. Anesthesias of the skin commonly occur, and subsequently trophic and traumatic lesions develop in the anesthetic areas. Paralyses result in deformities (e.g., claw hands). Neural involvement also leads to gradual atrophy and resorption of bone with resultant shortening of digits.

These two forms of leprosy are regarded as the "polar" types, representing extremes of tissue sensitivity to the mycobacterial antigens. The tissue response in the tuberculoid type appears to limit and overcome the invading organisms, whereas the tissue response in lepromatous leprosy does not limit the growth

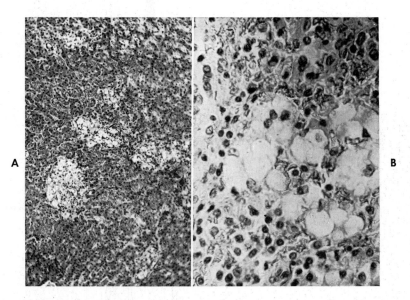

Fig. 7-10. **A,** Lepromatous leprosy. Miliary lepromas in liver, composed of vacuolated histiocytes, often containing lepra bacilli. **B,** Higher magnification of section shown in **A.** (**A,** ×80; **B,** ×360; from Koppisch, E.: Leprosy. In Anderson, W. A. D., editor: Pathology, ed. 4, St. Louis, 1961, The C. V. Mosby Co.)

of the bacilli. Impairment of cell-mediated immune responses has been demonstrated in patients with lepromatous leprosy (p. 84).

Lepra bacilli and tubercle bacilli are distinguished by the following characteristics: the lepra bacilli are numerous in the lesions (at least in the lepromatous type), are intracellular, are arranged in masses or bundles, are straight and plump, and contain coarse granules; the tubercle bacilli are scarce in skin lesions, occur singly or in small groups, and are slender, bent, and finely granular.

Sarcoidosis (Besnier-Boeck-Schaumann disease)

Originally described as sarcomalike nodular lesions of the skin, sarcoidosis is now recognized as a generalized systemic granulomatous disease in which there is most commonly involvement of the lymph nodes, lung, bone marrow (phalanges), spleen, liver, eye, parotid gland, and other organs. The lesions consist of nodular accumulations of epithelioid cells similar in appearance to the epithelioid cells in tuberculosis, with which the condition is most easily confused. Necrosis is absent or minimal, and when present, it is not true caseation necrosis.

The clinical manifestations depend on the organs involved. Most patients are between 20 and 40 years of age and have a benign but sometimes prolonged course. Death from sarcoidosis per se is uncommon. Death usually results from extensive lung involvement with pulmonary insufficiency and cor pulmonale. Occasionally, frank tuberculosis supervenes. The frequency of the disease appears to be greater in the southeastern area than in other parts of the United States, and the incidence is higher in black than in white patients and in women than in men.

Etiology. The etiology of sarcoidosis is unknown. It frequently has been considered an atypical form of tuberculosis, although characteristically it is impossible to demonstrate the tubercle bacillus in the lesion by staining or animal inoculation, and the patients often do not react to tuberculin injection. It may be an exaggerated nonspecific response to a lipid fraction of varied organisms or other irritants.

Some epidemiologic studies have led to the investigation of forest products as possible etiologic factors in sarcoidosis. Pollen from pine (and other gymnosperms) has been shown to contain waxes similar to those of tubercle bacilli and to produce similar epithelioid lesions on injection. Direct evidence of an etiologic retationship is not available. In addition to pine pollen, other agents that have been incriminated in the etiology of sarcoidosis are viruses, acid-fast mycobacteria, and fungi, but a definite association with these agents has not been proved. Among the viruses considered to be responsible is a herpeslike virus (p. 172). Genetic factors have also been considered in view of the observation of familial sarcoidosis involving several families. A common opinion is that an immunologic abnormality, involving sensitivity to a variety of agents, is responsible.

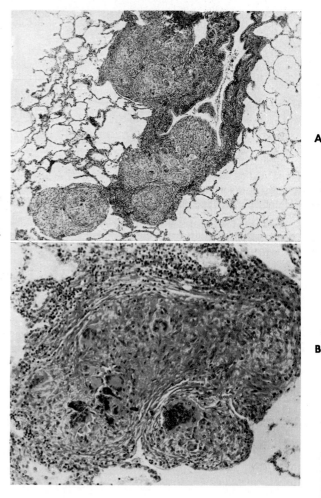

A

B

Fig. 7-11. Sarcoidosis of lung. **A,** Nodular granulomas surround bronchiole and small vein (low magnification). **B,** Giant cells and other cellular components of fused cluster of nodules, shown at higher magnification. (From Gunn, F. D.: Lung. In Anderson, W. A. D., editor: Pathology, ed. 4, St. Louis, 1961, The C. V. Mosby Co.)

Clinical features. The clinical features of sarcoidosis are variable. In addition to the pulmonary manifestations already mentioned, the following features may be present:

1 Lymphadenopathy, involving any group of nodes, especially intrathoracic and cervical

2 Radiolucent lesions in the bones, particularly in the phalanges, as seen by x-ray examination

3 Involvement of the uveal tract in the eye and of the parotid gland (uveoparotid fever, or Heerfordt's syndrome)

4 Skin lesions (papules, nodules, infiltrating plaques, and erythema nodosum)

5 Hepatomegaly caused by lesions in the liver

6 Symptoms resulting from direct myocardial involvement, although less common than cor pulmonale related to lung disease

7 Sometimes, constitutional symptoms with no significant evidence of organ involvement (e.g., fever, weight loss, malaise)

8 An immunologic deficiency characterized by impaired cell-mediated immunity (T cell defect); yet frequently there is evidence of B cell overactivity (e.g., increased serum immunoglobulins)

Structure. The sarcoid lesion consists of dense nodular accumulations of the epithelioid type of large mononuclear cells (Fig. 7-11). Necrosis is absent or minimal, reticulum remains relatively intact throughout the nodule, and giant cells, commonly of the Langhans' type but also of the foreign body type, are usually present. Inclusions, often of stellate (asteroid body), conchoidal (Schaumann body), or irregular bizarre shape, sometimes are seen in the giant cells (Fig. 7-12). Fibrosis develops with aging and healing of the lesions. The Kveim, Nickerson-Kveim, or Kveim-Siltzbach skin test, using a suspension of hu-

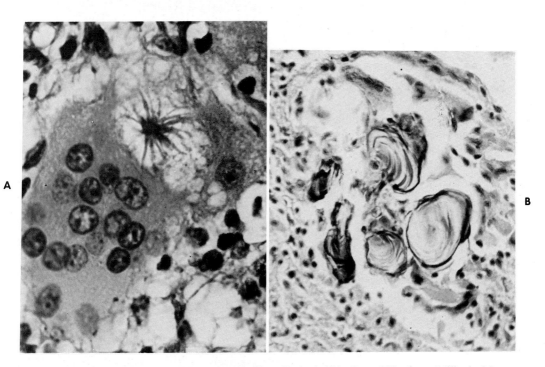

Fig. 7-12. A, Asteroid. **B,** Schaumann bodies. (**A,** ×1,026; **B,** ×390; from Millard, M.: Lung, pleura, and mediastinum. In Anderson, W. A. D., and Kissane, J. M., editors: Pathology, ed. 7, St. Louis, 1977, The C. V. Mosby Co.)

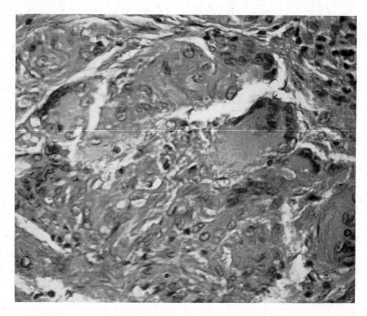

Fig. 7-13. Silica granuloma. Sarcoidlike nodule with multinucleated foreign body giant cells, which occasionally contain small crystalline structures. (From Haukohl, R. S., and Anderson, W. A. D., editors: Pathology seminars, St. Louis, 1955, The C. V. Mosby Co.)

man sarcoidal tissue, is positive when a papule develops, which histologically consists of a sarcoidlike granuloma. This skin reaction is likely to be negative in long-standing inactive disease and in patients without lymph node involvement. It is usually positive in early or active sarcoidosis and particularly when lymphadenopathy is prominent. It has been reported in patients with lymphadenopathy due to diseases other than sarcoidosis. Lesions of berylliosis and the granulomatous reaction to silica crystals simulate those of sarcoidosis (Fig. 7-13).

In summary, the typical (but not pathognomonic) lesions of sarcoidosis resemble those of noncaseating tuberculosis, but without acid-fast bacilli. The occasional report in the literature that describes acid-fast bacilli in "sarcoid" lesions leads to some confusion, since it is generally believed that the inability to demonstrate acid-fast organisms in the lesions is one of the important differences between sarcoidosis and tuberculosis.

Biochemical changes in Boeck's sarcoid include hyperproteinemia, hyperglobulinemia, and elevated serum calcium and blood alkaline phosphatase levels. Hypercalcemia is thought by some investigators to result from increased sensitivity to vitamin D.

REFERENCES

Auerbach, O.: Am. J. Dis. Child. **75:**555-569, 1944 (tuberculosis in children).
Auerbach, O.: Am. J. Pathol. **20:**121-136, 1944 (miliary tuberculosis).
Auerbach, O., and Green, H.: Am. Rev. Tuberc. **42:**707-730, 1940 (healing of tuberculosis cavities).
Binford, C. H.: South. Med. J. **51:**200-207, 1958 (leprosy).
Brown, R. C.: Int. Pathol. **6:**86-92, 1965 (atypical mycobacteria).
Browne, S. G.: Int. J. Lepr. **33**(suppl.):400-403, 1965 (clinical patterns of leprosy).
Chapman, J. S.: The atypical mycobacteria and human mycobacteriosis, New York, 1977, Plenum Medical Book Co.
Clough, P. W.: Ann. Intern. Med. **51:**174-178, 1959 (editorial —Boeck's sarcoid).
Cochrane, R. G., and Davey, T. F., editors: Leprosy in

theory and practice, ed. 2, Bristol, 1964, John Wright & Sons, Ltd.

Cummings, M. M., and Hudgins, P. C.: Am. J. Med. Sci. **236:**311-317, 1958 (sarcoidosis and pine pollen).

Cunningham, J. A.: In Sommers, S. C., editor: Pathology annual, vol. 2, New York, 1967, Appleton-Century-Crofts, p. 31 (sarcoidosis).

Damsker, B., Bottone, E. J., and Schneierson, S. S.: Am. Rev. Respir. Dis. **110:**446-449, 1974 (human infections with *Mycobacterium bovis*).

Davson, J.: J. Pathol. Bacteriol. **49:**483-490, 1939 (pulmonary apical scars).

Doege, T. C.: J.A.M.A. **192:**1045-1048, 1965 (tuberculosis mortality, United States).

Hoeprich, P. D., editor: Infectious diseases, ed. 2, New York, 1977, Harper & Row, Publishers, Inc.

Israel, H. L., and Goldstein, R. A.: N. Engl. J. Med. **284:**345-349, 1971 (Kveim-antigen reaction and lymphadenopathy).

Job, C. K.: Int. J. Lepr. **33**(suppl.):533-541, 1965 (pathology of leprosy).

Kataria, Y. P.: Clinical notes on respiratory diseases. **14**(3):2-6, 10-14, 1975 (sarcoidosis—an overview).

Lefford, M. J.: Am. Rev. Respir. Dis. **111:**243-246, 1975 (delayed hypersensitivity and immunity in tuberculosis).

Middlebrook, G.: In Dubos, R. J., and Hirsch, J. G., editors: Bacterial and mycotic infections of man, ed. 4, Philadelphia, 1965, J. B. Lippincott Co., pp. 490-529 (mycobacteria).

Mitchell, D. N., and Scadding, J. G.: Am. Rev. Respir. Dis. **110:**774-802, 1974 (sarcoidosis).

Monthly vital statistics report: Final mortality statistics, 1972, vol. 23, no. 6, supp. 2, November 6, 1974, U.S. Department of Health, Education, and Welfare, p. 4 (death rate for tuberculosis).

Myers, J. A.: J.A.M.A. **194:**1086-1092, 1965 (natural history of tuberculosis).

Rich, A. R.: The pathogenesis of tuberculosis, Springfield, Ill., 1944, Charles C Thomas, Publisher.

Schepers, G. W. H.: Am. J. Cardiol. **9:**248-276, 1962 (pericarditis).

Selkon, J. B.: Tubercle **50**(suppl.):70-78, 1969 (atypical mycobacteria).

Siltzbach, L. E., editor: Ann. N.Y. Acad. Sci. **278:**1-751, 1976 (Seventh International Conference on Sarcoidosis and Other Granulomatous Disorders).

Storrs, E. E., et al.: Am. J. Pathol. **92:**813-816, 1978 (lepromatous leprosy in armadillos).

Vanek, J., and Schwarz, J.: Am. Rev. Respir. Dis. **101:**430-431, 1970 (sarcoidosis and acid-fast bacilli).

8

Rickettsial, viral, and chlamydial diseases

Rickettsial and viral diseases are considered together because they are closely related biologically. Viruses and rickettsiae, with the exception of *Rickettsia quintana,* are obligate intracellular parasites that multiply only when they are in living cells by utilizing the enzyme systems of these cells. Because of their complex growth requirements, they cannot be cultivated on lifeless media. They may be propagated in living animals, in tissue cultures, or in the cells of the membranes of the developing chick embryo. *Rickettsia quintana,* the cause of trench fever, behaves differently than the other pathogenic rickettsiae in that it multiplies extracellularly and can be cultivated on cell-free media. In contrast to viruses and rickettsiae, bacteria generally are able to live independently, so that they exist and multiply extracellularly within the tissues of a host, and they can be cultivated on cell-free media. There are a few bacteria with partial enzyme deficiencies that often grow within cells, but even these can be grown on special cell-free media (e.g., *Bartonella bacilliformis*).

Rickettsiae are considered to be intermediate between bacteria and viruses in regard to morphologic features and independent metabolic activity, but they are more closely related to bacteria, resembling them in several respects. They are visible by light microscopy (when appropriate stains are used), appearing as small, pleomorphic coccobacillary forms.

Also, like bacteria, they are retained by the Berkefeld filter, reproduce by binary fission, contain both nucleic acids (RNA and DNA), possess certain metabolic enzymes, and are susceptible to antibiotics. However, although they possess a certain degree of independent metabolic activity, they are greatly dependent on the intracellular enzymes of the host for much of their metabolism.

Viruses, on the other hand, are devoid of any enzymes for their own metabolic functions and are totally dependent on the enzymes of the infected cells. A virus, in its simple form, consists of an outer coat of protein and an inner core of nucleic acid—either RNA or DNA, not both. The protein portion is antigenic and is responsible for most of the immunologic reactions induced by viruses. Because of their very small size, viruses can be seen only with the electron microscope, with the exception of some of the large viruses that are just barely visible with the light microscope (e.g., the intracytoplasmic "elementary bodies" of smallpox).

The causative agents of psittacosis, lymphogranuloma venereum, trachoma, inclusion conjunctivitis, and possibly cat-scratch disease were formerly classified as viruses but are now grouped separately, between the rickettsiae and the viruses. These obligate intracellular parasites, sometimes called "pseudoviruses," bear a resemblance to the rickettsiae in size,

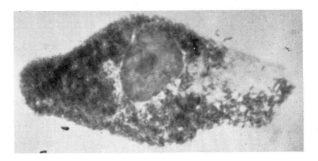

Fig. 8-1. Typhus rickettsiae. Photomicrograph showing serosal cell almost completely filled with *Rickettsia prowazekii*. (Giemsa-stained film preparation from scrotal sac of infected guinea pig; courtesy Dr. H. Pinkerton.)

staining characteristics, reproduction by binary fission, possession of both RNA and DNA, and susceptibility to antibiotics, but they have a more limited capacity for independent metabolic activity. This psittacosis-lymphogranuloma-trachoma group of agents has been named the *bedsoniae* after Bedson, who made the first comprehensive study of the psittacosis agent. They also are referred to as *chlamydiae* (genus *Chlamydia*).

Rickettsial diseases

The rickettsiae, except for *Rickettsia quintana*, lead an intracellular existence in the tissues of many arthropods. These organisms usually do not injure their arthropod hosts and in several instances are transmitted from generation to generation by inclusion in the ova. Of the many rickettsiae inhabiting arthropod tissues, those listed in Table 8-1 are known to be pathogenic for man. *Bartonella bacilliformis*, the cause of Carrión's disease, is not included with the rickettsiae but is closely related to them and will be discussed in this chapter for the sake of convenience.

Clinically, rickettsial diseases are acute fevers, usually with characteristic skin eruptions and with variable mortality in different outbreaks. Clinically variant forms are seen, partly as a result of variation in virulence and partly because of strain modifications from prolonged residence in different arthropod and mammalian hosts. Immunologic studies have shown, however, that all rickettsial diseases known at present fall into one or another of the groups noted in Table 8-1.

Typhus group. Numerically, *epidemic or human typhus* is the most important of the rickettsial diseases. About 15 million cases with over 3 million deaths occurred during and shortly after World War I. In World War II, devastating epidemics did not occur, a fact that probably may be attributed largely to improved delousing methods and prophylactic vaccination. The etiologic agent, *Rickettsia prowazekii* (Fig. 8-1), is carried from man to man by the infected louse, *Pediculus humanus*. The organisms, which multiply in the intestinal lining cells and are present in the feces of the louse, gain entrance to dermal capillaries through the puncture wound made by the louse in feeding.

Brill-Zinsser disease is a recrudescence or relapse of louse-borne (epidemic) typhus many years after a prior attack. It has been suggested that the microorganisms of the previous episode remain dormant and become activated when the host's defenses are diminished for some reason.

Endemic or murine typhus caused by *Rickettsia typhi (mooseri)*, with a reservoir in wild rats, is transmitted to man by the bite of the

Table 8-1. Rickettsial diseases of man

Disease	Etiologic agent	Vector	Distribution
1. Typhus group			
a. Epidemic	*Rickettsia prowazekii*	Human louse	Potentially worldwide
b. Brill-Zinsser disease	*Rickettsia prowazekii*	See text	Potentially worldwide
c. Murine	*Rickettsia typhi*	Rat flea	Worldwide
2. Spotted fever group			
a. Rocky Mountain spotted fever	*Rickettsia rickettsii*	Ticks	North and South America
b. North Asia tick-borne rickettsiosis	*Rickettsia siberica*	Ticks	Asiatic U.S.S.R., Mongolia
c. African tick "typhus"	*Rickettsia conori*	Ticks	Africa, India, Mediterranean area
d. Queensland tick "typhus"	*Rickettsia australis*	Ticks	Queensland, Australia
e. Rickettsialpox	*Rickettsia akari*	Mites	U.S.A., U.S.S.R., Korea
3. Tsutsugamushi disease	*Rickettsia tsutsugamushi*	Mites	South Asia, Western Pacific
4. Q fever	*Coxiella burnetii*	Airborne (ticks)	Worldwide
5. Trench fever	*Rickettsia quintana*	Human louse	Europe, U.S.S.R., Mexico

From Pinkerton, H.: Rickettsial, chlamydial, and viral diseases. In Anderson, W. A. D., and Kissane, J. M., editors: Pathology, ed. 7, St. Louis, 1977, The C. V. Mosby Co.

rat flea. This type is clinically milder, and slight but definite immunologic differences between it and epidemic louse-borne typhus have been demonstrated. Presumably, murine typhus may be transformed into epidemic typhus by repeated louse transfer, but this has not been proved.

The gross pathology of typhus is not impressive. No changes other than splenic enlargment and cloudy swelling of the organs are seen. Microscopically, there is found a generalized proliferative reaction of the endothelium of small blood vessels, often leading to thrombosis and caused by the growth of rickettsiae in the cytoplasm of the endothelial cells. Localized perivascular collections of mononuclear cells (so-called typhus nodules) also are characteristic. Demonstration of the organisms is difficult and requires perfect fixation and staining. Fixation in Regaud's fluid and staining by the Giemsa method are most satisfactory. Lesions are seen most strikingly in the skin, myocardium, and brain. In the myocardium, in addition to the vascular lesions, a diffuse infiltration of mononuclear cells between the muscle fibers is seen, with myocar-

dial fiber degeneration in some instances. In the brain, the characteristic focal lesions center around minute damaged capillaries. Petechial hemorrhages, perivascular cuffing, and glial nodes also are seen, so that the picture resembles that of the various types of viral encephalitis. Interstitial pneumonitis, characterized by the accumulation of mononuclear cells in the alveolar walls, often appears to be part of the picture of uncomplicated typhus.

Clinically, typhus is characterized by headache, mild chills, and fever, which reaches its height at the end of the first week and terminates by rapid lysis, in uncomplicated cases, on the fourteenth to sixteenth day. The characteristic rash appears between the fourth and eighth days. It consists of pink macules and papules 2 to 5 mm in diameter, which later become hemorrhagic because of thrombosis of the skin capillaries. In the second week, delirium, stupor, or even coma may be seen as a result of the encephalitis. Gangrene of the skin from vascular occlusion is occasionally seen. Death may be due to the myocarditis, to the encephalitis, to secondary bronchopneumonia, or to generalized toxemia. There is evidence that a shocklike condition with peripheral circulatory failure, hemoconcentration, and low blood pressure also may be important in many fatal cases. Contributing to the fatal outcome may be impairment of renal function resulting from vascular lesions, interstitial inflammation, and tubular damage in the kidneys.

The natural mortality is 20% to 70% in epidemic typhus and 2% to 3% in murine typhus. It is practically nil in young children and very high in the aged. Antibiotics such as chloramphenicol and the tetracyclines have improved the prognosis greatly.

Spotted fever group. In addition to Rocky Mountain spotted fever of the United States and Brazilian spotted fever (São Paulo typhus), which are essentially the same disease, the spotted fever group of rickettsial diseases includes North Asia tick-borne rickettsiosis, African tick typhus, Queensland tick typhus, and rickettsialpox. The clinical picture of Rocky Mountain spotted fever is similar to that of typhus, but the rash appears earlier (on the second to fifth day), is more hemorrhagic, appears first on the extremities, and involves the palms and soles. Cases have occurred in all sections of the United States. It is endemic in the South Atlantic states, where the largest number of infections are reported. The mortality in Rocky Mountain spotted fever in different localities varied greatly but averaged about 20% before the advent of specific antibiotic therapy. It has decreased since the institution of proper antimicrobial treatment, but deaths still occur and are frequently related to delay in instituting appropriate therapy. In African tick typhus, or fièvre boutonneuse, a local lesion at the portal of entry and regional lymphadenitis are reported.

All of these diseases except rickettsialpox are carried by ticks, and the rickettsiae are found in the cytoplasm and also in compact clusters in the nuclei of the cells of many tissues in ticks, including the salivary glands. Several varieties of ticks and several intermediate mammalian hosts are involved in the epidemiology of different varieties within this group.

Pathologically, the changes in spotted fever (Fig. 8-2) are much like those in typhus. Differential microscopic diagnosis can be made only by an experienced observer. Rickettsiae are found in the smooth muscle cells of arterioles as well as in the endothelial cells, whereas in typhus the organisms are confined to the endothelium. The pathologic physiology and modes of death are those already described for typhus.

Rickettsialpox is carried from the house mouse to man by a mite. The etiologic agent *Rickettsia akari,* localizes in the nuclei of infected yolk sac cells. The rash in this disease passes through a vesicular stage. Little is known of the systemic pathologic changes in man, since the disease has no mortality.

Tsutsugamushi group. The tsutsugamushi group of diseases occurs in Japan, China, Sumatra, Australia, and several other countries and islands along the western Pacific coast. Included in the group is "scrub typhus," which assumed military importance in World War II. The etiologic agent, *Rickettsia tsutsugamushi,* is carried by the larval form of the tropical mite, *Trombicula akamushi.*

Tsutsugamushi disease is an exanthematic febrile illness, often difficult to differentiate clinically from typhus and spotted fever. In most strains, a necrotic lesion occurs at the site of attachment of the vector, together with regional lymphadenitis. The mortality without chemotherapy is high (20% to 60%). The disease has a reservoir in mice and other rodents and is readily transmitted to mice and guinea pigs by the injection of blood from human patients.

The pathologic changes are essentially like those in typhus and spotted fever, with the addition of mild rickettsial peritonitis, pleuritis, and pericarditis. Interstitial pneumonitis (Fig. 8-3), probably of rickettsial origin, usually is found but often is complicated by bacterial bronchopneumonia. The tendency for thrombosis to occur is much less than in typhus and spotted fever, and for this reason the rash does not become hemorrhagic and resembles more the eruption seen in measles. The cerebral and myocardial lesions resemble those of typhus and of spotted fever.

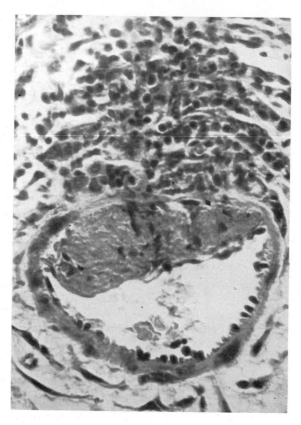

Fig. 8-2. Rocky Mountain spotted fever, showing characteristic vascular lesion. Fibrin thrombus partially occludes lumen of vessel, and there is focal perivascular collection of lymphocytes and macrophages. (Courtesy Dr. H. Pinkerton.)

Q fever. Australian Q fever, described in 1936, is probably identical with American Q fever and "Balkan grippe," which have been discovered more recently. The etiologic agent, *Coxiella (or Rickettsia) burnetii*, has been isolated from ticks in Montana. Unlike other rickettsiae, it passes through porcelain filters. Clinically, there is usually no rash, but an atypical bronchopneumonia, discoverable at times only by x-ray examination, seems to be a constant finding. The mortality is low.

The epidemiology is not yet clear. In Australia and the United States, slaughterhouse and stockyard workers have become infected, either directly or by the inhalation of tick feces. Epidemiologic studies of "Balkan

grippe" suggested the inhalation of dust contaminated by animals rather than person-to-person transfer as the mode of transmission. In fatal cases, the lungs show firm consolidaton and, microscopically, an interstitial pneumonia, with inflammatory cells in the alveolar walls, while the alveolar spaces contain fibrin with only a few mononuclear cells.

Diagnosis. The Weil-Felix reaction, carried out much like the Widal reaction in typhoid, is of value in the diagnosis of typhus, spotted fever, and tsutsugamushi disease. The organisms used are strains of *Proteus* bacilli isolated from patients. Although these organisms are unrelated to the etiologic rickettsiae, agglutination occurs frequently in high titers for some

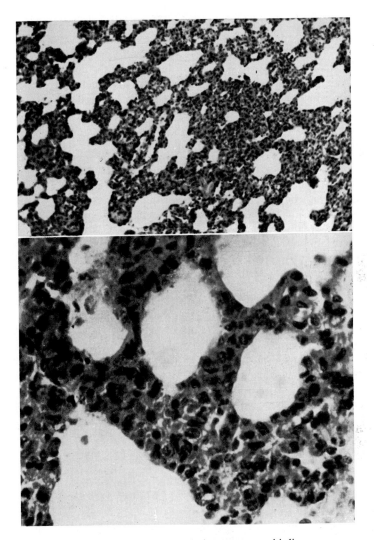

Fig. 8-3. Interstitial pneumonia in tsutsugamushi disease.

unknown reason. In the typhus group, agglutination in high titer with *Proteus* OX19 is characteristically obtained (although it is less often positive in Brill-Zinsser disease), whereas in tsutsugamushi disease, the principal agglutinins are against *Proteus* OXK. In Rocky Mountain spotted fever, agglutinins for OX19 and OX2 are commonly present. Q fever, rickettsialpox, and trench fever are not associated with agglutinins for *Proteus*.

Injection of guinea pigs with blood from suspected cases is often necessary for the accurate diagnosis of sporadic cases of typhus, spotted fever, and Q fever. After the strain has been established in guinea pigs, cross-immunity tests with known strains are carried out. Complement fixation tests also are valuable.

Vaccination. Although the rickettsiae refuse to grow on cell-free bacteriologic media, vaccines of undoubted value have been prepared against typhus, spotted fever, and Q fever. Of the various sources of rickettsiae, the infected yolk sac membrane of the developing chick embryo has proved most suitable for large-scale production of vaccine. The rickettsiae grow freely in the cells lining the yolk sac and are readily freed from their host cells and from the yolk to form the emulsion used for vaccination.

Bartonellosis (Carrión's disease)

Carrión's disease is of considerable importance in Peru, Ecuador, Chile, and Colombia but has not been reported elsewhere. It is caused by a rickettsialike bacterium, *Bartonella bacilliformis,* which is carried by sandflies of the genus *Phlebotomus.* It occurs in two stages: an acute febrile anemia. (Oroya fever) and a nodular cutaneous eruption (verruga peruana). The anemic stage is caused by the growth of the organism in the red blood cells. In severe cases, the red cell count falls rapidly and death occurs in a few days. The cutaneous eruption occurs during convalescence from the anemic stage or may occur in persons who have passed through a mild anemic stage with-

out clinical illness or with only mild illness.

The organism, which grows in special cell-free media, is found in proliferating endothelial cells of the cutaneous lesions as well as in the red blood cells. In fatal cases, not only the red cells but also the reticuloendothelial cells in almost all organs are filled with organisms. Microscopically, the cutaneous lesions resemble rapidly growing hemangioendotheliomas, but eventually they heal without leaving scars. Diagnosis is made by finding the organism in red blood cells in Giemsa-stained blood smears (Fig. 8-4) or by blood culture.

Infections caused by bacteria that parasitize erythrocytes *(hemotropic bacteria),* other than *Bartonella bacilliformis,* have recently been recognized in a few patients in the United States.

Viral diseases

Several of the larger viruses are nearly as large as rickettsiae and some of the smaller bacteria, whereas the smaller viruses approach molecular size (8 mμ). Nucleic acid (RNA or DNA) appears to be the infectious heart of the·

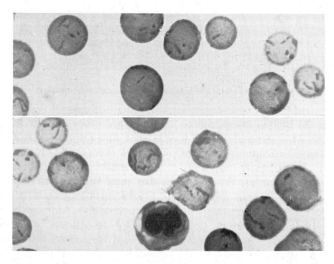

Fig. 8-4. Oroya fever, showing bacillary and coccoid forms of *Bartonella bacilliformis* in erythrocytes. (Giemsa-stained blood film.)

virus particle and is concentrated in the interior, within a protein exterior part. This simple form, however, may be modified in some viruses. The inner core may consist of a nucleoprotein (nucleic acid combined with protein), as in the influenza virus, and the protein coat in more complex animal viruses may be surrounded by an envelope consisting of lipid, protein, and sometimes carbohydrate.

In association with many viral infections, *inclusion bodies* are seen in the infected cells. The bodies occur either in the nucleus or in the cytoplasm. They vary considerably in shape and size but usually are roughly spherical, and their average size is about that of the erythrocyte. They usually are eosinophilic with ordinary staining methods but may be basophilic or amphophilic, and they tend to be surrounded by a clear zone in the nucleoplasm or cytoplasm in which they are embedded.

The inclusion bodies of several of the larger viruses, such as those of smallpox, are clusters of small rickettsialike structures known as *elementary bodies*. Such inclusions are granular in appearance when suitably stained. The inclusion bodies associated with the smaller viruses are homogeneous or coarsely vacuolated. They may be aggregates of elementary bodies, too small to be seen as individuals, or they may arise from the damaged cytoplasm or nucleoplasm of cells. It has been suggested that in the early stages inclusion bodies are basophilic because of the presence of nucleic acid in the viruses, and that in the later stages they become eosinophilic because they lack infectious viruses and represent only the altered site they once occupied.

The important properties of viruses are as follows:

1 Viruses grow only within cells, often only within certain types of cells and in certain species of animals (cell and host specificity). They cannot be cultivated in cell-free media. They can be grown only in media containing living cells or in the membranes of the developing egg embryo.

2 There may be a formation of inclusion bodies (see previous discussion). In many viral diseases, however, these structures are not seen.

3 Many viruses lie dormant in tissues for long periods (latent infection), producing neither symptoms nor lesions. Under certain circumstances, the infection may flare up. Latent infections may be established in utero and may remain so for a long time after birth. It is not certain what causes this latency, but contributing factors may be the presence of antibodies or other viral inhibitors (e.g., *interferon*, a protein produced by viral-infected cells). Interferon is probably produced by all cells of the body but particularly by cells of the reticuloendothelial system and lymphocytes. In addition to viruses, other agents also have been shown to be inducers of interferon. Because of the ability of interferon to inhibit viral multiplication, there is presently interest in trying to produce sufficient amounts of interferon for possible use in the prevention and treatment of viral infections. (See p. 87 for the relationship between interferon and the immune system.)

4 Viruses are sensitive to environmental conditions (e.g., temperature, radiation, nutritional changes), which affect intracellular enzyme functions.

5 Viral infections tend to pave the way for bacterial infection, which is often the true cause of death.

6 Immunity of high degree and long duration characteristically follows viral infections. Exceptions to this are the common cold, influenza, and herpes simplex.

7 Many viruses are transmitted to man by insect vectors.

8 Viral infections, in general, do not respond to usual antibacterial chemotherapeutic agents such as the sulfonamides, chloramphenicol, the tetracyclines, and penicillin. This is probably because of their intracellular location and metabolic dependence on their host cells.

The microscopic changes produced by viral infection are almost as varied as those produced by bacteria, including degeneration and necrosis of cells, inflammatory cell reaction (chiefly mononuclear), fusion giant-cell formation, and hyperplasia. Sometimes cellular inclusion bodies accompany these lesions. Of particular interest is the fact that certain tumors of lower animals are apparently caused by viruses, notably the Rous chicken sarcoma, the Shope rabbit papilloma, leukemia in fowl and mice, and Lucke's carcinoma of the frog kidney. In the last tumor, nuclear inclusions are seen. The possible relationship of viruses to human cancer is discussed on p. 258.

For the isolation of viruses, the intracerebral or intranasal injection of mice and the intranasal injection of ferrets have proved particularly successful, but in certain viral disease the monkey is the only animal that has been successfully infected. The propagation of viruses in tissue cultures and on the chorioallantoic and yolk sac membranes of the chick embryo also has been of great value. In tissue cultures, cytopathogenic agents have been isolated that are not yet associated with specific diseases. Growth of viruses on mammalian cells cultivated in vitro has been an important technique in the recent increase of knowledge of viruses and viral infection.

The inoculation of animals and tissue cultures is a useful diagnostic laboratory procedure for identifying an individual virus as the cause of a disease. The specimen used for inoculation may be blood, cerebrospinal fluid, feces, throat secretion, vesicle fluid, or tissue (e.g., brain). Other diagnostic procedures include demonstration of characteristic intracellular inclusions in tissue specimens or scrapings of cutaneous vesicles, detection of viral antigens in infected tissues by means of fluorescent antibody technique, and detection of a rising antibody titer in the patient's serum during the course of the illness.

The classification of viruses is based on the chemical composition, morphologic features, and antigenicity of the mature virus particle *(virion)*. Generally, two major groups are considered, depending on the nucleic acid content—RNA or DNA viruses. These are further subclassified as to size of the virion, morphologic features of the subunits *(capsomeres)* of the protein coat *(capsid)*, presence or absence of an envelope, and antigenic types. In the following discussion, the viral diseases are grouped according to the system of the body

in which the chief clinical manifestations are seen.

VIRAL DISEASES OF THE CENTRAL NERVOUS SYSTEM

The viral diseases of the central nervous system form a group of great clinical importance. In addition to those in which a viral etiology has been proved by transmission to experimental animals, there are several conditions of probable viral etiology.

Viruses produce a diffuse inflammation of brain or cord substance (encephalitis or myelitis) or cause lesions in both brain and cord (encephalomyelitis). Meningitis is a common accompanying feature and, in some cases, may be the predominant lesion (e.g., lymphocytic choriomeningitis). For the most part, the viruses develop within ganglion cells of the brain and cord and in neuroglial cells. Nervous tissue responds to the necrosis of these cells by an inflammatory reaction, essentially like that in other tissues but with certain special features. Since the lesions produced by different viruses have many histologic features in common, certain general types of lesions may first be described.

Capillary congestion and petechial hemorrhages into the perivascular spaces and surrounding brain substance are often seen in viral infections. Accumulations of lymphocytes and plasma cells around blood vessels (perivascular cuffing) is another common type of lesion. Early degenerative changes in ganglion cells are difficult to recognize, but nuclear degeneration, especially when accompanied by the accumulation of large mononuclear phagocytes around the damaged cells, is clear evidence of cell death. This phenomenon is called *neuronophagia*. The mononuclear phagocytes are derived from the microglial cells, which are believed to be of mesenchymal origin and members of the reticuloendothelial system.

Focal collections of neuroglial cells (glial nodes) appear to be an attempt at repair and correspond to fibroblastic proliferation outside of the nervous system. Swelling, sometimes with proliferation, of capillary endothelium occurs much as it does in inflammatory lesions elsewhere but rarely is accompanied by thrombosis. Focal areas of demyelination and encephalomalacia may be seen, but extensive demyelination is likely to occur only in so-called postinfection encephalomyelitis.

Rabies. Rabies is a viral disease that up until a short time ago has been invariably fatal once clinical symptoms have developed. Recently, a 6-year-old child, bitten by a rabid bat, was reported to have recovered from an illness diagnosed as clinical rabies on the basis of epidemiologic, clinical, and laboratory investigations. Apparently, this is the first documented case of recovery from this disease in man.

Rabies usually is acquired by the bite of a rabid dog, but it also may be transmitted to human beings by the bite of infected bats, wolves, foxes, skunks, squirrels, and other animals. The virus is introduced into the wound with the saliva and travels slowly along the peripheral nerves to reach the brain. The long incubation period in most cases (often several months) allows time for preventive vaccination. When a dog suspected of having rabies has bitten a human being, the dog should be captured alive. If the dog has rabies, the animal will die in a few days, and a positive diagnosis can be made by finding the characteristic intracytoplasmic inclusion bodies (Negri bodies) in the ganglion cells of the brain. Intracranial injection of emulsified dog brain into mice may give a positive diagnosis in some cases in which Negri bodies cannot be found. Staining tissue from the brain or salivary glands of the dog with fluorescent antibody is regarded as a reliable diagnostic technique.

Clinically, the disease is manifested by muscle spasm, excitement, generalized convulsions, and eventual coma. The pathologic lesions are confined to the brain and spinal cord. Grossly, no striking changes are seen. Microscopically, there may be areas of petechial hemorrhage, perivascular accumulations of lymphocytes, and ganglion cell degeneration with the accumulation of phagocytic cells (neuronophagia). In the ganglion cells are found the pathognomonic, eosinophilic, intracytoplasmic Negri bodies. Often, however, the inflammatory reaction is minimal, and the only evidence of the disease is the presence of these Negri bodies. Goodpasture believed that the Negri bodies are composed largely of degeneration products of the neurofibrillae, but others have shown evidence that they are the sites of virus replication. With ordinary staining methods, the Negri bodies appear homogeneous or vacuolated rather than granular. Recently, the diagnosis of rabies in a child bitten by a dog was confirmed by virus isolation and rising antibody titers before the death of the patient, whose clinical course was prolonged by intensive supportive treatment.

Poliomyelitis (infantile paralysis). Poliomyelitis is an acute viral infection in which the most important lesions are those involving the spinal cord. It is primarily a disease of children. The relative immunity of adults is probably the result of mild unrecognized or asymptomatic infections during childhood. During epidemics, which occur in the late summer and fall, many children who do not show paralysis suffer from mild upper respiratory or gastrointestinal symptoms, with or without minor neurologic findings. The virus may be isolated from the throat washings of such children. These mild or abortive cases are much more common than those with frank paralysis and probably play an important part in the epidemiology of the disease. There is some evidence that apparently healthy people may act as carriers of the virus.

Experimentally, the disease may be transmitted to monkeys by intranasal injection of the virus, and some strains have been adapted to mice. The high concentration of the virus in human stools and its isolation from sewage suggest that under natural conditions the gastrointestinal route of infection may be important. It is possible that the virus may also enter the body by way of the oropharynx. The evidence suggests that the bloodstream is the principal route by which the virus reaches the central nervous system. Paralytic disease can be prevented by an antibody barrier in the bloodstream.

The cultivation of the virus in tissue culture has led to the development of a vaccine that has reduced the incidence of paralytic poliomyelitis.

Clinically, the disease is characterized by fever, malaise, headache, vomiting, and occasionally neck rigidity. Spinal fluid examination usually shows 10 to 200 cells per cubic millimeter, with lymphocytes predominating, although neutrophils may be more conspicuous in the early stages. Within 2 or 3 days, flaccid paralysis of the arms and legs commonly occurs. This lower motor neuron type of paralysis is caused by necrosis of the ganglion cells in the anterior horns of the spinal cord. Involvement of the respiratory center leads to sudden death. In certain cases, the brain is involved, giving a clinical picture suggesting encephalitis.

Grossly, the spinal cord and, in the superior type, the brainstem and dentate nucleus may show edema and petechial hemorrhages.

The microscopic lesion consists essentially of degeneration and necrosis of the ganglion cells, followed by inflammation, and usually is best seen in, but not limited to, the anterior horns of the spinal cord. Intranuclear inclusions are said to be present in the ganglion cells in the early stages, but they are difficult to find in human autopsy material. Such inclusions have been demonstrated in experimental infection in monkeys. The various changes occurring in the ganglion cells include swelling and chromatolysis (dissolution of Nissl substance); nuclear alterations such as displacement, loss of staining, fragmentation, pyknosis, and disappearance; and fragmentation and shrinkage of cells. Often, the ganglion cells have largely disappeared. The various types of reaction described earlier (perivascular mononuclear-cell cuffing, petechial hemorrhage, neuronophagia, and glial nodes) are characteristically seen (Fig. 8-5). Neutrophils usually are present in considerable numbers,

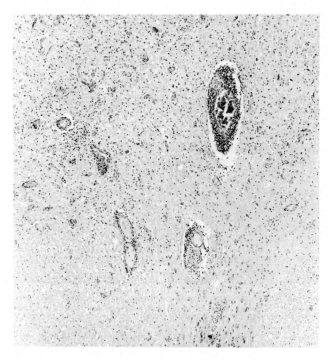

Fig. 8-5. Spinal cord in acute poliomyelitis, showing perivascular accumulation of lymphocytes ("perivascular cuffing"). Lymphocytes are scattered throughout, and ganglion cells are depleted.

often in focal collections, and their presence is important in differentiating the superior type from encephalitis lethargica, since the inflammatory cells are almost all mononuclears in the latter disease. In poliomyelitis, a slight lymphocytic infiltration of the meninges commonly occurs. Also, lesions may be present in the cerebellum and cerebrum. Lesions sometimes seen outside the nervous system include parenchymatous degeneration of the liver and kidneys, myocarditis, slight splenomegaly, and generalized lymphadenopathy (lymphoid hyperplasia).

In unrecovered cases, the paralyzed muscles show atrophy and replacement by fatty tissue and connective tissue.

Encephalitis lethargica. Encephalitis lethargica (epidemic encephalitis, Economo's disease) is a disease of unknown cause that was common after World War I but is now rarely diagnosed. The establishment of the viral origin of St. Louis encephalitis, Japanese B encephalitis, equine encephalomyelitis, and Murray Valley encephalitis, formerly known as Australian X disease, all of which resemble epidemic encephalitis pathologically, is probably the most important reason for believing in the viral nature of epidemic encephalitis. The herpesvirus has been suspected of causing encephalitis lethargica but rarely was recovered by animal inoculation and, on the whole, the evidence was far from conclusive.

The clinical picture was variable and characterized by various combinations of somnolence, excitement, diplopia, and reflex changes. The mortality during the acute stage was 20% to 40%. Lethargy often persisted for many months. Dementia, permanent cranial nerve paralysis, and other neurologic symptoms sometimes occurred. Paralysis agitans (parkinsonism), with slow speech, expressionless face, and pill-rolling tremor, was a common sequela, even when the initial attack was mild. The spinal fluid, in the actue stage of the disease, showed a normal or slightly increased cell count (lymphocytes), and neutrophils were absent.

The gross and microscopic lesions were seen in the cerebral cortex, basal ganglia, midbrain, and pons and, in general, were similar to those of poliomyelitis except for their different distribution, less severe degeneration of ganglion cells, and the absence of neutrophils, already commented on. Perivascular collections of lymphocytes were the most constant and conspicuous microscopic feature. Inclusion bodies have not been described.

St. Louis encephalitis. St. Louis encephalitis shows only minor clinical and pathologic differences from encephalitis lethargica but is readily transmissible to mice by the intracerebral injection of brain tissue from fatal cases. Evidence of mosquito transmission of this type of encephalitis has been obtained. The usual transmission cycle in nature involves birds and mosquitoes, and man is an incidental host when bitten by an infected mosquito. The virus has been recovered from chicken mites.

Lesions are most prominent in the midbrain and brainstem, but they occur to a lesser degree in the cerebral cortex, cerebellum, and spinal cord. Microscopically, they are similar to those of encephalitis lethargica, although meningeal infiltration by lymphocytes tends to be more striking in St. Louis encephalitis. Inclusion bodies have not been demonstrated. Serious sequelae of the type following encephalitis lethargica occur only rarely.

Equine encephalomyelitis. Equine encephalomyelitis is of particular interest as an example of a disease that was thoroughly studied in a lower animal (the horse) before there was reason to suspect its importance in human pathology. Two strains were first recognized in the United States, the eastern and western, which only partially cross-immunize. The disease is immunologically distinct from St. Louis encephalitis and other known types of viral encephalitis.

The pathologic lesions involve the brain and spinal cord and microscopically resemble those of encephalitis lethargica, but neutrophils are more prominent. Inclusion bodies are not seen.

The disease is almost certainly conveyed to man by mosquitoes. The eastern form in man is more severe and has a higher mortality than the western form. Another equine disease,

Venezuelan equine encephalomyelitis, so named because the causative virus was first isolated in Venezuela, is self-limited when it occurs in man and rarely is fatal.

Lymphocytic choriomeningitis. Lymphocytic choriomeningitis is characterized by headache, nausea, vomiting, and rigidity of the neck. In some cases, the clinical picture resembles that of influenza. The disease has a low mortality, and the pathologic picture in man has not been sufficiently studied. In mice and guinea pigs, which are readily infected by the inoculation of spinal fluid from a human case, there is a severe lymphocytic reaction in the meninges, and interstitial pneumonia also is found.

The infection occurs naturally in lower animals, particularly the mouse. Inhalation of dusts contaminated by secretions or excreta of infected mice may be a means of transmission of the disease to man. Spread from animals to man is suggested by appearance of the disease in laboratory personnel following contact with infected animals, including hamsters, and by recent reports of outbreaks of human infection among owners of pet hamsters.

Acute disseminated (postinfectious) encephalomyelitis. Acute disseminated encephalomyelitis occurs after certain infectious diseases (notably measles, mumps, smallpox, and chickenpox) and vaccination for smallpox or rabies. It also occurs spontaneously. Some workers believe that the viruses of the antecedent diseases or those introduced by vaccination are etiologically involved, either directly or by inducing cerebral anoxia. The evidence for this is not conclusive, but in some instances the virus has been isolated from the brain, or inclusion bodies have been demonstrated. The most widely held theory, however, is that an autoimmune mechanism is responsible for the disease (p. 89).

Microscopically, there is some perivascular lymphocytic and other mononuclear cell infiltration, but the essential feature is extensive perivascular demyelination, best demonstrated by a special stain, such as the Weigert stain. This stain colors the normal myelin sheaths black, and areas of demyelination stand out clearly.

Slow-virus infections. In contrast to the more familiar acute viral infections, there are certain diseases of the central nervous system in which the virus remains in the tissues for a long time, even several years, prior to the appearance of clinical manifestations. Because of the long incubation period, these diseases are called "slow-virus infections." They are prolonged degenerative disorders and include *kuru* (a disease among natives of the New Guinea Highlands), *progressive multifocal leukoencephalopathy, subacute sclerosing panencephalitis,* and *Creutzfeldt-Jakob disease.*

There are a number of other diseases in which there is a suspicion of a relationship with slow-virus infections, although further study is necessary to prove such a relationship. Among these diseases are multiple sclerosis, postencephalitic parkinsonism, amyotrophic lateral sclerosis, Schilder's disease, and Altzheimer's presenile dementia.

VIRAL DISEASES OF THE RESPIRATORY SYSTEM

The lung, like the central nervous system, reacts to viral infections in a rather characteristic manner, so that the viral cause of a pulmonary lesion may be strongly suspected from histologic evidence alone. Viral pneumonias are of the interstitial type. Inflammatory cells are largely of the mononuclear variety and accumulate chiefly in the alveolar walls and the peribronchial and septal connective tissue. The alveolar lining cells often undergo cuboidal metaplasia, and mitotic figures are seen in them. The alveoli either remain free from exudate or contain a serous or protein-containing exudate, with only a few inflammatory cells, chiefly mononuclear. Condensation of this exudate by inspired air often forms a hyaline eosinophilic membrane that lines the alveoli. These features, although suggestive, are not pathognomonic of viral infection, since they occur in infections with other intracellular parasites (*Rickettsia* and *Toxoplasma*) and probably in certain bacterial and allergic inflammations of the lung.

The damage inflicted by viruses often makes

the lung susceptible to bacterial invasion. Secondary bacterial pneumonia, with its usual picture of exudation into the air spaces, is often present in fatal cases and may obscure the characteristic picture of the original viral pneumonia. There is evidence, for example, that a preceding infection of the lung with the influenza virus is of etiologic importance in certain epidemics of staphylococcal pneumonia.

Influenza. Numerically, influenza is the most important of the viral diseases. During the pandemic of 1918-1919, it is estimated that 500 million cases occurred, with 15 million deaths. In 1933, Smith and associates reproduced the disease in ferrets by the intranasal injection of filtered washings from the nose and throat of human cases, thus demonstrating the viral nature of the disease. Mice also are susceptible, and the virus may be propagated in the fertile egg. Several antigenically different strains are known. There are three types, A, B, and C, with type A being subdivided into A, A_1, and A_2 (Asian). The A_2 virus was responsible for the 1957-1958 and the 1968-1969 "Hong Kong" pandemics. Variants of this Hong Kong virus have caused recent outbreaks in England, the United States, and elsewhere. In 1974, swine influenza virus was isolated from the lung of a patient who had received chemotherapy for Hodgkin's disease. In 1976, this virus, which is believed to be closely related to the strain that caused the 1918-1919 pandemic, was serologically identified in patients in the New Jersey area. Vaccination against influenza is available but presents some problems because of strain differences resulting from antigenic drifts of the virus and the short duration of immunity.

The influenza viruses have been designated as to type, place of origin, serial number of strain, and year of isolation, e.g., A/England/1/53, A_2/Hong Kong/1/68, and B/Hong Kong/5/72. Recently, a new notation was recommended for the influenza A virus. It is similar to the previous designation but omits the subtype of the strain and describes the character of the antigens hemagglutinin (H) and neuraminidase (N). The hemagglutinin is subdivided into types H0, H1, H2, and H3 and the neuraminidase into types N1 and N2. Examples, of the new designation are A/Hong Kong/1/68 (H3N2), A/Singapore/1/57 (H2N2), and A/Denver/1/57 (H1N1). The swine influenza virus identified in 1976 has been designated A/New Jersey/8/76 (HswiN1).

Clinically, the disease is a respiratory infection with fever, prostration, and muscle pains. Clinical diagnosis is difficult in sporadic mild cases. Reliable laboratory diagnosis can be made by isolating the virus or by demonstrating antibodies in the blood of the patient. The serologic procedures commonly used are the hemagglutination inhibition and complement fixation tests. In its uncomplicated form, the disease lasts for only 2 or 3 days and recovery is rapid. Fatalities are largely caused by bacterial pneumonia resulting from secondary infection with the influenza bacillus, pneumococci, streptococci, staphylococci, and other organisms. The conditions that initiate and terminate epidemics and pandemics are unknown.

Pathologically, influenza is characterized by an acute inflammation of the nasopharynx, trachea, and bronchioles, with congestion, edema, and necrosis and desquamation of the epithelial lining cells. Mucosal epithelial cells may exhibit hyperchromatism and pleomorphism. Metaplasia frequently occurs. Grossly, the lungs most frequently show patchy areas of firm, deep red consolidation, giving the picture of hemorrhagic bronchopneumonia. Occasionally the picture is that of lobar pneumonia. Acute splenitis and other visceral changes characteristic of sepsis are seen. Alveolar emphysema is present in the less involved areas, and severe interstitial emphysema is occasionally seen, even spreading to the subcutaneous tissues in the neck (p. 426).

Microscopically, the picture of viral pneumonia, as just described, is seen only in cases with early fatal termination and usually is obscured by a superimposed purulent bacterial pneumonia. Often, however, the viral type of pneumonia may still be seen in the less involved areas. In the pandemic of 1918-1919, the pneumonic lesions showed a striking tendency to heal by organization rather than by resolution, probably because of severe damage to the alveolar lining cells. Inclusion bodies are not found in association with either human or experimental influenza. However, electron microscopy has revealed aggregates of intranuclear particles and the presence of the same particles in the cytoplasm, the exact nature of which has not been determined.

Common cold. The common cold, sometimes referred to as "acute coryza," is characterized by catarrhal inflammation of the upper respiratory tract, usually confined to the nasopharynx, pharynx, larynx, and trachea. The most important etiologic agents are the rhinoviruses, of which there are more than 75 serotypes. Other agents, which are not exclusively common cold viruses, may cause the symptoms of common colds in some patients. These include parainfluenza viruses, the respiratory syncytial virus, influenza A and B viruses, coxsackievirus A21, adenoviruses, some echoviruses, and *Mycoplasma pneumoniae*. A similarity to influenza is seen in the fact that secondary bacterial invaders are responsible for the formation of mucopurulent exudate and for the distressing symptoms that appear after the first 2 or 3 days. Immunity is of a very transient nature, perhaps partly because of the occurrence of immunologically different strains of virus.

Pathologically, one sees hyperemia and swelling of the involved mucous membranes, with an exudate that is at first serous but rapidly becomes mucopurulent with the advent of secondary bacterial infection. Hyperplasia and increased secretion of the mucous glands may persist for many weeks after recovery. Involvement of the mucosa lining the accessory nasal sinuses may prolong the infection because of the imperfect drainage of these cavities. Pneumonia is of rare occurrence.

Diseases caused by adenoviruses. Adenoviruses cause catarrhal inflammations of the pharynx and eye (pharyngoconjunctival fever, acute febrile pharyngitis, acute follicular conjunctivitis, and epidemic keratoconjunctivitis) and have caused epidemic acute respiratory disease in military recruits. Characteristic intranuclear inclusions have been observed in

the lungs of patients dying from severe adenovirus pneumonia. Adenovirus types 12, 18, and 31 produce undifferentiated sarcoma when inoculated into newborn hamsters.

Viral pneumonias in infants and children. Several types of fatal pneumonia occur in infancy and childhood that have microscopic features that are so distinctive that they suggest the etiologic diagnosis. One of these is *Adams' epidemic pneumonitis of infants,* characterized by interstitial pneumonia, often with syncytial giant cells, and with cytoplasmic inclusions in the epithelium of the bronchi, in lining cells of the alveoli, and in the giant cells. Unlike measles pneumonia, nuclear inclusions are not apparent. The etiologic agent has been identified as the respiratory syncytial (RS) virus, formerly named "chimpanzee coryza agent" because it was first isolated from chimpanzees with coryza. Respiratory syncytial virus infections appear to be uncommon in the neonatal period during the first 4 weeks of life, but a recent outbreak among newborn infants has been reported in which it was noted that the disease was often atypical and overlooked, especially in infants under 3 weeks of age.

In 1939, Goodpasture and associates described a type of infantile pneumonia associated with intranuclear inclusions in the lungs. Today, this is believed to have been *adenovirus pneumonia.* Other distinctive forms of pneumonia in infants and children are *measles giant cell pneumonia* and the pneumonia of *cytomegalic inclusion disease.*

Measles giant cell pneumonia. In 1910, Hecht described a distinctive type of pneumonia of infancy and childhood (Hecht's giant cell pneumonia). It is an interstitial pneumonitis, characterized by large, multinucleated giant cells formed by proliferation and fusion of cells that line alveoli (Fig. 8-6), alveolar ducts, and bronchioles (syncytial giant cells). Intracytoplasmic and intranuclear inclusions also are present. For some years, the etiologic agent was not known. In 1959, Enders and co-workers isolated measles virus at autopsy from materials obtained from patients with typical giant cell pneumonia (see Fig. 15-22).

Cytomegalic inclusion disease. A virus in

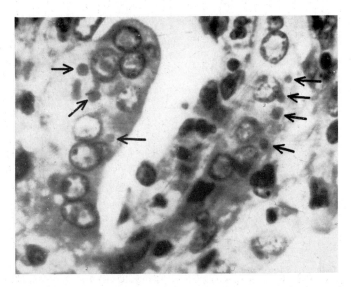

Fig. 8-6. Cytoplasmic inclusion bodies in multinucleated cells lining pulmonary alveoli. Several faintly stained nuclear inclusions are also present (from case of giant cell pneumonia).

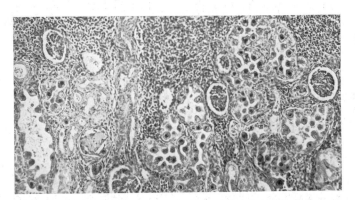

Fig. 8-7. Kidney. Cytomegalic inclusion disease of infancy showing intranuclear inclusion bodies.

the salivary gland that probably infects many persons subclinically may cause an intrauterine infection that produces symptoms in early infancy. In fatal cases, large intranuclear inclusion bodies and occasionally smaller, less conspicuous intracytoplasmic inclusions may be found disseminated in many organs (Figs. 8-7 and 8-8). Interstitial inflammation (e.g., in the lungs and kidneys) is likely to be present, characterized by lymphocytic, plasma cell, and macrophagic infiltration. Intestinal

ulcerations and encephalitis also have been reported. Periventricular calcification in the brain of infants may occur. The characteristic large inclusions also may be found incidentally in the salivary glands or various organs of children or adults who have been ill with other diseases (e.g., leukemia, various malignant tumors, and severe anemias) or as a complication of steroid and antibiotic therapy and the administration of cytotoxic drugs. Obvious clinical evidence of the viral infection in older

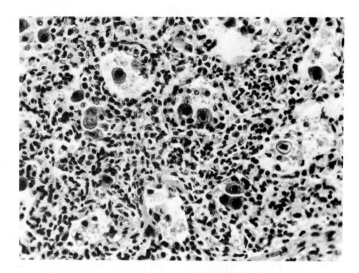

Fig. 8-8. Lung. Intranuclear inclusion bodies in cytomegalic inclusion disease of infancy, associated with interstitial inflammation.

children and adults is not common. The inclusions have been recognized occasionally in renal epithelial cells contained in urinary sediment.

Cytomegalovirus infection is known to develop as a complication of renal, cardiac, or bone marrow transplantation. Although it commonly appears without symptoms in the recipients, serious illness and even death can occur. It may be due to reactivation of a latent endogenous virus, or it may be a primary infection. The source of the latter is likely to be the donor transplant. Some investigators claim that primary cytomegalovirus infections in transplant recipients are more severe than endogenous reinfections. It has been shown that cytomegalovirus causes immunosuppression of humoral and cellular defenses in animals and man. Therefore, when cytomegalovirus infection, particularly the primary form, occurs in transplant recipients, it may further predispose the already immunosuppressed patients to bacterial or fungal infections.

Primary atypical pneumonia. Primary atypical pneumonia is an epidemic disease with very low mortality, occurring chiefly in young adults. It has been of frequent occurrence in army camps. Clinically, it is characterized by coryza, fever, sore throat, headache, and dry cough with little sputum. Leukopenia, rather than the leukocytosis that accompanies bacterial pneumonia, is the rule. Roentgenograms show consolidation of the lung, spreading outward from the hilus.

Grossly, the lungs show patchy, deep red, firm consolidation. Microscopically, the picture is that of an interstitial pneumonia, with accumulation of mononuclear cells in the alveolar walls and peribronchial connective tissue. Cuboidal metaplasia of the alveolar lining cells and hyaline membrane formation are seen in some cases.

The etiology of this condition is not yet clear. The term *virus pneumonia* has been applied to the condition, but *atypical pneumonia* seems preferable at the present time. The relation of the disease to Q fever, to benign histoplasmosis, and to certain mild infections of the psittacosis group requires further study. Some cases are associated with the development of cold agglutinins and infection with *Mycoplasma pneumoniae,* the Eaton agent.

CUTANEOUS VIRAL DISEASES

Smallpox (variola). The etiologic agent of smallpox is characterized by its affinity for the epidermis. Transmission is either by direct contact or by droplet infection from the respiratory tract. The skin lesions begin as papules, which later become vesicles, then pustules, and finally crusts. The lesions may be discrete, confluent, or hemorrhagic, the last type being almost always fatal. Healing with pitting of the skin is characteristic of the confluent form. A mild form of the disease, known as alastrim, or para-smallpox, is also recognized. The historic aspects of vaccination with cowpox (vaccinia) are too well-known to require discussion here.

Clinically, the disease is characterized by severe headaches and high fever. The fever usually subsides with the appearance of the papular skin lesions but returns with the vesicular and pustular stages of the lesions.

The specific changes of smallpox are seen in the epithelial cells of the skin and mucous membranes. Typical eosinophilic inclusion bodies (Guarnieri bodies) are seen in the cytoplasm of these cells. These inclusions, originally believed by Guarnieri to be protozoa, are now known to consist of closely packed elementary bodies, each having a diameter of about 0.2 μ. Intranuclear inclusion bodies occasionally occur. As a result of the presence of the virus, the epithelial cells undergo swelling (ballooning degeneration) and necrosis. Vesiculation and pustule formation occur, but on mucous surfaces the lesions become punched-out ulcers rather than pustules, probably because of the lack of a horny layer.

A fatal outcome may result from secondary bacterial infection in the form of pneumonia, which may lead to septicemia, the etiologic agent being most often a streptococcus or a pneumococcus. It is probable that this bacterial pneumonia is preceded by pneumonia of the viral type. In some instances, however, signs of bacterial infection are not present, and death is believed to be caused by the overwhelming viral infection. Occasionally, acute disseminated encephalitis is a complication.

Chickenpox (varicella). Chickenpox is a mild viral infection of childhood characterized by a typical skin eruption. The disease is acquired either by direct contact or through the upper respiratory tract. The cutaneous lesions are most numerous on the face and trunk but eventually have a generalized distribution, often including the buccal and pharyngeal mucosa. They pass through macular and papular stages and become vesicular, with a surrounding bright red erythematous ring. Eventually, crusts form, beneath which epithelial repair takes place. Fresh crops of lesions appear in the same skin areas on successive days, so that lesions in various stages of development may appear side by side. This is in contrast to the lesions of smallpox, which evolve simultaneously.

Microscopic examination of the lesions shows congestion and edema of the corium, with mononuclear cell infiltration. Vesicles containing fluid are found in the epidermis. Vesicle formation is preceded by ballooning degeneration and disruption of epidermal cells. Some of the affected cells become multinucleated (Tzanck giant cells). Nuclear eosinophilic inclusions are found in many of the epidermal cells, including the multinucleated ones.

The rare fatalities that occur are usually associated with disseminated infection, in which case similar inclusions are found in the viscera. Varicella pneumonia has been described in adults and may be fulminant and fatal. The complication of postinfectious (acute disseminated) encephalomyelitis is a rare occurrence.

Herpes zoster. Herpes zoster (shingles) is characterized by the formation of an erythematous and vesicular eruption along the course of sensory nerves. The lesions occur on the trunk or face and usually are associated with pain, discomfort, fever, and malaise. Involvement of the eye (zoster ophthalmicus) may have serious results unless treated promptly.

The cutaneous vesicular lesions are microscopically similar to those of varicella and also show acidophilic nuclear inclusion bodies. The basic lesion, however, is degeneration in the posterior root ganglia with associated perivascular mononuclear cell infiltration. In the process of healing, portions of the ganglia may be converted into scar tissue. It is generally agreed that varicella and herpes zoster are different manifestations of an infection caused by a single virus known as the varicella-zoster (VZ) virus.

• • •

Patients with malignant lymphomas and leukemias and those receiving immunosuppressive therapy are particularly susceptible to herpes zoster and chickenpox, and under these circumstances the viral diseases are likely to be progressive and attended by serious complications. Also, the patients are more likely to have serious complications after smallpox vaccination. It is probable that disturbed immunity, particularly cellular immunity, is the major factor responsible for the breakdown of the antiviral defense in these situations. A decrease in the level of interferon has been demonstrated in the fluid of chicken pox and herpes zoster vesicles in some cancer patients, suggesting that a depression of interferon formation may be a factor causing decreased resistance to viral infection in these patients.

Herpes simplex. Herpes simplex is the common "cold sore" or "fever blister" that occurs most often on the lips but may involve the mouth (herpetic stomatitis), genital mucosa, conjunctiva, skin of the face, or other regions. It may occur spontaneously but most often appears during the course of some febrile illness. There is reason to believe that the virus often lies dormant in tissues and is stimulated to produce lesions by some unknown mechanism that commonly acts in the presence of fever. The lesions of the skin, mouth, and conjunctiva are commonly caused by the herpes simplex virus type 1. Genital lesions are usually caused by herpesvirus type 2, which differs serologically from type 1. It should be noted that herpes simplex virus (HSV) affecting man is also referred to as *Herpesvirus hominis* (HVH) to distinguish it from the herpesvirus of nonhuman primates.

If fluid from a human vesicular lesion is rubbed into the scarified cornea of a rabbit, a specific viral conjunctivitis is produced. The virus is relatively large and causes granular nuclear inclusion bodies, which usually fill but do not distend the nuclei. Intracranial injection in mice causes an encephalitis that may be serially transmitted. The histologic appearance of this lesion in mice resembles that of encephalitis lethargica. Rare cases of human encephalitis occur that show nuclear inclusions resembling those of cutaneous herpes and in which herpesvirus has been recovered from the brain.

Histologic examination of the cutaneous lesions shows epithelial degeneration and necrosis, with vesicle formation. The vesicles resemble those of varicella microscopically. The nuclear inclusions already described are present in many of the epithelial cells.

It has become clear that "hepatoadrenal necrosis," a fatal infection of newborn infants, is generalized herpes simplex infection ("herpes simplex neonatorum"). Typical inclusions are found in the focal necroses in the liver and adrenal glands. The mothers of the infants usually show mild herpetic lesions of the vagina but are otherwise asymptomatic. Type 2 herpesvirus usually is isolated from lesions of the neonatal disease, which apparently is contracted from the mother's genital herpetic lesions. Disseminated herpesvirus infection occurs rarely in adults and is associated with high mortality. The type 2 virus also is suspected as a possible cause of carcinoma of the cervix uteri.

A herpeslike virus (EBV), first discovered in cell cultures from tissue of a Burkitt's lymphoma, has been linked serologically with several diseases in man, e.g., nasopharyngeal carcinoma, infectious mononucleosis, and sarcoidosis, in addition to Burkitt's tumor. However, except for infectious mononucleosis, it has not been definitely established that this virus is the cause of these diseases.

Measles (rubeola). For years it has been possible to transmit measles only to monkeys but not to other laboratory animals, and for this reason the study of its virus has been difficult. In subsequent investigations, it appears that the measles virus has been adapted to suckling mice and possibly to suckling hamsters. There are morphologic and immunologic similarities between measles in human beings and distemper in animals.

Measles is highly communicable and is spread chiefly by droplet infection through the upper respiratory tract. Clinically it is characterized by fever, cough, coryza, conjunctivitis, and a distinctive type of nonhemorrhagic macular or maculopapular rash that is most severe on the face but involves the entire body. Koplik's spots, which are of early diagnostic significance, occur in the mouth, usually opposite the first molars. They consist of minute white flecks, formed by necrotic epithelial cells and surrounded by a bluish areola, outside of which is a red areola.

The cutaneous lesions show vacuolar degeneration and eventual necrosis of the epithelial cells and considerable perivascular lymphocytic infiltration, with endothelial proliferation in the capillaries, arterioles, and venules. The capillaries are greatly congested and occasionally rupture to form minute areas of hemorrhage in the corium. Koplik's spots show an essentially similar picture. Epidermal syncytial giant cells, as well as intranuclear and intracytoplasmic inclusions in some of these cells, have been demonstrated in the lesions of the skin and oral mucosa (Koplik's spots). By electron microscopy, the inclusions were identified as viral, microtubular aggregates resembling those seen in tissue cultures infected with measles virus.

In fatal cases, death usually is caused by bronchopneumonia. It is difficult to separate the lesions caused by bacterial pneumonia from those produced by the initial viral infection. Most fatalities occur late in the course of the disease, and although the bronchopneumonia seen then is often of the interstitial type, it has no particularly characteristic features. In patients dying early in the course of the illness, a peculiar type of pneumonia with giant cell formation and nuclear and cytoplasmic inclusions has been described (p. 168). In addition to bronchopneumonia, other bacterial infections may complicate measles, especially otitis media. Postinfection encephalitis is a rare and serious complication. Giant cell pneumonia and encephalitis with viral inclusions and multinucleated giant cells in the brain in fatal measles have been noted especially in patients with impaired immunity.

In prodromal measles, large multinucleated cells have been observed in the lymphoid tissue of lymph nodes, tonsils, adenoids, Peyer's patches, and appendix (Fig. 8-9). These cells in lymphoid tissue, believed by some to be formed by fusion of lymphocytes and possibly plasma cells, are known as Warthin-Finkeldey giant cells. Occasionally, the finding of these giant cells in routine examination of surgically removed appendices has enabled the pathologist to make a diagnosis of measles before the appearance of the rash or Koplik's spots. Cytologic examination of nasal smears from children with catarrhal symptoms may enable early diagnosis by recognition of these characteristic giant cells of measles.

German measles (rubella). German measles is a mild exanthem affecting children and young adults. A macular rash develops rapidly on the head and trunk and disappears in a few days. The rubella virus has been isolated and found to be an RNA virus that is distinct from the measles virus.

The most important aspect of this otherwise rather trivial infection is the occurrence of congenital abnormalities in some infants born of mothers who acquired the disease in the early months of pregnancy. The virus may interfere with normal fetal development, the most common defects being microcephaly, deaf-mutism, cardiac abnormalities, cataract, and dental defects. In one carefully conducted prospective study, it was noted that *major* defects occurred in 15% of children of mothers who had rubella during the first 16 weeks of pregnancy and that *minor* abnormalities were seen in an additional 16% of children. The term "rubella syndrome" is used in reference to those infants born with congenital anomalies following intrauterine infection with rubella virus. Other features of this syndrome include thrombocytopenic purpura, icterus, anemia, hepatosplenomegaly, low birth weight, and

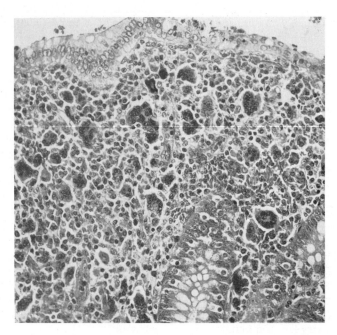

Fig. 8-9. Warthin-Finkeldey giant cells in lymphoid tissue of mucosa of appendix in measles.

radiolucent areas in the metaphyses of long bones.

Molluscum contagiosum. Molluscum contagiosum is a benign skin disease characterized by the occurrence of raised, umbilicated, waxy cutaneous nodules. The lesions may be multiple, in which case the diagnosis usually is made clinically, or single, in which case the lesion may be suspected of being neoplastic and often is excised for diagnosis. The lesions heal spontaneously, usually after a few months, and are not associated with constitutional symptoms.

The prickle cells of the epidermis undergo hyperplasia and degeneration, with the development of rounded hyaline masses (molluscum bodies) in their cytoplasm. These eosinophilic (sometimes basophilic) inclusion bodies, as seen by electron microscopy, are aggregations of the minute elementary bodies of the virus.

MISCELLANEOUS VIRAL INFECTIONS

Mumps. The virus of mumps has an affinity for the salivary glands and the testis (or ovary). The outstanding symptom is painful swelling of the parotid gland. Orchitis is rare before puberty but occurs in about one fifth of the male adults with mumps. The infection may be transmitted serially in monkeys by the injection of saliva directly into Stensen's duct and has been cultivated in embryonated eggs.

Histologically, the parotid gland shows severe congestion and edema, catarrhal inflammation of the excretory duct, degenerative changes in the glandular epithelium, and leukocytic infiltration of the tubules and interstitial tissue. Repair takes place without permanent obstruction of the ducts or formation of scar tissue. In the testis, one finds a similar acute inflammatory reaction, probably dependent on primary injury to the tubular epithelium. Repair may be associated with a reduction in size of the affected testis. Impotence and sterility are rare, since the condition is usually unilateral and even when bilateral, does not often cause enough permanent damage to interfere with normal function. Sterility may occur in bilateral disease if testicular atrophy is severe enough.

Meningoencephalitis may occur during or after parotitis or even in the absence of symptoms of salivary gland disease. Oophoritis, pancreatitis, and subacute thyroiditis are other possible manifestations of mumps. Characteristic inclusion bodies have not been observed in tissues of patients with mumps. Giant cells with eosinophilic cytoplasmic inclusion bodies may form in tissue culture cells infected with mumps virus.

Yellow fever. Yellow fever is a highly fatal, mosquito-borne viral disease of great clinical importance in the tropics, particularly in Africa and South America. The outstanding clinical features are fever, severe jaundice, hematemesis, hemorrhage into the gastrointestinal tract, hematuria, and evidences of severe renal damage, including uremia in fatal cases. Unfortunately, although the control of the mosquito vector, *Aedes aegypti,* has greatly reduced the disease, it has not completely eradicated it, since there is a reservoir in monkeys and perhaps other wild jungle animals from which forest mosquitoes, particularly of the genus *Haemagogus,* may transmit the infection to man. The endemic form of the disease in South America is called "jungle yellow fever." Human vaccination is carried out by injecting virus that has been modified by cultivation in chick embryos (i.e., a live attenuated virus).

Liver disease is the key feature of yellow fever and is manifested by abnormalities of serum bilirubin and a prothrombin deficiency. The degree of prothrombin deficiency and its rate of recovery indicate the extent and duration of the hepatic lesion. A hemorrhagic tendency, caused by the prothrombin deficiency, may result in a secondary lesion of hemoglobinuric nephrosis. Death may result either from severe liver damage or from renal failure.

Postmortem examination shows hemorrhage into the gastrointestinal tract, a yellow liver often mottled with red areas, pale swollen kidneys, and a friable dark red spleen. Microscopically, there is extensive necrosis of liver tissue with fatty infiltration that at first has a midzonal distribution but later becomes more diffuse. The damaged liver cells appear swollen, eosinophilic, and finely granular, with intracytoplasmic hyaline areas (Councilman bodies). Nuclear inclusions, less prominent and less easy to recognize than those of other viral infections, are found occasionally in human liver and almost constantly in fatal yellow fever in the monkey. This type of inclusion ("Torres body") forms a small irregular diffuse eosinophilic mass adjacent to or partially surrounding the nucleolus. The necrosis of liver cells is so extensive that one might expect repair by fibrous tissue, but hepatic cirrhosis as a sequela to yellow fever has not been reported. In the kidneys, severe hemoglobinuric (lower nephron) nephrosis is found. Other lesions that have been described include myocardial degeneration and petechial hemorrhages in the brain as well as on serous surfaces.

Viral hepatitis. There are certain well-known viruses that can produce infection in the liver (e.g., yellow fever virus, cytomegalovirus, herpes simplex virus). The term *viral hepatitis,* however, when not qualified further, usually refers to inflammation of the liver caused by other viruses. Two forms of viral hepatitis that have been recognized for many years are hepatitis A (infectious hepatitis, IH, MS-1, or epidemic or short-incubation type) and hepatitis B (serum hepatitis, SH, MS-2, or long-incubation type). It appears that the two forms of viral hepatitis are immunologically distinct, although they are similar morphologically. The morphologic features are discussed on p. 443.

Hepatitis A (infectious hepatitis) tends to occur in children and young adults, usually in epidemics, and is characterized by a relatively short incubation period (15 to 50 days). Most commonly, it is acquired through the oral route. Apparently, the virus is excreted in the feces and is transmitted by fecal-oral contact among individuals, particularly in circumstances where poor sanitation or overcrowding exists. Ingestion of infected raw or partially cooked mollusks (e.g., clams and oysters) harvested from polluted waters may be the means of transmission in some instances. Occasionally, hepatitis A may follow inoculation (parenteral route).

Hepatitis B (serum hepatitis) occurs at any

age and has a longer incubation period (50 to 160 days) than type A hepatitis. Usually, it is transmitted by parenteral injection of human blood products originating from latent infected donors or by injection of other substances using contaminated needles or syringes. However, it also may be transmitted by nonparenteral means. There is evidence that hepatitis B is an important occupational hazard for health-care personnel, e.g., those working in hemodialysis units and in other hospital units in which patients have received multiple blood product transfusions. Although transmission of the infection could occur through an inapparent percutaneous inoculation of blood or serum (e.g., through a minor break in the skin), nonparenteral transmission of the virus via body fluids, such as urine, feces, or saliva, has been suggested.

Viruslike particles have been identified electron microscopically in the serum of some patients with viral hepatitis (type B), but as yet the specific virus of hepatitis A or B has not been isolated and grown in tissue culture. In 1965, a new antigen was found in the serum of an Australian aborigine, referred to as *Australia antigen,* that subsequently was found to be associated with viral hepatitis. The antigen may be detected by immunodiffusion, complement fixation, and electron microscopy. The antigen, later named *hepatitis associated antigen* (HAA), has been found to be associated specifically with hepatitis B (serum hepatitis). The evidence suggests that the antigen is closely associated with the hepatitis virus and may be on the virus. It is present on the surface of the viruslike (Dane) particles found in hepatitis B. This antigen is also known as *hepatitis B surface antigen* (HB$_s$Ag) and has been detected in various body fluids in addition to serum (e.g., urine, feces, saliva, pleural and ascitic fluids and semen) in patients with acute hepatitis B and in asymptomatic carriers. Several subtypes of HB$_s$Ag have been described.

Investigators have been searching for some time for an antigenic marker in patients with hepatitis A that is comparable to HB$_s$Ag. In a study of epidemics of infectious (short-incubation) hepatitis in Italy and England, the sera of the affected patients were negative for Australia antigen, but a new antigen was said to have been detected that was called *epidemic hepatitis-associated antigen* (EHAA). However, other investigators have suggested that this antigen is not specifically related to the virus of type A hepatitis since it may be found also in the serum of patients with other liver disorders. Recently, viruslike particles that appeared to be distinct from hepatitis B virus have been described in fecal extracts of patients in the acute phase of hepatitis A. Subsequently, investigators were able to identify antibody to the viruslike antigen (by immune electron microscopy) in the serum of patients convalescing from hepatitis A, and they regarded the antigen as the etiologic agent of hepatitis A. The antigen has been designated HA Ag. Also, specific complement fixation and immune adherence tests and radioimmunoassay methods have been developed recently for identification of hepatitis A antibody.

Currently, there is interest in a third form of viral hepatitis. Evidence has been presented showing that certain hepatitis cases are not caused by HB virus or hepatitis A agent and that another hepatitis virus may be the cause. This disease is usually called *non-A, non-B hepatitis*. It has also been referred to as "type C (viral) hepatitis" and is usually transmitted by administration of blood or blood products. In some instances, however, the method of transmission is not known. Recently, evidence for an infectious agent was suggested by the transmission of non-A, non-B hepatitis to chimpanzees with sera from affected persons. Furthermore, some investigators, using immunodiffusion techniques, have identified an antigen in sera of patients with non-A, non-B posttransfusion hepatitis. The antigen was shown to be distinct from antigens of hepatitis A and B. Several investigators have reported electron microscopic evidence of viruslike particles in patients with this form of hepatitis and in experimentally infected chimpanzees. In view of the differences in the description of these particles in the individual reports, it is possible that there may be more than one non-A, non-B hepatitis agent.

Infections caused by coxsackieviruses.
Viruses of the coxsackie group belong to the larger group of enteroviruses. They have been isolated from throat washings and feces of patients with a variety of human diseases as well as asymptomatic persons. The 30 types fall into two groups, A and B.

The study of the coxsackieviruses is incomplete. Strong evidence indicates, however, that Group A viruses cause *herpangina,* a mild febrile illness of infancy characterized by vesicular and ulcerative lesions on the soft palate and in the faucial areas. Occasionally, the common cold is associated with one of the Group A viruses. Group B viruses apparently cause *epidemic pleurodynia* (Bornholm disease), a febrile illness in which the outstanding symptom is severe pain in the abdomen and chest, with painful respiration. The disease is of short duration and has never been fatal. Both of these diseases have been recognized clinically for many years. There is some evidence that certain strains of Group A and Group B coxsackieviruses may cause a nonfatal type of aseptic meningitis and occasionally a paralytic disease. Coxsackieviruses, especially Group B, also cause myocarditis of newborn infants and acute nonspecific pericarditis.

Diseases caused by echoviruses. The echo (enteric cytopathogenic human orphan) viruses became recognized when tissue cultures were used for viral isolation from stools. More than 20 types have been identified. Some types have been recognized as causing epidemics of diarrheal disease in infants and children. Other types appear to cause an aseptic meningitis without paralysis or sequelae. A variety of other clinical effects have been attributed to these viruses. Little is known about the pathologic features of diseases caused by the echoviruses because fatalities are rare.

Infectious mononucleosis. A common disease of teenagers and adults, infectious mononucleosis is generally considered to be viral in origin (see p. 480 for discussion of features of the disease). Certain evidence (e.g., the identification of the EB virus in throat washings and the demonstration of EBV-specific antibodies in patients with this disease) suggests that the Epstein-Barr virus is the cause. Interestingly, this is the virus that has been incriminated as the possible etiologic agent of Burkitt's lymphoma and nasopharyngeal carcinoma in human beings.

Epidemic hemorrhagic fever. Epidemic hemorrhagic fever, described by Japanese workers in 1943 and probably recognized 10 years earlier by the Russians, first appeared in United States troops in Korea in 1951. The viral agent only recently has been isolated. Some evidence suggests a mite as the vector and a rodent (field mouse) as the reservoir.

The clinical picture is dominated by fever, hemorrhage, and severe renal involvement, with associated changes in fluid balance. Early deaths have been ascribed to shock and late deaths (up to the thirtieth day of illness) to renal failure.

The characteristic pathologic features are as follows:

1 Hemorrhagic lesions, particularly in the renal medullae, right atrium of the heart, and gastrointestinal submucosa
2 A peculiar type of necrosis in the renal medullae, anterior lobe of the pituitary gland, and adrenal glands
3 Mononuclear cell infiltration of the heart, pulmonary alveoli, pancreas, spleen, and liver

The renal lesions, because of the areas of coagulative necrosis and hemorrhage, somewhat resemble infarcts grossly. Microscopically, the changes include those of lower nephron nephrosis, but the total picture in the kidney is almost pathognomonic of the disease. The basic change appears to be increased vascular permeability with edema and hemorrhages.

Chlamydial diseases

As mentioned previously, the group of obligate intracellular parasites causing such diseases as psittacosis, lymphogranuloma venereum, trachoma, and inclusion conjunctivitis are no longer considered to be viruses. These agents are intermediate between the rickettsiae and the viruses and are named *chlamydiae (bedsoniae)*. Cat-scratch disease is included in this discussion because it is generally believed to be caused by one of these agents, although the organism has not been isolated. The chlamydiae have also been considered by certain investigators to be an etiologic agent in nongonococcal (nonspecific) urogenital infections (e.g., urethritis).

Ornithosis (psittacosis). Ornithosis is acquired by inhalation of a rickettsialike agent *(Chlamydia)* present in dried urine and feces from infected birds. The disease was originally named *psittacosis* because it was thought at first that only psittacine birds (parrot family) harbored the causative organisms. However, it has been shown that several birds other than those of the parrot family, including pigeons and the fulmar petrel (a sea gull), may harbor the agent and cause human infection. Since the causative agent has been isolated from different species of birds, the more general name *ornithosis* has been proposed for the disease.

Clinically, ornithosis is an acute febrile illness with intense headache and physical signs of an atypical pneumonia. Leukopenia, instead of the leukocytosis that accompanies bacterial pneumonia, is an important diagnostic feature.

Pathologically, one finds splenomegaly and congestion and cloudy swelling of the viscera, as in any acute infection, but the characteristic changes are in the lungs, where patchy pneumonic consolidation is found. Microscopically, the picture is that of a pneumonia in which mononuclear cells rather than neutrophils predominate. At first, an alveolar exudate with fibrin and leukocytes is prominent, but during resolution an interstitial component of the inflammation is apparent. The alveolar lining cells are stimulated and appear to have become cuboidal in type with frequent mitoses.

Spherical clusters of minute coccoid elementary bodies of rather characteristic appearance are found with great difficulty in sections of human lungs but are very conspicuous in the brain tissue of mice after intracerebral injection of the agent and also may be found in mononuclear cells in the lung during the early stages of experimentally induced pneumonia.

Lymphogranuloma venereum. Structurally and antigenically, the agent producing lymphogranuloma venereum is like that of the other chlamydiae (bedsoniae). The disease is discussed on p. 194.

Trachoma. The agents causing trachoma and inclusion conjunctivitis are similar and are referred to as TRIC agents. In film preparations from the infected conjunctiva, spherical clusters of coccoid elementary bodies are commonly found in the cytoplasm of the epithelial cells. The cytologic picture somewhat resembles that seen in psittacosis and lymphogranuloma venereum. Trachoma can be reproduced in the monkey.

The lesion is characterized by subepithelial congestion, newly formed capillaries, and focal collections of lymphocytes and macrophages with lymphoid follicle formation, causing granular elevations of the conjuctiva. Necrosis and scarring of the lesions may occur. A serious complication is corneal involvement with necrosis and ulceration.

Inclusion conjunctivitis. Inclusion conjunctivitis (swimming pool conjunctivitis) initially is similar pathologically to trachoma, but recovery takes place without necrosis and other complications. The reservoir of infection is in the genitourinary tract. Newborn infants are infected during passage through the birth canal, and adults are infected by bathing in unchlorinated pools or lakes.

Cat-scratch disease. Cat-scratch disease is a self-limited type of granulomatous and suppurative lymphadenitis, possibly caused by chlamydiae, although a viral cause has not been excluded. Attempts to isolate the agent have been unsuccessful. It has been suggested in an occasional report that atypical mycobacteria may be responsible, since photochromogenic acid-fast bacilli have been isolated from lymph nodes of patients diagnosed as having cat-scratch disease. In almost all instances, the disease is associated with contact with cats. A history of a claw scratch or bite may be obtained.

A transient papule occurs at the site of entry (usually on the hand or arm), and the regional lymph nodes become greatly swollen. Fever is variable. Over a period of weeks or months, the lesions slowly subside, with or without suppuration. In excised lymph nodes, one finds focal areas of suppuration, or cores of necrotic debris containing relatively few neutrophils, surrounded by wide bands of epithelioid cells, with a few giant cells. The picture resembles that of lymphogranuloma venereum and even may be mistaken for chronic tularemia or tuberculosis. A specific cutaneous test with antigen prepared from purulent material of patients known to have the disease is helpful in establishing the diagnosis.

REFERENCES

Andrewes, C. H.: Med. Clin. North Am. **51:**765-768, 1967 (common cold).

Archer, G. L., et al.: N. Engl. J. Med. **301:**897-900, 1979 (infection caused by erythrocyte-associated bacterium).

Armstrong, R. W., et al.: N. Engl. J. Med. **283:**1182-1187, 1970 (interferon production in varicella and vaccinia).

Balfour, H. H., Jr.: Arch. Intern. Med. **139:**279-280, 1979 (cytomegalovirus and transplantation).

Bhatt, D. R., et al.: Am. J. Dis. Child. **127:**862-869, 1974 (human rabies).

Biggar, R. J., et al.: J.A.M.A. **232:**494-500, 1975 (lymphocytic choriomeningitis and pet hamsters).

Blumberg, B. S.: Ann. Intern. Med. **87:**111-115, 1977 (non-A, non-B hepatitis).

Blumberg, B. S., and Melartin, L.: Arch. Intern. Med. **125:**287-292, 1970 (Australia antigen and hepatitis).

Blumberg, B. S., et al.: J.A.M.A. **207:**1895-1896, 1969 (Australia antigen and hepatitis).

Breitfeld, V., et al.: Lab. Invest. **28:**279-291, 1973 (fatal measles infection, leukemia, and altered immunity).

Chatterjee, S. N., et al.: J.A.M.A. **240:**2446-2449, 1978 (cytomegalovirus in renal transplant recipients).

Coursaget, P., et al.: Lancet **2:**92, 1979 (viruslike particles in non-A, non-B hepatitis).

Deibel, R., et al.: J.A.M.A. **232:**501-504, 1975 (lymphocytic choriomeningitis and pet hamsters).

DelPrete, S., et al.: Lancet **2:**579-581, 1970 (new serum antigen in infectious hepatitis).

Dudgeon, J. A., et al.: Br. Med. J. **2:**155-160, 1964 (rubella).

Editorial: Lancet **2:**1007-1008, 1973 (type A hepatitis).

Elton, N. W., et al.: Am. J. Clin. Pathol. **25:**135-146, 1955 (yellow fever).

Enders, J. F., et al.: N. Engl. J. Med. **261:**875-881, 1959 (measles and giant cell pneumonia).

Feinstone, S. M., Kapikian, A. Z., and Purcell, R. H.: Science **182:**1026-1028, 1973 (viruslike antigen in hepatitis A).

Ferris A. A., Kaldor, J., and Gust, I. D.: Lancet **2:**243-244, 1970 (fecal antigen in viral hepatitis).

Ginsburg, C. M., et al.: J.A.M.A. **237:**781-785, 1977 (infectious mononucleosis and EBV).

Gocke, D. J.: N. Engl. J. Med. **291:**1409-1411, 1974 (type B hepatitis).

Golden, W.: J.A.M.A. (Medical News) **242:**2517-2518, 1979 (news item—studies of non-A, non-B hepatitis virion by C. Trepo et al.).

Goodpasture, E. W.: J. Pediatr. **18:**440-446, 1941 (pathology of viral disease).

Goodpasture, E. W., Auerbach, S. H., Swanson, H. S., and Cotter, E. F.: Am. J. Dis. Child. **57:**997-1011, 1939 (description of adenovirus pneumonia).

Hall, C. B., et al.: N. Engl. J. Med. **300:**393-396, 1979 (neonatal respiratory syncytial virus infection).

Hattwick, M. A. W., et al.: Ann. Intern. Med. **76:**931-942, 1972 (recovery from rabies).

Hattwick, M. A. W., et al.: J.A.M.A. **240:**1499-1503, 1978 (fatal Rocky Mountain spotted fever).

Hawley, H. B., et al.: J.A.M.A. **226:**33-36, 1973 (coxsackievirus B epidemic at boys' summer camp).

Henle, G., and Henle, W.: Hosp. Pract. **5:**33-41, July 1970 (EB virus in infectious mononucleosis).

Hersh, T., et al.: N. Engl. J. Med. **285:**1363-1364, 1971 (nonparenteral transmission of viral hepatitis type B).

Hirschman, R. J., et al.: J.A.M.A. **208:**1667-1670, 1969 (Australia antigen and viral hepatitis).

Hirshaut, Y., et al.: N. Engl. J. Med. **283:**502-506, 1970 (herpeslike virus in sarcoidosis).

Ho, M.: N. Engl. J. Med. **283:**1222-1223, 1970 (editorial—interferon and herpes zoster).

Hoeprich, P. D., editor: Infectious diseases, ed. 2, New York, 1977, Harper & Row, Publishers, Inc.

Hoofnagle, J. H., et al.: Ann. Intern. Med. **87:**14-20, 1977 (non-A, non-B hepatitis).

Horsfall, F. L., Jr., and Tamm, I., editors: Viral and rickettsial infections of man, ed. 4, Philadelphia, 1965, J. B. Lippincott Co.

Josey, W. E., et al.: Am. J. Obstet. Gynecol. **101:**718-729, 1968 (genital infection and herpesvirus type 2).

Kalter, S. S., et al.: Nature (Lond.) **224:**190, 1969 (herpeslike virus particles in cat-scratch disease).

Krugman, S., and Giles, J. P.: J.A.M.A. **212:**1019-1029, 1970 (viral hepatitis).

Krugman, S., et al.: J.A.M.A. **217:**41-45, 1971 (viral hepatitis).

Lander, J. J., et al.: N. Engl. J. Med. **285:**303-307, 1971 (viral hepatitis type B, MS-2 strain).

Lennette, E. H.: N. Engl. J. Med. **297:**884-885, 1977 (Rocky Mountain spotted fever).

London, W. T., et al.: N. Engl. J. Med. **281:**571-578, 1969 (Australia antigen).

Manz, H. J.: Hum. Pathol. **8:**3-26, 1977 (viral infections of the central nervous system).

McGavran, M. H., et al.: Am. J. Pathol. **40:**653-670, 1962 (psittacosis).

Med. World News **12:**25-28, April 2, 1971 (slow viruses).

Melnick, J. L., and Rawls, W. E.: Hosp. Pract. **4:**37-41, Feb. 1969 (herpesvirus in induction of cervical carcinoma).

Miller, W. J., et al.: Proc. Soc. Exper. Biol. Med. **149:**254-261, 1975 (immunologic identification of hepatitis A antibody).

Nahmias, A. J., and Roizman, B.: N. Engl. J. Med. **289:**667-674, 719-725, 781-789, 1973 (infection with herpes simplex viruses 1 and 2).

Niederman, J. C.: N. Engl. J. Med. **294:**1355-1359, 1976 (infectious mononucleosis and EBV).

Pinkerton, H., et al.: Am. J. Pathol. **21:**1-23, 1945 (giant cell pneumonia).

Prince, A. F., et al.: Lancet **2:**241-246, 1974 (possible hepatitis C virus).

Recavarren, S., and Lumbreras, H.: Am. J. Pathol. **66:**461-470, 1972 (pathogenesis of verruga of Carrión's disease).

Rhodes, A. J., and van Rooyen, C. E.: Textbook of virology, ed. 5, Baltimore, 1968, The Williams & Wilkins Co.

Ristic, M., and Krier, J. P.: N. Engl. J. Med. **301:**937-939, 1979 (hemotropic bacteria).

Robinson, W. S., and Lutwick, L. I.: N. Engl. J. Med. **295:**1168-1175, 1232-1236, 1976 (virus of hepatitis B).

Schachter, J.: N. Engl. J. Med. **298:**428-435, 490-495, 540-548, 1978 (chlamydial infections).

Sheehy, T. W., Hazlett, D., and Turk, R. E.: Arch. Intern. Med. **132:**77-80, 1973 (scrub typhus).

Shimizu, Y. K., et al.: Science **205:**197-200, 1979 (EM study of non-A, non-B hepatitis agents).

Shirachi, R., et al.: Lancet **2:**853-856, 1978 (non-A, non-B hepatitis viral antigen).

Sigel, M. M., and Beasley, A. R.: Viruses, cells, and hosts, New York, 1965, Holt, Rinehart & Winston, Inc.

Smith, W., et al.: Lancet **2:**66-68, 1933 (transmission of influenza virus to ferrets).

Sobonya, R. E., et al.: Arch. Pathol. Lab. Med. **102:**366-371, 1978 (fatal measles pneumonia in adults).

Spaulding, W. B., and Hennessy, J. N.: Am. J. Med. **28:**504-509, 1960 (cat-scratch disease).

Suringa, D. W. R., et al.: N. Engl. J. Med. **283:**1139-1142, 1970 (measles virus in skin and Koplik's spots).

Tamm, I., editor: Am. J. Med. **38:**649-766, 1965 (symposium on viruses).

Tamm, I., and Sehgal, P. B.: Am. J. Med. **66:**3-5, 1979 (interferons).

Top, F. H., Sr., and Wehrle, P. F., editors: Communicable and infectious diseases, ed. 8, St. Louis, 1976, The C. V. Mosby Co.

Villarejos, V. M., et al.: N. Engl. J. Med. **291:**1375-1378, 1974 (role of saliva, urine, and feces in transmission of type B hepatitis).

Vitvitski, L., et al.: Lancet **2:**1263-1267, 1979 (antigen in non-A, non-B hepatitis).

Weiner, L. P., et al.: N. Engl. J. Med. **288:**1103-1110, 1973 (viral infections and demyelinating diseases).

WHO Report: A revised system of nomenclature for influenza viruses, Bull. WHO **45:**119-124, 1971.

Wolbach, S. B., Todd, J. T., and Palfrey, F. W.: The etiology and pathology of typhus, Cambridge, Mass., 1922, Harvard University Press.

Young, E. J.: J.A.M.A. **235:**2731-2733, 1976 (disseminated herpesvirus infection).

9

Spirochetal and venereal diseases

SYPHILIS

Syphilis, caused by the spirochete *Treponema pallidum,* is one of the most important of the venereal diseases. Although much is known about the control of syphilis and gonorrhea, the other very important venereal disease (p. 126), their incidence is of such proportions that they still have to be considered among the major national health problems. Syphilis causes disability and death mainly from involvement of the heart, blood vessels, and nervous system, but any organ may be affected. The clinical manifestations are extremely variable, and latent periods occur in which there are no clinical signs other than positive serologic reactions. The course of the disease is described in three stages.

The characteristic lesion of the primary stage (chancre) is a hard ulcer that develops at the point of entrance of the organisms and hence is usually on the genitalia. The secondary stage, developing about 6 weeks after the chancre, is characterized by maculopapular skin rashes, mucous patches on the oral mucosa, and generalized slight lymph node enlargement. Tertiary lesions develop after a latent period of months or years. They may be localized areas of specific, granulomatous inflammation with gummy necrosis (gumma) or a chronic nonspecific inflammation with gradual destruction of tissue and development of fibrosis. This latter type of reaction is more common. Penicillin is effective in the treatment of early syphilis (primary and secondary lesions).

In contrast with the varied clinical and gross manifestations, the microscopic features of syphilis are relatively simple and constant but rarely pathognomonic. Lesions of the skin in any stage of syphilis may show considerable and irregular epithelial hyperplasia and sometimes, as in certain gummatous ulcers, may simulate a cancerous change (pseudocarcinomatous hyperplasia). The inflammatory cells in syphilitic lesions are predominantly lymphocytes and plasma cells, situated around small blood vessels and later more diffusely spread throughout the tissue. Fibroblastic proliferation and fibrosis accompany the process. Small blood vessels in syphilitic lesions exhibit changes, frequently an intimal thickening (endarteritis) and luminal narrowing or obstruction. In addition to the factor of hypersensitivity, this vascular change and consequent ischemia probably contribute to the necrosis of the gumma. Final proof of the syphilitic nature of a lesion depends on demonstration of the spirochete. Spirochetes are numerous in primary and secondary lesions but are scarce in tertiary lesions.

The *Treponema pallidum (Spirochaeta pallida)* is a slender organism, 5 to 15 μ in length, i.e., usually about once or twice the diameter of a red blood cell. It is characterized by its thinness and by the closeness and regularity of its corkscrewlike spirals, which average about 12 in number. It is stained only with great difficulty and is best demonstrated in smears from syphilitic lesions by dark-field examination or against a black

Table 9-1. Spirochetal diseases

Disease	Spirochete	Morphology of spirochete	Main features of disease
Syphilis	*Treponema pallidum*	5 to 15 μ long; about 12 slender, tightly wound regular coils	Venereal; widespread
Yaws (frambesia)	*Treponema pertenue*	Resembles *T. pallidum*	Nonvenereal; lesions and stages similar to syphilis
Pinta	*Treponema carateum*	Indistinguishable from *T. pallidum*	Nonvenereal; bluish pigmented and depigmented areas of skin
Relapsing fever	*Borrelia recurrentis, Borrelia duttonii*	7 to 20 μ long; easily stained; 5 to 10 loosely wound, wavy spirals	Spread primarily by lice and ticks; organism found in blood smears during febrile period
Spirochetal jaundice (Weil's disease) Spirochetosis ictero-haemorrhagica	*Leptospira icterohaemor-rhagiae*	6 to 15 μ long; fine, tightly wound spirals enclosing axial filament, prolonged to form straight or hooked ends	Hemorrhages in various organs, particularly lungs; degeneration and necrosis in liver and kidney; spirochetes excreted in urine
Vincent's angina	*Borrelia vincentii*	5 to 10 μ long; 3 to 8 irregular shallow spirals; constantly found with long fusiform bacilli *(Bacillus fusiformis)*	Symbiotic infection, associated with gangrenous and sloughing lesions of mouth, throat, and respiratory tract
Rat-bite fever (sodoku)	*Spirillum minus*	2 to 5 μ long; broad spiral organism; regular spirals; blunt ends with flagella	Febrile infection caused by bite of infected rat; primary lesion at point of inoculation; recurring chills and fever; spirochete sometimes demonstrated in blood but better isolated by injection of blood into mice

background of India ink. In tissues, it may be demonstrated by Levaditi's method, or some modification of it, in which the spirochete is impregnated with silver. Methods for staining the organism in tissues are technically difficult and uncertain. Serologic tests for syphilis include demonstration of detectable levels of reagin in the serum and the *Treponema pallidum* immobilization (TPI) test, i.e., progressive immobilization and death of the spirochetes by serum of a syphilitic patient in the presence of complement.

Primary stage

The *chancre,* or primary syphilitic lesion, appears at the point of inoculation of the spirochete after an incubation period of 1 to 6 weeks. An abrasion of the skin or mucosa facilitates entry of the organism but probably is unnecessary for penetration of the genital mucosa. The chancre is on the genitalia in more than 90% of the patients, the next most common location being the lips or mouth. In 20% or more of the patients, no primary lesion develops, or it is hidden in the urethra or vagina and passes unnoticed. Syphilis has been transferred by blood transfusion, the spirochete being directly inoculated with the donor's blood. In such cases, there is no primary lesion.

Very soon after penetration, the organisms spread to the regional lymph nodes and then, by way of the bloodstream, become widely distributed in tissues of the body. Hence, prophylactic treatment must immediately follow exposure.

After the incubation period (average time, 3 weeks), the chancre begins as a thickening

Table 9-2. Course of syphilis

Stage	Time	Lesions	Pathologic background	Result
Incubation period	Average 3 weeks	No clinical signs	Reproduction of organisms locally at site of inoculation and widespread distribution throughout body	Development of chancre
Primary stage	6 weeks	Chancre; local lymph node enlargement	Hard ulcerative lesion at point of inoculation, with many organisms; serologic tests for syphilis become positive	Heals spontaneously with slight scarring
Secondary stage	1 to 3 years; latent periods and recurrences	Eruptive lesions on skin and mucous membranes; generalized lymph node enlargement	Localized areas of congestion with perivascular round cell infiltrations; minimal tissue destruction; lesions rich in spirochetes and highly infective; serologic tests for syphilis positive	Heals spontaneously with minimal scarring
Latent periods *Tertiary stage*	6 months to 20 years Lasts for remainder of life	Present but not evident clinically Chronic destructive fibrosing lesions and/or gummas may involve any organ; aortitis with aortic valve involvement and regurgitation, coronary ostial narrowing, aneurysm; meningitis, meningovascular lesions, general paresis, and tabes dorsalis	Progressive destruction of parenchymatous tissue and replacement by scar tissue, producing eventual functional breakdown; serologic tests for syphilis may be positive or negative	Partial healing with fibrosis, producing functional and anatomic disturbances of organs

and hardening of the surface tissue. The epithelium of this area becomes necrotic and sloughs off, leaving a shallow ulcer a few millimeters to a centimeter in diameter. The ulcer is single, round, and characterized by painlessness and hardness. The induration extends to form a flat hard mass that exudes clear serum but no pus. Secondary infection may occur and change the characteristic features. Histologically, the lesions show fairly dense granulation tissue with many small vessels and an infiltration of lymphocytes and plasma cells. These chronic inflammatory cells at first surround the small blood vessels but later spread out and become diffuse. The hardness of the lesion results from connective tissue formation and the accumulation of inflammatory cells. Necrosis is absent except on the surface. Secondary infection may change the histologic picture. There is nothing absolutely characteristic about the lesion, and certain diagnosis depends on demonstration of the abundant spirochetes.

The chancre heals in 3 to 8 weeks. The induration disappears, the area is re-covered by epithelium, and healing leaves only slight fibrosis or scarring. The serologic tests for syphilis usually becomes positive about 1 or 2 weeks after the appearance of the chancre.

With development of the chancre, the regional lymph nodes (usually inguinal) become enlarged, firm, and shotty but are not painful. In the enlarged nodes, there is hyperplasia of the cells lining the sinuses, which are filled with mononuclear cells. Small areas of focal necrosis may occur, but there is no tendency for the glands to suppurate.

Secondary stage

Secondary lesions appear 6 to 10 weeks after the development of the chancre and are characterized by simultaneous appearance over the whole body, insignificant tissue reaction with little tissue destruction, and richness in organisms. Serologic tests for syphilis are almost invariably positive and are most dependable during this stage.

During the incubation period and the period of the chancre, spread has occurred throughout the whole body by the lymphatics and bloodstream. Multiplication in these new foci results in the breaking out of innumerable lesions. On the skin, they most commonly take the form of a macular or papular rash, but any type of skin eruption may be imitated. Sore throat is common, and elevated white "mucous patches" involve the oral mucosa. There is a generalized slight lymph node enlargement, the glands being hard, discrete, and shotty. Histologically, the lymph nodes may show marked follicular hyperplasia, simulating giant follicular lymphadenopathy. Flat condylomas (condylomata lata) develop in moist areas about the genitalia or anus. These are broad lobulated elevations in which epithelial overgrowth is a marked feature.

In all secondary skin lesions, the histologic change is essentially a perivascular accumulation of lymphocytes and plasma cells, with varying amounts of vascular dilatation and congestion. In macular lesions, cells are few in number. In papular lesions, they are numerous in deep layers of the epithelium and in the corium. Focal epidermal abscesses occur in pustular lesions, but ulceration is not particularly common. The epithelium shows little change except in the condylomas, in which papillomatous overgrowth may be marked. Healing occurs without scars. Milder recurrences of secondary lesions, separated by latent periods of apparent health, are characteristic of the usual course in untreated patients.

Less common manifestations of secondary syphilis include iritis, periostitis, arthritis, meningismus (rarely acute meningitis), nephropathy, and hepatitis. The nephropathy is considered to be a form of immune complex disease. Changes in the liver may be insignificant, but in some instances there may be Kupffer cell and endothelial cell hyperplasia, portal and lobular collections of inflammatory (particularly mononuclear) cells, sparse liver cell necrosis, and lipid deposits or lipofuscin in some hepatocytes. Occasionally, spirochetes have been identified in properly stained liver sections.

Tertiary stage

A latent period of a few months to 5 or as long as 20 years occurs between secondary and tertiary lesions. During this period, the person appears well, and the presence of active syphilis is recognizable only by serologic tests. Nevertheless, a slow, mild, chronic inflammation progresses in various invaded tissues, particularly the cardiovascular system or nervous system. This slow destruction and fibrosis may lead to eventual functional breakdown or may be evident only by gross or microscopic examination after the death of the individual.

Gumma is a less common type of tertiary lesion characterized by great destruction of tissue and relatively few organisms. The gumma may be found in almost any organ or tissue. It is usually a solitary nodule of necrotic tissue (Fig. 9-1), varying from microscopic size to a diameter of several centimeters. The opaque necrotic material has an elastic or "gummy" consistency. Microscopically, it presents features of coagulation and caseation necrosis, because in some areas "ghost" or "shadow" forms of underlying tissue architecture can be seen and in others amorphous, granular debris is evident. About the necrotic material are lymphocytes, plasma cells, and macrophages. Multinucleated giant cells occur less frequently than in tuberculosis. Proliferating con-

nective tissue cells encapsulate the lesion, and vascularized connective tissue may extend a considerable distance into the necrotic center, whereas fibrous tissue is usually absent in the center of a tubercle. Although there are differences between gummas and tubercles, the histologic differentiation of single lesions is not always possible without demonstration of organisms. The history of associated lesions usually must be considered in diagnosis.

When a gumma involves skin or mucous membrane, there is sloughing of necrotic material, so that an ulcer results. Gummatous ulcers have irregular sharp walls, a punched-out appearance, and an irregular base. The palate is a common site and may be completely perforated. Gummas heal with absorption of the necrotic material and formation of dense fibrous distorting scars. The distortion is particularly well seen in the liver, where deep contracted scars produce a peculiar irregular lobed appearance *(hepar lobatum)*.

Occasionally, there is involvement by numerous miliary gummas, which begin as the usual perivascular involvement but in which necrosis is slight or never complete. Healing occurs with diffuse and irregular fibrosis of the tissue.

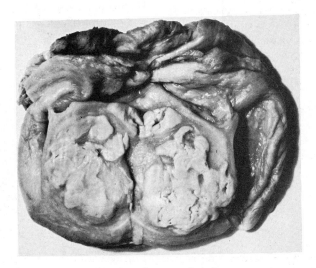

Fig. 9-1. Gumma of testis.

Although syphilis may affect practically any organ or tissue, only the more important are considered here.

Circulatory system

The aorta is involved more commonly than any other organ, probably in every patient with active syphilis. Especially affected are the ascending aorta and arch, parts that possess a particularly rich lymph supply. This area of major involvement is in contrast to that in atherosclerosis, in which the lower abdominal portion is very considerably involved.

All layers of the aorta are affected. The adventitia shows perivascular collections of lymphocytes and plasma cells and later is scarred and thickened. The most important damage is to the media, in which destruction of elastic fibers and muscle and scar formation so weaken the wall as to allow aneurysmal bulging. The intima is involved by an irregular fibrous thickening, which appears as an irregular wrinkling and pitting. The resulting tree bark appearance (linear furrowing) is grossly characteristic (Fig. 9-2) but not pathognomonic. More distinctive are the small, puckered stellate fissures, which are the result of underlying medial scars. The intimal change causes little functional damage, except when it involves the sinuses of Valsalva, where it may result in narrowing or occlusion of coronary openings, an important complication of syphilitic aortitis. Similar syphilitic lesions, also with aneurysm formation, less commonly involve other arteries. Proximal portions of the coronary arteries may be stenosed or obliterated by syphilitic endarteritis.

Heart

Syphilis may involve the region of the aortic valve and sometimes the myocardium. Changes in the valves may be dilatation of the aortic ring, thickening and shortening of the cusps, and separation of the cusps at the commissures (Fig. 9-3). These three types of change, which may occur singly or in combination, all produce insufficiency of the aortic valve. The extra burden of diastolic regurgitation into the left ventricle causes a work hypertrophy of that part.

The myocardium may be affected by the narrowing or occlusion of the proximal portions or openings of the coronary arteries. The resultant myocardial ischemia may cause angina pectoris and myocardial fibrosis. Granulomatous myocarditis with formation of gummas occurs rarely. There is a dispute as to whether a primary nonspecific myocarditis characterized by interstitial infiltration of lymphocytes and plasma cells followed by fibrosis is caused by syphilitic organisms. Conducting bundles may be involved by any of the myocardial lesions associated with syphilis and give rise to heart block.

Nervous system

Syphilitic involvement of the nervous system may appear as meningeal and/or vascular

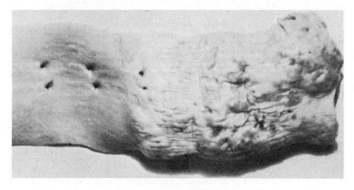

Fig. 9-2. Syphilitic aortitis. Note longitudinal striation and ''tree bark'' appearance.

lesions, general paresis (dementia paralytica), or tabes doralis (locomotor ataxia). Also, a gumma may develop in any part of the brain and simulate a tumor in its manifestations.

Meningeal involvement. Meningeal involvement in syphilis is usually chronic and, rarely, acute meningitis. The usual form is associated with considerable thickening and adherence of all layers. The tissues are infiltrated with lymphocytes, plasma cells, and macrophages (Fig. 9-4). The blood vessels are involved, and perivascular infiltration and fibrosis give rise to the meningeal thickening. Varying degrees of degeneration of underlying nerve cells accompany the meningitis.

Meningeal changes may involve the cranial nerves or produce obstructive hydrocephalus. Narrowing of the cerebral vessels (syphilitic

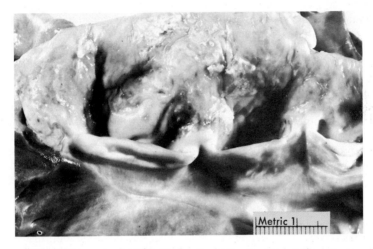

Fig. 9-3. Syphilitic aortitis and valvulitis. Note separation of aortic valve cusps at commissures.

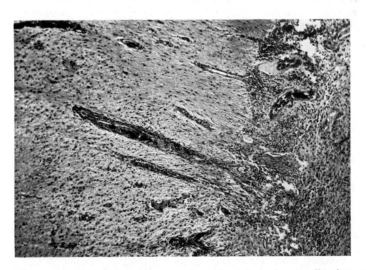

Fig. 9-4. Syphilitic meningitis. Inflammatory exudate of meninges is extending into cerebral tissue, particularly around vascular spaces.

endarteritis) may lead to cerebral atrophy or arterial thrombosis and infarcts of the brain (meningovascular syphilis).

General paresis. General paresis is usually a late manifestation of syphilis. Treponemas have been demonstrated in the involved tissue. The disease is manifested by disturbances of memory, personality changes, visual disturbances, incoordination (particularly in the hands and tongue), and psychotic episodes. Varying degrees of atrophic change affect the cerebral convolutions, the ventricles are dilated, and there is usually some accompanying meningeal involvement, with thickening and adhesions.

Microscopic changes include degeneration and reduction in number of nerve cells and fibers in the cerebral cortex, especially in the frontal region, and proliferation of cortical neuroglia. Collections of plasma cells and lymphocytes are present about blood vessels. Storage in the microglia of a large amount of iron-containing substance, which gives a Prussian blue reaction, is a most characteristic finding.

Tabes dorsalis. Tabes dorsalis (locomotor ataxia) is characterized by a degeneration of the posterior roots and posterior columns of the spinal cord as a result of syphilis. The reason for the degenerative process is not clear. Injury to the nerve fibers has been attributed to meningitis about the dorsal roots, to direct inflammation in the dorsal root ganglia, to a toxin, or to the presence of the spirochete itself.

Varying degrees of meningeal inflammation and thickening accompany the cord changes, which usually are most pronounced in the lumbar portion of the cord. The posterior columns are shrunken and retracted and pale gray on the cut surface. In these degenerated areas, axons and myelin sheaths have disappeared, and there is increased neuroglial tissue (gliosis). In the posterior roots, there is also demyelination and a decrease in the number of nerve fibers. Frequently, the optic nerve also is involved. Occasionally, there is a round cell infiltration where the posterior roots penetrate the arachnoid. Apparently as a result of loss of

proprioceptive sensation, certain joints (particularly the knees) may be subjected to unusual trauma related to weight bearing. Destructive changes may occur in the cartilage and adjacent bone, causing the joints to become hypermobile *(Charcot's joints)*.

Congenital syphilis

Syphilis is frequently congenital, but it is not hereditary. Placental and fetal tissues are a particularly good soil for growth of the spirochete, and congenital infection probably occurs whenever the mother has active syphilitic infection. The maternal infection may be old and clinically latent, or it may have been acquired just before or during pregnancy.

Infection of the fetus may result in death in utero and abortion, in premature labor and stillbirth, or in a live child with active syphilitic lesions. In some cases, the infant appears well at birth but later develops evidence of syphilis (lues tarda). The fetus probably does not become infected before the fifth month of pregnancy. The Langhans' layer of cells of the placental villi, which does not disappear until after 16 weeks, apparently protects against intrauterine infection until that time.

Placenta. In syphilitic stillbirths and in neonatal active syphilis, the placenta is abnormally large. It often shows changes caused by the infection but infrequently so great as to be diagnostic. Thickening of the intima and adventitia of the vessels of the placenta and umbilical cord and the enlargement of the villi by new connective tissue formation about the central blood vessels have been ascribed to syphilis.

Skin lesions. Syphilitic infants frequently exhibit mucocutaneous lesions. These are usually in the form of a maculopapular rash, blebs or bullae on the hands and feet, and desquamation. Rhinitis, with snuffles, and fissures about the lips and anus (rhagades) may occur. The infant appears small and undernourished, but the liver and spleen are enlarged.

Organ involvement. Often, there is faulty development of organs, which appear enlarged, dense, and fibrous. The lung, liver, spleen, pancreas, and kidney frequently are involved. The change in the lung is commonly called white pneumonia (pneumonia alba). The pulmonary alveoli are not fully developed, being lined by cubical epithelial cells, and their walls are greatly thickened by fine connective tissue and small round mesoblastic cells. An interstitial infiltration by mononuclear cells also occurs. In the enlarged liver, there is an increase of connective tissue, particularly around portal areas but generally extending diffusely throughout the liver. Focal areas of gummatous necrosis and many focal collections of small, round, dark, blood-forming cells may be seen. Similar excess hematopoietic activity is evident in the spleen. Fibrosis or undifferentiated mesoblastic tissue is also prominent in the pancreas and kidney. In the latter organ, a prominent neogenic zone at the outer edge of the cortex indicates the delayed development. Spirochetes usually are demonstrated in the involved organs.

Osteochondritis. Osteochondritis is the most constant lesion of congenital syphilis. It may be the sole lesion and is a valuable aid in roentgenologic diagnosis. In long bones, the line of ossification between cartilage and bone is wide, irregular, yellowish, and opaque instead of a normal thin, even, gray translucent line. There is irregular and incomplete ossification in this area, with development of a cellular granulation tissue. Osteoblastic activity is diminished, with disturbance of normal resorption and alteration in the growth of cartilage. Periostitis with thickening frequently accompanies the osteochondritis but seldom occurs alone.

Other effects. Later forms of congenital syphilis produce various scars and deformities, some of which are characteristic stigmas of the disease. These include gummatous destruction of the nasal bones (saddle nose), bulbous or tapered incisors with a notch in the center of the biting edge (Hutchinson's teeth), interstitial keratitis producing corneal opacity, and saber shin resulting from periostitis. Lesions of the central nervous system are not uncommon, but cardiovascular lesions are rare. The combination of nerve deafness, interstitial keratitis, and Hutchinson's teeth is known as Hutchinson's triad or syndrome.

OTHER SPIROCHETAL DISEASES

Yaws (frambesia). Yaws is a tropical disease closely similar to syphilis and is caused by the spirochete Treponema pertenue, which is almost indistinguishable from the syphilitic spirochete. In yaws, the serologic tests for syphilis are positive, and treatment with penicillin is effective. Yaws is not a venereal disease—it spreads by direct contact, mainly to children.

An initial primary lesion develops at the point of inoculation (usually on a leg or arm), at first as a papule and then developing into a larger papillomatous lesion (raspberrylike; thus, the term frambesia). It may heal or persist and ulcerate. Weeks later, this is followed by generalized scattered scaly macules, which progress to the development of papules and frambesiform, papillomatous lesions. The initial lesion exhibits severe epithelial hyperplasia, with lymphocytes and plasma cells in the dermis. Usually, the spirochete is found only in the epidermis. The predominant involvement of the epidermis in yaws is in contrast to that in syphilis, in which the main changes and the spirochetes are found in the corium. In the scaly macular lesions, epithelial proliferation is slight and cellular infiltration scanty. Late tertiary lesions may ulcerate and show epithelial hyperplasia. Histologic differentiation of the cutaneous and subcutaneous lesions of yaws and syphilis is unreliable. In addition to skin ulcers, destructive lesions of the bones occur in the tertiary stage.

Yaws differs from syphilis in that (1) the initial lesion is extragenital, (2) the infection is acquired most often in childhood but is never congenital, (3) mucous membrane lesions usually are absent in the secondary stage, and (4) macular eruptions (roseola), iritis, and alopecia are uncommon. A long latent period between secondary and late manifestations is unusual in yaws, but the tertiary lesions are similar to those of late syphilis. Skeletal involvement is common, with a high incidence of osteoporosis. Yaws is a milder disease than syphilis, and there is less frequent involvement of the cardiovascular and nervous systems. *Gangosa* (a destructive nasopharyngitis), *goundou* (an exostosis of nasal bones), and *juxta-articular nodes* have been considered sequelae of yaws.

Pinta (carate; mal de los pintos). Pinta is a nonvenereal infection caused by the spirochete *Treponema carateum (Treponema herrejoni)*, which is morphologically indistinguishable from the spirochete of syphilis. It is common among dark-skinned peoples of Central and South America, particularly in Mexico and Columbia. The exact method of transmission is undetermined but probably is by direct contact. Insect transmission also has been suggested. The serologic tests for syphilis are positive in most cases, especially in the late stages, and penicillin is effective in therapy.

The initial lesion is a persistent nonulcerating papule, followed in 5 or more months by secondary lesions (pintids) in the form of macules and papules. At first these are red, and then they show varying degrees of pigmentation, some being slaty blue in color. The terminal stage is a disfiguring white area of complete depigmentation. The lesions tend to be symmetrically arranged and usually are on the extremities (Fig. 9-5). Except in the terminal stage, spirochetes are demonstrable in lymph extracted from the lesions by dark-field examination and in the epidermis by silver impregnation of histologic sections.

The earlier lesions of the skin show a thickened epidermis with elongated papillary processes, edema, infiltration of lymphocytes, and scanty basal pigment. The corium shows an abundant perivascular leukocytic infiltration, mainly plasma cells and lymphocytes, and numerous melanophores. The late lesions are characterized by epidermal atrophy with absence of basal pigment, with many melanophores and lymphocytic accumulation in the corium. The final stage is one of epidermal atrophy with loss of papillae, complete ab-

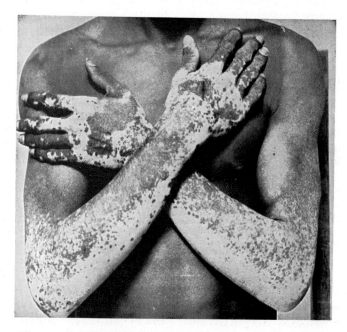

Fig. 9-5. Pinta. (Courtesy Dr. Howard Fox; from Sutton, R. L., and Sutton, R. L., Jr.: Diseases of the skin, ed. 10, St. Louis, 1939, The C. V. Mosby Co.)

sence of pigment, and fibrosis of the corium. There are lymph node lesions similar to those of syphilis but with the constant presence of melanin pigment. Aortitis and cerebrospinal fluid changes similar to those of syphilis have been described clinically in some cases.

Weil's disease (spirochetosis icterohaemorrhagica). Weil's disease (spirochetal jaundice) is a severe prostrating infection caused by the spirochete *Leptospira icterohaemorrhagiae* and characterized by sudden onset, fever, jaundice, hemorrhagic tendencies, muscle pain, and renal involvement. Spread occurs to man principally from rats, although other animals may harbor the organisms (e.g., mice, dogs, pigs, and horses). The organism is excreted in the rat's urine, and human infection occurs through the skin. The condition occurs mainly in crowded communities with unhygienic, damp living conditions, as in trenches during war. Laboratory diagnosis is most easily made by inoculation of blood into guinea pigs. Generalized jaundice is usually but not invariably present.

Damage to capillaries is shown by widely distributed minute hemorrhages. The liver is slightly enlarged and bile stained. Microscopically, one sees biliary stasis in central portions of the lobule, dissociation of hepatic cords, and degeneration of hepatic cells. Focal necrosis may be present. Regeneration of hepatic cells, particularly late in the disease, also is noted. The kidneys exhibit degeneration and necrosis in convoluted tubules and interstitial lymphocytic infiltration. Degenerative, inflammatory, and reparative changes are common in muscle fibers, particularly those of the calf or pectoral region.

Similar but much rarer leptospiral diseases are canicola fever, caused by *Leptospira canicola,* and Fort Bragg or pretibial fever, caused by *Leptospira autumnalis.*

Fusospirochetosis. A symbiotic infection caused by a spirochete *(Borrelia vincentii)* and a long fusiform bacillus *(Bacillus fusiformis)* is often referred to as Vincent's infection. The mouth is most commonly affected (trench mouth), with the production of necrotizing lesions, particularly on the pharyngeal or tonsil-

lar areas or gums. The same organisms often are associated with gangrenous bronchial and pulmonary lesions and may be found in lung abscesses, probably as secondary invaders. Genital fusospirochetal lesions also occur, particularly in persons with low resistance to infections. The genitalia and perineum are involved by ulcerative and destructive lesions, which give rise to intense local pain and foul discharge. The genital lesions are commonly considered to be venereal in nature, but there is some doubt about this. Most of the cases are probably the result of autoinoculation.

Relapsing fever. Relapsing fever is a widespread acute spirochetal disease characterized by recurring paroxysmal attacks of fever and prostration and disseminated by lice and ticks.

The louse-borne type, caused by *Borrelia recurrentis,* is spread in epidemic fashion from man to man by *Pediculus humanus.* Usually, there are one to three febrile relapses, each lasting 4 to 6 days. Spirochetes are numerous in the peripheral blood. The mortality is low in otherwise healthy persons, but it has reached 50% in epidemics during periods of famine.

The tick-borne form of relapsing fever is epizootic among rats and other rodents, and the causative spirochete, *Borrelia duttonii,* may be transmitted incidentally to man by the bite of a tick of the genus *Ornithodoros.* There are usually four or more febrile relapses, lasting 2 to 4 days. During febrile periods, spirochetes are demonstrable in the peripheral blood, and the mortality is very low.

There are no very characteristic pathologic changes. Around the malpighian bodies the spleen shows zones of hemorrhagic congestion and infiltration of neutrophilic leukocytes and mononuclear cells. Foci of necrosis are also present. Spirochetes are abundant and easily demonstrated by silver stains. The liver, kidneys, and heart show degenerative changes, and the liver also exhibits focal necrosis.

Rat-bite fever (sodoku). Rat-bite fever is usually the result of a bite by a wild rat in which the organism *Spirillum minus* is commonly parasitic. Dogs, cats, and mice also have been reported to transmit the infection. A primary lesion develops at the portal of entry, followed by recurring attacks of chills and fever, a cutaneous eruption, lymph node enlargement, leukocytosis, muscle pains, and prostration. The organism may sometimes be demonstrated in blood smears, but it is more commonly isolated from blood by inoculation of mice. The condition responds to treatment with penicillin. A clinically similar condition that also may follow a rat bite is caused by *Streptobacillus moniliformis* (Haverhill fever).

NONSPIROCHETAL VENEREAL DISEASES

Chancroid (soft chancre). Chancroidal infection, caused by *Haemophilus ducreyi,* is an acute venereal disease characterized by soft genital ulcers, which often are followed by enlargement and suppuration of inguinal lymph nodes.

Microscopically, the primary ulcer shows a superficial layer of necrotic debris, neutrophils, fibrin, and red blood cells, fringed by a zone rich in plasma cells, macrophages, and neutrophils. Small, newly formed vessels show severe endothelial swelling and proliferation in this zone. Fibroplastic proliferation is slight. The underlying deepest zone shows dense infiltration by lymphocytes and plasma cells.

Gonorrhea. See p. 126.

Granuloma inguinale. Granuloma inguinale (granuloma venereum) is a chronic ulcerative granulomatous infection involving the skin and the subcutaneous tissues of the external genitalia and the inguinal region but occasionally occurring on other parts of the body. The spread is probably by venereal means. Small intracellular coccobacillary forms *(Donovania granulomatis),* called Donovan bodies (Fig. 9-6), are present in the lesions and apparently represent the causative agent. They have been cultivated in the yolk of developing chick embryos.

The lesions show luxuriant granulation tissue, massively infiltrated by macrophages and plasma cells, with only a few lymphocytes and neutrophilic leukocytes. The pathognomonic cell in the lesion is a large mononuclear cell, 25 to 90 μ in diameter, with many intracytoplasmic clear areas filled with the deeply staining round or rodlike Donovan bodies. These bodies stain intensely with silver salts, giving a closed safety pin appearance because of their ovoid shape and intense bipolar staining. Nonspecific regional lymphadenopathy sometimes occurs. In lesions with severe fibroblastic reaction, interference with lymphatic drainage may result and lead to elephantiasis of the genitalia. Rarely, lesions may

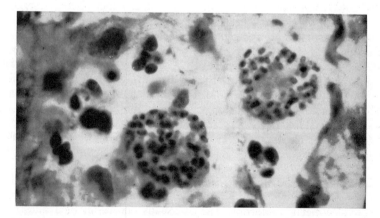

Fig. 9-6. Donovan bodies of granuloma inguinale (venereum). Those within macrophages are stained with silver. (×1900; from Torpin, R., Greenblatt, R. B., and Pund, E. R.: Am. J. Surg. **44**:551-556, 1939.)

Table 9-3. Differential features of chancre, soft chancre, lymphogranuloma venereum, and granuloma inguinale

	Etiology	Diagnostic tests	Inguinal nodes	Gross features	Microscopic pathology
Chancre	Syphilis (*Treponema pallidum*)	Demonstration of spirochete. Serologic tests for syphilis + 1 to 2 weeks after appearance of chancre	Slight enlargement, discrete, shotty	Hard, painless ulcer	Not pathognomonic; certain diagnosis depends on demonstration of spirochetes
Soft chancre chancroid	*Haemophilus ducreyi*	Intradermal test + after third week	Large, suppurative	Soft, ulcerative lesion, often multiple	Not pathognomonic, but three ill-defined zones are present
Lymphogranuloma venereum	Ornithosis-lymphogranuloma venereum agent (*Chlamydia*)	Frei test	Large (more usual in males than in females), often appear after primary lesion has subsided	Primary lesion is small, painless, nonindurated, and papular; later, may be elephantiasis and secondary ulceration and rectal stricture, especially in females	Lymph nodes show multiple stellate abscesses surrounded by mononuclear cells, including macrophages of epithelioid type
Granuloma inguinale	Donovan bodies, bacilli (*Donovania granulomatis*)	Demonstrations of Donovan bodies in smear or tissue section	Ulceration may involve inguinal region (nonspecific regional lymphadenopathy sometimes occurs)	Irregular spreading areas of ulceration (scarring may cause obstruction of lymphatics and elephantiasis of genitalia)	Specific large, mononuclear cell, with intracytoplasmic clear spaces and Donovan bodies

develop in more distant sites as a result of hematogenous spread.

Lymphogranuloma venereum. Lymphogranuloma venereum (lymphogranuloma inguinale; lymphopathia venereum) is an infection of worldwide distribution and is quite common in the United States, particularly among black people. The causative agent is not a virus, as formerly thought, but an agent similar to that responsible for ornithosis, an organism *(Chlamydia* or *Bedsonia)* intermediate between rickettsiae and viruses. Venereal spread is probably most common. An evanescent and often unnoticed primary lesion on the genitals is followed later by a variety of manifestations, such as inguinal lymph node enlargement (buboes), genital elephantiasis, rectal stricture, and warty polypoid growths about the anus, vulva, and urethra and in the rectum or the vagina. The disease has a marked predilection for lymphatic structures, with resulting lymph stasis, elephantiasis, and ulceration. Constitutional symptoms are common in the acute stage. An immunologic skin test (Frei test) and a complement fixation test are valuable diagnostic aids.

Lymphatic spread from the primary lesions leads, in males, to the formation of inguinal buboes. In females, lymphatic drainage from deeper parts of the vagina and the cervix is to pararectal and parasacral glands, and this commonly leads to inflammatory stricture of the rectum. This is the most serious manifestation of lymphogranuloma venereum. Some investigators disagree with the lymphatic theory of origin of proctitis and rectal stricture in the female and suggest other possible modes of development of these lesions: (1) anal coitus, (2) infection by way of the anal canal resulting from spillage of infected material from the vulva during coitus, and (3) direct spread of the causative organisms from the posterior wall of the vagina to the rectum. In males, rectal stricture is uncommon but may occur as a result of anal coitus.

Acute changes in the involved lymph nodes are characteristic. Minute miliary abscesses may be evident grossly. Microscopically, there are circumscribed masses of large mononuclear cells, the centers of which become necrotic with the formation of irregular or stellate-shaped abscesses containing many neutrophilic leukocytes and surrounded by densely packed mononuclear cells (Fig. 9-7). Among the latter cells are macrophages that resemble epithelioid cells and tend to be arranged in palisade fashion. An occasional Langhans' giant cell may be seen. In vulvar ele-

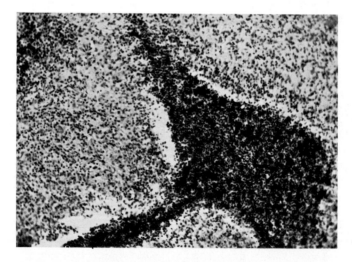

Fig. 9-7. Lymphogranuloma inguinale. Characteristic stellate abscess in lymph node. Irregular necrotic center containing neutrophilic leukocytes is surrounded by mononuclear cells.

phantiasis (esthiomene), the essential change is a thrombotic lymphangitis, with chronic edema and sclerosing fibrosis resulting in induration and enlargement of involved parts. Similar lymphangitis is present in rectal stricture, with the addition of miliary infiltrations of the muscularis by lymphocytes and plasma cells and ulceration of the mucosa. Rarely, systemic lesions have been described, apparently caused by hematogenous dissemination.

On transmission of the causative agent to mice by the intracranial route, clusters of elementary bodies similar to those of ornithosis may be seen in mononuclear cells composing the exudate in the meninges and in the substance of the brain. The infective agent may be grown in the yolk sac of the chick embryo, smears from which show the elementary bodies.

REFERENCES

American Medical News **13:**4, 1970 (editorial—VD pandemic).

Black-Schaffer, B., and Rosahn, P. D.: Am. J. Syph. Gon. Vener. Dis. **28:**27-43, 1944 (syphilis).

Brooks, S. E. H., et al.: Arch. Pathol. Lab. Med. **103:**451-455, 1979 (hepatic changes in secondary syphilis).

Brown, T. M., and Nunemaker, J. C.: Bull. Johns Hopkins Hosp. **70:**210-327, 1942 (rat-bite fever).

D'Aunoy, R., and von Haam, E.: Arch. Pathol. **27:**1032-1082, 1939 (lymphogranuloma venereum).

De Brito, T., et al.: Virchows Arch. [Pathol. Anat.] **342:**61-69, 1967 (liver in human leptospirosis).

Ferris, H. W., and Turner, T. B.: Arch. Pathol. **24:**703-737, 1937 (yaws).

Fleming, W. L., et al.: J.A.M.A. **211:**1827-1830, 1970 (venereal disease in 1968).

von Haam, E.: Am. J. Trop. Med. **18:**595-608, 1938 (venereal fusospirochetosis).

Harris, W. D. M., and Cave, V. G.: J.A.M.A. **194:**1312-1313, 1965 (congenital syphilis).

Hoeprich, P. D., editor: Infectious diseases, ed. 2, New York, 1977, Harper & Row, Publishers, Inc.

Kowal, J.: N. Engl. J. Med. **264:**123-128, 1961(rat-bite fever).

Lee, T. J.: J.A.M.A. **242:**1187-1189, 1979 (discussion of diagnostic serologic tests for syphilis).

Marshall, A., and Brown, J.: Br. J. Surg. **48:**340-341, 1960 (genital fusospirochetosis).

Nicholas, L., and Beerman, H.: Am. J. Med. Sci. **254:**549-569, 1967 (late syphilis).

Olansky, S.: Med. Clin. North Am. **48:**653-665, 1964 (syphilis).

Rosahn, P. D., and Black-Schaffer, B.: Am. J. Syph. Gon. Vener. Dis. **28:**142-164, 1944 (syphilis).

Rosahn, P. D., and Black-Schaffer, B.: Arch. Intern. Med. **72:**78-90, 1943 (syphilis).

Sheldon, W. H., and Heyman, A.: Am. J. Pathol. **22:**415-425, 1946 (chancroid).

Sigel, M. M., editor: Lymphogranuloma venereum, Coral Gables, Fla., 1962, University of Miami Press.

Top, F. H., Sr., and Wehrle, P. F., editors: Communicable and infectious diseases, ed. 8, St. Louis, 1976, The C. V. Mosby Co.

Wright, D. J. M., and Doniach, D.: Proc. R. Soc. Med. **64:**419-422, 1971 (immunology of syphilis).

10

Mycotic, protozoan, and helminthic infections

Mycotic infections

Fungi are cellular filamentous plants belonging to a division called Thallophyta. Because of the absence of chlorophyll, they must obtain food from organic material already synthesized. They may be saprophytic or parasitic, i.e., they may obtain their food from dead organic material or from a living organism. Fungal infections are not rare in man and frequently are serious. Yeasts and fungi may be stained prominently in tissue sections by means of the periodic acid–Schiff, methenamine silver, mucin (for capsules of some organisms, e.g., cryptococci), and acridine orange fluorescent stains. Superficial involvement of skin or mucous membrane is a common type of fungal infection, as in athlete's foot and thrush. The more serious types of parasitic fungi produce widespread chronic destructive lesions. In some of the fungal infections, the inflammatory response and tissue damage are the result of hypersensitivity to the fungal antigens. Fungi that are ordinarily saprophytic, such as *Aspergillus, Mucor,* and *Candida,* are producing infection with increasing frequency in patients receiving prolonged antibiotic, immunosuppressive, or steroid therapy and in those with predisposing diseases such as diabetes mellitus and leukemia.

Dermatomycosis. The term *dermatomy-*

cosis literally means "cutaneous fungal infection." Although it suggests any fungal infection of the skin, whether superficial or associated with deep or systemic mycoses, the term is generally used for the fungal infections affecting primarily the epidermis and/or its appendages (hair and nails). These are usually caused by fungi of the dermatophyte group *(Trichophyton, Microsporum,* and *Epidermophyton)* but also may be caused by *Candida* organisms, which are considered later, or by a few other fungi, such as *Malassezia furfur,* the agent responsible for *pityriasis (tinea) versicolor.*

Dermatophytosis refers to the group of infections caused by the dermatophytes, i.e., the common "ringworm" infections or "tineas," so designated in antiquity because of the circular or ringlike appearance of many of the lesions and the mistaken idea that the cause was a worm or insect (L. *tinea,* worm, larva, or grub). The tineas are usually named according to the site of the lesions, e.g., *tinea pedis* (athlete's foot), *tinea capitis* (scalp), *tinea corporis* (general body surface), *tinea unguium* (nails), and *tinea cruris* ("jock itch" of groin). Microscopically, the fungi are demonstrated in the keratinized portion of the epidermis, the nails, and within or on the external surface of the hair shafts, and a nonspecific type of inflammatory response of varying degree or no inflammation at all may be present. In some patients, hypersensitivity to the fungus leads to the development of sterile papular and vesicular lesions on the hands (dermatophytids).

Actinomycosis. Actinomycosis is a chronic suppurative infection caused by *Actinomyces bovis* (principally in cattle) and *Actinomyces israelii* (common in man). In cattle, the disease is known as "lumpy jaw." *Actinomyces* organisms are normally present in the mouth. Although related to the true bacteria, they also exhibit some features similar to those of the higher filamentous fungi. The organism grows in the tissues in colonies composed of a tangled, felted mass of filaments, surrounded by radiating projections known as "clubs" (hence, the term *ray fungus*). Club formation occurs only in tissues, not in culture, and is thought to be a reaction on the part of the organism to the surrounding tissues. A protein substance encasing the terminal clubs makes them eosinophilic. When pus from a lesion is spread in a thin layer on a glass slide, the actinomycotic colonies may be seen grossly as yellow "sulfur granules." Infection caused by the aerobic, partially acid-fast *Nocardia asteroides* are relatively rare but result in a similar disease. A granulomatous nocardiosis caused by an intracellular organism has been described.

Some break in skin or mucous membrane is apparently necessary to allow entrance of the actinomycetes into the body. A direct contagion has not been proved. The infection is geographically widespread. The mouth, jaws, and face are most commonly affected, with the intestinal tract the next most frequently involved area, particularly the ileocecal region and appendix. In the latter, the infection may be mistaken clinically for chronic appendicitis and after surgery may leave a chronic sinus. The liver often becomes involved in any type of abdominal actinomycosis. Occasionally, the fallopian tubes are infected. Pulmonary actinomycosis may simulate a chronic abscess, caused by ordinary pyogenic bacteria, or tuberculosis.

The characteristic lesions are chronic abscesses resulting from progressive penetration and destruction of tissue. Many leukocytes are present in the zone of suppuration, surrounded by a wall of granulation tissue containing many mononuclear cells and occasional giant cells. In older areas, there is distinct connective tissue formation. Histologic diagnosis depends on finding the ray fungus in the abscesses.

In the cervicofacial type, the lesion usually starts in the gums and spreads to the submaxillary region, where there may be tumorlike masses or soft suppurating lesions and chronic sinuses from which pus escapes. Occasionally, the primary lesion is in the skin. Intestinal involvement produces a chronic inflammatory mass and may lead to suppurating sinuses. Spread to the liver by the portal bloodstream results in multiple, small, ragged abscess cavities. The thoracic type begins in the bronchioles and subsequently involves the pulmonary parenchyma and pleura, with eventual perforation of the chest wall.

Spread is rarely through lymphatics but is usually by direct extension or occasionally by the bloodstream. Actinomycotic septicemia may result in metastatic abscesses in various organs and tissues.

Mycetoma pedis (Madura foot). Mycetoma pedis is a chronic suppurative infection of the foot caused by a variety of fungi or funguslike organisms that may be differentiated by cultural studies. Granules representing colonies of the organism are found in the tissues and in discharged pus. About half the cases are caused by certain members of the order Actinomycetales, such as *Nocardia brasiliensis, Nocardia caviae,* or *Streptomyces* sp. (actinomycetoma), and the remainder are caused by a variety of true fungi, e.g., *Madurella mycetomi, Madurella grisea,* or *Monosporium apiospermum* (maduromycosis or Madura foot).

Aspergillosis. Most members of the genus *Aspergillus* are saprophytic and nonpathogenic. Some are found as harmless invaders of the external auditory canal, nasal sinuses, and external genitalia and as secondary invaders in lung abscesses.

In involvement of the ear, the external auditory canal may be partly filled with foul moist material spotted with black granules. The lung appears to be the most common site of important infection. The pulmonary lesion may be in the form of a bronchopneumonia, abscesses, small infarcts (resulting from thrombosis caused by vascular invasion by organisms), or a mass of *Aspergillus* mycelia ("fungus ball") in a cavity that may be newly formed or may be a preexisting inflammatory (e.g., tuberculous) or carcinomatous cavity. Chronic granulomatous reaction to the organisms in the lungs also has been reported.

A primary fatal disseminated infection is uncommon, but generalized aspergillosis as a secondary complication is more frequent and tends to occur in patients with debilitating disease and in those who have received steroid or antibiotic therapy. The resulting disease in various tissues or organs is characterized by abscesses, necrotizing lesions, and sometimes chronic granulomatous inflammation.

Candidosis (moniliasis). The *Candida* species of fungi (formerly called *Monilia*) are commonly found in the mouth, intestinal tract, and vagina of normal individuals. *Candida albicans* is the most common cause of candidosis.

A common form of the disease known as *thrush* affects the oral mucosa (tongue, gums, lips, and cheeks) or the pharynx and is most often seen in debilitated infants and children. The lesions, which appear as white patches on the mucosa, consist of an abundant growth of yeast cells and hyphae, with a nonspecific acute or subacute inflammation in the underlying tissue. Similar lesions occur on the vulvovaginal mucosa, particularly in diabetic and pregnant women. The skin may be affected, especially in moist areas, e.g., the perineum, the inframammary folds, and between the fingers.

Lesions of the nails (onychia) and about the nails (paronychia) may occur. Occasionally, esophageal (Fig. 10-1), bronchopulmonary, and widely disseminated forms of candidosis are observed. Invasiveness is favored by lowered resistance of the host, as may occur in

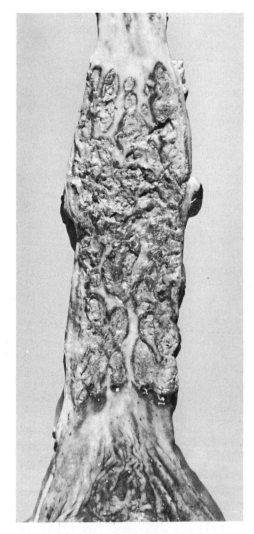

Fig. 10-1. Esophageal candidosis in patient with leukemia. (Courtesy Dr. J. F. Kuzma.)

association with various debilitating illnesses and intensive antibiotic, immunosuppressive, or steroid therapy. Candidial endocarditis has been reported in drug addicts, following the intravenous injection of narcotics, and as a complication of cardiac surgery.

Phycomycosis. Phycomycosis is an uncommon infection of the lungs, ears, nervous system, and intestinal tract caused by a fungus that is more commonly encountered as a saprophyte or contaminant. The lesions may show an intense necrotizing and suppurative inflammatory process in which the irregularly branching coenocytic or nonseptate filaments of the fungus are seen. Although this infection is commonly called "mucormycosis," there are several species of Phycomycetes that may be causative, including *Mucor, Rhizopus,* and *Absidia*. These fungi have a tendency to invade vessels, causing thrombosis and infarction.

Phycomycosis is especially seen in patients with uncontrolled diabetes mellitus, leukemia, and other debilitating diseases and in those receiving antibiotics, corticosteroids, chemotherapeutic agents for cancer, and irradiation.

Histoplasmosis. Histoplasmosis (reticuloendothelial cytomycosis) is an infection caused by an oval, yeastlike organism (1 to 4 μ in diameter), *Histoplasma capsulatum*. The disease was discovered and named by Darling in 1906. The causative organism was recognized as a yeast by Rocha-Lima in 1912 and was cultured by DeMonbreun in 1933. Widespread occurrence of the disease and prevalence in the United States have been recognized, as evidenced by positive histoplasmin skin tests, which indicate past or present infection, and by specific serologic tests that indicate active disease. Positive diagnosis depends on finding the organisms in cultures of the sputum, blood, or bone marrow or in biopsied tissue such as lymph nodes.

The infection is not spread between individuals but appears to be from soil contaminated by fecal material of chickens, pigeons, starlings, other birds, and bats. In South Africa, most of the recognized benign pulmonary infections seem to have been acquired from contaminated caves (cave disease). Endemic areas of histoplasmosis have been found in many parts of the world, particularly near large rivers and where there is high humidity with warm temperatures. In some endemic areas of the United States, histoplasmin skin tests have indicated that 70% to 85% of the population have had an infection. Fewer than one in 1,000 develop active progressive disease, perhaps from endogenous reinfection. The lungs are believed to be the usual portal of entry of the organisms.

From developing knowledge of the disease, it appears that histoplasmosis can be roughly categorized into four forms: acute pulmonary, chronic pulmonary, acute disseminated, and chronic disseminated.

The *acute pulmonary* form may be asymptomatic or symptomatic. The basic reaction in the lungs and lymph nodes consists of foci of tuberculoid granulomas that tend to heal. Most instances of histoplasmosis are benign, asymptomatic pulmonary infections, with positive histoplasmin skin test and healed calcified nodules in the lung and peribronchial lymph nodes, often resembling the healed primary complex of tuberculosis. The symptomatic pulmonary infections may be either mild and "flulike" or more severe, resembling atypical pneumonia. Usually the prognosis is good. Multiple pulmonary infiltrations, with or without hilar lymphadenopathy, may be demonstrated in roentgenograms of the chest and, in the more prolonged cases, tend to calcify and simulate healed miliary tuberculosis. In some patients, a localized pulmonary tuberculoid granulomatous lesion with caseation necrosis, calcification, and fibrotic border (histoplasmoma) may occur, appearing in the roentgenogram of the chest as a "coin" lesion. This lesion is sometimes removed surgically because of the clinical suspicion of lung cancer.

The *chronic pulmonary* form of histoplasmosis is progressive, forming granulomatous inflammation with caseation necrosis and cavitation, and frequently is misdiagnosed as pulmonary tuberculosis, or it may occur in association with tuberculosis. It is seen most commonly in middle-aged and elderly men and has a poor prognosis.

The *acute disseminated* form of the disease may be either benign or progressive, the latter being fatal, and may occur at any age, but particularly in the young and elderly. The spleen, lymph nodes, and liver are enlarged. There is a septic-type fever, with anemia and leukopenia. Bone marrow smears may reveal the organisms or granulomas, and sometimes the organisms may be found in mononuclear cells in blood smears.

The *chronic disseminated* form occurs mainly in elderly people and is usually fatal.

The characteristic pathologic change in disseminated forms is a widespread reticuloendothelial hyperplasia, with a large number of the oval organisms within phagocytic cells (Fig. 10-2). A clear halo about the organisms produces a capsulelike effect. Organs most commonly involved are the spleen, liver, lymph nodes, lungs, bone marrow, oral mucosa, adrenal glands, and intestines. Hyperplasia of endothelial cells lining small blood vessels may lead to partial or complete occlusion of their lumina. Ulcerations of the colon, tongue, larynx, and pharynx and a patchy

pneumonitis are also common. Vegetative endocarditis has occurred. In certain organs, particularly the adrenal glands, caseation necrosis may occur. Organisms in these necrotic areas are often atypical, being distorted and larger than the usual *Histoplasma*. Adrenal involvement has eventuated in Addison's disease.

Cryptococcosis. Cryptococcosis (torulosis; European blastomycosis) is a mycotic disease caused by *Cryptococcus neoformans (Cryptococcus hominis; Torula histolytica),* a budding, yeastlike, nonmycelial fungus characterized by a mucinous capsule. Although not a frequent infection, it is geographically widespread, affects all ages (two thirds of cases are between the ages of 30 and 60 years), and is the commonest cause of mycotic meningitis. The meninges, brain, and lungs are most of-

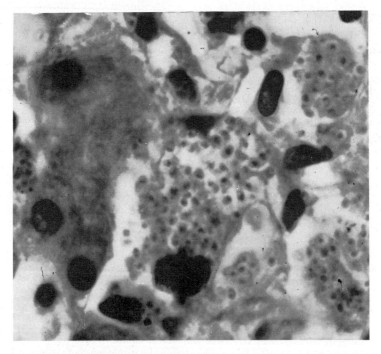

Fig. 10-2. Histoplasmosis of liver. Oval or round form of *Histoplasma capsulatum* in reticuloendothelial cells (Kupffer cells and macrophages). From fatal case of progressive systemic histoplasmosis in infant. (From Baker, R. D.: Fungal, actinomycetic, and algal infections. In Anderson, W. A. D., and Kissane, J. M., editors: Pathology, ed. 7, St. Louis, 1977, The C. V. Mosby Co.)

ten involved, but skin, mucous membranes, and other organs occasionally are affected. Nervous system involvement is usually fatal, whereas a localized lesion elsewhere may be amenable to surgical excision. *Cryptococcus neoformans* has been isolated from soil and pigeon droppings. The portal of entry into the body is not apparent but is believed to be usually the respiratory tract, from which the organisms make their way to the central nervous system and other sites.

Meningeal cryptococcosis is characterized by pale, grayish, mucoid, translucent nodules or a diffuse exudate. In about half the patients, there are intracerebral lesions. The basal ganglia and the midbrain, as well as the cortex, may be involved. There is little cellular reaction to the infection, particularly in the nervous system, where the organisms are in small cystlike spaces filled with the mucoid material of the capsular polysaccharide (Fig. 10-3). Less common are granulomatous lesions. In the lungs, there may be widespread involvement or localized lesions. Histiocytic cells may be numerous, and the organisms may be within macrophages or may be extracellular. Older lesions may be more granulomatous, with some giant cells and fibrosis.

Skin lesions are usually the result of systemic infection, but sometimes they are isolated, suggesting that the organisms occasionally may enter the body through the skin. These lesions may remain localized or may spread to the central nervous system. Systemic cryptococcosis may develop as a terminal infection in patients with leukemia or malignant lymphoma.

The *Cryptococcus* organism appears in tissues as a spherical or ovoid budding cell, 5 to 10 μ in diameter, with a mucinous capsule up to five times the diameter of the cell proper. The capsule, which fails to stain by usual histologic methods and appears as a clear halo, may be stained by mucicarmine or by certain stains for acid mucopolysaccharides. No mycelia are formed. In pulmonary and meningeal infections, the organisms may be found in fresh unstained preparations of sputum and spinal fluid, and the capsule may be rendered prominent by mixture with India ink.

North American blastomycosis (Gilchrist's disease). Infection with *Blastomyces dermatitidis,* a yeastlike organism, is largely restricted to the North American continent. It most commonly involves the skin and lungs but also may be more widely systemic. The

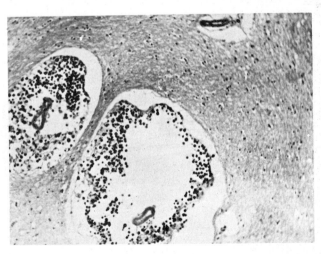

Fig. 10-3. Cerebral cryptococcosis. Cystic areas in cerebral tissue contain numerous small, round, yeastlike organisms.

primary site of the infection is almost always pulmonary. The cutaneous type forms a chronic or subacute ulcer. In systemic blastomycosis, there may be widespread involvement of the lungs, subcutaneous tissue, nervous system, internal organs, bones, and joints.

Blastomycetes are round or oval unicellular organisms about 20 μ in diameter and have a thick, refractile, double-contoured cell wall (Fig. 3-4). Reproduction takes place in the tissues by budding (Fig. 10-4).

The cutaneous lesions occur most frequently on the face, hands, and legs. They begin as papules, which slowly ulcerate and extend at the margin. Minute abscesses, frequently showing individual organisms within them, are present in and beneath the epidermis, and the surrounding tissue is infiltrated by lymphocytes, plasma cells, macrophages, fibroblasts, and neutrophilic leukocytes. Giant cells are often present and may contain organisms in their cytoplasm. Certain diagnosis depends on seeing the organisms in the tissue. The epidermis often undergoes pronounced hyperplasia with irregular extensions downward into the dermis, simulating carcinoma *(pseudoepitheliomatous* or *pseudocarcinomatous hyperplasia).* Pulmonary disease is characterized by chronic suppurative and granu-lomatous inflammation, sometimes with foci of caseation necrosis. Blastomycetes are found within and outside of giant cells.

South American blastomycosis (paracoccidioidal granuloma) is similar to the North American blastomycosis, but the organisms in the tissues show multiple buds, and lesions of lymph nodes and mucous membranes are prominent.

Coccidioidomycosis and coccidioidal granuloma. Infection with the fungus *Coccidioides immitis* is endemic in the southwestern United States, particularly California, but a few cases have been reported in other parts of the Americas. Warm, dry, and dusty areas apparently are suitable for spread of the infective arthrospores. The portal of entry is the respiratory tract, but abrasions of the skin are believed to have been the site of entry of the organisms in exceptional cases. In most patients, the infection is focalized in the lungs, is self-limited, and is asymptomatic. More severe but self-limited infections may be manifested by an acute respiratory illness (influenzal or pneumonic form). This is the form sometimes referred to as valley fever or San Joaquin fever. Sensitivity to the fungus, as manifested by a skin test with coccidioidin, develops 10 to 40 days after infection, and transient humoral antibodies (precipitins and

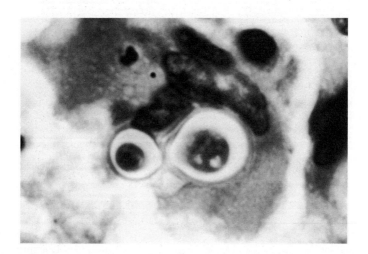

Fig. 10-4. *Blastomyces dermatitidis* in giant cell, reproducing by budding (see also Fig. 3-4).

complement fixation) may be detectable. The allergy as shown by reaction to coccidioidin remains, and the patient, after recovery, is highly resistant to reinfection. In a few patients, manifestations of erythema nodosum or erythema multiforme develop.

In a small proportion of infections, instead of arrest there is a progressive or disseminated coccidioidomycosis (coccidioidal granuloma), and in such cases the mortality is high. The lungs, skin, bones, and lymph nodes are involved most frequently. The central nervous system also may be affected. The condition is easily mistaken for tuberculosis or blastomycosis. Diagnostic proof depends on demonstrating the fungus either by culture and animal inoculation or microscopically in tissue. In tissues, the organism may be found free or in giant cells as a rounded body (spherule), 5 to 70 μ in diameter, with a highly refractile, double-contoured wall. Some organisms contain endospores. Reproduction by endosporu-

lation differentiates the organisms from blastomycetes, which reproduce by budding.

Morphologically, the lesions in the lungs resemble those of tuberculosis, with tubercle-like foci and varying degrees of caseation necrosis. Although predominantly granulomatous, a suppurative reaction with micro-abscesses is often a concomitant feature. Organisms may be seen in the lesions, some of which show endospores (Fig. 10-5). Fibrocaseous foci may undergo cavitation. Pleural involvement and regional lymphadenopathy occur. Healed or arrested disease is evidenced by residual nodules in the lung and mediastinal lymph nodes, similar to the primary complex of tuberculosis, or by a single solid parenchymal lesion (coccidioidoma), or by a thin-walled cavity. In progressive disease, the active lesions in the lungs become more widespread, and with dissemination, abscesses and granulomatous foci (tuberclelike lesions) appear in many organs. These lesions may sim-

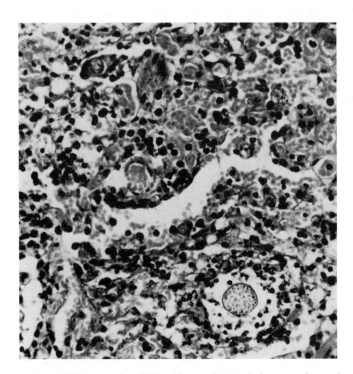

Fig. 10-5. Coccidioidomycosis of lung. Note endosporulating organism at bottom.

ulate those of blastomycosis, but differentiation is possible by recognition of the endosporulating organisms. In the skin lesion, as in blastomycosis, pseudoepitheliomatous or pseudocarcinomatous hyperplasia of the epidermis occurs.

Rhinosporidiosis. Rhinosporidiosis is a chronic infection with *Rhinosporidium seeberi,* an endosporulating organism that produces polypoid or pedunculated tumorlike masses on the nasal mucosa. The condition is rare in the United States and is reported most commonly from Ceylon and India.

Sporotrichosis. The fact that sporotrichosis, an uncommon fungal infection, occurs mainly in farmers and nurserymen suggests that spread may be from plants. The primary lesion is usually on the skin of the arms or hands, and apparently it is related to a minor puncture wound, such as a thorn prick. The inflammation is a combined granulomatous and suppurative type. The skin lesions are usually multiple, ulcerative, and easily mistaken for gummas (Fig. 10-6). Frequently, they are situated along the course of the lymphatics, which become thickened. The fungus, *Spo-*

rothrix (Sporotrichum) schenckii, appears in the involved tissue as a small, spindle-shaped, single-celled gram-positive organism. Only rarely does dissemination occur throughout the body to cause visceral lesions. In the disseminated forms, it is possible that the respiratory and intestinal tracts are portals of entry.

The causative organisms are few and difficult to demonstrate in the tissues in the usual case of human sporotrichosis, but they tend to appear in large numbers and are more readily demonstrated in lesions of human disseminated disease, as well as in the experimental disease in mice.

Chromoblastomycosis. Relatively uncommon but occurring in widely distributed areas, chromoblastomycosis is an infection by moldlike pigmented fungi belonging to the genera *Hormodendrum* and *Phialophora.* It occurs mainly in farmers or persons having contact with vegetation and affects the skin, usually of an extremity, producing a verrucous dermatitis. It does not become systemic.

The lesions may be papular, verrucous, or ulcerative. Microscopic diagnosis is made by

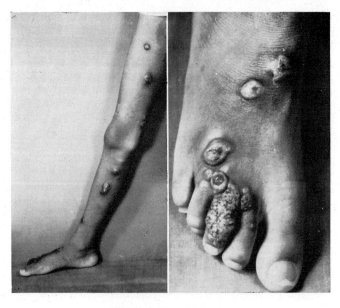

Fig. 10-6. Sporotrichosis.

finding the brown, thick-walled, rounded septate cells of the fungus in the lesion (Fig. 10-7). Epithelial proliferation, sometimes pseudoepitheliomatous, may be prominent, and a cellular reaction with plasma cells, macrophages, and multinucleated giant cells commonly occurs. Microabscesses also are frequently present.

Protothecosis. Protothecosis is an uncommon disease that is worthy of mention since it is being recognized more frequently and the etiologic agent in the tissues may be mistaken for certain of the common fungi. It is caused by unicellular, achlorophyllous organisms of the *Prototheca* species, which morphologically bear a close resemblance to certain unicellular algae. Generally, they are regarded as achloric algae, although some investigators have considered them to be fungi or funguslike. In man, protothecosis has been observed to be of the cutaneous type, whereas in lower animals a systemic form with cutaneous involvement has been found. The human lesions have been confined to the epidermis and dermis and are usually characterized by hyperkeratosis and chronic granulomatous inflammation with minimal cellular reaction consisting of lymphocytes, histiocytes, a few neutrophils, and eosinophils. The etiologic agents may be demonstrated in the tissues by Gomori methenamine silver or Gridley stains or by fluorescent antibody stain. Characteristic endosporulating cells, which differ from those of *Coccidioides immitis,* may be seen, but if they are not present the *Prototheca* cells may resemble nonsporulation cells of well-known fungi (e.g., *Blastomyces dermatitidis, Cryptococcus neoformans,* and nonreproductive stages of *Coccidioides immitis).*

Protozoan infections

The main protozoan diseases in man are amebiasis (caused by *Entamoeba histolytica),* malaria (caused by sporozoa of the genus

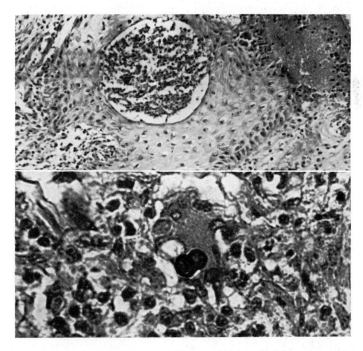

Fig. 10-7. Chromoblastomycosis. Note dark, thick-walled organisms in tiny epidermal abscess (top) and in giant cell (bottom).

Plasmodium), trypanosomiasis, and leish-maniasis.

Amebiasis. The pathogenic *Entamoeba histolytica* is an actively motile and phagocytic organism 20 to 30 μ in diameter. It has a single, delicate, barely distinguishable nucleus. The trophozoite (not the cyst) form penetrates the tissue of the large intestine, causing characteristic chronic ulcers (Fig. 10-8). Its presence may or may not be associated with the clinical symptoms of amebic dysentery. Metastasis of the amebae through the portal vein to the liver results in liver "abscess."

Human infection results from ingestion of mature amebic cysts, usually in contaminated food or water. After ingestion, the cysts pass through the stomach, unchanged, into the small intestine. Excystation of the cysts, which begins in the terminal ileum, is followed by development of a colony of trophozoites in the cecum and their establishment throughout the colon. It is possible that trophozoites may remain as commensal organisms in the lumen of the intestines without giving rise to clinical disease, although some investigators believe that in all cases there is tissue penetration by the trophozoites, associated with varying degrees of clinical and pathologic manifestations. According to the latter view, asymptomatic cases may occur in

which the lesions are too small to be detected. Some of the trophozoites become encysted in the lumen of the colon. At first, the cysts are immature and contain one nucleus, but by successive nuclear division they become quadrinucleated, and it is the latter mature form that is transmissible to man.

When trophozoites invade the mucosa of the intestine, they produce lysis of the tissue by means of their enzymes. At first, the lesions are minute, almost pinpoint-sized. The amebae then penetrate the submucosa and extend laterally, producing large, characteristically undermined and flask-shaped ulcers (Figs. 10-9 and 10-10). The ulcers have shaggy, yellowish brown edges and a floor formed by submucous or muscular coats. Initially, there is very little inflammatory cell infiltration except for a few mononuclear cells. Secondary bacterial infection from the intestine is usual, and this results in further tissue destruction and leukocytic infiltration. Granulation tissue appears later in the bases of the ulcers. A fibrinous serositis may be caused by amebae migrating through the wall of the colon to the serosal surface. In severe cases, there may be perforation of muscular and serous coats and general peritonitis or adhesions to neighboring structures. The cecum, flexures, and rectum are common sites, but any portion of the large

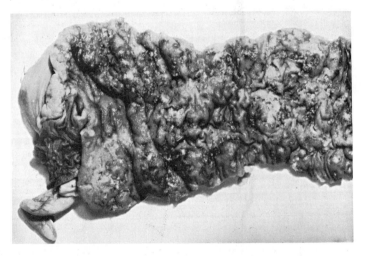

Fig. 10-8. Amebic colitis. Note shaggy and irregular areas of ulceration.

bowel, including the appendix, may be involved. The small intestine is rarely affected. Occasionally, a localized mass of granulation tissue may occur in the wall of the colon, secondary to amebic ulceration. Such a lesion, known as "amebic granuloma" or "ameboma," may be mistaken for carcinoma of the colon clinically or, when in the cecum, may simulate simple appendicitis. Microscopically, the ameboma consists of fibrous tissue, lymphocytes, plasma cells, and eosinophils.

Liver "abscess" is the most frequent complication. It may be single or multiple and have a diameter of a few millimeters or many centimeters. The lining is rough and shaggy, and in older "abscesses" there is a connective tissue wall. The contents are grumous, semifluid, and yellowish red or chocolate colored. Microscopically, the amebae are found in the edge of living tissue and in the adjacent necrotic material. True pus is not present, unless secondary bacterial infection occurs, but the term *abscess* is commonly used for these liquefied, necrotic, amebic lesions. Occasionally, transportation of the organisms by hepatic veins results in a similar lung "abscess." However, the most frequent cause of these pulmonary lesions is direct extension of an hepatic "abscess" through the diaphragm.

***Balantidium coli* infections.** See p. 547.

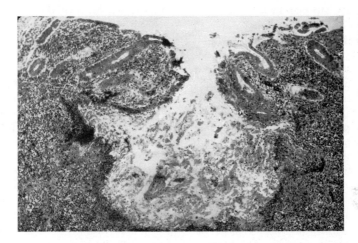

Fig. 10-9. Amebic ulcer of colon. Note undermining of edges and characteristic shape. (AFIP.)

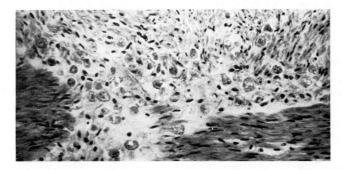

Fig. 10-10. Amebic colitis. Amebae in submucosa and invading muscularis. Note absence of any significant tissue reaction. (AFIP.)

Malaria. Malaria is an infection with a protozoan parasite that has an asexual cycle in man and a sexual cycle in the *Anopheles* mosquito. The parasite is a sporozoan, and three common species infect man, causing three types of the disease: *Plasmodium vivax* (vivax or tertian malaria), *Plasmodium malariae* (quartan malaria), and *Plasmodium falciparum* (falciparum, estivoautumnal, or malignant tertian malaria). A rare fourth type is that caused by *Plasmodium ovale* (ovale malaria). They differ in the interval of time required for the completion of a cycle in man, with paroxysms of chills occurring at the time of sporulation.

Life cycle. The parasite (in the form of sporozoites) is injected into man by the bite of an infected female *Anopheles* mosquito. After an exoerythrocytic phase of 7 to 10 days within hepatic cells, the parasite reaches the bloodstream and invades a red blood cell, where it enlarges and matures, producing a characteristic large form (schizont) that can be identified by appropriate stains of a blood smear. The intracellular parasite makes use of the hemoglobin in the red cell, using up the protein fraction and leaving the "heme" portion as a brownish, granular "malarial" pigment, which is a form of hematin and not melanin. By intracellular division, the large form breaks up into a number of small forms (merozoites). Rupture of the red cell releases the pigment and merozoites into the bloodstream. Each of these attacks a new red cell, and the asexual cycle (schizogony) is repeated. The time taken for completion of this cycle is quite uniform and constant for the particular type of parasite. Consequently, large numbers mature and rupture into the bloodstream at about the same time and produce the characteristic malarial chill, which recurs at regular intervals.

A few of the intracellular parasites develop male and female sexual forms, called microgametocytes and macrogametocytes, respectively. These forms, when released into the bloodstream, do not reenter new red cells but perish unless taken into the stomach of an anopheline mosquito along with its blood meal. Here, they undergo maturation into microgametes and macrogametes during the early phase of the sexual cycle (sporogony). Subsequently, the microgametes and macrogametes fuse to produce a motile fertilized form (zygote), which penetrates the wall of the stomach and forms a cyst (oocyst). Large numbers of spores (sporozoites) develop within this cyst, eventually reach the salivary glands of the mosquito, and are ready to infect the next person bitten.

General pathology. Pathologic changes in malaria are dependent on the following factors:

1 Large numbers of red cells are parasitized and destroyed, with the production of a secondary anemia.

2 The malarial pigment (hematin) is a peculiar breakdown product of hemoglobin and is produced in large amounts. It does not occur normally in the body and is not an intermediate product in the breakdown of hemoglobin and the formation of bile pigment. The pigment is taken up by phagocytic cells of the reticuloendothelial system. The resulting reticuloendothelial hyperplasia contributes to enlargement of the spleen and liver. The deposited pigment imparts a slaty gray or grayish black color to the enlarged spleen and, to a lesser extent, discolors the liver.

3 Obstruction of small blood vessels is probably the most important factor in the pathology of malaria. This is seen particularly in *Plasmodium falciparum* malaria and is mainly caused by the formation of small agglutinated masses of parasitized and pigmented erythrocytes. An undue stickiness of the surfaces of the parasitized red blood cells is apparently responsible for the agglutination, and the malarial pigment may be a factor in the pathogenesis of this process. The vascular obstructions result in insufficient blood supply to various tissues. In certain organs (e.g., the brain), this ischemia may result in dysfunction or even the development of small areas of necrosis.

Lesions in individual organs. In addition to the characteristic changes in the spleen, liver, bone marrow, nervous system, and kidneys in malaria as noted in the following paragraphs, the plasmodia may be demonstrated in properly stained sections of tissues, e.g., in the parasitized erythrocytes in capillaries and in phagocytic cells of the spleen, liver (Kupffer cells), bone marrow, and other organs.

The *spleen* may be greatly enlarged and is discolored a slaty gray or grayish black. Microscopically, an enormous amount of pigment is seen in phagocytic cells. The *liver* is usually only slightly enlarged and discolored. Microscopically, pigment is seen in the Kupffer cells lining the sinusoids. Occasionally, small focal areas of necrosis are present. In the *bone marrow,* some hyperplasia and retention of pigment are evident microscopically.

In the *nervous system,* tiny areas of hemorrhage and focal necrosis with softening may be found in the brain and cord. Cerebral involvement occurs particularly with severe *Plasmodium falciparum* infections. Small blood vessels here, as in other tissues, appear congested and obstructed with agglutinated masses of parasitized red cells. In cases not too rapidly fatal, the so-called malarial granuloma of Dürck may be found. Around a central occluded capillary is an area of necrotic tissue, surrounded in turn by a zone of extravasated red cells and proliferating neuroglial cells. The necrotic material is removed, and a cellular nodule of neuroglial cells remains. The effects of cerebral lesions in malaria depend on their position and extent.

Usually, no gross changes are evident in the *kidneys.* Mild microscopic changes occur constantly. These are mainly tubular degenerations and blockage of tubules by casts. In certain cases, as in the complication called blackwater fever, the renal changes are severe. *Blackwater fever,* associated particularly with malignant malaria, is characterized by sudden, massive intravascular hemolysis. There is an intense hemoglobinuria, with the passage of red or reddish black urine. This complication is usually fatal. The reason for its development in certain cases is unknown, although an immunologic explanation for the massive hemolysis has been suggested. The kidneys show marked degeneration, particularly of the convoluted tubules, and many tubules contain pigment casts. The renal changes

are similar to those of hemoglobinuric nephrosis (p. 352).

Leishmaniasis. Leishmaniasis is a tropical condition caused by protozoan parasites with a complex life cycle. Transmission is by the *Phlebotomus* fly (sandfly). The four main types of *Leishmania (donovani, tropica, mexicana,* and *brasiliensis)* are morphologically indistinguishable.

Leishmania donovani produces the disease kala-azar (visceral leishmaniasis), prevalent in India and parts of China but also occurring in the Mediterranean region, east Africa, and parts of Central and South America. The organism can be seen in phagocytic cells of the reticuloendothelial system. The intracellular parasites in tissue sections resemble *Histoplasma* but can be differentiated by the presence of the kinetoplast. The spleen is greatly enlarged.

Leishmania tropica produces the oriental sore (Old World cutaneous leishmaniasis), a chronic granulomatous ulcer, prevalent in areas of central Asia and the Middle East, in the Mediterranean region, and in parts of Africa. In this disease, one or more cutaneous ulcers appear on the extremities or face. *Leishmania mexicana* produces a similar disease (New World cutaneous leishmaniasis) that occurs widely in Central and South America. In Mexico (Yucatan) and northern Guatemala, the disease commonly involves the ear, especially among chicle workers (Chiclero ulcer).

Leishmania brasiliensis (American leishmaniasis; mucocutaneous leishmaniasis) results in chronic granulomatous ulcers similar to the oriental sore. There is a distinct tendency to involvement of the skin and mucosa of the mouth, nose, and pharynx. It occurs in Central and South America.

Trypanosomiasis. Trypanosomes are large, flagellated protozoan parasites, closely related to the *Leishmania.* The African strains, *Trypanosoma gambiense* and *Trypanosoma rhodesiense,* are spread by the bites of *Glossina* (tsetse) flies and cause African sleeping sickness. Trypanosomes are found in the blood and often in cerebrospinal fluid. The lymph nodes in general are enlarged and soft, but those of the neck and groin are most strikingly so. Chronic meningoencephalitis and meningomyelitis are present, most severe about the pons and medulla. Microscopically, there is a perivascular infiltration of small round cells.

The American type of trypanosomiasis (Chagas' disease), caused by *Trypanosoma cruzi*, is found in various parts of Central and South America. Spread to man is by various triatomid bugs. The infective forms, which are passed in the "kissing" bug's excreta, contaminate the bite wound or other abrasions of the skin. Bats, armadillos, rats, and other animals act as reservoir hosts. In man and other mammals, the trypanosomes leave the blood and enter tissue cells, in which they assume leishmanial forms. The heart, brain, and liver are most commonly involved, but almost any tissue may be invaded. The heart is enlarged and microscopically shows a diffuse myocarditis and leishmanial forms in the muscle fibers. Most acute cases occur in children.

Toxoplasmosis. Toxoplasmosis is caused by the protozoan *Toxoplasma gondii*. Congen-

ital disease results from transplacental transmission, the mother having acquired the infection at the time of or after conception. Acquired toxoplasmosis results from ingestion of the cyst forms of the organism in raw or undercooked meat or from ingestion of the mature oocysts expelled in cat feces.

The congenital form of the disease in infants is an acute or subacute granulomatous encephalitis, with hydrocephalus, convulsions, and a characteristic type of bilateral chorioretinitis. Presumptive clinical diagnosis is based on the recognition of this ocular lesion by ophthalmoscopic examination, with evidence of hydrocephalus and focal intracerebral calcification on roentgenologic examination, and on the presence of several hundred lymphocytes and erythrocytes per cubic millimeter in the spinal fluid. Definite diagnosis during life may be made by finding the organisms in the spinal fluid or by transmitting the disease to guinea pigs (Fig. 10-11, *A*) or mice by the injection of spinal fluid or blood.

In fatal cases of the congenital type, hydro-

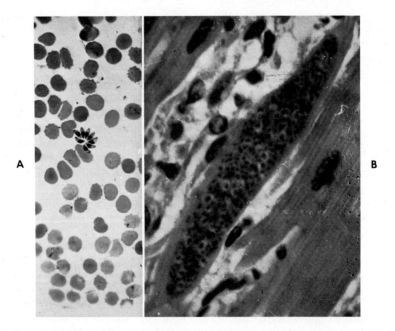

Fig. 10-11. Toxoplasmosis. *Toxoplasma* in Giemsa-stained preparation from omentum of guinea pig, **A,** and in human heart muscle, **B.** (From Pinkerton, H., and Henderson, R. G.: J.A.M.A. **116:**807-814, 1941.)

cephalus is found with necrotic granulomatous foci in the brain that range from microscopic size to 1 cm or more in diameter. These lesions are numerous in the walls of the dilated ventricles, and *Toxoplasma* organisms are found in them. Calcification may be seen in some of the lesions. Myocardial fibers may be distended with large, compact clusters of protozoa (Fig. 10-11, *B*), and focal lesions with organisms are sometimes present in the liver and elsewhere.

Acquired toxoplasmosis is frequently asymptomatic, although it is frequently detected serologically. Mild disease may be attended by the presence of lymphadenopathy affecting single or multiple lymph nodes, particularly the cervical nodes. Clinical manifestations, such as fever, malaise, myalgia, maculopapular rash, and hepatosplenomegaly, may be observed in some patients with lymphadenopathy. The enlarged lymph nodes show follicular hyperplasia with normal mitoses and much nuclear debris from necrotic cells. Small clusters of pale histiocytic or epithelioid cells are scattered throughout the node, particularly toward the periphery. Lymph sinuses are packed with macrophages and some neutrophils. Rarely, toxoplasmic cysts are found in the nodes. Toxoplasmic lymphadenitis is distinctive but not diagnostic, and confirmation is obtained most frequently by serologic tests for toxoplasmosis in suspected cases.

Chorioretinitis, frequently granulomatous, also occurs in acquired toxoplasmosis, but its presence in adults may also represent a reactivation of a latent congenital infection. Severe disseminated disease, characterized by serious organ system involvement, such as myocarditis, pneumonitis, hepatitis, or meningoencephalitis, may also occur. This form is often fatal, particularly in immunologically deficient patients.

Pneumocystosis. Infection caused by the protozoon *Pneumocystis carinii* is usually limited to the lungs, being known as "pulmonary pneumocystosis," *Pneumocystis* pneumonia, or "interstitial plasma cell pneumonia." Only rarely has widespread dissemination of the organisms to other organs been observed. The pneumonia is characterized by a foamy, pale,

eosinophilic substance in the alveoli and infiltration of the alveolar septa by lymphocytes, histiocytes, and plasma cells. The foamy alveolar material is made up of masses of minute oval organisms, which are not clearly defined in hematoxylin-eosin sections. The organisms, which are about 1 μ in diameter, are found in cysts. The latter, measuring about 6 to 8 μ or more in diameter, are well demonstrated by Gram-Weigert or silver methenamine stain. The intracystic organisms may be demonstrated by Giemsa stain. *P. carinii* have usually been identified by histologic examination of lung tissue obtained by biopsy or at autopsy. However, in some instances they have been demonstrated by examination of pulmonary secretions in the living patient.

The disease occurs most frequently in debilitated infants. It also may occur in older children and adults afflicted with leukemia, lymphoma, cytomegalic inclusion disease, or other disorders that are debilitating or accompanied by depressed immune response (p. 411).

Helminthic infections

The three large groups of parasitic worms are the Nematoda (roundworms), Trematoda (flukes), and Cestoda (tapeworms). Some worms have developed a complex life cycle, and most of them have an animal host in which they pass a larval phase and are parasites of man during their adult stage. One type, *Echinococcus granulosus,* passes its larval stage in man and its adult life in the dog or other animals. The same is true of *Echinococcus multilocularis.*

DISEASES DUE TO ROUNDWORMS

Ascaris lumbricoides infection. *Ascaris lumbricoides,* the common roundworm, is a long, cylindrical, nonsegmented worm with separate male and female forms. Its average length is about 20 to 23 cm. Infection is acquired by the ingestion of fertilized eggs, which hatch and free their larvae in the upper small intestine. Here, the larvae penetrate the lymphatics and are carried to the blood and thence to the lungs. In the lung, they penetrate alveoli and are coughed up in sputum. Some are swallowed with the sputum and develop into mature worms in the small intestine. About 2 months are required for the complete cycle. The female may produce as many as 200,000 eggs daily. In severe infections, the migrating larvae may cause an acute pneumonia, often with numerous eosinophils. The presence of the adult worms in the intestine may cause slight irritation of the gut, but more often their presence is symptomless. A large mass of worms may produce intestinal obstruction. Also, because of their wanderlust, the worms may migrate into and obstruct natural passages (e.g., bile ducts, pancreatic ducts, appendix). The eggs are passed in the feces and undergo a period of incubation (about 2 weeks) in the soil before they become infective.

Enterobius vermicularis infection. *Enterobius vermicularis (Oxyuris vermicularis,* pinworm) is a tiny worm 5 to 12 mm in length. It is especially common in children. Infection results from ingestion of fertilized eggs, which hatch and release their larvae in the duodenum. Maturation of larvae occurs as they pass down to the cecum; the adult worms copulate, after which the males die and the females migrate down the large bowel to the perianal region, where they lay their eggs about the anus. Itching in the anal region is a common symptom. Occasionally, female pinworms in the appendix cause irritation, inflammation, and obstruction, simulating appendicitis (p. 551). Hand-to-mouth transmission from the perianal area is a principal means of acquiring the infection.

Hookworm infection. Two species of hookworms cause disease in man—*Ancylostoma duodenale* and *Necator americanus.* The latter is the more prevalent species in the United States. Since the ova of each of these is similar, a study of the adult obtained from the intestinal tract would be necessary for identification of the species. The mouth has cutting plates *(Necator americanus)* or teeth *(Ancylostoma duodenale),* by which the worm attaches itself to the intestinal mucosa. The

small intestine, its habitat, may show numerous bleeding spots as a result of injury thus produced. Ova are passed in the feces and, if deposited in warm moist soil, hatch and produce larvae. In about 5 days, the larvae are infectious for man and are able to penetrate skin with which they come in contact. At the site of penetration, usually between the toes, there is a mild local inflammation *(ground itch).* The larvae enter the circulation through the lymphatics or venules, pass to the lung, and then, by way of trachea and esophagus, pass to the small bowel. The condition is often accompanied by severe anemia, eosinophilia, and evidence of general intoxication.

The larvae of the dog and cat hookworm, *Ancylostoma brasiliense,* can penetrate the human skin. They produce an irritating skin lesion (creeping eruption or cutaneous larva migrans) but do not proceed to maturity. This must be distinguished from the form of visceral larva migrans caused by the ingestion of embryonated eggs of *Toxocara canis* (an ascarid of dogs and cats). In this condition, *toxocariasis,* the larvae penetrate the small intestine and migrate throughout the viscera, producing fever, eosinophilia, hepatomegaly, pulmonary symptoms, and allergic granulomas in various organs.

Strongyloidiasis. *Strongyloides stercoralis* is a nematode that may have a free-living direct cycle in soil or a parasitic indirect cycle. In the latter, noninfective rhabditiform larvae, passed in the stool to the soil, develop into infective filariform larvae, which penetrate the skin or buccal mucosa, enter vessels, and reach the lungs, where they undergo some maturation. They pass into the alveoli, travel through the bronchi and trachea, and then enter the gastrointestinal tract. A focal acute colitis may result, with areas of reddening and swelling of the mucosa and submucosa (Fig. 10-12). The female worm deposits eggs in the mucosa, where they hatch and produce rhabditiform larvae. The latter are passed in the stool but occasionally can transform to filariform larvae in the colon, so that reinfection can take place by penetration of the infective larvae into the colonic mucosa.

Trichuriasis. *Trichuris trichiura,* or whip-

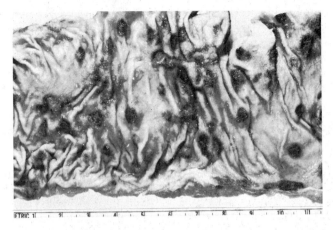

Fig. 10-12. Lesions of intestinal mucosa associated with *Strongyloides* infection.

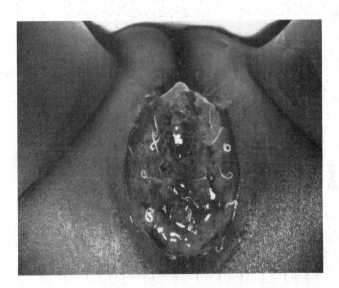

Fig. 10-13. Rectal prolapse in child, showing *Trichuris trichiura* infection.

worm, is one of the common intestinal parasites. Infection is acquired by swallowing eggs that have matured in the soil. The larvae are hatched in the small intestine, where they are attached to the mucosa and undergo maturation, and then descend to the cecum to become adults.

The adult worms are found in the cecum and colon, sometimes in tremendous numbers.

The mucosa may be congested or may show small focal areas of inflammation. Occasionally, diarrhea and rectal prolapse may occur (Fig. 10-13). Eosinophilia is a frequent accompaniment.

Filariasis. The filariae are roundworms that live in the lymphatics or tissues of man. The infective filariform larvae are transmitted to man by a biting insect. In *Bancroftian fila-*

riasis, the larvae migrate out of the insect's labium onto the skin to enter the lymphatic system, and the larvae mature to adults in the regional lymph nodes or more frequently in their larger lymphatic trunks. The cause is *Wuchereria bancrofti,* which is the most widespread filarial nematode, being found in parts of Central and South America, Africa, India, Asia, and various Pacific islands. At one time, there was a focus of cases in South Carolina.

The adult worms live in the lymphatics of man, mainly in the pelvic region and male genitalia (Fig. 10-14), causing an obliterative granulomatous lymphangitis. Eventually, this may result in lymphatic obstruction and consequent elephantiasis of the scrotum or limbs. It has been suggested that the obstructive lymphedema is preceded by dependent lymphedema that occurs earlier as a result of incompetent dilated varicose lymphatics caused by an immunopathologic reaction induced by the adult and developing worms. About a year after infection, larvae (microfilariae) appear in the blood, usually with nocturnal periodicity. The microfilariae, when taken up by various culicide and anopheline mosquito vectors, develop into infective larval forms. Infections with *Brugia (Wuchereria) malayi* are similar, although the microfilariae are somewhat different.

Onchocerca volvulus is a filarial nematode that causes *onchocerciasis.* It is found in circumscribed areas of Guatemala and Mexico (at elevations of 1,100 to 5,000 feet) and in Africa. It has recently been identified also in Colombia, Brazil, and Yemen. Spread is by the gnat or black fly, *Simulium.* The adult worms are found in localized inflammatory fibrous nodules (onchocercomas; Fig. 10-15), most common in American onchocerciasis in subcutaneous tissue of the head region. Microfilariae are found in superficial parts of the skin and are particularly abundant near the nodule, but also at a distance. An erysipeloid dermatitis, eosinophilia, and ocular disturbances are

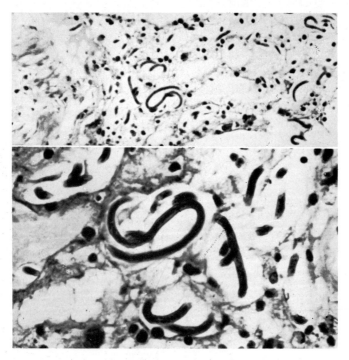

Fig. 10-14. Microfilariae of *Wuchereria bancrofti* in epididymis.

common manifestations. Invasion of the eye by microfilariae frequently produces visual disturbances and blindness.

Trichinosis. In man, *Trichinella spiralis* has been found to have infected 4% of bodies examined at autopsy in various parts of the United States during the period 1951 to 1970, a considerable reduction from the approximately 15% incidence noted during the years 1931 to 1950. The frequency of reported instances of clinical trichinosis in the United States is much lower than that encountered at autopsy. Regulations and laws prohibiting use of raw garbage as swine feed helped considerably to reduce the incidence of trichinosis.

The infection is common in rats, from which pigs and other flesh-eating mammals may become infected. Pigs, however, are more commonly infected by eating uncooked garbage containing infected pork scraps. Ingestion by man of partially cooked or raw pork containing the larvae in muscles frees the encysted larvae in the small bowel. Here, they mature in the intestinal mucosa. The adults copulate, and the fertilized females give birth to larvae, which invade tissues, penetrate blood vessels, and reach the voluntary muscles, in which they become encysted (Fig. 10-16). The extraocular muscles, masseter muscles, tongue, larynx, diaphragm, cervical

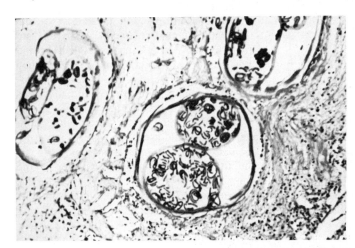

Fig. 10-15. Onchocercoma. Adult worm, containing many microfilariae, embedded in inflammatory nodule.

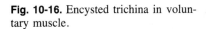
Fig. 10-16. Encysted trichina in voluntary muscle.

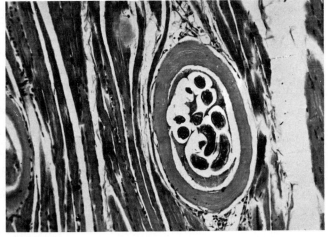

muscles, and intercostal muscles are most frequently and heavily involved. Sites of tendinous insertions especially are affected. Occasionally, a massive encystment in muscles is accompanied by myositis, with swelling, pain, and tenderness. Muscle fibers degenerate, and focal inflammatory reactions occur about the larvae. After a time, the encysted larvae die and become calcified. Interstitial myocarditis, with infiltrations of neutrophilic and eosinophilic leukocytes, is common in trichinosis. Although the larvae often invade the myocardium during the acute phase of trichinosis, they do not encyst in the muscle of the heart. Inflammatory and hemorrhagic foci also may be found in the central nervous system. Clinical trichinosis may have allergic manifestations.

DISEASES DUE TO TREMATODES

The trematodes, or flukes, are nonsegmented flatworms that live in the blood or tissues and have complicated life cycles. Those most important in man are the blood flukes (schistosomes), the liver flukes *(Clonorchis sinensis* and *Fasciola hepatica),* and the lung fluke *(Paragonimus westermani).*

Schistosomiasis (bilharziasis). The male and female blood flukes live in various parts of the portal bloodstream, and the eggs are excreted with feces or urine. The eggs hatch in fresh water, and the resulting free-swimming organisms (miracidia) attack and infect appropriate species of snails. After a period of development and multiplication in the molluscan host, fork-tailed, free-swimming forms (cercariae) are discharged and can penetrate human skin coming into contact with the infected water. Transient local irritation or an urticarial rash may appear at the site of entry in the skin. Having penetrated peripheral venules or lymphatics of the dermis, the larvae are carried in the bloodstream, and those that reach the portal circulation survive and mature. The important lesions that develop are caused by the deposition of eggs in the liver, the walls of the bowel and urinary bladder, and other tissues.

Schistosoma haematobium is most prevalent in Africa. The pelvic veins, particularly the vesiculoprostatic plexus, are the frequent location of the parasites, and the terminal-spined ova are deposited in the wall of the bladder and passed in the urine. The irritation of the ova in the bladder wall gives rise to cystitis, hematuria, and sometimes carcinoma of the bladder. The rectal wall also may be affected.

Schistosoma mansoni infections are widely distributed in Africa, northern South America, and the Caribbean region. The mature worms locate mainly in the lower colonic and rectal branches of the portal veins. The lateral-spined eggs extruded into the intestinal wall cause a chronic inflammatory reaction. Pseudotubercles and small abscesses form around the ova, and fibrosis and thickening of the bowel wall eventually develop. Many ova are carried by the portal stream to the liver and deposited around portal spaces, where they cause formation of pseudotubercles (granulomas) and fibrous nodules. Eventually, this may lead to a progressive "pipestem" cirrhosis, with obstruction of the portal circulation, splenomegaly, and ascites (p. 453).

Schistosoma japonicum infections are common in the Far East, particularly in the Yangtze Valley of China and in areas of Japan, Formosa, and the southern Philippines. The adult worms are most commonly in branches of the superior mesenteric vein draining the small intestine. The eggs, which have only a small rudimentary lateral spine, are extruded through the wall of the small bowel, in which they cause much irritation, dysenteric symptoms, chronic inflammation, and fibrous thickening. Many eggs are carried to the liver, where they cause pseudotubercle (granuloma) formation, periportal fibrosis, portal obstruction, splenomegaly, and ascites.

Nonhuman varieties of schistosome cercariae have caused severe dermatitis *(swimmer's itch)* in some areas of the United States, although the parasites are incapable of developing to maturity in man.

DISEASES DUE TO TAPEWORMS

A tapeworm is a long hermaphroditic worm consisting of a series of proglottids and a small scolex (''head'') (Fig. 10-17) provided with

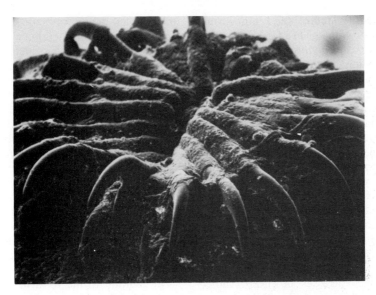

Fig. 10-17. Head of human tapeworm as seen by scanning electron microscopy. (Original magnification, ×500; from Klainer, A. S., and Perkins, R. L.: Hosp. Pract. **6:**88-91, 95-97, 1971.)

suckers or grooves. Hooklets may or may not be present. Each mature proglottid may produce a large number of eggs. With the exception of the dog tapeworm *(Echinococcus)* and sometimes the pork tapeworm *(Taenia solium),* man harbors the mature worm, and larval forms occur in an intermediate host.

Hymenolepis nana (dwarf tapeworm) infection. *Hymenolepis nana* is the smallest human tapeworm and the most common in the United States. The adults are 10 to 40 mm long and may be numerous in the upper ileum. Infection occurs chiefly in children and is usually acquired by the ingestion of eggs from human or rodent sources.

Taenia saginata (beef tapeworm) infection. Living cysticerci (larval forms) of *Taenia saginata* are ingested with insufficiently cooked beef. It is the second most common tapeworm in the United States. Maturation of the larva takes place in the intestine after it has attached itself to the mucosa. The adult worm has a small pyriform head with four lateral suckers and a body with 1,000 to 2,000 proglottids, which extend for many feet. Symptoms may be slight and are caused by irritations due to the large size of the worms.

Taenia solium (pork tapeworm) infection. In *Taenia solium* infection, the intermediate host is the hog. The worm is 8 to 12 feet long, has a small globular head with four sucking disks and a number of hooklets, and has about 1,000 proglottids. Although uncommon in the United States, the pork tapeworm is particularly important, because the larvae, as well as the adult, can develop in man. Hence, when infection is present, precautions to prevent the ingestion of eggs are essential.

Intestinal infection in man occurs by the ingestion of poorly cooked pork containing living cysticerci (larvae), which attach themselves to the mucosa and become adult worms. If eggs are ingested by man, embryos (oncospheres) liberated by action of gastric juice migrate into the body tissues and become encysted larvae, or cysticerci *(cysticercosis).* The brain, eyes, muscles, heart, liver, and lungs have been involved by the cysticerci, with disturbances resulting from the space that they occupy and the surrounding inflammatory reaction.

Diphyllobothrium latum (fish tapeworm) infection. *Diphyllobothrium latum,* also known as *Dibothriocephalus latus,* undergoes two stages in intermediate hosts: a procercoid larval stage in a cyclops and a plerocercoid larval stage in freshwater fish. Infection in man occurs by the ingestion of raw fish containing the plerocercoid larvae, which mature in the intestine. The adult worm is long and has an almond-shaped head with two lateral sucking grooves but no hooklets. A possible complication of this infection is megaloblastic anemia, apparently due to some interference with vitamin B_{12} and the intrinsic factor.

Echinococcosis (hydatid disease). In the case of *Echinococcus granulosus,* the adult worm is found in the dog and doglike animals and other mammals. Dogs acquire the infection from eating carcasses of sheep, cattle, and hogs in endemic areas. The adult worm is small, measuring 3 to 5 mm in length. The head is distinctive with four sucking disks and a circle of hooklets. Three proglottids constitute the body.

Man may be infected by swallowing the ova in dust, food, or water contaminated by the feces of an infected animal, usually a dog, or by hand-to-mouth transmission after close contact with (e.g., petting) an infected dog. Oncospheres (embryos) are liberated in the intestine, penetrate the wall into blood vessels, and pass to the liver and other organs. Lodged in an organ, they form cystic structures known as unilocular hydatid cysts, which vary up to 20 cm or even more in diameter. The cysts have a white outer layer and a granular inner germinal layer. From this inner layer, new cysts develop, and scolices (or heads) of new worms are formed. These can be recognized by seeing the row of hooklets. Eventually, the larvae die out, and the cyst becomes converted into a puttylike mass with calcification of the capsule. This capsule, seen in liver but not bone cysts (Fig. 10-18), is the result of fibrosis accompanying the host's inflammatory response to the cyst. Material from hydatid cysts, used as antigen, results in a skin reaction (Casoni test). This intradermal reaction and also a complement fixation test may be helpful in clinical diagnosis.

In addition to the form of hydatid disease caused by *Echinococcus granulosus,* there is a more serious type, characterized by invasive, alveolar, or multilocular cysts (echinococcosis alveolaris), that is produced by *Echinococcus multilocularis.* The alveolar cyst, appearing most frequently in the liver, consists of a spongy mass of minute, irregular cavities. It is not encapsulated, tends to grow peripherally into the adjacent tissue, often undergoes necrosis, and evokes a granulomatous inflammatory response in the tissue. The adult tapeworm of *Echinococcus multilocularis,* which is similar to that of *Echinococcus gran-*

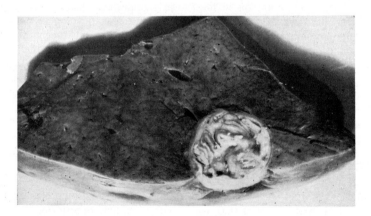

Fig. 10-18. *Echinococcus* cyst of liver. Note convoluted membranous content.

ulosus, is found in the fox, dog, and cat, and the chief sylvatic intermediate hosts are the microtine rodents.

Hydatid disease caused by *Echinococcus granulosus* is not commonly acquired by man in the United States, with only a few indigenous cases being reported. It occurs more frequently in northwestern Canada and Alaska and has a high incidence in Australia, New Zealand, Uruguay, Argentina, northern and southern Africa, and parts of Europe. Alveolar cysts of *Echinococcus multilocularis* are prevalent in central Europe, Russia, Siberia, and Alaska.

REFERENCES

Anderson, W. A. D., and Morrison, D. B.: Arch. Pathol. **33**:667-686, 1942 (malaria).

Anderson, W. A. D., et al.: Am. J. Clin. Pathol. **11**:344-355, 1941 (histoplasmosis).

Arean, V. M.: In Sommers, S. C., editor: Pathology annual, vol. 1, New York, 1966, Appleton-Century-Crofts, pp. 68-126 (schistosomiasis).

Ash, J. E., and Spitz, S.: Pathology of tropical diseases, Philadelphia, 1945, W. B. Saunders Co.

Baker, R. D., editor: Human infection with fungi, actinomycetes, and algae, New York, 1971, Springer-Verlag New York Inc.

Baum, G. L., and Schwartz, J.: Am. J. Med. Sci. **238**:661-684, 1959 (North American blastomycosis).

Beck, J. W., and Davies, J. E.: Medical parasitology, ed. 2, St. Louis, 1976, The C. V. Mosby Co.

Binford, C. H., and Connor, D. H., editors: Pathology of tropical and extraordinary diseases, Washington D.C., 1976 (vol. 1) and 1978 (vol. 2), Armed Forces Institute of Pathology.

Blumenthal, D. S.: N. Engl. J. Med. **297**:1437-1439, 1977 (intestinal nematodes in the United States).

Boyd, J.: J. Trop. Med. Hyg. **64**:1-13, 1961 (amebiasis).

Burke, B. A., and Good, R. A.: Medicine **52**:23-47, 1973 *(Pneumocystis carinii* infection*).*

Chandler, F. W., et al.: Arch. Pathol. Lab. Med. **102**:353-356, 1978 (differences between *Prototheca* and green algae).

Connor, D. H.: N. Engl. J. Med. **298**:379-381, 1978 (onchocerciasis).

dos Santos, Neto, J. G.: Am. J. Clin. Pathol. **63**:909-915, 1975 (toxoplasmosis).

Emmons, C. W., Binford, C. H., Utz, J. P., and Kwon-Chung, K. J.: Medical mycology, ed. 3, Philadelphia, 1977, Lea & Febiger.

Georg, L. K., et al.: J. Bacteriol. **88**:477-490, 1964 (actinomyces).

Gould, S. E., editor: Trichinosis in man and animals, Springfield, Ill., 1970, Charles C Thomas, Publisher.

Gray, G. F., Jr., et al.: Am. J. Pathol. **69**:349-358, 1972 (lymph nodes in toxoplasmosis).

Hoeprich, P. D., editor: Infectious diseases, ed. 2, New York, 1977, Harper & Row, Publishers, Inc.

Hutter, R. V. P.: Cancer **12**:330-350, 1959 (mucormycosis).

Katz, A. M., and Pan, C.: Am. J. Med. **25**:759-770, 1958 (*Echinococcus* disease).

Koppisch. E.: Puerto Rico J. Public Health Trop. Med. **16**:395-455, 1941 (schistosomiasis).

Koppisch, E.: J.A.M.A. **121**:936-942, 1943 (schistosomiasis).

Krick, J. A., and Remington, J. S.: N. Engl. J. Med. **298**:550-553, 1978 (toxoplasmosis).

Krogstad, D. J., et al.: N. Engl. J. Med. **298**:262-265, 1978 (amebiasis).

Lau, W. K., et al.: J.A.M.A. **236**:2399-2402, 1976 (*Pneumocystis carinii* in respiratory secretions).

Littman, M. L., and Zimmerman, L. E.: Cryptococcosis, New York, 1956, Grune & Stratton, Inc.

Mahmoud, A. A.: N. Engl. J. Med. **297**:1329-1331, 1977 (schistosomiasis).

Marcial-Rojas, R. A., editor: Pathology of protozoal and helminthic diseases, Baltimore, 1971, The Williams & Wilkins Co.

Marsden, P. D.: N. Engl. J. Med. **300**:350-352, 1979 (leishmaniasis).

Morrison, D. B., and Anderson, W. A. D.: Public Health Rep. **57**:90-94, 161-174, 1942 (malaria).

Most, H.: N. Engl. J. Med. **298**:1178-1180, 1978 (trichinosis).

Mostofi, F. K., editor: Bilharziasis, New York, 1967, Springer-Verlag New York Inc.

Naji, A. F.: Arch. Pathol. **68**:282-291, 1959 (aspergillosis).

Nelson, G. S.: N. Engl. J. Med. **300**:1136-1139, 1979 (filariasis).

Neva, F. A.: N. Engl. J. Med. **277**:1241-1252, 1967 (malaria).

Prystowsky, S. D., et al.: N. Engl. J. Med. **295**:655-658, 1976 (invasive aspergillosis).

Rahimi, S. A.: Arch. Pathol. **97**:162-165, 1974 (disseminated *Pneumocystis carinii* in thymic alymphoplasia).

Sanger, P. W., et al.: J.A.M.A. **181**:88-91, 1962 (*Candida* infection).

Schantz, P. M., and Glickman, L. T.: N. Engl. J. Med. **298**:436-439, 1978 (toxocaral visceral larva migrans).

Smith, J. W., and Bartlett, M. S.: Lab. Med. **10**:430-435, 1979 (diagnosis of *Pneumocystis* pneumonia).

Stansfeld, A. G.: J. Clin. Pathol. **14**:565-573, 1961 (toxoplasmic lymphadenitis).

Straatsma, B. R., et al.: Lab. Invest. **11**:963-985, 1962 (phycomycosis).

Sudman, M. S.: Am. J. Clin. Pathol. **61**:10-19, 1974 (protothecosis).

Teutsch, S. M., et al.: N. Engl. J. Med. **300**:695-699, 1979 (toxoplasmosis associated with infected cats).

Wartman, W. B.: Medicine **26**:333-394, 1947 (filariasis).

11

Chemical poisons, radiation injuries, and nutritional disturbances

Chemical poisons

Poisons are chemical agents that injure tissue by their reaction with it. With many poisons, the effects depend on the quantitative factor of dosage. Many substances that are innocuous or even necessary to the body in small doses are harmful when concentrated or in large quantities. Although use of poison is an ever-popular method of suicide, more than 50% of poisonings appear to be accidental and less than 1% homicidal. A large number of accidental poisonings involve children who, unfortunately, manage to ingest a variety of toxic household substances, poisonous plants, and drugs. Many poisonings are the result of industrial hazards. Direct contact with chemicals commonly causes injury to the skin of workers (e.g., dermatitis), and inhalation of dusts and fumes or absorption of noxious materials through the skin may induce more serious illness.

A matter of grave concern today is the ever-increasing number of hazardous substances being demonstrated in our environment. Although some effects of air and water pollution have been recognized, others undoubtedly will be revealed by current and future investigations.

Poisons may be classified as follows, realizing, of course, that some of the poisons could be listed in more than one category:

corrosives acids and alkalies, including sulfuric acid, lye, phenol, and formaldehyde, which destroy cells at the point of contact (mouth, esophagus, stomach, etc.)

inorganic metals and nonmetals mercury, arsenic, lead, phosphorus, cadmium, beryllium, fluorides, silica, chromates, etc.

gases chemical asphyxiants such as carbon monoxide, irritants such as nitrogen dioxide, and "war gases"

volatile organic poisons alcohols, cyanides, chloroform, carbon tetrachloride, etc.

nonvolatile organic poisons alkaloids, petroleum products, etc.

pesticides DDT, parathion, 2,4-D, 2,4,5-T, paraquat, and other harmful ingredients of insecticides, rodenticides, herbicides, etc.

bacterial toxins and food poisons staphylococcal and botulinus toxins, poisons from certain foods (e.g., mushrooms, fish)

plant and animal poisons toxins from poisonous plants (including mushrooms), snakes, spiders, scorpions, fish, stinging marine invertebrates (e.g., jellyfish), etc.

drugs barbiturates, other hypnotics and sedatives, analgesics, antibiotics and other antiinfection drugs, cancer chemotherapeutic agents, tranquilizers, hallucinogens, etc.

The two poisons most frequently found in fatal cases are carbon monoxide and barbiturates. Other hypnotics and sedatives, analgesics, and alcohols (methyl and ethyl) also are relatively common.

Corrosive poisons. The chief effect of corrosive strong acids and alkalies is local destruction of tissues. Sulfuric, nitric, and hydrochloric acids produce rapid destructive effects on mucous membranes when ingested. Similar effects may be produced by contact with the skin. Corrosive action is often evident on the mucosa of the lips, mouth, and pharynx as well as the esophagus and stomach. The lesions are reddish brown or black from sulfuric acid, grayish white from hydrochloric acid, and yellowish brown from nitric acid. In the stomach and intestine, the crests of mucosal folds are most severely affected. With sulfuric acid the stomach may be intensely red or have a black tarry appearance (carbonization). The stomach wall feels hardened, rough, and dry. With nitric acid there is no hardening, but extensive ulceration and sloughing of the mucosa occur. With hydrochloric acid the tissue is white or grayish brown and shriveled. The strong acids acting on blood form acid hematin, with widespread brownish black discoloration.

Ingestion of a corrosive alkali such as lye produces softening, swelling, and often ulceration of the mouth, esophagus, and stomach. The stomach feels soapy. If the poisoning is not fatal, healing occurs with marked fibrosis, severe stricture of the esophagus being a common result.

Phenol (carbolic acid) produces fixation and partial detachment of mucosa. These areas are whitish and of leathery consistency. The characteristic odor of phenol aids in identification.

Mercury. Poisoning may be caused by the ingestion of inorganic compounds of mercury, such as mercuric chloride (corrosive sublimate). The effects depend on dosage and length of survival time. In the acute cases, there is corrosion of the stomach and duodenum, the mucosa of which appears white and opaque. In the colon, there is an intense hemorrhagic and membranous inflammation. Vomiting and diarrhea (often bloody) may lead to severe loss of fluid, with dehydration and early death due to shock. If there is survival for a few days or weeks, severe destruction of renal tubular epithelium occurs, with calcium deposition in the necrotic tubules (Fig. 11-1).

Anuria is likely to occur, and in such cases death usually results from uremia. It is apparent that the lesions are produced in the sites where the metal is absorbed (upper gastrointestinal tract) and excreted (colon and kidneys).

A different clinicopathologic picture is observed in poisoning by methylmercury and other alkylmercury compounds. These organic forms of mercury affect the nervous system, producing paresthesias of the extremities, mouth, and lips; ataxia; slurred speech; concentric constriction of visual fields (which may progress to blindness); loss of hearing; mental deterioration; and even death. In fatal cases, pathologic changes have been described in the brain, including cerebral cortical atrophy, particularly in the visual cortex of the occipital lobe, and cerebellar cortical atrophy. Outbreaks of this type of poisoning have occurred after ingestion of grain seeds treated with mercury-containing fungicides or of animals fed on such seeds. In 1956, a disease was encountered in Minamata, Japan that was characterized chiefly by neurologic manifestations and some fatalities. It was subsequently discovered that the disease was methylmercury poisoning caused by the ingestion of fish caught in contaminated waters of Minamata Bay and neighboring seas. Since then, some investigators have referred to methylmercury poisoning as *Minamata disease.* In 1964 and 1965, a similar outbreak occurred in Niigata, Japan. The waters in the Minamata and Niigata areas were polluted by methylmercury that came from nearby chemical plants.

Methylmercury can pass through the placenta and may induce fetal injury, as evidenced by the findings of the Minamata Bay incident. In a cytogenetic analysis of human subjects exposed to methylmercury through ingestion of contaminated fish, there was a statistically significant relationship between frequency of cells with evidence of chromosomal damage and blood-cell mercury levels.

Chronic mercury poisoning has been described in workers exposed to mercury vapors and is characterized by stomatitis, salivation, blue gum line, diarrhea, tremors, neuropa-

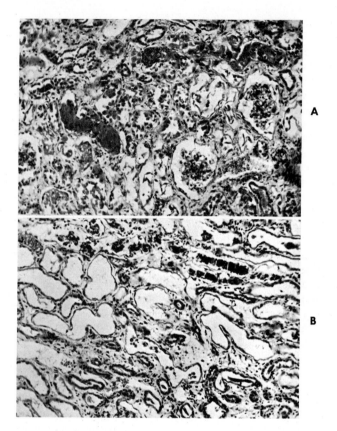

Fig. 11-1. Kidney in mercury bichloride poisoning. **A,** Seven days after ingestion of poison. Note destruction and desquamation of tubular epithelium. **B,** Eleventh day. Note loss of tubular epithelium, flattened tubular lining, and dark calcium masses deposited on necrotic debris in tubular lumina.

thy, muscle weakness, and mental disturbances.

Arsenic. Poisoning is usually caused by inorganic arsenicals, the most toxic form being the trivalent arsenic trioxide. Inorganic arsenic may be found in pesticides, paints, and certain medicines. Arsenic may produce acute poisoning with effects on the stomach, nervous system, and vascular endothelium elsewhere. Shock may cause early death, so that no striking anatomic changes may be evident. In patients surviving a few days, there will be congestion, edema, and hemorrhages in the gastric mucosa and degenerative changes in the heart, liver, and kidneys. There also may

be purpuric hemorrhages in various tissues, including the subendocardial layer of the heart.

Chronic arsenic poisoning may be characterized by skin pigmentation and hyperkeratosis of the plantar surfaces of the hands and feet, peripheral nerve degeneration, and hepatic damage. Also associated with chronic arsenicalism are epithelial carcinomas of the skin that develop after a latent period of 3 to 40 years or more. On the basis of epidemiologic data, arsenic is suspected of causing internal cancers, especially in the lungs (p. 397). In a recent study, an arsenic-containing pesticide was used to induce lung cancer in rats, but more study is needed to evaluate the role of arsenic alone. Arsenic has produced chromosomal breaks in human leukocytes cultured in vitro and has been shown to be teratogenic in certain animals by inducing birth defects, but such abnormalities have not been observed in human subjects.

Lead. Acute lead poisoning occurs infrequently, but chronic lead poisoning (plumbism) appears commonly as an industrial disease in adults engaged in work in which lead or compounds of lead are used. Poisoning also may result from drinking water carried in lead pipes and from inhaling fumes from battery casings burned as fuel. Occasionally, it has resulted from the ingestion of liquids containing lead released from the lead glaze of earthenware jugs in which the liquids were stored. In children, lead poisoning occurs quite frequently as a result of an abnormal appetite for nonedible substances (pica), including lead-containing paint peelings, and from chewing on objects painted with lead-pigment paints. An important source of lead, particularly for children since they are more vulnerable than adults to lead, may be the atmosphere in the vicinity of industrial plants and in communities with heavy traffic where there is a significant output of lead in automobile emissions. Lead has also been identified in "moonshine" whiskey distilled through automobile radiators, in the decorative decals on drinking glasses, and in certain foodstuffs. At least one instance of lead poisoning was reported to have occurred in a patient who was ingesting a prescribed health food, a calcium supplement made from horse bone. The bones of horses, particularly old ones, contain a considerable amount of lead.

Characteristics of lead poisoning are intestinal colic; weakness or paralysis of the extensor muscles (e.g., wrist or foot drop); secondary anemia with reticulocytes, polychromasia, and basophilic stippling prominent in the blood smears; a blue line on the gums; and mental disturbances. Lead becomes deposited chiefly in bones as a lead phosphate, apparently by a mechanism similar to that causing calcium deposition. Parathyroid hormone will mobilize the lead from the bones. Lead also can be demonstrated in the brain, liver, and kidneys.

The most constant lesions due to lead are the blue line of the gums and the anemia with stippling of red cells. Other findings frequently present are degenerative changes in the brain (encephalopathy) and peripheral nerves (neuropathy), muscular atrophy and fibrosis, degeneration of the male gonads with impaired spermatogenesis, and blue patches on the mucosa of the intestine. Acid-fast intranuclear inclusion bodies may be found in the liver cells and tubular epithelium of the kidneys. Most of the reports in the literature concerning the effects of lead on the heart have referred to electrocardiographic abnormalities considered to be lead-induced, although in one report interstitial fibrosis of the myocardium was described in a child with chronic lead poisoning. Ultrastructural changes have been observed in the myocardium of lead-intoxicated laboratory mice. The most important target organ in children is the brain. There is concern about the possibility that certain functional cerebral disturbances may result from intrauterine lead exposure during pregnancy, since lead has been shown to cross the placenta. Teratogenic effects of lead have been reported in some species of laboratory animals.

Phosphorus. Poisoning usually results from the ingestion of the toxic yellow or white form of phosphorus, an ingredient of certain insecticides and rodenticides. Acute phosphorus poisoning causes death by failure of the circulation. Fatty degeneration and necrosis develop in the liver, and milder fatty changes develop in the heart and kidney. Chronic phosphorus poisoning, which occurs rarely today, produces necrosis of the jaws, particularly around infected teeth. This complication, the "phossy jaw," was particularly prevalent among workers in the match industry, who continually inhaled phosphorus vapor. Today, this source of poisoning has been eliminated since the nontoxic red phosphorus is now used instead of the yellow or white phosphorus in match heads.

Cadmium. Inhalation of cadmium fumes is

an occasional industrial hazard. It may produce an acute pneumonitis that is sometimes fatal. Repeated short exposures may result in severe emphysema. The ingestion of salts of cadmium may cause gastrointestinal irritation followed by degenerative changes in the kidneys, liver, and myocardium.

Beryllium. Exposure to beryllium dusts or fumes may occur in the manufacture of fluorescent light materials and beryllium alloys of copper, and it has resulted in distinctive pulmonary disease (berylliosis). However, most manufacturers of fluorescent light bulbs have discontinued the use of beryllium in their products.

In the acute form of berylliosis, there is extensive pulmonary consolidation with exudate of fluid and mononuclear cells in the alveolar spaces and of lymphocytes and plasma cells in the alveolar walls. The chronic form is an extensive irregular and nodular pulmonary fibrosis that results from healing of granulomatous lesions. The granulomas have a center of fibrinoid or granular debris surrounded by zones of mononuclear cells, some lymphocytes and plasma cells, and fibrous tissue that extends into the lesions. Multinucleate giant cells similar to those of tuberculosis and also basophilic "conchoidal" bodies may be present in the granulomas. The extensive pulmonary fibrosis may lead to marked dyspnea and right-sided heart failure. Berylliosis has been noted to cause more bronchiolar and vascular damage than seen in sarcoidosis, from which differentiation is difficult. Demonstration of beryllium in involved tissue may be necessary for definite diagnosis.

Similar granulomatous lesions may occur in the skin following penetration of skin by beryllium particles (Fig. 11-2). These nodular lesions are extremely chronic and persistent, and permanent healing may result only when the tissues containing the foreign material are excised.

Carbon monoxide. Carbon monoxide poisoning is due to the inhalation of illuminating

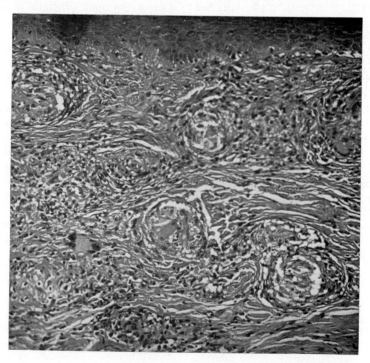

Fig. 11-2. Beryllium granuloma of skin.

gas, exhaust of automobiles, or gas from a defective stove or heater. The carbon monoxide has a much greater affinity for hemoglobin than has oxygen, so that death is due to asphyxia.

In patients dying soon after exposure to carbon monoxide, the blood, tissues, and organs are colored a bright cherry red. Following prolonged exposure and death in a few days, there may be marked vascular dilatation and congestion, hyaline thrombi, perivascular "ring" hemorrhages, and minute foci of demyelination or necrosis in the white matter of the brain (Fig. 11-3), all due to anoxemia. Petechial hemorrhages also may be seen in the myocardium. Morever, in persons surviving 48 hours or more, anoxemia may result in symmetric areas of softening of the brain involving the lenticular nuclei, mainly in the globus pallidus. Anoxic necrosis in the myocardium, particularly in the papillary muscles of the left ventricle, has been observed in

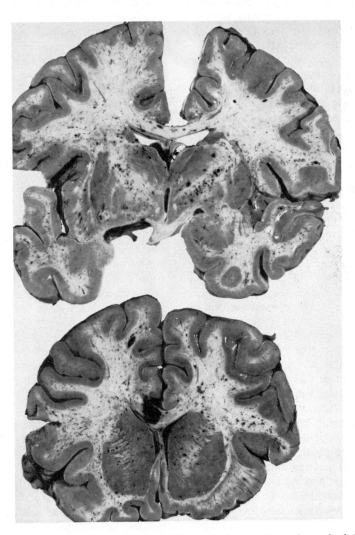

Fig. 11-3. Carbon monoxide poisoning with petechial hemorrhages in cerebral tissue.

those surviving the exposure 36 hours or more.

It has been suggested that carboxyhemoglobin increases vascular permeability, permitting greater deposition of cholesterol, a factor predisposing to atherosclerosis. Since cigarette smoking raises the carboxyhemoglobin level, this may be a means by which smoking produces or aggravates atherosclerotic coronary heart disease.

Nitrogen dioxide. Silo-filler's disease is a fibrosing and obliterating bronchiolitis due to the inhalation of irritating fumes from freshly filled silos. The toxic agent appears to be nitrogen dioxide, some of which is partially polymerized to nitrogen tetroxide.

Alcohol. *Methyl alcohol* (wood alcohol or methanol) causes poisoning by oxidation to formaldehyde and formic acid, injuring particularly the highly specialized tissues of the retina, brain, liver, and kidneys. If there is recovery from acute poisoning, blindness may follow due to atrophy of optic nerves. It is probable that the metabolite, formaldehyde, is responsible for the toxic injury to the retina with subsequent changes in the optic nerve, whereas production of formic acid is likely the major factor causing metabolic acidosis, the more serious general toxic effect of methanol poisoning.

Alcoholism due to *ethyl alcohol* may be either acute or chronic. In *acute alcoholism,* death frequently is due to some complication of the intoxication, such as trauma or suffocation, rather than the result of alcoholism itself. However, when the alcohol blood level is sufficiently high, depression of the central nervous system may be the cause of death. The mucosa of the stomach is hyperemic, with small petechial hemorrhages or erosions. The brain is wet and edematous, and the cerebrospinal fluid appears to be in excess. *Chronic alcoholism* is associated with several pathologic changes. The gastric mucosa is involved by a mild chronic catarrhal inflammation. One of the most constant findings is enlargement or marked fatty metamorphosis of the liver. A more severe and sometimes fatal form of liver disease may occur that is characterized by cellular necrosis and inflammation ("alcoholic hepatitis"). Portal cirrhosis of the liver is present in 5% to 8% of alcoholics, and 50% to 80% of patients with this lesion have a history of alcoholism (p. 447). Many alcoholics suffer nutritional deficiencies, a possible factor in hepatic changes and in other possible complications, such as peripheral polyneuropathy and Wernicke's encephalopathy.

Acute pancreatitis, varying from mild to severe necrotizing forms, and chronic pancreatitis may develop in alcoholics. Cardiac disease of the beriberi type may occur in chronic alcoholics because of accompanying nutritional disturbance (thiamine deficiency). However, a more frequent form of heart disease is that attributed to the direct effects of alcohol on the myocardium, so-called alcoholic cardiomyopathy (p. 327).

According to recent studies, excessive use of alcohol by women during pregnancy may result in congenital abnormalities in the offspring. A wide spectrum of effects of ethyl alcohol on the fetus has been reported, the most severe of which is a group of anomalies referred to as the *fetal alcohol syndrome.* Studies in experimental animals have demonstrated the teratogenic properties of ethyl alcohol, some of the anomalies being similar to those observed in human subjects.

Cyanides. *Hydrocyanic acid* and *cyanides* cause very rapid death without leaving diagnostic morphologic changes. The characteristic odor of peach kernel or bitter almonds assists in detecting the poison. Cyanides are respiratory enzyme poisons. A controversial drug, *Laetrile,* which is used by some individuals for the treatment of cancer, is actually amygdalin, a glycoside that contains cyanide. A young child was reported to have developed cyanide poisoning following the accidental swallowing of Laetrile tablets.

Chloroform and carbon tetrachloride. *Chloroform* in excess may produce degeneration and necrosis in the liver, initially affecting the central regions of the lobules. *Carbon tetrachloride* similarly damages the liver and also produces a severe acute tubular degeneration of the kidneys, which may cause death from renal failure.

Petroleum products. Petroleum products such as kerosene, gasoline, and lighter fluid produce central nervous system depression and pulmonary lesions. The latter are often more serious, with the development of a bronchopneumonia in which a mononuclear leukocytic infiltration and hyaline membranes are prominent features.

Food poisoning. Whereas poisons such as arsenic are sometimes added to food by accident or design, food poisoning usually refers to the effects of pathogenic bacteria growing in the food or to poisons in plant tissues, such as in certain mushrooms. A number of infections by bacteria and worms may be spread by food, but food poisonings with acute gastrointestinal symptoms are mainly due to infection of the food with organisms of the paratyphoid B (Salmonella) group. Local superficial inflammatory lesions develop in the intestine. Botulism is the toxemia resulting from the ingestion of the exotoxin of Clostridium botulinum with food, and its principal effects are on the nervous system. Proper cooking of food will destroy the toxin. The ingestion of preformed enterotoxin, produced by staphylococci growing in certain foods, is another cause of food poisoning.

Mushroom poisoning is associated most commonly with Amanita phalloides, the ingestion of which causes acute gastrointestinal symptoms and a high mortality (45% to 70%). Fatty degeneration in the liver, heart, kidneys, and voluntary muscles is the most prominent autopsy finding. Some gastroenteritis and also degenerative changes in the brain may be present.

Poisonous fish may be harmful in several ways: through their bite or sting, through bacterial contamination or allergens, or through specific toxic effects of their flesh, liver, or roe (ichthyosarcotoxism). Certain species (e.g., barracuda) appear to be toxic in certain seasons or geographic areas. The fish family Tetraodontidae (blowfish, toadfish, puffer, etc.) appears to be inherently poisonous, and death may occur in less than an hour or up to 20 hours after ingestion (mortality, 60%). The poison tetrodotoxin is an aminoperhydroquin-azoline compound. One of the most striking effects of this toxin is severe hypotension, which appears to result from peripheral vasodilatation. The effect has been attributed to a release of vasomotor tone due to blockade of the vasomotor nerves. However, some investigators believe that another factor may be the direct relaxant action of the toxin on vascular smooth muscle, which may act in combination with the neural effect.

Arachnidism. The venom of the female La-trodectus mactans (black widow spider) is a potent poison that appears to be a toxalbumin. Apparently, it acts on nerves or nerve endings, producing painful muscle contractions. Fatal cases have shown an acute hemorrhagic nephritis, and areas of necrosis in the liver, kidneys, spleen, and adrenal glands have been seen in experimental animals.

Drugs. Drugs serve a useful purpose in the treatment of various diseases but, under certain circumstances, may produce harmful effects. The term "iatrogenic disease" applies to any disorder in a patient resulting from treatment by a physician, including drug therapy. Adverse effects of drugs may result because of an overdose, either intentional or accidental, a primary example of which is acute barbiturate poisoning, with depression of the central nervous system, coma, and even death.

Certain drugs, even in normal doses, produce detrimental side effects. In some instances, these reactions result after a drug is given over an extended period. For example, corticosteroids may produce gastric erosions, peptic ulcers, retention of sodium and water with edema, and depressive psychosis; salicylates (e.g., aspirin) may produce gastric hemorrhage; potassium chloride may induce jejunal and ileal ulcers; phenothiazine drugs can cause hypotension, parkinsonism, and depression; phenacetin and other analgesics are considered a cause of interstitial nephritis and renal papillary necrosis in some patients; some of the antimicrobial agents, such as the penicillins, certain cephalosporins, sulfonamides, polymyxins, and amphotericin, may induce various forms of nephrotoxicity; antimetabolites may cause depression of bone marrow; and dinitrophenol and triparanol (MER-29) have been reported to be cataractogenic. Certain side effects are indirect consequences of the drug, e.g., antibiotics may predispose to mycotic infections after changing the bacterial flora of the intestine.

Some patients exhibit an *intolerance* to drugs, even at lower than usual doses, with effects resembling overdosage. For example, elderly individuals are more susceptible to the effects of phenothiazine drugs and barbiturates; drugs normally excreted by the kidneys (e.g., streptomycin and kanamycin) are not tolerated well by patients with renal disease; and drugs normally detoxified by the liver (e.g., steroids) are not tolerated by patients with hepatic disorders.

Some drugs may cause *allergic reactions* (e.g., anaphylaxis, skin eruptions, necrotizing vasculitis, hepatitis, myocarditis, hematologic disorders). Drugs in this category include penicillin, the sulfonamides, phenylbutazone, and antitetanus serum. Recently, instances of necrotizing vasculitis were reported in a group of drug abusers who used a variety of hallucinogens, opiates, stimulants, and sedatives. Methamphetamine was a drug commonly used by these patients. Autoimmune responses following drug therapy have been observed, apparently due to the formation of antibodies that react against the proteins of the host's own cells. Examples of such autoimmune responses are hemolytic anemia, thrombocytopenia, and manifestations resembling systemic lupus erythematosus (p. 686).

Certain drugs are considered to be *teratogenic* in man. Among these is the well-known teratogen, thalidomide, which characteristically produces *phocomelia* as well as other deformities. Presently, there is concern about the possibility that intrauterine exposure to sex hormones during the vulnerable period of embryogenesis may result in congenital anomalies. This concern results from the observation of various malformations in offspring of mothers who received hormones, such as progesterone/estrogen compounds or progesterone alone, during the early stage of pregnancy. It should be noted that there are many drugs and chemical agents, including certain pesticides, that have been shown to be teratogenic in animals but have not been definitely established as causes of birth defects in man.

Of interest is the possible *tumorigenic* or *carcinogenic* effect of some drugs. The possible relationship of benign tumors or tumorlike lesions in the liver to oral contraceptives is referred to on p. 456. Recently, *vaginal* and *cervical clear cell adenocarcinoma*, as well as *adenosis* (a nonneoplastic proliferation of glands), has been observed in young female patients who have been exposed in utero to stilbestrol, which was administered to their mothers during pregnancy (p. 661). There is some suggestion that patients with neoplasms, such as Hodgkin's disease, are at a greater risk of developing a second primary neoplasm, frequently acute leukemia, following chemotherapy. Some of the antineoplastic drugs used effectively in the treatment of tumors have been shown to be carcinogenic in experimental animals.

Drug abuse is an important cause of illness and death. *Alcoholism,* resulting from excessive intake of ethyl alcohol, is a common and serious form of drug abuse. Medical problems associated with alcoholism are many and some of these have been referred to earlier. Ethyl alcohol, a depressant of the central nervous system, decreases mental acuity and impairs motor coordination. Alcohol intoxication frequently results in physical injury to oneself, but more important, it is a major factor in the great number of injuries and deaths that occur on our nation's highways. It also creates behavioral problems, interferes with one's ability to work or to socialize, and often leads to marital and family difficulties.

Physical dependence may be associated with alcohol abuse and may appear as the *alcohol withdrawal syndrome*. This is one of the most serious effects of alcoholism and often occurs within hours after cessation of prolonged high alcohol intake. It consists of tremors, weakness, sweating, anxiety, intestinal cramps, and hyperreflexia, sometimes followed by visual hallucinations and even convulsive seizures. In some alcoholics a more serious form of withdrawal illness occurs, i.e., "delirium tremens," which includes auditory, visual, and tactile hallucinations, mental confusion, restlessness, insomnia, excessive perspiration, tachycardia, and generalized tremors. Death may occur during an attack of delirium tremens, although the majority of patients usually recover. However, in some individuals, persisting medical or psychologic sequelae may be observed.

A number of other drugs also produce physical dependence with the development of withdrawal symptoms when the drug is discontinued abruptly after prolonged use. Among the physically addicting drugs, in addition to ethyl alcohol, are the opiates, barbiturates, minor tranquilizers, and some of the nonbarbiturate sedatives.

Psychologic dependence is essentially a need or craving for a drug to which one has been accustomed. It is a mental state that drives one back to using the drug after having abstained from it for a time. In its most serious form, an individual is dominated by compulsive behavior directed toward obtaining and using the drug and often will perform immoral and illegal acts in order to obtain the money to purchase the drug. A variety of drugs may be associated with psychologic dependence, although some have a greater tendency to be psychologically habit-forming than others. Among the drugs that produce psychologic dependence are the opiates, synthetic narcotics, barbiturates, ethyl alcohol, minor tranquilizers, amphetamine, cocaine, LSD, and marihuana.

Some of the drugs subject to abuse may produce certain psychiatric disorders, such as persistent psychosis, although in some instances it may be difficult to exclude the possibility that the psychotic state developed, because there was already a preexisting psychiatric illness. Another problem among drug users is overdosage, which sometimes results in death, particularly in narcotic addicts for whom intravenous injection is a common method of administration of the drug. Medical problems not caused by the drugs themselves may also appear as a result of drug abuse.

These may develop because of the irritant properties of the substances other than the drug (e.g., the diluents) that are present in the preparation injected or because of infections that may develop as a result of unsterile injection procedures. The following are some examples of these medical problems: skin infection (abscess and cellulitis) and scars at the site of injection, the scars sometimes involving muscle and causing permanent muscle contractures; serum hepatitis; tetanus; bacterial or fungal endocarditis and its serious complications; bacterial pneumonia; thrombophlebitis; and septicemia.

Environmental pollution. *Air pollution* is an important cause of aggravation of preexisting cardiac and respiratory illnesses, particularly chronic respiratory conditions (e.g., bronchial asthma, chronic bronchitis, and emphysema). Less severe effects include irritation of the eyes and upper respiratory tract. It has not been determined what specific diseases are caused by air pollutants, although the latter have been incriminated in the etiology of bronchogenic carcinoma. Pollutants include particulate matter (ash, soot, smoke, and radioactive dust), oxides of nitrogen, hydrogen sulfide, hydrocarbons, sulfur dioxide, pollens, carbon monoxide, certain metals, and singlet oxygen (electrically stimulated form of molecular oxygen with greater than normal energy).

The problem of air pollution is increasing because of the expansion of industrialization and the heavy automobile traffic with resultant emission of automobile exhaust containing large amounts of carbon monoxide, unsaturated hydrocarbons, nitrogen oxides, and carbon dioxides. Photochemical smog (which occurs in some of our big cities) is produced from these emission compounds in the presence of sunlight.

Water pollution has altered our waterways, making them unsuitable for agriculture, recreation, wildlife, and fish and as sources of municipal and industrial water supply. Pollutants include sewage, infectious agents, dissolved mineral substances that enhance the growth of algae, synthetic organic compounds (from household detergents, insecticides, and weed killers and other pesticides), inorganic chemicals and metals (e.g., salts, acids, and mercury from industrial plants), and radioactive substances.

Soil pollution also presents a hazard to health. Such pollution may be contributed to by synthetic agricultural chemicals (e.g., pesticides and fertilizers) and infectious agents.

Although certain pollutants are distributed initially in one or another environmental compartment (air, water, or soil), there often is a crossing-over of pollutants between compartments. Of importance, also, is the fact that *foods* may be contaminated accidentally by environmental pollutants (e.g., pesticides, heavy metals, and plasticizers), and at times, certain potentially hazardous chemical substances may intentionally be added to foods (e.g., antioxidants and dyes).

The adverse effects of environmental pollutants include the usual acute or chronic effects known to be associated with the particular chemical, physical, or infectious agent involved. Some of these effects are discussed elsewhere in this chapter and in other chapters. In addition, there is great concern about the possibility that some pollutants may be responsible for the production of cancer (carcinogenic effect), developmental defects (teratogenic effect), or mutations (mutagenic effect).

One of the most effective environmental mutagens is radiation, although some of the other environmental agents, including chemicals, also appear to be mutagenic. Many of the genetic studies have involved experimental animals and even *Drosophila*. However, the study of chromosomal aberrations in human subjects known to be exposed to environmental pollutants also provides considerable information concerning their mutagenic potential.

A great deal of the information regarding the teratogenic effect of ionizing radiation in man came from a study of the offspring of mothers exposed to radiation from the atomic bomb explosions at Hiroshima and Nagasaki and also from a study of infants born of mothers who received intensive pelvic radiotherapy

during early pregnancy in the 1920s. Much information pertaining to the teratogenic potential of other environmental agents, including metals and chemicals (e.g., pesticides), comes from data obtained from experimental studies in laboratory animals. One of the examples of teratogenicity of environmental chemicals in man is methylmercury, as evidenced by the studies of the offspring of women who were exposed to the chemical during the Minamata incident (p. 221). In Minamata, Japan, the pregnant women were exposed by eating fish taken from water polluted by methylmercury that came from a nearby chemical plant.

The relationship between environmental agents and carcinogenesis, including the role of radiation, infectious agents, and chemicals, is discussed on pp. 257-262.

It has been found that a number of the environmental chemicals are contaminated by toxic chlorine-containing compounds, the chlorinated dibenzofurans and/or the chlorinated dibenzodioxins. In such instances, it is important to conduct investigations to determine whether the toxic effects attributed to the chemical are caused by the chemical itself, its contaminants, or a combination of both. One of the most toxic compounds is the chlorinated dibenzodioxin TCDD (2,3,7,8-tetrachlorodibenzo-*p*-dioxin). TCDD recently received much publicity in the lay press when, in the summer of 1976, a considerable quantity of the compound was released into the atmosphere in Saveso, Italy following an explosion in a chemical plant, endangering the health of many people in the town and adjacent areas.

Although the general population is constantly exposed to potentially hazardous pollutants, it is usually the workers who are most heavily exposed to hazardous substances since they are using or producing them in their occupation. There have been many instances of illness resulting from exposure to dangerous compounds in the occupational environment. The following are just a few examples: neurologic disorders caused by the pesticides kepone and leptophos; carcinoma of the lung resulting from exposure to asbestos or to bis(chloromethyl) ether; angiosarcoma of the liver in workers exposed to vinyl chloride; pulmonary disease in workers exposed to silica, beryllium, coal dust, or cotton dust; lead poisoning in workers in smelting and battery plants; and bladder cancer resulting from exposure to benzidine.

Much information about the adverse effects of occupational and environmental agents, including their teratogenic and oncogenic potential, is obtained by epidemiologic investigations and by in vivo animal testing. In recent years, there has been a major effort to develop inexpensive, reliable, short-term bioassays to be used as predictors of carcinogenicity. One of the most popular short-term bioassays is the so-called Ames test, which is based on the concept that there is usually a correlation between mutagenicity and carcinogenicity. In this test, mutant strains of *Salmonella typhimurium* are exposed in vitro to a minute amount of a chemical. Since many chemicals require enzymatic activation for them to become mutagenic or carcinogenic, microsomal enzymes of rat or human liver are added. The tester strains of bacteria were chosen for their sensitivity and specificity in being reverted by mutagens from a histidine requirement to growth on a histidine-free medium. A positive reaction consists of the growth of revertant bacteria around the site of the test material. Among the various applications of this test is its use as a prescreening technique for identifying potentially hazardous chemicals that require further testing for carcinogenicity by means of the conventional animal bioassay. Another short-term carcinogenesis bioassay is an in vitro test that has as its end point chemically induced transformation of mammalian cells in culture. An interesting variant of this test utilizes both in vivo and in vitro systems, i.e., pregnant hamsters are treated with the suspected carcinogen and cells obtained from their fetuses are cultured and examined for transformation. There are other short-term bioassays that have different end points.

Radiation injuries

All living cells are damaged by ionizing radiation and may be destroyed by sufficient dosage, but the degree of susceptibility varies. Radiation has its main therapeutic usefulness in the treatment of malignant tumors (p. 246). Radiosensitivity and radioresistance of various cells and tissues are only relative. Immature or poorly differentiated cells and those undergoing mitosis are particularly radiosensitive. The relative degree of radiosensitivity of normal tissues and of some neoplastic lesions is noted in Table 11-1. The effect of ionizing radiation on cells does not appear to be recognizable as of a specific type but is a degeneration that, if sufficiently severe, leads to death of the cell.

Effects of ionizing radiation on surviving cells include mutations or permanent alterations in their physiologic capabilities. An important delayed or late effect is a tendency of cells injured by radiation to undergo malignant change. Cancers of skin and of bone have been the most frequent neoplasms produced by localized irradiation, and leukemia has been the most frequent malignancy following whole body irradiation.

The *effects of whole body irradiation* depend on dosage and on whether it is a single large exposure or repeated doses. A single large dose of total body irradiation (e.g., atomic bomb exposure) causes depletion of cells, particularly in tissues in which the cell population is normally renewed by continued cell division and maturation. Intestinal epithelium, bone marrow, and the testes are particularly affected. Early loss of intestinal epithelium leads to diarrhea, with dehydration and loss of body sodium. A lesser dose with survival for several days shows effects on hematopoietic tissues, with depletion of leukocytes, platelets, red blood cells, and lymphocytes. Purpuric and hemorrhagic manifestations develop, with decreased resistance to infections. An increased incidence of *leukemia* has been noted in atomic bomb victims who survived the immediate effects. The *effects of low-dosage whole body irradiation* that is repeated or spread out

Table 11-1. Relative radiosensitivity of normal cells and select tumors

Radiosensitivity	Normal cells	Tumors
Very high	Lymphocytes Immature hematopoietic cells Intestinal epithelium Spermatogonia Ovarian follicular cells	Leukemia Most forms of lymphoma Dysgerminoma Seminoma Granulosa cell tumor

High	Urinary bladder epithelium
	Esophageal epithelium
	Gastric mucosa
	Mucous membranes of mouth
	  and pharynx
	Epidermal epithelium
	  (including hair follicles and
	  sebaceous glands)
	Epithelium of optic lens
		Transitional cell carcinoma of
		  bladder
		Adenocarcinoma of stomach
		Epidermoid carcinoma of
		  skin, oropharynx,
		  esophagus, and cervix

Intermediate	Endothelium
	Growing bone and cartilage
	Fibroblasts
	Glial cells
	Glandular epithelium of breast
	Pulmonary epithelium
	Renal epithelium
	Hepatic epithelium
	Pancreatic epithelium
	Thyroid epithelium
	Adrenal epithelium
		Vascular and connective tissue
		  components of most tumors
		Osteogenic sarcoma
		Astrocytoma
		Chondrosarcoma
		Epidermoid carcinoma of lung
		Liposarcoma
		Adenocarcinoma of breast,
		  kidney, thyroid, colon,
		  liver, and pancreas

Low	Mature hematopoietic cells Muscle cells Mature connective tissues Mature bone and cartilage Ganglion cells	Rhabdomyosarcoma Leiomyosarcoma Ganglioneuroma

From Anderson, R. E.: Radiation injury. In Anderson, W. A. D., and Kissane, J. M.: Pathology, ed. 7, St. Louis, 1977, The C. V. Mosby Co.

over a long time are under intensive investigation. The important effects may be in *carcinogenesis* and *genetic changes*.

Nutritional disturbances

Adequate dietary intake is necessary for the maintenance of health. Not only is an adequate caloric content necessary, but certain proteins, minerals, and vitamins also are essential. Slight deficiency may be difficult to recognize pathologically as well as clinically. The problem is further complicated by the rarity in man of pure deficiencies such as may be produced in carefully controlled experimental animals. Inadequate diets for human beings often lack several essentials so that the resulting lesions are a mixture. The role of dietary factors in the pathogenesis of atherosclerosis, cirrhosis of the liver, and other diseases is discussed elsewhere.

Vitamins are organic compounds essential in the diet for normal growth and maintenance of life. They are active in the regulation of metabolism and transformation of energy but do not themselves furnish energy or building material, and they are effective in small amounts. Several vitamins, particularly thiamine, riboflavin, and nicotinic acid, are

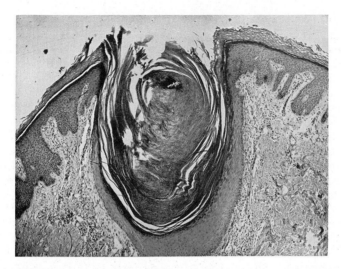

Fig. 11-4. Hyperkeratosis of hair follicle in vitamin A deficiency. (Courtesy Dr. Chester N. Frazier; from Sutton, R. L., and Sutton, R. L., Jr.: Diseases of the skin, ed. 10, St. Louis, 1939, The C. V. Mosby Co.)

closely concerned with intracellular respiration, providing chemical groupings essential for intracellular oxidations and reductions.

VITAMIN A

Vitamin A is a fat-soluble, unsaturated alcohol and has as its precursor certain vegetable pigments known as carotenes. Deficiency results in night blindness, dermatosis, and xerophthalmia.

One of the diagnostic features of vitamin A deficiency is subnormal dark adaptation. Vitamin A is an essential constituent of retinal pigments used to register visual stimuli. When it is deficient, the regeneration of visual purple is delayed and dark adaptation is poor.

The primary effect of vitamin A deficiency is on epithelium, which undergoes atrophy and replacement by a keratinizing type of epithelium. In man, the specific lesions are found in the eyes, conjunctiva, lining epithelium of various organs and ducts, and the skin and its appendages. The commonest and earliest appearance of metaplastic squamous epithelium is in the trachea and bronchi, and next in the pelvis of the kidney. The eye changes also consist of a metaplasia of the corneal and conjunctival epithelium, followed by corneal infection. The skin is rough, scaly, and dry because of hyperkeratosis of skin and hair follicle epithelium (Fig. 11-4) and metaplasia of sweat gland epithelium.

Vitamin A can be demonstrated in microscopic sections by fluorescence microscopy. Ultraviolet light is used, the vitamin A exhibiting a fading greenish fluorescence in the dark field. By this method, vitamin A has been found distributed in the lipids of the epithelial and Kupffer cells of the liver, in the epithelial cells of the adrenal cortex, in the tubular and Leydig cells of the testis, in the granulosa, theca, and stroma cells of the ovary, in the fat cells, in gland cells of the lactating breast, and in kidneys with abnormal glomerular permeability.

Vitamin A and its naturally occurring derivative, all-*trans*-retinoic acid, are used in the treatment of acne, and one of the newer analogs (synthetic retinoids), 13-*cis*-retinoic acid, appears to be effective in the management of severe, chronic, treatment-resistant forms of acne. The mechanism of action of the latter drug is probably its ability to inhibit the synthesis of sebum by the sebaceous glands.

Hypervitaminosis A. Hypervitaminosis A occurs in young children and adults because of an excessive intake of vitamin A, usually through ingestion of large amounts of vitamin concentrates. Affected adults usually complain of fatigue, loss of appetite, and bone pain and have spotty alopecia, skin lesions including generalized desquamation and pigmentation, and hepatomegaly. Microscopically, the liver may show little or no change, but occasionally there is hepatic fibrosis or cirrhosis as well as an accumulation of lipid-storing cells. Some of these manifestations also may occur in infants, but, in addition, there may be increased intracranial pressure, bulging fontanels, hypoprothrombinemia with hemorrhagic diathesis, cortical thickening of bones, premature closure of epiphyseal growth plates, and retardation of bone growth.

Acute toxicity has been reported in adults after ingestion of liver rich in vitamin A (e.g., polar bear or bearded seal liver). Symptoms include nausea, vomiting, irritability, headache, lethargy, and drowsiness. Various anomalies of the bones of the head, including cleft palate and skull defects with exencephaly, have been produced in offspring of female animals treated with excess vitamin A during pregnancy.

Vitamin A and cancer. According to the August-September 1978 issue of the FDA Drug Bulletin, the natural derivative of vitamin A, retinoic acid, which is used widely as a topical medication in the treatment of acne, enhanced the cancer-inducing effects of ultraviolet radiation on the skin in some animal experiments.

On the other hand, evidence is accumulating that the natural forms and the synthetic analogs of vitamin A (the retinoids), which control cell differentiation in many epithelial tissues, inhibit the biologic process that leads to cancer formation in these tissues. It has been shown in experimental animals that deficiency of dietary retinoids enhance the development of chemically induced epithelial tumors and that high oral doses of retinoids are useful in preventing epithelial cancers. The synthetic retinoids appeared to be less toxic and more potent in the prevention of the cancers than the natural retinoids. The potential usefulness of synthetic retinoids for the prevention of cancer in man (referred to as "chemoprevention" in contrast to "chemotherapy") is being investigated, particularly in patients with premalignant lesions. It is postulated that this pharmacologic approach may result in the arrest or reversal of the progression of premalignant cells toward invasive cancer.

VITAMIN B COMPLEX

Vitamin B has been found to contain a number of specific factors. Since the chemical nature of most of these factors is known, they are more properly designated by their correct chemical names rather than referred to as B_1, B_2, etc. The factors in the B complex include thiamine hydrochloride, riboflavin, nicotinic acid, pantothenic acid, pyridoxine hydrochloride, folic acid, and cyanocobalamin. The B complex is found in yeast, whole grain cereals, wheat germ, rice polishings, etc.

Thiamine hydrochloride (B₁)

Thiamine is a water-soluble vitamin, the deficiency of which results in beriberi. Thiamine is important in the intracellular metabolism of glucose, with the pyrophosphate of thiamine acting as a coenzyme (with carboxylate) in the breaking down of pyruvic acid. Thiamine deficiency also is believed to be the factor causing *Wernicke's disease.*

Beriberi. The main clinical features of beriberi are loss of appetite, peripheral neuritis with muscle tenderness and changes in reflexes, tachycardia, cardiac failure, and edema. The disease occurs in acute and chronic forms. At autopsy, the findings in chronic forms are usually complicated by an infection. The more acute and uncomplicated forms are characterized by dilatation and moderate hypertrophy of the heart, generalized edema, hydrothorax, hydropericardium, and congestion of viscera. Microscopically, the heart shows edema, with hydropic degeneration of muscle fibers. Microscopic nerve lesions are seen most frequently in nerves supplying the lower extremities, although cranial and vagus nerves also are affected frequently. There is vacuolar degeneration of Schwann cells, followed by fragmentation of axis cylinders and myelin sheath degeneration.

Riboflavin (B_2 or G)

Deficiency of riboflavin (ariboflavinosis) is said to produce in man a lesion called *cheilosis*, characterized by superficial cracks or fissures at the angles of the mouth. A nasolabial seborrheic skin lesion, glossitis, and circumcorneal congestion also may be present. Riboflavin appears to be important in tissue respiration, for combined with phosphoric acid it unites with specific proteins to form enzymes that act as dehydrogenases.

Nicotinic acid (niacin)

Considerable evidence indicates that deficiency of nicotinic acid is an important factor in pellagra, although probably in most cases multiple deficiencies are present. Nicotinic acid (niacin) is an essential component of the pyridine-protein intracellular enzyme systems, which are important in carbohydrate metabolism.

Pellagra. Pellagra is characterized by brown, scaly, patchy skin eruptions, soreness of the mouth, redness of the tongue, indigestion, diarrhea, and nervous disturbances. The skin lesions tend to appear particularly in areas exposed to sunlight.

Pathologic changes are found in the skin, gastrointestinal tract, and nervous system. The skin lesions begin with edema of the papillae, dilatation of the papillary blood vessels, and degeneration of the connective tissue of the superficial part of the corium. This is followed by epidermal hyperplasia and hyperkeratosis with an increase in pigment. The lesions are similar to sunburn or x-ray dermatitis. In late stages, the epidermis is thin and atrophic and the corium is fibrosed. The oral mucosa may be affected in a similar fashion.

The intestinal lesions are more characteristic. The colon is thick-walled and reddish, and there may be a patchy pseudomembranous

change in its mucosa. The mucosa may be infiltrated by chronic inflammatory cells, but most pathognomonic is a cystic dilatation of the crypts of Lieberkühn.

The nerve lesions appear late and are more prominent in the central nervous system than in peripheral nerves. Patchy degeneration may be present in the cerebrum, and irregular patches of myelin degeneration in the spinal cord most commonly involve posterior columns.

Pantothenic acid and pyridoxine (B_6)

The role of pantothenic acid and pyridoxine in human pathology is still uncertain. Pyridoxine-deficient monkeys have been shown to develop atherosclerosis, and the possibility has been suggested that pyridoxine deficiency may be a factor in the pathogenesis of some instances of atherosclerosis in man.

Certain drugs (e.g., isoniazid for treatment of tuberculosis) interfere with utilization of pyridoxine, causing a deficiency, with development of cheilosis and peripheral neuritis. Some types of microcytic anemia and convulsive seizures in infants have responded to treatment with pyridoxine.

Folic acid and cyanocobalamin (B_{12})

Folic acid (pteroylglutamic acid) deficiency leads to megaloblastic anemia. Folic acid is used in the treatment of sprue and megaloblastic nutritional anemias in man. It corrects the red blood cell deficiency of pernicious anemia but, unlike vitamin B_{12}, does not improve the degeneration in the spinal cord that is characteristic of this disease. Vitamin B_{12} is the extrinsic factor necessary for cure of pernicious anemia. Its absorption appears to be dependent on an intrinsic factor in the gastric mucosa.

ASCORBIC ACID (VITAMIN C)

Ascorbic acid is a water-soluble vitamin, the deficiency of which leads to scurvy. This vitamin is essential for the production and maintenance of intercellular substances of mesenchymal origin, i.e., collagen of fibrous tissue and the matrices of bone, dentine, and cartilage. Mesenchymal tissues (fibroblasts, osteoblasts, etc.) grow in the absence of vitamin C, but they cannot produce intercellular substance. Hemorrhages and changes in bone are the prominent features of scurvy. In vitamin C–deficient animals, fractured bones cannot be restored to functional integrity. The broken ends are united by fibroblasts, but neither collagen nor osseomucin is produced. There is little evidence that excess of vitamin C promotes healing of wounds or fractures, but deficiency of vitamin C appears to have serious effects and prevents formation of scars of normal strength. Deficiency of vitamin C interferes with the production of acid mucopolysaccharides, which occurs in the early stages of normal wound healing.

The ascorbic acid levels of plasma and urine can be quantitatively determined, but analysis of the ascorbic acid content of the white cell–platelet layer of centrifuged blood is a more useful indicator of the vitamin C status of the body. Scurvy does not occur until this is almost entirely depleted.

Scurvy. Human scurvy is more common in children (Barlow's disease) than in adults. The essential features are hemorrhages, changes in bones and teeth, and anemia.

The hemorrhages may be in any organ or tissue and vary from small petechiae to massive hematomas. Any injury or trauma to a tissue predisposes to hemorrhage, which is due to changes in the integrity of capillary walls. Petechial hemorrhages in the skin are most prominent clinically. In infants, very painful subperiosteal hemorrhage is common.

The skeletal lesions are most prominent at the costochondral junctions, the ends of the femurs and tibias, and at the wrists. Grossly, there is a curved, yellowish, widened zone at the junction of the diaphysis and cartilage. Microscopically, this zone shows evidence of disordered growth and interruption of the process of ossification. Fragile connective tissue fibers are formed, a watery zone appears about the osteoblasts, and osteoid tissue is defective. Also, elsewhere in the bones, new bone formation is lacking, whereas bone resorption

goes on at a normal rate. The result is rarefaction of bone, similar to that which occurs in senility.

Lesions in the teeth may occur before skeletal lesions are prominent. The gums become swollen and bleed easily. The teeth tend to loosen and may even fall out as a result of rarefaction of alveolar bone. Degenerative and atrophic changes also develop in the substance of the teeth themselves.

VITAMIN D

Vitamin D (calciferol, D_2; 7-dehydrocholesterol, D_3) is a fat-soluble vitamin that not only is available in food but also may be formed from ergosterol in the skin by ultraviolet radiation. It is important in calcium and phosphorus metabolism, the part it plays being to increase calcium absorption from the intestine or to increase phosphorus retention and, in turn, calcium retention. Thus, for action of this vitamin, adequate mineral intake is essential. Vitamin D is essential for prevention of rickets (see below) and osteomalacia (p. 703). It is also important for prevention of hypocalcemic tetany. Some investigators also believe that it participates in the prevention of osteoporosis and muscle weakness.

Rickets. Deficiency of vitamin D leads to rickets in growing children. The corresponding condition in adults is termed osteomalacia. Rickets is most common in infancy, but an adolescent form also occurs. Adequate mineral intake and solar radiation, as well as dietary vitamin D, are important in the prevention of rickets.

Rickets is fundamentally a deficient calcification of osteoid tissue and an abnormal involution of cartilage in growing bones. Endochondral bone growth is disturbed. The excess of uncalcified osteoid tissue results in unusual softness of the bones, which become bent and deformed near the joints. Such deformities are common about the knees (bowlegs), costochondral junctions (rachitic rosary; Fig. 11-5), and thorax (pigeon breast). The most significant gross changes are seen on the cut surface of an epiphyseal region. The tissue is softened, and the normally sharp narrow line of

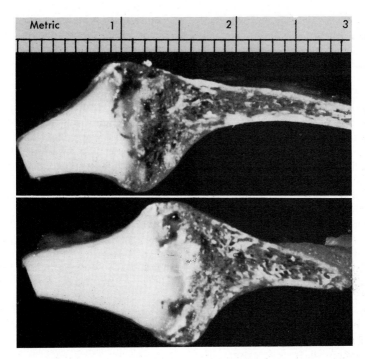

Fig. 11-5. Costochondral junction of ribs in rickets. Junctional zone is wide and irregular in contrast to normal appearance of narrow sharp line of ossification.

ossification is replaced by a wide irregular zone of soft gray tissue. Histologically, the area shows great disorder of growth with excess osteoid tissue and failure of its calcification. In all parts of the bones, there is an excess formation of bone matrix, which remains uncalcified or eventually is poorly calcified (Fig. 25-2, *B*). The bone marrow becomes fibrous.

The teeth suffer from the same lack of calcification as occurs in bones. The lesions are in the permanent dentition. Dimpling of the enamel, furrows, and other types of defects may result.

Hypervitaminosis D. Vitamin D overdosage is known to result in deleterious effects. A very large intake is necessary in man before damage occurs. Hypercalcemia is likely to occur as a result of increased absorption of calcium through the intestinal wall and mobilization of calcium from the bone. The demineralization of bone is followed by deos-

sification. Metastatic calcification occurs, with calcium deposits in various sites, particularly the kidneys.

VITAMIN E (TOCOPHEROL)

Little is known about the pathology of vitamin E deficiency in man. In experimental animals, it leads to degenerative and atrophic changes in the testes and also to severe degenerative changes in skeletal muscles, accompanied by marked cellular infiltrations. Focal myocardial necrosis with calcification of necrotic myocardial fibers may occur. A ceroid-type pigment is present in the tissues of some of the animals.

Lesions in the muscle similar to those described in animals on deficient vitamin E diets, along with ceroid pigment in certain tissues, have been reported in patients with cystic fibrosis. It has been shown that tocopherol plasma levels are low in patients with absorptive defects, such as cystic fibrosis and congenital biliary atresia. A definite relationship of vitamin E deficiency to primary muscle diseases or myocardial lesions in man has not been determined. There is some suggestion that erythropoiesis and erythrocyte survival time may be influenced by tocopherol. A macrocytic megaloblastic anemia in malnourished children has responded to tocopherol therapy. Severe anemia caused by ineffective erythropoiesis, along with muscular wasting, has been described in monkeys given a diet deficient in vitamin E. Anemias related to vitamin E deficiency in other animal species are caused by other mechanisms.

Vitamin E and *selenium* have closely related functions in normal metabolism in animals, although this relationship is not clearly understood. In certain spontaneously developing myopathies and related conditions in animals that have been attributed to vitamin E deficiency, a lack of selenium has been implicated. Some of these disorders respond to either vitamin E or selenium, others only to vitamin E, and others only to selenium. This group of disorders is generally referred to as *selenium/vitamin E responsive diseases*.

VITAMIN K

Vitamin K is necessary for the formation of prothrombin, an essential in the clotting mechanism. Absorption of vitamin K from the intestine is favored by the presence of the bile salts. Lack of vitamin K causes a hemorrhagic tendency, as noted in obstructive jaundice and in the hemorrhages of newborn infants.

KWASHIORKOR

A nutritional deficiency of infancy and childhood prevalent in West Africa and elsewhere has been called kwashiorkor. It appears to be a protein deficiency, although it is inexactly known whether it results from deficiency of protein as a whole or of certain specific amino acids. Deficiency of certain minerals, such as magnesium, also may be important. Affected children develop rashes and ulcerations of the skin, edema, an enlarged fatty liver, and sometimes hepatic necrosis. Acinar atrophy and apparent relative fibrosis of the

pancreas are prominent findings. Infections are important as a precipitating factor and as a cause of death.

MARASMUS

Marasmus is a form of protein malnutrition that is characterized by marked weight loss and wasting of subcutaneous fat and muscle but without the edema and impaired hepatic function seen in kwashiorkor. Marasmus and kwashiorkor are related and may represent different aspects of the same disease. In some instances, marasmus may undergo transition to kwashiorkor.

REFERENCES

Adelson, L.: Am. J. Clin. Pathol. **22:**509-519, 1952 (common poisons).
Appel, G. B., and Neu, H. C.: N. Engl. J. Med. **296:**663-670, 722-728, 784-787, 1977 (nephrotoxicity of antimicrobial agents).
Arena, J. M.: Poisoning, ed. 4, Springfield, Ill., 1978, Charles C Thomas, Publisher.
Benson, J.: J. Forensic Sci. **1:**119-125, 1956 (poisonous fish).
Bingham, E.: The Sciences **18**(6):6-7, 30-31, 1978 (occupational environmental hazards).
Braigo, K. T., et al.: N. Engl. J. Med. **300:**238-240, 1979 (Laetrile intoxication).
Campbell, J. A. H.: Arch. Dis. Child. **31:**310-314, 1956 (kwashiorkor).
Citron, B. P., et al.: N. Engl. J. Med. **283:**1003-1011, 1970 (necrotizing angiitis in drug abusers).
Clark, L.: Aust. Vet. J. **47:**568-571, 1971 (hypervitaminosis A).
Clarren, S. K., and Smith, D. W.: N. Engl. J. Med. **298:**1063-1067, 1978 (fetal alcohol syndrome).
Committee on Medical and Biologic Effects of Environmental Pollutants: Arsenic, Washington, D.C., 1977, National Academy of Sciences.
Crosby, W. H.: J.A.M.A. **237:**2627-2629, 1977 (lead-contaminated health food).
Deichmann, W. B., and Gerarde, H. W.: Toxicology of drugs and chemicals, New York, 1969, Academic Press, Inc.
DeLuca, H. F.: Arch. Intern. Med. **138:**836-847, 1978 (vitamin D).
Dimijian, G. G.: Contemporary drug abuse. In Goth, A.: Medical pharmacology, ed. 9, St. Louis, 1978, The C. V. Mosby Co.
Editorial: J.A.M.A. **163:**118-119, 1957 (poisonous fish).
Epstein, S. S.: Am. J. Pathol. **66:**352-373, 1972 (environmental pathology).
Epstein, S. S.: Cancer Res. **34:**2425-2435, 1974 (environmental determinants of human cancer).
FDA Drug Bulletin **8:**26, August-Sept. 1978 (retinoic acid and sun-caused skin cancer).

Fielding, J. E., and Russo, P. K.: N. Engl. J. Med. **297:**943-945, 1977 (exposure to lead).

Finck, P. A.: Milit. Med. **131:**1513-1539, 1966 (carbon monoxide).

Fitch, C. D.: Ann. N.Y. Acad. Sci. **203:**172-176, 1972 (hematopoiesis in vitamin E deficiency).

Follis, R. H., Jr.: Deficiency disease, Springfield, Ill., 1958, Charles C Thomas, Publisher.

Geelen, J. A. G.: Teratology **7:**49-56, 1973 (malformations due to hypervitaminosis A).

Goldsmith, J. R.: Hosp. Pract. **5:**63-71, May 1970 (air pollution and disease).

Goldwater, L. J.: Human toxicology of mercury. In Matsumura, F., et al., editors: Environmental toxicology of pesticides, New York, 1972, Academic Press, Inc., pp. 165-175.

Goodhart, R. S., and Shils, M. E., editors: Modern nutrition in health and disease, ed. 6, Philadelphia, 1980, Lea & Febiger.

Hay, A.: Nature **262:**636-637, 1976 (dioxin exposure in Saveso, Italy).

Hofmann, F. G., and Hofmann, A. D.: Handbook on drug and alcohol abuse, New York, 1975, Oxford University Press.

Hruban, Z., et al.: Am. J. Pathol. **76:**451-468, 1974 (liver in hypervitaminosis A).

Ivankovic, S., et al.: Int. J. Cancer **24:**786-788, 1979 (arsenic-containing pesticides and lung cancer in rats).

Janerich, D. T., et al.: N. Engl. J. Med. **291:**697-700, 1974 (oral contraceptives and birth defects).

Jenkins, K. J., and Hidiroglou, M.: Can. J. Anim. Sci. **52:**591-620, 1972 (selenium/vitamin E: a review).

Kahn, E.: N. Engl. J. Med. **285:**49-50, 1971 (editorial—mercury-contaminated tuna fish).

Kao, C. Y.: Fed. Proc. **31:**1117-1123, 1972 (pharmacology of tetrodotoxin and saxitoxin).

Kark, R. A. P., et al.: N. Engl. J. Med. **285:**10-16, 1971 (mercury poisoning).

Khan, M. Y., et al.: Arch. Pathol. Lab. Med. **101:**89-94, 1977 (lead cardiomyopathy in mice).

Klein, M., et al.: N. Engl. J. Med. **283:**669-672, 1970 (earthenware containers as source of lead poisoning).

Kraybill, H. F., and Mehlman, M. A., editors: Environmental cancer, New York, 1977, John Wiley & Sons, Inc.

Lancranjan, I.: Arch. Environ. Health **30:**396-401, 1975 (reproductive ability in workmen exposed to lead).

Louria, D. B., et al.: Ann. Intern. Med. **76:**307-319, 1972 (human toxicity of certain trace elements).

Lowry, T., and Schuman, L. M.: J.A.M.A. **162:**153-160, 1956 (silo-filler's disease).

Nelson, N., et al.: Environ. Res. **4:**1-69, 1971 (hazards of mercury: special report to the Secretary's Pesticide Advisory Committee, Dept. of Health, Education, and Welfare, Nov. 1970).

Nora, A. H., and Nora, J. J.: Arch. Environ. Health **30:**17-21, 1975 (syndrome of multiple congenital anomalies associated with teratogenic exposure).

Odom, E. T., and Capel, W.: Milit. Surg. **113:**460-466, 1953 (arachnidism).

Pease, C. N.: J.A.M.A. **182:**980-985, 1962, (hypervitaminosis A).

Peck, G. L., et al.: N. Engl. J. Med. **300:**329-333, 1979 (treatment of severe acne with 13-*cis*-retinoic acid).

Penney, J. R., and Balfour, B. M.: J. Pathol. Bacteriol. **61:**171-178, 1949 (vitamin C).

Rao, K. S. J.: Lancet **1:**709-711, 1974 (kwashiorkor and marasmus).

Reuhl, K. R., and Chang, L. W.: Neurotoxicology **1:**21-55, 1979 (effects of methylmercury on the development of the nervous system).

Richter, R. W., editor: Medical aspects of drug abuse, New York, 1975, Harper & Row, Publishers, Inc.

Saffiotti, U., and Wagoner, J. K., editors: Ann. N.Y. Acad. Sci. **271:**1-516, 1976 (occupational carcinogenesis).

Schepers, G. W. H.: Int. Arch. Gewerbepath. **19:**1-26, 1962 (berylliosis).

The Sciences: **10:**5-8, 34-36, Oct. 1970 (air pollution); **10:**5-9, Dec. 1970 (water pollution).

Seixas, F. A., Williams, K., and Eggleston, S., editors: Ann. N.Y. Acad. Sci. **252:**1-399, 1975 (medical consequences of alcoholism).

Skerfving, S., et al.: Environ. Res. **7:**83-98, 1974 (methylmercury-induced chromosome damage in man).

Smith, J. P., et al.: J. Pathol. Bacteriol. **80:**287-296, 1960 (cadmium).

Sporn, M. B.: CA **29:**120-125, 1979 (retinoids and cancer prevention).

Sporn, M. B., and Newton, D. L.: Fed. Proc. **38:**2528-2534, 1979 (prevention of cancer by retinoids).

Tephis, T. R., et al.: In Hayes, W. J., Jr., editor: Essays in toxicology, vol. 5, New York, 1974, Academic Press, Inc., pp. 149-177 (biochemical toxicology of methanol).

Tsubaki, T., and Irukayama, K., editors: Minamata disease, Tokyo, 1977, Kodansha Ltd.

van Vleet, J. F.: J. Am. Vet. Med. Assoc. **166:**769-774, 1975 (experimental vitamin E–selenium deficiency in dogs).

Wellings, S. R.: Lab. Invest. **24:**455, 1971 (editorial—ecologic pathology).

Wilson, J. G.: Teratology **7:**3-16, 1973 (drugs as teratogens in man).

Wilson, J. G.: Fed. Proc. **36:**1698-1703, 1977 (teratogenic effects of environmental chemicals).

Yeh, S.: Hum. Pathol. **4:**469-485, 1973 (skin cancer in chronic arsenicism).

12

Disturbances of growth

The process of growth of cells, tissues, and organs and of the body as a whole presents unsolved problems of great complexity. The disturbances in growth of the body as a whole (i.e., dwarfism, gigantism, etc.) are hormonal, metabolic, or congenital developmental disturbances and are considered elsewhere (p. 700). The repair of tissue after injury and replacement of tissue lost through normal wear and tear are processes that proceed continuously. The cells and tissues that are least highly organized and differentiated in function and structure (e.g., connective tissues) are most easily replaced. Highly organized structures, such as renal glomeruli or ganglion cells of the central nervous system, are irreplaceable. Between these extremes are all gradations in capacity for regeneration, repair, and growth response to normal or abnormal stimuli.

Growth disturbances involving tissues or organs are neoplastic or nonneoplastic in nature. Neoplastic growths (neoplasms or tumors) will be considered later in this chapter. Among the nonneoplastic growth disturbances are those characterized by:

1. Diminished growth
   a. Acquired (e.g., atrophy), which has been discussed previously (p. 22)
   b. Congenital failure of development (e.g., hypoplasia, aplasia, and agenesis), which has been mentioned previously (p. 22)
2. Excessive growth of cells (e.g., hypertrophy and hyperplasia)

3. Disturbance of cellular differentiation (e.g., metaplasia)
4. Developmental tumorlike masses (e.g., hamartomas and heterotopias)

HYPERTROPHY AND HYPERPLASIA

Hypertrophy refers to an increase in size of constituent cells of a tissue or organ, and hyperplasia refers to an increase in number of the constituent cells. Either of these processes, or both occurring simultaneously, may cause enlargement of the involved tissue or organ. In hypertrophied cells, there may be some increase in size of nuclei, but the enlargement is caused primarily by a greater than normal production of cytoplasmic components, such as endoplasmic reticulum, mitochondria, and (in muscle cells) myofilaments. Enlargement resulting from increased water content (cellular hydration) is not hypertrophy. Hyperplasia occurs in tissues whose cells are capable of mitotic division.

Factors that induce hypertrophy or hyperplasia include increased functional demand and endocrine stimulation. Examples of the former are (1) cardiac hypertrophy resulting from a greater work load placed on the heart because of increased peripheral resistance (hypertension) or abnormal valvular function and (2) enlargement of the residue of an organ or tissue when a portion is removed or destroyed ("compensatory" hypertrophy and/or hyperplasia; regenerative hyperplasia). Similarly, in the case of paired organs (e.g., the kidneys), removal of one may be followed by enlargement of the other. Among the hormones that induce hypertrophy or hyperplasia, or both, are those of the pituitary gland and the gonads. For example, in regard to the hyperplastic changes in the breasts and endometrium during the menstrual cycles and in pregnancy, stimulation by hormones from the ovaries appears to be the controlling mechanism.

Certain tissue cells that lose their ability to undergo mitosis, such as the myocardial fibers in the adult heart, respond to etiologic factors only by hypertrophy, as in the example of "work hypertrophy" mentioned previously (although it has been suggested by several investigators that hypertrophied muscle fibers in the adult heart, beyond a certain point, may proliferate by amitotic division, i.e., by longitudinal splitting). On the other hand, organs such as the liver, endocrine glands, and lymphoid tissues readily respond by hyperplasia, with or without hypertrophy. An excess of growth hormone of the pituitary gland produces hypertrophy of heart muscle fibers, but it causes hyperplasia in the thymus gland and a combination of hypertrophy and hyperplasia in the liver. During pregnancy, there are different responses by the uterine tissues, e.g., the myometrium undergoes hypertrophy mainly (with some increase in the number of smooth muscle cells) and the endometrium exhibits hyperplasia predominantly.

Although hyperplasia is a nonneoplastic process, it may be the site of development of a neoplasm. In some instances a malignant tumor *(cancer)* may ensue, particularly when the hyperplasia is abnormal or atypical in nature, e.g., the areas of *dysplasia (atypical hyperplasia)* in the epithelium of the cervix uteri (p. 658) and the focal *adenomatous (atypical) hyperplasia* and the more extensive *cystic glandular hyperplasia* noted in the endometrium (pp. 643-646).

METAPLASIA

Metaplasia is a change from one type of cell to another. It may be the result of chronic inflammation or irritation, impairment of nutrition and function, or demand for altered func-

tion. A common example is a change from columnar or secretory epithelium to a squamous type. This change may be observed in bronchial mucosa, the gallbladder, or the endocervix as a result of chronic inflammation. Vitamin A deficiency produces a similar metaplasia (p. 233). Metaplasia is common also in cells of the connective tissue type, with the appearance of cartilage or bone in unusual situations such as scars, arteriosclerotic blood vessels, injured and sightless eyes, or degenerated areas of a goiter.

HAMARTOMA

Hamartomas are tumorlike malformations or inborn errors of tissue development composed of an abnormal mixture of tissues normally present in the involved area. Frequently, there is an excess of several tissues, but sometimes one type of tissue is predominant or is the only one represented. The excessive tissues tend to be mature but are arranged in a disorganized fashion. Hamartomas lack the capacity of true neoplasms for limitless proliferation, although they tend to grow with the part affected. Although they are not neoplastic, they occasionally give rise to true neoplasms. Examples of hamartomatous lesions are some angiomas (e.g., the common "birthmark" or hemangioma), benign pigmented nevi ("moles"), and growths in the kidneys consisting of a mixture of smooth muscle, fibrous, and adipose tissues.

HETEROTOPIA

Heterotopia (aberrance or ectopia) refers to the presence of tissues or organs in sites in which they are not normally found. Although heterotopias may be acquired occasionally (e.g., displacement of tissue as a result of trauma or inflammation), they usually are congenital in origin. During prenatal development, an organ or part of it may be displaced and develop in unusual areas, e.g., adrenal cortical tissue in the kidney or retroperitoneal tissue and multiple foci of splenic tissue ("accessory spleens") in extrasplenic sites. (Rarely, accessory spleens are not congenital abnormalities but result from dissemination and peritoneal implantation of splenic tissue following injury or rupture of the spleen.) Another form of heterotopia is the malformation resulting from a primary abnormal differentiation occurring in a developing tissue *(heteroplasia),* e.g., gastric mucosa in part of the mucosa of a Meckel's diverticulum or an island of cartilage in the hypoplastic kidney. Heteroplasia is distinguished from metaplasia, for the abnormal differentiation occurs in developing tissues in the former and in already differentiated or adult tissues in the latter. The term *choristoma* is sometimes used for tumor-like masses of heterotopic tissue. On rare occasions, a true neoplasm may develop in heterotopic tissue, e.g., an islet cell tumor or a pancreatic carcinoma arising in aberrant pancreatic tissue situated in the wall of the stomach or intestine.

NEOPLASMS (TUMORS)

Willis has defined a tumor or neoplasm as "an abnormal mass of tissue, the growth of which exceeds and is uncoordinated with that of the normal tissues, and persists in the same excessive manner after cessation of the stimuli which evoked the change."* The abnormal, excessive, and indefinitely progressive multiplication of cells in neoplasms is unlike that which occurs in inflammation, repair, and hyperplasia; for in these nonneoplastic conditions, the extent of cellular proliferation is limited by certain regulatory controls. It should be noted that, although an increase in number of cells is a distinctive feature of tumors, the term hyperplasia generally is not applied to it. As Willis has pointed out, it is best to restrict the term hyperplasia to the nonneoplastic cellular proliferation that occurs as a response to loss of tissue or to increased functional demand or as a result of endocrine stimulation (p. 240). Tumors are composed of cells and intercellular substances such as may be found in embryonic or mature tissues. Growth activity predominates over function, although the latter is not necessarily lacking.

*From Willis, R. A.: Pathology of tumours, ed. 4, London, 1967, Butterworth & Co. (Publishers) Ltd.

In certain tumors, such as those from endocrine glands, functional activity may be an important feature. Endocrine activity also occurs in some tumors of nonendocrine origin. Tumors act as parasites, absorbing nourishment from the blood, growing with enhanced vitality at the expense of normal tissues, and yet performing no useful work for the body. The designation *benign* or *malignant* is given to tumors in accordance with their clinical behavior and morphologic features, which will be discussed in detail later. The essential differences between these types may be stated briefly as follows.

Benign tumors are those that tend to grow slowly and expansively, and unless they are in some vital spot or interfere with an important organ, they are well tolerated and do not necessarily interfere with the person's well-being or shorten his life. They usually are composed of well-differentiated mature types of tissue.

Malignant tumors generally are more rapidly growing than benign tumors, tend to infiltrate and extend into normal structures, and, unless effectively treated, interfere with health and eventually cause death. They usually are composed of cells less differentiated than the normal. Another term for a malignant tumor is *cancer.*

Today, cancer ranks second among the causes of death in the United States, the first being heart disease. The leading cause of cancer deaths among men, numbered according to rank, are cancers arising in (1) the lung, (2) the colon and rectum, and (3) the prostate; whereas, among women, they are cancers in (1) the breast, and (2) the colon and rectum. Until recently, cancer of the uterus ranked as the third major cause of cancer deaths among women, but according to the American Cancer Society's Facts and Figures 1975, uterine cancer has dropped to fourth place largely because of earlier detection of the disease, particularly by the Papanicolaou smear test (p. 255). Lung cancer has become the third major cause of cancer deaths among women, probably related to the increase in the number of women smokers. Malignant tumors are not limited to any age group, although most of them occur in older persons. Cancer is a leading cause of death in children in the age group 1 to 14 years, ranking second to accidents. The common types of cancer in childhood include leukemia, malignant lymphomas, neurogenic tumors (neuroblastoma, brain tumors, retinoblastoma), Wilms' tumor of the kidney, and sarcoma of bones and other connective tissues.

Classification

Neoplasms are classified according to structure and origin, since etiology is too uncertain to form a satisfactory basis. No grouping seems entirely satisfactory, but the simplest and most common classification divides tumors into the following varieties:

Tumors of mesenchymal origin
    Benign
    Malignant—sarcoma
Tumors of epithelial origin
    Benign
    Malignant—carcinoma
Mixed tumors and teratomas
    Benign
    Malignant

In the first group (tumors of mesenchymal origin) are included not only fibroblastic tumors but also those of cartilage, bone, fat, blood vessels, lymphatic tissue, mesothelium, muscle, and blood-forming tissues. The mixed tumors are those arising from multipotential cells and containing more than one type of tissue. Teratomas arise from totipotential cells, often contain representatives of all three germ layers, and show attempts at organ formation.

The tumors of particular organs are considered with the other lesions of those organs, where details of classification and structure are presented.

Characteristics

Benign tumors. Benign tumors do not endanger life unless they are so situated as to interfere with some vital organ or function. They usually grow slowly and after reaching a certain size may remain stationary. Their growth is expansive. They push aside normal tissues but do not invade and hence appear as circumscribed, well-demarcated growths that may be surrounded by a fibrous capsule caused by pressure on the adjacent tissue. They do not metastasize, i.e., secondary tumors are not formed in other organs. Necrosis and ulceration occur less frequently than in malignant tumors. Local removal is usually successful and not followed by recurrence.

Histologically, benign tumors usually are composed of a well-differentiated, mature type of tissue closely imitating the normal tissue of their origin. Rarity of mitotic figures reflects their slow growth.

Malignant tumors. Malignant tumors are those neoplasms whose unhindered progression is likely to cause death of the person. They often grow rapidly, not only by expansion but also by infiltration and invasion of surrounding tissues, so that they are unencapsulated and poorly demarcated. However, it should be noted that occasionally a malignant tumor may appear to be localized and even encapsulated. Cancers have a tendency to develop metastases in distant organs. Local removal of a malignant tumor, unless absolutely complete, is followed by recurrence at the same site. Malignant tumors are more prone to degeneration and ulceration than are benign tumors.

Histologically, the cells and structural organization of malignant tumors exhibit inadequate maturation or lack of differentiation of varying degree that at times is so pronounced that the tissue of origin is not identifiable. The degree of *anaplasia,* the term applied to the loss of cellular and organizational differentiation, tends to parallel the degree of malignancy of a neoplasm. Pleomorphism of cells and their nuclei (i.e., variation in size and shape), enlargement of nuclei with an increased nucleocytoplasmic ratio, clumping of chromatin, hyperchromatism of nuclei, and prominent nucleoli are other common histologic features of malignant neoplasms (Fig. 12-1). Relative frequency of mitotic figures reflects their rapid growth, and abnormal forms of mitotic nuclei may be present (Fig. 12-2).

Although in most instances the differences between benign and malignant neoplasms are

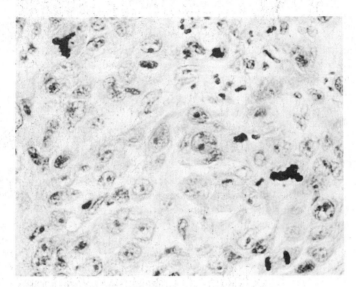

Fig. 12-1. Histologic appearance of malignant tumor—undifferentiated carcinoma. Note variation in size and shape of nuclei and mitotic figures, including abnormal tripolar mitoses.

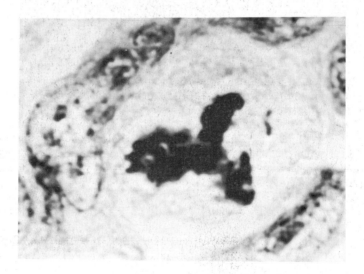

Fig. 12-2. High-power view of abnormal, tripolar mitotic figure.

distinctive, there are certain tumors in which the features are not so clear-cut. Borderline cases occur that may be difficult to classify.

Stroma of tumors. In addition to the neoplastic cells themselves, a tumor has a supporting connective tissue stroma with blood supply, on which the growth of a tumor depends. The amount of stroma in a tumor varies considerably. Some neoplasms are composed mostly of tumor cells with very little stroma and are soft (e.g., medullary carcinoma of the breast). Other tumors, particularly carcinomas, stimulate formation of an abundance of fibrous stroma, causing the neoplasm to be hard or *scirrhous* (e.g., scirrhous carcinoma of the breast). The formation of excessive stromal fibrous tissue often is referred to as *desmoplasia*.

Recent evidence indicates that tumor cells liberate a substance, known as *tumor angiogenesis factor* (TAF), that stimulates the growth of new capillaries in the host, so that the tumor becomes vascularized *(tumor angiogenesis)*. This is one means by which progression of tumors may occur. Currently, there is interest in identifying factors that inhibit angiogenesis as an approach to the control of tumor growth.

Electron microscopic features. Electron microscopy is useful in the diagnosis of neoplasms, particularly when a tumor is poorly differentiated and identification of its type is not clearly established by light microscopy. The presence of certain distinctive cytoplasmic organelles, filaments, or inclusions frequently aids in the interpretation of the nature of tumors. Examples of the characteristic ultrastructural features that provide clues for correct diagnosis are the following: (1) secretory granules and vesicles, such as zymogen granules in acinic cell carcinomas, mucin granules in poorly differentiated adenocarcinomas, distinctive granules in certain endocrine tumors (e.g., carcinoid and islet cell tumors) and in neuroblastomas, pinocytotic vesicles in neurogenic and smooth muscle tumors, and melanin granules (premelanosomes and melanosomes), in malignant melanomas, (2) cytofilaments, such as tonofilaments (often associated with desmosomes) in squamous cell carcinomas and myofilaments in muscle tumors, (3) glycogen deposits in Ewing's sarcoma, differentiating it from lymphoreticular malignant neoplasms, and in other tumors (e.g., hepatocellular, renal cell, and squamous cell carcinomas, and (4) microvilli in glandular tumors.

Estimation of malignancy and prognosis

The factors that must be considered in estimating the result of a cancer include (1) type of tumor, (2) its situation, (3) duration, size, spread, and presence or absence of metastasis, (4) age and condition of the patient, (5) rate of clinical growth, (6) histologic structure, and (7) radiosensitivity.

The *type of tumor* is important, since cancers vary in their degree of malignancy and course. Certain tumors, such as the basal cell carcinoma of the skin, grow slowly and rarely metastasize. At the other extreme are tumors of rapid growth and early extension, such as myeloma of bone and lymphosarcoma.

The *situation* of a tumor influences the outcome because it may interfere with vital structures or may be such as to make operative removal difficult, e.g., gliomatous tumors of the brain and carcinoma of the esophagus.

The *duration* of the tumor influences prognosis, for it allows time for spread. Thus, a tumor that is easily curable in an early stage may be hopeless later. *Extensive local spread* or *metastasis* to other organs suggests an earlier and more inevitable end. On the other hand, a tumor of long duration with only slight increase in size and no metastasis suggests slow growth, low malignancy, and a relatively favorable outcome.

Age is of some importance, in that certain tumors seem to progress more rapidly in younger persons. *Pregnancy* and *lactation* cause more rapid growth in cancer of the breast.

Histologic structure is of importance in indicating the type of tumor, rapidity of growth, and degree of anaplasia or differentiation. Systems of histologic grading have been evolved.

Radiosensitivity of a tumor is often important in determining how long life may be prolonged or if cure is possible.

Microscopic grading of cancer. Many factors other than histologic structure influence the degree of malignancy, but among tumors of the same type and arising at the same site, there are variations in malignancy that can be correlated roughly with the degree of anaplasia or undifferentiation. Such microscopic grading of the malignancy of a tumor, if put on a numerical and standardized basis, is helpful in predicting the course of the disease when used in conjunction with the factors noted previously, such as size, degree of extension, etc.

It may also be of help in determining the type of treatment likely to give the best results. In general, the greater the anaplasia of a tumor (i.e., the higher the microscopic grade of malignancy), the greater its radiosensitivity. Numerical systems of histologic grading, if used alone, may have limited prognostic value for individual cases.

Broders originated and popularized a method of grading according to which tumors are divided into four grades of malignancy*:

  Grade I: Tumors showing a marked tendency to differentiation, with three fourths or more of their cells differentiated

  Grade II: Three fourths to one half of the cells differentiated

  Grade III: One half to one fourth of the cells differentiated

  Grade IV: One fourth to none of the cells differentiated

While this system of grading is generally useful, it often is extended and modified in the case of tumors of certain organs, e.g., cervix uteri or rectum. The various modifications are noted later as these tumors are considered. Statistics regarding the duration of life in untreated cancer (i.e., the natural history of the disease) must be known to evaluate methods of therapy.

Clinical stage classification of cancer. The clinical staging of cancer is the division of cases of cancer into groups according to a plan based on extent of the disease. One such plan, known as the TNM system, uses three components: the size or extent of the primary tumor (T), the involvement of regional lymph nodes (N), and the presence or absence of distant metastasis (M). Carcinoma in situ is designated as TIS. Increasing involvement of each element may be denoted by combining the letter with a number from 0 to 4, so that a shorthand system of designating extent of a cancer of a particular site may be used. Categorization into stages may then be made according to classification agreed on for each site.

Carcinoma in situ. In some tissues, partic-

ularly the epidermis of the skin, the squamous epithelium of the exocervix, the endometrium, and the bronchial epithelium, an area of atypical proliferation occurs affecting usually the entire thickness of the epithelium and exhibiting the cytologic features similar to those of invasive cancer but no demonstrable penetration into the subepithelial stroma. It is generally believed that this lesion, *carcinoma in situ,* is a true intraepithelial cancer that frequently becomes invasive carcinoma if left untreated. The lesion is also known as "preinvasive carcinoma." There is some controversy as to whether it is a reversible process. A less extensive involvement of the epithelium by atypical cells is referred to as *dysplasia* or "atypical hyperplasia." In itself, dysplasia is not a neoplastic change, but some pathologists believe that it may progress to carcinoma in situ, although the frequency of such a transformation is not known.

Effects of radiation

In the treatment of tumors by ionizing radiation, roentgen rays (or x-rays) and gamma rays are the ones particularly used. All tissues, normal and neoplastic, are affected by radiation so that radiosensitivity is a relative term. Cells that are actively proliferating or that are of a primitive type are more sensitive than normal tissues, so that there is usually a considerable margin between the doses that are damaging to neoplastic and to normal tissue.

The effects of x-rays or gamma rays on growing cells vary with the intensity and duration of exposure and consist of (1) destruction of some cells, (2) inhibition of imminent mitosis, followed by abnormal mitosis and disruption of the cells, and (3) damage to resting cells so that continued proliferation fails. Cells in a premitotic phase are believed to be particularly susceptible, although this has been questioned.

Radiation also may affect the cells indirectly. Action on blood vessels supplying tumor tissue may be of importance. An early effect of radiation is extreme hyperemia due to distention of capillaries, and this may be followed by thrombosis or rupture. Larger blood

*Broders, A. C.: Surg. Clin. North Am. **21:**947-962, 1941.

vessels may be completely obliterated. The effect on the tumor bed contributes to the effects of radiation on tumor tissue.

Radiosensitivity of tumors. Since all tumors can be affected by radiation, the terms *radiosensitivity* and *radioresistance* are relative. Radiosensitivity does not necessarily imply curability by radiation. Easy accessibility and tolerance of surrounding structures are important factors in curability. Radiation may be valuable in relief of pain (e.g., in skeletal metastasis from carcinoma of the breast), even though not curative.

Radiosensitivity varies with the reproductive activity of the tissue (law of Bergonié and Tribondeau) and increases with increasing anaplasia and embryonal quality of tumor cells. The tumor bed is also important—a bed of slight vascularity or of fat, bone, or cartilage is unfavorable. Tumor recurrences tend to be more resistant than was the original tumor. The presence of infection in the tissue appears to decrease sensitivity.

The relative degree of radiosensitivity of some tumors is noted in Table 11-1 (p. 232).

Spread and metastasis

Malignant tumors spread by direct invasive growth into surrounding tissues and by the formation of secondary tumors not connected with the original neoplasm. This latter process, called metastasis, is due to extension by lymphatics, by the bloodstream, and by implantation. The distribution of metastatic tumors appears to be determined by the number of tumor emboli that reach and lodge in various organs and tissues, as well as by differences in suitability of different tissues for the growth of tumor cells. Metastatic tumors are most common in lymph nodes, lungs, liver, bones, kidneys, and adrenal glands. The spleen and skeletal muscle are relatively infrequent sites of metastasis.

The *invasiveness of malignant tumors* may be associated with certain characteristics of cancer cells, particularly *decrease in cohesiveness* and *loss of contact inhibition*. A low concentration of calcium within cancer tissue may be one factor that contributes to the decrease

in cohesiveness of cancer cells, although in some types of cancer imperfect formation of intercellular junctions may play a role. Inhibition of growth and movement of cells when in contact with each other is a characteristic of normal tissue cells (contact inhibition). On the other hand, such inhibition is not evident among cancer cells (loss of contact inhibition), and as a result, they continue to proliferate and spread. Certain investigators, using intracellular electric techniques to determine whether intercellular communication is involved in control of tissue growth, have shown that in normal cells the junctional membrane surfaces are freely permeable to varying-sized ions and molecules, whereas the cells of cancerous growths are impermeable even to small ions. The implication is that intercellular communications permit possible growth-controlling substances to flow from one cell to another in normal tissues but not in malignant neoplasms. It has been proposed that alterations in the proteins and glycoproteins of surface and internal membranes of transformed cells may set into motion a series of functional changes that impart to the cells the characteristics of malignancy, such as those just discussed.

Of uncertain or speculative importance in the mechanism of invasion of malignant tumors are such factors as *rapidity of growth* of a tumor, *increased motility* of cancer cells, and *elaboration of hydrolytic enzymes* or *other lytic products* by cancer cells. The old hypothesis of Ribbert that there is a loss of growth restraint on the part of the surrounding tissues has little to support it.

Lymphatic metastasis. Extension by the lymphatics is the common method of spread of carcinoma. Tumor cells grow into lymphatic channels and are broken off and carried as *emboli* to a lymph node (Figs. 12-3 and 12-4). Here, the tumor cells lodge and often can be seen initially in the subcapsular space or peripheral sinus. Thus, a secondary tumor is started that may eventually overwhelm the node, break through the capsule, and spread locally as well as onward in the lymphatic system.

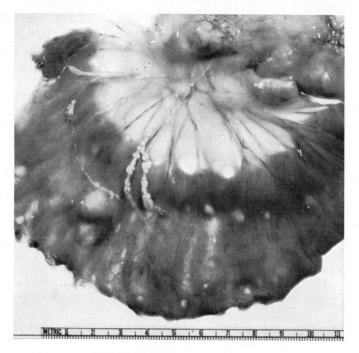

Fig. 12-3. Lymphatic extension of carcinoma in mesentery with metastasis in lymph nodes.

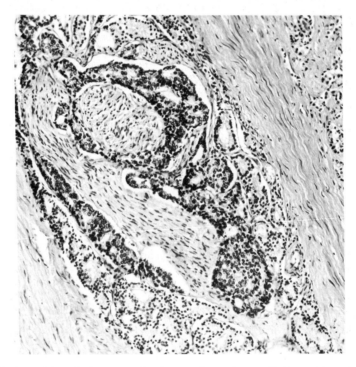

Fig. 12-4. Perineural lymphatic metastasis of prostatic carcinoma. Perineural lymphatic space is filled with glandular tumor.

There also may be lymphatic spread by *permeation,* i.e., by direct and continuous growth along a lymphatic channel. However, lymphatic permeation appears to occur less commonly than lymphatic embolism.

Lymph nodes draining the area of a primary carcinoma occasionally contain granulomas of a tuberculoid or sarcoidlike appearance, apparently stimulated by irritant materials absorbed from the neoplastic area. Intracellular asteroid bodies or other inclusions may be present. The draining lymph nodes may contain paramyloid material or may show marked sinusoidal and follicular histiocytic change. Some investigators consider sinusoidal histiocytosis to be a defensive reaction to an antigenic stimulus and regard it as a favorable prognostic sign.

Metastasis by bloodstream. Extension by the bloodstream is the common method of spread of sarcoma, but many carcinomas spread in this fashion as well. Tumor cells penetrate the thin wall of a vein, are broken off, and are carried away as emboli. Tumor emboli that enter branches of the portal vein lodge in the liver, and that organ is the common site for metastasis from tumors of the intestinal tract (Fig. 12-5). Tumor emboli from systemic veins tend to lodge in the lung, or they may be carried by the paravertebral venous system to reach the bones of the vertebral column, shoulder girdle, and pelvis (Fig. 12-6). Undoubtedly, some tumor cells reach the arterial circulation directly or by passage through pulmonary capillaries. Probably many

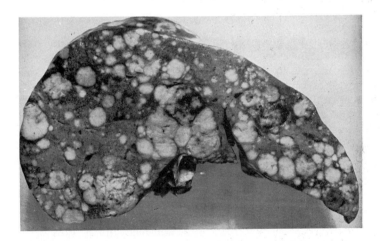

Fig. 12-5. Metastatic carcinoma of liver. Primary tumor in stomach.

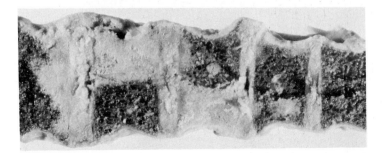

Fig. 12-6. Metastatic carcinoma (from prostate gland) in vertebral column. Dense, grayish masses represent metastatic tumor.

tumor emboli fail to survive. The tissues in which the emboli lodge must be capable of rapidly supplying adequate blood or nourishment for the tumor tissue. It is possible that some tumor cells enter the bloodstream after having first passed through the lymphatic circulation.

Metastatic tumors are uncommon in certain tissues and organs, such as voluntary muscle, heart, and spleen. Blood-borne metastasis involves mainly lung, liver, and bone. Metastatic tumors of the brain are most commonly from the lung, breast, stomach, prostate gland, and adrenal gland. Those tumors that metastasize to bone with particular frequency are hypernephroma of the kidney and carcinomas of the prostate gland, lung, ovary, breast (Fig. 12-7), testis, and thyroid gland. Most metastatic tumors in bone are characteristically destructive, so that they appear as radiolucent areas in roentgenograms *(osteolytic metastases)*. Certain neoplasms, however, such as prostatic carcinoma in men and carcinoma of the breast in women, tend to produce skeletal metastases that are accompanied by formation of new bone at the metastatic site, appearing as radiopaque areas in roentgenograms *(osteoplastic metastases)*. These tumors, of course, also may produce osteolytic metastases.

Metastasis by implantation. Extension by implantation occurs when tumor cells involving a serous or mucous membrane become detached and are later implanted on other areas. Carcinoma of the ovary commonly spreads throughout the peritoneal cavity in this fashion (Fig. 12-8). When cancer involves a serosal surface, considerable fluid is usually present in the cavity and often is of a hemorrhagic character. Tumor cells may be demonstrable in such fluids by centrifuging and making smears and paraffin sections of the cellular material thus thrown down. Implantation of malignant cells also may occur in operative wounds and along the track of a needle puncture.

Effects of tumors

Local and systemic effects. Benign neoplasms can produce serious effects as a result of their location and expansive growth by compressing vital structures and causing obstructions of visceral lumina. Benign tumors near a surface may become ulcerated and bleed, or infection may be superimposed. Those that are pedunculated may become twisted, leading to interference with the blood supply, followed by infarction. Some benign tumors of endocrine organs may cause harmful effects by producing excessive hormones.

Malignant neoplasms may produce the same effects as benign ones, but, because of their more rapid growth and invasiveness, local effects tend to be more pronounced, and metastases appear. Anemia may occur as a result of hemorrhage, depression of hematopoiesis (associated with superimposed infections or involvement of bone marrow by primary or metastatic tumors), or disturbed nutrition (due to suppression of appetite or obstruction of the alimentary tract). Loss of weight, sometimes

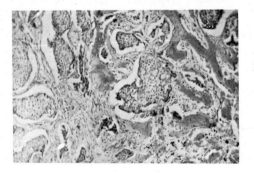

Fig. 12-7. Metastatic carcinoma from breast in bone marrow.

with severe wasting (cachexia), has been attributed to starvation, hemorrhage, ulceration, infection, necrosis of tissue with release of toxins, diversion of body nutrition in favor of the neoplastic growth, pain, sleeplessness, and anxiety, but often the cause is not apparent.

The secretion of hormones by neoplasms arising in endocrine organs is a feature that is more characteristic of well-differentiated benign tumors than cancers. The production of hormones by these tumors tends to be unregulated and may be excessive, so that symptoms of hyperfunction of the involved organs may occur. Examples are (1) hyperinsulinism (hypoglycemia) resulting from islet cell tumor of the pancreas, (2) acromegaly in the adult or gigantism in the child due to acidophil adenoma of the pituitary gland, (3) hyperparathyroidism due to parathyroid tumor, and (4) hyperestrinism (precocious puberty in girls or endometrial hyperplasia, and sometimes carcinoma, with vaginal bleeding in adult women) due to granulosa–theca cell tumor of the ovary. However, in some instances, nonfunctioning tumors arising in or metastasizing to endocrine organs may cause sufficient destruction of the latter, so that symptoms associated with hypofunction of the involved organs may develop; e.g., an expanding, nonfunctioning chromophobe adenoma of the pituitary gland may compress and destroy adjacent normal pituitary tissue, resulting in hypopituitarism.

Paraneoplastic syndromes. There are various less usual, and sometimes peculiar, clinical manifestations of malignant neoplasms that are not accounted for by the anatomic position of the primary tumor or its metastases or by iatrogenic effects of therapy. These disorders, often referred to as *paraneoplastic syndromes,* may be the result of identifiable endocrine, metabolic, or other types of activity of the cancer, but at times the clinical manifestations are unexplained. It sometimes happens that these less usual disorders become clinically evident long before the more typical manifestations of cancer appear. Among these disorders are those related to the elaboration of hormones by tumors originating from tissues that normally do not produce them (so-called *ectopic hormone-secreting tumors* or *paraendocrine tumors*). The following are examples of the paraneoplastic syndromes and some of the tumors with which they are associated.

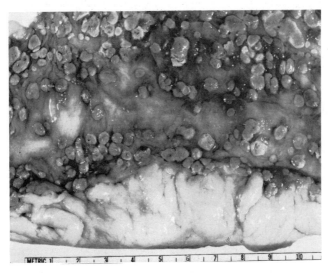

Fig. 12-8. Carcinomatous nodules on peritoneal surface of colon.

1 Endocrine and other metabolic disorders
  a Inappropriate secretion of antidiuretic hormone (bronchogenic carcinoma—oat cell type)
  b Hyperadrenocorticism with or without classical features of Cushing's syndrome (bronchogenic carcinoma—oat cell type and thymoma)
  c Gonadotropin secretion (carcinomas of bronchus, liver, breast)
  d Hypercalcemia and hypercalcinuria (not due to osseous metastases), possibly related to secretion of parathyroid hormone or parathyroid hormone–like substance or to other bone-resorbing factors, such as vitamin D–like substances, osteoclast-activating factor (OAF), and prostaglandins (bronchogenic carcinoma—squamous cell type; carcinomas of breast, kidney, ovary, pancreas, colon)
  e Hypoglycemia, possibly due to secretion of insulinlike substance, deficient glucogenesis, or increased utilization of glucose by large size of tumor (large intrathoracic or retroperitoneal fibrosarcoma; hepatocarcinoma)
  f Increased serum acid phosphatase (prostatic carcinoma)
2 Neuromuscular disorders
  a Peripheral neuropathy (carcinomas of bronchus, breast, ovary, and gastrointestinal tract; Hodgkin's disease)
  b Degenerative brain disorders (bronchogenic carcinoma)
  c Myopathy (carcinomas of bronchus, breast, ovary, colon, prostate)
3 Vascular and hematologic disorders
  a Migratory phlebothrombosis, nonbacterial thrombotic endocarditis, disseminated intravascular coagulation (consumption coagulopathy), occurring separately or in combination, due to release of clotting factor (carcinomas of pancreas, bronchus, gastrointestinal tract, prostate, ovary)
  b Erythrocytosis due to secretion of erythropoietin or similar substance (renal cell carcinoma and hepatocarcinoma, but also by a benign tumor—a large uterine leiomyoma)
  c Red cell aplasia due to hypofunction of bone marrow, possibly related to immunologic factor (e.g., damage to bone marrow erythroblasts by antibody or immune complex) or to secretion of inhibitor of erythropoietin (thymoma)
4 Cutaneous and skeletal disorders
  a Dermatomyositis, possibly resulting from autoimmune reaction initiated by tumor antigens (carcinomas of bronchus, breast, gastrointestinal tract, and ovary; malignant lymphoma)
  b Pigmented verrucous lesions of skin, i.e., acanthosis nigricans (intra-abdominal carcinomas, e.g., stomach)
  c Hypertrophic osteoarthropathy (bronchogenic carcinoma)

Causes of death in cancer patients. Despite advances in therapy that have resulted in remissions and prolonged survival among many cancer patients, there is still a substantial number of patients with malignant tumors whose life span is shortened. In a recent study at the M. D. Anderson Hospital and Tumor Institute, Houston, Texas, the following primary causes of death in cancer patients were identified: infection (47%), organ failure (25%), infarction (11%), carcinomatosis (10%), and hemorrhage (7%).

The most common fatal *infections* were pneumonia (24%), septicemia (18%), and peritonitis (3%). Among the other infections (2%), pyelonephritis was the major one. Most of the infections occurred in relation to cancer of the genitourinary tract. Pneumonia occurred most frequently in patients with bronchogenic carcinoma, cancer of the head and neck, and malignant melanoma. Septicemias were seen most commonly in patients with genitourinary and gastrointestinal cancers. The factors that were responsible for the development of fatal infections in most patients (67%) were necrosis or ulceration of tumors and compression or obstruction of the urinary, alimentary, or respiratory tracts by tumor masses. Another factor was neutropenia, resulting from chemotherapy or radiotherapy, that predisposed 14% of the patients to fatal infections. Other contributing factors were radiation-induced mucositis, necrosis, perforations or adhesions, and operative procedures, which resulted in wound dehiscence and peritonitis. Gram-negative bacteria, i.e., *Escherichia coli*, *Klebsiella* species, and *Pseudomonas aeruginosa*, were the commonest organisms causing infection. Others included *Staphylococcus aureus*, *Clostridium* species, enterococci, and fungi.

Organ failure, which consisted of respiratory failure, cardiac insufficiency, central nervous system failure, hepatic coma, and renal insufficiency, usually resulted from invasion by the tumor, although in more than half of the patients with cardiac insufficiency, arteriosclerotic heart disease was responsible.

The most frequent sites of *infarction* were the lungs and heart. Slightly more than half the infarcts in the lungs were related to interference of the circulation by the tumor, and the other were related to pulmonary embolism from a distant venous thrombus. The vast majority of myocardial infarcts were caused by atherosclerosis; relatively few were due to the tumor.

Fatal *hemorrhage* occurred most frequently in the gastrointestinal tract and the brain but was seen also in the region of the head and neck, the lungs, and the peritoneal cavity. Bleeding was caused by the underlying tumor in most of the patients. Among the other factors responsible for the hemorrhage was thrombocytopenia, resulting from radiotherapy or chemotherapy or less often from replacement of the bone marrow by tumor.

The remaining patients had *carcinomatosis,* i.e., advanced metastatic malignant disease, without evidence of any other pathologic process. Death in these patients was contributed to by severe emaciation (cachexia) and electrolytic imbalance. Most often, carcinomatosis was seen in patients with malignant melanoma and breast cancer.

Immune response to tumors. A relationship between the immune defense system of the host and neoplastic disease is suggested by a number of observations in both man and animals, among which are the following: (1) Patients with certain immune deficiency diseases and organ transplant patients receiving immunosuppressive therapy seem to be more prone to develop primary malignant neoplasms, particularly of the reticuloendothelial system (i.e., lymphomas). (2) Animals with immune deficiency produced by immunosuppressive therapy or by neonatal thymectomy are more susceptible to the induction of neoplasms. (3) In man, spontaneous regression of a neoplasm, regression of metastases after surgical excision of the primary tumor, or failure of metastatic growth by malignant cells that entered the circulation during an operation occurs occasionally. (4) Experimentally, rejection of transplanted tumors occurs in animals

previously immunized against the neoplasm by exposure to small, sublethal doses of tumor tissue. (5) In certain human cancers, there appears to be an antitumor reaction, as evidenced by a lymphocytic and histiocytic infiltration in the stroma or by a sinusoidal histiocytic proliferation in adjacent lymph nodes.

The ability of the host to mount an immunologic defense against cancer is related to the fact that cancer cells acquire new surface antigens (on or in the plasma membrane) that are not present in normal cells. It is commonly believed that the host maintains a constant immunologic surveillance, whereby the immune system detects and destroys newly formed malignant cells, and that the appearance of a tumor suggests a breakdown or inadequacy of the host's immunologic defense system. In this regard it is of interest to note that a major effort in current immunologic research in the treatment of malignant tumors is the use of nonspecific stimulants, such as the attenuated tuberculosis vaccine, BCG, to increase the ability of the immune system to react against cancer (p. 90).

Cell-mediated mechanisms are believed to play a greater role in the host's defense against tumors than humoral immunity. There are at least four ways by which cell-mediated mechanisms may be involved in the destruction of tumor cells.

T lymphocyte cytotoxicity. Cytolysis of tumor cells by T lymphocytes occurs without involvement of antibodies or complement following direct contact and interaction of the lymphocytes with the antigen-bearing target cells. The T cells are capable of directly lysing the tumor cells. As a result of the contact with the effector T lymphocytes, the tumor cells undergo progressive changes in membrane permeability followed by osmotic swelling and eventual rupture. It has been suggested that a cytotoxic factor (i.e., lymphotoxin), which is liberated by the stimulated lymphocytes, may contribute to the lysis.

Macrophage-mediated cytotoxicity. Macrophages have been shown to be cytotoxic to tumor cells. It was noted previously (p. 87) that macrophages may be "activated" by a lymphokine, the *macrophage-activating factor* (MAF), which is liberated by immunologically active lymphocytes. Other agents also may activate macrophages, e.g., interferon, bacteria and their products, endotoxin, Freund's adjuvant, and BCG. The "activated" macrophages exhibit an immunologically nonspecific cytotoxicity to tumors, i.e., they destroy various types of tumor cells. However, they apparently recognize and do not destroy normal cells in the area. In some situations, macrophages may be acted upon by a product of immunologically active lymphocytes known as *specific macrophage arming factor* (SMAF). These "armed" macrophages show a specific cytotoxicity to the particular tumor cells that had stimulated the T lymphocytes that were involved in "arming" the macrophages, and they do not destroy other types of tumor cells. The antitumor activity of macrophages may be inhibited by certain factors secreted by cancer cells. Recently, an inhibitor substance has been identified in extracts of certain cancer cells that impairs chemotactic activity of macrophages. In some patients with Hodgkin's disease, a naturally occurring inhibitor, the *chemotactic factor inactivator,* has been discovered in the serum.

Antibody-dependent cell-mediated cytotoxicity. Tumor cells may be coated with antitumor antibody so that they can be lysed by cells that have Fc receptors, including lymphocytes and macrophages. The lymphocytes are non-T cells, such as K or null cells.

NK cell cytotoxicity. Recently, it has been shown that normal (nonsensitized) lymphocytes derived from non–tumor bearing mice, which are termed "natural killer" (NK) cells and lack the surface markers of mature mouse lymphocytes, are capable of lysing tumor cells, although the mode of cytotoxic action of the NK cells has not been clearly defined yet. NK cell reactivity has been shown to be increased by certain agents, such as BCG.

• • •

As for the role of humoral immunity, cytotoxic circulating antibodies can be detected, but it is only under special circumstances that the immune response against neoplasms seems to be accomplished by humoral antibodies. The presence of complement is usually required for cytolytic action. An apparent paradox is that some neoplasms tend to grow better in the presence of specific circulating antibodies, probably because the latter interfere with the cell-mediated tumor destruction. Some investigators suggest that the antibodies form complexes with antigen that block the activity of sensitized cytotoxic lymphocytes. This immunologic enhancement may be the mechanism by which progressive growth of a tumor occurs in vivo despite the fact that its cells are inhibited by immunologically reactive cells in vitro.

There is no question about the existence of tumor-specific antigens in animal neoplasms produced experimentally by means of viruses, chemicals, or x-radiation. In these animals, all neoplasms induced by a given virus share the same tumor antigens, whereas the tumors induced by a given chemical or by x-radiation are antigenically distinct. In human beings, the evidence of tumor antigenicity is not so striking. However, with the development of new techniques for the detection of tumor-induced immune reactions, cell-mediated and/or humoral immunity to a variety of tumors in patients has been demonstrated (e.g., malignant melanoma; acute leukemia; neuroblastoma; choriocarcinoma; Hodgkin's disease; Burkitt's lymphoma; cancer of the gastrointestinal tract, breast, and prostate gland; and sarcomas, including osteosarcoma).

Certain human cancer antigens are similar to those found in embryonic and fetal tissues, such as the carcinoembryonic antigen (CEA), associated with colorectal carcinoma, and α_1-fetoprotein (AFP), associated with hepatocarcinoma and testicular embryonal carcinoma. The detection of these antigens in the serum of patients, particularly by radioimmunoassay, has been used as a laboratory procedure for the diagnosis of these cancers. However, circulating CEA has been identified in patients with other types of carcinoma and nonmaliganant inflammatory bowel disease, including ulcerative colitis and granulomatous diseases, although the nonmalignant disorders yield low titers. Although the determination of CEA serum values may not be an absolute test for malignancy or specific type of cancer, it may be used for assessing the prognosis and management of patients with colorectal carcinoma, particularly in monitoring for tumor recurrence following resection. It has been found that elevated levels of circulating AFP may occur with cancers other than those in the liver and testis and also in patients with nonmalignant hepatic disease (e.g., viral hepatitis and chronic active hepatitis), but the levels of AFP are much higher in association with hepato-carcinoma and embryonal carcinoma of the testis.

A biologic cloning technique has been developed recently that may lead to large-scale production of monoclonal antibodies specific for tumor antigens as well as other antigens (e.g., viral). The expectation is that this procedure will have important clinical applications, including the diagnosis and treatment of cancer and other diseases. In the monoclonal antibody technique, antibody-producing lymphocytes are obtained from the spleen of laboratory mice immunized with foreign (e.g., tumor) cells; then the splenic lymphocytes are fused in vitro with mouse myeloma or lymphoma cells, which are malignant. The resulting cells, called *hybridomas,* proliferate and produce antibodies as long as they are maintained in cultures. (Hybridomas contain genetic material from each cell used in the fusion process, including the genes from the splenic lymphocytes that control antibody production and the genes from the mouse malignant tumor cells that are responsible for continuous proliferation. Ordinarily, the antibody-producing lymphocytes would not grow well in the in vitro cultures in the absence of fusion with the malignant mouse cells.) Since different lymphocytes produce antibody against only one of the various antigens on the surface of a cell, the next phase of this technique is to separate the hybridomas into individual clones in tissue culture dishes. In this way, antibody directed against a single antigenic determinant is produced by each clone. The monoclonal anti-

body made by each cell line is collected and matched against its antigen.

Cytologic diagnosis of malignancy

Papanicolaou demonstrated, in smears made from vaginal secretions, that cells shed from the cervix, endometrium, and vagina showed characteristics that reflected hormonal, inflammatory, and neoplastic conditions of the tissue from which the cells originated. Of particular importance was the finding that early carcinoma of the cervix, at a stage when its visual examination might reveal no abnormality, could be detected by microscopic study of the cells.

The recognition of malignant cells from the cervix is based on nuclear characteristics, which are enlargement, variations in size, shape, and structure, and hyperchromasia (Fig. 12-9). Less frequently, macronucleoli and mitoses are important features. These nuclear alterations are also found in cancer cells shed from other tissues. The certainty of identification as malignant cells increases with the number of distinguishing features that are recognized. The presence of two or more characteristics is necessary to safely identify a cell as a cancer cell. Interpretation of the presence of cancer is also more accurate when based on the changes in many cells, although under some circumstances a few seriously altered cells may be of great significance.

In addition to the morphologic characteristics of the nucleus of the malignant cells, the application of cytochemical methods shows increased DNA and RNA as characteristic of rapidly growing cells.

Nuclear enlargement. Nuclear enlargement or increase of the nucleocytoplasmic ratio is an important characteristic of malignant cells, although it also may be found in cells with certain degenerative changes and in cells of benign proliferative reactions. Change in nuclear size can best be appreciated when it can be compared with a normal, nonmalignant cell of the same origin.

Variations in nuclear size, shape, and structure. *Variation in nuclear size* also is observed in the cells of some malignant tumors

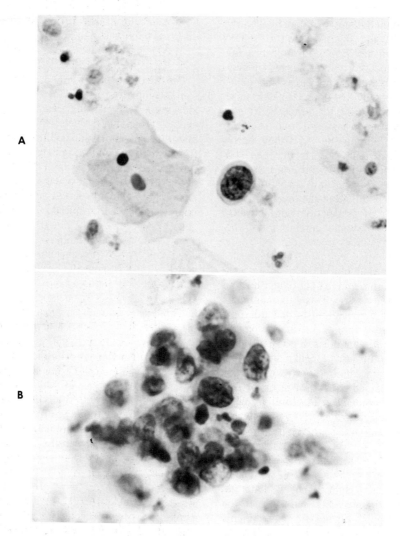

Fig. 12-9. A, Single undifferentiated cancer cell from uterine cervix obtained by vaginal irrigation smear method. Compare with mature squamous cell on left. **B,** Cluster of cancer cells in smear of uterine cervix. (From Anderson, W. A. D., and Gunn, S. A.: Cancer **20:** 1587-1593, 1967.)

and is more significant when of marked degree. *Variation in nuclear shape* may be related to cellular shape or may be unrelated. Observed in many malignant cells, and more commonly associated with rapidly growing cancers, it may be seen as bizarre or lobulated nuclear forms or other abnormal configurations.

Alterations in nuclear structure as compared with the chromatin pattern of the normal interphase nucleus characterize many malignant cells. The chromatin may be aggregated in coarse masses or may vary from one site to another in the nucleus. Many and varied aberrations of chromatin pattern are encountered on examination of many different cancer cells.

Hyperchromasia. Hyperchromasia, an increase in intensity of nuclear staining, may be caused by an increase in the amount of chromatin material or by a change in its character. Although an important feature of malignant cells, it may be simulated by overstaining, so it is important to compare with normal cells in the same preparation.

Macronucleoli. Macronucleoli are enlarged, circumscribed, acidophilic nuclear bodies, one or more of which are found in some malignant cells. Abnormality of shape of the nucleoli in addition to enlargement is of added significance. Large basophilic intranuclear masses may occur but also are seen in the nuclei of cells from benign proliferative processes.

Mitosis. Mitosis is uncommonly seen in isolated tumor cells, but the occurrence of an abnormal cell division is significant.

• • •

The importance of cytologic diagnosis lies in its ability to detect cancer in an organ at an early stage. Because of anatomic location, most organs are not accessible for cytologic examinations in a practical screening or case-finding procedure for the detection of early cancer. Most useful for the uterine cervix, cytologic examination may be applied also to the endometrium, mouth, lung, urinary tract, prostate gland, and skin. Obtaining suitable cells from the stomach or other parts of the intestinal tract requires special methods or instruments, but cytologic examination may be a diagnostic aid in patients with symptoms related to these areas.

The original Papanicolaou method involved examination of cells obtained by vaginal aspiration. For detection of cancer of the uterine cervix, smears of cells obtained by direct scraping of the region of the squamocolumnar junction of the cervix have been found to be more advantageous. Papanicolaou divided his cytologic findings into five groups. This classification, which has been rather widely used, is as follows:

Class I: Absence of atypical or abnormal cells

Class II: Atypical cytology but no evidence of malignancy

Class III: Cytology suggestive of malignancy but not conclusive

Class IV: Cytology strongly suggestive of malignancy

Class V: Cytology conclusive for malignancy

In some laboratories a modification of this classification may be used; e.g., a cytologist may simply report that a smear is positive, doubtful, negative, or unsatisfactory.

Estimating the degree of malignancy of a cancer, as is frequently attempted in grading tumors by histologic examination, is not done on cytologic examinations.

Cytologic evidence of malignancy should be confirmed whenever possible by biopsy and histologic examination.

Etiology and pathogenesis

Cancer should be regarded not as single disease but as a group of diseases in which there may be etiologic multiplicity. The etiology of tumors has to be considered as a separate problem for each organ. Many causative factors and tumor-producing agents are known, but a single ultimate cause of all forms of tumors has so far eluded discovery. Among the causes of neoplasms are exogenous agents, referred to as "oncogenic" (tumor-producing) or "carcinogenic" (cancer-producing), such as viruses, chemicals, and x-radiation. In addition, there are endogenous (host) factors that may be responsible for the origin of neoplasms or, at least, serve as contributing or predisposing factors, e.g., heredity, sex, hormonal imbalance, and age.

Viruses. Viral etiology of tumors was first realized by the discovery of the chicken leukemia virus in 1908 by Ellerman and Bang and the chicken (Rous) sarcoma virus by Peyton Rous in 1911. Subsequently, other viruses were found to be oncogenic, in a variety of animals. The oncogenic viruses, their proteins, and their antibodies may be identified by various techniques, including electron microscopy, cell culture, immunologic methods (such as immunofluorescent, cytolytic, and neutralizing antibody studies), and techniques of biochemistry and molecular biology. Although viruses are established as a cause of some neoplasms in animals, there is no definitive proof yet that viruses cause cancer in man. There is only circumstantial evidence that they play an etiologic role in human cancers.

There are approximately 600 known viruses in animals. Of these, about 150 are considered to be oncogenic, about 50 of which are DNA viruses (having complete sets of genes or genomes composed of DNA) and about 100 of which are RNA viruses (genomes composed of RNA). The oncogenic DNA viruses include (1) herpesviruses, which are mainly associated with naturally occurring cancer in animals (e.g., Lucke's renal carcinoma in the frog and Marek's [lymphomalike] disease in chickens), (2) polyoma virus, (3) simian virus 40 (SV40), and (4) adenoviruses. The oncogenic RNA viruses, also known as "leukoviruses" or "oncornaviruses," include (1) type B viruses (associated with mammary tumors in mice and monkeys) and (2) type C viruses (associated with leukemias and sarcomas in vertebrates). Examples of type C viruses are Rous sarcoma virus, feline leukemia virus, and simian sarcoma virus from a fibrosarcoma of a woolly monkey. In the RNA virus–induced tumors, viral particles may be observed in tumor cells by electron microscopy. The type B virus particles have an eccentrically located nucleoid and appear to originate from preformed intracytoplasmic structures by budding through the cell membrane. Type C virus particles have a centrally located nucleoid and appear to develop and mature as infectious viruses by a budding process at the surfaces of infected cells.

In man, there is a benign skin growth, the common wart, that is viral in origin, although this is considered by some investigators to be a hyperplastic lesion rather than a true neoplasm. The view that some human cancers may be caused by viruses is supported by certain findings in various clinical and laboratory studies. An infectious cause of leukemia has been hinted at by the observation of "leukemia clusters" (i.e., small communities with a high incidence of the disease), and a possible relationship to a virus was suggested by the finding of particles resembling RNA type C virus in human leukemia cells. In addition, evidence of a link between these particles and known type C viruses in animals has been reported. There are also reports of oncornavirus-like B and C particles in some tissue specimens of human breast cancer. A virus resembling herpesvirus hominis type 1 (HVH-1), also known as herpes simplex virus type 1, which causes oral herpetic lesions (fever blisters), has been found in association with certain human cancers. This virus, known as Epstein-Barr virus (EBV), has been identified by electron microscopy in tissue culture cells obtained from Burkitt's lymphoma, and antibodies of the virus have been found in high titers in many patients affected by this disease. Nasopharyngeal carcinoma is also associated with EBV as evidenced by the demonstration of viral antibodies in a high percentage of patients with this lesion. Herpesvirus hominis (herpes simplex virus) type 2 (HVH-2), the agent responsible for genital herpetic infection, has been incriminated as a possible cause of carcinoma of the cervix uteri. Epidemiologic evidence suggests that the cause of this cancer is sexually transmitted. Antibodies to HVH-2 have been demonstrated in the vast majority (80% or more) of women with cervical cancer but in only about one third of control women. Hodgkin's disease is another malignant lesion that may be related to a herpes-type virus, since the latter has been identified in tissue culture cells obtained from this neoplasm.

Some of the spontaneous tumors occurring in animals may be induced by viruses transmitted naturally from other infected animals. The *oncogenic action* of these exogenous viruses depends on the integration of the viral genome into the genetic structure of the host cell, causing an alteration of the cell's genetic code, that is transmitted to the cell's progeny. The resulting cells assume characteristics whereby they escape the tissue's growth-restricting controls and eventually become fully developed cancer cells. With regard to DNA oncogenic viruses, the viral DNA is inserted into the genome of the host cell and is replicated with it. Instead of undergoing lysis, the affected cells are stimulated to proliferate, but replication of the infectious virus does not occur in the transformed cells. This is in contrast to another possible effect of DNA viruses, i.e., "productive infection." This occurs in permissive cells of a natural host, in which replication of the virus takes place, followed by lysis of the cells. On the other hand, oncogenic RNA viruses can replicate themselves within the host cells as they transform them, without causing lysis of the cells. Investigations have shown that RNA oncogenic viruses contain an enzyme, an RNA-directed DNA polymerase (or *reverse transcriptase*), that reverses the usual direction of information in a cell (DNA to RNA). It has been suggested that because of this enzyme, viral RNA may serve as a template for synthesis of viral DNA (termed *provirus*), which then may be integrated into the genome of the host cell.

A different mechanism, i.e., activation of normally repressed genetically transmitted endogenous virogene information, instead of infection from animal to animal, has been proposed to explain the spontaneous occurrence in animals of tumors caused by some RNA type C tumor viruses. According to the *oncogene theory,* the genome of normal cells from their inception contains the genes for the production of RNA type C virus, being transmitted from parent to offspring through germ cells. These genes are referred to as "endogenous virogenes," a portion of which is responsible for transforming a normal cell into a tumor cell, ie., the "oncogene." The endogenous virogenes and oncogenes are maintained in an unexpressed form by repressors in normal cells. Various intrinsic factors (e.g., genetic, hormonal) or extrinsic factors (e.g., chemical agents, radiation, other infecting viruses) may initiate oncogenesis by destroying the repressors that control the oncogenic information in these cells, thus activating the virogenes and oncogenes. This hypothesis differs from the *protovirus theory.* The latter proposes that

modifications of the original genetic information of cells are caused by successive transfers from DNA to RNA to DNA. As a result, cells containing genetic information that is independent of the cell genome are produced, giving rise to the protovirus, which directs the synthesis of RNA type C virus. Protovirus formation is distinguished from endogenous type C virogenes of the oncogene theory in that it involves gene sequences not originally in the genome of the host.

Other living agents. Biologic agents other than viruses generally are not considered to be important in the etiology of tumors, yet some of them may play a role in the development of certain cancers. *Schistosoma haematobium*, a parasite common in Egypt, produces chronic irritation of the urinary bladder and is associated with a high incidence of cancer in this organ. The fungus *Aspergillus flavus* produces carcinogenic aflatoxins, such as aflatoxin B_1, which is hepatocarcinogenic in rats and is suspected of being one of the causes of the high incidence of human hepatocarcinoma in Africa and elsewhere. The aflatoxin is a common contaminant of certain foods eaten by the people in these areas. Presently, there is much interest concerning the possible role of bacteria in the cause of colorectal carcinoma in man. It has been postulated that bacteria in the colon may produce carcinogens or cocarcinogens from components in the diet (e.g., fats and proteins) or from compounds in the endogencous secretions (e.g., bile acids).

Chemical agents. The production of cancer by chemical irritation or stimulation was achieved in 1915 by Yamagiwa and Itchikawa, who found that repeated painting of the skin of rabbits with coal tar resulted in carcinoma. Previous knowledge of occupational cancers suggested that such a result might be expected. Paraffin and tar workers and chimney sweeps were known to be peculiarly subject to the development of squamous cell carcinoma of the skin. Frequently cited as the first report of the carcinogenic effect of environmental chemicals in man was that by Percival Pott in 1775, who observed the occurrence of scrotal cancer in a high percentage of chimney sweeps in England. However, 14 years before Pott's observation, there was another report that also could be characterized as dealing with environmental chemical carcinogenesis, although it was not concerned with any occupation. In 1761, Dr. John Hill described lesions in the nasal mucosa that he considered to be cancer and related them to the patients' use of snuff, a form of tobacco.

The first pure substance found to possess carcinogenic activity was 1,2,5,6-dibenzanthracene, one of the *polycyclic aromatic hydrocarbons,* the discovery being made by Kennaway and Hieger in 1930. Later, in 1933, Cook, Hewett, and Hieger isolated the carcinogenic aromatic hydrocarbon 3,4-benzpyrene from coal tar. Since then, other potent carcinogenic polycyclic aromatic hydrocarbons have been identified, including 20-methylcholanthrene, 7,12-dimethylbenzanthracene, and 3-methylcholanthrene.

It is of interest that these carcinogens have a chemical relationship to certain naturally occurring substances, such as deoxycholic acid, estrogen, and other steroids, some of which have produced tumors in experimental animals. The aromatic hydrocarbons induce cancers in a variety of tissues at the site of primary contact. For example, if the agent is painted on the skin, carcinoma of the squamous epithelium is produced; if it is injected beneath the skin, a subcutaneous sarcoma develops; and if it is given orally, carcinoma of the gastrointestinal tract occurs. This is in contrast to other types of chemicals that induce cancer in a site remote from the point where they are applied or enter the body, such as certain aromatic amines, which produce cancer of the urinary bladder, even though they may be introduced into the body through the skin, orally, or by way of the respiratory tract. Since polycyclic aromatic hydrocarbons have been identified in cigarette smoke and polluted air, it has been suggested that inhalation of these chemicals may, in some way, be responsible for respiratory cancer (bronchogenic carcinoma) in man.

Other chemical carcinogens include the following: *aromatic amines,* e.g., 2-naphthylamine, benzidine, 4-aminobiphenyl, auramine, and magenta, which are associated with an increased incidence of bladder cancer in persons exposed to them, and 2-acetoaminofluorene and 2-aminofluorene, which are commonly used in the experimental production of cancer in animals; *nitrosamines,* which are carcinogenic for experimental animals and are suspected of producing cancer in man by the ingestion of foods containing them or by the endogenous formation of these substances through combination of nitrate and amine in the gastrointestinal tract; *azo compounds,* e.g., dimethylaminoazobenzene ("butter yellow"), which produces liver cancer in the rat; *alkylating agents,* e.g., betapropriolactone and propanesultone, which are carcinogenic for experimental animals; *ethyl carbamate (urethan),* which induces lung adenomas in mice; *aflatoxins,* metabolites of *Aspergillus flavus,* which were referred to earlier; and certain other substances, such as the *halo ethers* [chloromethyl methyl ether and bis (chloromethyl) ether], *nickel* and *chromium* compounds, and *asbestos,* which are associated with lung cancer. Recently, *vinyl chloride,* used in making polyvinyl chloride, has been incriminated as a cause of a rare neoplasm of the liver (angiosarcoma) in workers exposed to this chemical. Similar lesions and other cancers have been reported in rats experimentally exposed to vinyl chloride.

The *polychlorinated biphenyls* (PCBs) have been found to produce hepatocellular carcinoma in rats and hyperplastic gastric lesions in monkeys and are suspected cancer agents in man. The PCBs have been used commercially for nearly 50 years, being used in insulating fluids in heavy duty electrical equipment, such as transformers and capacitors, and in liquid seals, hydraulic fluids, lubricants, adhesives, paints, printing ink, duplicating machine paper, and other items. In recent years, the PCBs have been identified as a significant contaminant in the environment and have thus become one of the most serious potential health hazards.

Other substances (cocarcinogens) may augment the effect of the known carcinogenic agents, even though alone they may have little or no carcinogenic activity. Croton oil acts as an effective cocarcinogen in producing tumors of the skin by painting with tar. This and other experimental studies have suggested a *two-stage hypothesis of carcinogenesis:* an *initiating stage,* in which cells exposed to a carcinogenic agent are altered without visible evidence of neoplastic transformation, and a *promoting* stage, during which there is a change to progressive growth that is stimulated by various factors. The initial change that occurs in the host's cells is transmitted to their progeny. The time that elapses between the first exposure to a carcinogenic agent and the appearance of a tumor varies, depending on the nature and dose of the carcinogen and certain host factors, including tissue susceptibility. This "latent period," which may be months to many years, is a feature not only of chemically-induced tumors but also of tumors caused by other oncogenic agents.

It has been shown that many chemical carcinogens must be metabolized in order to exert their carcinogenic activity. The parent unreactive carcinogen (precarcinogen) is metabolized to an intermediate form (proximate carcinogen), which is then converted to a final reactive form (ultimate carcinogen). The ultimate carcinogen has been described as a reactive electrophile (i.e., molecule with electron-deficient atoms) that initiates the carcinogen process by reacting with nucleophiles (i.e., molecules with electron-rich atoms) in crucial tissue components, such as the nucleic acids and proteins.

The hypotheses that have been proposed to explain how chemical carcinogens induce cancer include genetic and nongenetic mechanisms: (1) fixation of the carcinogen to host cells' DNA, resulting in alterations of the genetic information (somatic mutation), (2) carcinogenic modification of RNA, which (by means of reverse transcription) leads to a modified DNA (somatic mutation), (3) activation of a latent oncogenic virus or an "oncogene" (gene of RNA type C virus that some investigators believe to be an integral part of the DNA of a normal cell), and (4) alteration of the cellular environment (e.g., changes in the immunologic capacity or hormonal balance) that permit preferential proliferation of the altered cells.

Physical agents. *Radiant energy* is a well-known cause of cancer in man and experimental animals. *Excessive exposure to sunlight* (ultraviolet rays) is an important causative factor in many cancers of the skin. The lesions occur after many years of overexposure and chronic sunburn and so are seen mainly in sailors and farmers or others who spend a great deal of time outdoors, particularly in sunny southern areas. Fair-skinned persons are more susceptible to this injury. Experimentally, skin tumors have been produced in rodents by means of ultraviolet (actinic) rays. The wavelengths of the carcinogenic rays are between 2,600 and 3,300 Å.

Ionizing radiation is known to produce cancer in man and animals. Pioneer workers with roentgen rays developed irritative lesions of the skin that eventually became cancers resulting from prolonged and repeated overexposure to radiation. Some watch dial painters, who used luminous paint containing radioactive materials and inadvertently ingested some of it, developed bone cancer (osteosarcoma). An increase in incidence of bronchogenic carcinoma has been noted among miners of radioactive ores (e.g., uranium). Thyroid tumors, including cancer, have been observed in Japanese exposed to fallout and atomic bomb radiation at Hiroshima and Nagasaki. An increased incidence of thyroid cancer has been found in persons who have had radiation of the thymus in infancy. A high incidence of leukemia has been demonstrated in mice exposed to whole body irradiation. In the past, there was a greater frequency of leukemia among radiologists as compared with other physicians. A high incidence of leukemia was noted among the Japanese survivors of the atomic bomb explosion, the peak in frequency being reached 6 years after the explosions; however, the rates have declined markedly since then. Currently, there is concern that there may be a relationship between irradiation and breast cancer. A higher rate of incidence of breast cancer has been recently reported among women survivors of the atomic bomb explosions in Japan compared with nonexposed women.

The mechanisms by which radiation induces cancer very likely are similar to those related to chemical carcinogens, i.e., altering the genetic code of the target cell, thus causing somatic mutation, or activating a latent oncogenic virus or an oncogene, or changing the cellular environment in such a way as to enhance proliferation of the altered cells.

The role of *physical trauma* as an oncogenic agent is controversial. There does not appear to be sufficient evidence that a single uncomplicated physical trauma produces cancer. Usually, the injury only calls attention to a tumor already present but previously unrecognized.

Hormones. *Hormonal imbalance* has been effective in causing certain types of tumors in experimental animals, e.g., estrogen administration has produced tumors of the mammary gland, uterus, pituitary gland, and testis and castration has led to the development of tumors in the adrenal glands. In man, hormonal imbalance may play a role in the development of some neoplasms, particularly carcinoma of the endometrium and breast in women and carcinoma of the prostate gland in men. Altering the hormonal environment in cancer patients may control the growth of malignant tumors in some instances. For example, some premenopausal women who have advanced breast cancer show regression of their cancer following ovariectomy, and regression of prostatic cancer may occur in men after castration. Similar hormone dependency is observed in certain experimentally produced tumors in animals. The tendency for breast cancer to occur in single women, infertile married women, and late-married women suggests the possible role of unopposed estrogen activity during the long reproductive life span. There is a lower risk of breast cancer in fertile women, particularly those with three or more children, probably because the pregnancies result in interruption of the ovarian cycle, thus causing less exposure to estrogens. The association of cancer of the endometrium or breast in postmenopausal women with ovarian cortical hyperplasia or endocrine tumors of the ovary, which produce estrogens, suggests a hormonal influence. Oral contraceptives, which contain steroid sex hormones, have been implicated in the development of primary liver tumors in women.

Recently, Herbst and associates reported the development of an uncommon neoplasm, vaginal adenocarcinoma, in young women. In most cases it appeared 14 to 22 years after their mothers had received stilbestrol therapy for threatened abortion during pregnancy. Similar cases have been observed since the report. Apparently this observation, which represents the first evidence of transplacental chemical carcinogenesis in man, not only shows a relationship of hormones to neoplasia but also raises the question as to what other chemicals or drugs may be involved in transplacental carcinogenesis. Cervical clear cell adenocarcinoma has also been found in young women as a result of intrauterine exposure to stilbestrol.

Sex. There is an obvious difference in the incidence of certain types of tumors in men and women, apart from those in organs of reproduction. Some investigators have suggested that this sex difference may be related to endogenous host factors, such as a difference in effectiveness of the immune system in the two sexes and the presence of specific sex hormones. However, the role of extrinsic factors, such as smoking, occupational exposures, and other environmental factors, cannot be excluded. For example, lung cancer, the number one cause of cancer death among men, is becoming a more frequent type of cancer among women, apparently because more teenage girls and women have acquired the smoking habit.

Age. Malignant tumors are not restricted to any age group, although most of them occur in older individuals. The association of cancer with aging may be a reflection of a long latent period during which the carcinogenic-stimulated cells and their progeny undergo the various sequential changes leading to definite characteristics of cancer. The tendency for aging cells to develop a large number of mutations may be a factor. Also, there is evidence of a decrease in humoral and cellular immune response in man and animals as they become older, so that an impaired immune defense system may contribute to the increased incidence of tumors in older persons. It should be remembered, however, that certain types of tumors tend to occur particularly in childhood, e.g., leukemia, neuroblastoma, and Wilms' tumor of the kidney.

Diet. Experimentally, it has been shown that restriction of caloric intake in mice reduces the occurrence or slows the time of appearance of certain types of tumors. Also, high levels of dietary casein or high levels of riboflavin have been found to protect the rat liver from carcinogenesis by 4-dimethylaminoazobenzene. Apparently, the protein improves the resistance of the liver to the hepatotoxic agent and also increases the storage and utilization of riboflavin. Riboflavin is beneficial because it is an essential constituent in an enzyme system that detoxifies azo compounds.

Benzpyrene has been identified in smoked fish and charcoal-barbecued (charred) meat, both of which have been suggested as possible causative factors in carcinoma of the stomach in man. Mention has already been made of other carcinogenic substances in foods, such as aflatoxin B_1 and nitrosamines. Currently, various intentional or unintentional constituents of food and beverages are under investigation to determine their carcinogenic potential, including additives, hormones used for fattening food animals, and pesticides.

On the basis of epidemiologic evidence, the dietary pattern has been implicated in the etiology of colorectal cancer, but there is a difference of opinion as to which component of the diet is responsible. Some investigators claim that high animal protein and high fat diets are more likely to develop the cancer, whereas others believe that diets high in unrefined carbohydrate and low in fiber content are associated with cancer. Among the hypotheses that have been proposed to explain the etiologic relationship of the diet to cancer is one that stresses the action of intestinal bacteria on dietary components or on secretions produced in response to the diet. Such action may result in the production of carcinogens or cocarcinogens from the dietary proteins and fats or from the bile acids, the secretion of which is stimulated by the dietary fat. One suggestion is that a low-residue (fiber-depleted) diet results in fecal stasis, which may allow more time for growth of bacteria, for their action on the bile salts or dietary components, and for contact between the intestinal mucosa and any carcinogens that may form by this action.

Heredity. Experimentally, heredity has been shown to be important as a factor in the development of tumors. By selective inbreeding it has been possible to increase or decrease the incidence of certain types of spontaneous tumors within a given strain of animal. In man heredity has been suspected as a factor in the etiology of tumors because of an increased incidence of cancer in certain families (e.g., breast, colorectal, and stomach cancer), although this in itself is not definitive evidence of a hereditary factor. There probably is no general overall hereditary predisposition to cancer, but such hereditary tendencies toward cancer as may exist operate independently for different tumor types. Stronger evidence that heredity plays a role in cancer is noted in the observation that the same type of cancer (e.g., leukemia) occurs in identical twins more commonly than by chance.

The influence of heredity is best seen in certain of the less common types of neoplasms, such as retinoblastoma, familial polyposis of the colon, and neurofibromatosis, which are inherited as autosomal dominant traits. One of these tumors, retinoblastoma, is a malignant neoplasm. The other two are benign in themselves, but they may give rise to cancers and are often referred to as precancerous conditions. A much greater predisposition to cancer occurs in familial polyposis of the colon than in neurofibromatosis. Xeroderma pigmentosum, a condition in which there is an abnormal sensitivity to sunlight, is another inherited (autosomal recessive) precancerous disease. It gives rise to skin cancer. Also, there is a strong familial incidence of multiple adenomas arising in more than one endocrine gland in the same patient (polyendocrine or multiple endocrine adenomatosis). This condition occurs as an autosomal dominant trait.

Immunologic factors. Several immunologic concepts have been proposed to explain the origin of neoplasms. Among these is a long-held view that, as an effect of the action of various tumor-inducing agents, normal cells lose certain tissue-specific antigens that are responsible for keeping these cells in restraint. As a result, the cells become uninhibited so that they proliferate and extend beyond their usual limits. However, the recognition that tumor cells also acquire new antigens that were not present in the tissue of origin (tumor-specific antigens) has led to another concept. It has been postulated that in most instances the newly formed antigens of transformed cells induce immune responses that prevent further growth of the cells, but occasionally a tumor develops because of a breakdown in the immunologic control system. Among the theories advanced as to the immunologic mechanisms of tumor production are the following: (1) Tumor-specific antigens are responsible for production of enhancing antibodies, i.e., those that offer protection against the destructive effect of sensitized cells, or the antibodies combine with antigen to form "blocking" antigen-antibody complexes that inhibit the activity of sensitized cytotoxic lymphocytes. (2) An excess of the newly formed antigens causes immunologic paralysis or tolerance. (3) The antigens initiate an immunologic mechanism that produces chromosomal abnormalities conducive to development of tumors. (4) The carcinogenic agent causes suppression of immunologic reactions. (5) Early in the evolution of a tumor, the immune response is weak and, by some means, is able to stimulate rather than inhibit growth of tumor cells ("immunostimulation of tumor growth").

Mechanism of carcinogenesis. The carcinogenic process begins with the initial interaction between a carcinogenic stimulus and the target tissue of a susceptible host (the *initiation phase*). As to the subsequent steps in the development of cancer, two major possibilities have been suggested. According to one hypothesis, the initiation process induces cancer cells in the target tissue that remain dormant for varying periods. Many or all of the properties of cancer are already present in the neoplastic cells. There is then a *process of emergence,* caused by noncarcinogenic stimuli *(promoting agents),* which exert a proliferative response that encourages growth of the transformed dormant cells. According to the second hypothesis, which is the more widely accepted view, the initiation process induces altered nonneoplastic cells, followed by an evolutionary progression to cancer involving multiple cell populations. The initial changes produced by carcinogenic stimuli are transmitted to subsequent generations of cells, with possibly other changes occurring in each new cell population until, eventually, there is complete transformation to malignant neoplastic cells. Proliferation of the altered cells may be stimulated by a number of factors that serve as promoting agents, such as changes in the immune system or in hormonal balance, chronic irritation, and chronic inflammation. In some instances, repeated exposures to a carcinogenic agent may be necessary for transformation to malignant cells. In such cases, it is possible that the carcinogen acts as both an initiating and promoting agent.

Several hypotheses have been proposed to explain the nature of the initiating event in carcinogenesis. One of these is the *somatic mutation* hypothesis, according to which neoplasia results from an alteration in genetic material of somatic cells that is transmissible to subsequent generations of cells. This alteration (mutation) may be brought about by (1) direct modification of the existing DNA, or (2) fixation to DNA of alterations that first occurred in RNA. The latter mechanism involves reverse transcription.

Consistent with the mutation theory is the frequent appearance of certain chromosomal aberrations in many cancers. Commonly, there is a variation from the normal (diploid) number of chromosomes. Sometimes the number may be irregularly increased, resulting in an odd number (aneuploidy). Several neoplastic conditions have consistent chromosome patterns. For example, the Ph[1] chromosome is seen in most patients with chronic myelocytic leukemia, i.e., a chromosome number 22 that is lacking most of its long arm. Recently, it has been shown that the deleted material from this chromosome may be translocated to another chromosome, usually a chromosome number 9. In meningioma, the characteristic cytogenic feature is loss of a chromosome number 22, and in Burkitt's lymphoma, there is extra material at the end of a chromosome number 14. There is some question as to whether these karyotypic changes are the cause or the effect of carcinogenesis, although the prevalent opinion seems to be that they are the latter.

An alternative hypothesis regards neoplasia as arising by *differentiation* of the stem cells in normal tissues *without a fixed change in the genome* as the initial event. Since the genome is unaltered, it is assumed that the malignant expression of the nucleus is under the control of the cytoplasm. The genome is believed to contain all the information needed for the phenotypic expression of cancer, but it is repressed in normal cells. The initial process in carcinogenesis, then, may be an alteration in certain cytoplasmic components causing removal of the repressors of the genetic information. The stem cells from which neoplasms arise are those involved in tissue renewal and should not be confused with the undeveloped embryonic cells ("fetal rests"), which Cohnheim believed to be the origin of tumors (see below). Another hypothesis that considers control of genetic information to be by repressors is the *oncogene theory* discussed on p. 259.

Mention should be made of the hypothesis proposed some years ago by Cohnheim that related the origin of tumors to the existence of *"rests of fetal cells."* According to this theory, misplaced or superfluous embryonic cells failed to proceed to full development, remained dormant for a period, and then with recommencement of growth resulted in a tumor. The current opinion is that these fetal rests are not a common source of neoplasms, although they may give rise to certain tumors, such as chordomas and pituitary craniopharyngiomas, and to certain tumorlike developmental abnormalities (hamartomas).

Mesenchymal tumors

The benign mesenchymal tumors are named according to their type of tissue, e.g., fibroma (fibrous connective tissue), lipoma (fat), and myoma (muscle). The malignant connective tissue tumors, or sarcomas, may be undifferentiated or may be so well differentiated that their tissue of origin is recognizable (e.g., fibrosarcoma and liposarcoma). Various forms of connective tissue tumors are listed in Table 12-1 for purposes of description.

Fibroma. Fibromas are derived from and composed of fibrous connective tissue and are of wide distribution. Most commonly they are found in connection with the skin, subcutaneous tissue, fascia, or tendons, but they also occur in certain organs, such as the ovary, kidney, breast, and intestine. With slow and expansive growth, they tend to encapsulation. Microscopically, they are composed of interlacing bundles and fibers of collagenous connective tissue.

Desmoid is a fibroma arising in musculoaponeurotic structures, particularly frequent in the lower anterior abdominal wall. Trauma seems to be a predisposing factor, and most cases have occurred in women who have borne children. There may be local infiltration of muscle, but sarcomatous transformation and metastases do not develop.

Keloid is an excessive formation of a fibrous scar resulting in a tumorlike mass resembling a fibroma. Certain persons, particularly blacks, are prone to this excessive fibrosis following injuries of the skin. Microscopically, the keloid consists of dense bundles of collagenous and hyalinized connective tissue.

A benign growth, possibly reactive or inflammatory in nature, that simulates a sarcomatous lesion has been called *nodular fasciitis* or *pseudosarcomatous fibromatosis*. It grows rapidly, usually in subcutaneous tissues, and affects children as well as adults. The bulk of the tumor is composed of myxoid fibroblastic proliferation, with many capillaries, and some

Table 12-1. Mesenchymal tumors

Origin or type of cell	Benign form	Malignant form
Fibrous connective tissue	Fibroma	Fibrosarcoma
Peripheral nerve sheaths	Neurofibroma	Neurogenic sarcoma; neurofibrosarcoma
	Schwannoma or neurilemoma	Malignant schwannoma
Fatty tissue	Lipoma	Liposarcoma
Myxomatous tissue	Myxoma	Myxosarcoma
Cartilage	Chondroma	Chondrosarcoma
Bone	Osteoma	Osteogenic sarcoma (osteosarcoma)
Muscle	Myoma	Myosarcoma
Smooth	Leiomyoma	Leiomyosarcoma
Striated	Rhabdomyoma	Rhabdomyosarcoma
Notochord	Chordoma (rare)	Chordoma
Lymphoid tissue		Malignant lymphoma
Serous linings	Benign mesothelioma	Mesothelial sarcoma (malignant mesothelioma)
Blood or lymph vessels	Angioma	Angiosarcoma
Neuroglia	Glioma	Glioma
Cell origin undetermined		Undifferentiated sarcoma
		Small round cell sarcoma
		Large round cell sarcoma
		Mixed cell sarcoma

lymphoid and histiocytic cells. Typical mitoses may be numerous. There is lack of encapsulation, and irregular extension occurs into adjacent tissues.

Fibrosarcoma. Fibrosarcoma is a malignant tumor tending to differentiate in the direction of fibrous connective tissue. It occurs at any age, but the highest incidence is in the fifth and sixth decades. The most common site of origin is in the extremities, particularly the lower, but the origin may be from connective tissue in any region. Fibrosarcoma appears as a rounded, lobulated tumor, often appearing circumscribed or encapsulated and either hard and fibrous or soft and friable, depending on the amount of collagenous tissue that has been formed. Areas of degeneration, necrosis, myxomatous change, or cyst formation may be present.

Simple excision is often followed by recurrence. Following repeated recurrences, death may result from visceral metastasis or from infection and hemorrhage of the ulcerating tumor. The degree of malignancy tends to be proportional to the number of mitotic nuclei and tumor giant cells and to the scarcity of collagen fibers.

Tumors composed of two or more mesen-

chymal derivatives that ordinarily are not found together in a single tumor have been called *mesenchymomas*. With rare exceptions, such tumors are malignant.

Large fibrosarcomas, particularly of the abdomen, pelvis, retroperitoneal area, and thorax, occasionally are associated with attacks of hypoglycemia. The hypoglycemic episodes, with simulate hyperinsulinism, cease on removal of the tumor. Insulin is not demonstrable in the tumor tissue, and the mechanism of the hypoglycemia is not known. (See paraneoplastic syndromes, p. 252, for suggested mechanisms.)

Neurofibroma and neurilemoma. Neurofibromas and neurilemomas *(schwannomas)* (Fig. 12-10) arise from the sheaths of peripheral nerves. Among the intracranial nerves, the eighth is the most commonly involved, the tumor being found in the cerebellopontine angle (acoustic neurinoma). The exact origin of the peripheral nerve sheath tumors (e.g., from the sheath of Schwann, endoneurium, perineurium) has been a subject of discussion, and the terminology used has varied depending on the favored theory.

Recklinghausen's disease is a familial form of *multiple neurofibromatosis*. Neurofibromas

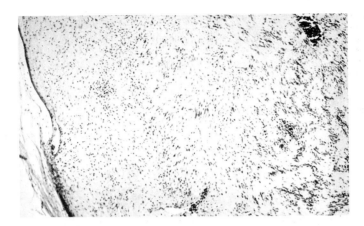

Fig. 12-10. Neurilemoma. Palisading of nuclei is evident on right.

are found on branches of the cutaneous nerves and along nerve trunks of the thorax, brachial and lumbar plexus, and extremities (Fig. 12-11). Cranial nerves and spinal nerves within the spinal canal are sometimes involved as well. Coffee-colored areas of skin pigmentation are common stigmas of this disease. The tumors are benign nonencapsulated focal lesions or may diffusely involve the nerves from which they grow. In a small proportion of patients, one or more of the tumors may become malignant. A loose wavy arrangement of fibrils, sometimes with formation of whorls, is characteristic of neurofibroma. Mucoid degeneration of the collagen of the tumor is common. In addition to this multiple form, neurofibromas sometimes are seen as *solitary lesions* (e.g., in the skin).

Neurilemomas, which often are included in the general family of neurofibromas, are most often single but may be multiple. Occasionally, they occur along with the neurofibromas in Recklinghausen's neurofibromatosis. Palisading of nuclei is characteristic of neurilemomas, and often a double palisade encloses a space (Verocay body). Malignant change in a neurilemoma does not occur or is very rare. In contrast to neurofibromas, the neurilemomas are encapsulated.

Neurogenic sarcoma (neurogenous sarcoma). Sarcomatous tumors of soft tissue may be found in distinct relation to nerves. More often such relationship is not demonstrable, and in such cases the features suggesting a neurogenous origin are (1) arrangement of the cells in definite bundles with an interlacing pattern of the herringbone type, (2) wavy, fine, elongated nuclei that tend to line up in parallel fashion to form rows (palisading), and (3) fibrils, demonstrable by silver stains, distributed in pericellular fashion.

The proportion of sarcomas of skin and subcutaneous tissues that are of neurogenous origin is a matter of debate. Ewing and others have held that the majority of such spindle cell sarcomas arise from peripheral nerves. From a practical standpoint, the criteria of degree of malignancy and the prognosis are the same for neurogenic sarcoma and fibrosarcoma, varying with the number of mitoses and tumor giant cells and the scarcity of fibers. It may be difficult to determine whether a neurogenic sarcoma is derived from fibroblastic elements of the sheath (neurofibrosarcoma) or from Schwann cells (malignant schwannoma or malignant neurilemoma).

Lipoma. Lipomas are benign, circumscribed masses of an adult type of fat tissue. They occur in many situations but especially in the subcutaneous tissues of the back or shoulder region. In some cases, they are multiple, grow to a large size, and appear to have

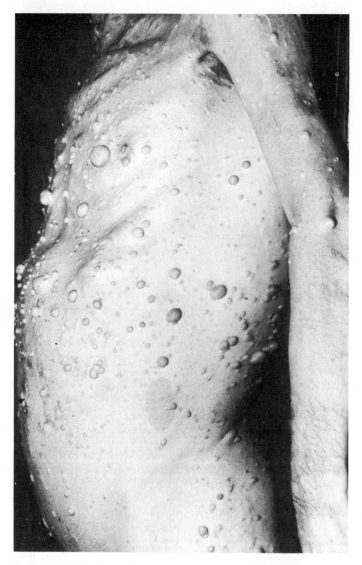

Fig. 12-11. Multiple neurofibromatosis. Note also dark areas just above thigh (coffee-colored or café au lait spot).

a familial factor in their causation. In certain rare instances, they show a connection with nerves and are painful. Microscopically, they are composed of fat cells of the usual type found in adipose tissue, although of a larger average size.

Hibernoma is a rare type of fatty tumor that arises from a structure in human beings that is homologous to the so-called hibernating gland of animals and that develops from persistent brown multilocular fat.

Liposarcoma. Liposarcoma apparently arises from undifferentiated mesenchymal cells that develop into malignant lipoblasts with the capability to differentiate. Some liposarcomas are well differentiated, consisting predomi-

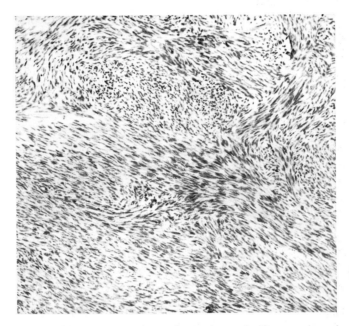

Fig. 12-12. Leiomyoma. Intertwining bundles of smooth muscle fibers run in various directions, and some are cut transversely.

nantly of mature fat cells with mucoid or myxomatous areas and occasional undifferentiated bizarre lipoblasts. Other tumors are less differentiated and quite cellular, consisting chiefly of myxomatous tissue with fusiform and spindle cells as well as a varying number of immature, sometimes bizarre and multinucleated, lipoblasts and relatively few mature fat cells. These liposarcomas are usually highly vascular. Another type of liposarcoma is pleomorphic, highly undifferentiated (anaplastic), and sometimes difficult to differentiate from other anaplastic mesenchymal tumors.

The well-differentiated liposarcomas are infiltrative and tend to recur after excision, but relatively few of them metastasize. The poorly differentiated liposarcomas are locally destructive and frequently develop metastases. Liposarcomas occur most often about the buttocks and lower limbs and in the retroperitoneum.

Myxoma. Myxoma is a mesenchymal tumor in which a mucoid intercellular substance (probably hyaluronic acid) separates stellate embryonic connective tissue cells so as to resemble in appearance primitive mesenchyme or the tissue of the umbilical cord. A pure myxoma is rare, but a myxomatous change or degeneration in a portion of some other type of connective tissue tumor is not uncommon.

Myxosarcoma. Myxosarcoma, like myxoma, is very rare as a pure tumor.

Tumors of cartilage and bone. *Chondroma, chondrosarcoma, osteoma,* and *osteogenic sarcoma (osteosarcoma)* are tumors that usually arise in connection with skeletal structures and are considered in Chapter 25.

Tumors of muscle. The benign muscle tumors are of two types: *rhabdomyoma,* an extremely rare tumor of striated muscle, and *leiomyoma,* a very common tumor composed of smooth muscle (Fig. 12-12). Leiomyomas occur most frequently in the uterus, where they have an abundant fibrous stroma and are commonly called ''fibroids'' (p. 647). They also occur in many other situations where smooth muscle is normally found, as in the intestinal tract.

Malignant transformation of a uterine

myoma to a *leiomyosarcoma* may occur, although most of the leiomyosarcomas arise de novo. A pure *rhabdomyosarcoma* is relatively uncommon, but striated muscle fibers sometimes are found in malignant mixed tumors such as those of the kidney (p. 372) and uterus (p. 653). Pleomorphic rhabdomyosarcomas occur mainly in the extremities of older persons. An alveolar type of rhabdomyosarcoma has been described in adolescents and young adults. Embryonal or botryoid rhabdomyosarcomas occur chiefly in infants or young children and are located mainly in the orbital region or the urogenital tract.

The so-called *granular cell myoblastoma* (granular cell tumor) is an uncommon tumor that has been interpreted as derived from primitive myoblasts, although some writers have considered other origins (e.g., Schwann cells). Most examples have been found in the tongue, but some have appeared in the skin, skeletal muscle, and other sites. They are composed of large polyhedral cells with small nuclei and an abundant, pale, granular cytoplasm. Cross-striations and structures resembling myofibrils have been observed in some cases. The tumor may be encapsulated, but in most instances it appears to be locally infiltrative. It is benign and often is associated with pseudocarcinomatous hyperplasia of the overlying epithelium.

Another granular cell tumor that formerly was considered to be a malignant "organoid" variety of granular cell myoblastoma most often arises in the upper thigh. Its true nature is debatable, but it is a distinctly different tumor, and origin from nonchromaffin paraganglia rather than a myoblastic origin has been suggested. Because of uncertain histogenesis, others have referred to this tumor by the noncommittal term of *"alveolar soft part sarcoma."* The tumor is slow in its growth but may metastasize by the bloodstream to the lung, brain, or elsewhere.

Chordoma. Chordoma is a rare tumor that arises from notochordal remnants at the upper or lower ends of the vertebral column. It is composed of large, clear, closely packed cells having a vacuolated cytoplasm (p. 719).

Lymphomatous tumors. *Lymphocytic lymphosarcoma, reticulum cell sarcoma,* and other malignant lymphomas are considered in Chapter 17. Plasma cell tumors occur as solitary or multiple tumors of bone marrow (myeloma) and also as extramedullary tumors, mainly in the nasopharyngeal region (p. 718).

Mesothelioma. Mesothelioma is a primary tumor arising from serous surfaces such as the pleura, pericardium, and peritoneum (p. 432).

Vascular tumors. Growths composed of endothelial cells tending to form blood or lymphatic channels consist of both benign and malignant forms. Specialized varieties are glomus tumors and hemangiopericytomas. The vascular tumors are considered on p. 295.

Glioma. The gliomas are tumors arising from the neuroglial or supporting cells of the central nervous system (p. 737).

Undifferentiated sarcoma. Many of the malignant mesenchymal tumors fail to differentiate into recognizable types of cells. They often are given descriptive designations such as small round cell sarcoma, large round cell sarcoma, mixed cell sarcoma, and spindle cell sarcoma, although there may be little practical advantage in such labels. Mitoses are numerous in these highly malignant growths.

Small round cell sarcoma arises in a variety of sites and tends to be rapid in growth and metastasis. It forms a fairly well demarcated, pinkish white, fleshy mass in which areas of degeneration and hemorrhage are common. Microscopically, it is composed of small, round, uniform cells, among which are abundant thin-walled blood vessels. The *large round cell sarcomas* are similar grossly but are composed of cells that are larger, are less uniformly round, and have more abundant cytoplasm. Many of the tumors designated as small and large round cell sarcomas are, in reality, lymphosarcomas and reticulum cell sarcomas. The *mixed (polymorphic) cell sarcomas* are made of cells of variable size and shape, often with bizarre tumor giant cells.

Spindle cell sarcoma shows some differentiation toward recognizable fibroblastic cells. The tumor is somewhat harder, less prone to degenerative changes, and less malignant than the round cell forms. It is composed of bundles of elongated spindle-shaped cells with oval nuclei. When the elongated cells are cut transversely, they appear rounded and show only scanty cytoplasm.

General characteristics of sarcoma. Malignant mesenchymal tumors are more prone to occur at any age throughout life than are carcinomas. During the first few decades of life, they have a much higher relative frequency than malignant epithelial tumors. They tend to be soft and of fleshy appearance and consistency, except in the highly differentiated types. Hemorrhages and degenerative changes are common in the tumor tissue. The tumors usually have abundant, thin-walled blood vessels that are intimately associated with the tumor cells, whereas in epithelial tumors the blood vessels are contained in the stroma that separates groups of tumor cells. The thinness and intimacy of vessels in sarcomas readily enable the tumor cells to grow through their walls. Hence, they commonly metastasize by way of the bloodstream, the lung being the most frequent site for secondary tumors. Lymph node metastasis also occurs in 5% to 10% of sarcomas.

Epithelial tumors

Tumors derived from and made up of epithelial tissues may be classified into two groups, the benign and the malignant (carcinoma). An epithelial tumor, like normal epithelial tissue, has a connective tissue stroma that supports the epithelium and contains blood and lymphatic vessels. Insufficiency of this stroma, on which nutrition depends, results in degenerative changes and necrosis in the tumor. On the other hand, the stroma may progress equally with the growth of the epithelial elements or even exceed it, producing fibroepithelial tumors or, in the case of carcinoma, scirrhous tumors.

Benign epithelial tumors

Benign epithelial tumors are of two main types: *papilloma,* which grows outward from an epithelial surface (such as cutaneous or mucosal), and *adenoma,* which is derived from

and imitates glandular epithelium. The benign tumors progress slowly. By their expansile growth, they compress surrounding tissue but do not infiltrate and never form metastases. The cells tend to conform closely to a normal appearance.

Papilloma. A papilloma is a pedunculated or sessile tumor growing outward from a surface, consisting of fingerlike processes of varying length, thickness, and number. Microscopically, the neoplastic epithelial cells are situated externally around a branching core of connective tissue containing blood vessels. The type of epithelium is that of the surface of origin, i.e., squamous (skin, palate, and larynx), transitional (urinary tract), columnar (intestine), or cuboidal (lining of a cyst). The surface of a papilloma is exposed to injury by pressure or friction, so that ulceration, infection, and inflammatory changes are common. The main features distinguishing them from carcinoma is that the tumor cells do not penetrate the underlying tissues.

Cutaneous papillomas may be true tumors, but a group of inflammatory growths of the skin are also loosely called papillomas. The latter include venereal warts (condylomas), the common warts of children (verruca vulgaris), which are of infectious origin, and pyogenic granulomas, or excessive growths of granulation tissue.

The true papilloma of the skin is a hard, rough tumor with a broad base that may be several centimeters in diameter. The surface is rough and fissured, often with marked keratinization of the superficial cells. When keratinization is excessive, these may be called cutaneous horns.

Some papillomatous tumors of the skin are pigmented and may be confused with true melanomas. They have the structure of an ordinary cutaneous papilloma, but there is abundant melanin in the epidermal cells.

Papillomas from mucous surfaces often have long delicate processes attached around a thin central stalk. This type is seen in its typical form in the bladder. A sessile papillary growth occurs in the large intestine that consists of multiple fingerlike processes covered by proliferating columnar epithelium of the mucosal surface and is known as a villous papilloma. This lesion differs from the pedunculated adenoma, which is referred to later.

Intracystic papilloma, in which the projection of the tumor is into the cavity of a cyst, is seen particularly in cystic lesions of the ovary and the breast.

Adenoma. An adenoma is a benign tumor derived from glandular or secretory cells. It usually has a slow rate of growth and a well-defined margin and tends to reproduce the tissue from which it is derived. The tumor cells may function and produce a secretion similar to, or the same as, that produced by the normal glandular tissue. Thus, mucin tends to be produced in intestinal growths, colloid in thyroid adenomas, and bile in liver adenomas. In the case of adenomas made up of endocrine tissue, excessive secretory activity may result in clinical evidence of hyperactivity of the particular endocrine gland. Distention with secretory material and cyst formation is also a common result of functional activity (cystadenoma).

Since any glandular tissue may give rise to tumor, adenomas are of extremely varied structure. Those that grow within the substance of a gland tend to be rounded and encapsulated. Those that grow from the secretory cells of a mucous membrane, such as endometrium or intestine, tend to be polypoid and pedunculated. Pedunculated adenomas, which often are referred to as polyps, commonly occur in the intestine as single or multiple lesions. There are several hereditary disorders characterized by multiple polyposis of the intestine (Fig. 12-13). It should be noted that the term "polyp" is not restricted to this type of growth, for it frequently is applied to any lesion projecting from a mucosal surface, whether neoplastic or nonneoplastic, including inflammatory or hyperplastic masses.

Malignant epithelial tumors

Carcinoma. Malignant epithelial tumors form a most important group because of their numerical frequency and serious effects. They vary widely in rate of growth, degree of ana-plasia or differentiation, and gross and microscopic appearance. They are distinguished from benign epithelial tumors in that they invade and destroy normal tissue and usually will spread by metastasis.

Carcinomas differ in the degree to which they imitate their tissue of origin. In some cases, the resemblance to normal tissue is very close, with well-formed glands, tubules, or lining epithelium. At the other extreme, there may be so much anaplasia or resemblance to an embryonic type of tissue that the origin of the tumor or even its epithelial nature is difficult to determine.

The stroma likewise is variable. Invading carcinoma cells utilize the existing stroma of the destroyed tissue. When the tumor growth is rapid, the connective tissue and blood vessels are often inadequate to support and nourish the tumor, so that degeneration and death of tumor cells result. Other tumors tend to stimulate the growth of the connective tissue stroma (desmoplasia), sometimes to exceed the development of the epithelial elements.

A number of terms are used in the classification and description of carcinomas. *Squamous cell carcinoma* arises from surface epithelium such as the skin, mouth, lip, or cervix, and it is made up of squamous epithelial cells. It also may arise from the esophagus, anus, larynx, nose, sinuses, renal pelvis, ureters, bladder, and bronchi (Fig. 12-14). It is most easily identified by the presence of prickle cells or keratinization. *Adenocarcinoma* is a tumor with cells having a glandular arrangement or origin (Fig. 12-15). The terms *scirrhous, medullary,* and *mucoid* or *gelatinous,* as used here, refer to gross and microscopic appearance. A *scirrhous carcinoma* is hard and fibrous because of abundant stroma. A *medullary carcinoma* is soft and brainlike in consistency because it has little connective tissue stroma. *Mucoid* or *gelatinous carcinomas* are soft and translucent as a result of an accumulation of a mucoid or colloid material. Carcinomas are frequently not uniformly scirrhous, medullary, or mucoid throughout their whole substance. *Carcinoma simplex* is a carcinoma of glandular tissue in which the cells

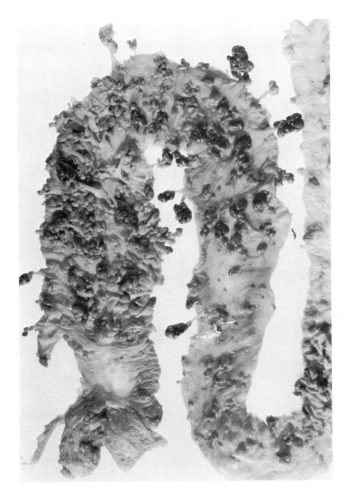

Fig. 12-13. Multiple polyposis of large intestine. (Courtesy Dr. J. F. Kuzma.)

do not form glandular structures but are arranged in solid cords and masses separated by a connective tissue stroma.

Other types of neoplasms

In addition to the usual mesenchymal and epithelial tumors just described, there are those arising from embryonic precursors of tissues *(embryonic tumors)* and those composed of tissues of different character in the same growth *(mixed tumors* and *teratomas).*

Embryonic tumors. Embryonic tumors arise in early life from tissues that are still undiffer-

entiated and that continue to proliferate at the embryonic level. They include Wilms' tumor of the kidney (nephroblastoma), retinoblastoma (retinal neuroepithelioma), embryonic tumors of the liver, and embryonic sarcomas of the urogenital organs of children.

Mixed tumors. Mixed tumors are derived from pluripotential cells, i.e., cells capable of differentiation into more than one type of tissue. Such tumors are often embryonic tumors that show differentiation into tissues that are not normally seen in the same adult organs but that can be derived from immature mesen-

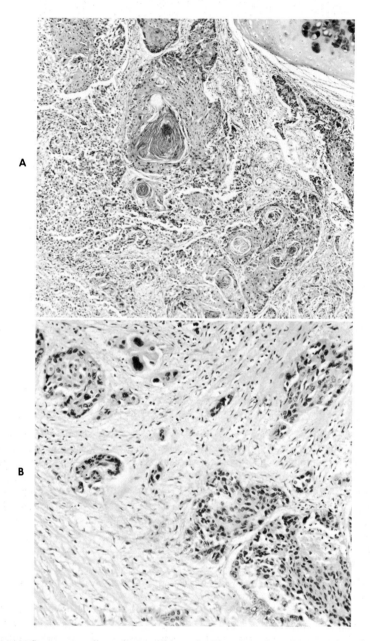

Fig. 12-14. A, Squamous cell carcinoma of bronchus (portion of cartilage in upper right corner). Note areas of differentiation of cancer with formation of keratinized masses in center of nests of tumor cells ("keratin pearls"). **B,** Undifferentiated area of squamous cell carcinoma shown in **A** with invasion and associated fibrous tissue proliferation (desmoplasia).

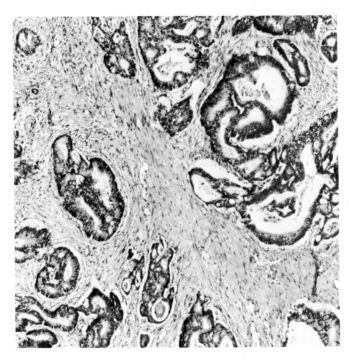

Fig. 12-15. Adenocarcinoma of colon. Atypical glands invading wall of colon associated with proliferation of fibrous tissue of stroma.

chyme. They differ from teratomas in that they are derived from one germ layer. In such tumors of the kidney (Wilms' tumor or embryoma, p. 370) and liver, both epithelial and connective tissue elements are commonly present, but organ development is not found.

Mixed tumors containing a mixture of tumor forms derived from mesenchyme have been termed *mesenchymomas*. They are found most frequently in the urogenital tract (uterus, p. 653) and breast but also occur in other soft parts. The malignant mesenchymoma arising in the uterus, commonly referred to as *mesodermal mixed tumor*, occasionally includes an epithelial *(carcinomatous)* element along with the usual mesenchymal *(sarcomatous)* tissue. The so-called mixed tumor of the salivary glands is regarded by many not as a true mixed tumor but as an epithelial neoplasm referred to as *pleomorphic adenoma* (p. 519).

Teratomas. A teratoma is a type of mixed tumor made up of various kinds of tissue representing the three primitive layers of blastoderm, the neoplastic tissues being foreign to the part in which the tumor arises. Willis, among others, supports the hypothesis that teratomas arise from foci of totipotential cells that have escaped the influence of the "primary organizer" during early embryonic development. The common occurrence of teratomas in midline or near-midline sites suggests that the disturbance emanates from the region of the embryonic primitive streak.

Teratomas occur most frequently in the ovaries and testes but also may involve the anterior mediastinum, sacrococcygeal and retroperitoneal regions, and base of the skull. Rarely, they arise in other sites such as the brain, pineal gland, and neck. The tumors consist of a mixture of tissues at varying stages of differentiation, from the most undifferentiated embryonic tissue to the most ma-

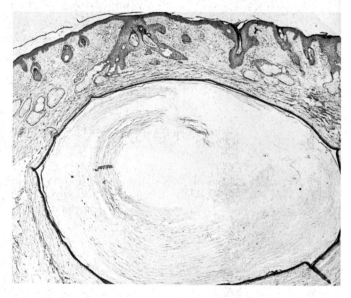

Fig. 12-16. Epidermal cyst of skin lined by thin layer of squamous epithelium and filled by layered mass of keratin.

ture adult type, including highly organized structures (e.g., skin and its appendages, teeth, digits, portions of nerves, nerve ganglia, brain, intestines).

Teratomas may be benign or malignant. The former tend to be mostly cystic (e.g., "dermoid" cysts), with tissues that are usually of the mature, adult type, whereas the latter tend to be solid and may continue to proliferate at the embryonic level, producing tissues of all degrees of immaturity. Occasionally, one type of cell in a teratoma becomes malignant, and metastases are made up of this type of cell alone.

CYSTS

A cyst is a cavity that may contain fluid or semisolid material and is surrounded by a definite wall (Fig. 12-16). There is usually a lining of cells (e.g., epithelial, mesothelial).

Classification

The many varieties of cysts can be fitted into the following classification:

retention cysts due to blockage of ducts or tubules, with cystic distention of the proximal portion; cysts of the kidney and pancreas are usually of this type; some cysts of the skin may be of this type, and some may be of traumatic origin (inclusion cysts)

cysts due to developmental errors those arising from the branchial clefts, the thyroglossal duct, and the remains of the wolffian duct (hydatids of Morgagni); also of developmental origin are some sebaceous cysts of the skin, cystic hygromas (p. 296), and the cysts associated with spina bifida (p. 746)

cystic tumors or cystomas (cystadenomas) those that arise very commonly from the ovary and other organs

cysts from serous cavities those that arise by outpouchings from bursae and tendon sheaths (e.g., "Baker's cyst" in the popliteal space)

parasitic cysts those due to the *Echinococcus granulosus* (hydatid cysts) and amebiasis

pseudocysts those formed as a result of hemorrhagic material (hematoma) that has become encapsulated; also to be included here are the cyst-like spaces formed as a result of mucinous degeneration

REFERENCES

Ackerman, L. V., and Rosai, J.: CA **22:**41-54, 1972 (various aspects of tumors).

Allen, D. W., and Cole, P.: N. Engl. J. Med. **286:**70-82, 1972 (viruses and human cancer).

Ashley, D. J. B.: Evans' histologic appearances of tumours, ed. 3, New York, 1978, Churchill Livingstone, Inc. (general reference).

Baston, O. V.: Am. J. Roentgenol. Radium Ther. Nucl. Med. **78:**195-212, 1957 (vertebral vein system).

Berenblum, L.: Arch. Pathol. **38:**233-244, 1944 (irritation, trauma, and tumor formation).

Bosman, H. B., and Hall, T. C.: Proc. Natl. Acad. Sci. U.S.A. **71:**1833-1837, 1974 (enzyme activity in cancers).

Boyd, W.: The spontaneous regression of cancer, Springfield, Ill., 1966, Charles C Thomas, Publisher.

Burnet, F. M.: Progr. Exp. Tumor Res. **13:**1-27, 1970 (concept of immunologic surveillance).

Busch, H., et al.: Cancer Res. **23:**313-339, 1963 (nucleolus of cancer cell).

Castro, J. E., editor: Immunological aspects of cancer, Baltimore, 1978, University Park Press.

Conney, A. H.: N. Engl. J. Med. **289:**971-973, 1973 (carcinogen metabolism and human cancer).

Creech, J. L., and Johnson, M. N.: J. Occup. Med. **16:**150-151, 1974 (vinyl chloride).

del Regato, J. A., and Spjut, H. J.: Ackerman and del Regato's cancer; diagnosis, treatment, and prognosis, ed. 5, St. Louis, 1977, The C. V. Mosby Co. (general reference).

Dmochowski, L.: Am. J. Clin. Pathol. **60:**3-18, 1973 (molecular mechanisms in viral neoplasia).

Dmochowski, L., and Bowen, J. M.: Am. J. Clin. Pathol. **62:**167-172, 1974 (immunology and neoplasia).

Editorial: J.A.M.A. **161:**66-67, 1956 (keloids).

Everson, T. C., and Cole, W. H.: Spontaneous regression of cancer, Philadelphia, 1966, W. B. Saunders Co.

Farber, E.: Cancer Res. **33:**2537-2550, 1973 (carcinogenesis).

Fialkow, P. J.: Blood **30:**388-394, 1967 ("immunologic" oncogenesis).

Fisher, B.: Adv. Surg. **5:**189-254, 1971 (present status of tumor immunology).

Fisher, B., and Fisher, E. R.: Ann. Surg. **150:**731, 1959 (factors influencing metastases).

Foulds, L.: J. Chronic Dis. **8:**2-37, 1958 (natural history of cancer).

Gallo, R. C., editor: Recent advances in cancer research—cell biology, molecular biology, and tumor virology, vols. 1 and 2, Cleveland, 1977, CRC Press, Inc.

Goodall, C. M.: Int. J. Cancer **4:**1-13, 1969 (paraendocrine cancer syndromes).

Green, H. N., Anthony, H. M., Baldwin, R. W., and Westrop, J.: An immunological approach to cancer, New York, 1967, Appleton-Century-Crofts.

Green, I., Cohen, S., and McCluskey, R. T., editors: Mechanisms of tumor immunity, New York, 1977, John Wiley & Sons, Inc.

Gyorkey, F., et al.: Hum. Pathol. **6:**421-441, 1975 (electron microscopy in diagnosis of tumors).

Haddow, A.: Br. Med. Bull. **21:**133-139, 1965 (immunology of cancer cell).

Hall, T. C.: Cancer Res. **34:**2088-2091, 1974 (paraneoplastic syndromes).

Henney, C. S., et al.: Am. J. Pathol. **93:**459-468, 1978 ("natural killer" cells).

Herbst, A. T., et al.: N. Engl. J. Med. **284:**878-881, 1971 (stilbestrol and vaginal adenocarcinoma).

Hiatt, H. H., Watson, J. D., and Winsten, J. A., editors: Origins of human cancer, vols. 1, 2, and 3, Cold Spring Harbor, N.Y., 1977, Cold Spring Harbor Laboratory.

Hobbs, C. B., and Miller, A. L.: J. Clin. Pathol. **19:**119-127, 1966 (endocrine function in tumors).

Holtz, F.: Cancer **11:**1103-1109, 1958 (liposarcoma).

Hueper, W. C., and Conway, W. D.: Chemical carcinogenesis and cancers, Springfield, Ill., 1964, Charles C Thomas, Publisher.

Inagaki, J., et al.: Cancer **33:**568-573, 1974 (causes of death in cancer patients).

Jamakosmanović, A., and Loewenstein, W. R.: J. Cell Biol. **38:**556-561, 1968 (intercellular communications in thyroid cancer).

Klein, G., and Oettgen, H. F.: Cancer Res. **29:**1741-1746, 1969 (immunologic factors involved in growth of primary tumors).

Knudson, A. G.: Am J. Pathol. **77:**77-84, 1974 (heredity and human cancer).

Köhler, G., and Milstein, C.: Nature **256:**495-497, 1975 (cultures of fused cells secreting antibody).

Kraybill, H. F., and Mehlman, M. A., editors: Environmental cancer, Washington, D.C., 1977, Hemisphere Publishing Corporation.

Laurent, J., Debry, G., and Floquet, J.: Hypoglycaemic tumours, Amsterdam, 1971, Excerpta Medica Foundation.

Lawrence, W., et al.: Cancer **17:**361-376, 1964 (embryonal rhabdomyosarcoma).

Lieberman, P. H., et al.: J.A.M.A. **198:**1047-1051, 1966 (alveolar soft-part sarcoma).

Loewenstein, W. R., and Kanno, Y.: J. Cell Biol. **33:**225-234, 1967 (intercellular communications in cancer growth).

McIntire, K. R., et al.: Cancer Res. **32:**1941-1946, 1972 (α-fetoprotein in hepatocellular carcinoma).

Medical News: J.A.M.A. **242:**2161-2163, 1979 (monoclonal antibodies).

Melchers, F., Potter, M., and Warner, N. L., editors: Lymphocyte hybridomas (current topics in microbiology and immunology), New York, 1978, Springer-Verlag.

Miller, J. A., and Miller, E. C.: J. Natl. Cancer Inst. **47**(3):V-XIV, 1971 (chemical carcinogenesis).

Miller, R. W.: J. Natl. Cancer Inst. **47:**1169-1171, 1971 (transplacental chemical carcinogenesis in man).

Miller, R. W.: J. Natl. Cancer Inst. **49:**1221-1227, 1972 (radiation-induced cancer).

Mizejewski, G. J.: Am. J. Med. Sci. **266:**359-369, 1973 (humoral responses in tumor immunity).

Monkman, G. R., et al.: Mayo Clin. Proc. **49:**157-163, 1974 (trauma and oncogenesis).

Morton, D. L.: J. Reticuloendothel. Soc. **10**:137-160, 1971 (human tumor antigens).

Nelson, N.: N. Engl. J. Med. **288**:1123-1124, 1973 (carcinogenicity of halo ethers).

Nicholson, G. W. de P.: Studies on tumor formation, St. Louis, 1950, The C. V. Mosby Co. (general reference).

Order, S. E., et al.: N. Engl. J. Med. **285**:471-474, 1971 (tumor-associated antigen in Hodgkin's disease).

Pierce, G. B.: Fed. Proc. **29**:,1248-1254, 1970 (differentiation).

Pierce, G. B.: Am. J. Pathol. **77**:103-118, 1974 (neoplasms, differentiation, mutations).

Piessens, W. F.: Cancer **26**:1212-1220, 1970 (evidence for human cancer immunity).

Pilch, Y. H., and Golub, S. H.: Am. J. Clin. Pathol. **62**:184-211, 1974 (lymphocyte-mediated responses in neoplasia).

Pitot, H.: Am. J. Pathol. **87**:443-472, 1977 (carcinogenesis and aging).

Prehn, R. T.: J. Natl. Cancer Inst. **59**:1043-1049, 1977 (immunostimulation in tumors).

Prehn, R. T., and Prehn, L. M.: Am. J. Pathol. **80**:529-550, 1975 (pathobiology of neoplasia).

Purtilo, D. T., et al.: Am. J. Pathol. **91**:607-688, 1978 (genetics of neoplasia).

Redmond, D. E., Jr.: N. Engl. J. Med. **282**:18-23, 1970 (tobacco and cancer in 1761).

Regezi, J. A., and Batsakis, J. C.: Arch. Pathol. Lab. Med. **102**:8-14, 1978 (electron microscopic diagnosis of head and neck tumors).

Report and Commentary: The carcinogenic hazard of radiation to the breast, CA **20**(1):24-31, 1970.

Roulet, F. C., editor: The lymphoreticular tumours in Africa, Basel, 1964, S. Karger.

Schottenfeld, D.: CA **20**(1):35-43, 1970 (medical syndromes associated with malignant tumors).

Searle, C. E., editor: Chemical carcinogens, Washington, D.C., 1976, American Chemical Society.

Schuster, J., et al.: Am. J. Clin. Pathol. **62**:243-257, 1974 (immunologic diagnosis of human cancers).

Silver, H. K. B., et al.: Proc. Natl. Acad. Sci. **70**:526-530, 1973 (human α-fetoprotein).

Silverberg, E.: CA **30**:23-38, 1980 (cancer statistics).

Smith, R. R., and Hilberg, A. W.: J. Natl. Cancer Inst. **16**:645-657, 1955 (seeding in operative wounds).

Smith, R. T.: N. Engl. J. Med. **278**:1207-1214, 1268-1275, 1326-1331, 1968 (tumor-specific immune mechanisms).

Sorokin, J. J., et al.: J.A.M.A. **228**:49-53, 1974 (carcinoembryonic antigen assays).

Spector, B. D., et al.: Clin. Immunol. and Immunopathol. **11**:12-29, 1978 (immunodeficiency diseases and malignancy).

Stout, A. P.: Tumors of the peripheral nervous system. In Atlas of tumor pathology, Sect. II, Fasc. 6, Washington, D.C., 1949, Armed Forces Institute of Pathology.

Symposium: Third Conference on Embryonic and Fetal Antigens in Cancer, Cancer Res. **34**:2021-2137, 1974.

Tannenbaum, S. R., et al.: J. Natl. Cancer Inst. **53**:79-84, 1974 (nitrosamines).

Tashjian, A. H., Jr.: N. Engl. J. Med. **290**:905-906, 1974 (hypercalcemias of cancer).

Temin, H. M.: Proc. Natl. Acad. Sci. U.S.A. **69**:1016-1019, 1972 (RNA tumor viruses).

Todaro, G. J., and Huebner, R. J.: Proc. Natl. Acad. Sci. U.S.A. **69**:1009-1020, 1972 (oncogene theory).

Warren, L.: Am. J. Pathol. **77**:69-76, 1974 (malignant cell and its membranes).

Weber, G.: N. Engl. J. Med. **296**:486-493, 541-551, 1977 (enzymology of cancer cells).

Weinstein, R. S., and McNutt, N. S.: N. Engl. J. Med. **286**:521-524, 1972 (cell junctions).

Wells, H. G.: J.A.M.A. **114**:2177-2183, 2284-2289, 1940 (lipoma).

Willis, R. A.: Bull. N.Y. Acad. Med. **26**:440-460, 1950 (teratoma).

Willis, R. A.: Teratomas. In Atlas of tumor pathology, Sect. III, Fasc. 9, Washington, D.C., 1951, Armed Forces Institute of Pathology.

Willis, R. A.: Pathology of tumours, ed. 4, London, 1967, Butterworth & Co. (Publishers) Ltd. (general reference).

Willis, R. A.: The spread of tumours in the human body, ed. 3, London, 1973, Butterworth & Co. (Publishers) Ltd.

Wynder, E. L., and Reddy, B. S.: Cancer **34**:801-806, 1974 (metabolic epidemiology of colorectal cancer).

13

Cardiovascular system

The circulatory system, which includes the heart, blood vessels, and lymphatics, is concerned with the essential nutrition of tissues. Disease of this system is a major cause of illness and disability and is the leading cause of death in the United States.

Blood vessels and lymphatics

Generally speaking, lesions of blood vessels are important in proportion to the degree to which they reduce circulation to vital tissues. Such an effect is most commonly produced by a hardening and thickening of arterial walls, referred to as arteriosclerosis. Arteries and veins are also subject to inflammations (arteritis and phlebitis), dilatation (aneurysm and varicosity), and neoplasms. Thrombosis, embolism, and hemorrhage are important accompaniments to vascular diseases.

STRUCTURE OF ARTERIES

Arterial vessels are composed of three coats: intima, media, and adventitia. The *intima,* or inner layer, consists of a lining of endothelial cells, beneath which are smooth muscle, elastic, and collagen fibers, along with a few mesenchymal cells, in a background of acid mucopolysaccharide. The *media* is formed by smooth muscle and elastic tissue. A conden-

sation of the elastic tissue at the inner margin of the media forms the internal elastic lamella. This inner elastic band frequently appears wavy because of postmortem contraction of the vessel. A less definite outer condensation of elastic tissue sometimes forms an external elastic lamella. The *adventitia,* or outer wall, contains a loose network of connective tissue and elastic fibrils, carrying blood vessels (vasa vasorum) and nerves to supply the vessel wall.

The vascular supply to the wall of blood vessels is richer and more extensive than was previously suspected. Small vessels supplying arterial walls are much more numerous in older persons and in the presence of atherosclerosis. Intimal vasa vasorum are common in atherosclerotic vessels, but their presence in normal intima is not apparent.

The arterial system may be divided into three main types of vessels according to size and structural variations: elastic arteries, muscular arteries, and arterioles. The group of elastic arteries includes the largest vessel, the aorta, and its immediate branches. In this group, the vessel wall contains elastic tissue in greatest proportion. Elastic recoil of these vessels maintains blood flow and pressure during diastole. The second group, the muscular distributing arteries, are the medium-sized vessels, such as the brachial, radial, and femoral arteries. In these vessels, elastic tissue is present in smaller amount and muscle tissue in greater amount than in elastic arteries. The third group, the arterioles, includes the small arteries of organs, down to the size of capillaries. In these vessels, muscle tissue is most abundant and elastic tissue is relatively slight. Their contraction is important in the regulation of blood pressure and flow.

ARTERIOSCLEROSIS

The term *arteriosclerosis* literally means "hardening of the arteries" and is sometimes used synonymously with "atherosclerosis." However, according to present usage, arteriosclerosis is a generic term that includes three diseases of the arterial tree: (1) atherosclerosis, (2) Mönckeberg's medial sclerosis, and (3) arteriolosclerosis. In the first disease, the principal change is in the intima; in the second, the media; and in the third, the intima, the media, or both.

Atherosclerosis. Intimal thickening and regressive changes are the characteristic features of atherosclerosis. It affects mainly the large elastic vessels, the aorta being most severely involved. It also affects the coronary, renal, and cerebral arteries and the larger arteries of the extremities. The intimal lesions range from small, slightly raised, longitudinal yellow streaks ("fatty streaks") to larger, pearly gray or gray-yellow nodules or plaques containing lipid and hyalinized connective tissue ("fibrous plaques") and advanced lesions with ulceration, thrombosis, hemorrhage, and calcification ("complicated lesions")

There has not been complete agreement among investigators concerning the *pathogenesis* of atherosclerosis in man, particularly with regard to the nature of the events that initiate the process. As a result, several hypotheses have been proposed that present different concepts as to what the early events of the atherosclerotic process may be. Among these hypotheses are the following:

1 The earliest change consists of fatty streaks in the intima caused by lipids infiltrating from the blood plasma. The lipids appear within mesenchymal cells, which generally are considered to be smooth muscle cells, although recent investigators regard them as multipotential, smooth musclelike cells capable of producing collagen, elastic, and muscle fibers (so-called myointimal cells). Some of the lipid-containing cells may be macrophages. The lipids filter through the endothelium along with plasma, usually as free molecules or possibly also carried in macrophages, and the larger lipoprotein complexes are trapped in the intima. Prior damage to the intima is not apparent, but an excess amount of lipids in the plasma, nutritional disturbances, hormonal factors, or hemodynamic factors may enhance lipid infiltration.

2 Local alterations in the vascular wall resulting from some form of injury (hemodynamic, endocrine, metabolic, immunologic, hypoxic, etc.) precede lipid deposits. The alterations may consist of increased vascular permeability and certain changes in the mesenchymal tissue of the intima, particularly the mucopolysaccharide component (e.g., an increased production of sulfated glycosaminoglycans). It has been suggested that the altered vascular permeability permits passage of large molecules, such as β- and pre-β-lipoproteins and fibrinogen, which react with the altered mucopolysaccharide component, leading to their entrapment within the intima. The possibility also has been considered that local lipid synthesis may play a role in the accumulation of lipids in the intima.

3 Mural thrombi occur on the endothelium, become organized and incorporated into the intima, and are then infiltrated by lipid.

4 Platelets agglutinate over areas of endothelial damage and then disintegrate and release vasoactive amines that increase permeability to lipids and proteins, allowing these substances to accumulate in the intima. Some studies suggest that platelets penetrate the intima and, upon disintegration, release lipids contained in their cytoplasm.

5 Recent hypotheses emphasize proliferation of smooth muscle cells in the intima as the significant early event in the formation of atherosclerotic lesions, the proliferating cells being capable of producing connective tissue matrix (collagen, elastic proteins, and proteoglycans).

a According to one view, this proliferation

occurs in response to some form of injury to the arterial endothelium (e.g., by chronic hyperlipidemia, infections, or chemical, immunologic, or mechanical factors). The injury results in desquamation of endothelium, followed by platelet adherence and aggregation and release of factors from the platelets, which, together with plasma constituents (e.g., lipoproteins and/or hormones), enter the arterial wall and induce migration of smooth muscle cells from the media to the intima, as well as proliferation of the cells, and/or proliferation of preexisting intimal smooth muscle cells. The intimal proliferation is accompanied by formation of new connective tissue and deposition of intracellular and extracellular lipid.

b Some investigators have proposed that the focal proliferations of smooth muscle cells in the intima represent monoclonal growths resembling benign neoplasms. As with neoplasms, there is an initiation phase during which intimal cells are altered by certain factors (e.g., chemical mutagens, radiation, viruses), followed by a promotion phase during which proliferation of the altered cells is brought about by various chemical, nutritional, or mechanical factors. It has been suggested that low density proteins of the serum, which are taken up by the intimal smooth cells, may be carriers of mutagenic or potential mutagenic agents.

It is generally agreed that no matter what the initial events, excessive accumulation of lipids, principally cholesterol and its esters, in the arterial intima is an essential feature of atherosclerotic lesions and plays an important role in their development and progression. In the early lesions (fatty streaks), the lipids appear mainly intracellularly, within smooth muscle cells and macrophages, but also as extracellular deposits. The principal source of cholesterol in the intima is probably the blood plasma, but it is also possible that the plasma lipids are hydrolyzed and re-esterified by the cells that have taken them up. With progression of the lesions, fibrous plaques form that consist of lipid-laden smooth muscle cells, increasing amounts of extracellular lipid, and newly formed connective tissue. Although connective tissue components may be derived from the intimal smooth muscle cells, the organization of mural thrombi with incorporation into the intima may contribute to the formation of the connective tissue. In larger lesions, the central portion is frequently soft, containing degenerated and necrotic tissue, free fat, and visible cholesterol crystals. Microscopically, the cholesterol appears as clear, elongated, fusiform clefts, because the crystals have been dissolved out in preparation of the section (Fig. 13-1). The soft, yellow nodule is an atheroma (''porridgelike'' mass). In advanced lesions, ulceration of atheromas and superimposed thrombi may be seen. The internal elastic lamina is frayed and fragmented, and in places it may be absent. Calcium salts become deposited in the atheromatous lesions and form thin, brittle, calcified plates, which may crack easily. When an atheromatous plaque is large, it may encroach upon and cause thinning of the media. Progressive loss of elasticity accompanies atherosclerosis, but much of this may be an aging effect.

The atheromatous lesions are much more prevalent in the abdominal than in the thoracic aorta. Their distribution is patchy, they are eccentrically placed, as a rule, and they are found at points of stress, e.g., on the posterior wall of the aorta, especially about orifices of the intercostal and lumbar arteries, and at the point of branching of major vessels. Atherosclerosis may be superimposed on syphilitic lesions in the thoracic aorta.

Complications of atheromatous plaques include the following:

1 Narrowing of the lumen, resulting in ischemia
2 Thrombosis over the plaque, with possible occlusion of the lumen, or, in the case of small thrombi, the thrombi may organize, become incorporated into the intima, and contribute to growth of the plaque
3 Hemorrhage into the plaques, which, in some instances (e.g., coronary artery),

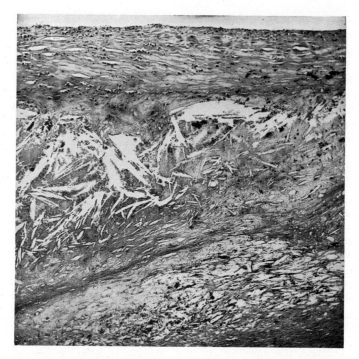

Fig. 13-1. Section through advanced atheromatous plaque. Numerous cholesterol clefts may be seen in pale central part. Small dark spots are caused by calcium deposits. (Courtesy Dr. E. M. Hall.)

may contribute to luminal occlusion and may also initiate thrombosis

4 Rupture of soft atheromatous material into the lumen, which may cause occlusion at the site (in a small vessel), give rise to an atheromatous embolus, or initiate thrombosis

5 Formation of an aneurysm because of thinning and weakening of the media adjacent to the large plaque

Obstruction of certain vessels, caused by the plaque itself or one of its complications, may lead to serious ischemic effects, e.g., sudden death or myocardial infarct with involvement of the coronary arteries, infarct of the brain in cerebral atherosclerosis, and hypertension with renal arterial disease. The Leriche syndrome, occurring chiefly in men and characterized by ischemic effects in the lower limbs (e.g., pallor, coldness, cramps, and claudication), an inability to maintain a penile erec-

tion, and impotence, is the result of a progressive atheromatous thrombotic occlusion of the abdominal aorta at or above its bifurcation.

The *etiology* of atherosclerosis involves a complex interrelationship between multiple factors, both endogenous and environmental. The actual cause or causes are unknown, but there are various *predisposing* or *contributing factors*. In many studies, the role of *plasma* and *dietary lipids* has been emphasized. There is evidence that an increase in serum β-lipoproteins, hypercholesterolemia, and an increased cholesterol-phospholipid ratio in the blood are significant in the development of atherosclerosis. An increase in serum triglycerides also may be important. People whose diet contains large amounts of saturated animal fat and cholesterol have a higher serum cholesterol level and an increased incidence of coronary atherosclerotic heart disease than those whose diet is low in these fats. It is interesting to note, however, that some birds that do not have animal fats in their diet (e.g., certain species of pigeons) develop spontaneous atherosclerosis similar to that in man. Certain diseases associated with hypercholesterolemia, such as *diabetes mellitus, hypothyroidism,* and *familial hypercholesterolemia,* frequently are associated with atherosclerosis. *Hereditary predisposition* is a factor, but it is not certain whether this is related to familial patterns of lipid metabolism.

Cholesterol feeding in rabbits is a well-known experimental method of producing atherosclerosis. Similarly, atherosclerosis has been produced in the dog, rat, mouse, and other animals, but, in certain of these, other procedures are necessary, e.g., the use of antithyroid drugs or surgical removal of the thyroid gland. In monkeys, atherosclerosis can be produced by pyridoxine deficiency without any special fat diet. Hyperlipemia also appears to increase the tendency toward thrombosis. Heparin, in addition to its anticoagulant effect, helps to correct the abnormal lipoprotein pattern often found in atherosclerotic patients.

The influence of *sex* is evident in the observation that atherosclerosis is much less likely to occur in women before menopause, although the incidence increases progressively after menopause. It is not clear which factors in the premenopausal period are protective to women. There has been a suggestion that certain *hormones,* e.g., estrogens, may play a role in this regard. In some studies, women whose ovaries were removed developed coronary atherosclerosis more often and at an earlier age than those with intact ovaries. Also, the incidence and severity of the disease have been observed to be less in men treated with estrogens for carcinoma of the prostate than in nontreated men. However, not all investigators have found a difference in incidence of coronary atherosclerotic heart disease in castrated women compared with noncastrated women. Furthermore, recent studies strongly suggest that women who use oral contraceptives are at a greater risk of developing myocardial infarction (a manifestation of coronary heart disease) than nonusers.

Age is considered by some investigators to be important, but it should be noted that atherosclerosis is not a disease limited to advanced age. Atherosclerosis can also occur in the young, as evidenced by the autopsy finding of coronary atherosclerosis in young men killed in military action in Korea and Vietnam. Proponents of the aging theory point out that there is a progressive intimal thickening in the arteries from the time of birth, although this may be related to continued intravascular mechanical stress. It also has been suggested that intimal plaques are essentially compensatory phenomena in response to underlying medial weakness resulting from degenerations associated with aging. *Emotional stress, physical inactivity, obesity,* and *cigarette smoking* are other possible predisposing or contributing factors.

Local hemodynamic forces in the bloodstream (e.g., turbulence of flow and sites of increased wall tension) are undoubtedly important in the development of atherosclerosis. This is suggested by the fact that atheromatous plaques are most prevalent at or just beyond the orifices or bifurcations of arteries and at points where vessels are relatively fixed. *Hypertension* is apparently not a primary cause of atherosclerosis but may aggravate the lesion by accentuating the local hemodynamic factors, or when hypercholesterolemia exists in a hypertensive patient, the high intravascular pressure probably accelerates infiltration of lipid through the arterial wall.

Medial sclerosis (Mönckeberg's sclerosis). Medial sclerosis occurs particularly in the medium-sized muscular arteries, such as the femoral, radial, and temporal, usually in elderly persons. There are degeneration, swelling, and fragmentation of medial muscle fibers, followed by calcium deposition (Fig. 13-2). Occasionally, bone is formed in the vessel wall. The vessels become hard and tortuous, so that palpable vessels such as the radial artery can be felt as rigid tubes.

The medial changes alone do not narrow the lumen and have little effect on the circulation. However, the medial sclerosis may be associated with intimal atheromatous lesions that

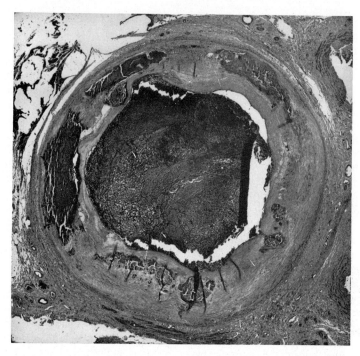

Fig. 13-2. Mönckeberg's medial sclerosis. Note dark calcified plaques in media. Recent thrombus fills lumen. (Courtesy Dr. E. M. Hall.)

could interfere with blood flow. Vasotonic influences may be causative factors in the development of medial sclerosis. In experimental animals, similar lesions are produced by the administration of epinephrine, nicotine, or other agents that produce prolonged spasm of the vessels.

Arteriolosclerosis. There are two types of arteriolar change characterized by thickening of the vessel wall and narrowing of the lumen: hyaline arteriolosclerosis and hyperplastic arteriolosclerosis, both of which are characteristic but not pathognomonic of hypertension.

In *hyaline arteriolosclerosis,* the wall is thickened and hyalinized as a result of deposition of a hyaline material in the intima and media, with obliteration of the underlying cellular details. There is a controversy as to the origin of the vascular hyalin. Some investigators have demonstrated by electron microscopy

that the hyalin is deposited primarily in intimal spaces, possibly derived from excessive infiltration of plasma proteins, and that larger deposits tend to infiltrate the adjacent elastic tissue and media. Others interpret the ultrastructural features of hyaline arteriolosclerosis as evidence that the hyaline material is derived from increased basement membrane substance of endothelial and smooth muscle origin. Hyaline arteriolosclerosis is seen especially in the kidneys and other organs of patients with benign hypertension (Fig. 13-3).

Hyperplastic arteriolosclerosis usually affects larger arterioles and is associated with severe hypertension, particularly accelerated (or malignant) hypertension. It is characterized by cellular proliferation of the intima, hypertrophy of the muscle cells of the media, and fibrosis of the adventitia. The intimal change consists of concentric lamellae of fibroblasts and elastic fibers (''onionskin'' appearance) as-

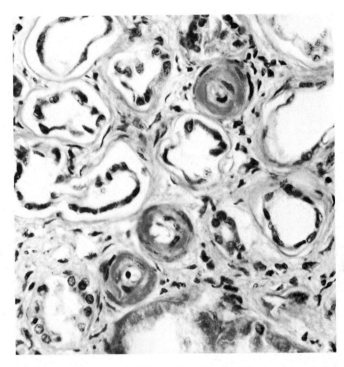

Fig. 13-3. Hyaline arteriolosclerosis in kidney of patient with benign (essential) hypertension.

sociated with luminal narrowing. In some electron microscopic studies, it was concluded that the increased cellularity of the intima results from the presence of smooth muscle cells migrating from the media and that there is a proliferation of smooth muscle cells in the media.

Both forms of arteriolosclerosis may coexist in a tissue (e.g., in a patient who has had benign hypertension for years and then suddenly develops acceleration of the hypertension). Fibrinoid necrosis of the arterioles ("necrotizing arteriolitis") also may be noted in arteriolosclerosis, particularly in patients with malignant hypertension.

Endarteritis obliterans. The use of the term *endarteritis obliterans* is not really correct, since it implies an inflammatory process, which is not present in the conditions so designated. The term applies to a localizing process affecting small arteries that is character-

ized by intimal thickening and narrowing or obliteration of the lumen. Such may be seen in atherosclerosis involving the muscular arteries of the lower extremities, often associated with superimposed thrombosis. Known as "arteriosclerosis obliterans" (Fig. 13-4), this may interfere with the flow of blood and, if collateral circulation is inadequate, may cause serious ischemic changes. Intimal proliferative thickening may be seen in small arteries in areas of chronic inflammation (e.g., adjacent to tuberculous cavities of the lung or in the base of a peptic ulcer). It also develops in the blood vessels of a region in which active circulation is no longer needed, i.e., as an involutionary change in vessels whose capillary beds have been reduced by tissue atrophy. Hence, it occurs in the hypogastric arteries and ductus arteriosus after birth, in the arteries of the uterus and ovaries in old age, and in involution of uterine arteries after pregnancy.

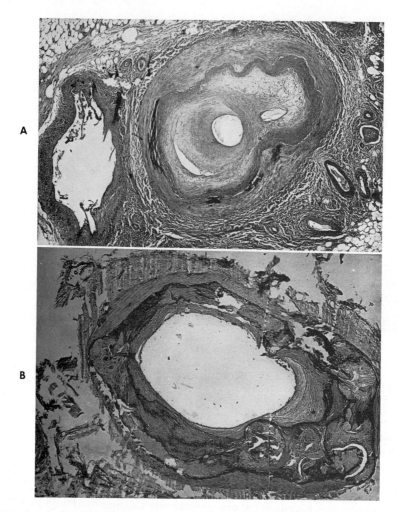

Fig. 13-4. Arteriosclerosis obliterans. **A,** Significant intimal proliferation ("endarteritis") of anterior tibial artery. Organized thrombus surrounds larger luminal opening. Dry gangrene of great toe in 73-year-old black woman. **B,** Note excessive medial calcification of tibial artery. Gangrene and cellulitis of great toe and dry gangrene of fourth and fifth toes in 82-year-old white man. (From Gore, I.: Blood and lymphatic vessels. In Anderson, W. A. D., editor: Pathology, ed. 6, St. Louis, 1971, The C. V. Mosby Co.)

INFLAMMATION OF ARTERIES

Acute nonspecific arteritis. Acute inflammation of an artery may arise from local *bacterial infections* that spread to involve vessel walls. It also may result from intravascular spread of infections, as in septicemia or embolism. Complications of infectious arteritis include thrombosis, rupture with hemorrhage, and aneurysmal formation (so-called mycotic aneurysms).

Other microorganisms (e.g., *rickettsiae*) and noninfectious agents (e.g., *trauma* and *chemicals*) also may produce acute nonspecific arteritis.

Chronic arteritis. Chronic arteritis of the granulomatous type may be seen in *tuberculo-*

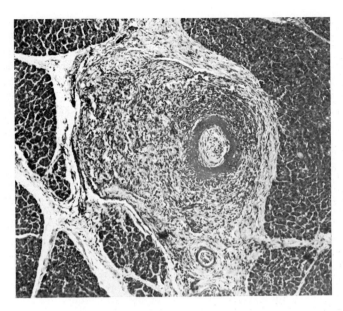

Fig. 13-5. Polyarteritis nodosa of pancreas.

sis and *syphilis*. The important lesion in syphilis is aortitis, characterized mainly by a chronic necrotizing and fibrosing inflammation, although small gummatous granulomas are sometimes seen (p. 186).

Necrotizing arteritis. Acute arteritis associated with necrosis of the vascular wall, usually of the fibrinoid type, is a characteristic of certain hypersensitivity reactions (as with sulfonamides, other drugs, and foreign serum).

A similar type of vasculitis may be seen in the group of so-called collagen diseases, in which altered immunity plays a role, e.g., in rheumatic fever, systemic lupus erythematosus, polyarteritis nodosa, and rheumatoid arthritis.

Polyarteritis nodosa. Polyarteritis nodosa (periarteritis nodosa) is an acute inflammation with degeneration and necrosis involving the walls of medium-sized and small arteries (Fig. 13-5). Various organs and tissues may be involved, but most frequently affected are the kidneys, heart, liver, gastrointestinal tract, muscles, and peripheral nerves. These tissues may be involved together or successively. The variety of organ involvement produces clinical

pictures that are of great variability and are difficult to diagnose. Biopsy of a nodule from skin or muscle frequently enables clinical recognition. The condition may occur at any age. It is estimated that recovery occurs in about 10% of cases.

The etiology of polyarteritis nodosa has been variously ascribed to a specific virus, rheumatic fever, streptococci, and allergy. Frequent association of the condition with asthma or other allergic states and similarity to vascular changes in known hypersensitivity reactions favor the hypothesis that it may be a severe manifestation of hypersensitivity. Certain studies support the view that polyarteritis nodosa is an immune complex disease associated with the presence of a virus-related antigen in the serum, viz., Australia antigen (p. 176). The evidence suggests that the vascular damage is caused by deposits in the vessel walls of immune complexes consisting of Australia antigen, homologous IgM antibody, and complement.

In some instances, the inflammatory changes have been thought to begin in the adventitia and in other cases, in the intima or innermost part of the media. Acute, subacute, chronic and healed stages have been described. The earliest, or acute, phase is characterized by fibrinoid necrosis, usually beginning in the media. In the subacute stage, there is cellular exudation. Eosinophils are the most characteristic cells of the inflammatory reaction, but lymphocytes, plasma cells, and neutrophilic leukocytes may be present. The occurrence of plasma cells, in view of their role in antibody production, may be evidence of the hypersensitivity mechanism. Exudation is followed by proliferative changes around the vessel and also of the intima. Thrombosis often occurs. Occlusion of the lumen and infarction are common results. In the chronic phase, granulation tissue develops and healing begins. Absorption of exudate and fibrosis result in the final healed condition. When various organs are involved successively, the several stages may be evident in the different organs.

Yellowish red nodules, which occur in the affected vessels, usually are caused by small localized dilatations or aneurysms at points of degeneration, inflammation, and weakening of the vessel wall. Nodules may be formed also by the localized cellular infiltration and proliferation. Rupture of one of the aneurysmal nodules may result in serious hemorrhage.

Temporal arteritis. Temporal or cranial (giant cell) arteritis is a granulomatous inflammatory process affecting mainly temporal or other cranial arteries. It occurs chiefly in older age groups, is usually self-limited, and has a better outlook than polyarteritis nodosa, but it may be complicated by blindness in one or both eyes because of involvement of the retinal arteries.

The affected vessels show an inflammatory infiltrate, chiefly lymphocytes, in the intima and inner part of the media and a disruption of the internal elastic lamina associated with multinucleated giant cells. Eosinophils are usually absent from the exudate. There may be patchy necrosis of the media. Fibrous healing of the inflammation causes luminal narrowing. Thrombosis may occur.

Thromboangiitis obliterans. Buerger introduced the term *thromboangiitis obliterans* to describe an inflammatory condition of the vessels of the extremities in which thrombosis and, later, fibrosis interfere with the blood supply to the limbs. The condition occurs almost exclusively in males who are tobacco smokers. The etiology is uncertain. Some investigators have considered it to be a specific infection, and others believe that allergy to tobacco plays an important role. It is often referred to as *Buerger's disease*.

Buerger's disease usually begins before 35 years of age and appears unrelated to the occurrence of arteriosclerosis. It may affect the arms as well as the legs, produces severe pain in the involved extremities, and is closely correlated in its progression with a continuation of smoking or in lack of progression with abstinence from smoking. Small and medium-sized vessels of the upper and lower extremities are segmentally involved. Evidence of atherosclerosis is usually lacking. Migratory thrombophlebitis is associated in some cases.

An acute lesion has been described as a fresh or incompletely organized thrombus containing multiple tiny abscesses (microabscesses). These are foci of neutrophilic leukocytes, usually surrounded by mononuclear epithelioid cells and sometimes multinucleated giant cells. Later, the neutrophilic leukocytic foci disappear, although the epithelioid cell nodules may remain.

In this early stage, an inflammatory infiltrate may involve all coats of a segment of a deep artery and adjacent vein. There is rarely any necrosis in the vessel wall. The inner elastic lamina is intact. The process advances to a proliferative stage with organization (Fig. 13-6) and healing by fibrosis. Usually, arteries, veins, and nerves become bound together in a dense fibrous scar. Some recanalization of the lumen often develops. Venous valves are damaged and disrupted by the inflammation and organization of thrombi. The early acute phase may give little clinical evidence of its presence. After thrombosis and organization, insufficient blood supply to the extremity may result in pain on exercise (intermittent claudication) or even gangrene of the ischemic tissues. The degree of circulatory disturbance is

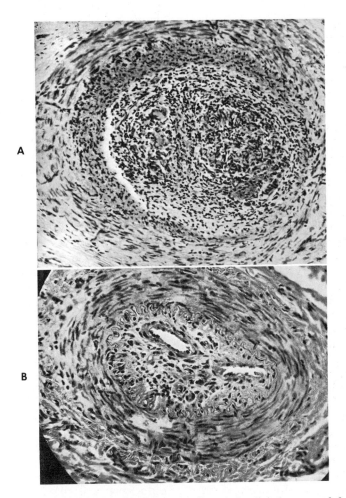

Fig. 13-6. Thromboangiitis obliterans (Buerger's disease) in digital artery of finger. **A,** Early proliferative phase in organization of thrombus. Note presence of giant cells. **B,** Canalization of organized thrombus. Lymphocytes, fibroblasts, and endothelial cells are present in central mass. Note characteristic wavy internal elastic membrane. Gangrene and ulceration of thumb in 30-year-old white man. (From Gore, I.: Blood and lymphatic vessels. In Anderson, W. A. D., editor: Pathology, ed. 6, St. Louis, 1971, The C. V. Mosby Co.)

largely influenced by the amount of collateral circulation that can be established.

NEUROGENIC ARTERIAL DISEASE

Raynaud's disease. Raynaud's disease or syndrome is characterized by symmetric pallor of both hands (rarely the feet), accompanied by numbness, tingling, and burning sensations, caused by functional vasospasm of the arterioles. Cyanosis, redness, and even ischemic necrosis may ensue. The disease occurs chiefly in young women. The cause is unknown, but exposure to cold and emotional stimuli may initiate the attacks.

Raynaud's phenomenon. Raynaud's phenomenon, in which there are symptoms caused by vascular spasm similar to those in Raynaud's disease, is secondary to known diseases or conditions, e.g., Buerger's disease, arteriosclerosis obliterans, trauma (in typists, pianists, and pneumatic hammer operators), Sudeck's bone atrophy, cervical rib syndrome, progressive systemic sclerosis (generalized scleroderma), systemic lupus erythematosus, ergotism, and polyarteritis nodosa.

ANEURYSM

An aneurysm is a localized, abnormal, persistent dilatation of a vessel, usually an artery. The dilatation, resulting from a weakness of the vessel wall, may be saccular, fusiform, or cylindrical. In the typical aneurysm, all layers of the vessel wall are included. Certain lesions, called false aneurysm and arteriovenous aneurysm, are not true aneurysms in the sense of the foregoing definition. A dissecting aneurysm is not a typical aneurysm in that there is not a dilatation including all layers of the vascular wall, but there is some distention of the outer portion of the wall.

The *causes* of arterial aneurysms include atherosclerosis, syphilis, cystic medial necrosis, acute bacterial infections, congenital weakness of the wall, and trauma. The aorta is the most common site of aneurysms. Aneurysms also may arise in the heart wall, usually the left ventricle, as a result of a myocardial infarct.

Atherosclerotic aneurysm. Today, atherosclerotic aneurysm is the most common form of aortic aneurysm because of the lowered incidence of syphilis (which formerly was the commonest cause) and because of the increasing life span of man. It occurs most commonly in men, usually in the sixth or seventh decade or beyond. Aneurysms result when the atheromatous lesions are severe enough to produce destruction and weakening of the underlying media. They are usually of the fusiform type, less frequently saccular, and often contain laminated thrombi. The thrombus may not completely obstruct the lumen of a large vessel such as the aorta, although it may occlude the ostia of its branching vessels, but it may obstruct the lumen of a small artery (e.g., popliteal artery) affected by an aneurysm.

By far the commonest site of an atherosclerotic aneurysm is the abdominal aorta (Fig. 13-7), especially the infrarenal segment, although the thoracic aorta and other arteries (e.g., popliteal artery) may be sites. The serious complications include compression of adjacent structures and rupture with hemorrhage and, in some instances, thrombotic occlusion and thromboembolism.

Syphilitic aneurysm. Syphilitic aneurysm, a late manifestation of syphilis, usually involves the first portion or the arch of the aorta, although the abdominal aorta or other vessels occasionally are affected. The localized dilatation is caused by weakening of the media by destruction of the elastic tissue. Disruption and loss of elastic fibers are evident microscopically in the wall of the aneurysm (Fig. 13-8). The media of the vessel is partially replaced by connective tissue.

The saccular variety is most common. It increases progressively in size, causing atrophy and erosion of any structure on which it impinges, including bony tissue. Thrombosis in successive layers occurs in the aneurysmal sac. This serves to strengthen the wall to some extent, although there is little organization of the thrombus.

Symptoms usually result from the pressure and erosion of adjacent structures. The outcome is commonly perforation and death from hemorrhage. The aneurysms often coexist with other effects of syphilitic aortitis, i.e., aortic insufficiency and coronary ostial narrowing, and if they occur in the aortic arch they may cause inequality of blood pressure in the upper extremities.

Dissecting aneurysm. Dissecting aneurysm is produced by penetration of circulating blood into the wall of a vessel and its subsequent extension for varying distances along its length. It is simply a hemorrhage into the vessel wall itself, which, by its force, splits or "dissects" the wall, causing a widening of the vessel. The aorta is the vessel commonly involved.

The dissection is through the media of the vessel, at the junction of the outer one-third and inner two-thirds (Fig. 13-9) and extends for short or long distances proximally or distally. At the end of its dissection, it may rup-

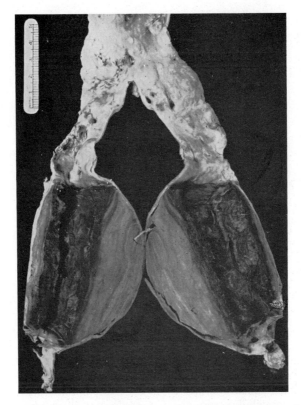

Fig. 13-7. Atherosclerotic aneurysm of abdominal aorta. Aorta and aneurysm have been bisected lengthwise to show laminated thrombus almost filling sac. Note channel kept open by force of bloodstream. (From Gore, I.: Blood and lymphatic vessels. In Anderson, W. A. D., editor: Pathology, ed. 5, St. Louis, 1966, The C. V. Mosby Co.)

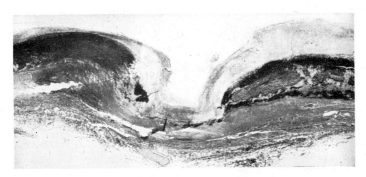

Fig. 13-8. Syphilitic aortitis with beginning aneurysm. Elastic tissue (stained black) of media is destroyed in a local area, with bulging at weakened point.

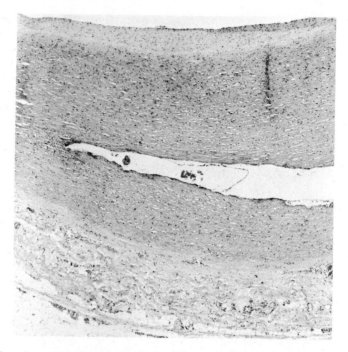

Fig. 13-9. Dissecting aneurysm of aorta. Hemorrhage dissects media at junction of its outer one third and inner two thirds.

ture externally by tearing through the outer portion of the wall. Less commonly, it perforates again into the lumen. Sudden death results from perforation externally into surrounding tissues or into the pericardial sac (producing cardiac tamponade) when the first portion of the aorta is involved. Rupture back into the lumen occasionally leads to recovery, either through lining of the channel by endothelium or, more rarely, by thrombosis, organization, and fibrous obliteration of the channel.

About 70% of dissecting aneurysms begin in the ascending aorta. The primary intimal tear at this point is usually transverse, irregular, and 1 or 2 cm in length. Dissection distal to the primary tear is longer than that proximal to the rupture, although some proximal dissection almost always occurs. In a few instances, a primary intimal tear is absent. Since a large proportion of primary tears are 1 or 2 cm above the aortic valve, the frequency of rupture into the pericardial sac is easily under-

stood. Dissection distally may progress to the aortic bifurcation and beyond. Extension of the dissection into the origins of the branching arteries may cause obstruction of these vessels. If the hemorrhage ruptures back into the original aortic lumen, it does so through a secondary intimal (reentry) tear. Dissection in the vicinity of the aortic valve ring may lead to aortic insufficiency.

The underlying cause of dissecting aneurysm in most instances is some degenerative change or defect of the media, although occasionally such alteration is not readily demonstrable. The degenerative lesion resembles that observed in *Erdheim's disease,* so-called *idiopathic cystic medionecrosis of the aorta.* Microscopically, there are areas in the media showing loss of muscle and elastic fibers and accumulation of a mucoid material filling the spaces created by this loss. The degenerative changes are not associated with inflammatory reaction. Syphilis is not an etiologic factor in dissecting aneurysm, but hypertension is present in a very high proportion of cases. Aortic dissection occurs most commonly in the fifth and sixth decades. One fourth of the cases occur before the age of 40 years and sometimes with pregnancy. There is also an association with Marfan's syndrome and with coarctation of the aorta.

The exciting cause is usually a sudden increase of blood pressure because of mental or physical stress. Trauma is rarely a factor, although dissecting aneurysm is an occasional complication of carotid arteriography. The primary tear of the intima may start at an atheromatous ulcer, but this is unusual. Most investigators believe that rupture of the vasa vasorum in the weakened media is the initial event causing intramural hemorrhage and that the primary intimal tear is secondary to this.

Mycotic aneurysm. Aneurysms may occur in small arteries in which localized inflammation has produced sufficient weakening of the vessel wall. Such a process produces nodules in polyarteritis nodosa. When the vascular inflammation is caused by infection, the resultant aneurysm is called "mycotic." The term "mycotic" is a misnomer, since literally it refers to fungal infection and the aneurysm referred to here is caused by various microorganisms, particularly bacteria.

In mycotic aneurysm, the inflammation usually is caused by lodgment of an infected embolus or by infection of the wall by way of vasa vasorum. Occasionally, extension of infection from inflamed aortic valves affects the sinuses of Valsalva or adjacent portions of the aorta, producing a mycotic aneurysm in that area that is often referred to as an "erosive aneurysm."

Congenital aneurysm. Congenital aneurysms occur particularly in superficial cerebral vessels, sometimes in miliary fashion. They are caused by a muscle defect in the media at points of bifurcation, with a small saccular ("berry") aneurysm developing in the angle. In addition to the muscle defect, degeneration of the internal elastic membrane as a result of continued overstretching from blood pressure is necessary before aneurysm develops. The muscle defect, and not the aneurysm itself, is

congenital. Rupture of such an aneurysm is an important cause of subarachnoid hemorrhage. Congenital aneurysms occasionally occur in the aorta (e.g., in the sinus of Valsalva).

Traumatic aneurysm. Weakening of the arterial wall caused by a penetrating or blunt injury may result in an aneurysm, usually saccular. The most common site is the thoracic aorta, frequently related to the compression chest injuries sustained in automobile accidents.

False aneurysm. False aneurysm is a paravascular encapsulated hematoma that communicates with the lumen of a blood vessel, i.e., the wall of the saclike structure is not composed of elements of the blood vessel wall. It occasionally follows a traumatic rupture of a small vessel, as by a knife or bullet.

Arteriovenous aneurysm. Arteriovenous aneurysm is really a fistula, or an abnormal communication, between an artery and a vein. Its usual cause is traumatic penetration of an adjacent artery and vein. It may arise from rupture of an arterial aneurysm (e.g., aorta) into an adjacent vein (e.g., superior or inferior vena cava). Less commonly, it may be a developmental anomaly or occur in a vascular neoplasm (glomus tumor). If vessels of a considerable size are involved, the direct arteriovenous shunt produces disturbance in circulation that may lead to cardiac hypertrophy. The artery and vein proximal to the fistula may become dilated.

PHLEBITIS

Inflammation of veins is often an extension of a local infection to involve their walls. Thrombosis usually develops in the infected veins, and spread of the infection may thus occur by infected emboli as well as directly along the vein wall.

Phlebitis occasionally complicates acute systemic infectious diseases. Acute noninfectious phlebitis may occur in hypersensitivity angiitis and as a result of trauma or chemical injury. Chronic nonspecific and granulomatous forms of phlebitis exist. Idiopathic phlebitis also occurs. An obliterative endophlebitis of small hepatic veins (veno-occlusive disease of the liver), probably caused by the ingestion of *Senecio* alkaloids, has been reported in Jamaica and elsewhere.

VENOUS THROMBI

A thrombus may form in a vein as a result of phlebitis *(thrombophlebitis)* or may be caused by factors other than inflammation *(phlebothrombosis)*. Obstruction of a major vein may cause chronic venous insufficiency. In a lower limb, this may result in edema, induration, sometimes ossification, eczematous dermatitis, pigmentation, and ulceration. A rare complication, and one that occurs only when there is massive venous obstruction, is gangrene. Frequent, recurrent formation of thrombi in the same segment of a vein or, more often, in widely scattered areas of the body or the extremities is known as "thrombophlebitis migrans" (as occurs in thromboangiitis obliterans) or "phlebothrombosis migrans" (such as that related to visceral cancer).

The association of visceral carcinoma with thrombosis in one or more major veins or with phlebothrombosis migrans is referred to as *Trousseau's syndrome*. The release of thromboplastin or proteolytic enzymes from the cancer site is regarded as the cause of thrombosis in this syndrome.

VARICOSE VEINS

Abnormally tortuous and dilated veins *(varicose veins* or *varicosities)* are produced by increased intravenous pressure and weakness of the vein walls. The condition is seen most frequently in the veins of the lower extremities, the hemorrhoidal veins, and the veins at the lower end of the esophagus.

Varicosities of the lower extremities, involving principally the superficial veins, are either *primary,* developing as a result of inherent weakness of the vein walls and a relative increase in intravenous pressure, or *secondary* to venous obstruction (e.g., thrombosis or extrinsic pressure by tumors). Heredity may play a role in the incidence of varicose veins. Defects of venous valves are not usually the primary cause, except in rare cases of congenitally absent valves. Distortion

of valves in thrombophlebitis may be contributory. Loss of supporting perivenous tissues (as in emaciation or advanced age) may contribute to varicosities. Thrombosis and chronic venous insufficiency are possible complications of varicose veins in the lower limbs.

Hemorrhoids are varicosities of hemorrhoidal veins. Varices at the lower end of the esophagus are common where there is obstruction in the portal circulation, as in cirrhosis of the liver. Rupture of one of these distended vessels with hemorrhage is a common terminal event in cirrhosis of the liver.

SUPERIOR VENA CAVA OBSTRUCTION

Obstruction of the superior vena cava interfering with the return flow of blood to the heart results in elevated venous pressure in the upper extremities and thorax, delayed circulation time in the upper half of the body, cyanosis and edema of the face, neck, and upper extremities, and distention of collateral venous channels (azygos, internal mammary, lateral thoracic, and vertebral collateral routes) in the upper portion of the body. The obstruction is caused most frequently by intrathoracic neoplasms, lymphomas, and aortic aneurysms. Bronchogenic carcinoma is a relatively frequent basis of the obstruction caused by invasion of the venous wall by the tumor.

LYMPHANGITIS

Inflammation of the lymphatics may appear in infections, and spread may occur from a local area along the lymphatics to the lymph nodes. When such inflammation is superficial (e.g., on the arm), the lymphatic involvement may be seen as reddish, painful streaks, and the lymph nodes of the axilla become enlarged and tender (lymphadenitis, p. 480).

LYMPHATIC OBSTRUCTION

Obstruction of lymphatic flow from an area results in retention of fluid in the part, which becomes enlarged and hard. Marked degrees of the enlargement are called elephantiasis and are most common when the lymphatic obstruction is caused by filariasis with its inflammatory involvement of lymphatics. Idiopathic lymphedema (noninflammatory) occasionally occurs. It may be congenital (p. 98) or may develop later in life.

Operative procedures may interfere with normal lymph drainage, and in the case of radical amputation of the breast, an enlargement and brawny edema of the arm may result. Lymphangiosarcoma may complicate a severe prolonged lymphedema of either idiopathic or postoperative origin.

TUMORS

Angiomas. Angiomas are growths made up of blood or lymph vessels (hemangiomas and lymphangiomas). They are often congenital and probably arise from embryonic rests of mesodermal tissue. Some may be simply vascular malformations, but others are true neoplasms. Angiomas are common in childhood. *Lindau–von Hippel* disease is a hereditary de-

velopmental defect in which hemangiomas occur in the brain, retina, and elsewhere. Also frequently found in this condition are cystic lesions of the kidneys and pancreas and hypernephroma of a kidney.

Hemangioma. There are several types of hemangiomas. *Capillary hemangioma* is composed of well-differentiated, thin-walled capillaries (Fig. 13-10). It may appear as a dark red, elevated mass ("strawberry nevus") of the skin in infants, which tends to disappear spontaneously in later childhood, or it may show up as the typical "port wine stain," especially of the face and neck.

Cavernous hemangioma, in which the vascular spaces are dilated, engorged blood sinuses (Fig. 13-11), also occurs in the skin and is the common type in internal organs such as the liver.

Hemangioendothelioma is a form of capillary hemangioma in the young that consists of solid masses of proliferating endothelial cells,

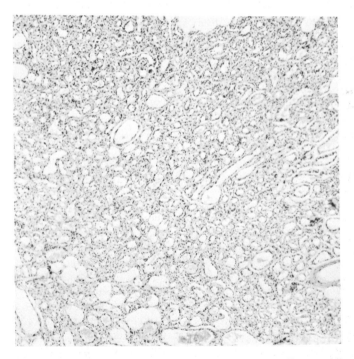

Fig. 13-10. Capillary hemangioma of skin. Most of vessels are small, resembling capillaries. Compare with Fig. 13-11. (×62.)

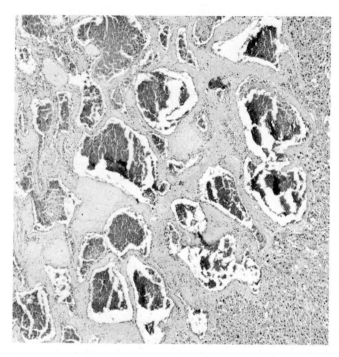

Fig. 13-11. Cavernous hemangioma of liver. Large, dilated vascular spaces filled with blood, separated by thick fibrous walls. (×48.)

with only a few patent vessels. This type is seemingly locally invasive in its growth and may be misdiagnosed as a malignant tumor.

Sclerosing hemangioma is a blood vessel tumor in which there is overgrowth of the collagenous connective tissue framework of the tumor (Fig. 13-12). This results in occlusion of the vessels and breakdown of trapped red cells. Phagocytes containing hemosiderin pigment may be sufficiently numerous to give the tissue a brownish color. Other macrophages contain lipid material. A few giant cells usually are present.

Kaposi's idiopathic hemorrhagic sarcoma is considered on p. 692.

Lymphangioma. The three main types of lymphangioma are the simple or *capillary,* the *cavernous,* and the *cystic (hygroma).*

The *capillary* and *cavernous* types are similar to the corresponding hemangiomatous tumors but differ in the absence of red cells in their channels and in the frequent presence of lymph follicles and lymphocytes.

The *cystic* type of lymphangioma or hygroma occurs in the neck or axilla and is designated respectively as *hygroma colli cysticum* (Fig. 13-13) and *hygroma axillare.* Originating from lymphatic nests, which retain embryonic power of irregular growth, they grow to be large, multilocular cystic tumors. Their cavities are lined by endothelium and contain straw-colored fluid (Fig. 13-14). Lymphoid tissue is often abundant in the cyst walls.

Glomus tumor (angiomyoneuroma). The glomus is an arteriovenous anastomosis found normally in the skin and concerned with temperature regulation. The glomus tumor, or angiomyoneuroma, arising from this structure occurs in the extremities and is characterized clinically by intense pain and tenderness. Va-

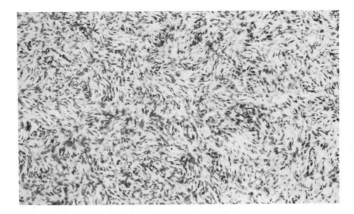

Fig. 13-12. Sclerosing hemangioma (xanthofibroma) of skin. Elongated cells form characteristic irregular curled pattern with many small vascular channels.

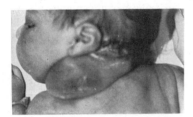

Fig. 13-13. Cystic hygroma of neck.

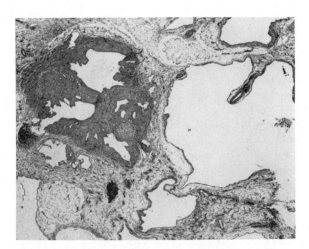

Fig. 13-14. Cystic hygroma. Irregular channels and cystic spaces containing lymph have connective tissue stroma, which is mainly loose, but with denser areas and occasional accumulation of lymphocytes.

somotor phenomena and atrophic changes in the involved extremity are sometimes associated.

The tumors are composed of a tangled mass of blood vessels enclosed within a capsule (Fig. 13-15). In the vessel walls are masses of cuboid or rounded epithelioid glomus cells, probably derived from pericytes, and smooth muscle cells. Bundles of myelinated nerves are recognizable in or near the capsule of the tumor, from which slender, nonmyelinated fibers pass among the glomus cells and become continuous with their cytoplasm.

Hemangiopericytoma. Hemangiopericytoma is a vascular tumor composed of endothelial tubes surrounded by rounded or elongated cells believed to be derived from pericytes, as are the epithelioid cells of the glomus tumor. Pericytes, described by Zimmerman, are contractile cells wrapped about capillaries that function in changing luminal size. Most examples have been benign, but local invasion and even metastases have been reported.

Angiosarcoma. In contrast to the benign angiomatous tumors, angiosarcomas are rare. Sometimes referred to as malignant hemangioendotheliomas, angiosarcomas occur mainly in adults, but they also appear in childhood.

Recently, an unusual number of these tumors have been observed in the liver of workers exposed to vinyl chloride (p. 457). Lymphangiosarcoma is practically unknown in children. In adults, lymphangiosarcoma may develop in an area of severe persistent lymphedema of an extremity. This may occur as a rare complication of radical mastectomy for cancer of the breast.

Heart

CARDIAC FAILURE

Cardiac failure is a clinical state in which the heart is unable to maintain an adequate circulation for bodily needs. It may be acute or chronic.

Acute heart failure may be the result of sudden failure of the myocardium because of infarction, rapid pericardial hemorrhage (cardiac tamponade), obstruction to outflow as in massive pulmonary embolism, or inadequate venous return to the heart (as in various forms of shock). In acute failure caused by myocardial injury or massive pulmonary embolism, there is a sudden reduction in cardiac output, the cardiac chambers dilate, and acute venous congestion ensues (acute congestive heart fail-

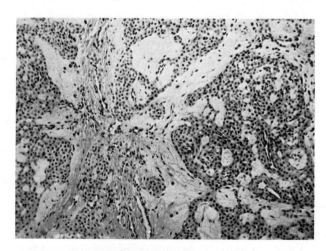

Fig. 13-15. Glomus tumor.

ure). In acute heart failure associated with various forms of shock, the fall in cardic output is evident, but acute venous congestion usually is not a manifestation, except in cardiac shock, such as that caused by myocardial injury (e.g., infarction), in which acute congestive failure may also be present.

Chronic (congestive) heart failure is the consequence of progressive diseases that weaken the heart directly or cause an increased demand on the heart, occurring most commonly in association with atherosclerotic coronary heart disease, hypertensive cardiopathy, and valvular deformities. The clinical picture is related to hemodynamic changes (viz., those concerned with blood flow and pressure relations throughout the cardiovascular system) and disturbances in the body fluids and electrolytes.

To explain the development of the manifestations of congestive heart failure, two mechanisms have been suggested in the past and are known as "backward failure" and "forward failure." According to the *backward failure* theory, there is an increase in diastolic pressure within the failing ventricle or ventricles followed by a rise in atrial pressure, which is transmitted backward, producing an elevated pressure in the veins. In *forward failure,* the manifestations result from failure of the heart to pump a sufficient output, causing a diminished flow of blood to the tissues, particularly to the kidneys. Actually, these two mechanisms do not function independently of each other, since in a continuous circulation one does not occur without the other. Whenever the cardiovascular system makes sufficient adjustments to maintain adequate output, a state of *compensation* is reached. The principal compensatory phenomena are tachycardia, cardiac dilatation, and cardiac hypertrophy. When the adjustments are inadequate, a state of cardiac *decompensation* is said to exist.

Heart failure may involve either side of the heart separately or the entire heart, but in the latter the features frequently are predominantly those of right-sided heart failure. In *left-sided heart failure,* the major manifestations are those associated with passive congestion and edema of the lungs. In more severe cases, pulmonary hypertension results, leading to failure of the right side of the heart. *Right-sided heart failure* is frequently combined with that of the left, although there are instances in which it is isolated. The manifestations of right-sided heart failure include subcutaneous edema (particularly in the dependent parts of the body), hydrothorax, ascites, passive congestion of the liver and spleen, generalized venous congestion, cyanosis, and usually increased blood volume. The cardiac output in typical congestive heart failure is usually reduced, although in some patients at rest it may be normal. Cardiac failure associated with diminished output is called "low output heart failure." Cardiac failure associated with hyperthyroidism, arteriovenous shunts (including arteriovenous fistulas and the vascular shunts in the bones in Paget's disease or osteitis deformans), and severe anemias may be accompanied by an elevated cardiac output—thus, it is given the designation "high output heart failure."

The pathogenesis of edema in cardiac failure is an intriguing problem that has held the interest of investigators for a long time but still is not completely solved. For many years, the edema has been explained as a consequence of increased venous pressure, leading to a rise in capillary blood pressure, increased filtration, and edema. Although increased venous pressure plays a part in the development of edema, the emphasis today is on the importance of retention of sodium and water in the body. The role of intrinsic renal mechanisms and hormonal or neural factors (e.g., reduction in glomerular filtration rate, enhanced renal tubular reabsorption of sodium, hypersecretion of aldosterone or a decrease in the rate of inactivation of aldosterone by the liver, and an increased release of antidiuretic hormone) has been discussed in Chapter 5.

CONGENITAL HEART DISEASE

Congenital malformations of the heart are usually (1) abnormalities of the great vessels or their valves, (2) failure of completion of the septa between atria or ventricles, or (3) anomalies of the size or position of the heart.

Frequently, two or more cardiac anomalies occur in association. In 10% to 15% of patients with congenital heart disease, anomalies exist in other parts of the body. Defects that cause a shunt of blood from the venous to the arterial side (i.e., from right to left) are commonly associated with cyanosis. The main factor in the cyanosis is the admixture of venous and arterial blood in the peripheral circulation. The oxygen deficiency gives rise to a compensatory increase of red cells in the blood both in number (polycythemia) and in average size. Clubbing of the ends of fingers and toes is also common in such cases. Other manifestations of congenital heart disease are dyspnea on exertion, poor feeding, lack of weight gain, and cardiac murmurs. Serious complications include congestive heart failure, bacterial endocarditis, paradoxical embolism, cerebral abscess (even in the absence of bacterial endocarditis), pulmonary tuberculosis, rupture of the aorta or cerebral arteries, cerebral embolism and infarction, and sudden death.

Congenital heart disease occurs in about five per 1,000 live births. Most cardiac anomalies have their inception during the fifth to eighth weeks of embryonic life. Intrinsic factors of faulty germ plasm or hereditary tendencies are important etiologically in some cases. Marfan's syndrome (arachnodactyly) frequently is associated with abnormalities of the great vessels or heart. In mongolism and Turner's syndrome, both related to chromosomal aberrations, cardiovascular anomalies often are seen. Extrinsic factors such as viral infections and the ingestion of certain drugs by the mother appear to be etiologically important in other cases. German measles (rubella) in the mother during the first 2 months of pregnancy is associated with a significant incidence of congenital cardiac effects. Thalidomide, taken during the early weeks of pregnancy, is associated with cardiac septal defects as well as with phocomelia, a deformity of the limbs.

Following is an anatomic classification of congenital heart disease*:

---

*Modified from Abbott, M. E.: Atlas of congenital cardiac disease, New York, 1936, American Heart Association.

Anomalies of heart as a whole
  Ectopia cordis
  Dextrocardia
  Congenital idiopathic hypertrophy
  Endocardial fibroelastosis
  Congenital rhabdomyoma
Defects of atrial and ventricular septa
  Patent foramen ovale
  Defects of atrial septum
  Persistent ostium atrioventriculare commune
  Localized defects of ventricular septum (maladie de Roger)
    Eisenmenger's complex
  Congenital aneurysms of ventricular septum
Truncus arteriosus or anomalous development of great vessels
Transposition of arterial trunks
Pulmonary stenosis and atresia
  Tetralogy of Fallot
Aortic and mitral atresia with rudimentary left ventricle
Tricuspid atresia with rudimentary right ventricle
Anomalies of chordae and endocardium
  Chiari's network
  Fenestration of semilunar valves
  Subaortic stenosis
  Bicuspid aortic valve
Patent ductus arteriosus
Coarctation of aorta
Anomalies of the coronary arteries

Some of the most common forms of clinical congenital heart disease, which frequently are amenable to surgical treatment, are discussed in the following paragraphs.

Pulmonary stenosis. Isolated pulmonary stenosis is usually valvular and associated with an intact ventricular septum. Less frequently, there is stenosis of the infundibulum of the right ventricle. The right ventricle becomes hypertrophied, and there often is poststenotic dilatation of the pulmonary trunk. If a patent foramen ovale or an atrial septal defect is present, a right-to-left shunt and cyanosis may develop. Sometimes, a defect of the ventricular septum or a patent ductus arteriosus may be associated with pulmonary stenosis. An uncommon cause of obstruction to the flow of blood from the right ventricle is stenosis of the main pulmonary artery or its branches.

Patent ductus arteriosus. Normally during fetal life, blood passes from the pulmonary artery through the ductus arteriosus to the aorta, thus bypassing the lungs. Obliteration of the channel occurs a few weeks after birth. When it remains open, it is often associated with other defects, such as pulmonary stenosis or patent septa. The abnormal left-to-right shunt at the ductus level causes increased work of the left ventricle and hypertrophy of that chamber, as well as enlargement of the pulmonary artery and its branches. If pulmonary hypertension develops, hypertrophy of the right ventricle, a reversed shunt (right to left), and cyanosis result.

Aortic stenosis and coarctation of aorta. Narrowing of the aortic opening (valvular, subvalvular, or supravalvular) is less common than pulmonary stenosis and causes left ventricular hypertrophy. Narrowing of the aorta beyond the valve (coarctation of the aorta) occurs in infantile and adult types.

In the infantile type of coarctation, there is a narrowing of the aorta between the origin of the left subclavian artery and the insertion of the ductus arteriosus. This narrowing is an exaggeration of the normal fetal condition. This form is associated with other cardiovascular anomalies and is fatal early in infancy.

In the adult type, there is a sharp constriction of the aorta just proximal to, at, or immediately distal to the insertion of the ductus arteriosus. This form is compatible with long life. Compensatory collateral circulation develops through internal mammary and intercostal vessels, and the left ventricle hypertrophies. In some cases, the ductus arteriosus may be patent.

Atrial septal defects. Frequently, it is found that the foramen ovale has remained open but with a competent although unfused valve. In such cases, no important transseptal leakage occurs. However, with a widely patent, inadequately guarded foramen ovale, a shunt of blood from left to right occurs, with enlargement of the right atrium, the right ventricle, and the pulmonary artery. The left ventricle remains relatively small.

Other types of atrial septal defects are a persistent ostium primum in the lower end of the septum, a defect high in the septum (sinus venosus type), or an absence of the entire atrial septum.

When a septal defect is complicated by pulmonary hypertension, the shunt may be reversed (right to left). An atrial septal defect combined with mitral stenosis (acquired or congenital) is known as *Lutembacher's syndrome*.

Ventricular septal defects. Patency of the ventricular septum, usually in its upper membranous portion, is a common anomaly. Small defects may cause little disturbance. Large defects cause hypertrophy of the left and right ventricles as a result of a left-to-right-shunt. The defect may be associated with cyanosis if pulmonary hypertension and reversal of the shunt occur as a result of increased pulmonary vascular resistance. In some instances, it is believed that the pulmonary vascular resistance is caused by an abnormal persistence of the fetal vascular pattern rather than by increased pulmonary blood flow.

Sometimes, the term "Eisenmenger's complex" is applied to hearts showing a high ventricular septal defect with an overriding aorta, hypertrophy of the right ventricle, and a normal or dilated pulmonary artery.

A basal ventricular septal defect combined with a persistent ostium primum (atrial septal defect) produces an undivided common orifice for the mitral and tricuspid orifice. The common orifice (persistent ostium atrioventriculare commune) has a valve consisting of four or five leaflets. (Fig. 13-16). This cardiac anomaly is seen frequently in patients with Down's syndrome (mongolism).

Tetralogy of Fallot. The tetralogy of Fallot is a common association of defects that includes (1) a patent ventricular septum, (2) pulmonary stenosis (infundibular or valvular), (3) relative displacement of the aorta to the right (dextroposition) so that it tends to lie above the patent part of the ventricular septum, and (4) hypertrophy of the right ventricle.

Depending on whether the pulmonary stenosis is severe or mild, the patient may be cyanotic or acyanotic. Pulmonary artery atresia may be present in some cases. In severe pulmonary stenosis or pulmonary artery atresia,

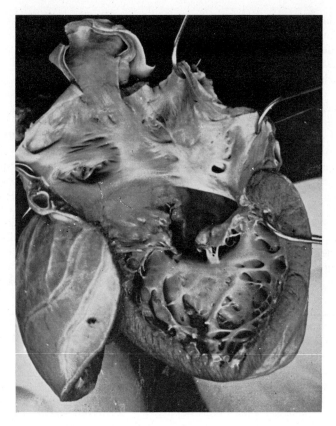

Fig. 13-16. Congenital defect of ventricular and atrial septa (ostium atrioventriculare commune). (Courtesy Dr. V. Moragues.)

collateral circulation to the lungs is through the bronchial arteries or other aortic branches. A patent ductus arteriosus may be present.

PERICARDIAL LESIONS

Abnormalities of the pericardium are frequently secondary to diseases elsewhere, but they may be primary.

Serous atrophy of pericardial fat. In any chronic disease with severe emaciation, the subepicardial fat may be reduced in amount, and it acquires a watery, translucent, gelatinous character.

Hydropericardium. The pericardial sac normally contains about 30 to 50 ml of fluid. The presence of more than 100 ml is called hydro-pericardium, and amounts as large as 1 to 2 liters may accumulate. The usual cause is cardiac failure. It also occurs in the nephrotic syndrome, in hypoproteinemic states, and as a result of mediastinal lesions obstructing pericardial venous circulation. Large amounts of fluid present some interference with the heart's action and reduce inflow by pressure on incoming veins.

Hemopericardium. Petechial hemorrhages of the pericardium are common in many toxic, infectious, and asphyxial conditions. Actual hemorrhage into the pericardial sac (hemopericardium) may result from cardiac rupture after infarction, rupture of a saccular or dissecting aneurysm of the aorta into the pericardium

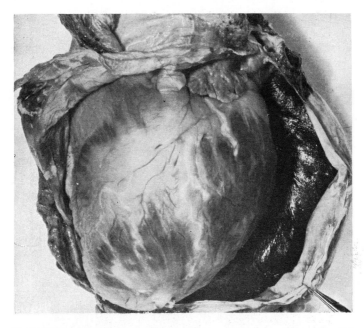

Fig. 13-17. Hemopericardium caused by rupture of aneurysm into pericardial sac.

(Fig. 13-17), or trauma of the heart and great vessels. The effect depends on the rate of hemorrhage as well as on the amount.

Acute hemorrhage with rapid accumulation in the sac of 150 or 250 ml may interfere with cardiac action and cause death from acute heart failure (cardiac tamponade). The hemorrhage causes a rapid rise of pressure outside the heart that, when it exceeds the venous pressure, prevents the heart's filling in diastole. At autopsy, the pericardial sac and the great veins are distended with blood, but the heart is contracted and empty. Slow leakage of a liter or more of blood into the sac may interfere less with the heart's action.

Acute pericarditis. Frequently encountered in clinical practice is acute nonspecific (or "benign") pericarditis, which is usually serofibrinous. In most cases, the cause is undetermined, but some may have a viral origin. There is usually an antecedent respiratory infection, and recovery from the pericarditis is the rule. The condition may recur, and rare fatalities have been reported.

Acute pericarditis also may be caused by rheumatic fever, pyemia, certain infectious diseases, and spread from adjacent inflammations of pleura, lung, mediastinum, and myocardium. Mild pericarditis is usual in association with myocardial infarctions and sometimes occurs in uremia. These various causes usually produce a fibrinous or serofibrinous exudate, except for pyogenic infections, which tend to produce fibrinopurulent or purulent pericarditis. When the exudate is predominantly fibrinous, movements of the heart form the fibrin into cords or villi, and the surface of the heart and parietal pericardium have a peculiarly shaggy appearance (Fig. 13-18). This is often referred to as "bread and butter" appearance.

Tuberculous pericarditis. Tuberculous pericarditis usually is caused by an extension from adjacent lung, pleura, or mediastinal lymph node infection. It is a chronic serofibrinous pericarditis characterized by very distinct thickening of visceral and parietal layers (Fig. 13-19). Tuberculous granulomatous lesions are

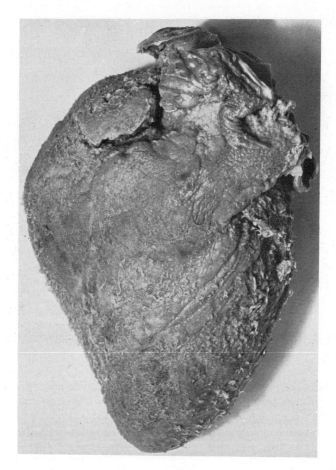

Fig. 13-18. Acute fibrinous pericarditis. Note shaggy coat of fibrin covering surface of heart.

seen in the thick pericardial walls at the base of the exudate. Organization of the exudate often results in firm pericardial adhesions, but localized pockets of fluid or liquefied caseous debris may be present.

Chronic pericarditis and pericardial scars. True chronic pericarditis does exist, but more commonly seen are the scars or adhesions of a previous acute pericarditis. The scars are usually whitish irregular areas of fibrosis on the anterior surfaces of the ventricles and often are called "soldier's spots" or "milk plaques." They represent areas of organized and scarred pericardial exudate.

Adhesions between visceral and parietal layers of pericardium may vary from just a few bands to complete obliteration of the sac (Fig. 13-20). *Adherent pericardium* (so-called chronic adhesive pericarditis) seldom, if ever, causes embarrassment or hypertrophy of the heart, except possibly in some instances where prominent adhesions extend to adjacent structures, e.g., mediastinum and thoracic cage ("chronic mediastinopericarditis").

Chronic constrictive pericarditis (Pick's disease) is a condition in which fibrous thickening of the pericardium mechanically interferes with the heart action and sometimes causes constriction of entering veins. The main effect is interference with diastolic filling of the ven-

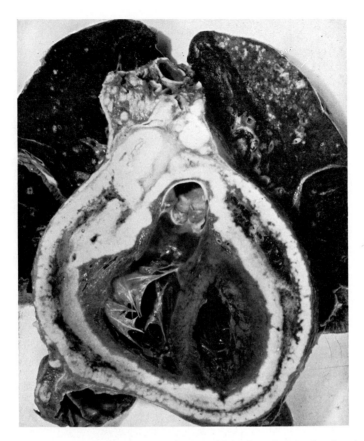

Fig. 13-19. Tuberculous pericarditis. Note tremendous thickening of visceral and parietal pericardium, massive caseation of mediastinal lymph nodes, and tuberculous areas in lung tissue.

tricles, and increased systemic venous pressure, chronic hepatic congestion, ascites, and hydrothorax develop. Similar progressive hyaline thickening and adhesions may involve the serosa over the spleen, liver, and undersurface of the diaphragm. The cause in most cases is unknown (idiopathic). Of the known causes, tuberculous pericarditis is probably the most frequent, although its incidence is diminishing. Other causes include purulent pericarditis, hemopericardium of various causes, and, rarely, acute nonspecific pericarditis, rheumatoid pericarditis, and other lesions.

Polyserositis of unknown cause *(Concato's disease)* is characterized by large effusions into the various serous cavities, including the pericardium. It may terminate in constrictive pericarditis.

RHEUMATIC FEVER

Rheumatic fever is a systemic, poststreptococcic, nonsuppurative inflammatory disease that seriously affects the heart and also involves arteries, joints, tendons, subcutaneous tissues, and the nervous system. It usually is acquired in childhood (especially between the ages of 4 and 15 years). It is the chief cause of heart disease in persons under 40 years of age. (See also p. 90.)

Etiology. The cause of rheumatic fever is still not completely solved. It generally is

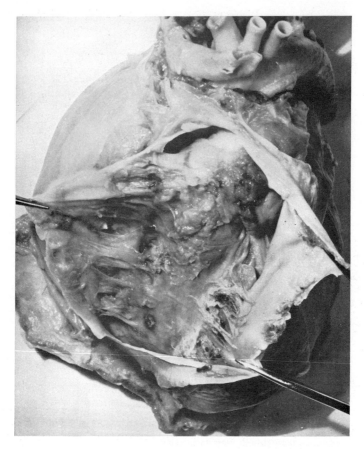

Fig. 13-20. Adhesive pericarditis. Pericardial sac has been opened, and fibrous bands joining visceral and parietal pericardium are evident.

agreed that it occurs after infection (frequently nasopharyngitis) with Group A β-hemolytic streptococci. The lesions of rheumatic fever are not the result of direct infection by these organisms but represent an allergic or hypersensitivity reaction. Experimental cardiac lesions similar to those of rheumatic fever have been produced by sensitization of animals to foreign proteins. The human disease occurs usually after a latent period of 2 or 3 weeks after the streptococcal infection, and elevated titers of antibodies to antigens of Group A β-hemolytic streptococci can be demonstrated. The prevalent view is that the organisms have the ability, in some way, to stimulate production of antibodies in the host that react with its own tissue (autoantibodies). Certain investiga-

tors have suggested that a virus or a virus acting in synergy with streptococci may be the cause of rheumatic fever. In addition to age, mentioned previously, there are other predisposing factors that may play a role in increasing the incidence of rheumatic fever, including poor socioeconomic conditions (overcrowding and poor nutrition) and possibly hereditary susceptibility.

Characteristic lesions. Characteristic lesions of rheumatic fever are innumerable minute foci of injury to interstitial and supporting tissues, i.e., collagen and its supporting ground substance throughout the body. The heart and blood vessels especially are susceptible. In the early phases, the inflammatory reaction is exudative (edema and increased acid

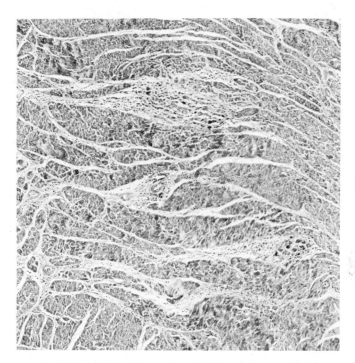

Fig. 13-21. Aschoff bodies of myocardium (low power). Note interstitial and perivascular position.

mucopolysaccharide), but there may follow a degenerative and proliferative type of reaction. In the most severe foci of injury, there is a degenerative change in connective tissue (swelling and fragmentation of collagen and fibrinoid degeneration) and proliferation of histiocytic cells, forming a "submiliary" granuloma. In their characteristic form, as may be seen in the myocardium, each of these minute nodules of proliferative inflammation is known as an Aschoff body. The eventual result is fibrosis.

Rheumatic heart disease. Death may occur during the acute phase of rheumatic fever, but most deaths occur years after the acute attack and are caused by valve deformities. The cardiac involvement is a *pancarditis*, i.e., pericardium, myocardium, and endocardium are injured.

Pericarditis is important mainly in acute phases. It is a fibrinous, sometimes serofibrinous, sterile form. Healing results in fibrous adhesions with partial or complete obliteration of the pericardial cavity.

The *myocarditis* is characterized by the presence of specific Aschoff bodies, widespread damage to the interstitial collagen framework of the myocardium, and the development of areas of fibrosis. Foci of nonspecific myocarditis and of necrosis of muscle fibers also may be seen in the active disease. The myocardial fibrosis partly results from the involvement of coronary vessels, as well as from fibrous change in Aschoff nodules, producing a weakened heart muscle.

The *endocarditis* very commonly leads to mitral and aortic valve deformities, but only occasionally does it deform the tricuspid or pulmonary valve. These serious valvular deformities, along with myocardial involvement, result in a failure of the circulation.

The Aschoff body, as it occurs in the myocardium, is an oval or elongated nodule of microscopic size, situated interstitially between muscle fibers and often adjacent to a small blood vessel (Fig. 13-21). Swelling, degeneration, and fragmentation of collagenous fibers and the presence of Aschoff cells are characteristic features (Fig. 13-22). The Aschoff cells are large, elongated, and irregular, often have multiple vesicular nuclei, and have granular basophilic cytoplasm. These proliferative cells usually are considered to be derived from cardiac (Anitschkow) histiocytes or primitive resting mesenchymal cells, although certain investigators have suggested that they may be derived from injured myocardial fibers. Lymphocytes, plasma cells, or even neutrophilic leukocytes also may be present in acute phases. Gradual replacement of the Aschoff cells by fibroblasts results in a tiny fibrous scar in which lymphocytes may persist for many months.

Aschoff bodies occurring in the heart elsewhere than in the myocardium are composed of the same elements but are less regularly arranged and are of a different shape and distribution, hence, they are less easily recognized.

Granulomatous foci in extracardiac lesions may be suggestive of, but should not be confused with, Aschoff bodies.

In *rheumatic endocarditis,* the mitral valve is involved most frequently, the mitral and aortic valves combined next most frequently, the aortic valve alone less frequently, and the tricuspid and pulmonary valves still less frequently. The earliest changes occur in the subendothelial layers, with degeneration of connective tissue and proliferative activity. The inflammation spreads throughout the whole valve substance, and histologically it shows edema, alteration of collagen, fibrinoid change, an exudate of macrophages, plasma cells, and lymphocytes, with occasional neutrophils, and the formation of young capillaries. Aschoff cells may be seen, but seldom are well-formed Aschoff bodies noted. The endothelium is destroyed. Vegetations form at the line of contact of the leaflets (i.e., areas of

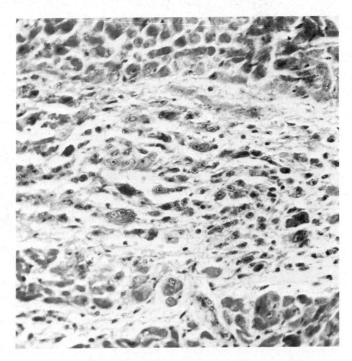

Fig. 13-22. Aschoff body of myocardium (high power). Multinucleated dark cells are Aschoff cells. Fraying of collagen fibers in background.

trauma), usually 1 to 5 mm from the free margin (Fig. 13-23). These vegetations are multiple, firm, small, smooth, warty masses that consist mainly of platelets and fibrin; bacteria are absent. Being firm and not crumbly, they do not give rise to emboli. Areas of hyalinization and necrosis develop within the inflamed tissue.

Healing of the inflammation often results in a thick, distorted, retracted, and insufficient valve, e.g., mitral or aortic insufficiency. Varying degrees of stenosis are a particularly common result in the mitral valve but also may involve the aortic valve. Calcification of the dystrophic type may be superimposed on the healed valves, sometimes quite prominently (e.g., calcific aortic stenosis). Bacterial endocarditis or nonbacterial thrombotic endocarditis may be superimposed on healed valvular lesions. These complications, as well as mural thrombi in the left atrium or its appendage (especially in mitral stenosis), may give rise to emboli. Frequently, the mural endocardium also is involved. The endocardium of the left atrium, just above the posterior leaflet of the mitral valve, often is thickened and irregular (MacCallum's patch). The microscopic picture is similar to that seen in the valves. Chordae tendineae also are involved and eventually become shortened and fibrous. Biopsy of the left atrial appendage at the time of surgical valvulotomy for mitral stenosis frequently shows Aschoff bodies, even in cases that clinically have not appeared to be active.

Extracardiac rheumatic lesions. "Growing pains," a frequent minor manifestation of rheumatic fever in children, result from synovitis of the hamstring tendons. Heel pain is caused by synovitis of the bursa of the Achilles tendon. Fibromyositis also occurs. Small subcutaneous nodules are often present and consist of a central necrotic area with fibrinoid change, surrounded by histiocytes and fibroblasts in a radial palisade arrangement.

In joint involvement (rheumatic polyarthritis), the synovial membranes are swollen and hyperemic. The increased fluid in the joint is cloudy but not purulent. Degenerative and necrotic changes and granulomatous formations are present in deeper structures. These are somewhat similar to Aschoff bodies. The ankles, knees, and wrists are most often affected.

Involvement of the nervous system, clinically called *Sydenham's chorea* (St. Vitus' dance), is a diffuse meningoencephalitis that is rarely fatal. Aschoff bodies are not found in the nervous system, but one sees congestion and thrombosis of small vessels, endothelial proliferation, and perivascular round cell infiltration.

Pleural involvement is very common in

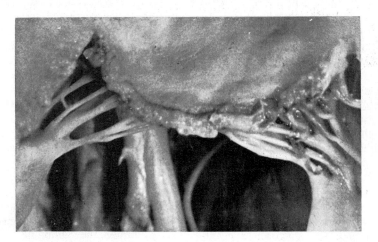

Fig. 13-23. Rheumatic vegetations on mitral valve. (Courtesy Dr. V. Moragues.)

rheumatic fever. Rheumatic pleurisy is usually associated with effusion of sterile serofibrinous fluid. Sometimes, the exudate is highly fibrinous and heals with fibrous pleural adhesions. The lung may have characteristic rheumatic involvement of small blood vessels, but a specific rheumatic pneumonia also has been described (p. 416).

Cardiac lesions in rheumatoid disease. Rheumatoid arthritis may be accompanied by cardiac lesions. Focal granulomatous nodules with fibrinoid necrosis may be found in the pericardium, valve leaflets, or myocardium. These nodules resemble those seen in the subcutaneous tissue in this disease and in rheumatic fever. In ankylosing (formerly "rheumatoid") spondylitis, one may see aortitis with aortic valvulitis, simulating syphilitic cardiovascular disease.

SYPHILITIC HEART DISEASE

Syphilitic heart disease is described on p. 186.

INFECTIVE ENDOCARDITIS

Infection of the valvular or mural endocardium may be caused by a variety of organisms, including bacteria and fungi and only rarely other organisms, such as rickettsiae. The usual form is *bacterial endocarditis,* which is caused by bacteria other than the tubercle bacilli or the spirochetes. *Fungal endocarditis* is much less common but is still important and sometimes produces a clinical and pathologic picture that resembles the bacterial form. *Tuberculous endocarditis* occurs rarely, and *syphilitic endocarditis (valvulitis)* has been referred to in an earlier chapter.

Bacterial endocarditis. Bacterial endocarditis is essentially a disease of the cardiac valves, although there may be extension to the adjacent mural endocardium. The disease may occur on normal valves, but commonly it involves previously damaged valves, particularly those affected by old rheumatic valvulitis or congenitally deformed valves, such as bicuspid aortic valves and aortic or pulmonary stenosis. In recent years, atherosclerotic valvular disease has been observed as a fairly common underlying lesion. Bacterial endocarditis also may occur at the site of ventricular septal defects but seldom involves atrial septal defects. Patency of the ductus arteriosus and coarctation of the aorta also predispose to bacterial infection, in which instances the lesion affects the endothelium ("bacterial endarteritis"). Infective endocarditis may occur at the site of implantation of heart valve prostheses.

Depending on the virulence of the causative organism, bacterial endocarditis may be characterized by an acute fulminant clinical course *(acute bacterial endocarditis)* or a protracted course *(subacute bacterial endocarditis).* Usually the former is caused by highly pathogenic organisms and the latter by organisms of low virulence. However, it is not always possible to determine what the severity of the disease will be on the basis of the etiologic agent. In some instances, organisms that are usually of low virulence may produce a clinically acute disease, whereas certain virulent pathogens may induce a more indolent form of the disease. Some patients with the subacute form of the disease may suddenly develop serious complications, such as valvular ulceration and rupture, resulting in a rapid downhill course, although it is not possible to predict which patients will do so.

Etiology. Streptococcus viridans, an organism of relatively low virulence, is the most common cause of bacterial endocarditis, although it has decreased somewhat in importance during the antibiotic era. *Staphylococcus aureus,* a highly virulent organism, is also a common offender and has increased in importance in recent years. Generally, the organisms of low virulence affect previously diseased valves, whereas the more pathogenic ones, such as the staphylococci, not infrequently involve normal heart valves. Pneumococci and gonococci, which were once prominently associated with endocarditis, have been observed infrequently as causative agents since the advent of antibiotics. Among the less common organisms that may cause endocarditis, some of which have increased in importance during the antibiotic era, are other strains of streptococci and staphylococci, gram-negative enteric bacilli (*Enterobacter* species, *Klebsiella* species, and *Pseudomonas* species), *Listeria,* and *Haemophilus influenzae.* Fungi also are being observed more frequently as causes of endocarditis (p. 313). Some of the less usual organisms are found particularly in patients who are severely debilitated as a result of other diseases, in those who are receiving immunosuppressive therapy, and in drug addicts who administer the narcotic intravenously to themselves.

In some instances, the offending organisms reach the heart from a significant infection elsewhere, e.g., lung, skin, or kidneys, the endocarditis being a complication of another serious disease. However, often there is no other serious infection, and a transient bacteremia is apparently an important etiologic factor. This may occur under various circumstances, e.g., in association with infected teeth, mild upper respiratory tract infections, dental manipulations, operative genitourinary procedures (such as catheterization), normal deliveries, abortions, and even cardiac catheterizations. Also, the organisms may be introduced intravenously by drug addicts through self-injections, and sometimes they may be introduced into the heart inadvertently during cardiac surgery (e.g., implantation of valve prostheses). Organisms arising from serious infections elsewhere or associated with self-injection of narcotics are usually highly pathogenic and tend to produce clinically acute disease; those related to a transient bacteremia without severe infection in other sites tend to cause subacute illness; and valvular infections following cardiac surgery may be either acute or subacute.

Cardiac lesions. As noted previously, bacterial endocarditis is a disease that mainly affects the heart valves, although the lesions that occur elsewhere are similar to those on the valves. The valvular lesions are seen most frequently in the left side of the heart, usually with involvement of either the mitral or aortic valve but often with involvement of both mitral and aortic valves. The pulmonary and tricuspid valves are much less frequently affected. The characteristic feature is the presence of vegetations, which occur on the atrial surfaces of the atrioventricular valves and on the ventricular surfaces of the semilunar valves. The vegetations consist of masses of fibrin, platelets, and bacteria.

Grossly, the vegetations vary in size and shape, but they are usually larger than the vegetations of rheumatic endocarditis. Sometimes, they are quite large and polypoid or globose (Fig. 13-24). They tend to be friable, so that they give rise to emboli, in contrast to the rheumatic lesions, which do not. Extension of the vegetations to the adjacent endocardium and to the chordae tendineae may be seen. Destruction of a valve leaflet with perforation may occur (Fig. 13-25).

Microscopically, there is nonspecific inflammation of the underlying valve. In acute fulminant cases, neutrophils are prominent and there may be extensive necrosis with abscess formation. The abscess may extend to the valve rings. In prolonged cases, varying degrees of granulation tissue and fibroblastic proliferation with mononuclear inflammatory cells are seen (Fig. 13-26). In the myocardium there may be minute foci of nonspecific inflammation (so-called Bracht-Wächter bodies) and sometimes abscesses.

Healing of a vegetation occurs by the process of organization. This is accompanied by endothelialization of the surface of the vegetation and calcification. Viable bacteria may persist for a long time in the middle of a healing vegetation. The fibrosis and calcification that take place during the healing process may lead to distortion and deformity of valves, so that valvular insufficiency may occur or may accentuate that already present. Aneurysmal formation and perforation of healed valve leaflets also can occur.

Extracardiac lesions. In bacterial endocarditis, pathologic changes in organs other than the heart frequently result from the breaking away of small portions of the friable valvular vegetations. The effects of *embolism* give rise to varied symptoms. Embolism is evidenced in the kidney by hematuria and infarcts, in the spleen by pain caused by infarction, in the skin by petechiae, in the retina by hemor-

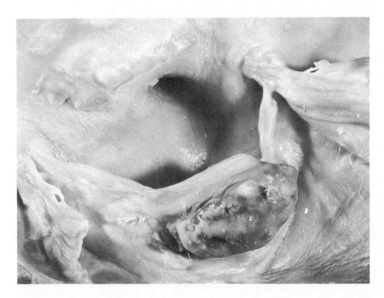

Fig. 13-24. Bacterial endocarditis with large vegetation on ventricular side of aortic cusp.

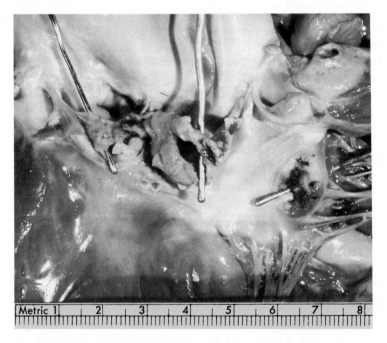

Fig. 13-25. Bacterial endocarditis of aortic valve with perforation of cusps.

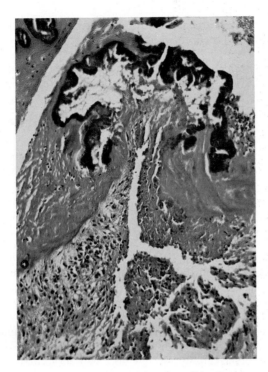

Fig. 13-26. Vegetation on mitral valve in bacterial endocarditis. Dark masses of bacteria at top are partially embedded in fibrin. Thickened valve leaflet (below) is diffusely infiltrated by large mononuclear cells and fibroblasts and is involved by necrosis. Few neutrophilic leukocytes are seen in fibrin. (From Scotti, T. M.: Heart. In Anderson, W. A. D., and Kissane, J. M., editors: Pathology, ed. 7, St. Louis, 1977, The C. V. Mosby Co.)

rhages and blindness, in the brain by hemiplegia or other evidence of cerebral infarction, and in blood vessels themselves by the formation of mycotic aneurysms. Abscesses may occur, particularly when the emboli contain highly virulent organisms.

One type of renal lesion associated with bacterial endocarditis *(focal necrotizing glomerulonephritis)* usually has definite peculiarities. The smooth surface of the slightly swollen kidneys is covered by punctate hemorrhages—thus, the expression "flea-bitten kidneys." Microscopically, the focal nature of the change is characteristic; only certain glomeruli are involved, and the rest are normal (p. 341). This lesion is thought to be an immunoallergic, rather than an embolic, phenomenon.

Small, raised, red tender areas on the hands and feet, particularly the fingertips *(Osler's nodes),* are characteristic lesions that result from toxic or allergic inflammation of small vessels. Painless, hemorrhagic, slightly raised areas *(Janeway lesions)* occurring usually in the palms may also be present.

While bacteremia is usually demonstrable throughout the disease and is a useful feature in diagnosis, bacteria-free periods may occur even though there are repeated emboli to various organs.

Fungal endocarditis. Endocarditis caused by fungi occurs much less frequently than bacterial endocarditis. In recent years, however, there has been an increased incidence of fungal endocarditis, due particularly to *Candida albicans* and *Aspergillus,* as a result of the widespread use of antibiotics and adrenal corticoids. Fungal endocarditis also is observed in narcotic addicts who use unsterile procedures in introducing the drug intravenously and in some patients subjected to cardiac surgery (e.g., valve replacement). Clinically, fungal endocarditis may simulate bacterial endocarditis.

NONINFECTIVE ENDOCARDITIS

Rheumatic endocarditis. Rheumatic endocarditis is discussed on p. 308.

Atypical verrucous endocarditis (Libman-Sacks disease). Warty mural and valvular vegetations, which represent neither the rheumatic nor bacterial types of endocarditis, have been described by Libman and Sacks. This disease is found in association with 40% to 60% of cases of systemic lupus erythematosus (p. 686). The vegetations often occur on both valve surfaces and also in the valve pockets. Embolic phenomena are not a characteristic feature. The essential change is a hyaline swelling of subendothelial collagen with fibrinoid degeneration, followed by an inflammatory reaction with macrophages, plasma cells, capillary proliferation, and later fibrosis. *Hematoxylin-staining bodies* that are remnants of the nuclei of mesenchymal cells may be present.

Nonbacterial thrombotic endocarditis. Another form of noninfective endocarditis is that formerly called "terminal," "cachectic," or "marantic" because it was believed to be a clinically insignificant lesion occurring as a terminal event in patients with wasting diseases. It is now known to occur in association with a variety of diseases, not necessarily marantic types, and the lesion is clinically important.

The nonbacterial vegetations form along the line of closure of valves, with a tendency to affect previously deformed valves (e.g., healed rheumatic valvulitis). Swollen collagen and fibrinoid change in the underlying valve are present, but inflammatory cells are not conspicuous—thus, the condition is often called "degenerative verrucal endocardiosis." These vegetations may give rise to embolism

and also may serve as a nidus for the development of bacterial endocarditis.

Lambl's excrescences, small filiform processes on the noduli Arantii of the aortic cusps, may represent healed vegetations of this nonbacterial type.

VALVULAR DEFORMITIES

Deformities of cardiac valves result from a healed or chronic valvulitis or, occasionally, are congenital malformations. The results of inflammation in the valves are seen as thickening, adhesions, retraction, and shortening of the leaflets. There may be a narrowing of the valve opening (stenosis), or closure of the valve may be insufficient so that leakage (regurgitation) occurs through it. Valvular insufficiency and stenosis may be produced by the same deformity. Valve deformities are common on the left side of the heart (aortic and mitral) but are uncommon on the right side (tricuspid and pulmonary).

Aortic stenosis. Aortic stenosis may occur as a pure lesion, but frequently it is associated with aortic insufficiency. Noncalcific valvular stenosis usually is caused by rheumatic fever. Congenital valvular or subaortic stenosis also occurs.

Bicuspid aortic valve is sometimes associated with aortic stenosis. Calcific aortic stenosis (Fig. 13-27) is attributed mainly to rheumatic fever. However, when it occurs in advanced age, particularly in the absence of lesions in other valves, it is regarded as atherosclerotic in origin (Mönckeberg's aortic sclerosis). Healed bacterial endocarditis, especially related to *Brucella* organisms, is a possible cause.

Left ventricular failure, hypertrophy, and dilatation result from aortic stenosis. Angina pectoris appears frequently because of a reduced coronary blood flow. Sudden death may occur.

Aortic insufficiency. Regurgitation through the aortic valve during diastole may result from dilatation of the aortic ring or from changes in the leaflets themselves. Dilatation of the ring may accompany dilatation of the rest of the heart, or it may result from disease such as syphilitic aortitis. Changes in the leaf-

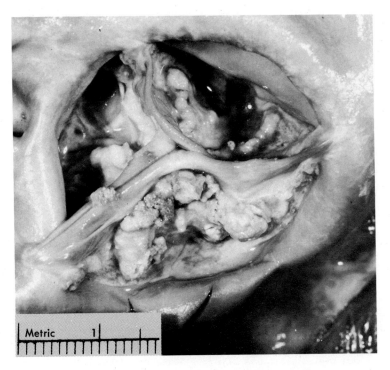

Fig. 13-27. Aortic valve showing calcific stenosis.

lets are commonly caused by syphilis or rheumatic fever. The leaflets may be simply affected or distorted at the commissures, but often the whole leaflet is thickened, with rounded edges and distinct shortening and retraction. Among other causes of aortic insufficiency are bacterial endocarditis with or without valvular rupture and dissecting aneurysm involving the ascending aorta.

Diastolic regurgitation through the aortic valve is accompanied by a significant fall in systemic diastolic pressure and hence a high pulse pressure. Severe hypertrophy and dilatation of the left ventricle result from the extra work. Fibrosis of the endocardium, with formation of endocardial "pockets" caused by the regurgitating blood, is a characteristic feature. Angina pectoris may result from coronary insufficiency (related to low diastolic pressure) and an increased demand of the hypertrophied heart for more oxygen.

Mitral stenosis. Mitral stenosis is one of the most common valve deformities and almost in-variably is caused by rheumatic inflammation. Thickening, adhesions, and retraction of valve leaflets and chordae tendineae may produce all degrees of stenosis (Fig. 13-28). The orifice may be narrowed to a tiny slit or "buttonhole." The rigidity and retraction usually cause some insufficiency of the valve as well. Calcification is frequently present. Occasionally, mitral stenosis is caused by other endocardial diseases such as bacterial endocarditis, particularly if the latter is healed.

Increased work of the left atrium will compensate for a mild mitral stenosis. A more severe uncompensated stenosis results in increased pressure and stasis in the pulmonary circulation and increases the work of the right ventricle. Thus, left atrial dilatation, chronic passive congestion of the lungs, and right ventricular hypertrophy constantly accompany any great degree of mitral stenosis. In pure stenosis, the left ventricle is normal or small in size.

Mitral insufficiency. Regurgitation through

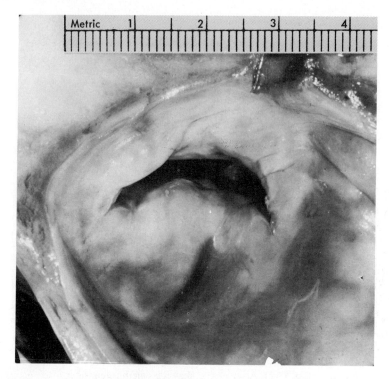

Fig. 13-28. Mitral stenosis with "fishmouth" orifice. (From Scotti, T. M.: Heart. In Anderson, W. A. D., and Kissane, J. M., editors: Pathology, ed. 7, St. Louis, 1977, The C. V. Mosby Co.)

the mitral valve is most often a relative insufficiency resulting from the dilatation of the mitral ring accompanying a dilatation of the left ventricle, but insufficiency also may be caused by shortening and retraction of the leaflets and chordae tendineae, which are usually caused by rheumatic valvulitis. Bacterial endocarditis may also cause mitral insufficiency by destruction of the leaflets or by chordal rupture. If regurgitation is severe, one finds left atrial dilatation along with hypertrophy of the left and right ventricles.

Tricuspid stenosis. Tricuspid stenosis is uncommon but usually results from rheumatic inflammation or congenital disease.

Tricuspid insufficiency. Tricuspid insufficiency usually is caused by dilatation of the right ventricle, with associated dilatation of the valve ring. Insufficiency may also result from valvular involvement, as in rheumatic

valvulitis or occasionally in the carcinoid syndrome (p. 565).

Pulmonary stenosis. Pulmonary stenosis most often is caused by congenital deformity of the valve rather than inflammatory scarring. It results in right ventricular hypertrophy. It also may occur as part of the carcinoid syndrome (p. 565).

Pulmonary insufficiency. Leakage through the pulmonary valve is very rare. It usually is caused by dilatation of the right side of the heart.

Myxomatous transformation of valves. There is a deformity of cardiac valves characterized by a myxomatous change in the valvular connective tissue, resulting in thickening, stretching, and redundancy of the cusps or leaflets. Inflammation and calcification are not part of the process. The lesion involves the aortic and mitral valves most frequently and is

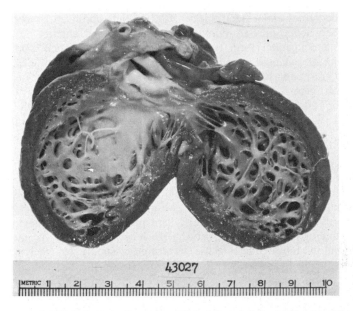

Fig. 13-29. Endocardial fibroelastosis (7-month-old black female infant). Heart weight, 77 g. Left ventricle hypertrophy and dilatation. (From Scotti, T. M.: Heart. In Anderson, W. A. D., and Kissane, J. M., editors: Pathology, ed. 7, St. Louis, 1977, The C. V. Mosby Co.)

referred to as *myxomatous transformation* or *mucoid degeneration of heart valves* or as *blue valve* or *floppy valve syndrome*. The cause is not known, but in some instances the lesion is regarded as an incomplete expression *(forme fruste)* of Marfan's syndrome and may be seen in some patients with congenital or rheumatic heart disease. Frequently, no other cardiac disease is present, and the deformity is not associated with symptoms, although a midsystolic click and/or late systolic murmur may be detected on physical examination. However, sometimes there may be serious effects, such as valvular insufficiency, rupture of valve or chordae tendineae, predisposition to infective endocarditis, or, rarely, sudden death.

ENDOCARDIAL FIBROELASTOSIS

Endocardial fibroelastosis is an endocardial thickening resulting from the proliferation of collagenous and elastic tissue elements. It is commonly generalized but is most prominent in the left ventricle and sometimes involves the valves. Most cases are seen in infancy, with evidence of cardiac dysfunction or fail-

ure, but in some cases the cardiac disability is not present until childhood or adult life. Mural thrombosis with thromboembolism is more characteristic of the adult form of the disease.

The heart usually is greatly enlarged, chiefly because of hypertrophy and dilatation of the left ventricle (Fig. 13-29). In addition to the thickened endocardium, there may be a patchy myocardial fibrosis, which, in some cases, has been attributed to a thickening and narrowing of thebesian vessels.

The disturbance of function and production of symptoms may be related to interference with normal contraction by the thickened endocardium, interference with the vascular supply of the underlying myocardium, producing anoxia, or impairment of conduction.

The etiology is obscure. Infantile endocardial fibroelastosis is congenital in origin and probably is a developmental abnormality. Other theories incriminate intrauterine endocardial anoxia, congenital metabolic disturbance, lymph stasis, organizing endocardial fibrin deposits, and mechanical stress. The cases in which symptoms first appear in adulthood usually have a lesser degree of endocardial thickening. It is not clear whether they are etiologically related to the congenital form of the disease. Histochemical changes similar to those of collagen diseases have been described. Some investigators consider impairment of cardiac lymph flow to be important in the pathogenesis.

ENDOMYOCARDIAL FIBROSIS

In some areas, particularly in Africa, endomyocardial fibrosis (an idiopathic disease) is a relatively frequent form of cardiac disturbance, with circulatory failure and death. It consists of a massive, destructive, scarring process involving one or both ventricles, usually in the apices and the inflow tracts. Dense, white, fibrous tissue replaces the endocardium and adjacent myocardium.

In contrast to endocardial fibroelastosis, there is little or no increase of elastic tissue. The papillary muscles and chordae tendineae are affected and fused, and the posterior leaflet of the atrioventricular valve often is sealed to the mural endocardium. Mural thrombi may be evident. The atria may be involved. Cardiac hypertrophy may or may not be present.

Theories concerning the etiology of endomyocardial fibrosis include viruses, malnutrition, and autoimmunity as possible causative factors.

CORONARY HEART DISEASE

Coronary circulation. Right and left coronary arteries supply the heart, taking their origin from a protected position in the aortic sinuses of Valsalva. Tiny accessory openings occasionally occur adjacent to the main openings.

The right coronary artery curves to the right in the atrioventricular groove as the right circumflex artery and then descends in the posterior interventricular sulcus as the posterior descending branch. The right coronary artery supplies the posterior half of the interventricular septum, a portion of the posterior part of the wall of the left ventricle, the posterior wall and almost all of the anterior portion of the right ventricle, and the right atrium.

The left coronary artery early divides into circumflex and anterior descending branches. The circumflex branch supplies the left atrium and the left margin of the left ventricle, including part of its posterior wall. The anterior descending branch of the left coronary artery runs toward the apex in the anterior interventricular sulcus and supplies the anterior wall of the left ventricle, the immediately adjacent part of the anterior wall of the right ventricle, and the anterior half of the interventricular septum.

In normal hearts, anastomotic communications between coronary vessels are small and are probably of little functional significance. However, when there is interference with the coronary supply by atherosclerotic narrowing or occlusion, the anastomotic channels enlarge where needed and become functional. Such anastomotic development may provide some compensation for arteriosclerotic changes. The size (circumference) of the main coronary arteries in proportion to the weight of the heart provides a rough index of the functional capacity of the myocardium.

The thebesian vessels are minute channels that open directly into the cardiac chambers. Under certain circumstances, flow in these channels may be reversed, and they may assist in nutrition of the myocardium. Their assistance possibly contributes to the comparative rarity of infarction of the muscle of the atria or the right ventricle, which are relatively thin walled.

Coronary atherosclerosis. Arteriosclerosis involving coronary vessels is of the atherosclerotic intimal type (p. 280). Intimal fibrous thickening (Fig. 13-30), lipoid deposits, and often calcium deposition, all of which narrow the lumen of the vessel, are the main features. The larger vessels on or near the surface of the heart are particularly involved. Small arteries within the myocardium rarely show significant sclerosis. The left coronary artery, particularly the anterior descending branch, is usually more severely affected than the right coronary artery.

The intima of normal coronary arteries is without demonstrable vasa vasorum, but in

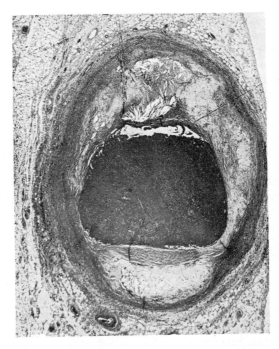

Fig. 13-30. Coronary atherosclerosis and thrombosis. Intima is irregularly thickened and media thinned because of advanced atheromatosis. (From Scotti, T. M.: Heart. In Anderson, W. A. D., and Kissane, J. M., editors: Pathology, ed. 7, St. Louis, 1977, The C. V. Mosby Co.)

and around atherosclerotic lesions may be found capillaries that take their origin from the intimal endothelium of the artery or from the medial vasa vasorum. The importance of hemorrhage from these delicate channels in the initiation of coronary thrombosis has been emphasized.

The *pathogenesis, etiology,* and *morphologic aspects* of atherosclerotic lesions were reviewed previously in the general discussion of atherosclerosis on pp. 280-283.

Complications of coronary atherosclerosis are (1) narrowing of the arterial lumen by progression of the plaque, (2) thrombosis, (3) intimal hemorrhage, (4) rupture of an atheromatous plaque, and (5) rarely, aneurysmal formation.

Coronary arterial occlusion is most often caused by an atherosclerotic plaque itself or by one of its complications, particularly thrombosis. In a few cases, intimal hemorrhage

(into a plaque) causes complete occlusion of the lumen and also may predispose to thrombus formation, as already mentioned. Rupture of the plaque may cause occlusion at the site, form an atheromatous embolus, or initiate thrombosis. Another important cause of occlusion is narrowing of the coronary ostia by lesions of syphilitic aortitis. Less commonly, coronary occlusion is produced by other lesions, such as embolism, polyarteritis nodosa, other forms of arteritis, and dissecting aneurysm.

Diseases of the coronary arteries in themselves are not necessarily accompanied by clinical or morphologic evidence of heart disease. However, when a sufficient degree of myocardial ischemia is produced to disturb the metabolism and performance of the heart, manifestations occur. The result is *ischemic* or *coronary heart disease.* Coronary heart disease, especially the atherosclerotic type, is the chief form of fatal cardiac disease in the United States. The effects of coronary artery disease include angina pectoris, myocardial fibrosis, myocardial infarction, congestive heart failure, cardiac hypertrophy and dilatation, and sudden death. A significant factor that may modify these effects, or may even prevent the development of myocardial ischemia, is an adequate collateral circulation through anastomotic channels.

Various environmental, biochemical, physiologic, and pathologic factors are associated with a considerable increase in susceptibility to coronary heart disease and are known as "risk factors." The usually accepted risk factors for coronary heart disease are hypertension, obesity, diabetes mellitus, cigarette smoking, family history of coronary heart disease, and elevated levels of cholesterol, β-lipoproteins, and triglycerides. Age, sex, and race are also important factors. In general, the risk of the disease increases with age, and white men are more susceptible to it than white women. Coronary atherosclerosis tends to occur less frequently in American blacks than in whites, except perhaps in black women as compared with white women. However, sex difference is not as significant among blacks as it is among whites. Of course, the incidence of coronary artery disease is increased in women in the presence of other risk factors (e.g., hypertension, diabetes mellitus, hypercholesterolemia). It has also been shown that women using oral contraceptives are at a greater risk of developing myocardial infarction than nonusers and that oral contraceptives seem to act synergistically with other risk factors, such as cigarette smoking, hypertension, and hypercholesterolemia. Emotional stress and physical inactivity also appear to be associated with an increased incidence of coronary heart disease.

Angina pectoris is characterized by paroxysmal pain in the chest provoked by an increase in the demands of the heart (e.g., by exertion, emotions) and is relieved by a decrease in the work of the heart. A transient myocardial ischemia (acute coronary insufficiency) is the cause, brought on by a dispro-

portion between the oxygen requirements of the myocardium and the coronary arterial blood flow. The underlying coronary disease is usually coronary atherosclerosis with narrowing or occlusion of one or more branches of the coronary arteries. Other diseases causing angina pectoris, by reducing coronary blood flow or increasing the oxygen needs of the heart, are syphilitic coronary ostial narrowing, aortic stenosis or insufficiency, cardiac hypertrophy, and severe anemias.

Sudden death may be the termination of coronary artery disease in patients who have experienced anginal attacks, or it may occur in persons who appear healthy and have had no previous symptoms of cardiovascular disease. Commonly, these patients have severe coronary atherosclerosis, with or without old organized thrombi, or recent coronary thrombosis may be the cause. The mechanism of sudden death is thought to be cardiac arrest or ventricular fibrillation.

Fibrosis of the myocardium, focal or diffuse, characteristically occurs in patients with a chronic, progressive type of myocardial ischemia, as in severe coronary atherosclerosis and stenosis of the coronary ostia. The myocardial lesion usually is found in patients who have had a history of attacks of angina pectoris or who died suddenly as a result of coronary insufficiency without myocardial infarction. The lesions are considered to represent fibrous replacement of atrophic muscle fibers, but some writers attribute them to healing of minute infarcts. If sufficient myocardial damage occurs, cardiac insufficiency, hypertrophy, and dilatation may ensue.

Myocardial infarction. A consequence of sudden myocardial ischemia is myocardial infarction, although this does not always happen. Muscle necrosis may be prevented if collateral circulation is adequate, or the patient may die too soon after the sudden onset of ischemia. In most patients with myocardial infarction, moderate to severe coronary atherosclerosis, with luminal narrowing or old organized atherosclerotic thrombi, is found and considered to play an important role in the pathogenesis of the infarct. In some cases, an acute thrombotic occlusion is superimposed. In those instances in which an acute occlusion is not detected, it is assumed that acute myocardial ischemia is the result of coronary insufficiency brought on by factors that increase the demand of the myocardium for oxygen. When a thrombus is present it is likely to be found at the site of greatest narrowing of the vessel, usually within 3 or 4 cm of the coronary ostia. The vessel most frequently occluded is the anterior descending branch of the left coronary artery, with the right coronary artery next most frequently affected and the left circumflex least often involved. Rarely are other lesions responsible for sudden coronary occlusion, e.g., embolism, hemorrhage in a plaque without thrombosis, dissecting aneurysm, and arteritis.

It has been noted that infarction of the myocardium can occur in the absence of sudden permanent coronary occlusion. Instances of myocardial infarction have been reported in which normal or nearly normal coronary arteries have been demonstrated. In such cases the possibility has been considered that a temporary coronary occlusion has occurred, e.g., arterial spasm or thrombosis followed by canalization and reestablishment of the lumen.

Until recently, it was generally held that when a coronary arterial thrombus is found in association with a myocardial infarct, it is the immediate cause of the infarct. However, a number of investigators have presented evidence contrary to this view. Their studies suggest that coronary thrombosis is usually the result rather than the cause of infarction. They postulate that the thrombus forms in the already narrowed atherosclerotic vessel as a result of the circulatory disturbances brought on by the myocardial infarct, viz., diminished cardiac output and consequent slowing of the coronary blood flow.

Myocardial infarction usually is accompanied by prolonged substernal oppression or pain, shock, electrocardiographic changes, fever, leukocytosis, increased transaminase activity of the serum, and increased sedimentation rate. The pathologic changes in an infarct of the myocardium have much in common with infarcts elsewhere, but certain features are peculiar because of the nature and function of the heart. The relative infrequency of infarction involving the atria or the right ventricle has been mentioned.

There is a characteristic *position* occupied by the myocardial changes after coronary occlusion. Occlusion of the anterior descending branch of the left coronary artery produces an infarct of the anterior part of the interventricular septum and of the apical and anterior part of the wall of the left ventricle. Obstruction of the circumflex branch of the left coronary artery affects the wall of the left ventricle in its lateral portion or in its posterolateral aspect. Obstruction of the right coronary artery produces an infarct that involves the posterior half of the interventricular septum and a portion of the posterior wall of the left ventricle.

Although the aforementioned are the usual and typical areas of myocardial infarction, the location of the coronary occlusion and the site of infarction do not always have a constant relationship. Blumgart and associates have demonstrated "infarction at a distance," i.e., an infarct caused by sudden obstruction of an artery that had been supplying anastomotic channels and adequate nutrition to the affected area, which formerly was supplied by another coronary artery that had undergone gradual occlusion in the past. It also has been shown that ventricular infarcts show patterns similar to the known patterns of cardiac muscle bundles. Thickness of an infarct appears to be related to the complications of aneurysm and rupture of the myocardium.

The *appearance* of an infarct of the myocardium varies with its age. A visible infarct does not have time to develop if death rapidly follows acute myocardial ischemia. In early stages, an infarcted area may be dark red or hemorrhagic in appearance. Later, the area becomes yellowish and opaque (Fig. 13-31). Microscopically, the necrotic muscle fibers are swollen, hyalinized, and lacking their striations and nuclei. Leukocytes abundantly infiltrate the area (Fig. 13-32).

The infarcted area undergoes softening (myomalacia cordis), which results in weak-

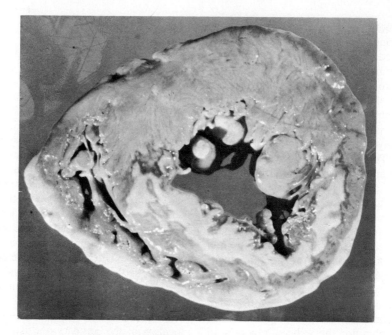

Fig. 13-31. Recent myocardial infarct of left ventricle, anteroseptal. (From Scotti, T. M.: Heart. In Anderson, W. A. D., and Kissane, J. M., editors: Pathology, ed. 7, St. Louis, 1977, The C. V. Mosby Co.)

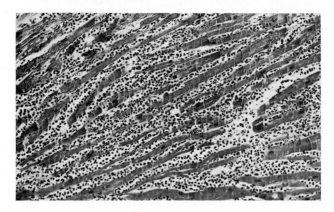

Fig. 13-32. Myocardial infarct. Muscle fibers are necrotic, and there is abundant leukocytic infiltration.

ening of the area and sometimes rupture. Rupture is most common in the first week and is rare after the third week. Localized pericarditis is present over the area of infarction, and mural thrombi (Fig. 13-33) form on the injured endothelium lining the region of infarction.

The *healing* of myocardial infarcts is by scar tissue replacing the destroyed muscle, which does not regenerate. Necrosis of muscle and leukocytic infiltration are predominant features of the first week. In the second week, one sees removal of necrotic muscle and re-

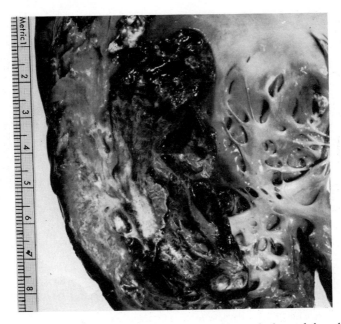

Fig. 13-33. Myocardial infarct of left ventricle with attached mural thrombus.

placement by connective tissue. This is evident grossly as a zone of red depressed tissue surrounding pale brown areas of necrotic muscle. The new connective tissue lays down increasing amounts of collagen until the area is converted into a firm, grayish, fibrous scar that forms in about 5 weeks to 3 months, depending on the size of the infarct. After 3 months, the scar becomes firmer and whiter.

In very early myocardial infarcts, before any gross or microscopic alterations are recognized by conventional methods of examination, certain chemical, histochemical, and electron microscopic changes can be demonstrated. Decreased enzyme activity within the myocardium seems to be a finding that is useful in the detection of early myocardial infarcts.

The *complications* and *causes of death* include (1) cardiac failure, left and/or right ventricular, (2) coronary failure or episodes of acute coronary insufficiency during convalescence from the recent infarct, (3) cardiac shock, (4) mural thrombi with thromboembolism, and (5) rupture of the heart with hemopericardium (cardiac tamponade).

Sudden death may be related to cardiac rupture, massive pulmonary embolism, or coronary failure. Ventricular aneurysms or calcification may develop in healed infarcts (so-called sequelae).

HYPERTROPHY AND DILATATION

Increase in size of the heart is the result of increased work thrown on the organ and an enlargement of the individual muscle fibers. Hyperplasia by mitotic division and regeneration of muscle fibers do not occur in the adult heart. Some investigators suggest that in hearts weighing more than 500 g ("critical heart weight"), thickened muscle fibers split longitudinally, causing an increase in the number of fibers.

The average normal heart weighs 300 g in men and 250 g in women. In cases of great hypertrophy, weights may range from 700 to 1,000 g or more. In normal hearts the left ventricle averages 10 to 12 mm and the right ventricle 3 to 4 mm in thickness. In hypertrophied hearts the thickness is greater and varies with the degree of hypertrophy.

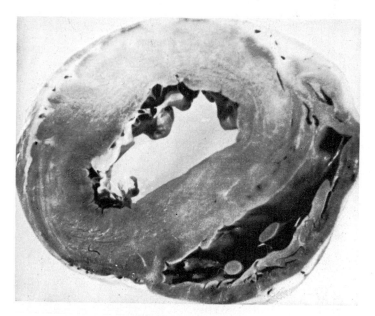

Fig. 13-34. Hypertrophy of left ventricle in chronic hypertension. Note excessive thickening of wall of left ventricle as compared with wall of right ventricle. Heart has been cut transversely through ventricles.

When an unusual amount of work is thrown on the heart muscle, it attempts to compensate by enlarging the muscle fibers. The portion of the heart that hypertrophies is determined by the location of the circulatory stress or burden imposed on it.

Hypertrophy of the left ventricle commonly results from (1) hypertension (Fig. 13-34), either primary or secondary, such as that associated with chronic glomerulonephritis, (2) aortic regurgitation or stenosis, (3) mitral regurgitation, and (4) coronary atherosclerosis.

Hypertrophy of the right ventricle is caused by (1) mitral stenosis, (2) pulmonary stenosis or regurgitation, (3) increased resistance in the pulmonary circulation (cor pulmonale), perhaps from emphysema or severe pulmonary arteriosclerosis, and (4) coronary atherosclerosis. Also, failure of the left ventricle throws increased work on the right ventricle and may cause hypertrophy.

Often, dilatation of the cardiac chambers precedes and accompanies hypertrophy (Fig. 13-35). One form of dilatation results from toxic effects on the myocardium, as in the degenerative cardiomyopathies and various types of myocarditis. Another form occurs when there is an excessive demand imposed on the heart by structural defects (e.g., valvular disease) or increased peripheral resistance (hypertension). A localized dilatation may occur in a weakened area of infarction.

Cases of hypertrophy without obvious cause ("idiopathic cardiac hypertrophy") are seen in young adults as well as in infants and children. A variant of this lesion is "familial cardiomegaly," in which a familial tendency extends over several generations. Usually, the hypertrophy and dilatation affect all chambers. In some patients, there is a localized area of unusually severe hypertrophy in the outflow tract of the left ventricle, producing manifestations of subaortic stenosis (so-called familial muscular subaortic stenosis, a form of "obstructive cardiomyopathy"). Other forms of idiopathic hypertrophy of the heart have already

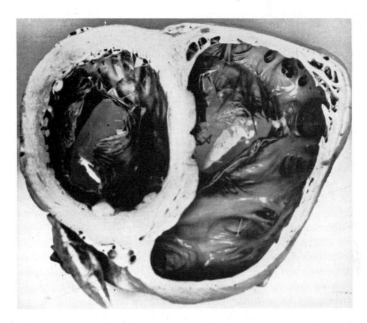

Fig. 13-35. Dilatation of ventricles.

been mentioned, i.e., endocardial fibroelastosis and endomyocardial fibrosis.

In the past, the diagnosis of "idiopathic hypertrophy" was made loosely and included such entities as glycogen storage (Pompe's) disease and Fiedler's myocarditis.

HYPERTENSIVE HEART DISEASE

Peripheral hypertension produces hypertrophy of the left ventricle because of its increased load. The hypertension is a disturbance of peripheral arterioles, however, and the cardiac effects are secondary (p. 345). Coronary atherosclerosis or other cardiac lesions are not infrequently associated. Eventually, the heart may be unable to cope with its increased work so that dilatation and congestive circulatory failure result. Congestive heart failure causes a considerable proportion of deaths from hypertension.

COR PULMONALE

Cor pulmonale or pulmonary heart disease is a condition in which the right side of the heart is subject to excessive strain because of some abnormality of the pulmonary circulation or lesion of the lungs. Enlargement of the right ventricle (dilatation and/or hypertrophy), with or without failure, is the essential feature.

Acute cor pulmonale may result from a massive pulmonary embolism that obstructs a major portion of the pulmonary circulation and is characterized by rapid dilatation of the pulmonary trunk, conus, and right ventricle. Multiple smaller emboli with organization may lead to chronic cor pulmonale. Other more common causes of chronic cor pulmonale are chronic bronchitis with chronic obstructive emphysema and widespread pulmonary fibrosis arising from a variety of conditions. Primary pulmonary arteriosclerosis is a rare cause of cor pulmonale.

The mechanism of production of chronic cor pulmonale appears to involve not only an obstruction in the pulmonary circulation but also a failure of oxygenation, which induces a reflex vasoconstriction and rise of pulmonary blood pressure. In chronic obstructive emphysema, a pulmonary insufficiency results from disturbed gas exchange because of ineffective alveolar ventilation and abnormal alveolar perfusion. Dyspnea, cyanosis, and polycythemia are common clinical accompaniments. The right ventricle becomes hypertrophied, and there may be some dilatation. With right-sided failure, hypertrophy of the right atrium may occur.

MYOCARDITIS

Acute myocarditis frequently is associated with bacterial endocarditis, and other bacterial infections may be associated with direct invasion of the myocardium by pathogenic organisms. The nonspecific acute inflammation may be predominantly interstitial with little parenchymal damage, or degeneration and necrosis of muscle may be prominent with only slight interstitial inflammation being in evidence. Abscesses occur in pyogenic infections. Granulomatous myocarditis is seen in tuberculosis, brucellosis, and tularemia. Myocardial abscesses also may be present in brucellosis. Sarcoidosis produces tuberculoid granulomatous lesions in the heart and may even be a cause of sudden death. Rare gummatous lesions occur in tertiary syphilis. Fibrosis associated with narrowing of the coronary ostia in syphilis is sometimes mistaken for "chronic myocarditis." The same applies to the myocardial fibrosis associated with coronary sclerosis.

Myocarditis also occurs in rickettsial infections such as typhus fever and in parasitic infections such as Chagas' disease (*Trypanosoma cruzi*). In trichinosis, a severe myocarditis may be present, although the larvae do not encyst in the myocardial fibers. Fungal infections produce lesions of the myocardium similar to those seen in other tissues and organs. Certain drugs or poisons cause toxic effects on the myocardium (degenerations and focal necrosis), followed by nonspecific inflammation. Serum sickness has been reported to have an associated myocarditis. Interstitial myocarditis with prominent eosinophils may follow sulfonamide administration, apparently due to hypersensitivity.

Certain collagen diseases, including rheumatic fever, are associated with myocarditis. Rheumatoid arthritis frequently is accompanied by valvular and myocardial lesions similar to those of rheumatic heart disease or to the granulomatous lesions in subcutaneous rheumatoid nodules. Adhesive pericarditis is also common with rheumatoid arthritis.

In some instances, pheochromocytomas are associated with myocardial lesions, which may be patchy areas of degeneration and necrosis of myocardial fibers followed by nonspecific inflammation and fibrosis. Presumably caused by secretion from the pheochromocytoma, the change has been called "norepinephrine myocarditis." It may be associated with unexpected death from myocardial failure. Experimentally, multiple, small necrotic lesions accompanied by inflammatory cell infiltration have been produced by the administration of epinephrine and norepinephrine. With administration of isoproterenol, however, more severe necrosis, which is actually infarctlike, has been produced.

Isolated, primary, or *Fiedler's myocarditis* is a severe myocarditis of unknown etiology that occurs unassociated with a disease process elsewhere to which it might be secondary. There may be either a diffuse infiltration of the interstitial tissue of the heart by lymphocytes, plasma cells, and eosinophils or focal granulomatous lesions with destruction of muscle fibers.

OTHER MYOCARDIAL DISEASES

Fatty metamorphosis (degeneration), fatty infiltration, basophilic (mucinous) degeneration, and *glycogen infiltration* of the myocardium, *atrophy* of the heart, and cardiac involvement in *hemochromatosis* have been discussed in Chapter 2.

Amyloidosis of the heart occurs as a feature of primary systemic amyloidosis and of amyloidosis associated with multiple myeloma. It also occurs as a distinctive type in elderly patients, in their seventh to ninth decades, with amyloid deposits largely restricted to the heart. Since it seems to be a manifestation of senescence, it often is referred to as "senile cardiac amyloidosis."

Nutritional disturbances also affect the heart. *Beriberi,* induced by a lack of vitamin

B₁ (thiamine), is characterized by cardiac enlargement chiefly caused by dilatation, especially of the right ventricle. Excessive intake of alcohol may produce a similar nutritional disturbance, but it also can cause a direct effect on the myocardium, resulting in degenerative changes and fibrosis—so-called *alcoholic cardiomyopathy*. A form of myocardial degenerative disease has been described in patients who drank large quantities of beer ("beer drinkers' myocardosis"). Cobalt, used to improve beer's foam or "head," may have been responsible for the myocardial disease.

Endocrine disturbances are seen in *hyperthyroid heart disease, hypothyroidism* (myxedema heart), and *acromegaly* (cardiac hypertrophy). The effect of *catecholamines* ("norepinephrine myocarditis") has been mentioned. *Carcinoid heart disease* is associated with the "carcinoid syndrome." In metastasizing carcinoids of the intestine, the increased serum levels of serotonin (5-hydroxytryptamine), or possibly other substances, cause typical fibrotic lesions of the endocardium of the heart—chiefly affecting the right side and especially the pulmonary and tricuspid valves. The most common effects are pulmonary stenosis and tricuspid regurgitation.

Myocardial lesions have been reported in patients dying suddenly and unexpectedly who had been receiving treatment with tranquilizers (phenothiazine compounds). The lesions consisted of foci of myocardial degeneration, associated with hyperplastic changes in the arterioles and increased acid mucopolysaccharide in and about these vessels.

TUMORS AND CYSTS

Both primary and secondary tumors of the heart are uncommon. The most common primary tumor of the heart is the *myxoma,* a polypoid mass arising from the endocardium of one of the atria, particularly the left atrium (Fig. 13-36). This benign lesion, which oc-

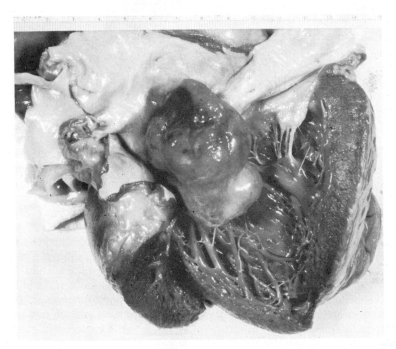

Fig. 13-36. Myxoma of heart. Note smooth glistening tumor attached to septal wall of left atrium and partly blocking mitral orifice. (From Scotti, T. M.: Heart. In Anderson, W. A. D., and Kissane, J. M., editors: Pathology, ed. 7, St. Louis, 1977, The C. V. Mosby Co.)

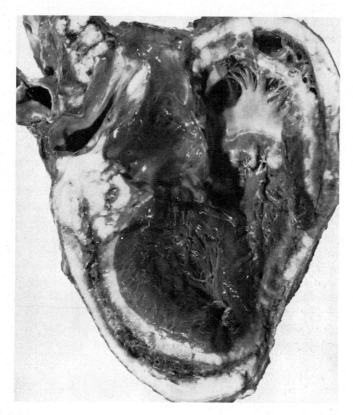

Fig. 13-37. Metastasis of bronchogenic carcinoma to heart. There is extensive invasion of pericardium and myocardium.

curs predominantly in adults, must be differentiated from edematous mural thrombi. A congenital, benign, striated muscle tumor *(rhabdomyoma)* is seen chiefly in infants, often in association with tuberous sclerosis. The myocardial fibers forming the tumorlike nodules are distended with glycogen. While some regard this lesion as the most common primary tumor of the heart in infants and children, others believe that it is a developmental anomaly or hamartoma. Other benign, but infrequent, intracardiac and pericardial tumors include *fibroma, lipoma,* and *angioma*.

Primary malignant neoplasms also originate in the heart or pericardium, such as *rhabdomyosarcomas* and other *intracardiac sarcomas* and *pericardial mesotheliomas* and *fibrosarcomas*. Among *metastatic tumors* of the heart,

the most frequent originate from bronchogenic carcinoma (Fig. 13-37), malignant lymphoma, leukemia, and malignant melanoma.

Various types of cysts also may occur in the heart and pericardium. *Blood cysts* are minute, round, red-brown nodules in the valves of infants, appearing chiefly on the atrial surfaces of the mitral and tricuspid valves. They are believed to result from blood being pressed into crevices on the surface of the cusps, followed by fusion of the mouths of the crevices. *Pericardial cysts* and the rare *intramyocardial epithelial cysts* are forms of congenital malformations that may be found in persons of all age groups.

REFERENCES

Abbott, M. E.: Atlas of congenital cardiac disease, New York, 1936, American Heart Association.

Adelson, L., and Hoffman, W.: J.A.M.A. **176:**129-135, 1961 (sudden death from coronary disease).

Alexander, C. S.: Br. Heart J. **29:**200-206, 1967 (alcoholic myocardiopathy).

Anderson, W. A. D., and Dmytryk, E. T.: Am. J. Pathol. **22:**337-349, 1946 (tumors of heart).

Becker, C. G., and Murphy, G. E.: Am. J. Pathol. **55:**1-37, 1969 (Aschoff bodies—suggested muscle origin).

Benditt, E. P.: Circulation **50:**650-652, 1974 (neoplastic-like proliferations in atherosclerosis).

Benditt, E. P.: Am. J. Pathol. **86:**693-702, 1977 (monoclonal origin of atherosclerotic plaques).

Bloor, C. M.: Cardiac pathology, Philadelphia, 1978, J. B. Lippincott Co.

Blumgart, H. L., et al.: Am. Heart J. **19:**1-91, 1940 (coronary artery disease).

Braunstein, H.: Circulation **28:**1071-1080, 1963 (pathogenesis of dissecting aneurysm).

Chandler, A. B.: Mod. Concepts Cardiovasc. Dis. **44:**1-5, 1975 (coronary thrombosis and myocardial infarction).

Chase, R. M., Jr.: Med. Clin. North Am. **57:**1383-1393, 1973 (infective endocarditis today).

Chatgidakis, C. B., and Barlow, J. B.: Med. Proc. **7:**377-385, 1961 (primary mural endocardial disease).

Cortes, F. M., editor: The pericardium and its disorders, Springfield, Ill., 1971, Charles C Thomas, Publisher.

Engel, H. J., et al.: J.A.M.A. **230:**1531-1534, 1974 (coronary artery disease in young women).

Evans, W.: Progr. Cardiovasc. Dis. **7:**151-171, 1964 (alcoholic myocardiopathy).

Friedberg, C. K.: Diseases of the heart, ed. 3, Philadelphia, 1966, W. B. Saunders Co.

Friedman, M.: Pathogenesis of coronary artery disease, New York, 1969, McGraw-Hill Book Co.

Getz, G. S., et al.: Am. J. Med. **46:**657-673, 1969 (dynamic pathology of atherosclerosis).

Gocke, D. J., et al.: Lancet **2:**1149-1153, 1970 (polyarteritis and Australia antigen).

Gore, I.: Arch. Pathol. **53:**142-153, 1952 (dissecting aneurysm).

Gould, S. E.: Pathology of the heart, ed. 3, Springfield, Ill., 1968, Charles C Thomas, Publisher (general reference).

Grinvalsky, H. T., and Fitch, D. M.: Ann. N.Y. Acad. Sci. **156:**544-565, 1969 (beer drinkers' myocardosis).

Hirst, A. E., Jr., et al.: Medicine (Baltimore) **37:**217-279, 1958 (dissecting aneurysm).

James, T. N., and Keyes, J. W., editors: The etiology of myocardial infarction, Boston, 1963, Little, Brown & Co.

Jick, H., et al.: J.A.M.A. **240:**2548-2552, 1978 (myocardial infarction and estrogens).

Jones, R. J., editor: Evolution of the atherosclerotic plaque, Chicago, 1963, University of Chicago Press.

Kahn, D. S., et al.: Ann. N.Y. Acad. Sci. **156:**285-293, 1969 (isoproterenol-induced cardiac necrosis).

Kaplan, M. H., and Svec, K. H.: J. Exp. Med. **119:**651-656, 1964 (immunologic relation of streptococcal and tissue antigens).

Kline, I. K., et al.: Circulation **30:**728-735, 1964 (chronic impairment of cardiac lymphatics).

Lev, M.: Autopsy diagnosis of congenitally malformed hearts, Springfield, Ill., 1953, Charles C Thomas, Publisher.

Lie, J. T., et al.: Mayo Clin. Proc. **46:**319-327, 1971 (histochemical method for detecting early myocardial infarcts).

MacAlpin, R. N.: N. Engl. J. Med. **291:**470-471, 1974 (coronary occlusion).

Mann, J. I., and Inman, W. H. W.: Br. Med. J. **2:**245-248, 1975 (myocardial infarction and oral contraceptives).

Mann, J. I., et al.: Br. Med. J. **2:**241-245, 1975 (myocardial infarction and oral contraceptives).

Mann, J. I., et al.: Br. Med. J. **2:**445-447, 1976 (myocardial infarction and oral contraceptives).

Marshal, C. E., and Shappell, S. D.: Arch. Pathol. **98:**134-138, 1974 (sudden death and myxomatous posterior leaflet of mitral valve).

McCarthy, L. J., and Wolf, P. L.: Am. J. Clin. Pathol. **54:**852-856, 1970 (mucoid degeneration of heart valves).

McGee, W. G., and Ashworth, C.T.: Am. J. Pathol. **43:**273-299, 1963 (hypertensive arteriopathy—fine structure).

McGill, H. C.: Lab. Invest. **18:**560-564, 1968 (fatty streaks in atherosclerosis).

McNamara, J. J., et al.: J.A.M.A. **216:**1185-1187, 1971 (coronary artery disease in young soldiers).

Minick, C. R., et al.: Am. J. Pathol. **96:**673-706, 1979 (virus-induced atherosclerosis).

Morales, A. R., and Fine, C.: Arch. Pathol. **82:**9-14, 1966 (histochemical study of myocardial infarcts).

More, R. H., and Movat, H. Z.: J. Pathol. Bacteriol. **75:**127-132, 1958 (arteritis).

Movat, H. Z., et al.: Am. J. Pathol. **34:**1023-1031, 1958 (arteriosclerosis).

Murphy, G. E.: Medicine (Baltimore) **42:**73-117, 1963 (Aschoff bodies—suggested muscle origin).

Pascoe, H. R.: Arch. Pathol. **77:**299-304, 1964 (myocardial sarcoidosis).

Paterson, J. C.: Arch. Pathol. **25:**474-487, 1938 (coronary artery disease).

Paterson, J. C.: Am. Heart J. **18:**451-457, 1939 (coronary artery disease).

Peery, T. M.: Postgrad. Med. **19:**323-327, 1956 (brucellosis and heart disease).

Pomerance, A., and Davies, M. J., editors: The pathology of the heart, Oxford, 1975, Blackwell Scientific Publications Ltd. (general reference).

Richardson, H. L., et al.: J.A.M.A. **195:**254-260, 1966 (intramyocardial lesions in sudden death).

Ritterband, A. B., et al.: Circulation **27:**237-251, 1963 (gonadal function and coronary heart disease).

Robbins, S. L.: Hum. Pathol. **5:**9-24, 1974 (cardiac pathology—a look at the last 5 years).

Roberts, W. C.: Circulation **45:**215-230, 1972 (coronary arteries in fatal acute myocardial infarction).

Rona, G.: Can. Med. Assoc. J. **95:**1012-1019, 1966 (pathogenesis of human myocardial infarction).

Rona, G., et al.: Arch. Pathol. **67:**443-445, 1959 (infarctlike necrosis produced by isoproterenol).

Ross, R., and Glomset, J. A.: Science **180:**1332-1339, 1973 (smooth muscle cells in atherosclerosis).

Ross, R., et al.: Am. J. Pathol. **86:**675-684, 1977 (injury, intimal smooth muscle cells, and atherogenesis).

Rubin, E.: N. Engl. J. Med. **301:**28-33, 1979 (alcoholic cardiomyopathy).

Schechter, M. M.: Am. J. Med. Sci. **227:**46-56, 1954 (superior vena cava syndrome).

Schettler, F. G., and Boyd, G. S., editors: Atherosclerosis, New York, 1969, American Elsevier Publishing Co., Inc.

Scotti, T. M., and McKeown, C. A.: Arch. Pathol. **46:**289-300, 1948 (sarcoidosis).

Shaper, A. G.: Br. Med. J.**3:**743-746, 1972 (endomyocardial fibrosis).

Spiro, D., et al.: Am. J. Pathol. **47:**19-49, 1966 (hyperplastic arteriolar sclerosis).

Stout, A.P.: Cancer **2:**1027-1054, 1949 (hemangiopericytoma).

Stout, A. P.: Lab. Invest. **5:**217-223, 1956 (hemangiopericytoma).

Strong, J. P., and McGill, H. C., Jr.: Am. J. Pathol. **40:**37-49, 1962 (natural history of coronary atherosclerosis).

Szakács, J. E., and Cannon, A.: Am. J. Clin. Pathol. **30:**425-434, 1958 (l-norepinephrine myocarditis).

Thomas, W. A., et al.: N. Engl. J. Med. **251:**327-338, 1954 (endomyocardial fibroelastosis).

Walton, K. W.: Am. J. Cardiol. **35:**542-558, 1975 (pathogenetic mechanisms in atherosclerosis).

Weinstein, L.: J.A.M.A. **233:**260-263, 1975 ("modern" infective endocarditis).

Wissler, R. W., and Geer, J. C., editors: The pathogenesis of atherosclerosis, Baltimore, 1972, The Williams & Wilkins Co.

14

Kidneys, lower urinary tract, and male genitalia

Kidneys

RENAL STRUCTURE AND FUNCTION

The kidneys are composed of units (nephrons), each consisting of a glomerulus and its associated tubule (Fig. 14-1). A normal human kidney contains about 1.25 million nephrons, sufficient for a considerable reserve. The glomerulus is composed of a group of capillaries (capillary tuft) coming off an afferent arteriole and draining into an efferent arteriole. Consisting of about eight lobules, each of which is made up of an anastomosing capillary network, the tuft projects into a capsule-lined space that opens into the proximal convoluted tubule. A flattened epithelium lines the capsule (Bowman's capsule). The capsular epithelium and basement membrane are continuous with the epithelium and basement membrane of the proximal convoluted tubule, and at the hilus of the glomerulus they are reflected over the tuft, where they become continuous with the epithelium and basement membrane of the capillaries.

The electron microscope reveals that the glomerular capillaries are lined by a fenestrated endothelium, the fenestrations measuring up to 1,000 Å in diameter. The capillaries are supported by a basement membrane that differs from ordinary collagen in that it is homogeneous rather than fibrillar, and there is a marked increase in carbohydrate linked to hydroxylysine in the protein. The basement membrane consists of a central dense part (lamina densa) with less dense layers on either side (lamina rara interna and externa). The major source of the basement membrane material appears to be the visceral epithelial cells, which are seen along the outer side of the membrane (Fig. 14-2). The epithelial cells, or podocytes, have branching and interdigitating foot processes, or pedicles, which are attached to the outside of the basement membrane and separated by filtration slits 200 to 500 Å in width. The slits are bridged by a thin plasma membrane (filtration slit membrane) that, together with the basement membrane, serves as a filtration barrier to macromolecules such as proteins.

In the central portion of the glomerular lobules, the basement membrane thickens and encloses the mesangium. The latter serves as a supporting stalk for the glomerulus, extending from the hilus into the center of each lobule. It consists of an amorphous substance (mesangial matrix) that encloses mesangial cells. The latter, which have been shown to be phagocytic, are separated from capillary lumina by endothelial cells.

At the hilus of the glomerulus is a specialized structure, the juxtaglomerular apparatus (p. 346).

331

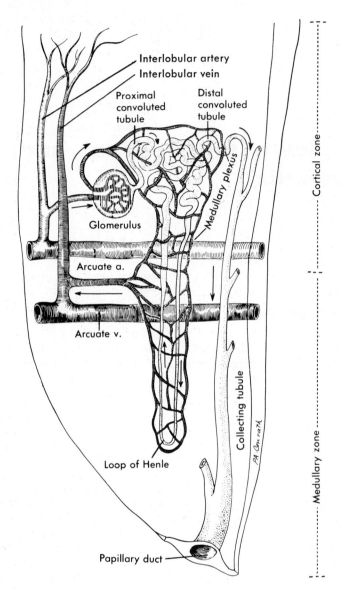

Fig. 14-1. Nephron. Diagrammatic representation of renal unit, showing circulatory relationships.

The total surface of a glomerular tuft is very large, and the aggregate surface of all tufts is enormous. The glomerulus acts as a filter, and from blood flowing through its capillaries, a practically protein-free filtrate of the plasma collects in the glomerular space and flows down the tubule. During this tubular passage, there is active resorption of water, glucose, chloride, sodium, and other substances. Active secretion by tubules of certain substances, notably creatinine and ammonia, also may occur. For this mechanism to function normally in the nephron, there must be (1) a free flow of blood through the capillaries of the tuft, (2)

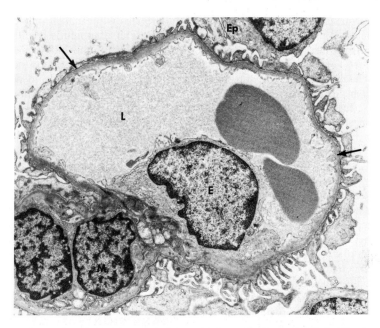

Fig. 14-2. Electron micrograph of normal glomerular loop showing epithelial cell, *Ep,* with delicate foot processes abutting on lamina densa (arrows). Mesangial cells, *M,* have darker cytoplasm and are separated from capillary lumen, *L,* by endothelial cell cytoplasm, *E.* (×5,300; courtesy Dr. V. Pardo.)

a normal filter, i.e., water, salt, urea, and other waste products must be allowed to filter through, but certain substances such as plasma proteins must be held back, and (3) a normal epithelial lining of the tubule and an unblocked lumen. Lesions in the kidney can produce functional disturbance by three corresponding types of qualitative change. Each may occur alone, but combinations of varying degrees of each are the usual occurrence. The large numerical reserve of identical units is such that a fraction of their number can maintain adequate function. Consequently, functional changes in relation to renal lesions must be considered on a quantitative as well as a qualitative basis. When functional deficiency occurs in chronic glomerulonephritis and nephrosclerosis, values for urea and creatinine clearance are closely correlated with the number of functioning glomeruli.

The vessels of the glomerular tuft, after, forming the efferent arteriole, again break up into capillaries, which supply the tubule.

Hence, obstruction of flow through the glomerulus also interferes with tubular blood supply. Destruction of a glomerulus usually results in atrophy and disappearance of the corresponding tubule, although aglomerular tubules have been demonstrated. Glomeruli do not regenerate. No new glomeruli are formed during adult life, although some compensation may result from hypertrophy of those remaining. Tubular epithelium, on the other hand, regenerates readily, provided the basement membrane is intact. Hence, injurious agents that affect the tubular epithelium alone (e.g., mercury bichloride) lead either to death of the person or to complete recovery, i.e., the injury is neither chronic nor progressive. After injury, regenerative tubular epithelial cells may have an atypical flattened form and are most resistant to injury.

UREMIA

Uremia is the complex clinical condition marking the final stage of renal insufficiency.

No particular substance or toxin is known to be causative, but it is probably an autointoxication resulting from the retention of various metabolic products ordinarily eliminated by the urinary mechanism. Azotemia, the retention of nitrogenous metabolites, also may be extrarenal (i.e., caused by diseases other than those of the kidneys).

Failure of function is denoted by an inability of the kidneys to produce a concentrated urine and to adapt to increased work. In final stages of failure, the specific gravity of the urine tends to be fixed at about 1.010, the urine being almost isotonic with serum. Urea, creatinine, uric acid, sulfate, chloride, ammonia, and phosphate are retained. The hydrogen ion concentration of the urine can no longer be varied to suit the body's need, and there is frequently a retention acidosis, which may be lessened by increased breathing and loss of acid through vomiting. The blood phosphorus level increases greatly, and the calcium level falls, resulting in nervous hyperirritability and muscle twitchings. Convulsions may occur when the uremia is associated with hypertension.

Other than the damaged kidneys, there are no constant anatomic changes in uremia. Edema of the brain is common. A mild sterile pericarditis is occasionally present, and degenerative changes have been described in outer portions of the myocardium. In some patients, electrocardiographic changes are indicative of hyperpotassemia. Necrotizing colitis is an occasional occurrence in uremia. Pulmonary edema, rich in fibrin, may occur, especially in hilar regions. Pulmonary hemorrhage originating from alveolar septa may be found in some patients with glomerulonephritis, particularly those with necrotizing glomerular or vascular lesions. In severe renal failure, there is an increased susceptibility to infection and a depression of the cellular immunity mechanism, with impaired ability to reject homografts.

RENAL EDEMA

Edema in renal disease is influenced principally by two factors: (1) loss of plasma albumin and (2) salt retention. If congestive heart failure also is present, it may contribute to the edema. The albuminuria results from increased permeability of the glomerular tufts, and the protein loss decreases the osmotic pressure exerted by plasma colloids to hold fluid within the vessels. The sodium chloride retention is caused by a lessened ability of the damaged kidney to excrete it. Loss of albumin is particularly important, because it exerts four times the osmotic force of globulin. In the "nephrotic" types of renal disease, a massive albuminuria and severe edema go hand in hand (p. 342).

The distribution of edema in renal disease often is independent of gravity and may appear first on the face rather than in dependent parts. The edema fluid has a low protein content and low specific gravity. In some patients with renal disease, cardiac failure develops and may contribute to the edema.

CLASSIFICATION OF RENAL DISEASES

Cardiovascular renal disease includes most conditions accompanying high blood pressure and is a very frequent cause of death in persons past middle age. Renal diseases of different origin and nature may produce similar disturbances of renal function and have much clinical similarity. Also, renal disturbances of different pathogenesis may reach late or end stages that are morphologically similar and difficult to differentiate.

The following classification of the main renal diseases is based on a combined consideration of the portion of the kidney primarily or most prominently affected and the type of involvement. Other parts of the kidney almost always show some secondary or less prominent pathologic change.

Glomerular disease
  Glomerulonephritis
    Diffuse
      Acute poststreptococcal
      Acute nonstreptococcal
      Subacute (or rapidly) progressive
      Chronic (or slowly) progressive
      Terminal (end-stage) chronic
      Hereditary nephritis
    Focal

Nephrotic syndrome
  Minimal change glomerular disease (lipoid nephrosis)
  Idiopathic membranous nephropathy
  Membranoproliferative glomerulonephritis
  Congenital (infantile) nephrotic syndrome
  Systemic lupus erythematosus
  Diabetic glomerulosclerosis
  Amyloidosis
  Renal vein thrombosis
  Infections
  Toxemia of pregnancy
  Extrarenal malignant neoplasms

Vascular disease
  Nephrosclerosis
    Atherosclerotic
    Arteriolosclerotic
  Hypertension
  Renal artery stenosis
  Infarction
  Bilateral cortical necrosis
  Systemic lupus erythematosus
  Diabetic glomerulosclerosis
  Polyarteritis nodosa
  Hemolytic-uremic syndrome

Tubular disease
  Acute tubular necrosis
  Reversible tubular lesions
  Chronic tubular disease
  Genetic or acquired tubular dysfunction (Fanconi syndrome)

Interstitial disease
  Acute diffuse interstitial nephritis
  Chronic diffuse interstitial nephritis
  Focal suppurative interstitial nephritis (pyemic kidney; abscesses of kidney)
  Pyelonephritis
  Necrosis of renal papillae (necrotizing renal papillitis)
  Pyonephrosis
  Radiation nephritis
  Tuberculosis

Metabolic disease
  Hyperparathyroid renal disease
  Nephrocalcinosis
  Calculi
  Oxalosis
  Urate deposits

Obstructive disease
  Hydronephrosis

Congenital malformations and anomalies
  Agenesis
  Hypoplasia
  Fusion
  Duplication of ureters or double pelvis

  Ectopia
  Anomalous renal vessels

Cysts

Tumors
  Benign
    Adenoma
    Fibroma
    Lipoma
    Hamartoma
    Juxtaglomerular cell tumor
    Leiomyoma
  Malignant
    Renal cell carcinoma (hypernephroma)
    Wilms' tumor
    Sarcoma
  Tumors of renal pelvis
  Metastatic

GLOMERULAR DISEASE

The forms of glomerular disease will be discussed under the headings of (1) glomerulonephritis (diffuse and focal) and (2) nephrotic syndrome.

Glomerulonephritis

Glomeruli may be injured by physical agents such as ionizing radiation, chemical agents, anoxia, and bacterial toxins. However, a major cause of inflammatory disease of the glomeruli is immunologic in nature. Two immunologic mechanisms that are frequently responsible for glomerular inflammation and scarring are referred to as *antiglomerular basement membrane disease* and *immune complex disease*. A third immunologic mechanism may be the *alternative complement pathway disease*.

According to the first concept, antibodies may form against glomerular basement membrane antigen, or antibodies that cross-react with the basement membrane may be produced by endogenous or exogenous antigens. This mechanism apparently is the basis of the kidney lesion in Goodpasture's syndrome, in some of the cases of rapidly progressive glomerulonephritis and chronic glomerulonephritis, and in experimental nephrotoxic serum nephritis. Fluorescence microscopy discloses a linear deposit of antiglomerular antibody along the glomerular basement membrane, and electron microscopy reveals a linear layer of material between the capillary endothelium and basement membrane.

In immune complex disease, antibody that is stimulated by foreign, nonglomerular antigen combines with the antigen, and this antigen-antibody complex, along with complement, is deposited in glomeruli. Fluorescent antibody studies reveal the immune complex as lumpy deposits in relation to the basement membrane and in the mesangium. The deposits are demonstrated by electron microscopy between epithelium or endothelium and basement membrane and in the mesangium. Deposits of this nature are demonstrated in the glomerular lesions of acute poststreptococcal glomerulonephritis, membranous nephropathy, some cases of subacute (or rapidly) progressive glomerulonephritis and chronic glomerulonephritis, and other diseases.

The alternative complement pathway disease is sometimes observed and occurs particularly in some instances of membranoproliferative glomerulonephritis. It is characterized by dense deposits in the glomeruli ("dense deposit disease"). The deposits show little, if any, immunoglobulin but prominent deposition of complement C3 as well as some properdin. Decreased serum complement C3 levels are usually observed. It is suggested that a circulating nephritic anticomplementary factor (C3NeF) is present that activates properdin factors and results in conversion of C3 to C3b (properdin or alternative complement pathway).

Diffuse glomerulonephritis

The forms of diffuse glomerulonephritis are (1) acute poststreptococcal glomerulonephritis, (2) acute nonstreptococcal glomerulonephritis, (3) subacute (or rapidly) progressive glomerulonephritis, (4) chronic (or slowly) progressive glomerulonephritis, (5) terminal (end-stage) chronic glomerulonephritis, and (6) hereditary nephritis.

Acute diffuse glomerulonephritis is characterized by an acute inflammatory process involving all glomeruli of both kidneys, resulting in blockage of many capillaries and cellular exudation, thus decreasing glomerular filtration. There is also increased capillary permeability, resulting in plasma proteins, red blood cells, and leukocytes in the urine. Most of the cases of acute diffuse glomerulonephritis follow hemolytic streptococcal infections, but some are apparently of nonstreptococcal origin.

Acute poststreptococcal glomerulonephritis. Epidemiologic, bacteriologic, and serologic studies indicate that acute diffuse glomerulonephritis may follow hemolytic streptococcal infections after a latent period of 1 to 4 weeks (average, about 10 days). The infections are usually of the upper respiratory tract but may be skin and wound infections. The nephritogenic strains of streptococci are types 12, 4, 1, and Red Lake. The microorganisms may be cultured during the infections, and later a rising titer of antibodies against streptococcal antigen (i.e., antistreptolysin [ASO] titer) may be demonstrated. However, the renal disease is not due to the presence of streptococci in the glomeruli. Immunologic, fluorescence, and electron microscopic studies indicate that acute poststreptococcal glomerulonephritis is an immune complex disease, with trapping of streptococcal antigen and human antibody in the glomeruli.

The disease occurs mainly in children and young adults, affecting males more frequently than females. Among the *clinical features* are hematuria (often described as smoky, rusty, or reddish brown urine), oliguria, proteinuria, edema, and hypertension. The *prognosis* usually is good. About 80% to 90% of children recover, although only 50% to 70% of adults have a good outcome. About 2% to 5% of patients with poststreptococcal glomerulonephritis die in the acute stage because of renal insufficiency (uremia), infection, or cardiac failure. Some patients who survive the acute disease may have persistent active progressive glomerulonephritis that either heals with some loss of nephrons or has a slow smoldering downhill course.

Grossly, the kidneys are swollen and are pale or congested, with smooth surfaces on which tiny hemorrhages are sometimes visible. *Microscopically,* the glomerular tufts appear

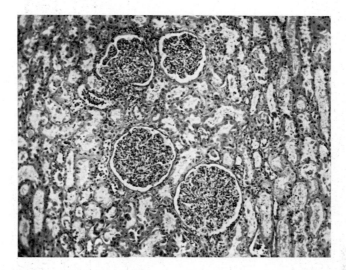

Fig. 14-3. Acute diffuse glomerulonephritis. Note large size and great cellularity of glomeruli.

enlarged, hypercellular, and bloodless (Fig. 14-3). The increased cellularity is due to proliferation of endothelial and mesangial cells and the presence of neutrophils and monocytes. The lobules of the glomeruli often are club shaped. Electron microscopic studies reveal characteristic deposits, so-called humps, between the basement membrane and epithelial cells that are believed to be immune complexes (Fig. 14-4). Focal fusion of epithelial foot processes may be seen. The width of the basement membrane usually is unaltered, although focal thickening may be noted. Tubular changes usually are not so marked as those in the glomeruli, but dilatation, cloudy swelling, hyaline droplet accumulation, or fatty degeneration may occur when inflammatory changes are severe.

The process is referred to as "acute exudative glomerulonephritis" when numerous neutrophils are present in most of the glomeruli and as "acute proliferative glomerulonephritis" when mesangial cells, endothelial cells, and monocytes predominate. In some instances, occasional glomeruli may show proliferation of epithelial cells lining Bowman's capsule, with early "crescent" formation. When damage is more severe, there may be rupture and throm-

bosis of capillaries with extravasation of red blood cells and fibrin in the capsular space, sometimes associated with epithelial crescents ("acute necrotizing glomerulonephritis").

The severity of the clinical picture and the eventual outcome may be correlated with the degree of glomerular inflammation and destruction as noted in renal biopsy. Acute exudative or proliferative lesions may resolve with only a slight increase in cellularity and mesangial thickening, whereas acute necrotizing lesions usually are irreversible.

Acute nonstreptococcal glomerulonephritis. Some patients with acute diffuse glomerulonephritis apparently have no evidence of preceding streptococcal infection, although it is possible that, in some instances, such infection existed previously but was undetected. Also, there have been reports of acute diffuse glomerulonephritis associated with various nonstreptococcal (bacterial and viral) infections.

Subacute (or rapidly) progressive glomerulonephritis. Subacute progressive glomerulonephritis, also referred to as *rapidly progressive glomerulonephritis,* has a rapid course and usually terminates in death from renal failure within 3 to 12 months. In a few patients,

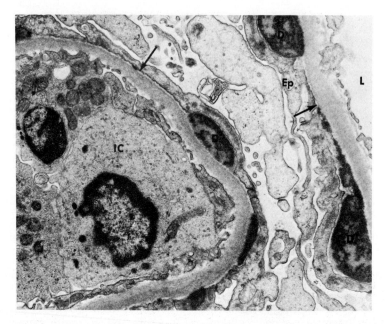

Fig. 14-4. Acute poststreptococcal glomerulonephritis. Electron micrograph showing proliferated intracapillary endothelial cells, *IC*, filling one of capillaries. Subepithelial electron-dense deposits, *D*, so-called humps, may be seen under swollen epithelial foot processes, *Ep*. Lamina densa (arrows) appears normal. *L*, Capillary lumen. (× 10,500; courtesy Dr. V. Pardo.)

the disease represents an active progression of an unresolved acute poststreptococcal glomerulonephritis. In other patients, however, the progressive lesions develop in the absence of a clinically evident acute stage and, commonly, without a history of preceding streptococcal infection.

Grossly, the kidneys are enlarged, pale, and soft ("large white kidneys"). There may be some irregularity of the surface and some adherence of the capsule. *Microscopically,* all of the glomeruli show changes. Capsular "crescents" caused by proliferation of the epithelium of Bowman's capsule are frequent and prominent, sometimes obliterating the tuft (Fig. 14-5). For this reason, the lesion is sometimes referred to as "crescentic glomerulonephritis." Red blood cells and proteinaceous material, including fibrin, may be seen in the capsular spaces. Cellular proliferation of the tufts is present but frequently is less pronounced than in acute glomerulonephritis. Scarring and foci of necrosis of tufts and adhe-

sions of tufts to capsules are common. Electron microscopy may disclose thickening of the basement membrane.

Goodpasture's syndrome refers to the association of glomerulonephritis with pulmonary hemorrhage. The renal lesions usually resemble those of rapidly progressive glomerulonephritis, although focal glomerulonephritis may be seen, particularly as an early lesion. The lungs show alveolar hemorrhage, hemosiderin-containing macrophages, and thickening of the alveolar walls. An immunologic basis for the pulmonary and renal lesions has been suggested by studies in some patients with this syndrome in whom antilung antibodies were demonstrated that cross-reacted with kidney glomerular basement membrane.

Chronic (or slowly) progressive glomerulonephritis. Patients with glomerulonephritis that pursues a slowly progressive course with smoldering activity over a period of years may be asymptomatic despite slight abnormal urinary findings (e.g., proteinuria and micro-

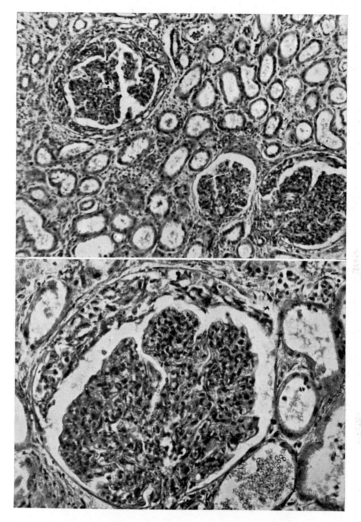

Fig. 14-5. Subacute (or rapidly) progressive glomerulonephritis with considerable epithelial proliferation. Note glomerular crescents resulting from proliferation of capsular epithelium.

scopic hematuria). Some patients develop marked proteinuria with hypoproteinemia and the nephrotic syndrome. Hypertension and eventually renal failure may appear in patients with progressive scarring of the kidney lesions. In some patients with chronic progressive glomerulonephritis, there is a history of an antecedent attack of acute poststreptococcal glomerulonephritis, but in most instances the disease appears insidiously without an antecedent acute attack.

Renal biopsy may disclose a chronic proliferative reaction with increase of mesangial cells and matrix (mesangial scarring), resulting in enlargement of glomerular lobules. Patients with this lesion, so-called chronic lobular glomerulonephritis, commonly develop the nephrotic syndrome. In others, focal sclerosis with recent and old glomerular scars may be seen. Some glomeruli appear normal by light microscopy, but in many of these glomeruli, electron microscopic study discloses focal thickening of the capillary basement membrane, focal subendothelial deposits, and flattening of foot processes. In all instances of chronic progressive glomerulonephritis, there is irregular atrophy of the tubules.

Terminal (end-stage) chronic glomerulonephritis. Terminal, or end-stage, chronic glomerulonephritis is characterized by chronic renal failure and hypertension. It may result from an acute diffuse glomerulonephritis, poststreptococcal or nonstreptococcal, that progresses to a chronic phase. Frequently, there is no history of an antecedent acute attack. The condition may progress over many years, with little clinical evidence except for a slowly progressive decrease of renal function. In other cases, there are long latent periods without serious impairment of renal function, punctuated by mild acute flare-ups. Other glomerular diseases that may give rise to end-stage chronic glomerulonephritis are lipoid nephrosis (rarely), idiopathic membranous glomerulonephritis, focal glomerulonephritis, and hereditary nephritis. The end result in each case is similar, i.e., failure of renal function, terminating in uremia, associated with small, contracted, scarred kidneys.

Grossly, the small, contracted kidneys are firm, with granular pitted surfaces and adherent capsules. The cortices are irregularly narrowed and scarred, with loss of normal architectural markings (Fig. 14-6). *Microscopically,* most of the glomeruli are partially or completely scarred, many being converted to hyaline masses. The number of glomeruli appears to be decreased, probably because of disappearance of some damaged glomeruli. Many tubules are atrophic or have disappeared. Fibrosis of the interstitial tissue is prominent, and there is an infiltration of the stroma by lymphocytes and sometimes by plasma cells and histiocytes. Medium-sized and small arteries commonly develop intimal and medial proliferation and thickening, mainly as a result of the hypertension that accompanies the nephritis. Fibrinoid necrosis and more marked proliferative changes in the vessels may occur in those instances in which hypertension is greatly increased. In some cases, the pathologic changes are not readily distinguishable from those caused by primary (essential) hypertension.

Hereditary nephritis. A hereditary chronic renal disease usually associated with nerve

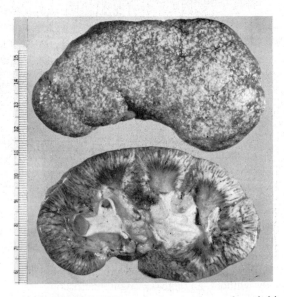

Fig. 14-6. Terminal (end-stage) chronic glomerulonephritis.

deafness has been studied in several families. The lesions have a mixture of features of chronic glomerulonephritis, pyelonephritis, and interstitial nephritis, and foam cells in the cortex may be a prominent feature. The foam cells are not pathognomonic, for they occur occasionally in various other renal diseases. In some instances, the foam cells can be identified as lipid-filled, degenerated, cortical tubular cells.

Focal glomerulonephritis

In contrast to the widespread glomerular involvement in diffuse glomerulonephritis, only some of the glomeruli are involved in focal glomerulonephritis (Fig. 14-7). Many of the glomeruli appear normal. The lesions in the affected glomeruli often are limited to one or two lobules, usually peripherally. Occasionally, an entire glomerulus is involved. The lesions are proliferative or necrotic, or both, and sometimes capillary thrombosis may be associated. Occasionally, an epithelial crescent lining the glomerular capsule is seen. The changes have sometimes been referred to as "glomerulitis." Focal glomerulonephritis occurs with a variety of diseases.

Bacterial endocarditis (mainly the *subacute* variety) is a well-known cause of focal glomerulonephritis. The focal glomerular lesion in this condition is usually fibrinoid necrosis, sometimes with capillary thrombosis, and has been referred to as "focal necrotizing glomerulonephritis." Proliferation of the tuft near the necrotic lesion or of the capsular epithelium (crescent formation) is sometimes evident. Because of the necrosis, petechial hemorrhages occur and may be seen on the subcapsular surface as tiny red areas, commonly referred to as "flea-bitten" appearance. Fibrosis (scarring) of the lesion is noted in endocarditis of longer duration. Formerly, the focal glomerular lesions were believed to be caused by tiny emboli from the infected cardiac valves (thus, the term "focal embolic glomerulonephritis"), but there is much evidence that this is not the correct pathogenesis, including the fact that bacteria usually are not demonstrated in the lesions. It is probable that the lesions represent an immunoallergic response to antigenic products of the bacteria. Since only a small proportion of glomeruli are altered, renal function usually is not affected, but hematuria may be manifested. If significant impairment of renal function occurs, it is likely to be due to an acute diffuse glomerulonephritis, which occasionally develops in bacterial endocarditis.

Focal glomerulonephritis is associated with

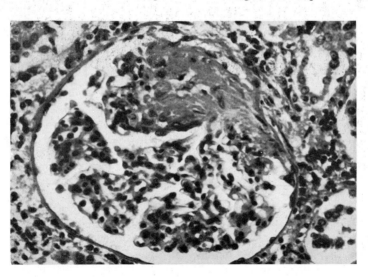

Fig. 14-7. Focal glomerulonephritis. (AFIP 80093.)

other clinical states, including *systemic bacterial infections* (other than bacterial endocarditis), other disorders producing immunologic injury of glomeruli (e.g., *Goodpasture's syndrome, polyarteritis nodosa, systemic lupus erythematosus,* and *Schönlein-Henoch syndrome*), and certain conditions characterized by disseminated intravascular coagulation (e.g., *endotoxin shock, amniotic fluid embolism,* and *thrombotic thrombocytopenic purpura*). In some instances, focal glomerulonephritis is *idiopathic* (as in patients with recurrent isolated hematuria or in persons with proteinuria discovered on routine urinalysis).

Nephrotic syndrome

The nephrotic syndrome is a clinical entity characterized by massive proteinuria, hypoproteinemia, edema, lipidemia (hypercholesterolemia), and lipiduria. Underlying the clinical complex may be one of a number of distinct diseases, although the condition they have in common is an increased glomerular membrane permeability that is evidenced particularly by the marked proteinuria. Edema in the nephrotic syndrome is due, in part, to the hypoproteinemia (lowered plasma colloid osmotic pressure) but also is related significantly to sodium retention due to increased aldosterone secretion (probably stimulated by low plasma volume incident to hypoproteinemia). There are a variety of conditions causing the nephrotic syndrome. It is sometimes associated with forms of glomerulonephritis already described, e.g., acute diffuse (proliferative) glomerulonephritis and chronic glomerulonephritis (especially the chronic lobular form). Other causes include lipoid nephrosis ("minimal change" or "foot process" disease), idiopathic membranous glomerulonephritis, congenital (infantile) nephrotic syndrome, systemic lupus erythematosus, diabetic glomerulosclerosis, amyloidosis, renal vein thrombosis, constrictive pericarditis, infections (syphilis, malaria), toxemia of pregnancy, and extrarenal malignant neoplasms.

Minimal change glomerular disease (lipoid nephrosis). Minimal change glomerular disease or "foot process" disease, also referred to as "lipoid nephrosis," is a major cause of the nephrotic syndrome, especially in young children (usually 1 to 3 years of age), although it may occur in older children and adults. As a rule, hypertension, hematuria, and azotemia do not accompany the features of the nephrotic syndrome except in the late stages in patients with unremitting disease. Generally, remissions and exacerbations are common in this disease.

The glomeruli show no significant change by light microscopy. Flattening and fusion of the epithelial foot processes are the most striking changes disclosed by electron microscopy. The basement membrane and the mesangium usually show no significant changes. Although immune deposits in the glomeruli have been noted in an occasional report, most investigators have reported their absence, so that a clear-cut immunologic mechanism for the development of the lesion has not been confirmed. The tubular epithelium may show hyaline droplets (evidence of proteinuria) and fatty droplets (evidence of lipiduria).

Intercurrent infection was a common cause of death in patients with lipoid nephrosis, but antibiotics have diminished the incidence of this complication. Response to adrenal steroids is generally good. The prognosis, therefore, is vastly improved today compared with former years. Only rarely has the disease been reported to progress to a chronic stage of renal insufficiency with hypertension and uremia (essentially, end-stage chronic glomerulonephritis).

Idiopathic membranous nephropathy. Another important cause of the nephrotic syndrome is idiopathic membranous nephropathy. This lesion is commonly referred to as "idiopathic membranous glomerulonephritis," but because of a lack of proliferation of cells or other inflammatory features, some investigators prefer the term "membranous nephropathy" or "membranous glomerulosclerosis" rather than "membranous glomerulonephritis." The major feature is a thickening of the glomerular basement membrane. The disease occurs particularly in adults but may appear in children. It has an insidious onset and its course tends to be prolonged. The prognosis is not as good as in lipoid nephrosis, and, unlike the latter, the disease does not respond well to steroid therapy. There may be progression to glomerular sclerosis with increasing renal insufficiency and uremia in the later stages, presenting the picture of end-stage chronic glomerulonephritis.

In addition to thickening of the basement membrane, electron microscopy discloses electron-dense deposits between the basement membrane and epithelial cells, the latter showing flattening and fusion of foot processes (Fig. 14-8). The deposits appear to project into the basement membrane, and the membrane next to the deposits may project outwardly in the form of "spikes." By immunofluorescence studies, gamma globulin corresponding to the subepithelial deposits may be demonstrated, suggesting an immunologic pathogenesis (immune complex disease).

Membranoproliferative glomerulonephritis. Membranoproliferative glomerulonephritis is also a cause of the nephrotic syndrome, although occasionally it may present as an acute hemorrhagic nephritic syndrome. The lesion is characterized by uniformly involved glomeruli with enlarged, hypercellular, club-shaped lobules (lobular configuration). There is an increase in mesangial cells and mesangial basement membrane material. The mesangium extends out to encircle the capillaries, producing thick, double-walled capillaries (so-called reduplication or splitting of the basement membrane). Neutrophils may be present in the glomeruli. Two forms of the lesion have been described. Type 1 is the more classic lesion, an immune complex disease, and is characterized by deposits of immune complexes in the capillary walls subendothelially and in the mesangium. In type 2, linear deposits of electron-dense material are seen in the peripheral capillary basement membrane lamina densa, with little evidence of deposits in the mesangium (so-called dense deposit disease). Complement (C3) is usually readily demonstrated

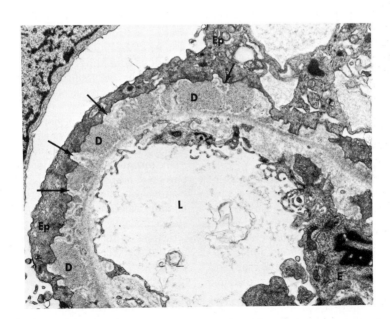

Fig. 14-8. Electron micrograph of renal lesion in idiopathic membranous glomerulonephritis. Spikelike areas of thickened lamina densa (arrows) may be seen between predominantly subepithelial electron-dense deposits, *D*. Epithelial foot processes, *Ep*, are fused and swollen. *E*, Endothelium. *L*, Capillary lumen. (×9,000; courtesy Dr. V. Pardo.)

in association with these deposits, but immunoglobulin deposits are slight or absent. Properdin may also be present.

Hypocomplementemia may occur in patients with membranoproliferative glomerulonephritis and tends to be more persistent in the type 2 form. The clinical picture of these two forms is similar, but the prognosis is poorer in type 2, which may result in progressive glomerular sclerosis and renal failure. Membranoproliferative glomerulonephritis may be idiopathic, but it can also develop in a variety of clinical states, including chronic bacteremia, chronic active hepatitis, parasitic infections, certain blood dyscrasias, and partial lipodystrophy.

Congenital (infantile) nephrotic syndrome. Congenital nephrotic syndrome occurs within the first few days or weeks of life. The disease, which has a high familial incidence, tends to be severe, and death results usually within the first year. In the glomerular tufts, the epithelial foot processes are flattened and fused as in lipoid nephrosis, and there may be patchy thickening of the basement membrane rather than the diffuse type seen in idiopathic membranous glomerulonephritis. There is a greater tendency to fibrosis of the glomeruli than in lipoid nephrosis. Gamma globulin and complement have been demonstrated in some glomeruli. A characteristic feature is cystic dilatation of the proximal convoluted tubules.

Systemic lupus erythematosus. See p. 349.

Diabetic glomerulosclerosis. See p. 351.

Amyloidosis. See p. 34.

Renal vein thrombosis. Increased pressure in the renal veins, such as that caused by venous thrombosis in adults, may result in the nephrotic syndrome. Severe forms of cardiac failure, as in chronic constrictive pericarditis, similarly may cause the nephrotic syndrome. Thickening of the basement membrane and subepithelial electron deposits may be demonstrated in the glomeruli, changes that are somewhat similar to those of idiopathic membranous glomerulonephritis. Diffuse or focal fusion of epithelial foot processes has been described. Some evidence suggests that renal vein thrombosis may be a frequent complication of the nephrotic syndrome rather than its cause.

Infections. Certain systemic infections, such as syphilis and malaria, may cause the nephrotic syndrome. Hypersensitivity may be important in the pathogenesis of the syndrome in some instances. Electron microscopy discloses subepithelial deposits and/or fusion of epithelial foot processes in the glomeruli.

Toxemia of pregnancy. Renal lesions regularly accompany the toxemias of late pregnancy (preeclampsia and eclampsia). The changes are more prominent in eclampsia.

Microscopically, the glomeruli are enlarged and bloodless and have narrowed capillaries. The capillary walls appear thickened because of a fibrinoid deposit. The mesangium and the endothelial cells are swollen. In addition to this swelling, electron microscopy reveals protein deposits between the endothelium and basement membrane and in the mesangium. The protein deposits are mainly fibrin, as demonstrated by fluorescent antibody studies. The deposition of fibrin, which apparently is related to a state of intravascular coagulation that occurs in toxemia of pregnancy, probably initiates the glomerular damage. Tubular changes, consisting of cloudy swelling, hyaline droplet accumulation, fatty change, and even necrosis, are secondary to glomerular lesions.

Usually, the renal lesions are reversible, although biopsy studies have shown permanent damage in some glomeruli in some patients.

Extrarenal malignant neoplasms. The nephrotic syndrome has been described in association with nonrenal malignant tumors, including carcinomas (e.g., bronchus, breast, stomach) and Hodgkin's disease and other lymphomas. In occasional instances, renal biopsy disclosed a membranous glomerulonephropathy with immunoglobulin deposition along the glomerular basement membrane. It is likely that a tumor-associated antigen induces the immune complex.

VASCULAR DISEASE

Sclerosis of renal arteries and intrarenal vessels is extremely important because of the association of these changes with high blood pressure. Ischemic renal tissue releases into the bloodstream a pressor substance that produces hypertension by constriction of peripheral vessels. Hypertension may be the result of atherosclerosis of a renal artery in those rare instances in which the lumen is constricted sufficiently to cause renal ischemia. In the usual case of hypertension, however, renal ischemia is associated with sclerosis of the smallest arteries or arterioles of the kidney. Sclerosis of the larger arteries within the renal substance is usually irregular and not generalized in its distribution. Hence, it rarely results in ischemia of sufficient renal tissue to produce hypertension, nor is there enough destruction to cause renal failure. It produces a few large, gross scars, similar to healed areas of infarction. Because it is a common finding in elderly persons, such a kidney is called a "senile arteriosclerotic kidney."

Senile arteriosclerotic kidney (atherosclerotic nephrosclerosis). The atherosclerotic involvement of large and medium-sized intrarenal arteries is a patchy change that results in irregular, depressed areas on the kidney surface. The kidney is not much decreased in size unless there is some other pathologic change. Microscopically, fibrous replacement of glomeruli and tubules is present in the scarred subcapsular portions of the cortex. There is some cellular infiltration by lymphocytes and plasma cells. These changes in the kidney rarely are associated with any severe hypertension or renal functional failure. Hypertension may occur, however, if an atherosclerotic plaque obstructs the renal artery or a major branch.

Hypertension

Cases of high blood pressure commonly are divided into *secondary* and *essential* types. The less common secondary type is the result of renal disease (such as chronic pyelonephritis and glomerulonephritis), renal artery stenosis, cerebral or cardiovascular disease, or endocrine lesions such as an adrenal or pituitary tumor.

Hypertension caused by unilateral renovascular disease (*renal artery stenosis*) is recognized clinically more frequently than in former years, mainly because of the ability to demonstrate lesions by aortography and renal angiography. It is the clinical counterpart of the classic Goldblatt experiment in dogs, in which clamping of the renal artery resulted in renal ischemia and hypertension. The causes of renal artery stenosis include atherosclerotic plaques, thrombosis, emboli, aneurysms, congenital malformations, fibromuscular dysplasia, and pressure from extrinsic tumors, scars, etc. Fibromuscular dysplasia consists of several types, including intimal fibroplasia, medial fibroplasia, and medial fibromuscular hyperplasia.

The common essential type of hypertension was so called because there seemed to be no primary lesion. It has been recognized that renal arteriolar sclerosis is an almost constant postmortem finding in essential hypertension. The arteriolar sclerosis is often a generalized change, particularly common in the spleen, pancreas, adrenal glands, and brain, but it is only in the kidneys that arteriolar sclerosis and hypertension seem to be closely associated. However, biopsy of the kidneys in hypertensive patients has shown that as many as 28% may have little or no vascular change. Early in essential hypertension, the renal blood flow is reduced by tonic muscle spasm of the renal arterioles. In this stage, the glomerular filtration rate and tubular functions are normal. Later, the renal ischemia is maintained and increased by structural narrowing or sclerosis of the arterioles and small arteries. Structural change with loss of nephrons is accompanied by reduction of glomerular filtration rate and tubular functions.

In a reported series of 2,300 renal biopsies from hypertensive patients, more than 80% had arteriolar nephrosclerosis, about 15% had chronic pyelonephritis, 1.3% had unilateral renovascular lesions, and 1% had chronic glomerulonephritis.

The importance of renal vascular changes in hypertension has been shown by Goldblatt, who produced renal ischemia by means of a clamp on the renal artery. It was demonstrated that the ischemic renal tissue released a pressor substance into the circulation that resulted in constrictive action on peripheral vessels and produced hypertension.

The substance secreted by the kidney (renin) is not, in itself, a pressor substance. Renin is an enzyme secreted into the blood, where it acts on a substrate, an alpha-2 globulin (hypertensinogen), to produce a decapeptide called angiotensin I. This, in turn, is acted upon by a converting enzyme to form angiotensin II. This substance constricts arterioles, elevates blood pressure, and stimulates the adrenal cortex to secrete aldosterone. It is probable that other factors in addition to angiotensin II are important in the sustained elevation of blood pressure in hypertensive patients. Hyperaldosteronism is present in some patients with hypertension. It is possible that both angiotensin II and aldosterone produce electrolyte changes that influence blood pressure. The role that aldosterone plays in sodium retention has been discussed.

Renin is secreted by specialized cells at the vascular pole of the glomerulus that form a functional structure called the *juxtaglomerular complex*. This consists of juxtaglomerular or granular epithelioid cells in the media of the afferent arterioles, a group of smaller cells situated in the angle formed by the two arterioles (lacis cells, or "polkissen"), and the macula densa, a specialized adjacent segment of the distal tubule.

The degree of granularity of the juxtaglomerular cells is an indication of their secretory activity. In severe arteriolar nephrosclerosis, the juxtaglomerular cells are hypertrophied, hyperplastic, and actively functioning. In unilateral renovascular hypertension, the juxtaglomerular cell change may be great. In hypertensive patients with mild arteriolar nephrosclerosis, pyelonephritis, Cushing's syndrome, and primary hyperaldosteronism, the juxtaglomerular cells do not appear to be hyperplastic and active.

Essential hypertension has been divided into "benign" and "malignant" clinical types. They appear to be fundamentally the same in nature. The malignant form more commonly

occurs in young adults. It is more rapidly progressive and has severe lesions. Death usually results from renal failure. Pathologically, the malignant form is characterized by hyperplastic arteriolosclerosis, usually with necrosis in the walls of small arteries and arterioles and small hemorrhages from the severely damaged vessels. These necrotizing vascular changes can be reproduced experimentally by renal ischemia sufficient to cause renal failure. Benign hypertension is the more common type, has a protracted course, and is less severe than the malignant form. Hyaline arteriolosclerosis is the typical vascular lesion in the benign form.

Common causes of death in hypertension are cerebral hemorrhage, renal failure (uremia), congestive heart failure, and coronary occlusion. Cardiac hypertrophy (left ventricle) is a constant finding in cases of hypertension. Retinal changes are also a constant part of hypertensive disease and consist of sclerosis of small retinal vessels, small hemorrhages, and edema. In the malignant phase, retinal changes are severe and may result in blindness.

The cause of essential hypertension is still unknown. Hereditary and racial tendencies are important. Body build and, to a lesser degree, obesity seem to have some association with hypertension. A high dietary intake of sodium chloride appears to predispose to hypertension. Experimental salt hypertension in the rat resembles human hypertensive disease in its evolution and lesions.

Kidney of hypertension (arteriolar nephrosclerosis). In benign hypertension, the most constant finding in the kidney is a sclerosis of small arteries and arterioles. Often, the smallest preglomerular vessels show the change most severely in the portion just proximal to the tuft. In many cases, the kidneys are of normal size and have smooth surfaces. With more severe or prolonged hypertension, any degree of atrophy may be found. The capsules are adherent, and the outer surfaces of the kidneys present a finely granular and scarred appearance. Tiny retention cysts are often present in the cortex. With such changes of vascular origin, the term *primarily contracted kidney* is used to differentiate this from the *secondarily contracted kidney* of glomerulonephritis. In practice, it is often impossible to distinguish grossly the contracted kidney of hypertensive nephrosclerosis from that of chronic glomerulonephritis.

Microscopically, the essential lesion in benign hypertension is a sclerosis of small arter-

ies and arterioles. Hyaline arteriolar sclerosis, which involves particularly the afferent arterioles, is a hyalinization and decreased cellularity of the wall, with a variable reduction in the size of the lumen (Fig. 14-9). Electron microscopy has indicated that this appearance is caused by deposition of a hyaline substance in the arteriolar wall. The vascular hyalin has been described previously (pp. 31 and 284).

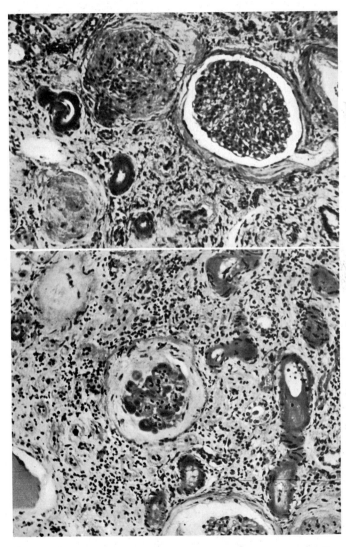

Fig. 14-9. Arteriolar nephrosclerosis in severe hypertension. Note extreme hyaline thickening of arteriolar walls and also glomerular changes.

Larger vessels, particularly the interlobular arteries, may show a laminated, eosinophilic intimal thickening, often with a prominent thickened and reduplicated internal elastic lamina (hyperplastic elastic sclerosis). Although the elastic tissue hypertrophy is prominent, the intima particularly is thickened with the production of fibrils and localization of small lipid particles.

The effects of the vascular changes are reflected in the glomeruli, which early show a thickening of the capillary basement membranes and later show varying degrees of hyalinization and atrophy. Hyaline deposits first appear beneath the endothelium but, with increase, later fill the capillary lumina. Glomerular capsules, as well as tufts, become thickened and hyalinized. The atrophy of glomeruli and associated tubules produces the renal shrinkage. In end stages with significant renal contraction, it is often difficult to distinguish chronic glomerulonephritis from arteriolar nephrosclerosis, even by microscopic examination. Remaining traces of a proliferative in-

flammatory process must be searched for as a distinguishing feature indicating glomerulonephritis.

In malignant hypertension, the kidneys often show little atrophy as a result of the rapid progress of the disease. Small hemorrhages on the outer surface of the kidney may cause it to resemble the "flea-bitten" kidney of focal glomerulonephritis. This is caused by acute necrotizing arteriolitis and arteritis. Hyperplastic arteriolar sclerosis of larger arterioles and small arteries may be prominent. The pathologic findings differ somewhat, depending on whether the hypertension was malignant from the beginning or whether it was benign with a superimposed malignant terminal phase. In the latter case, varying chronic changes with hyalinization and atrophy of glomeruli are present, but in addition to the usual arteriolar sclerosis, one sees a hyaline necrosis of vessel walls, some inflammatory cellular infiltration, and often hemorrhage about severely injured vessels (Fig. 14-10). The hyaline necrotic changes may extend to involve glomerular

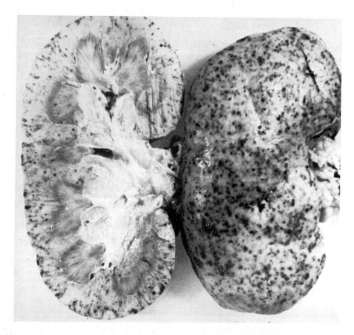

Fig. 14-10. Kidney in malignant hypertension, showing focal hemorrhages from arteriolonecrosis.

capillaries as well as arterioles and small arteries.

Primary reninism. Recently, a syndrome has been described consisting of hypertension, hyperreninemia, and secondary aldosteronism associated with a renin-producing tumor of the kidney *(primary reninism)*. In most of the patients, the tumor was composed of juxtaglomerular (JG) cells. Removal of the tumor resulted in cure of the patients with this syndrome. In one instance of primary reninism, a very small nonneoplastic lesion was detected in the kidney and was regarded either as a localized JG cell hyperplasia or a hamartoma with increase in the number of JG cells. An occasional renin-secreting Wilms' tumor has been reported to have caused hypertension.

Infarction

Renal infarcts are quite common as a result of *embolism* from the heart in cases of bacterial endocarditis, atrial fibrillation, and mural thrombosis after myocardial infarction. In rare cases, infarction has been sufficiently extensive to give rise to oliguria or anuria as well as to hematuria.

Thrombosis associated with *polyarteritis nodosa* may be a cause of renal infarcts (p. 352).

Renal vein thrombosis is an uncommon condition that may give rise to hemorrhagic infarction of the kidney, or if the main renal vein is occluded, there may be massive renal necrosis. In adults, renal vein thrombosis is usually a secondary extension from the thrombophlebitis of peripheral veins. In childhood, a primary renal vein thrombosis may be associated with ileocolitis accompanied by diarrhea and marked dehydration. Renal vein thrombosis may be associated with the nephrotic syndrome, particularly in adults (p. 344).

Bilateral cortical necrosis

There is an unusual condition of extensive necrosis of the peripheral layers of renal cortices that is of unknown cause but is sometimes associated with hemorrhage and toxemias of late pregnancy or acute infections. It also has been described in newborn infants, associated with maternal antepartum hemorrhage. A similar condition results from poisoning by dioxane or diethylene glycol, from injections of staphylococcal toxin, or from choline deficiency in experimental animals. The chief clinical feature is oliguria, and death usually results in a few days. Because of ischemia, irregular areas of necrosis involve the cortical portions of both kidneys. The surface is mottled by patchy, reddish yellow, opaque areas and has a soft consistency. The microscopic appearance is similar to that of infarction, with a zone of congestion and leukocytic infiltration about the margin of the necrotic areas (Fig. 14-11).

The ischemic necrosis of the renal cortices appears to be caused by a widespread organic or functional occlusion of the interlobular arteries and their branches, the terminal arteries, and the arterioles of the renal cortices. The actual mechanism of the vascular obstruction, whether by intense vasoconstriction, vasoparalysis, thrombosis, or necrosis of arterial walls, or a combination of these factors, may vary in different cases. Disseminated intravascular coagulation has been suggested as one of the basic factors in the pathogenesis of the diffuse cortical necrosis. The work of Trueta and associates suggests that there may be a vascular mechanism by which the cortex is bypassed, the blood being shunted through the medulla.

Systemic lupus erythematosus

In systemic lupus erythematosus, glomerular changes are common. Microscopically, the glomeruli may be normal, show minimal change (e.g., focal glomerulitis), or be markedly involved. When prominent, the lesions consist of thickening of the basement membranes of glomerular capillaries, often with fibrinoid change, producing the so-called wire loop appearance (Fig. 14-12). Foci of necrosis (sometimes with "hematoxylin bodies") and cellular proliferation (mesangial, endothelial, and epithelial) may be present. Occasional hyaline thrombi appear in capillary lumina. In later stages, glomerular scarring is seen. By

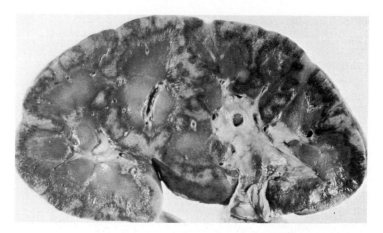

Fig. 14-11. Cortical necrosis of kidney. Reddened congestive zone outlines opaque necrotic cortical tissue.

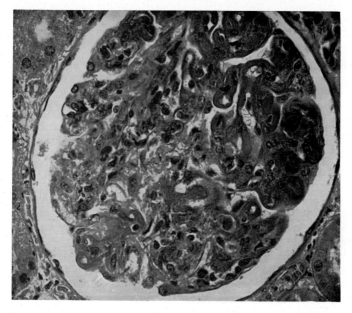

Fig. 14-12. Kidney in systemic lupus erythematosus showing "wire loop" lesions and fibrinoid necrosis of glomerulus.

electron microscopy, a "wire loop" lesion consists of thickening of the basement membrane, abundant subendothelial electron-dense deposit, and fusion of epithelial foot processes (Fig. 14-13). By immunofluorescence microscopy, deposits of immunoglobulin (mainly IgG) and complement are seen in the mesangium and basement membrane. Viruslike particles have been observed in the glomerular endothelium in electron micrographs, but their relationship to the disease is not clear (p. 686).

Some patients receiving certain drugs, such

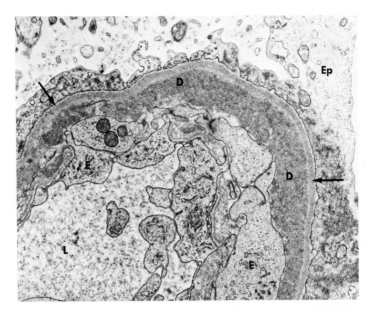

Fig. 14-13. Electron micrograph of renal glomerular lesion in systemic lupus erythematosus. Subendothelial dense deposits, *D*, may be seen under swollen endothelial cell cytoplasm, *E*. Epithelial cell, *Ep*, foot processes are fused. Lamina densa (arrows) is not thickened. *L*, Capillary lumen. (×10,500; courtesy Dr. V. Pardo.)

as hydrazides, anticonvulsants (Dilantin), and procainamide, develop antinuclear factors and manifestations similar to systemic lupus erythematosus.

Diabetic glomerulosclerosis

Diabetic glomerulosclerosis may be focal or diffuse. The typical lesion is nodular glomerulosclerosis *(Kimmelstiel-Wilson lesion)*, characterized by focal, nodular, hyaline areas usually appearing in central parts of glomerular lobules near the periphery (Fig. 14-14). It is generally held that the earliest changes occur in the mesangium, followed by gradual increase in the mesangial matrix. Thus, it is often referred to as "intercapillary glomerulosclerosis." Sometimes associated with these lesions is a so-called exudative lesion ("fibrin cap"), a deeply eosinophilic, homogeneous, electron-dense, fibrinoid material between the endothelial cells and basement membrane of the capillaries. Similar material may appear as a small, rounded, eosinophilic mass on the inner side of Bowman's capsule subepithelially ("capsular drop lesion").

Hyaline arteriolosclerosis, with involvement particularly of efferent glomerular arterioles, is often prominent in association with nodular glomerulosclerosis. The diffuse form of glomerulosclerosis is characterized by thickening of capillary membranes. This occurs more frequently than the nodular lesions and may appear alone or in combination with nodular glomerulosclerosis. In some patients with diabetic glomerulosclerosis, hypertension, albuminuria, edema (of the nephrotic type), and renal failure may occur.

Other renal lesions often associated with diabetes mellitus include arteriolosclerosis, pyelonephritis, and papillary necrosis. In uncontrolled diabetes, there may be glycogen accumulation in the cells of the distal straight portion of the proximal convoluted tubules and sometimes the contiguous portion of thin limbs of Henle's loops *(Armanni-Ebstein lesion)*.

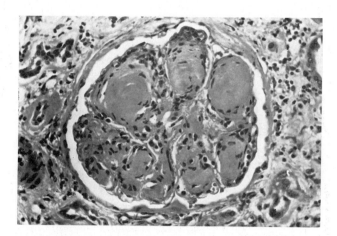

Fig. 14-14. Diabetic glomerulosclerosis. (AFIP.)

Polyarteritis nodosa

The kidneys are affected in 70% to 80% of patients with polyarteritis nodosa, an inflammatory disease of medium-sized and small arteries (p. 287). The renal lesions include cortical infarcts and glomerular changes. The glomeruli show focal glomerulonephritis (with foci of fibrinoid necrosis, inflammation, or epithelial crescents). Hypertension is common, and renal failure sometimes occurs.

Hemolytic-uremic syndrome

In recent years, there have been reports of a syndrome consisting of hemolytic anemia, thrombocytopenia, and renal insufficiency, referred to as the hemolytic-uremic syndrome. The essential feature in the kidneys is the formation of fibrin and platelet thrombi in the renal arterioles and glomerular capillaries. The vascular lesions are similar to those described in disseminated intravascular coagulation (p. 510). The syndrome occurs usually in children, particularly in association with various bacterial or viral infections. However, it may also occur in adults, e.g., in women as a complication of pregnancy.

TUBULAR DISEASE

The term *nephrosis* was coined originally to denote degenerative renal changes, as distinct from inflammation (nephritis) or vascular disease (nephrosclerosis). The older use of the term was in reference to degenerative changes in the tubules, particularly the sensitive convoluted tubules of the cortex. Today, however, it is used also to designate clinical conditions of glomerular origin (e.g., lipoid nephrosis, nephrotic syndrome). Tubular disease may be classified as (1) acute tubular necrosis, (2) reversible tubular lesions, (3) chronic tubular disease, and (4) genetic or acquired tubular dysfunction (e.g., Fanconi syndrome).

Acute tubular necrosis

Acute tubular necrosis (also referred to as acute nephrosis) is one of the major causes of acute renal failure, resulting in marked oliguria or anuria and a progressive rise in nitrogenous waste products in the blood. The lesion is associated with a variety of conditions that may be grouped into two major categories: those related to anoxia or ischemia (hemoglobinuric nephrosis, acute ischemic nephrosis, or lower nephron nephrosis) and those of toxic origin (toxic nephrosis). In some conditions, both anoxic and toxic factors play a role in causing tubular damage. Although necrotic lesions are not reversible, regeneration of tubular epithelium can occur if the patient survives the initial phase of acute renal failure.

Hemoglobinuric nephrosis (acute ischemic nephrosis; lower nephron nephrosis). A variety of conditions accompanied by

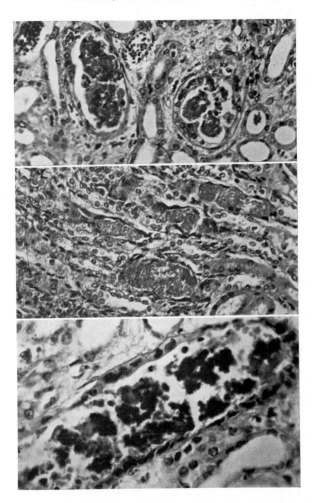

Fig. 14-15. Transfusion reaction in kidney. Tubules contain pigment casts, and their epithelial lining cells show degenerative changes.

a fairly massive destruction of blood or tissues and by shock may be followed by oliguria or anuria and by death from renal failure. The kidneys in such cases are characterized by degenerative changes of the tubules, pigmented casts in the tubular lumina, and edema of renal tissue (Fig. 14-15). Although the pathogenesis of the renal lesion has not been completely elucidated, it appears to be on the basis of a disturbance of renal blood flow (e.g., shock or renal arterial vasoconstriction), and hemoglobin or myoglobin and derived pigments may play a part in some cases. Al-

though the changes are often most prominent in the distal or lower portions of the nephrons, they are not limited to this area, so that the term *lower nephron nephrosis* has been described as "euphonious but erroneous."

Hemoglobinuric nephrosis is observed characteristically in cases of massive hemoglobinemia and hemoglobinuria, such as occur in blackwater fever and after transfusion with incompatible blood. Severe traumatic injuries involving crushing of muscle tissues or prolonged muscle ischemia also produce the condition (crush syndrome and posttraumatic anuria). Similar renal lesions may occur in cases of severe burns, heat stroke, uteroplacental damage, severe infections, and various poisonings. Shock and excessive vomiting often are associated with the conditions that lead to hemoglobinuric nephrosis. The development of renal functional failure is associated with oliguria, which often progresses to anuria. The urine excreted is highly acid, gives a positive benzidine reaction, and shows pigmented material or pigmented casts on microscopic examination.

The gross appearance of the kidneys is not specific. There is usually some swelling and enlargement, with increase of weight. The outer and cut surfaces of the cortex are pale, but the medulla is dark or dusky and shows accentuated striations.

Microscopically, the distal convoluted tubules are dilated and lined by flattened epithelium. Reddish or brownish casts (heme casts) are seen in the distal convoluted and collecting tubules. The tubular epithelium adjacent to the casts is often degenerated, showing focal cellular necrosis, and the basement membrane may be disrupted (tubulorrhexis). These casts may rupture into the interstitial tissue and lead to thrombosis of small veins nearby. The proximal convoluted tubules frequently are dilated and lined by flattened epithelium. Some investigators have described the tubulorrhexic lesion in the straight terminal portion of the proximal convoluted tubule. The glomeruli show no significant change. The interstitial tissue is edematous, showing focal infiltration by a variable number of leukocytes, mainly the mononuclear type. The oliguria or anuria may be mainly caused by a disturbance in renal circulation with inadequate glomerular filtration and may be contributed to by the blockage of tubular lumina with pigment casts and by excessive reabsorption or leakage of glomerular filtrate through the damaged tubular walls.

The pathogenesis of the renal lesion is not completely established, but much evidence suggests that it has a vascular basis, with disturbance of renal blood flow and ischemia. A renal vasomotor mechanism has been demonstrated that, on stimulation, causes renal cortical ischemia and diverts blood flow to the medulla. Hemoglobin and derived pigments may play some part in producing this vascular disturbance, in addition to the effect of tubular blockage.

Toxic nephrosis. Nephrotoxins are exogenous poisons that injure the kidney, most often by causing degeneration and necrosis of tubular epithelium. Mercury bichloride, a frequent example, causes a pure tubular injury of severe grade and results in oliguria, which usually progresses to anuria and death from uremia. Death occurs most frequently between the fifth and tenth days, at which stage the kidney is swollen and grayish white. The epithelium, particularly of the convoluted tubules, is necrotic, broken up, and irregularly desquamated. The interstitial tissue is edematous and often infiltrated by leukocytes. After 7 or 10 days, the kidney appears more red and congested, and calcium often is deposited in the degenerated and necrotic tubular epithelium. Evidence of epithelial regeneration and mitotic nuclei may be found at this time. (See Fig. 11-1.)

Other poisons that may produce toxic nephrosis include ethylene glycol (antifreeze), dioxane, diethylene glycol, carbon tetrachloride, phosphorus, and insecticides. *Ethylene glycol* causes a marked ballooning hydropic degeneration (vacuolar nephropathy) that may progress to focal hemorrhagic necrosis of the cortex. Calcium oxalate crystals are found in the tubular lumina. A similar picture, but without the oxalate crystals, is seen in *dioxane* and *diethylene glycol poisoning*. The tubular necrosis of *carbon tetrachloride poisoning* is associated with considerable amounts of neutral fat in the basal portions of the proximal convoluted tubules.

Bacterial toxins may cause tubular necrosis, usually accompanied by cloudy swelling, hydropic degeneration, or fatty change. *Cholemic nephrosis* is characterized by tubular degeneration and necrosis accompanying severe jaundice. Bile pigment is commonly seen, and leucine crystals may be present in the renal tubules. It is not certain whether the damage is caused by bile pigments, bile salts, or hepatic

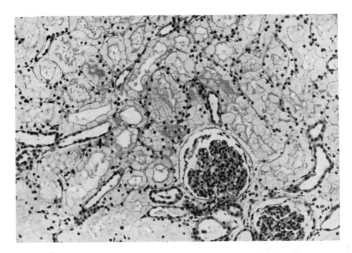

Fig. 14-16. Hydropic degeneration of kidney, caused by intravenous injection of hypertonic sucrose. (From Anderson, W. A. D.: South. Med. J. **34**:257-263, 1941.)

damage. *Hypersensitivity reactions* to sulfonamides, antibiotics, and other drugs may be accompanied by acute toxic nephrosis.

Reversible tubular lesions

The conditions causing acute tubular necrosis usually produce varying degrees of degeneration of tubular epithelium as well. In some instances when the injury is relatively mild, only degenerative changes (e.g., cloudy swelling, hydropic degeneration, and fatty change) may be seen, without obvious necrosis. Two other conditions associated with non-necrotic renal lesions are described in the following paragraphs.

A diffuse type of hydropic degeneration, characterized by numerous small pinocytic vesicles of the proximal tubules, results from the intravenous injection of hypertonic solutions of sucrose, mannitol, or similar substances (Fig. 14-16). The condition, known as *osmotic nephrosis,* is usually asymptomatic and readily reversible.

A distinctive vacuolar lesion, chiefly of the proximal convoluted tubules, is seen in severe potassium depletion (Fig. 14-17), as in chronic intestinal diseases with diarrhea (e.g., ulcerative colitis and regional enteritis). By electron microscopy, the vacuoles appear to represent marked distention of the basal infoldings of the tubular epithelial cells, apparently due to a disturbance of the electrolyte "pump" mechanism. This lesion, *hypokalemic (vacuolar) nephropathy,* is reversible following adequate potassium replacement.

Chronic tubular disease

Chronic atrophy of the renal tubules, resulting in abnormal tubular function, occurs in association with chronic glomerulonephritis, chronic interstitial nephritis, long-standing arteriolonephrosclerosis, and various lesions that result in obstruction of the outflow of urine in the tubules or from the kidney. The secondary effect on the tubules may be due to several factors, including direct injury related to the primary disease or ischemia produced by vascular changes.

Genetic or acquired tubular dysfunction (Fanconi syndrome)

Fanconi (or de Toni-Debre-Fanconi) syndrome is characterized by renal glycosuria, aminoaciduria, phosphaturia, often with acidosis, and a growth disturbance resembling rickets. A familial form, caused by a recessive gene, is usually evident in childhood. The basic disturbance appears to be a resorption

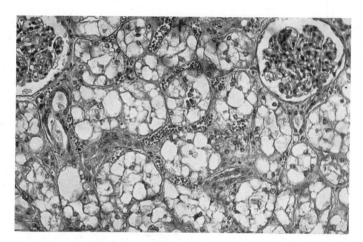

Fig. 14-17. Vacuolar nephropathy of potassium deficiency in regional enteritis. (Courtesy Dr. J. F. Kuzma.)

defect of the renal tubules, and microdissection shows a thin first part of the proximal convoluted tubules, described as a "swan neck" appearance. There is also a fibrosing chronic interstitial nephritis. In some cases, there is an associated cystinosis.

Adult, or acquired, Fanconi syndrome may result from an injury by heavy metals or degraded tetracyclines. It also has been reported with various cancers, including multiple myeloma. Cystinosis is not a usual feature.

INTERSTITIAL DISEASE

Interstitial nephritis, unlike glomerulonephritis, is essentially an exudative rather than a proliferative inflammation. Marked exudates of inflammatory cells may be present focally or diffusely in the interstitial tissue.

Acute diffuse interstitial nephritis. Acute interstitial nephritis occasionally occurs in association with certain acute infectious diseases (e.g., diphtheria, scarlet fever, Weil's disease). The inflammatory reaction usually consists of lymphocytes and plasma cells (even though the disease is regarded as clinically acute). In some instances, however, neutrophils or eosinophils may be seen. The tubules show degenerative changes, but the glomeruli usually are not affected.

Chronic diffuse interstitial nephritis.

Chronic interstitial nephritis is characterized by fibrosis of the interstitial tissue together with infiltration by lymphocytes and plasma cells and atrophy or loss of tubules. In many instances, it is not associated with any known disease or causative agent. It may occur, however, as a result of various types of renal injuries (e.g., chronic hyperparathyroidism, multiple myeloma). Association with analgesic abuse (e.g., phenacetin ingestion) has been reported, sometimes with accompanying necrosis of renal papillae (p. 357). Distinction of chronic interstitial nephritis from chronic pyelonephritis may be difficult.

Focal suppurative interstitial nephritis (pyemic kidney; abscesses of kidney). Lodgment of infected emboli, as part of a generalized pyemia, results in multiple abscesses throughout the kidney substance. The abscesses appear as small, rounded, yellowish opaque areas surrounded by a reddened hyperemic zone. They may be numerous, or a single large abscess (carbuncle) may be found. Staphylococci and *Escherichia coli* are the common organisms.

Pyelonephritis. The term *pyelonephritis* is used when both the parenchyma of the kidney and the renal pelvis are involved by interstitial inflammation caused by bacterial infection. Descending and ascending types are described.

In the former, bacteria reach the kidney by the bloodstream, primarily infecting renal tissue and "descending" to infect the pelvis. In the latter, the bladder and pelvis are infected first, and spread occurs by "ascending" to infect renal tissue. This may be upward spread via the lumen or by the lymphatics of the ureter. The relative frequency of ascending and hematogenous infection is uncertain and a point of debate.

The presence of renal scars appears to predispose to infection of the area by circulating bacteria. The susceptibility of the kidney to infection by organisms carried in the bloodstream is also enhanced by urinary tract obstruction. Ascending infection likewise may occur when there is obstruction with consequent stagnation of urine. Prostatic hyperplasia, strictures, stones, and tumors are among the various causes of urinary tract obstruction that predispose to pyelonephritis. Stagnation of urine may also be caused by vesicoureteral reflux, resulting in backflow of urine from the bladder (p. 374). Diabetes mellitus, pregnancy, and urethral catheterization or instrumentation are other factors that predispose to urinary tract infection. The so-called pyelitis common in children and pregnant women is really pyelonephritis.

The kidneys show wedge-shaped areas of inflammation extending through the cortex and medulla to the pelvis. Microscopically, such areas show interstitial infiltrations of inflammatory cells, often with some tubular destruction and abscess formation. In *acute pyelonephritis,* the cells are mainly neutrophilic leukocytes, and in *chronic pyelonephritis,* they are lymphocytes and plasma cells. In the chronic form, the mucosa of the pelvis is roughened, and masses of lymphocytes are found under the epithelium. In addition to the chronic inflammatory cells, collections of neutrophils may be present in the interstitial tissue and in tubular lumina *(active chronic pyelonephritis).* Continuation of low-grade interstitial inflammation results in gradual atrophy and destruction of tubules and in hyalinization of glomeruli by a process of periglomerular fibrosis and capsular thickening. Hyaline casts are present in enlarged tubules with atrophic epithelium, and some areas may have a thyroid-like appearance (Fig. 14-18). Eventually, there results a kidney that is coarsely pitted by shallow, often broad, U-shaped scars, greatly contracted, and of little functional value. Such a pyelonephritic contracture of the kidney may be unilateral and must be distinguished from unilateral renal hypoplasia. Since chronic pyelonephritis usually is bilateral, its end stages sometimes may be confused clinically with chronic glomerulonephritis. Morphologic differences between chronic pyelonephritis and chronic glomerulonephritis are noted in Table 14-1. Vascular changes and hypertension frequently are associated with chronic and healed stages of pyelonephritis.

Although many cases of chronic pyelonephritis can be traced from an acute onset, with persistent or recurrent bacterial infection, there is a significant number of chronic cases that are not related to an antecedent acute phase. It is noted especially that patients with chronic pyelonephritis not associated with urinary tract obstruction (nonobstructive chronic pyelonephritis) often have no evidence of past or current infection. Although in such instances one cannot exclude the possibility that prior asymptomatic bacterial infection may be involved, it has been suggested that damage may be produced by factors other than infection.

Necrosis of renal papillae (necrotizing renal papillitis). Necrosis of the renal papillae occurs as a complication of acute pyelonephritis, particularly in diabetic patients over 40 years of age, but also in nondiabetic patients with urinary tract obstruction (e.g., due to prostatic enlargement). Acute pyelonephritis is a fairly frequent complication of diabetes mellitus, and about 25% of patients show some necrosis of renal papillae, usually bilaterally. In some, the clinical course is fulminating, with death in a few days. The necrotic papillae stand out as pale, grayish yellow, infarctlike areas bordered by a reddish zone of inflammatory reaction (Fig. 14-19). Sequestration of the necrotic papillae occurs, and the necrotic material, in late stages, may be sloughed away and appear in the urine.

The pathogenesis of renal papillary necrosis

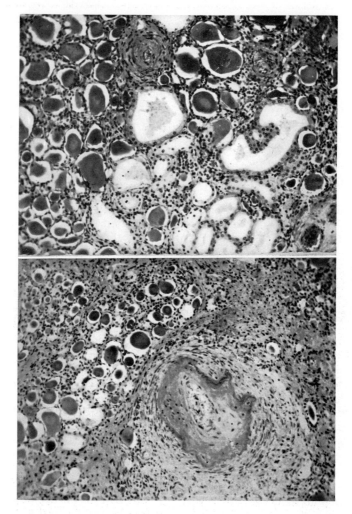

Fig. 14-18. Chronic pyelonephritis. Note dilated tubules filled with casts (thyroidlike appearance) and thickened blood vessels.

is not clear, although it appears to be related to interference with the blood supply to the tips of the medullary pyramids. Among the factors considered to cause ischemia are compression of the medullary vessels by inflammatory edema or by pressure of urine in the pelvis (in cases of urinary tract obstruction) and vasospasm associated with infection. Papillary necrosis seems to occur more commonly when infection is present in kidneys with sclerotic arteries.

Necrosis of renal papillae also has been de-

scribed in patients with a history of prolonged heavy use of analgesics. Previously, the lesion was thought to be caused by phenacetin, a common component of analgesics, and was referred to as "phenacetin nephritis." However, it was later observed that some patients with the lesion consumed analgesics that did not contain phenacetin. This observation, together with certain experimental evidence, suggests that analgesics other than phenacetin (e.g., aspirin) may also cause this lesion. The lesion is now referred to simply as *analgesic*

Table 14-1. Differentiating features of chronic pyelonephritis and chronic glomerulonephritis

	Chronic pyelonephritis	Chronic glomerulonephritis
Involvement	Unilateral, bilateral, or unequal	Bilateral
Gross	Nodularity or broad coarse scars	Fine granularity
Extent	Patchy	Diffuse
Glomerular changes	Focal or in scarred area	Diffusely involved
Membranous or proliferative glomerular lesions	Rare	Common
Tubular disappearance	In relatively large areas without glomerulosclerosis	Proportionate to sclerosed glomeruli
Dilated tubules with hyaline casts (thyroidlike areas)	Common	Small and uncommon
Hypertrophy of remaining tubules	Slight	Common and marked
Neutrophilic leukocytes	Common	Few
Plasma cells	Common	Infrequent
Vascular changes	Often severe	Usually moderate
Inflammation of pelvis	Usual	Infrequent
Necrosis of papillae	May be present	Absent

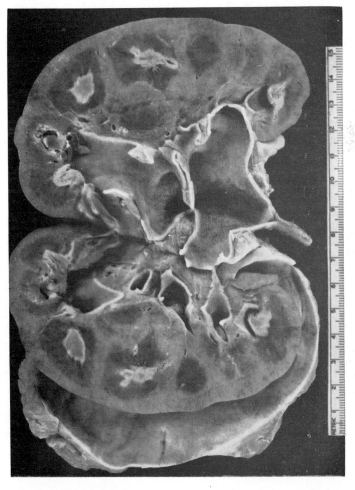

Fig. 14-19. Papillary necrosis of kidney in diabetes mellitus with ureteral stenosis and mild hydronephrosis.

nephropathy. The renal papillary necrosis usually is not accompanied by extensive neutrophilic exudate along the periphery as in pyelonephritis. The renal cortex may show varying degrees of chronic interstitial nephritis with fibrosis. In some recent studies, an unusual thickening of the small vessels in the lower urinary tract, including the renal pelvic and papillary vessels, has been described as an effect of analgesic abuse ("analgesic microangiopathy"), and the papillary necrosis in analgesic nephropathy has been attributed to ischemia resulting from this vascular lesion.

Papillary necrosis has also been observed in patients with *sickle cell anemia* and has been attributed to blockage of vasa recta by sickling red blood cells.

Experimentally, papillary necrosis of the kidney has been produced in rats by the intravenous administration of bromethylamine hydrobromide (BEA). Although it was originally thought that vasoconstriction was responsible for development of the lesion, it has been shown recently that medullary blood flow is not decreased following BEA administration. The possibility that BEA causes direct cytotoxic effect has been considered.

Pyonephrosis. When an obstructive factor is added to pyelonephritis, hydronephrosis and hydronephrotic atrophy are also present in variable degree. When the distended hydronephrotic pelvis is filled with pus, the condition is referred to as pyonephrosis. The end result may be a thin-walled sac filled with pus.

Radiation nephritis. When renal tissue is included in the field of therapeutic deep irradiation, renal damage may result, sometimes sufficiently severe to lead to hypertension or death from renal functional failure. Symptoms usually begin 6 to 12 months after the radiotherapy. The kidneys show thickened capsules and pericapsular fibrosis. Tubules are atrophic, with widespread interstitial fibrosis, glomerular damage, and fibrinoid necrotic lesions of arterioles.

Tuberculosis. Renal tuberculosis is secondary to an active tuberculous lesion elsewhere, the organisms reaching the kidney by hematogenous spread. The kidneys usually are involved along with other organs in acute miliary tuberculosis, but another form of renal tuberculosis also occurs in which there is a chronic ulcerative and spreading lesion. This form is usually unilateral, and the primary focus from which spread occurred is often not prominent. Embolic masses of organisms arrested in the kidney produce the first lesion in the cortex. By discharge of this lesion into a tubule, spread occurs to the medulla, where a caseous ulcerative tubercle appears on a renal papilla. From there, spread occurs to the mucosa of the pelvis, ureter, and bladder. Reinfection and extension to other portions of the kidney readily follow. Tuberculous strictures of the ureter and individual calices lead to stasis of the urine and hydronephrotic changes. There is a progression of the tuberculous process in the kidney tissue, with caseation, loss of tissue through ulceration, and hydronephrosis.

The appearance of the kidney depends on the state of the process. In an early period, a few yellowish opaque tubercles are seen in the cortex and near the tips of papillae. Later, caseous masses of varying size replace the renal tissue, and the ragged hydronephrotic cavities contain a thick, creamy pus.

The infected ureter becomes thick walled, rigid, and stenosed. The urinary bladder involvement begins at the ureteral opening and spreads as an irregular area of ulceration.

METABOLIC DISEASE
Hyperparathyroid renal disease

Renal hyperparathyroidism. Deficiency of renal function stimulates hyperplasia and hyperfunction of the parathyroid glands. The actual stimulating factor is probably some disturbance of calcium or phosphorus balance resulting from renal deficiency. Parathyroid hyperplasia and hyperfunction are present to some degree in all patients having severe deficiency of renal function.

Renal osteodystrophy. Various bone lesions have been described in association with chronic renal insufficiency with azotemia (renal or azotemic osteodystrophy). Retention of phosphates and low serum calcium are usual, although the latter may be normal, since it may be corrected by hypersecretion of the parathyroid glands, which become secondarily hyperplastic. The bone lesions may resemble rickets (in children) or osteomalacia (in adults). In severe cases, the changes are those of osteitis fibrosa cystica. Osteosclerosis has been reported in some patients. In children, the renal osteodystrophy has been referred to as "renal rickets," or, because it is associated with stunting of growth, it has been termed "renal dwarfism." The actual lesions in the urinary tract include those of a congenital nature (e.g., polycystic kidneys, hypoplasia, and abnormalities of the lower urinary tract resulting in dilatation of the ureters and hydronephrosis), chronic interstitial nephritis, chronic pyelonephritis, and chronic glomerulonephritis.

The cause of the skeletal changes in chronic renal insufficiency is obscure. The basic cause had been considered to be the metabolic disturbances initiated by hyperphosphatemia or by acidosis, but some investigators believe there is an acquired resistance to vitamin D accompanied by a compensatory hyperplasia and hypersecretion of the parathyroid glands.

Parathyroid nephritis. Hyperparathyroidism itself may produce renal lesions of a distinctive type and result in renal failure. The parathyroid hyperfunction may be caused by a localized adenomatous overgrowth of a single parathyroid gland or by a diffuse hyperplasia of all the parathyroid glands. The resulting disturbance in calcium metabolism appears to be the main cause of the damage to the kidney. Calcium deposits in the kidney are the characteristic feature.

In acute hyperparathyroidism the calcium may be mainly intratubular, but in chronic hyperparathyroidism it is interstitial and peritubular and is accompanied by interstitial fibrosis and cellular infiltration. Renal calculus formation is frequent and develops on the basis of a parenchymal calcium concretion (Fig. 14-20). Hyperparathyroidism is, however, the underlying cause of only a very small proportion of renal calculi.

Nephrocalcinosis

Calcification in the kidney (nephrocalcinosis) occurs not only with hyperparathyroidism, but also in the disturbance of calcium metabolism of the milk-alkali syndrome, sarcoidosis, and hypervitaminosis D. It also may be the result of skeletal involvement in multiple myeloma and some metastatic cancers, and it occurs in renal tubular acidosis, hy-

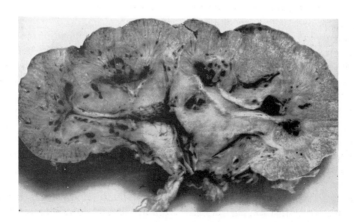

Fig. 14-20. Chronic interstitial nephritis and hyperparathyroid renal disease in hyperparathyroidism caused by parathyroid adenoma. Black calculous masses are evident in renal substance and in pelvis.

pochloremic alkalosis from excessive vomiting, and after tubular injury by nephrotoxins such as mercury bichloride.

Calculi

Stones, or calculi, formed in the urinary tract are caused by precipitation of chemical salts in the urine. Calculi frequently are classified as primary and secondary. The primary stones are those formed without apparent causal factors, such as infection, inflammation, or urinary obstruction and stasis. Secondary stones are those that follow evident inflammation or obstruction.

Etiology. The causes of stone formation are of two types: (1) those factors that cause increased urinary concentration of the crystalloids that compose stones and (2) changes of a physical or chemical nature in the urine or urinary tract that favor precipitation of crystalloids.

High concentration of crystalline salts in the urine favors precipitation. Colloids in the urine hold the crystalloids in solution in a supersaturated state. The balance is delicate and easily disturbed either by hyperexcretion of crystalloids, such as may occur in hyperparathyroidism, or by decrease of colloids, which may be caused by infection.

Encrustation of solid material with urinary salts is a factor of importance. A nidus for such precipitation may be bacteria, necrotic or degenerated tissue, or other foreign bodies. Encrustation frequently occurs on a small calcified plaque of a renal papilla.

Urinary reaction is important in the maintenance of urinary salts in solution and largely determines the composition of the stones. However, reaction alone (e.g., great alkalinity) is probably never the cause of stone formation.

Urinary obstruction acts by promoting stagnation and infection. It is rarely the sole factor.

Hyperparathyroidism has a known direct relationship to renal stone formation but probably accounts for 1% or less of renal calculi, although in some clinics up to 5% have been ascribed to hyperparathyroidism. The greatly increased excretion of calcium and phosphorus in the urine and the tendency to deposition of calcium salts in renal tissue result in calculus formation in 30% to 70% of patients with hyperparathyroidism.

Pathogenesis. A mechanism of primary stone formation has been described by Randall. Damage to a renal papilla results in calcium deposit in the injured tissue. When near the surface, this plaque of calcium becomes exposed by ulceration of overlying tissue and becomes a nidus on which any urinary salt may crystallize. Successive depositions produce a laminated stone, often of variable composition (Fig. 14-21). The plaque holds the stone in place until it has time to reach a considerable size before tearing away from its moorings.

Types. While stones often are composed of mixtures of uric acid, calcium oxalate, and phosphates, certain constituents predominate and give the stone distinctive character.

Uric acid stones (10% of renal stones) are brown, fairly smooth, and moderately hard and, on section, show concentric laminations. *Cystine stones* (less than 5% of renal stones) are yellowish and waxy. *Calcium oxalate stones* (15% to 30% of renal stones) are very hard, have a rough spiny surface of dark brown color, and are laminated. *Phosphate stones* (20% of renal stones) are soft, smooth, white, and friable. More than 50% of renal stones are composed of a mixture of calcium oxalate and phosphate.

Uric acid and cystine tend to precipitate in an acid urine, whereas phosphate stones are commonly associated with alkaline urines. Oxalate stones may form in urine at any pH.

Effects. Renal calculi may obstruct the outflow of urine, promote infection, and cause the pain of renal colic. The point of obstruction may be in the renal pelvis, ureters, or bladder. Partial or intermittent obstruction gives rise to dilatation of the ureter or renal pelvis (hydronephrosis) above the obstructed point. Stasis caused by obstruction promotes infection (pyelonephritis). Passage of a small stone through the ureter produces the severe pain of renal colic.

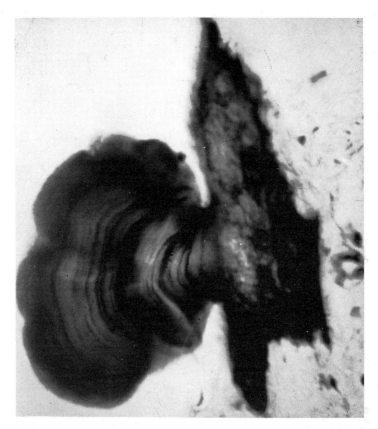

Fig. 14-21. Renal calculus. Calcium plaque in tissue of renal papilla with attached early stone. Note arrow necklike attachment of calculus and its laminated structure caused by successive deposits of precipitated material. (From Anderson, W. A. D.: J. Urol. **44:**29-34, 1940.)

Oxalosis

Oxalosis is a rare primary disturbance of oxalate metabolism, with the deposition of calcium oxalate in the kidneys and other tissues. Hyperoxaluria is accompanied by progressive calcium oxalate urolithiasis and nephrocalcinosis, usually beginning in early childhood. Renal damage occurs with recurrent urinary tract infection, and the cause of eventual death is usually renal failure. Oxalate also may be found in the myocardium, the walls of small arteries, and the rete testis.

Urate deposits

Uric acid infarcts and urate deposits in gout are considered on pp. 38-40.

OBSTRUCTIVE DISEASE

Hydronephrosis. Hydronephrosis is a dilatation of the renal pelvis and associated atrophy of renal tissue resulting from an obstruction to the outflow of urine (Fig. 14-22). Obstruction may result from a wide variety of causes (e.g., prostatic enlargements, calculi, congenital and inflammatory strictures, pregnancy, and tumors). Obstructions at or below the outlet of the bladder result in bilateral hydronephrosis. With obstruction of one ureter only, the corresponding kidney is hydronephrotic.

The degree of hydronephrosis depends on the degree and duration of the obstruction. Partial and intermittent obstructions result in a

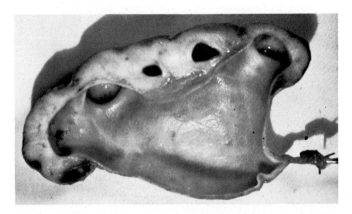

Fig. 14-22. Hydronephrosis caused by obstruction of upper end of ureter.

greater degree of hydronephrosis than do sudden complete obstructions. The latter tend to produce atrophy with relatively little hydronephrosis. In some cases, no mechanical obstruction can be demonstrated (nonobstructive hydronephrosis). Some of such cases may result from spinal cord lesions that cause paralysis of the bladder. Neuromuscular imbalance has been postulated as a possible explanation for others.

With distention of the renal pelvis, the calices flatten, the renal tissue becomes atrophic and thin (Fig. 14-23), and the dilated pelvis assumes a saccular and rounded form. In severe cases, the total size of the kidney and pelvis may be increased and the outer surface lobulated. The atrophy and fibrosis of the renal parenchyma affect tubules more rapidly than glomeruli. Hence, except in late stages, the tubular atrophy may seem to be out of proportion to the glomerular changes. Eventually, glomeruli become hyalinized. The occurrence of infection converts the condition into pyonephrosis. When hydronephrosis is unilateral, the opposite kidney may undergo a compensatory hypertrophy.

CONGENITAL MALFORMATIONS AND ANOMALIES

Agenesis and hypoplasia. Complete absence *(agenesis)* of both kidneys is rare and incompatible with life. In some instances, small nonfunctioning rudimentary kidneys may be found *(aplasia)*. Bilateral *hypoplasia* of severe degree likewise is incompatible with life. However, in less severe form, the child may live for months or a few years, in which instance there may be accompanying bone changes (renal rickets or osteodystrophy) and stunting of growth. Absence or hypoplasia of one kidney is more common, and the opposite kidney is larger than normal (compensatory hypertrophy).

Fusion. Congenital fusion of the kidneys, *horseshoe kidneys,* is most commonly a connection of the lower poles, either by a fibrous band or by actual renal tissue. The pelves are separate, and the ureters pass anteriorly across the lower poles of the kidneys (Fig. 14-24).

Duplication of ureters or double pelvis. The duplication of ureters and a double pelvis are common anomalies that usually are of no functional significance, although some investigators believe that they are more susceptible to complications. Persistence of some degree of fetal lobulation of the kidneys is also very common and harmless.

Anomalous renal vessels. Because of their abnormal position, anomalous blood vessels may produce compression of the ureter and cause hydronephrosis.

CYSTS

Cysts of the kidney are of three main types: *solitary cysts, retention cysts,* caused by tubular dilatation in vascular or inflammatory

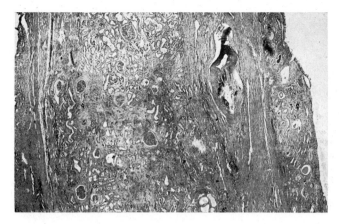

Fig. 14-23. Hydronephrotic atrophy of kidney. Full thickness of renal substance, with pelvic mucosa evident at right.

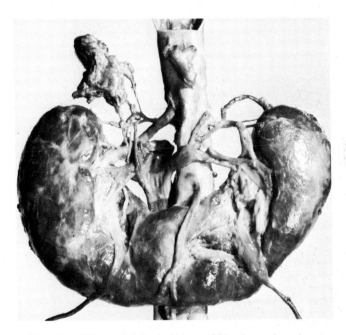

Fig. 14-24. Horseshoe kidney showing relations of blood vessels and ureters.

disease of the kidney, and the condition of *congenital polycystic kidneys*. A fourth variety, *peripelvic lymphatic cysts,* is rare.

The solitary cysts are usually serous, but they may be hemorrhagic. They vary from a few millimeters to several centimeters in di-

ameter. Some are congenital in origin, and others result from tubular obstruction. Occasionally, they are multilocular.

In advanced renal vascular disease or glomerulonephritis, there frequently are multiple small retention cysts, usually only a few mil-

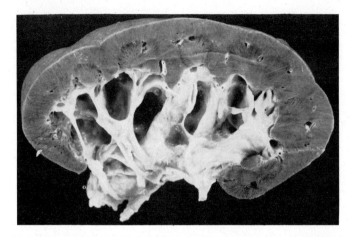

Fig. 14-25. Peripelvic cysts of kidney. (Courtesy Dr. J. F. Kuzma.)

limeters in diameter, resulting from tubular dilatation.

Peripelvic lymphatic cysts of the kidney are lymphatic distentions associated with obstruction of the lymphatic trunks of the hilus of the kidney (Fig. 14-25). They are usually small and unimportant, but rarely they have caused damage by pressure on renal vessels. They may distort the pelvic outline in roentgenograms.

Congenital polycystic kidneys. Polycystic kidney is a congenital maldevelopment. One or both kidneys may be involved by extremely numerous cysts of varying and often large size. The condition is present at birth, and absence of sufficient functioning renal tissue may result in death at that time or within the next few years. If renal functional tissue is sufficient, life may go on with little or no clinical evidence of the disease until the third, fourth, or fifth decade. At that time, renal failure results from the development of vascular disease, other accumulated injuries (e.g., infection) of the kidney, or progressive increase in the size of the cysts. The patients may have lumbar pain, a palpable mass in the kidney region, and hematuria, a picture simulating renal neoplasm. Other patients simply have acute or chronic renal failure with hypertension and cardiac hypertrophy, so that clinical differentiation from other types of renal dis-

ease may be very difficult. Attacks of hematuria are a quite distinctive finding and are caused by the rupture of blood vessels into cysts communicating with the pelvis.

The involved kidneys may be moderately or enormously enlarged, resulting from an increase in size of individual cysts rather than from an increase in their number. The kidneys have a knobby or irregular outline. The cysts are lined by cuboidal or, more commonly, flattened epithelium. In the newborn group, the remaining renal tissue is hypoplastic, the number of nephrons is reduced, and interstitial connective tissue is excessive. At a later age, in patients without clinical symptoms, the functional renal tissue between cysts is often abundant. The patients dying of renal failure show extreme atrophy of the renal tissue between the cysts, which is caused by progressive cystic enlargement and associated development of arterial disease.

Polycystic kidneys can be divided into several distinct types. Type 1, relatively uncommon, is found in newborn infants and usually is incompatible with continued life. The symmetrically enlarged kidneys have a spongy appearance (Fig. 14-26). The cysts are saccular or cylindrically enlarged collecting tubules. The disease appears to result from a hyperplasia of the interstitial portions of the collecting tubules developing from the ureteral buds. In-

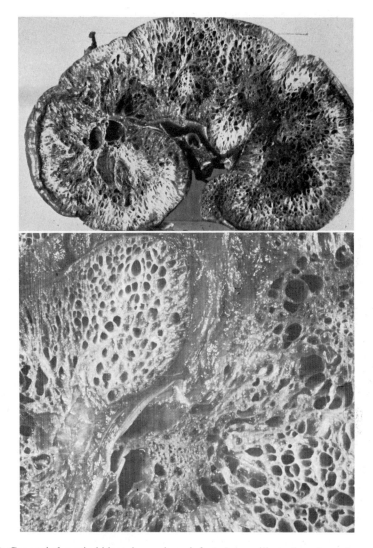

Fig. 14-26. Congenital cystic kidney in newborn infant. Lower illustration shows low magnification of cut surface.

trahepatic bile ducts usually are also cystic. The condition is apparently inherited as an autosomal recessive trait.

Type 2, seen at any age, may involve a portion of a kidney, one kidney, or both kidneys. Unilateral polycystic kidneys in adults are usually of this type. Bilateral involvement is usually fatal in infancy. The terminal or ampullar portion of collecting tubules is cys-

tic. The condition does not appear to be familial.

Type 3 is the common large bilateral polycystic disease of adults (Fig. 14-27). There is an irregular mixture of normal and abnormal tubules and nephrons. Cysts involve various parts of the nephron (Fig. 14-28). Connective tissue is increased. Cysts of other organs, particularly the liver, may be present. Occasion-

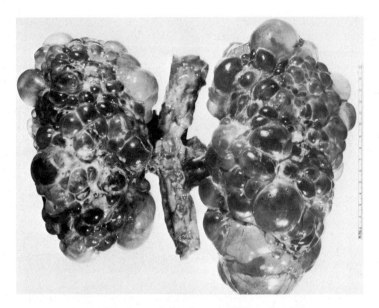

Fig. 14-27. Congenital polycystic kidneys in adult.

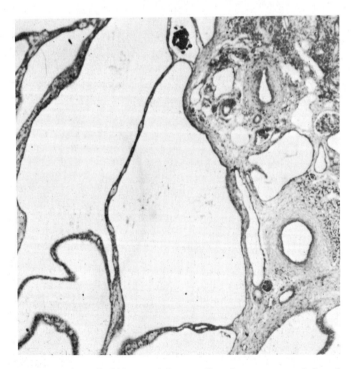

Fig. 14-28. Congenital polycystic kidney, adult type. Prominent cysts on left and atrophic renal tissue, with smaller cysts, on right.

ally, congenital (berry) aneurysms of cerebral arteries also may be present. There is sometimes a familial history, and it is believed to be inherited as an autosomal dominant trait with variable expression.

Type 4 is uncommon. The cysts are small, located mainly in the outer cortex, and are dilated Bowman's spaces. The condition appears to be caused by urethral or ureteral obstruction in early fetal development.

TUMORS
Benign tumors

Adenoma. Adenoma of the kidney is quite common and usually appears as a small (0.5 to 2 cm) gray or grayish yellow nodule in the cortex, at times projecting above the suface beneath the capsule of the kidney (Fig. 14-29). Microscopically, the epithelial cells, some of which may be vacuolated and contain lipid, form well-differentiated tubules, papillary structures, or solid masses. Some of the solid adenomas histologically may resemble certain renal carcinomas.

Fibroma. Fibroma is commonly found in the medulla, where it appears as a tiny grayish area. It is composed of irregularly arranged connective tissue fibers. The margin is usually irregular or ill defined, and a few tubules often are enclosed in the tumor. Many of them

may be of developmental origin or hamartomas. Fibromas are of little practical importance.

Lipoma. Lipoma of the kidney occurs rarely and may grow to a large size or undergo malignant change.

Hamartoma. *Angiomyolipomas* are often multiple, bilateral, and composed of an unorganized mixture of fibrous and fatty tissue, blood vessels, and smooth muscle fibers. Since they are often large, they may produce symptoms. These lesions are seen frequently in patients with tuberous sclerosis but may appear in the absence of the latter. A *leiomyomatous hamartoma* occurring in infants and young children has been observed that may be misdiagnosed as a Wilms' tumor. It consists of predominantly smooth muscle–type spindle cells.

Juxtaglomerular cell tumor. An unusual tumor composed of renin-producing JG cells of the kidney has been described in association with hypertension, aldosteronism, and hyperreninemia (p. 349). Electron microscopically, the JG cells contained rhomboid, polygonal, and round cytoplasmic granules. The rhomboid granules exhibited a crystalline substructure. In one report, mast cells were seen in association with the JG cells in the tumor, but their significance is not known.

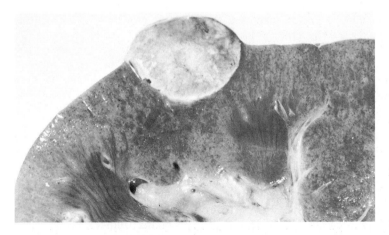

Fig. 14-29. Adenoma of kidney.

Malignant tumors

Malignant renal tumors are of unusual interest. They are of four types: (1) renal cell carcinoma (hypernephroma; Grawitz's tumor), which occurs particularly in the fifth and sixth decades, (2) embryonal adenosarcoma (Wilms' tumor), which occurs in infancy and early childhood, (3) carcinoma of the renal pelvis, and (4) sarcoma.

Renal cell carcinoma. Renal cell carcinoma, also known as hypernephroma, adenocarcinoma, or Grawitz's tumor, is the common malignant renal tumor of adults. It is called hypernephroma because it has been supposed to arise from "rests" of adrenal cells in the kidney. Small areas of adrenal cortical tissue often are found in the outer part of the kidney, just beneath the capsule. Adrenal heterotopia, with all or part of the adrenal glands within the capsule of the kidneys, is sometimes encountered. Also, adrenal tissue is not uncommon on the undersurface of the liver and in internal genitalia. Further, the adrenal nature of these tumors was suggested because of their microscopic resemblance to the adrenal cortex. They are composed of large, clear cells containing abundant, doubly refractive cholesterol esters, and the cells may be arranged in cords as in the adrenal cortex. However, this evidence is insufficient proof of their adrenal origin. Some areas of the tumor may show a papillary or tubular structure, and all gradations may be found between a close resemblance to adrenal cortex and clear-cut renal carcinoma. Hence, hypernephromas generally are considered to be simply renal carcinomas. Their origin is believed to be the convoluted tubular epithelium, as evidenced by electron microscopic studies of the tumor cells.

Renal cell carcinomas occur almost always after the age of 40 years. Their frequency in males is more than twice that in females. Occasionally, there is an associated polycythemia that disappears after nephrectomy. Erythropoietic-stimulating activity (erythropoietin) has been demonstrated in the tumor tissue or in the plasma in some instances. Hypercalcemia in the absence of bone metastases oc-

curs with some renal carcinomas because of secretion of a parathormonelike material by the tumors. Some renal carcinomas are accompanied by elevated urinary alkaline phosphatase activity and elevated urinary lactic dehydrogenase (LDH) activity. These enzyme changes are not specific for these lesions but are an aid in the diagnosis of renal carcinoma in the presence of a renal mass.

Renal cell carcinoma forms a large rounded tumor in the kidney (Fig. 14-30), at first well encapsulated and separated from the renal tissue. It is microscopically invasive, however, so that it is not easily shelled out or separated from surrounding tissue. The yellowish cut surface shows some connective tissue trabeculae coursing irregularly through the tumor. There is a great tendency to degeneration, necrosis, hemorrhage, and cyst formation.

Microscopically, the characteristic cells are large, with abundant pale, foamy cytoplasm (Fig. 14-31). In some areas, the cells may be smaller, with a denser, slightly granular, and more eosinophilic cytoplasm, more like ordinary renal tubular epithelium. The cells are arranged in solid sheets or as cords and papillary structures with a thin supporting stroma. The well-differentiated tumors of lower grade malignancy form tubular or papillary structures. Tumors of high malignancy have little tubular or papillary formation and show greater variation in size and staining of cells and nuclei and more frequent mitoses.

The growth of the tumor causes atrophy and fibrosis of adjacent tissue. In later stages, there is extensive invasion of renal substance. The tumor cells have a tendency to invade veins and grow along the blood vessels. Metastasis occurs by bloodstream, and the lungs, liver, and bones are the common sites for the secondary tumors.

Because of the relatively localized growth of this carcinoma in its early stages, it may attain considerable size with only painless hematuria as clinical evidence of its presence. Metastases in the lungs or bones may be the first indication.

Wilms' tumor. Wilms' tumor, also called *embryoma* or *embryonal adenosarcoma,* is a

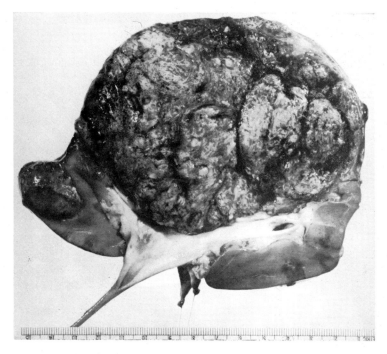

Fig. 14-30. Renal cell carcinoma (''hypernephroma'') of kidney.

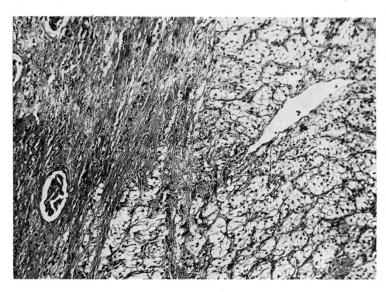

Fig. 14-31. Renal cell carcinoma (''hypernephroma'') of kidney. Compressed atrophic renal substance may be seen at left.

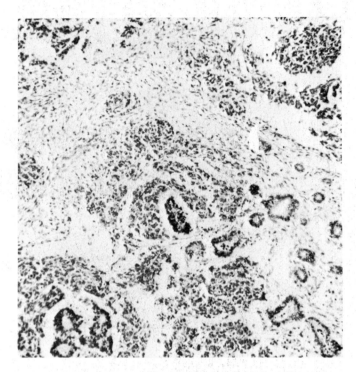

Fig. 14-32. Wilms' tumor of kidney. Solid epithelial masses and tubular structures with background of paler mesenchymal tissue.

rare mixed tumor of the kidney, the occurrence of which is almost entirely limited to the first 7 years of life (average age, 3 years), although a few cases have been reported in adults. These tumors account for about 20% of cancers in childhood. The origin is believed to be from mesodermal cells displaced during development but retaining the ability to grow and differentiate into various types of tissue. Other abnormalities, e.g., aniridia and chromosomal defects, may occur in Wilms' tumor patients.

At first, the tumor is surrounded by a dense connective tissue capsule and remains separated from the renal parenchyma until quite large. The kidney tissue is pushed into various shapes. Eventually, the capsule is ruptured and extension occurs to kidney tissue, omentum, and adjacent viscera. Blood-borne metastases are common in the lungs, but other organs, including the liver and brain, may be involved. Lymphatic spread to regional lymph nodes occurs frequently.

The tumor tissue is uniformly grayish white and moderately firm, but cysts or hemorrhage may be present. Microscopically, the predominant tumor elements are an abundant embryonic type of malignant connective tissue surrounding some glandlike tubules of variable size and shape. Epithelial cells also may form solid cords and strands of cells (Fig. 14-32). Occasionally, smooth or striated muscle, cartilage, or myxomatous tissue is present.

Sarcoma. Sarcoma may arise from connective tissue of the kidney, but this is uncommon. Examples of fibrosarcoma and liposarcoma have been reported. Instances of carcinosarcoma of the kidney in adults have been reported, the tumors differing from Wilms' tumor in that they lack embryonal features microscopically.

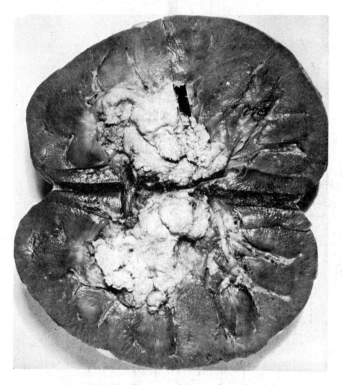

Fig. 14-33. Papillary carcinoma of renal pelvis.

Tumors of renal pelvis

The pelvis of the kidney gives rise to the same types of tumor as are found in the bladder, the common forms being transitional cell papilloma and papillary carcinoma (Fig 14-33). The papillary carcinomas may give rise to secondary implants lower down in the ureter. Poorly differentiated infiltrating forms, which extend into the renal substance, also occur. An infrequent variety is squamous cell carcinoma.

Lower urinary tract

URETER

The most important pathologic involvement of the ureters is *obstruction,* which may be caused by a calculus from the renal pelvis, by a stricture of congenital or inflammatory origin (Fig. 14-34), or, less frequently, by tumors either of the ureter itself or adjacent to and pressing on the ureter. Kinking of the ureter, which occurs when the kidney is abnormally movable, or an aberrant renal artery crossing the ureter causes some cases of partial or intermittent obstruction. Hydronephrosis is the common result unless the obstruction is transitory. Obstruction of the urinary tract below the ureters causes bilateral dilatation of the ureters (hydroureter).

Ureteritis cystica is a condition that may contribute to ureteral obstruction (Fig. 14-35). The cysts develop from the cell nests of von Brunn, which probably are focal downgrowths of mucosa occurring as a consequence of ureteritis. The upper portion of the ureter is most frequently involved, and there is frequent association with similar cystic lesions of the renal pelvis (pyelitis cystica) and the urinary bladder (cystitis cystica).

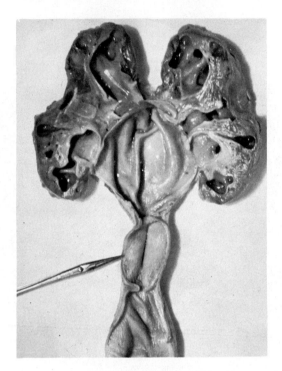

Fig. 14-34. Multiple strictures of ureter with hydronephrosis.

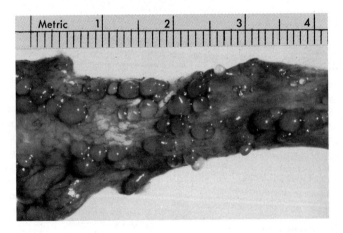

Fig. 14-35. Ureteritis cystica.

Tumors of the ureter are uncommon and are of the same gross and histologic types as those that arise in the bladder.

Vesicoureteral reflux is an abnormality characterized by a retrograde flow of urine from the bladder into the ureter and renal pelvis, a condition that predisposes to bacterial infection and is likely a factor leading to pyelonephritis in many children. The cause may be a congenital malimplantation of the ureter into

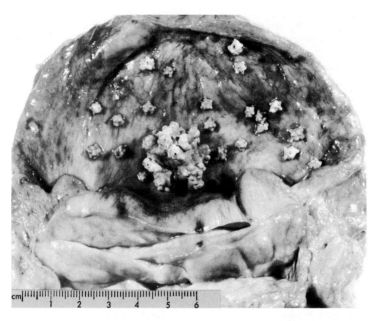

Fig. 14-36. Calculi in urinary bladder.

the bladder, but often it is due to an abnormal vesicoureteral sphincter mechanism. Vesicoureteral reflux can also occur when there is a bladder outlet obstruction with increased intravesical pressure.

URINARY BLADDER

Inflammation, obstruction, and tumors are the important lesions of the bladder. Congenital abnormalities and traumatic changes are less common.

Inflammation

Inflammation of the bladder *(cystitis)* may be acute or chronic. The infection may descend from a pyelonephritis, may reach the bladder by way of the urethra, or may be introduced by catheterization. The use of urinary antiseptics and the presence of calculi (Fig. 14-36) or other foreign bodies are factors that may induce inflammation. Obstruction of the bladder outlet, as by an enlarged prostate gland, is particularly likely to be associated with chronic inflammation. Important organisms in cystitis are pyogenic cocci and the colon bacillus.

Acute cystitis. In acute cystitis, the mucosa is congested and edematous. Congestion and inflammatory cells, particularly in the submucosa, are evident microscopically. More severe cystitis may be hemorrhagic, ulcerative, or gangrenous.

Chronic cystitis. Chronic cystitis is associated with considerable thickening of the bladder wall by granulation tissue and fibrosis unless an associated obstruction causes the wall to be dilated. Occasionally, the thickened mucosa shows small fluid-filled cystic cavities, the so-called cystitis cystica. Other special varieties of cystitis have been given the descriptive names of interstitial cystitis, gangrenous cystitis, follicular cystitis, bullous cystitis, etc.

Malakoplakia. Malakoplakia is an uncommon inflammatory condition characterized by soft, grayish yellow plaques involving the mucosa of the bladder. The etiology is not established, but it is associated with long-standing cystitis. The sessile plaques are formed by accumulations of cells in the mucosa and submucosa. Although there is a mixture of inflammatory cells, large mononuclear or histiocytic cells are most characteristic. Laminated, hematoxylin-staining structures (Michaelis-Gutmann bodies) may be present, and they are similar to the Schaumann bodies of sarcoidosis.

Obstruction

Obstruction to the outlet of the urinary bladder may be caused by prostatic hyperplasia, strictures of the urethra, tumor, calculus, or neurogenic disturbance. The bladder becomes distended and thin walled. Hypertrophy of muscle bundles follows if the obstruction is prolonged, so that the inner surface of the distended bladder is roughened by prominent muscular trabeculae. Distention of weak areas between the trabeculae may produce multiple small (false) diverticula.

Tumors

Tumors of the urinary bladder are more frequent in men and commonly occur in the age group of 50 to 70 years. Etiologic factors are not apparent in most instances. Industrial exposure to chemical agents (e.g., in aniline dye industry) is a factor in some cases. A higher incidence of bladder cancer is noted among those exposed to aromatic compounds, such as α- and β-naphthylamine, 4-aminodiphenyl, 4-nitrodiphenyl, and benzidine. The actual active carcinogenic substance may be a metabolic product of the chemical to which a person is exposed. Other factors suspected as causative in bladder cancer include cigarette smoking, certain food additives, chronic inflammations, vesical calculi, and infection with the parasite *Schistosoma haematobium*.

The common types of bladder tumors are papilloma and transitional cell carcinoma. Various other types, including squamous cell carcinoma, adenocarcinoma, and mucous carcinoma, occur only rarely. Some of the mucous adenocarcinomas appear to be of urachal origin and have a poor prognosis. Most bladder tumors appear in the trigone and lateral and posterior walls.

Papilloma. The papilloma is a delicate pedunculated tumor projecting from the mucosal surface. It has a narrow base and many fine villous processes that are not fused. Delicate branching villi compose the tumor, each having a thin connective tissue core containing blood vessels, separated by a definite basal membrane from a surface covering of transitional epithelium. The epithelium is well differentiated, and its cells are uniform in size, shape, and staining. Mitoses are rarely seen, if at all.

Papillomas may be single or multiple and frequently tend to recur. They are potentially malignant, although they may remain benign for months or years. Changes in the epithelial cells (such as an increase in the number of layers of cells, loss of polarity, atypical staining of nuclei, and some mitoses) and penetration of the cells through the basement membrane are evidence of transition of the papilloma to malignancy. Such a lesion is sometimes referred to as a "malignant papilloma."

Carcinoma. The usual form of bladder cancer is *transitional cell carcinoma*. Grossly, this tumor may be papillary, flat, or nodular and may be ulcerative or nonulcerative. The papillary carcinomas have a general architecture similar to histologically benign papillomas, but the villous processes tend to be shorter and fused. The tumors become bulky and cauliflowerlike with a tendency to hemorrhage and necrosis (Fig. 14-37). There is more irregularity of arrangement, size, and shape of the epithelial cells, and mitoses are more numerous than in histologically benign papillomas. The papillary carcinomas may be noninfiltrating or infiltrating. In the latter, there is invasion of the base of the tumor and the wall of the bladder. The sessile, flat, or nodular types of transitional cell carcinoma are infiltrating tumors. They may spread widely through the bladder wall and even to surrounding structures without forming a larger tumor in the bladder lumen. Microscopically, the tumors vary in the degree of differentiation, their cells ranging from those that maintain a resemblance to the transitional cell type to those that are highly anaplastic and pleomorphic, so that their cell type is difficult to recognize. Foci of squamous cell metaplasia may be seen in these tumors.

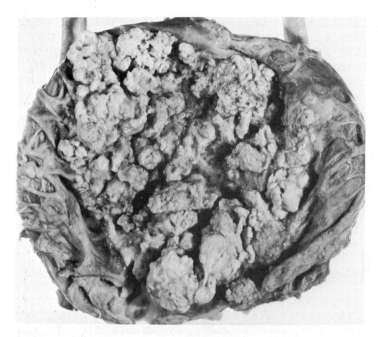

Fig. 14-37. Carcinoma of urinary bladder.

The much less common *squamous cell carcinoma of the bladder* is also an infiltrating tumor and tends to be flat, slightly elevated, and ulcerated. *Adenocarcinoma of the bladder* is rare, and its origin is not clear.

Bladder carcinoma spreads by contiguity through the vesical wall and then to adjacent structures (e.g., rectum, sigmoid, prostate, ureter, vagina, uterus, and pelvic wall). Spread by the lymphatics occurs commonly, with involvement of the pelvic and abdominal lymph nodes. Blood-borne metastases to the liver, lungs, bone, and other organs may occur later.

Male genitalia

PENIS

Phimosis. Phimosis is a condition in which the foreskin cannot be retracted.

Paraphimosis. In paraphimosis, a retracted foreskin cannot be brought forward. Paraphimosis, as well as phimosis, may be congeni-

tal or may be acquired and caused by inflammatory swelling and edema.

Balanitis. Balanitis is an inflammation of the glans. It is predisposed to by phimosis. The gonococcus and the colon bacillus are the common causative organisms.

Peyronie's disease. Peyronie's disease is a plastic induration or fibrosis of the penis. Its cause is unknown.

Hypospadias and epispadias. *Hypospadias* is a congenital malformation characterized by a urethral meatus on the underside of the penis due to imperfect closure of the urethral groove. It often is associated with other genital anomalies (e.g., cryptorchidism, bifid scrotum). *Epispadias* is a less common anomaly in which the urethral opening is located on the upper surface of the penis. It is commonly associated with cryptorchidism or extrophy of the urinary bladder.

Venereal lesions. The venereal lesions that may affect the penis are chancroid, syphilis (chancre), lymphopathia venereum, and granuloma inguinale. They have been considered in Chapter 9.

Erythroplasia of Queyrat. Erythroplasia of Queyrat affects chiefly the glans but may occur on the coronal sulcus or prepuce. It is a shiny, pink, slightly elevated, sharply demarcated lesion that microscopically shows irregular thickening of the epidermis, in which the proliferating epithelial cells often contain mitotic figures. Atypical cells are seen, and some are vacuolated. Subepithelial infiltration by lymphocytes and plasma cells is present. The lesion is regarded as precancerous by some and carcinoma in situ by others.

Since the histologic changes are similar to those seen in Bowen's disease of the skin (p. 692), some observers consider erythroplasia of Queyrat to be Bowen's disease of the penile mucosa, although others regard it as a separate clinicopathologic entity.

Squamous cell carcinoma. Squamous cell carcinoma is the most important tumor of the penis. It occurs on the glans or prepuce (less commonly), usually in patients past 50 years of age. It is particularly present among uncircumcised persons and often is preceded by chronic irritation from balanitis, phimosis, or retained smegma. It begins as a small warty growth, later developing into an ulcerative fungating mass. Metastasis occurs to inguinal and, later, retroperitoneal nodes.

URETHRA

Urethritis. Inflammation (urethritis) is the common lesion of the urethra and is usually of infectious origin. Acute urethritis may be gonococcal or nongonococcal. Some authors have suggested that the T-strain mycoplasmas are the primary cause of the nongonococcal form.

Stricture. Stricture of the urethra is a common result of infection, particularly gonorrhea, but its origin also may be traumatic or caused by a congenital fold of mucosa. The obstruction may cause dilatation of the bladder, ureters, and renal pelves.

TESTIS AND EPIDIDYMIS

Varicocele. Varicocele is a varicose dilatation of the veins of the pampiniform plexus of the spermatic cord. It may be primary (idio-

pathic) or secondary to venous obstruction, as by pressure.

Hydrocele. Hydrocele is the accumulation of clear watery fluid in the sac of the tunica vaginalis. It may be associated with trauma, infections, or neoplasms. A congenital form also occurs.

Hematocele. The presence of blood in the sac of the tunica vaginalis is referred to as a hematocele. It is most frequently related to trauma.

Spermatocele. Spermatocele is a cystic dilatation of the duct of the epididymis, containing fluid with spermatozoa.

Epididymitis. Inflammation (epididymitis) is most commonly caused by gonorrhea, the infection usually spreading from the seminal vesicles. One finds suppuration and the formation of small abscesses. Scarring, which follows the inflammation, often prevents the passage of spermatozoa, thus causing sterility, although testicular atrophy and sexual inactivity do not necessarily result. Nongonorrheal epididymitis is less common but may result from staphylococcal or colon bacillus infections.

Acute orchitis. Inflammation of the testis may result from trauma or from extension of an acute epididymitis or may be a complication in certain infectious diseases, particularly mumps, typhoid fever, and smallpox. It is the most serious feature of mumps in young adults. In some cases, it is followed by testicular atrophy and sterility.

Tuberculosis. Tuberculosis may involve the epididymis before the testis. Small conglomerate caseous tubercles are formed, similar in their gross and microscopic appearance to tubercles elsewhere. The lesions may be due to spread from tuberculous foci in the prostate gland or seminal vesicles or to hematogenous spread from lesions elsewhere (e.g., the lungs).

Syphilis. Syphilis more commonly involves the testis primarily and the epididymis secondarily. The syphilitic orchitis may be a gumma or a diffuse fibrosis.

Granulomatous orchitis. Granulomatous orchitis of a chronic nature and unknown pathogenesis is not uncommon. Trauma appears to be a factor in some cases.

Cryptorchidism. Cryptorchidism is a failure of descent of the testis into the scrotum. The testis is found in the peritoneal cavity or in the inguinal canal. The condition may be unilateral or bilateral. Microscopically, the undescended testis before puberty shows no significant change. After puberty, it shows evidence of atrophy of the seminiferous tubules, with absent or rare spermatogenesis. As a rule, the interstitial cells of Leydig persist, and their hormonal function is not disturbed. In some instances, these cells are increased in number. It is claimed by some investigators that cancer occurs more frequently in undescended testes as compared with normal scrotal testes.

Testicular atrophy. Causes of atrophy of the testes include cryptorchidism, old age (contributed to by sclerotic vessels), avitaminosis, malnutrition, hypothyroidism, hypopituitarism, cirrhosis of the liver (hyperestrinism), prolonged administration of estrogens (e.g., for prostatic cancer), ionizing radiation, and obstruction of the ductus epididymis. It also occurs as a late effect of some severe inflammations of the testis.

Torsion. Sudden twisting of the spermatic cord leads to obstruction of the veins and possibly the arteries, with circulatory disturbances in the testis and epididymis. There may be congestion and hemorrhage or, in more severe instances, definite infarction, which is often hemorrhagic. The cause may be violent exercise or straining. Torsion frequently affects undescended testes.

Klinefelter's syndrome. The features of Klinefelter's syndrome include masculine build, primary hypogonadism with failure of normal testicular development (seminiferous tubular dysgenesis) and azospermia, gynecomastia, increase in urinary gonadotropin, and often subnormal intelligence. The chromosomal patterns have been discussed previously (p. 12).

Tumors of testis

Almost all testicular tumors are malignant germ cell neoplasms and account for less than 1% of all cancer in males and about 5% of all genitourinary tumors. Some statistics show an increased incidence in the cryptorchid testis. Most testicular cancers occur between 20 and 35 years of age. The classification and terminology of testicular cancers are variable and confused. Ewing has regarded them all as teratomas, arising from sex cells and capable of reproducing any tissue. Commonly, they are divided into two groups only, seminomas and teratomas, but a more detailed classification includes (1) seminoma, (2) embryonal carcinoma, (3) choriocarcinoma, (4) teratoma, and (5) teratocarcinoma. An infrequent benign interstitial cell tumor also occurs.

Seminoma. The seminoma is the most frequent of the testicular cancers, occurs in an older age group, and is relatively less malignant than most of the other cancers. It is a circumscribed, firm, homogeneous grayish white mass varying up to the size of a grapefruit. The contour of the testis is usually maintained, since the tunica covering it is seldom invaded. Gray or yellowish opaque areas of necrosis may be present. Histologically, the seminoma is composed of uniform rounded or polygonal cells, with prominent round or oval hyperchromatic nuclei, arranged in diffuse sheets or in cordlike or tubular form (Fig. 14-38). A scanty stroma separates groups of cells and is sometimes infiltrated with small lymphocytes. This microscopic appearance is similar to that of dysgerminoma of the ovary (p. 628).

Embryonal carcinoma. The embryonal carcinoma may be of the adult or infantile type. The adult type is a more malignant, rapidly growing, and invasive tumor that usually shows more structural variation. Degeneration and necrosis are frequent in areas of the tumor, which tends to be soft, grayish, and opaque. The tumor cells may occur in solid sheets or may have a papillary or glandular structure. The cells tend to be larger and more variable than in the seminoma, with larger pleomorphic nuclei having coarsely clumped chromatin. The form that occurs in the infantile testis, also known as orchioblastoma or endodermal sinus tumor, has a some-

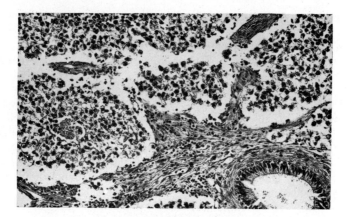

Fig. 14-38. Seminoma of testis.

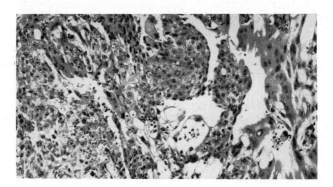

Fig. 14-39. Choriocarcinoma of testis.

what better prognosis than the adult type.

Choriocarcinoma. Testicular choriocarcinomas are usually small soft tumors with areas of hemorrhage and necrosis. Two types of cells—Langhans' and syncytial cells—occur, and villuslike structures may be formed (Fig. 14-39). The polyhedral Langhans' or cytotrophoblastic cells may form irregular sheets. The syncytial cells are large and multinucleated, with irregular hyperchromatic nuclei. Trophoblastic elements also may be seen in embryonal carcinomas.

Rare extragenital choriocarcinomas also occur in the male and, like the testicular tumor, are similar to the choriocarcinoma of the placenta. The choriocarcinomas are all highly malignant.

Teratoma. The teratoma is a moderate-sized tumor usually showing cysts of varying size containing keratohyaline material and sometimes mucin. The dermoid cyst, which is common in the ovary, is rare in the testes. Microscopically, a teratoma consists of a disorderly arrangement of fetal and adult structures of all three germ layers (Fig. 14-40). Well-differentiated tissues include cysts lined by squamous epithelium and filled with keratohyaline material, cartilage, smooth muscle, mucous glands, respiratory and gastrointestinal epithelium, and sometimes nerve tissue. The immature elements include primitive cartilage, mesenchyme, neuroectodermal canals, and primitive respiratory and intestinal tubules.

Teratocarcinoma. The teratocarcinoma is a

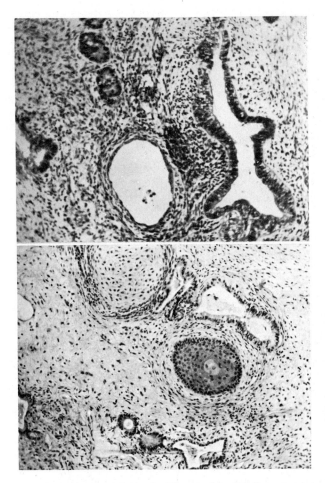

Fig. 14-40. Adult teratoma of testis. Note variety of cells and structures.

teratoma mixed with obviously malignant areas (e.g., seminoma, embryonal carcinoma, and sometimes sarcoma elements). Among the testicular cancers, it ranks second in frequency. The tumor is usually large, with a mixture of solid and cystic areas.

• • •

The major clinical manifestation of these tumors of the testis is the presence of a testicular mass. Some patients with cancer of the testis excrete increased amounts of gonadotropic hormone in the urine. Other hormones also may be demonstrated.

Metastasis occurs by blood and lymph channels. Lymphatic metastasis is found most frequently in the pelvis and abdominal retroperitoneal nodes. The lungs and liver are the organs most often the site of metastases. The 5-year survival rates tend to be as follows: seminoma, about 90% ; teratoma, about 70%; teratocarcinoma, about 50%; and adult embryonal carcinoma, about 30% (but about 70% for infantile embryonal carcinoma). The prognosis is very poor in choriocarcinoma, death occurring usually within 2 years.

Interstitial cell tumors. The interstitial (Leydig) cells of the testis are numerous in adults and appear increased in atrophic testes, as in elderly persons or in patients with undescended testes. Benign tumors composed of mature interstitial cells are of rare occurrence and have an endocrine function. In children, these are a rare cause of hypergenitalism and precocious development of secondary sexual characteristics due to androgenic secretion. In a few boys with this tumor, gynecomastia is observed in addition, and it also occurs in adult patients. Gynecomastia may be due to estrogen production or may be secondary to stimulation of the breasts by increased or altered androgens.

Tumors of epididymis

Primary tumors of the epididymis are very rare, and most are benign. The most common is the so-called adenomatoid tumor. This benign tumor is also found in the female genital tract, most often involving the fallopian tubes, uterus, or ovaries. It shows small glandlike spaces separated by an abundant fibrous and smooth muscle stroma (Fig. 14-41). Its origin is debatable, and it has been variously considered as epithelial, mesothelial, and lymphangiomatous and as a hamartoma of the mesonephros. Leiomyomas of the epididymis also occur.

PROSTATE GLAND

The prostate is a sexual gland. Its secretion is mixed with the sperm in the urethra at the time of ejaculation and functions to activate and prolong the motility of the spermatozoa. The gland has five lobes (median, two lateral,

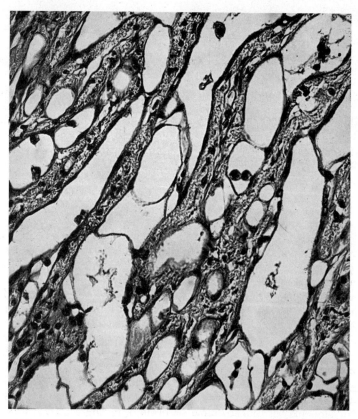

Fig. 14-41. "Adenomatoid tumor" of epididymis. Flattened cells line thin-walled spaces to give honeycomb appearance. (From Haukohl, R. S., and Anderson, W. A. D., editors: Pathology seminars, St. Louis, 1955, The C. V. Mosby Co.)

posterior, and anterior) and a group of gland acini in the midline of the urethral floor between the posterior vesical lip and the verumontanum (subcervical urethral glands of Albarran). The median lobe is that part dorsal to the urethra and between the converging ejaculatory ducts. The median lobe, the glands of Albarran, and the lateral lobes are particularly likely to undergo benign enlargement and cause obstruction.

The prostatic glands are lined by cuboidal or cylindrical epithelium and often contain concentrically laminated concretions, corpora amylacea. A hormonal secretion of the testis, activated by the pituitary gland, influences the prostate and causes its rapid maturation at puberty. Involution progresses during and after the fifth decade because of a decrease of hormonal stimulation. Estrogens appear to promote squamous metaplasia in the prostate gland.

Thrombosis of periprostatic veins is common in elderly bedridden patients. Focal infarctions often occur in enlarged prostate glands, and around them the glandular epithelium often undergoes squamous metaplasia. Small prostatic calculi are common in patients in older age groups.

The important lesions of the prostate gland are inflammation, hyperplasia, and carcinoma.

Inflammation

The common type of inflammation of the prostate gland is nonspecific prostatitis, but granulomatous forms also may occur.

Nonspecific prostatitis. Acute prostatitis may be caused by gonococci or other pyogenic organisms, such as streptococci, staphylococci, and colon bacilli. It may be due to spread from a urethritis but sometimes occurs as a complication of urethral catheterization or cystoscopy. The purulent material is confined within acini or extends and forms abscesses. The inflammation may clear up, but it commonly becomes chronic. Septicemias and pyemias also may result in multiple small abscesses of the prostate gland, *Staphylococcus aureus* being the most common causative or-

ganism. Chronic prostatitis is very common. A rare allergic prostatitis is sometimes seen in asthmatic patients.

Tuberculosis. Tuberculosis in the prostate is usually carried there by the bloodstream and in less than 20% of cases is secondary to foci elsewhere in urogenital organs. Typically, granulomatous and caseous lesions are formed that are similar to tuberculous lesions elsewhere.

Granulomatous prostatitis. In addition to tubercle bacilli, other organisms occasionally cause granulomatous prostatitis, e.g., fungi and atypical mycobacteria. Also, a granulomatous reaction with foreign body–type giant cells may be seen that apparently forms in response to secretions liberated from ruptured ducts that result from nonspecific inflammation (nonspecific granulomatous prostatitis).

Nodular hyperplasia (benign prostatic hypertrophy)

Benign enlargement is the commonest lesion of the prostate gland. It seldom occurs before the age of 50 years and is found in about 30% of men over the age of 60 years. About 17% have symptoms of urinary obstruction as a result, which is its main and important effect. The normal adult prostate gland weighs about 20 g. The enlarged gland is usually two to four times larger but seldom weighs more than 200 g, although heavier ones have been reported. There does not appear to be a transition between nodular hyperplasia and carcinoma.

The *anatomic changes* are the result of hyperplasia in the inner group of prostatic glands. Parts that may be involved include large portions of the lateral lobes, the median lobe, or the subcervical glands of Albarran. The hyperplasia includes a proliferation of periductal, periacinar, and periurethral stroma, including both connective tissue and smooth muscle fibers. Hyperplastic glandular growth also usually occurs, sometimes as a secondary phenomenon. Localized nodules of tumorlike or adenomatous tissue result (nodular hyperplasia), in which there are cystic dilations of acini with papillary infoldings lined by a single layer of high columnar epithelium and also areas with an increase in number of acini. Occasionally, there are nodules composed only of smooth muscle, or there are masses of lymphoid tissue. Prostatic median bar enlargement is predominantly caused by smooth muscle hypertrophy, associated with some interfascicular fibrosis and edema.

The *effect of prostatic enlargement* is to obstruct the outflow of urine. Enlargement of the lateral lobes compresses the urethra into a narrow and irregular slit. Enlargement of the median lobe or of the subcervical glands of Albarran results in a nodular mass that pushes up the floor of the bladder just inside the sphinc-

ter or in the proximal part of the urethra (Fig. 14-42). This midline enlargement is particularly effective in obstructing outflow of urine, acting as a plug to close the urethral orifice. A small sac forms behind the prostatic nodule, from which urine cannot be expelled, and contains the so-called residual urine.

Results of the obstruction may be seen in all parts of the urinary tract proximal to the prostate gland. The bladder becomes hypertrophied, with prominent muscular trabeculation evident on its mucosal surface. Diverticula may develop in weak areas between the trabeculae. The ureters and renal pelves undergo di-

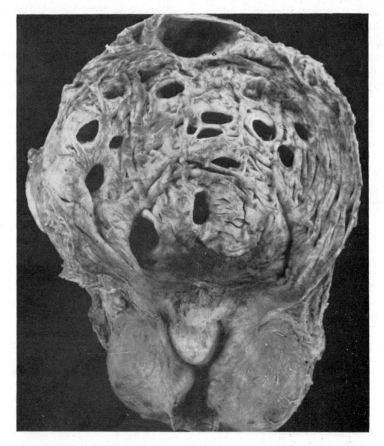

Fig. 14-42. Hyperplasia of prostate gland with obstruction of urethra by large middle lobe. Hypertrophied bladder with cellules and diverticula. (From Mostofi, F. K., and Leetsma, J. E.: Lower urinary tract and male genitalia. In Anderson, W. A. D., editor: Pathology, ed. 6, St. Louis, 1971, The C. V. Mosby Co.)

latation (hydroureter and hydronephrosis).

The *etiology* has been variously considered to be chronic inflammation, arteriosclerosis, and hormonal imbalance. The concept that the condition is one of true tumor formation has been rejected. A hormonal mechanism is believed by most investigators to be responsible for prostate hyperplasia, viz., an actual or relative increase in estrogens. It has been shown that the inner zones of the prostate gland are responsive to estrogens, and these are the sites of nodular hyperplasia.

Tumors

Carcinoma. Carcinoma of the prostate gland is an important cause of cancer deaths among men in the United States, being considered third in frequency (next to lung cancer, the most frequent, and cancer of the colon and rectum combined).

Carcinoma of the prostate gland seldom occurs before 50 years of age. At autopsy, it is observed as a microscopic finding in 14% to 46% of males over 50 years of age. In a large proportion of these cases, the cancer is occult or latent and has given rise to no clinical manifestations. The incidence of latent carcinoma increases with age. It is morphologically similar to the manifest carcinomas and shows the property of infiltration but lacks the capacity for rapid growth.

Whereas hyperplasia occurs in the inner mass of the prostate gland, the area that is responsive to estrogens, carcinoma arises in the outer mass or near the capsule, the area that is sensitive to androgens. Acid phosphatase of the serum is usually increased in patients with carcinoma of the prostate gland, particularly when metastases are present. If there are skeletal metastases, the alkaline phosphatase also may be increased.

The carcinomatous prostate gland tends to be firm or hard and to lack the elastic consistency of benign enlargement. Carcinoma may occur in a prostate that is the site of nodular hyperplasia, but apparently the two lesions are independent of each other, although some authors have suggested a possible relationship between them. Most cancers originate in the posterior lobe, next to the capsule. With invasion through the capsule, the gland becomes fixed to surrounding structures. Microscopically, the cancer is usually an adenocarcinoma with numerous acini that tend to be irregular and lined by several layers of epithelium (Fig. 14-43), but solid cords of epithelial cells also irregularly invade adjacent tissue. The latent or inactive carcinomas are not histologically distinguishable from the active and invasive cancers. Although an epidermoid carcinoma occasionally may be found in the prostate gland, adenocarcinoma is the common form. Invasion of the capsular perineural lymphatics occurs early. More distant lymphatic spread to the pelvic nodes is a late occurrence. Hematogenous metastasis to bones, lungs, and liver is common. In bone, an osteoplastic reaction frequently is induced by the tumor cells (p.

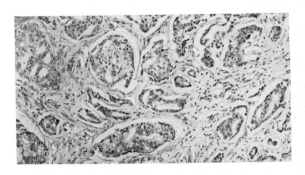

Fig. 14-43. Adenocarcinoma of prostate gland.

250). Treatment by castration or with estrogens causes metaplastic, degenerative, and atrophic changes in the tumor cells.

The cause of prostatic carcinoma is not known. The area in which cancer tends to occur, the androgen-sensitive outer subcapsular region, undergoes atrophy in older individuals as production of androgen is decreased. It has been postulated that biochemical alterations in these cells make them more susceptible to carcinogenic stimuli. Some have suggested that the tumor is initiated during the period of androgenic activity and remains quiescent during the time androgens are declining with advancing age. The dormant malignant cells are then stimulated to activity by other factors (e.g., pituitary, adrenal). Viral inclusions have been demonstrated in prostatic carcinoma in some studies.

Sarcoma. Sarcoma of the prostate gland is rare and easily confused with anaplastic carcinoma. Myosarcoma appears to be the most frequent type, but lymphosarcoma, spindle cell sarcoma, and other forms also occur.

REFERENCES

Abrahams, C.: Lancet **2:**346-347, 1976 (microangiopathy in analgesic nephropathy).

Abrahams, C.: N. Engl. J. Med. **301:**437-438, 1979 (microangiopathy in analgesic abuse).

Amador, E., et al.: J.A.M.A. **185:**769-775, 1963 (urinary enzymes in renal carcinoma).

Angell, M. E., et al.: N. Engl. J. Med. **278:**1303-1308, 1968 (active chronic pyelonephritis).

Armenian, H. K., et al.: Lancet **2:**115-117, 1974 (relation between prostatic hyperplasia and cancer of the prostate).

Balogh, F., and Szendroi, Z.: Cancer of the prostate, ed. 2. Budapest, 1968, Akadémiai Kiadó.

Bogdan, R., et al.: Cancer **31:**462-467, 1973 (leiomyomatous hamartoma of the kidney).

Burkholder, P. M., and Bradford, W. D.: Am. J. Pathol. **56:**423-467, 1969 (glomerulonephritis in children).

Burry, A., et al.: In Sommers, C., and Rosen, P. P., editors: Pathology annual, vol. 12, part 2, New York, 1977, Appleton-Century-Crofts, pp. 1-31, (analgesic nephropathy).

Churg, J., et al.: N. Engl. J. Med. **272:**165-174, 1965 (nephrotic syndrome).

Conn, J. W., et al.: Trans. Assoc. Am. Physicians **85:**353-368, 1972 (primary reninism).

Deichmann, W. B.: Bladder cancer, Birmingham, Ala., 1967, Aesculapius Publishing Co.

Dunnill, M. S.: Pathological basis of renal disease, Philadelphia, 1976, W. B. Saunders Co.

Franks, L. M.: J. Pathol. Bacteriol. **68:**617-621, 1954 (prostatic hyperplasia).

Franks, L. M.: J. Pathol. Bacteriol. **72:**603-611, 1956 (prostatic carcinoma).

Frimpter, G. W., et al.: J.A.M.A. **184:**111-113, 1963 (effect of degraded tetracycline).

Gluck, M. C., et al.: Ann. Intern. Med. **78:**1-12, 1973 (membranous glomerulonephritis).

Golden, A., and Maher, J. F.: The kidney; structure and function in disease, Baltimore, 1977, The Williams & Wilkins Co.

Graham, J. H., and Helwig, E. B.: Cancer **32:**1396-1414, 1973 (erythroplasia of Queyrat).

Grausz, H., et al.: N. Engl. J. Med. **283:**506-511, 1970 (viruslike particles in systemic lupus erythematosus).

Hagadorn, J. E., et al.: Am. J. Pathol. **57:**17-30, 1969 (Goodpasture's syndrome).

Hartroft, P. M.: Ann. Rev. Med. **17:**113-122, 1966 (juxtaglomerular complex).

Hartroft, P. M.: Bull. Pathol. **8:**165-167, 1967 (juxtaglomerular complex).

Heptinstall, R. H.: Pathology of the kidney, ed. 2, Boston, 1974, Little, Brown & Co.

Hirose, M., et al.: J.A.M.A. **230:**1288-1292, 1974 (primary reninism with hamartomatous renal lesion).

Holland, J. M.: Cancer **32:**1030-1042, 1973 (cancer of the kidney).

Jackson, G. G.: Arch. Intern. Med. **110:**663-675, 1962 (pyelonephritis).

Johnson, F. R., and Anderson, J. C.: J. Pathol. Bacteriol. **66:**39-46, 1953 (developmental remnants in kidney).

Jones, D. B.: Arch. Pathol. Lab. Med. **101:**457-461, 1977 (membranoproliferative glomerulonephritis).

Kaplan, B. S., and Drummond, K. N.: N. Engl. J. Med. **298:**964-966, 1978 (hemolytic-uremic syndrome).

Keslin, M. H., et al.: Arch. Intern. Med. **132:**578-581, 1973.

Kimmelstiel, P., and Wilson, C.: Am. J. Pathol. **12:**83-98, 1936 (diabetic glomerulosclerosis).

Kincaid-Smith, P.: The kidney; a clinico-pathological study, Oxford, 1975, Blackwell Scientific Publications Ltd.

Kleeman, C. R., editor: Arch. Intern. Med. **124:**261-321, 1969 (symposium on divalent ion metabolism and renal osteodystrophy).

Klein, L. A.: N. Engl. J. Med. **300:**824-833, 1979 (prostatic carcinoma).

Koffler, D., et al.: Am. J. Pathol. **54:**293-305, 1969 (Goodpasture's syndrome).

Kolata, G. B.: Science **207:**970-971, 1980 (chromosomal defects, aniridia, and Wilms' tumor).

Krickstein, H. I., et al.: Arch. Pathol. **82:**506-517, 1966 (hereditary nephritis).

Kurtzman, N. A., editor: Arch. Intern. Med. **131:**779-938, 1973 (symposium on renal pathophysiology).

Lannigan, R., and Insley, J.: J. Clin. Pathol. **18:**178-187, 1965 (focal glomerulonephritis).

Lee, L. W., et al.: J.A.M.A. **237:**2408-2409, 1977 (granulomatous prostatitis caused by atypical mycobacteria).

Llach, F., Arieff, A. I., and Massry, S. G.: Ann. Intern. Med. **83:**8-14, 1975 (renal vein thrombosis and nephrotic syndrome).

Lokich, J. L., et al.: Arch. Intern. Med. **132:**597-600, 1973 (nephrosis in Hodgkin's disease).

Loughridge, L. W., and Lewis, M. G.: Lancet **1:**256-259, 1971 (nephrotic syndrome in malignant disease of nonrenal origin).

Lucké, B.: Milit. Surg. **99:**371-396, 1946 (hemoglobinuric nephrosis).

Lundberg, G. D.: J.A.M.A. **184:**915-919, 1963 (Goodpasture's syndrome).

Lupton, C. H., Jr., and McManus, J. F. A.: Lab. Invest. **11:**860-866, 1962 (chronic pyelonephritis).

Maisel, J. C., and Priest, R. E.: Arch. Pathol. **77:**646-651, 1964 (phenacetin nephritis).

Mallory, T. B.: Am. J. Clin. Pathol. **17:**427-443, 1947 (hemoglobinuric nephrosis).

Maurer, H. S., et al.: Cancer **43:**205-208, 1979 (genetic factors in Wilms' tumor).

Mautner, W., et al.: Lab. Invest. **11:**518-530, 1962 (toxemia of pregnancy).

Mavromatis, F.: J.A.M.A. **193:**191-194, 1965 (tetracycline nephropathy).

McChesney, J. A.: J.A.M.A. **226:**37-39, 1973 (acute urethritis in male college students).

McGee, W. G., and Ashworth, C. T.: Am. J. Pathol. **43:**273-299, 1963 (hypertensive arteriopathy).

McGovern, V. J.: In Sommers, S. C., editor: Pathology annual, vol. 2, New York, 1967, Appleton-Century-Crofts (glomerulonephritis).

McKay, D. G.: Disseminated intravascular coagulation; an intermediary mechanism of disease, New York, 1965, Hoeber Medical Division, Harper & Row, Publishers, Inc. (bilateral cortical necrosis).

Merrill, J. P.: N. Engl. J. Med. **290:**257-266, 313-319, 374-381, 1974 (glomerulonephritis).

Mostofi, F. K.: Cancer **32:**1186-1201, 1973 (testicular tumors).

Mostofi, F. K., and Smith, D. E., editors: The kidneys, International Academy of Pathology monograph, Baltimore, 1966, The Williams & Wilkins Co.

Mostofi, F. K., et al.: Cancer **8:**741-758, 1955 (mucous adenocarcinoma of bladder).

Nanra, R. S., and Kincaid-Smith, P.: Br. Med. J.: **3:**559-561, 1970 (papillary necrosis in rats caused by aspirin).

Newman, D., and Vellios, F.: Am. J. Clin. Pathol. **42:**45-54, 1964 (carcinosarcoma of kidney in adult).

Osathanondh, V., and Potter, E. L.: Arch. Pathol. **77:**459-465, 466-473, 474-484, 485-502, 502-509, 510-512, 1964 (polycystic kidney).

Panner, B.: Arch. Pathol. **76:**303-317, 1963 (renal vein thrombosis and nephrotic syndrome).

Parker, J., and Kunin, C.: J.A.M.A. **224:**585-590, 1973 (pyelonephritis in young women).

Phillips, G., and Mukherjee, T. M.: Pathology **4:**193-204, 1972 (juxtaglomerular cell tumor of kidney).

Piering, W. F., et al.: Arch. Intern. Med. **137:**1625-1626, 1977 (infantile polycystic kidney disease in adult).

Ponticelli, C., et al.: Arch. Intern. Med. **140:**353-357, 1980 (hemolytic-uremic syndrome in adults)..

Quinn, E. L., and Koss, E. H., editors: Biology of pyelonephritis, Boston, 1960, Little Brown & Co.

Randall, A.: Ann. Surg. **105:**1009-1027, 1937 (renal calculi).

Randall, A.: Int. Abst. Surg. **71:**209-240, 1940 (renal calculi).

Reidenberg, M. M., et al.: Am. J. Med. Sci. **247:**25-29, 1964 (nephrotoxins).

Relman, A. S., and Schwartz, W. B.: Am. J. Med. **24:**764-773, 1958 (kidney in potassium depletion).

Reynolds, T. B., and Edmondson, H. A.: J.A.M.A. **184:**435-444, 1963 (phenacetin nephritis).

Riches, E. W., et al.: Br. J. Urol. **23:**297-356, 1951 (urinary tract tumors).

Routledge, R. C., et al.: Cancer **38:**1735-1740, 1976 (Hodgkin's disease and the nephrotic syndrome).

Schreiner, G. E., and Maher, J. F.: Am. J. Med. **38:**409-449, 1965 (toxic nephropathy).

Scowen, E. F., et al.: J. Pathol. Bacteriol. **77:**195-205, 1959 (renal calculi).

Sevitt, S.: Lancet **2:**135-141, 1959 (pathogenesis of uremia).

Sheehan, H. L., and Moore, H. C.: Renal cortical necrosis and the kidney of concealed accidental hemorrhage, Springfield, Ill., 1954, Charles C Thomas, Publisher.

Silverberg, E.: CA **30:**23-38, 1980 (cancer statistics).

Sniffen, R. C.: Arch. Pathol. **50:**259-284, 1950 (testicular atrophy).

Sniffen, R. C., et al.: Arch. Pathol. **50:**285-295, 1950 (testicular atrophy).

Solez, K., et al.: Am. J. Pathol. **76:**521-528, 1974 (experimental papillary necrosis of the kidney).

Sommers, S. C.: Henry Ford Hosp. Med. Bull. **14:**47-54, 1966 (renal factors in hypertension).

Spence, H. M., et al.: J.A.M.A. **163:**1466-1472, 1957 (cysts of kidney).

Spjut, H. J., and Thorpe, J. D.: Am. J. Clin. Pathol. **26:**136-145, 1956 (granulomatous orchitis).

Stanbury, S. W.: In Black, D. A. K., editor: Renal disease, ed. 2, Philadelphia, 1967, F. A. Davis Co. (bony complications of renal disease).

Teel, P.: Am. J. Obstet. Gynecol. **75:**1347-1353, 1958 (adenomatoid tumors).

Trueta, J., et al.: Studies of the renal circulation, Springfield, Ill., 1947, Charles C Thomas, Publisher.

Williams, H. E.: N. Engl. J. Med. **290:**33-38, 1974 (nephrolithiasis).

15

Upper respiratory tract, lungs, pleura, and mediastinum

Upper respiratory tract

NOSE AND SINUSES

Rhinophyma. The skin of the nose is subject to rhinophyma, a nodular enlargement characterized by hypertrophy of the sebaceous glands. Dilated sebaceous ducts and hypertrophied acini contain epithelial debris and inspissated sebaceous material. The glandular epithelium at times may undergo squamous metaplasia. The surrounding dermis may show some chronic inflammatory reaction and fibrosis.

Rhinitis. Rhinitis, an inflammation of the nasal mucosa, may show characteristics of an allergic inflammation with numerous eosinophils in the mucosa and surface exudate, or it may be nonallergic and infectious in origin. *Atrophic rhinitis (ozena)* is characterized by considerable crusting of the nasal mucosa.

Specific types of rhinitis include rhinoscleroma and rhinosporidiosis. *Rhinoscleroma* is characterized by nodular masses in the nose that are composed of granulation tissue with many lymphocytes and plasma cells and foamy mononuclear cells (Mikulicz's cells) (Fig. 15-1), which may contain an organism, *Klebsiella rhinoscleromatis*. *Rhinosporidiosis* is a specific fungal infection.

Polyps. Polyps of the nose and sinuses are predominantly inflammatory masses with edema, marked vascularity, a chronic cellular exudate, and sometimes cysts. Neoplastic polyps (epithelial papillomas) also occur.

Neoplasms. Tumors of the nose and sinuses, in addition to the epithelial papillomas, include angiomas, transitional cell carcinomas, squamous cell carcinomas, and adenocarcinomas. Various types of bone tumors may arise in the maxilla and involve the nose or sinuses. Mixed tumors of the salivary gland type, arising in the palate, may invade the nose or maxillary sinus.

LARYNX

Infectious inflammatory lesions of the larynx (laryngitis) are a common component of many respiratory infections, including tuberculosis. Tumors and tumorlike conditions are the most common serious lesions of the larynx.

Carcinomas of the larynx may arise from the epithelium lining the lumen of the larynx or from the mucous membranes of the orifice or pharyngeal surface of the larynx. By the clinical and topographic classifications commonly used, they have been divided into two general groups: intrinsic and extrinsic cancers. *Intrinsic* cancers are those arising from the interior of the larynx, and with these are included the subglottic growths as well as tumors of the vocal cords and ventricles. *Extrinsic* cancers are

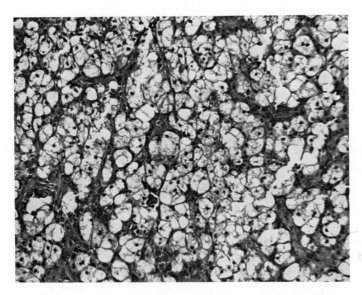

Fig. 15-1. Rhinoscleroma showing large pale Mikulicz's cells.

those arising from the mucous membranes of the hypopharynx, arytenoid folds, epiglottis, and piriform fossae. Laryngeal tumors also may be classified as supraglottic, glottic, and subglottic.

Benign lesions of the larynx that may simulate cancer include cysts, inflammations, keratoses, papillomas, and polyps.

Chronic obstruction of the larynx may be an important aspect of inflammations and neoplasms of the area. Acute obstruction may be allergic or may be caused by a bolus of food. Asphyxiation resulting from the obstruction of the airway by food ("the café coronary") is not uncommon.

Cysts. Laryngeal cysts are relatively uncommon. They may be acquired or congenital. Acquired cysts are retention cysts developing in a mucous gland, caused by inflammation or trauma, and may occur in the epiglottis, vocal cords, or lateral walls of the larynx. Congenital cysts occur in the epiglottis from inclusion of the lymphoepithelium of the entoderm (i.e., a branchial cyst) or may occur in the lateral walls of the pharynx or the aryepiglottic folds from displaced embryonal cells, which normally form the appendix of the ventricle. Laryngeal cysts may be lined by ciliated pseu-

dostratified columnar epithelium or by squamous epithelium.

Keratosis. Keratosis of the larynx, also called hyperkeratosis, leukoplakia, and pachyderma, occurs mainly in male adults as white elevations on the upper surface or edge of the vocal cords. There is hyperplasia of the squamous epithelium with varying degrees of hyperkeratosis and dyskeratosis. The irregularity of the epithelium may be such that distinction from carcinoma is difficult, and some cases appear to undergo transformation to carcinoma.

Papilloma. The papilloma is the most common benign tumor of the larynx. In children, papillomas may be of viral origin and usually disappear spontaneously. In adults, they are single or multiple and usually involve only the vocal cords. They tend to recur after removal, and about 3% become malignant. They are protruding tumors composed of a core of well-vascularized connective tissue, covered by hyperplastic and branched stratified squamous epithelium with variable amounts of keratin.

Polyps. A laryngeal polyp (laryngeal nodule or singer's node) is a thickening of the mucosa of the true vocal cord, most commonly found near the anterior commissure but sometimes it may appear in other areas. Laryngeal polyps occur in adults, affect men four times as frequently as women, and probably arise as a result of inflammation, trauma, or misuse of the voice. They usually are nodular, but sometimes are polypoid or even pedunculated, and may be seen in any one of four stages.

At first, there is a fibrous thickening of the stroma of the cord just beneath the squamous epithelium of the edge. In the second stage, it becomes polypoid because of edema and dilatation of vessels in the fibrous stroma. In the third stage, extreme dilatation of the thin-walled vessels may produce an angiomatous appearance (hemangioma). In the fourth stage, the stroma becomes hyalinized and amyloid-like in appearance (the so-called amyloid tumor) (Fig. 15-2). In any stage, the overlying epithelium may be atrophic, hyperplastic, or dyskeratotic. Only uncommonly does a laryngeal polyp undergo cancerous transformation.

Rarer benign tumors of the larynx include adenoma, chondroma, fibroma, neurofibroma, and myoblastoma.

Carcinoma. Carcinoma of the larynx constitutes 2% to 4% of all malignant tumors. Among cancers of the larynx, 98% or more are carcinomas. Men are affected ten to fourteen times as frequently as women. Most cases occur between the ages of 40 and 65 years, with the median age about 60 years.

A large majority of laryngeal carcinomas (96%) are squamous cell type, and most are fairly well-differentiated, slowly growing tumors. A few are basal cell carcinomas or adenocarcinomas. In the intrinsic group, two thirds are Grade I or Grade II squamous cell carcinomas, whereas the extrinsic carcinomas are more likely to be of higher grade or less differentiated. In recent years, squamous cell carcinoma in situ has been recognized more frequently than formerly, and it is likely that

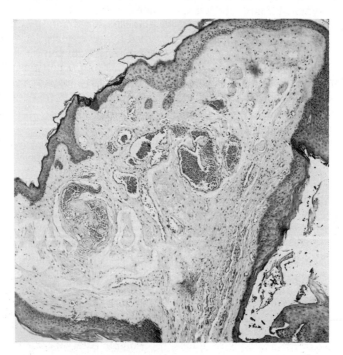

Fig. 15-2. Laryngeal nodule. Polypoid protrusion from vocal cord is covered by irregularly thickened and hyperkeratotic squamous epithelium. Central core contains dilated (angiomatoid) vascular spaces and hyalinized connective tissue. (×50.)

the invasive cancers often begin as in situ lesions.

Grossly, the cancers may appear simply as reddened, thickened areas or actual tumors varying from a few millimeters up to 6 cm or more in diameter (Fig. 15-3). They may be papillary or infiltrating and ulcerating. The papillary growths are raised above the surface, rough or granular, grayish white, and friable. Infiltrating growths produce a hard, ill-defined thickening, but eventually they tend to become elevated and ulcerated.

Histologically, the invasive carcinomas are composed of irregular infiltrating nests and cords of squamous epithelial cells, often with keratin masses. Mitoses vary in number. The stroma also is quite variable in amount. Some tumors are seen in an intraepithelial or carcinoma in situ stage.

Spread of laryngeal cancer may be by direct extension, by the lymphatics, and by the bloodstream. Lymphatic spread to lymph nodes of the neck and supraclavicular region is more common and earlier with extrinsic cancers than with the intrinsic growths. With spread by the bloodstream, which is relatively uncommon, metastases are found in the lungs and other organs.

The prognosis depends on the site, degree of extension, and histologic grading. Best prognosis is for carcinoma in situ, which should be cured by early and adequate therapy. Treated intrinsic invasive cancer limited to the vocal cord has a relatively good prognosis (approximately 80% 5-year survival), whereas supraglottic invasive lesions have a 5-year survival rate of 30% or less.

Lungs

The bronchi are involved in four main types of lesions: inflammation (bronchitis), obstructions (e.g., bronchial asthma), dilatations (bronchiectasis), and tumors (e.g., bronchogenic carcinoma). These types are frequently mixed, e.g., bronchiectasis and asthma have inflammatory changes as an integral part of the picture, and chronic bronchitis and bronchogenic carcinoma may be associated with obstruction of the bronchial lumen.

BRONCHITIS

Acute bronchitis. Acute bronchial inflammations have various causes, and a number of organisms may be found in the associated exudate. In many cases, the trachea and larynx also are involved, so that the condition is a laryngotracheobronchitis. Influenza is primarily a tracheobronchitis. Downward extension of diphtheria produces a fibrinous bronchitis. Pneumonic involvement of the lung has an associated acute bronchitis.

In acute bronchitis, the mucosa is thickened and reddened and eventually is covered by exudate, which may be mucoid, fibrinous, or

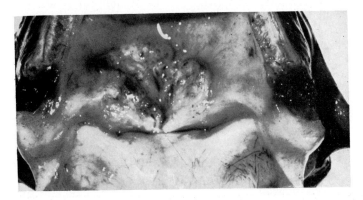

Fig. 15-3. Carcinoma of larynx. Neoplastic area is roughly nodular and irregularly thickened.

purulent. Microscopically, one finds congestion and infiltration of the mucosa, and often of deeper layers, by polymorphonuclear leukocytes. In severe cases, necrosis and desquamation of the epithelial surface may be evident, blending with the exudate on the surface. Dilatation (bronchiectasis) may result from the injury to bronchial walls, or abscess formation may follow spread of the infection.

Chronic bronchitis. Chronic inflammation of the bronchial tree occurs in association with a number of diseases of the lungs (e.g., tuberculosis and abscess) and bronchi (e.g., carcinoma and bronchiectasis). It also occurs in association with heart disease in which there is chronic passive congestion of the lungs.

The common form of chronic bronchitis, however, is that in which these bronchopulmonary or cardiac disorders are excluded as the sole cause of the manifestations. It is characterized by excessive mucus secretion in the bronchial tree associated with chronic or recurrent productive cough. The condition is most prevalent among men past 35 years of age and frequently in cigarette smokers, although it may occur in nonsmokers. Atmospheric pollution and occupational exposure to dust, fumes, and gases may be irritating factors in some patients. Infection may play a secondary role, usually viral and superimposed bacterial infection. Microscopically, in most instances, there is hyperplasia of the mucous glands and goblet cells of the mucosal epithelium. Infiltration by mononuclear cells and metaplastic epithelial change with loss of cilia may be seen. If infection is present, healing of the infection may result in fibrosis and deformity of the bronchial wall.

The disease may progress without further complications, but some patients develop reversible obstructive bronchopulmonary disease (bronchial asthma) and others eventually develop pulmonary emphysema (p. 423).

OBSTRUCTION OF BRONCHI

Obstruction of a bronchial lumen can be produced by (1) aspirated foreign material, (2) neoplasms, (3) pressure from without, as by enlarged lymph nodes, (4) inflammation or its sequelae, and (5) asthma. A complete obstruction leads to collapse (atelectasis) of the lung tissue supplied by the obstructed bronchus. Incomplete obstruction, or one that allows the entrance of air by active inspiration but blocks its exist on passive expiration, leads to dilatation of the alveoli. The aspiration of foreign substances into the bronchi often leads to an abscess of the lung.

Bronchial asthma. Bronchial asthma is a condition characterized by paroxysms of dyspnea and wheezing, with particular difficulty in expiration. In most instances, allergy is the basis for this disorder. The sensitivity may be to food, pollens, house dust, molds, animal dander, etc. Respiratory infections (viral or bacterial) may precipitate an asthmatic attack, either as an allergic response to the etiologic microorganism or as a nonspecific hyperreactivity of the bronchi to the infection. However, an allergic basis is not demonstrable in all patients with asthma. In some, heredity, emotional stress, or endocrine factors play an influential role.

Sputum produced in asthma is often distinctive because of a content of eosinphils, Curschmann's spirals, and Charcot-Leyden crystals. Excessive numbers of eosinophils may be found in the blood. Asthmatic attacks are characterized by spasm of bronchial muscles, mucosal edema, and overproduction of mucus by bronchial glands. Death during an attack is uncommon, although in prolonged attacks lasting for hours or days (status asthmaticus) or in chronic disease associated with impacted mucous plugs in the bronchi, death may result.

The lungs in asthmatics are voluminous and distended. Areas of atelectasis also may occur because of persistent bronchial obstruction by mucous plugs.

In the bronchiolar wall, there is (1) infiltration of eosinophils, (2) hypertrophy of muscle, (3) a thickened basement membrane and widened submucosal layer, and (4) enlargement and hyperactivity of mucous glands, which may be infiltrated by eosinophils. Excessive mucus secretion is present in the lumen, sometimes in the form of peculiar spiral plugs (Curschmann's spirals).

BRONCHIECTASIS

Bronchiectasis is a dilatation of the bronchi, either in a local area or generalized. The dilatation may be cylindrical, fusiform, or saccular if localized to one area. The lower lobes are more commonly involved than the upper, and the left lower lobe is involved more frequently than the right. The condition frequently is associated with chronic bronchitis or with multiple abscess formation resulting from the invasion of pyogenic and fusospirochetal organisms.

Etiology. The etiology and pathogenesis of bronchiectasis have been much debated, but a number of factors are considered causative, their relative importance varying in different cases. These factors (infection of the bronchial wall, traction on the bronchial wall from without, increased intrabronchial pressure, and congenital abnormality in bronchial development) are discussed in the following paragraphs.

Acute respiratory *infection involving the bronchial wall,* particularly in children, may injure or destroy muscle and elastic tissue. This most commonly follows bronchopneumonia or bronchitis complicating whooping cough, measles, and influenza. Infection may be associated with tuberculosis, mucoviscidosis (cystic fibrosis), or obstructive lesions such as tumors, aspirated foreign bodies, and compression of the bronchi by enlarged hilar lymph nodes (as in the middle lobe syndrome).

Traction on the bronchial wall from without may occur from either (1) atelectasis of lung tissue or (2) contraction of scar tissue resulting from inflammation of alveolar and bronchial tissue. Atelectasis brought about by an obstruction of the bronchial lumen exerts elastic pull on the bronchial wall because of the negative pleural pressure and the necessity for spatial adjustment in the thoracic cage. Fibrous contraction of pulmonary tissue, from tuberculosis, fibrosing pneumonia, etc., similarly may exert traction tending to dilate bronchi.

Increased intrabronchial pressure, such as produced by coughing may act to dilate bronchi when the wall is already weakened by an inflammatory and destructive process.

A *congenital abnormality in bronchial development,* particularly one involving the muscle and elastic components, may be an etiologic factor. There is a congenital type of bronchiectasis that includes the lesion referred to as congenital cystic disease of the lung. That a developmental factor may be important in the seemingly acquired cases has been suggested by the peculiar distribution of bronchiectasis, its frequent familial occurrence, and its association with other developmental abnormalities. The association of bronchiectasis with situs inversus and sinusitis is referred to as *Kartagener's syndrome.*

Lesions. The dilated bronchi are evident on the cut surface of the bronchiectatic lung. In the lower lobes, the dilatations are usually cylindrical, whereas in the less commonly involved upper lobes they tend to be saccular. When inflammation is severe, particularly with pyogenic and fusospirochetal infections, the bronchiectases appear grossly as multiple abscess cavities.

Microscopically, the essential change is absence, damage, or destruction of muscle and elastic elements of the bronchial wall (Fig. 15-4). This may be accompanied by variable degrees of inflammation. In slight and chronic bronchiectasis, there may be either atrophy or hypertrophy of the mucosa, with infiltration of lymphocytes and plasma cells in the bronchial wall and, eventually, fibrosis. Squamous metaplasia of the lining is sometimes seen. With severe inflammation, there may be necrosis of tissue, purulent exudate, and abscess formation. A focal necrotizing pulmonary lesion or abscess in the process of healing may become lined by a wall resembling that of a dilated bronchus, so that it often is mistakenly considered as a saccular type of bronchiectasis.

Mucoviscidosis. Cystic fibrosis (mucoviscidosis) commonly is accompanied by inspissated abnormal bronchial secretions with resultant obstruction, leading to secondary in-

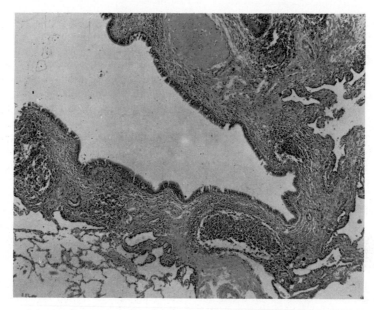

Fig. 15-4. Bronchiectasis showing bronchial dilatation, destruction of muscle, chronic inflammatory infiltrate, and fibrosis.

fections, atelectasis, emphysema, or bronchiectasis (p. 17).

Congenital bronchiectasis and congenital lung cysts. Congenital bronchiectasis is rare and frequently is spoken of as cystic disease of the lung. Anomalous bronchial or pulmonary development results in various-sized cysts that may or may not have an opening into a bronchus. The single or multiple cysts that form are lined by columnar epithelium, and some remnants of muscle and cartilage may be found in the wall. Numerous disseminated cysts, giving the lung a honeycomb structure, may be present. Complications of congenital cysts include infection, rupture with pneumothorax, and, sometimes with large lesions, respiratory embarrassment.

A rare type of congenital cystic disease of the lung appears to be a congenital lymphangiectasis. The small, thin-walled cysts are situated in connective tissue close to pulmonary blood vessels and are lined by endothelium.

TUMORS

Tumors of the lung constitute an extremely important group because of a high and increasing incidence of primary bronchogenic carcinomas. Tumors of the lung may be classified as follows:

Benign
Epithelial
    Papilloma of bronchus
    Tumorlets
    Peripheral adenoma
Mesodermal
    Vascular tumors (hemangioma)
    Bronchial tumors
        Fibroma
        Chondroma and osteochondroma
        Lipoma
        Leiomyoma
        Granular cell myoblastoma
Developmental
    Hamartoma
Malignant
Epithelial
    Bronchogenic
        Squamous cell (epidermoid) carcinoma
        Small cell (oat cell) carcinoma
        Large cell undifferentiated (anaplastic) carcinoma
        Adenocarcinoma
        Mixed types
    Bronchiolar carcinoma (pulmonary adenomatosis, alveolar cell carcinoma)

Bronchial "adenoma"
  Carcinoid type
  Cylindromatous (adenocystic) type
  Uncommon variants
    Oncocytoid
    Mucoepidermoid
    Papillary adenoma
Mesodermal (sarcoma)
  Undifferentiated sarcoma
  Fibrosarcoma
  Osteochondrosarcoma
  Leiomyosarcoma
  Lymphocytic lymphoma
Mixed epithelial and mesodermal tumors
  Carcinosarcoma
Reticuloendothelial tumors (involving lung as part of a generalized process)
  Hodgkin's disease
  Lymphocytic lymphoma
  Letterer-Siwe disease
Metastatic tumors
Pleural tumors
  Localized
  Diffuse

Benign tumors

Papilloma. Papillomas and papillomatosis of the bronchial tree are uncommon benign lesions similar to those that occur in the larynx. Except as a rarity, they do not undergo malignant change, but they may recur after bronchoscopic removal.

Tumorlets. *Atypical hyperplasias* of bronchiolar epithelium with extensions into the alveoli are common with chronic pulmonary inflammations. The proliferations may be of a variety of cell types—cuboidal, columnar, syncytial giant cell, or undifferentiated (reserve) cell. A number of infections (e.g., Hecht's giant cell pneumonia), chemical irritations (e.g., cadmium pneumonitis), and other chronic nonspecific inflammations may be accompanied by a proliferation of columnar bronchiolar epithelium extending to line alveolar spaces. Extensive cases may suggest or be confused with pulmonary adenomatosis.

Atypical hyperplasias in which the cells resemble undifferentiated (basal or reserve) cells of bronchial or bronchiolar epithelium occur at the periphery of the lung, frequently in relationship to scars, old infarcts, and bronchiectases. They form tumorlike masses *(tumorlets)*

in bronchiolar walls, alveolar spaces, or fibrous areas. Sometimes they are within spaces resembling lymphatic vessels (Fig. 15-5). They may resemble miniature undifferentiated (oat cell) carcinomas or suggest the appearance of bronchial adenoma and have been considered by some investigators to be minute peripheral carcinoids. Larger masses of such cells are similar to the tumors reported as "peripheral adenomas." Sometimes, they have been mistaken for and reported as early or small carcinomas (microcarcinomas). Although benign, their importance as precursors or their relationship, if any, to the numerous examples of "scar cancers," to cancers developing in old pulmonary infarcts, or to other carcinomas of the lung is unknown.

Hemangioma. Hemangiomas and other primary vascular tumors of the lung are very rare. Microscopic pulmonary "arteriovenous shunts" and arteriovenous fistulas have been described. Vascular lesions may occur as circumscribed *sclerosing hemangiomas* (histiocytoma and xanthoma) of the lung, an uncommon lesion showing many of the histologic features of sclerosing hemangiomas elsewhere. They may appear as localized "coin" lesions on roentgenographic examination and must be differentiated from a malignant tumor.

Hamartoma. Hamartomas are uncommon benign developmental tumorlike lesions. They contain representatives of the histologic components of bronchi or lung tissue, and cartilage is often the predominant tissue. They often appear as growths of connective tissue admixed with bronchial epithelium, cartilage, and sometimes adipose tissue. Most are peripheral or subpleural in position, but a few are endobronchial in origin.

These lesions are rounded, well-encapsulated masses that often shell out easily, are firm and grayish white, and have a rough nodular surface. They may be discovered at any age and occur more frequently in males than in females. Their chief importance lies in the difficulty of their clinical differentiation from cancer.

Other benign tumors. Fibromas, lipomas, chondromas, and leiomyomas are rare benign pulmonary tumors.

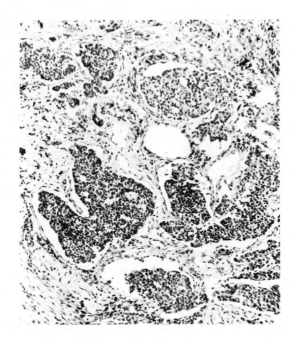

Fig. 15-5. Tumorlet. Cells appear to be in endothelial-lined spaces. (× 109.) (From Millard, M.: Lung, pleura, and mediastinum. In Anderson, W. A. D., and Kissane, J. M., editors: Pathology, ed. 7, St. Louis, 1977, The C. V. Mosby Co.)

Carcinoma

Primary carcinoma of the lung is mainly bronchogenic in origin. It is of frequent and rapidly increasing occurrence and ranks as the leading cause of mortality from cancer in males. It is more common in men than in women, but in recent years the incidence in women has been increasing. The highest incidence is between 50 and 60 years of age, but it is also common in the decades before and after. Tracheal carcinoma is rare, accounting for less than 0.1% of deaths from cancer. It is usually of squamous cell type.

Etiology and pathogenesis. The rapid increase in incidence of cancer of the lung during the last few decades appears only partially accounted for by better and newer methods of diagnosis. A real increase, in both sexes and involving the squamous cell and undifferentiated types of bronchogenic carcinoma, appears definitely established. The cause of this increase is a subject of intense interest and some debate.

A mass of evidence, chiefly statistical, indicts cigarette smoking, although the specific carcinogenic factor is unknown. Carcinogenic polycyclic aromatic hydrocarbons identified in cigarette smoke have been suspected. Squamous metaplasia, hyperplasia, and atypical proliferative changes of the bronchial epithelium have been found to occur more commonly in cigarette smokers compared with nonsmokers, and somewhat similar changes have been demonstrated in dogs subjected to inhalation of cigarette smoke through a tracheostoma for about 14 months. In dogs exposed to cigarette smoke in the same way for more than 2 years, tumors were found in the lungs, the majority being noninvasive or invasive bronchioloalveolar tumors. In two instances, an invasive bronchial squamous cell carcinoma of microscopic size was found. Invasive tumors were observed only in dogs smoking non–filter tipped cigarettes. Other lung lesions included fibrosis and emphysema. In mice, prolonged exposure to inhaled cigarette smoke

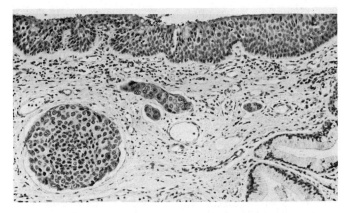

Fig. 15-6. Bronchial mucosa with squamous metaplasia and areas of carcinoma in situ. Underlying vascular spaces contain embolic masses of metastatic squamous cell carcinoma from elsewhere in lung.

increases the incidence of adenomatous lung tumors.

Other suggested etiologic factors include carcinogenic agents from atmospheric pollution in cities or tarring of roads and late effects of pneumonitis of viral origin. In certain industries, exposure to chromates, alpha halo ethers, and arsenicals and the development of asbestosis appear to cause increased incidence of pulmonary cancer. Such industrial exposures are insufficient to account for the large and widespread increase. Occupational pulmonary cancer has been long recognized among certain cobalt miners in central Europe (Schneeberg and Joachimstal), where radioactivity of the ores may be the important factor. Uranium miners in the United States who have had sufficient exposure to radiation have shown an increased incidence of lung cancer, mainly of the small cell (oat cell) type.

The relation of squamous metaplasia of bronchial epithelium to the development of carcinoma is still a debatable problem. Squamous metaplasia is a frequent occurrence in many chronic pulmonary irritations or in inflammatory lesions such as bronchiectasis. It is evident that it does not regularly proceed to the development of carcinoma. However, much evidence suggests that it may be a frequent precursor or accompaniment of broncho-

genic carcinoma. Detailed studies of the whole bronchial tree in cases of bronchogenic carcinoma, and in groups of smokers and nonsmokers, indicate a high frequency of squamous metaplasia and changes of carcinoma in situ (Fig. 15-6) in relationship to cancer development.

Natural history. Many lung cancers begin in large bronchi, soon obstructing them or interfering with their function and leading to emphysema, atelectasis, and pneumonitis. A later sequela may be bronchiectasis or abscess, or cavitation in a tumor itself may simulate abscess. Such secondary effects may hinder or obscure clinical and roentgenographic diagnosis. Common initial clinical symptoms are cough, hemoptysis, dyspnea, chest pain, wheezing, hoarseness, and persistent fever. The course of the disease is variable, depending on the type of tumor and its site.

Various extrapulmonary manifestations may be associated with bronchogenic carcinoma, particularly the undifferentiated small cell (oat cell) type, although certain manifestations, e.g., hypercalcemia, tend to be associated with squamous cell carcinoma. These manifestations, which sometimes precede the clinical evidence of the lung lesion, include:

1 Paraendocrine syndromes (e.g., Cushing's syndrome, hypercalcemia, excess ADH, and carcinoid syndrome)

2 Neuromuscular symptoms (e.g., peripheral neuropathy, cortical cerebellar degenerations, and myopathy)

3 Dermatomyositis

4 Pulmonary osteoarthropathy

5 Migratory phlebothrombosis

6 Nonbacterial thrombotic endocarditis

Gross types. Although extremely variable in gross appearance, most pulmonary carcinomas fall in one of three groups. The most common is a *hilar infiltrating form,* in which there are large tumor masses about the bronchi at the hilus of the lung, causing stenosis and ulceration of a bronchus and often massively involving mediastinal and peribronchial lymph nodes. In the less common *peripheral* or *nodular form,* there may be either a single peripheral tumor or multiple nodular tumor masses scattered throughout the lung. A *diffuse form,* simulating a pneumonia or organizing consolidation of the lung, may be difficult to recognize grossly. It is often of the terminal bronchiolar or alveolar cell type.

In the apex of the lung and at the thoracic inlet, the tumor may result in a distinctive clinical symptom complex *(Pancoast's syndrome),* characterized by pain around the shoulder and radiating down the arm, *Hor-*

ner's syndrome (unilateral enophthalmos, miosis, ptosis, and anhidrosis), and atrophy of the muscles of the arm and hand. Pancoast, after whom the syndrome is named, described the lesion in such cases as a *superior pulmonary sulcus tumor.* These apical tumors are apparently carcinomas of the terminal bronchioles that extend to involve the inferior cervical ganglion and the brachial plexus.

Microscopic types. Several histologic types are recognized. Although usually one cell pattern is observed in a single tumor, sometimes multiple sections of a tumor reveal a combination of cellular patterns.

Squamous cell (epidermoid) carcinoma. Most common is squamous cell carcinoma (Fig. 15-7), which constitutes 45% to 60% of carcinomas of the lung. Keratinization or intercellular bridges may be seen in the most mature forms, but most examples are less differentiated and may be quite pleomorphic. Variant forms may have areas with giant cells, spindle cells, or clear cells. Squamous cell carcinoma most often arises from larger bronchi near the hilus, but it also may be peripheral, where it tends to invade the body wall. Necrosis is frequent, and discharge of the necrotic material may result in cavitation. Com-

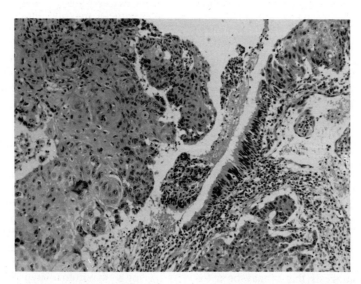

Fig. 15-7. Carcinoma of well-differentiated squamous type arising from bronchus.

pared with other types, the well-differentiated squamous cell tumors have a relatively slower metastatic potential and a somewhat better outlook if removed before the involvement of regional lymph nodes.

Small cell (oat cell) carcinoma. Small cell carcinomas constitute about 10% to 15% of pulmonary carcinomas. It has been proposed that they arise from "reserve cells" of the mucosa, which are small, dark cells between the basement membrane and the differentiated cells of the mucosal surface. Ordinarily, the tumors are composed of small, round, oat-shaped or spindle-shaped cells without structural formation. Mitoses are common. Such tumors, often called *oat cell carcinomas* (Fig. 15-8), but referred to by some authors simply as "small cell undifferentiated or anaplastic carcinomas," are easily mistaken for sarcoma and frequently were so considered in the past. Rapid growth and a tendency to early spread by the lymphatics (intrapulmonary and extrapulmonary) and by hematogenous metastasis

are characteristic, with a highly malignant rapid course and a poor prognosis.

The oat cell tumors tend to predominate in the stem bronchi and are uncommonly peripheral. Regional lymph nodes tend to be massively involved, often while the primary tumor is still small and before there is much bronchial obstruction. The tumor tissue is pale, translucent, and with only a slight tendency to necrosis.

Some investigators have produced electron microscopic evidence of neurosecretory-type granules in the cells of oat cell carcinomas that are similar to the granules in the Kultschitzky cells of the intestinal tract and in cells of bronchial carcinoid tumors. They suggest that oat cell carcinoma and bronchial carcinoid tumors are closely related and that oat cell tumors may be derived from Kultschitzky-type cells normally found in the bronchial mucosa rather than from the "reserve cells."

Large cell undifferentiated carcinoma. A large cell type of undifferentiated or anaplastic

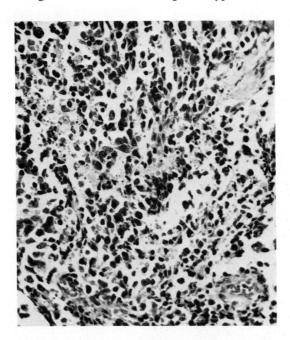

Fig. 15-8. Oat cell carcinoma, "usual" type. (×234; from Millard, M.: Lung, pleura, and mediastinum. In Anderson, W. A. D., and Kissane, J. M., editors: Pathology, ed. 7, St. Louis, 1977, The C. V. Mosby Co.)

carcinoma also occurs. It appears to be a form quite distinct from the small cell type and lacks epidermoid or glandular differentiation. Some of the large cell carcinomas are considered by certain writers to be undifferentiated adenocarcinomas.

Adenocarcinoma (columnar cell carcinoma). Adenocarcinoma constitues 9% to 12% of bronchogenic carcinomas and appears to be as frequent in women as in men. The tumors may arise from surface epithelium or from mucous glands, since mucus is demonstrable in some examples. They are composed of cuboidal or cylindrical cells and may be differentiated enough to form glandular or papillary structures (Fig. 15-9). Relatively, more occur peripherally than do other types. They often appear to be associated with lung scars, as many as two thirds in some series of cases. Growth tends to be rapid compared with squamous cell tumors, and hematogenous metastasis may be early and widespread.

Giant cell carcinoma. A giant cell carcinoma of the lung, which is characterized by numerous pleomorphic and bizarre cells of giant size (Fig. 15-10), has been noted for a relatively high degree of malignancy and a rapidly fatal course. It is an uncommon form of bronchogenic carcinoma that some authors regard as a variant of the large cell undifferentiated type. Most such cases are probably adenocarcino-

mas, and intracytoplasmic mucin is often demonstrable. Less frequently, there may be areas of recognizable squamous cell differentiation.

Mixed types. Mixed types of pulmonary carcinoma that contain some admixture of squamous, columnar, and undifferentiated cells are not uncommon. Varying methods of classifying such tumors lead to differences in percentage figures given for the common types.

Spread and metastasis. Spread of carcinoma of the lung is by direct extension, by the lymphatics, by the bloodstream, and by bronchial "embolism" or aspiration. Although any type of bronchogenic carcinoma may spread by any or all of these methods, squamous cell carcinoma is likely to extend by direct invasion, small cell (oat cell) carcinoma by the lymphatics, and adenocarcinoma by the bloodstream. Regional lymph nodes are involved in a high proportion of cases of bronchogenic carcinoma. Other common sites of metastasis are the liver, bones, adrenal glands, kidneys, and brain. Hematogenous metastasis is sometimes very widespread, and in some cases metastases produce clinical symptoms before the primary tumor does. Scalene node biopsy is sometimes a useful diagnostic procedure for carcinoma and other intrathoracic lesions, for it reflects the involvement of mediastinal lymph nodes. Enlarged medias-

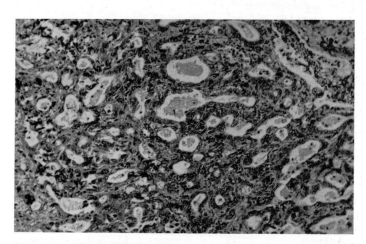

Fig. 15-9. Adenocarcinoma of lung.

tinal lymph nodes may compress or invade the superior vena cava to cause the "superior vena caval syndrome."

Prognosis. Unfortunately, most of the bronchogenic carcinomas are invasive and frequently unresectable and incurable by the time the diagnosis is made. Despite advances in therapy, there has been little improvement in the rather poor 6% to 10% overall 5-year survival rate. The prognosis has been found to be related to the histologic type, size, location, extension, and complications of the tumor. For example, in one series of cases in which the overall 5-year survival was 7%, the survival rate was 16% when the tumor was localized, 4% when there was regional spread, and 1% when there was distant spread. A better prognosis (34% 5-year survival rate) was noted when the cancer was asymptomatic (i.e., detected during a routine diagnostic test) as well as being anatomically localized and resectable by pneumonectomy. As to histologic types, the undifferentiated small cell (oat cell) cancer always has a very poor prognosis, even in apparently localized cases. A clinical stag-

ing system for carcinoma of the lung has been developed by the American Joint Committee for Cancer Staging and End Results Reporting (1973).

Bronchiolar carcinoma. About 3% of carcinomas of the lung are considered to arise from terminal bronchioles or alveolar lining cells *(alveolar cell tumors)*. The tumor cells line alveoli, their supporting stroma being the alveolar walls. The area of the tumor often is centered about a bronchiole, and evidence has suggested that bronchioles rather than alveoli are the source of these tumors. However, it is probable that most examples are simply variants of adenocarcinoma of the lung that have prominently adopted the alveolar fashion of intrapulmonary spread. What is sometimes considered a benign variant is referred to as *pulmonary adenomatosis,* although there is little evidence that this exists as an entity that can be distinguished from bronchiolar carcinoma.

Nodular and diffuse gross forms occur. The more common nodular form may be multiple and may simulate the appearance of metastatic carcinoma. The diffuse form may involve an

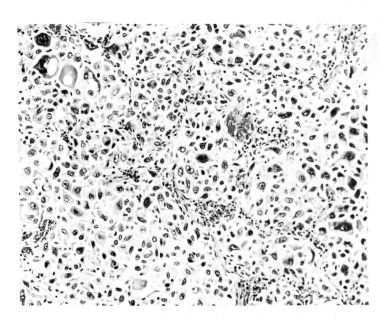

Fig. 15-10. Giant cell carcinoma of lung. Some of the giant cells contain intracytoplasmic mucin. ($\times 105$.)

entire lobe or occur as a single focus or as multiple foci and simulates the appearance of pneumonia. Whether there sometimes may be a multicentric origin is debatable, for some seeming multicentric tumors are explainable by aspirative or lymphatic spread. The tumor shows little or no necrosis, and the cut surface may be mucoid.

Microscopically, the tumor cells are tall, columnar, and usually mucus producing. They may regularly line alveolar spaces (Fig. 15-11) or may produce papillary protrusions into the lumen. The cells may be quite uniform, but sometimes hyperchromatic, irregular, and bizarre forms are present. Variations in appearance of the tumor cells do not correlate well with the clinical course. Rare ciliated cells may be found. Mitoses are infrequent. Calcified psammoma bodies are often present. The histologic appearance is similar to an infectious pulmonary adenomatosis of sheep (jagziekte), but an etiologic relationship has not been proved.

Bronchiolar carcinomas occur equally in men and women. There is a wide age distribution, although most cases occur between 40 and 60 years. The condition may be extensive before symptoms develop, which may be mainly dyspnea, cyanosis, and abundant watery or mucoid sputum. Death most often occurs from respiratory failure caused by progressive replacement of lung tissue, although at the time of termination, metastases are present in more than 50% of the patients, most often to regional lymph nodes, the liver, and the brain. Both lungs tend ultimately to be involved. Metastatic tumors from other organs (e.g., pancreas) may closely imitate and be mistaken for primary bronchiolar carcinoma.

Bronchial adenoma. "Adenomas" of a bronchus constitute 2% to 6% of primary tumors of the lung. Although not strictly benign, they are slow in growth and limited in their invasive, destructive, and metastasizing power. Hence, their malignant character is of low degree. They are of almost equal sex incidence, occur mainly under 50 years of age (average, 35 to 40 years), and have a slow course and a relatively good prospect of surgical curability.

They grow as polypoid or sessile tumors involving the subepithelial tissues of proximal bronchi, being derived from mucous glands and their ducts. They are more common on the right, involving the lower lobe or main stem bronchus, and are least common in the left upper lobe bronchus. Almost all are accessible to the bronchoscope. Although they may project

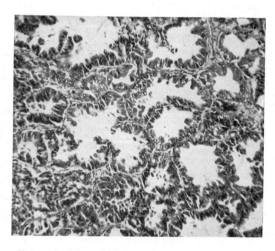

Fig. 15-11. Alveolar cell (terminal bronchiolar) carcinoma of lung. Alveolar spaces are lined by cancer cells.

into the lumen of a bronchus, causing partial or complete obstruction, most of the tumor is usually beneath the surface. Necrosis and ulceration are uncommon, but vascularity is considerable and hemorrhage may be a complication.

The carcinoid form is most frequent and histologically resembles the carcinoid tumors of the intestine, although argentaffin granules are only rarely demonstrable. Small uniform cells are arranged in strands, sheets, or masses situated about abundant, delicate sinusoidal vessels (Fig. 15-12). Mitoses are infrequent. Invasion and penetration of the capsule quite often occur, with metastasis to the tracheobronchial lymph nodes in about 9% and metastases to the liver, vertebrae, or kidney occasionally. The carcinoid tumors are resistant to radiation. Examples of carcinoid bronchial adenoma have been reported in which a metastasis in the liver was accompanied by the clinical functioning carcinoid syndrome.

The cylindromatous type (adenocystic basal cell carcinoma) constitutes about 15% of bronchial adenomas, tends to be more proximal than the carcinoid form (may involve the trachea), and more often has a sessile or diffuse form. Microscopically, cells are arranged in branching cylinders, tubes, or masses and may resemble basal cell tumors of the skin. They may have a secretion that stains with mucicarmine. As compared with the carcinoid form, they have less vascularity and tendency to hemorrhage, have a greater invasiveness, and are more radiosensitive. Metatasis may occur in almost one third of the patients, and prognosis for survival is poorer than with the carcinoid type.

The uncommon mucoepidermoid adenoma appears to have recognizable benign and malignant forms. It is composed of a mixture of sheets of squamous-type cells and mucus-secreting cells.

Other infrequent variant forms may be on-

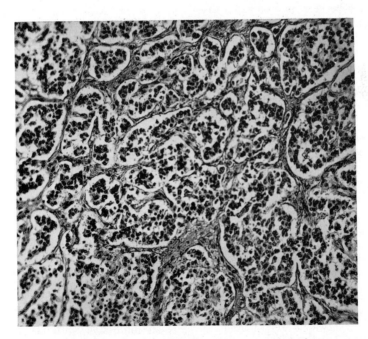

Fig. 15-12. Bronchial adenoma with characteristic trabecular and alveolar pattern. (From Haukohl, R. S., and Anderson, W. A. D., editors: Pathology seminars, St. Louis, 1955, The C. V. Mosby Co.)

cocytoid and papillary. The oncocytoid form, a variant of the carcinoid type, is composed of large eosinophilic cells and tends to occur at older ages.

Sarcoma

Although examples of hemangiosarcoma, fibrosarcoma, osteochondrosarcoma, and leiomyosarcoma of the lung have been reported, they are all extremely rare. Lymphocytic lymphoma originating in the lung is slightly less rare. It is similar to lymphocytic lymphoma elsewhere. The numerous sarcomas of the lung reported in older literature are now recognized as undifferentiated bronchogenic carcinomas.

Carcinosarcoma of the lung is composed of mixed malignant epithelial and mesodermal elements. Although a few examples have been reported, most cases appear to be anaplastic variants of squamous cell bronchogenic carcinomas.

Reticuloendothelial diseases occasionally involve the lungs as well as other organs. Such involvements may be seen in Hodgkin's disease, nonlipid reticuloendotheliosis (Letterer-Siwe disease), lymphocytic lymphoma, and leukemias. The process in the lung is similar to that in other organs.

International histologic classification

Because comparative and statistical studies have been hampered by a wide variation in criteria, classification, and terminology, a standard classification for such purposes has been proposed. Published by the World Health Organization,* it is as follows:

   I Epidermoid carcinomas
  II Small cell anaplastic carcinomas
     1 Fusiform cell type
     2 Polygonal cell type
     3 Lymphocytelike ("oat cell") type
     4 Others
 III Adenocarcinomas
     1 Bronchogenic
       a Acinar   } with or without mucin
       b Papillary }   formation

---

*Kreyberg, L.: Histological typing of lung tumours, Geneva, 1967, World Health Organization.

     2 Bronchiolo-alveolar
  IV Large cell carcinomas
     1 Solid tumors with mucinlike content
     2 Solid tumors without mucinlike content
     3 Giant cell carcinomas
     4 "Clear" cell carcinomas
   V Combined epidermoid and adenocarcinomas
  VI Carcinoid tumors
 VII Bronchial gland tumors
     1 Cylindromas
     2 Mucoepidermoid tumors
     3 Others
VIII Papillary tumors of the surface epithelium
     1 Epidermoid
     2 Epidermoid with goblet cells
     3 Others
  IX "Mixed" tumors and carcinosarcomas
     1 "Mixed" tumors
     2 Carcinosarcomas of embryonal type ("blastomas")
     3 Other carcinosarcomas
   X Sarcomas
  XI Unclassified
 XII Mesotheliomas
     1 Localized
     2 Diffuse
XIII Melanomas

Metastatic tumors

The lung is a common site for metastatic tumors, spread usually being by the bloodstream. Among the tumors that frequently produce metastases to the lungs are carcinomas of the breast, gastrointestinal tract, and genitourinary tract (e.g., uterus, prostate gland, and kidneys), malignant melanomas, and sarcomas of bone. Usually, multiple discrete nodular tumor masses are produced. Secondary metastatic spread elsewhere may occur from the metastatic tumors in the lung. Occasionally, a lymphatic extension to the lung may occur from cancer of the breast. A peculiar type of tumor metastasis to the lung has been described under the terms *lymphangitis carcinoma* and *diffuse infiltrative carcinoma*. The clinically inconspicuous primary tumor usually is an infiltrative scirrhous carcinoma of the stomach or colon. It should be differentiated from lymphatic spread of primary lung cancer (Fig. 15-13).

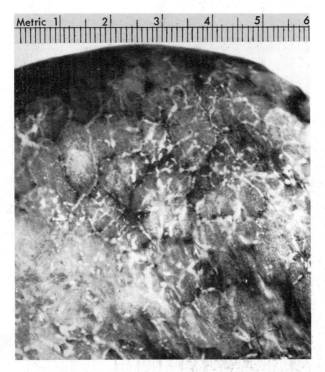

Fig. 15-13. Lymphangitic spread of carcinoma of lung.

PNEUMONIA

Inflammation of lung tissue is called pneumonia, although sometimes it is quite logically referred to as pneumonitis. Although commonly of bacterial origin, certain types (e.g., lipid pneumonia) are caused by other irritants. The anatomic types are known as lobar pneumonia, lobular pneumonia (bronchopneumonia), and interstitial pneumonia. Lobar pneumonia is almost always caused by pneumococcal infection, whereas bronchopneumonia is caused by a wide variety of organisms. Interstitial pneumonias are mainly nonbacterial (viral) or caused by *Mycoplasma, Rickettsia,* or related organisms.

Viral infections of the lung, including influenza, are considered on p. 166.

Lobar pneumonia

Lobar pneumonia is a diffuse, usually pneumococcal, consolidation affecting one or more lobes of the lungs. It occurs sporadically, at all ages, and often is preceded by an upper respiratory tract infection. The disease has a rapid onset with chills, cough, fever, and sometimes prostration. After a course of 1 or 2 weeks, recovery may occur by lysis or crisis, or it may be complicated by organization of the exudate, empyema, abscess formation, pericarditis, endocarditis, or meningitis.

In the earliest stage, the involved lobe is edematous and congested, followed rapidly by a stage of red hepatization (consolidation), in which a fibrinous exudate is added to the congestion. This, in turn, is followed by gray hepatization (Fig. 15-14), in which stage congestion is no longer present, and there is degeneration of cells of the exudate. In favorable cases, resolution follows, with increase in the proportion of macrophages and finally absorption of the exudate and restitution of the lung tissue to its previous healthy condition.

The classic features of lobar pneumonia as described here are not seen as frequently

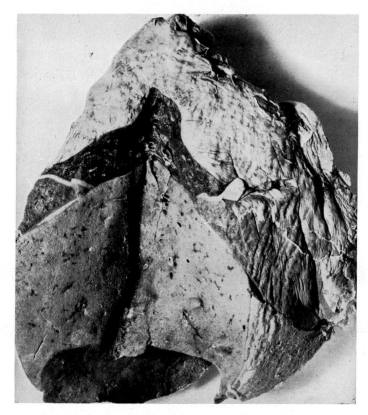

Fig. 15-14. Lobar pneumonia. Gray hepatization of lower lobe of lung. Pleural surface has thick fibrinous exudate.

today as in the past during the preantibiotic era.

Etiology. Lobar pneumonia is caused in almost all cases by pneumococci, but it may be caused by Friedländer's pneumobacillus and other bacteria. Pneumococci may be immunologically classified into about 82 serotypes. Although all types are pathogenic for man, the usual ones responsible for lobar pneumonia in adults are types 1, 3, 4, 5, 7, 8, 12, 14, and 19 and in children types 1, 6, 14, and 19.

Accessory etiologic factors believed of importance include anesthesia, inhalation of noxious gases, viral infection, cardiac failure, and trauma to the chest. These predisposing factors may play a role by inducing alveolar edema, which serves as a growth medium for the pneumococci. Patients who are debilitated by illness or alcoholism or who are exposed to chilly, wet weather seem to be especially susceptible.

Pathogenesis. Organisms reach the lungs by way of the respiratory passages. The bacteremia that often is present is believed to be secondary rather than primary to the pneumonia. Experimental lobar pneumonia has been produced in monkeys by the injection of pneumococci into the trachea. This resulted in an interstitial spread of the infection from the hilus to the periphery of the lung, with subsequent outpouring of exudate into the alveoli. Further clinical and experimental studies have suggested a different course of events in lobar pneumonia in human beings. A lobar pneumonia closely resembling that which occurs in

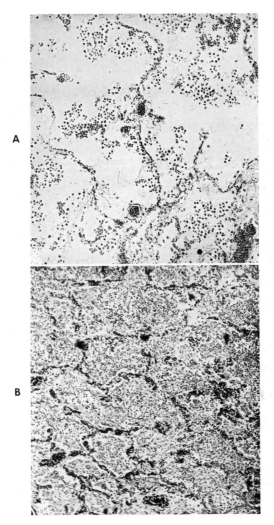

Fig. 15-15. Stages of lobar pneumonia. **A,** Stage of congestion. Edema and early leukocytic infiltration. **B,** Stage of red hepatization. Engorgement persists. Fibrin is scanty.

Continued.

human beings has been produced in the dog by implanting pneumococci suspended in a starch-broth paste into the terminal air sacs. A rapid outpouring of edema fluid quickly dispersed the organisms throughout the lobe by way of air passages and through the pores of Cohn in the alveolar walls, followed later by leukocytic exudation.

Morbid anatomy. The pneumonic process goes through a series of stages that are characteristic and roughly indicate the age of the process. There is no sharp dividing line between these stages, which merge into each other. Different stages are often evident in different portions of the involved lung. Acute inflammation in the lung has the characteristics of acute inflammation elsewhere, i.e., vascular congestion and outpouring of a fluid and cellular exudate.

The earliest stage, the *stage of congestion* (Fig. 15-15, *A*), is characterized by engorgement of blood vessels and outpouring of fluid

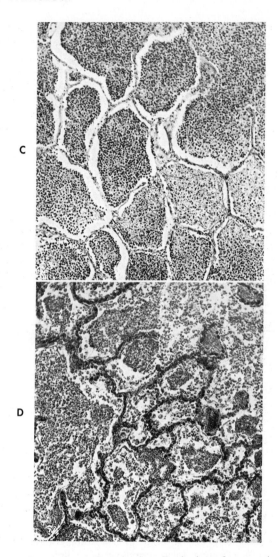

Fig. 15-15, cont'd. C, Stage of gray hepatization. Beginning of contraction of alveolar exudate. Alveolar walls are ischemic. **D,** Stage of resolution. Macrophages predominate. Masses of fibrin are free in alveolar spaces, and alveolar capillaries are engorged. (From Millard, M.: Lung, pleura, and mediastinum. In Anderson, W. A. D., and Kissane, J. M., editors: Pathology, ed. 7, St. Louis, 1977, The C. V. Mosby Co.)

into alveolar spaces. The involved lobe is heavier and less crepitant than normal, is red from the congestion and diapedesis of red cells, and oozes frothy, bloody fluid from its cut surface.

The *stage of red hepatization* rapidly follows. The lobe is consolidated by exudate fill-ing the air sacs and has the consistency of liver tissue. The cut surface is dark red and distinctly granular. Microscopically, the alveoli are filled by thin strands of fibrin mixed with red cells and neutrophilic leukocytes (Fig. 15-15, *B*). These cells are in a good state of preservation, and the vessels in the alveolar walls are congested. Many pneumococci are present in the alveoli. The pleura over the affected lobe is covered by a fibrinous exudate.

In the *stage of gray hepatization,* the lobe is still solid and of liverlike consistency, but it is somewhat softer than in the red stage and less granular. The gray color is caused by disappearance of the congestion and of the red cells in the alveoli and by an increased proportion of leukocytes in the alveolar exudate. Microscopically, the alveolar exudate contains a large proportion of neutrophilic leukocytes, a clumping of fibrin, and a decrease in number of red cells (Fig. 15-15, *C*). In later periods of this stage, the cells of the exudate show degeneration and disintegration. Pneumococci are still numerous in the exudate.

In the *stage of resolution,* the cut surface of the lung has a somewhat translucent jellylike appearance. At this time, many free macrophages are found in the alveoli (Fig. 15-15, *D*), arising from alveolar septal cells and blood monocytes. The macrophages engulf and destroy the organisms, which consequently are scarce in this stage. Neutrophilic leukocytes are less numerous and are disintegrating.

During recovery, the exudate is removed by being coughed up, by phagocytosis and removal by macrophages, and by liquefaction and absorption. The final result in the uncomplicated case of recovery is restoration of the lung to its previous condition with no residual scars.

Complications. Although most cases clear up without persisting lesions, a variety of complications may occur. *Empyema* is a persistent purulent pleurisy that follows the pneumonia. When the purulent effusion is large, the lung tissue collapses proportionately. Spread of pneumonia to cause *pericarditis* occasionally occurs. More rarely, there may be metastatic blood spread to cause pneumococcal *meningitis, arthritis,* or *endocarditis.*

In the involved lung tissue, several complications may develop. Only occasionally is there breakdown of tissue with localized *abscess formation.* Secondary infection of the abscess by fusospirochetal or putrefactive or-

ganisms results in *gangrene.* In rare cases, resolution of the alveolar exudate fails to occur, and it becomes organized. Such an *organizing pneumonia* is characterized grossly by a dense, solid, fleshy or elastic consistency, to which the term *carnification* of the lung often is applied. Microscopically, there are masses of fibrous tissue that fill the alveoli and join by fine strands passing through small openings in the alveolar walls (Fig. 15-16).

Bronchopneumonia (lobular pneumonia)

In bronchopneumonia, the inflammatory consolidation is patchy and irregular in distribution. It is usually secondary to or a complication of some other disease or infection, and the etiologic agents include a variety of bacteria and other irritants. The most common microorganisms involved are the staphylococcus, streptococcus, influenza bacillus, and pneumococcus. Specific types of bronchopneumonia occur in tuberculosis, tularemia, and plague.

In the pathogenesis of most cases, the infection reaches the lung by air passages, with the development of a bronchitis, and spreads to involve alveoli immediately adjacent to a bronchiole. Direct spread then may involve contiguous lobules. In some cases, this spread and confluence may be such that a whole lobe is involved, and distinction from lobar pneumonia is not obvious. Pyemia with numerous septic emboli to the lung setting up many small focal areas of inflammation may produce a condition that is grossly very similar to bronchopneumonia.

Examined grossly, both lungs usually are found to be involved, but unequally, and the lower lobes in their posterior and basal parts are particularly affected. Firm nodular areas of consolidation are palpable, and pus can be squeezed from the cut bronchioles in these areas. There is usually little or no exudate on the pleural surface, but it is likely to be mottled by alternating bluish and red areas. The cut surface of the lung is moist and red with some projecting reddish gray areas of consolidation. These areas often can be felt more eas-

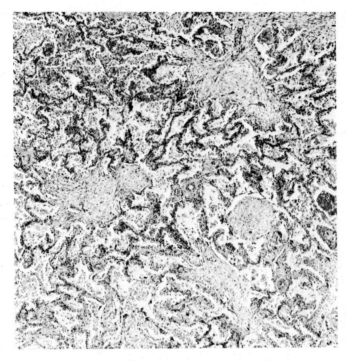

Fig. 15-16. Organizing pneumonia. Masses of young proliferating connective tissue can be seen passing from one alveolus to another.

ily than they can be seen. Some bluish areas of collapse and lighter areas of emphysema are often present as well. The moist and nongranular character of the cut surface differs from that of lobar pneumonia.

Microscopically, the consolidated areas show alveoli containing mononuclear and neutrophilic leukocytes. Fibrin and red cells are relatively scarce, although hemorrhagic types may be found, particularly in influenzal and staphylococcal pneumonias. Necrosis of tissue and abscess formation may be present in the cases caused by streptococci and staphylococci. The alveolar walls are congested. Bronchioles in the area contain exudate in their lumina and leukocytic infiltration in their walls that extends interstitially for a variable distance around them.

Types. Types of bronchopneumonia having a particular pathogenesis often are given dis-

tinctive names, although they have in common many of the features that have been noted.

Hypostatic, or *terminal, pneumonia* is that type found in patients with conditions such as heart disease or cerebral hemorrhage. The consolidation is found in lower and posterior parts of the lung where passive congestion and edema have been present.

Aspiration pneumonia is caused by the aspiration of material into the lung; e.g., septic material may be inhaled during an operation, particularly if the operation has involved the mouth, pharynx, or upper respiratory tract.

Postoperative pneumonia may be of the aspiration type, but often it is related to postoperative atelectasis of areas of lung tissue as a result of plugging of bronchi or bronchioles by secretion or exudate.

Suppurative pneumonia, in which necrosis

and pus formation are distinctive features, may be caused by staphylococci, hemolytic streptococci, or pneumococci.

Chemical pneumonias are those caused by irritating or poisonous gases.

Interstitial pneumonia

An interstitial reaction, particularly with mononuclear cells, occurs in the pneumonias that follow and complicate measles, influenza adenovirus infections, whooping cough, varicella, psittacosis, and other infectious diseases. This type of response has been regarded as the characteristic pneumonic reaction to a virus or to combined action of a virus and bacteria. Epidemics of viral pneumonia have exhibited interstitial reaction. Viral pneumonias, including the giant cell pneumonia of infancy (Fig. 15-22), are considered on pp. 166-170.

Deaths from an Asian influenza epidemic in 1957 and a Hong Kong influenza epidemic in 1968 have shown a severe laryngeal, tracheal, and bronchial inflammation associated with a variety of interstitial and secondary bacterial pneumonias that were similar to the changes found in the 1918 to 1920 influenza epidemic. Primary atypical pneumonia is caused principally by *Mycoplasma pneumoniae* (Eaton agent). In about 50% of the patients with *Mycoplasma* pneumonia, cold agglutinins develop to a titer of 1:40 or more during convalescence.

The gross features of interstitial pneumonia are not characteristic, but microscopically there is an interstitial thickening, particularly around the bronchi and bronchioles and in adjacent alveolar walls. This is caused by an increase in the number of mononuclear cells. The alveolar lumina frequently contain no exudate, but fibrin and a few leukocytes (chiefly mononuclear) may be present. The fibrin may appear as hyaline membranes lining the alveoli.

Farmer's lung is a granulomatous interstitial pneumonitis occurring in agricultural workers and resulting from the inhalation of dust from moldy hay or silage. Exposure may be followed by an acute febrile illness, but the course of the inflammation tends to be pro-

longed and chronic. The granulomatous pneumonitis is accompanied by varying degrees of focal obliterating bronchiolitis, interstitial fibrosis, and emphysema. The reaction is believed to be the result of hypersensitivity. An allergic interstitial pneumonitis or *hypersensitivity alveolitis* has been described also in pigeon breeders *(pigeon-breeder's lung)* and in others inhaling various organic dusts.

Other types of pneumonia

Pneumocystis pneumonia. Pneumonia caused by *Pneumocystis carinii* was first noted as occurring in premature and debilitated infants in central Europe. A plasma cell and lymphocytic infiltration of alveolar septa led to use of the term *interstitial plasma cell pneumonitis,* although it is an inconstant and often not a prominent feature.

This lesion has been recognized in widespread distribution, with cases reported from various areas of North America, and in adults as well as infants. Usually, but not always, it has occurred in persons debilitated by other conditions, including leukemia and malignant lymphomas. It also has occurred in patients with agammaglobulinemia and in patients receiving immunosuppressive therapy after renal transplantation, appearing to be related to long-term prednisone therapy.

The alveolar lumina contain a peculiar, foamy or vacuolated, lightly eosinophilic material in which the infective agent, *Pneumocystis carinii,* can be found (Fig. 15-17). There has been some question as to its nature, but today it is generally considered a protozoon. The organisms are not clearly seen in hematoxylin-eosin–stained sections, but special stains (e.g., methenamine silver) show the *Pneumocystis* cysts very well (p. 211). Hyperplasia of alveolar lining (septal) cells and sometimes hyaline membranes may be present. Diffuse interstitial fibrosis following an attack of *Pneumocystis carinii* pneumonia has been described.

Lipid pneumonia. The reactive lesions in the lung caused by oily and fatty substances introduced by way of the trachea have been termed *lipid pneumonia*. Cod-liver oil and liq-

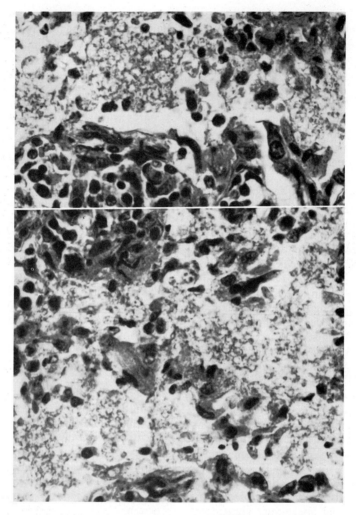

Fig. 15-17. Pneumocystis infection of lung. Masses of organisms in alveolar spaces have foamy appearance. Alveolar walls contain increased numbers of mononuclear cells, plasma cells, and lymphocytes.

uid petrolatum are the common causative agents, although olive oil, milk fat, and other substances may produce similar lesions. The fatty or oily materials gain entrance to the lung by way of the trachea because of forced feeding, disturbance of the swallowing mechanism, or excessive use of an oily (liquid petrolatum) base in nasal and laryngeal instillations. The condition is most frequent in infants, but an adult type also occurs in which

liquid petrolatum is usually the offending agent.

The fundamental lesion of lipid pneumonia is an interstitial proliferative inflammation, which is essentially a foreign body reaction. Macrophages laden with oil or fat, foreign body giant cells, and increased connective tissue are the essential features. Adult and infantile types have been described.

In lipid pneumonia of the infantile type,

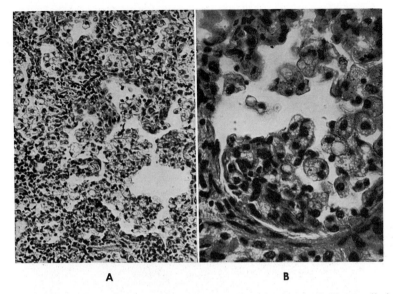

Fig. 15-18. Lipid pneumonia in infant. **A,** Low-power photomicrograph. **B,** Foam cells in alveolus and thickening of alveolar wall. (From Millard, M.: Lung, pleura, and mediastinum. In Anderson, W. A. D., editor: Pathology, ed. 5, St. Louis, 1966, The C. V. Mosby Co.)

there is pulmonary consolidation resulting from fat-laden macrophages and other inflammatory cells in the alveoli and alveolar walls, with little fibrosis (Fig. 15-18). Lipid pneumonia of the adult type (paraffinoma) is a nodular or tumorlike lesion in which fibrous scarring is prominent. The lesions are commonly located around the hilar region of the posterior and dependent portions of the lung. Vascular lesions with weakening of vessel walls may occur, and severe pulmonary hemorrhage has complicated bronchoscopy in some cases. Liquid petrolatum may be identified in tissue sections by its failure to stain black with osmic acid, although stainable by scarlet red. Cod-liver oil in the tissues is characterized by shredding of the oil and acid-fat staining by the Ziehl-Neelsen method.

Cholesterol pneumonitis. Chronic pneumonitis of the cholesterol type (foam cell pneumonitis) is characterized by alveolar spaces filled with vacuolated macrophages containing cholesterol-rich lipid, associated with necrotizing granulomatous and vascular lesions. Ulceration and obstruction of smaller branches of the bronchial tree, possibly a hypersensitivity phenomenon, have been proposed as the causative mechanism. Endogenous lipid pneumonia is also used as a term for the chronic obstructive lesions of the bronchi or bronchioles that are accompanied by lipid, chronic inflammation, and fibrosis. It may simulate the appearance of the aspiration type of lipid pneumonia.

Pulmonary alveolar proteinosis. Pulmonary alveolar proteinosis is a chronic disease characterized by the filling of distal air spaces (alveoli and bronchioles) with a granular and floccular proteinaceous and lipid-containing material (Figs. 15-19 and 15-20) that stains positively with the PAS technique. This material appears to be derived from proliferating septal cells, which become granular and undergo sloughing and necrosis. Acicular crystals and laminated bodies suggesting early stages of corpora amylacea may be present. The microscopic appearance must be distinguished from that of pulmonary edema, cholesterol pneumonitis, and *Pneumocystis* pneumonitis.

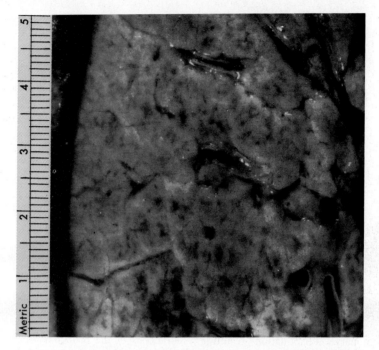

Fig. 15-19. Pulmonary alveolar proteinosis. Cut surface of lung shows diffuse grayish consolidation.

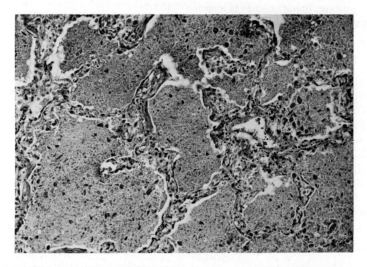

Fig. 15-20. Pulmonary alveolar proteinosis. Alveolar spaces are filled with granular eosinophilic material, with some darker eosinophilic condensation bodies. Alveolar walls contain little cellular infiltrate.

The cause is unknown. The clinical course is variable. It may or may not begin with a febrile illness and usually has a prolonged course associated with dyspnea and cough. Secondary fungal infection may occur.

Rats exposed to acute inhalation of quartz may develop a pulmonary lesion resembling alveolar proteinosis in man. The alveolar material in the experimental animals consists of protein and abundant lipid, and the lesion is referred to as ''alveolar lipoproteinosis.'' The alveolar walls show cellular hyperplasia affecting type II alveolar cells, which contain numerous, densely osmiophilic lamellar bodies.

A similar alveolar appearance has been observed in human patients with an acute form of silicosis.

Diffuse interstitial fibrosis of lung. In 1944, Hamman and Rich described an unusual condition of unknown etiology characterized by a diffuse and progressive fibrosis of alveolar walls. In the early stage, the process was marked by edema, fibrinous exudate, and inflammatory cells in the interstitial tissue (Fig. 15-21). Stainable bacteria were not demonstrated in the lesions. Progressive interstitial fibrosis followed, resulting in deficient aeration of the blood and manifested by dyspnea

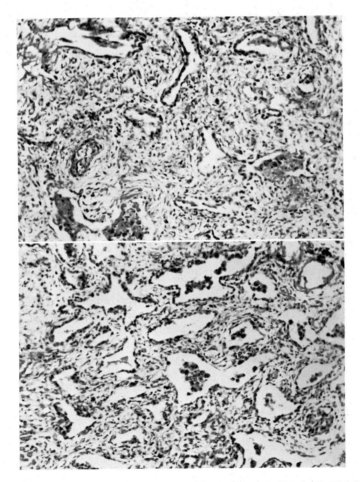

Fig. 15-21. Diffuse interstitial fibrosis of lung. (Courtesy Dr. A. R. Rich.)

and cyanosis. Enlargement and failure of the right side of the heart sometimes developed in a few weeks.

When Hamman and Rich described the lesion, they were impressed with the relatively rapid clinical course in their patients and they designated the lesion *acute diffuse interstitial fibrosis of the lungs*. Others have termed the entity *Hamman-Rich syndrome*. In subsequent years, patients with the disease have been observed in whom the clinical course was more prolonged, and the lesion has been referred to simply as diffuse interstitial fibrosis of the lungs. Other designations of this entity are *fibrosing alveolitis, usual interstitial pneumonia* (UIP), and *idiopathic pulmonary fibrosis.*

Although the cause is not known, the possibility that the condition belongs to the group of immunologic disorders of connective tissues has been suggested by the presence of a similar lesion in association with rheumatoid arthritis or in patients with the rheumatoid factor and by demonstration of immunoglobulins and complement in the lungs in some patients. A familial predisposition may exist in some instances, because the disease has been observed in several families. A similar pathologic picture has also been induced by certain drugs. Diffuse interstitial pulmonary fibrosis occurring in the late stages of other lung disorders, such as sarcoidosis, certain pneumoconioses, and obstruction to the outflow of pulmonary veins, may simulate the lesion seen in the Hamman-Rich syndrome.

Desquamative interstitial pneumonia. In recent years, a form of interstitial pneumonia of unknown cause has been observed that has been given the descriptive designation *desquamative interstitial pneumonia* (DIP). It is characterized by masses of desquamated type II alveolar cells and macrophages in the distal air spaces, focal interstitial thickening of the alveolar walls, proliferation of alveolar lining cells, and absence of necrosis and fibrinous exudate. The presence of lymphoid nodules in the interstitial septa, sometimes with plasma cells and eosinophils, also may be noted. Because of this histologic feature and certain clinical findings, some investigators have suggested that hypersensitivity may be a cause of desquamative interstitial pneumonia. It has been described in a few patients being treated with nitrofurantoin.

It is not clear whether DIP represents an early stage in the development of diffuse interstitial fibrosis of the lungs, described in the previous section, as suggested by some investigators. However, it appears to have a better prognosis than *usual interstitial pneumonia* and tends to respond favorably to corticosteroid therapy.

Lymphoid interstitial pneumonia. Another distinctive form of interstitial pneumonia differing from the usual types has been described and classified as *lymphoid interstitial pneumonia* (LIP), the principal feature being a heavy infiltration and proliferation of lymphocytes in both lungs. In certain reported instances, plasma cell infiltration is a prominent feature, sometimes with hypergammaglobulinemia.

Rheumatic pneumonia. Although cardiac lesions are of prime importance in rheumatic fever, pleurisy and pulmonary involvement are common. Mitral stenosis gives rise to a chronic passive congestion of the lung, resulting in brown induration. In addition to such changes, more specific primary rheumatic lesions have been described in the lung. This change is an interstitial pneumonitis, focal or widespread, with a tendency to recurrence.

In acute phases, congestion and hemorrhage are prominent. Focal areas of inflammation occur, with fibrinoid necrosis, fibrinous exudate in the alveoli, proliferation of mononuclear cells and fibroblasts, and eventual fibrosis. The peculiar focal areas of organizing inflammation have been referred to as Masson bodies. The specificity of the lesions is disputed. In subacute and chronic phases, the lung is of rubbery consistency, the toughness being caused by interstitial fibrosis and hyperplasia of elastic tissue. Such late changes may be difficult to separate from those resulting from passive congestion. Nodular pulmonary calcifications and ossification may be found in some long-standing cases of mitral stenosis, perhaps by organization of the exudate of rheumatic lesions.

Wegener's granulomatosis. Wegener's

granulomatosis, or necrotizing respiratory granulomatosis, appears to be a hypersensitivity disease involving primarily the respiratory tract but commonly affecting the kidneys and arteries elsewhere. Progressive, severe destructive or ulcerative lesions involve the lungs, with round or oval consolidations around affected bronchi. The lesions show angiitis and an inflammatory exudate in which eosinophils, plasma cells, mononuclear cells, and giant cells may be prominent. In the kidneys, focal glomerulitis with necrosis or fibrinoid change is most constant, although there may be some periglomerular granulomatous inflammation. Angiitis, involving medium-sized arteries, may be present elsewhere, e.g., in the spleen.

Although the severe cases have a short duration of a few months and may terminate in death, there is evidence that milder forms may occur. Possibly Loeffler's eosinophilic granuloma of the lung is a more benign form of a similar condition of hypersensitivity.

Loeffler's syndrome. Loeffler's syndrome is characterized by transitory pulmonary lesions, which are prominent in roentgenograms, an increase of eosinophilic leukocytes in the blood, and a mild clinical course. The lesion has been described as a bronchopneumonia with numerous eosinophilic leukocytes in the alveolar exudate, a tendency to organization, granulomatous foci, and necrotizing arteritis and arteriolitis. Bronchial changes may be similar to those in asthma. It has been considered an allergic reaction of pulmonary tissue, although a similarity to eosinophilic granuloma elsewhere and to the reticuloendothelioses has been suggested.

Granulomatous pulmonary lesions resulting from the inhalation of cosmetic aerosols have been reported and suggested by some as one cause of Loeffler's syndrome, but the frequency and importance are uncertain and debatable.

Legionnaires' disease. Legionnaires' disease is a newly recognized form of pneumonia that is so called because of a widely publicized outbreak of the disease at a convention of American Legionnaires at a hotel in Philadelphia in July 1976. At least 182 patients developed pneumonia, and 29 died as a result of this illness. Since then, several outbreaks have occurred in other parts of the country. Reexamination of previous epidemics of an unexplained respiratory illness in other cities has shown that Legionnaires' disease had occurred before the 1976 outbreak.

During and after the Philadelphia outbreak, an intensive search for the cause was instituted. The various causes that were considered included heavy metals, toxic gases, and infectious agents. Eventually, a bacterium (*Legionella pneumophila*) was identified in the tissues of patients with the disease and in peritoneal exudates of guinea pigs inoculated intraperitoneally with suspensions of patients' tissues. The organisms were difficult to detect in patients' tissues at first, since they stained faintly and inconsistently with Gram stains and did not grow in ordinary bacteriologic media. They are gram-negative, pleomorphic, rodlike bacteria that are best demonstrated by the Dieterle silver impregnation method of staining and exhibit specific immunofluorescent staining with sera from patients who survived Legionnaires' disease or from guinea pigs that were infected. The source of the bacteria in nature is not certain, although in recent outbreaks the organisms have been found growing in water of air-conditioning cooling towers or evaporative condensers and in nearby streams. The mode of spread of the disease has not been established, but it may be air-borne. One possibility is inhalation of bacteria in sprays of water from the evaporative condenser in air-conditioning systems. Person-to-person spread has been shown to be unusual or nonexistent but has not been ruled out.

Clinical features include malaise, myalgia, headache, rapidly rising fever with chills, cough, and chest pain, along with physical findings and roentgenographic evidence that are characteristic of pneumonia. Many of the patients have a preexisting illness that is sometimes serious. Apparently, the prognosis is worse if the underlying illness is debilitating or if the patient is elderly.

Grossly, the lungs exhibit varying degrees of consolidation that is often accompanied by a fibrinous pleuritis, with or without a serous or serosanguineous effusion. *Microscopically,* there is usually a dense intra-alveolar exudate consisting of varying proportions of neutrophils, macrophages, and fibrin, with varying degrees of necrosis of the inflammatory cells. Desquamation of alveolar lining epithelium is usually present. Sometimes edema of alveolar septa, with infiltration by inflammatory cells, is present. Alveolar septal necrosis is not a prominent feature, but focal necrosis may occur. The inflammation involves the respiratory bronchioles but not the larger bronchioles and bronchi. In some patients, a form of alveolar damage is seen that may occur in areas distant from the alveolar inflammation. This consists of regenerating alveolar epithelium, hyaline membranes, interstitial edema, occasionally sparse lymphocytic interstitial infiltration, and alveolar proteinaceous debris. It is possible that the cause of this alveolar damage is something other than the inflammatory disease itself, e.g., intensive oxygen therapy, shock complicating Legionnaires' disease, or recent chemotherapy or radiation of the chest for an underlying malignant tumor. The organisms are identified in the areas of alveolar inflammation in properly stained sections. They are found extracellularly or in phagocytes, chiefly macrophages and less frequently neutrophils. They are most numerous in areas where necrosis of inflammatory cells is most severe, and occasionally they are seen in the interstitial tissue.

Hyperplasia of the pulmonary alveolar lining. Electron microscopic study has suggested that alveoli are lined by a continuous cytoplasm of cells, with infrequent nuclei and few mitochondria. In a variety of pathologic conditions, alveolar lining cells appear in ordinary sections. The hyperplastic cells also may be derived from ''septal cells,'' which are normally found scattered in alveolar walls or in the niches between capillaries, or from downgrowth from terminal bronchioles. Such changes have been described in chronic passive congestion, in interstitial and lipid pneumonias, around tuberculous foci, in giant cell pneumonias of infancy (Fig. 15-22), and in pneumonia alba of congenital syphilis. Atypi-

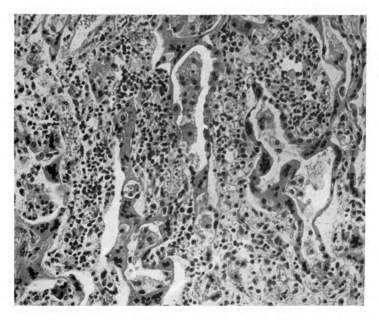

Fig. 15-22. Giant cell pneumonia in child. Alveolar spaces are lined by cells, some of which are fused to form giant cells.

cal hyperplasias of bronchiolar cells may form minute tumorlike masses (p. 395).

TUBERCULOSIS

Pulmonary tuberculosis, caused by the acid-fast *Mycobacterium tuberculosis,* is discussed in Chapter 7. In that chapter there is also a review of diseases caused by the atypical mycobacteria.

CIRCULATORY DISTURBANCES

Congestion. *Active* congestion in the lung accompanies acute inflammations or follows inhalation of irritants. *Passive* congestion is more common, the hypostatic form being found at almost every autopsy. The lower and posterior parts of the lungs are dark red and firmer than normal. More important is the *chronic passive congestion* that accompanies pulmonary hypertension and failure in the pulmonary circulation. This generalized pulmonary hyperemia may be present for an extensive period and gives rise to brown pigmentation and increased firmness, a condition called *brown induration of the lung.*

The most important cause of chronic passive congestion is mitral stenosis, but aortic stenosis, certain congenital cardiac defects, and other lesions associated with prolonged left ventricular failure occasionally give the same result. The brown color of the lung is caused by hemosiderin pigment, most of which is held in macrophages in alveolar spaces (heart failure cells). The hemosiderin may result from hemorrhages from the bronchopulmonary anastomoses in the mucosa of the terminal bronchioles. Iron pigment in adjacent stroma produces damage and reactive changes. Occasional cases of mitral stenosis may show minute foci of ossification in basal areas. The thickness of the alveolar walls, through which oxygen and carbon dioxide must diffuse, may be increased many times. The alveolar walls have increased collagenous interstitial tissue, thickening of capillary basement membranes, dilated capillaries, and edema. Alveolar lining cells tend toward cuboidal shape. Pulmonary vascular changes are common in such cases and consist of intimal thickening and athero-

sclerosis of arteries, hyperplastic arteriolar sclerosis, and, in some severe cases, even arteriolar necrosis. These vascular lesions are promoted by the high intravascular pressure, stagnation of blood, and edema.

Edema. Edema fluid in the lung may develop as a result of increased capillary blood pressure, as in passive congestion associated with left ventricular heart failure or mitral stenosis, or as a result of overloading of the circulation by administration of too much intravenous fluid. It also occurs in association with increased intracranial pressure, probably as a result of reflex stimulation. Another factor causing pulmonary edema is increased vascular permeability. This may be caused by inhaled irritating gases, inflammation in early stages of pneumonia, heroin overdosage, shock, hypoxia, etc. In shock, however, other factors may be operative in producing pulmonary edema.

The edematous lung is large, pale, and heavy and pits on pressure. Watery, frothy fluid flows or may be squeezed from the cut surface. In sections, the edema fluid appears as an eosin-staining material in the alveolar spaces. The intensity of the stain depends on the amount of protein present. Edema fluid with its protein content provides a medium favorable for bacterial growth and so promotes infection.

High concentrations of oxygen, as in mechanical ventilation, have been shown to cause pulmonary capillary congestion and edema, characterized by a proteinaceous exudate containing fibrin that commonly appears as "hyaline membranes" lining alveolar walls, alveolar ducts, and respiratory bronchioles. A later effect may be alveolar and interlobular septal edema, fibroblastic proliferation with early fibrosis, and prominent hyperplasia of alveolar lining cells.

High altitude acute pulmonary edema is found occasionally in persons who go to high altitudes for the first time, or it may occur in residents of high altitudes when they return home after some days or weeks at sea level. The edema is severe, with hyaline membranes. Increased capillary permeability, left sided cardiac failure, and increased pulmonary venous resistance may be important hemodynamic factors.

Pulmonary changes in uremia. A proportion of patients with uremia, hypertension, and left ventricular failure develop a central pulmonary edema that presents a characteristic roentgenologic appearance (hilar "butterfly pattern"). The periphery of the lungs tend to be spared. The combination of a rise in pulmonary capillary pressure resulting from cardiac failure and alteration in capillary permeability resulting from uremia produces a protein-rich or fibrinous type of pulmonary edema. However, the changes may occur in uremia with little or no evidence of heart failure. Improvement in the uremic condition by peritoneal dialysis may be accompanied by improvement in the pulmonary edema. There appears to be some correlation with the degree of acidosis, as indicated by depression of the blood carbon dioxide content.

Grossly, the lungs are rubbery and yield frothy fluid on firm pressure (solid edema). Microscopically, the alveolar walls are thickened and congested, and the alveolar spaces contain an eosinophilic fibrinous fluid with a tendency to hyalinization and formation of eosinophilic (hyaline) membranes lining alveoli (Fig. 15-23). The pathologic changes are similar to those seen in other conditions with cardiac failure and associated vascular damage, as in rheumatic pneumonitis.

Thrombosis, embolism, and infarction. Blockage of pulmonary arteries by embolism is common, but primary thrombosis is relatively rare. Thrombi that give rise to pulmonary embolism most commonly originate in veins of the lower extremities, pelvic veins, the prostatic venous plexus, vena cava, and right atrium. Pulmonary embolism is common in older age groups and in medical as well as surgical diseases. There is developing evidence that pulmonary embolization in surviving patients may be a precursor of pulmonary arteriosclerosis and pulmonary hypertension. Postoperative pulmonary embolism is most likely to follow abdominal or pelvic surgical procedures. If the embolus blocks the pulmonary artery or one of its large branches, it may cause rapid death and is easily clinically mistaken for coronary occlusion. The actual

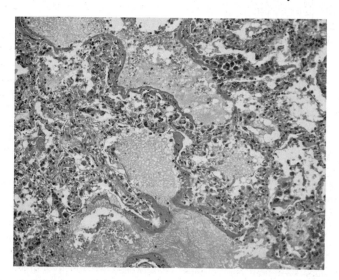

Fig. 15-23. Lung in fatal uremia (uremic pneumonitis). Alveolar spaces contain eosinophilic edema fluid with peripheral condensations forming hyaline membranes. Alveolar walls are thick and edematous, and there are some focal accumulations of macrophages containing hemosiderin pigment.

mechanism of death is not clearly understood but may be due to the sudden reduction of blood flow alone or combined with a sympathetic-inhibitory reflex or shock. There is insufficient time for development of an infarct of the lung in such rapidly fatal cases. Demonstration of the embolus at autopsy often can be facilitated by opening the pulmonary artery in situ before removal of the heart.

Blockage of smaller pulmonary arteries by emboli results in infarction of lung tissue if there is already some interference with the pulmonary circulation, such as passive congestion or edema. Embolism alone does not result in infarction of the normal lung, probably because blood supplied by bronchial arteries and by anastomoses of pulmonary intralobular arteries is sufficient to maintain nutrition. Pulmonary infarcts are almost always red and hemorrhagic. They form bulging, dark red, firm, conical areas, with their base at the pleural surface. Microscopically, the whole area of infarction, including alveolar spaces, walls, and capillaries, is stuffed with blood. In later stages, necrosis of the alveolar walls may be observed, and there is decolorization of the blood. Extensive pulmonary embolism with subsequent organization may lead to heart failure (cor pulmonale).

An embolus tends to be coiled, twisted, impacted, or riding a bifurcation. Its shape may not conform to that of the vessel in which it lies, and it may have freshly broken ends. A thrombus is usually attached to the vessel wall, has a sessile base, and is molded to the shape of the vessel.

Other forms of pulmonary embolism (e.g., fat, amniotic fluid, air) have been discussed before (pp. 113-116).

Blast injury. Pulmonary hemorrhage associated with thoracic trauma or asphyxia is common in both peace and war injuries.

In war experience, "blast injury" or pulmonary concussion caused by a nearby bomb or other high explosive may produce fatal pulmonary hemorrhage without external evidence of trauma. The lungs show bilateral and roughly symmetric hemorrhagic consolidation deep in their substance. There is an associated general pulmonary congestion, and the hemorrhage may be progressive. Microscopically, the appearance is similar to that of a recent infarct, but some areas may show fibrin and monocytes as well as red cells in alveolar spaces and so simulate in appearance the red hepatization stage of pneumonia.

In compression asphyxia, the lesion differs in that the hemorrhages are mainly subpleural and in the lines of the ribs, with emphysema outlining rib markings. In the pulmonary hemorrhage caused by the traumatic impact of a solid, the hemorrhage may be unilateral and related to the site of the blow, and around this point the lung is torn or contused.

Arteriosclerosis. Pulmonary arteriosclerosis of mild degree is common but rarely of clinical importance. In larger arteries, it is evident grossly as intimal atherosclerosis. Hypertension and congestion in the pulmonary circulation (e.g., in mitral stenosis) lead to vascular changes. There may be dilatation, atherosclerosis, and medial thickening of the larger elastic arteries. The muscular arteries show thickening of the media, due to vasoconstriction and/or hypertrophy, and marked intimal cellular proliferation that extends to the arterioles. As a consequence, there is marked vascular narrowing. Complications, such as thrombosis and necrotizing arteritis with fibrinoid change, may occur. Thromboembolic conditions with embolizations of smaller pulmonary vessels may contribute to the development of pulmonary sclerosis and hypertension.

There is an uncommon condition of primary sclerosis of pulmonary arteries, associated with hypertrophy of the right side of the heart and usually resulting in death from heart failure. Some of these cases, particularly when associated with severe cyanosis, are often designated as *Ayerza's disease.* However, the concept of Ayerza's disease has been variable. Ayerza did not describe the pathologic changes in his report, and probably most of his patients had pulmonary hypertension associated with congenital heart disease, although a few may have had idiopathic pulmonary hypertension.

PULMONARY CALCIFICATION

Calcification in the lung is most commonly a dystrophic calcification occurring in areas of necrosis and inflammation, most often as a result of tuberculosis, histoplasmosis, or other fungal infections. The lung also may be the site of metastatic calcification in severe cases of hyperparathyroidism, the alveolar walls and blood vessels being affected particularly.

Rounded laminated bodies (corpora amylacea) occasionally are seen in alveolar spaces where there has been chronic inflammation. They may be present in association with pulmonary alveolar proteinosis. Rarely, they may be present in enormous numbers and may be calcified *(microlithiasis alveolaris pulmonum)*, so that they produce widespread opacity in roentgenograms. The cause is unknown, but probably they result from the calcification of remnants of inflammatory exudate or necrotic material in alveolar spaces.

ATELECTASIS

Atelectasis is a term that strictly refers to an incomplete expansion of the lungs but also is commonly used for a collapse of lung tissue. The three main causes are (1) failure of expansion in the newborn infant (congenital), (2) compression of lung tissue, and (3) bronchial obstruction. Atelectasis does not interfere with respiratory function unless areas of considerable size are involved.

In many stillborn infants, the lungs are completely atelectatic and airless. Infants who live for a few days have lungs with patchy areas of atelectasis or incomplete expansion. Compression atelectasis results from pressure against lung tissue, as by air, transudate, or exudate in the pleural cavity or by tumors. Bronchial obstruction (e.g., by mucous plugs, tumors, or enlarged lymph nodes) results in atelectasis because the air is absorbed from the nonaerated portion of the lung. Atelectasis involving the middle lobe of the right lung *(middle lobe syndrome)* is related to extrabronchial compression by enlarged lymph nodes. However, in some patients, bronchoscopic or bronchographic evidence of obstruction of the middle lobe bronchus is not demonstrated.

Atelectatic lung tissue is dark red or blue because of congestion, and it is firm, noncrepitant, and depressed below the surrounding surfaces. Microscopically, the alveolar walls are pressed together, forming more or less parallel bands separated by narrow elongated alveolar spaces. If atelectasis is present for a considerable period, fibrosis may occur and reexpansion becomes impossible.

Acute massive collapse. Acute massive collapse refers to the rapid atelectasis of the whole lung or a large part of a lung. The mediastinum is displaced toward the affected side, and there is evidence of respiratory difficulty. It is an occasional complication of abdominal operations, peritonitis, and diaphragmatic pleurisy. Bronchial obstruction (by mucinous secretions) and interference with the cough reflex are believed to be the important factors in causation. There is some evidence that atelectasis may occur in the absence of obstruction ("contraction atelectasis") because of active contraction of smooth muscle elements in the lung distal to the terminal bronchioles.

Hyaline membrane disease. A condition in newborn infants of failure of pulmonary expansion or pulmonary collapse has as its most prominent microscopic feature hyaline membranes lining the bronchiolar and alveolar ducts.

Clinically, the condition is called "respiratory distress syndrome," or "pulmonary syndrome of the newborn." It is particularly common in premature infants, after cesarean section, and in infants of mothers with diabetes mellitus. The mortality is high.

The lungs are dark red, of liverlike consistency, edematous, and poorly aerated. Histologically, there is widespread atelectasis and prominent hyaline membranes of eosin-staining homogeneous material lining mainly respiratory bronchioles and alveolar ducts and occasionally alveoli (Fig. 15-24).

The hyaline membranes apparently result from increased plasma exudation. Fibrin has been demonstrated in the membranes by some investigators, but in a recent study it was observed only occasionally. Necrotic epithelial cells and amniotic fluid contents may be en-

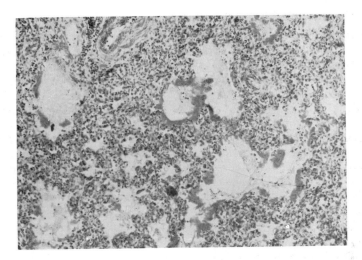

Fig. 15-24. Hyaline membrane disease of lung in newborn infant.

meshed in the membranes. Although the hyaline membranes may contribute to the respiratory difficulty, they apparently are not the primary cause. Pulmonary lymphatic vessels are enlarged and distended, but the mechanism of development of this lymphangiectasia is not clear.

The cause of the disease is not known, but it is generally believed that a deficiency of pulmonary surfactant, a surface-active substance capable of lowering alveolar surface tension, may be responsible for the atelectasis. Some have suggested that an inhibition of the fibrinolysin system accounts for persistence of the hyaline membranes. A pathogenetic mechanism that has been proposed recently is as follows: pulmonary vasoconstriction causes alveolar hypoperfusion, resulting in (1) deficiency of surfactant on alveolar surfaces with subsequent atelectasis and (2) increased alveolar wall permeability with effusion into air spaces.

Hyaline membranes of similar appearance may be found in the lungs of adults in a variety of conditions characterized by pneumonitis and edema, such as uremic pneumonitis, viral interstitial pneumonitis, irritation from inhaled chemicals, and after irradiation.

Hyaline membrane disease of infancy is to be distinguished from the *sudden infant death syndrome* (SIDS), which accounts for many deaths during the first year of life, particularly between 2 weeks and 4 months of age. The principal feature in SIDS is unexpected and unexplained death in apparently well infants, although a minor illness (e.g., slight upper respiratory tract infection) may have existed before death. Although minimal inflammatory changes in the lungs are sometimes observed in these infants, it is doubtful that they are responsible for the deaths (commonly referred to as "crib deaths"). Also noted in some of these infants is increased muscle in small pulmonary arteries. This lesion has been attributed to chronic alveolar hypoventilation and hypoxia, which are believed to be associated with recurrent episodes of sleep apnea.

PULMONARY EMPHYSEMA

Emphysema is the most common chronic disease of the lungs and a major cause of pulmonary disability. It is commonly included in the group of disorders referred to as nonspecific *chronic obstructive pulmonary disease* (COPD). In view of the frequent association of emphysema with chronic bronchitis, another common cause of chronic obstructive pulmonary disease, the designation *emphysema-bronchitis* complex is sometimes used. As mentioned before, however, chronic bronchitis may exist without pulmonary complications (p. 392). Also, there are instances of emphysema not associated with bronchitis. Yet many patients with chronic obstructive pulmonary disease have both a bronchitic and an emphysematous component, often with one or the other predominating.

There is considerable confusion in the literature concerning the definitions and concepts of pulmonary emphysema, and through the years they have been changing. Literally, the term *emphysema* means *inflation,* and it was originally used for any condition of inflation by air or gas in any tissue of the body. *Pulmonary emphysema* may be defined as *vesicular emphysema* when inflation involves the air spaces of the lungs (i.e., distal to the terminal bronchioles) and *interlobular (interstitial) emphysema* when inflation affects the tissue between the air spaces. Commonly, when the term "pulmonary emphysema" is used without a qualifying adjective, it usually implies the vesicular form. It should be noted, however, that some writers today regard "vesicular emphysema" as a synonym for one type of emphysema, viz., "panlobular emphysema." There is a tendency among some investigators, particularly in the United States, to limit the term "pulmonary emphysema" to those cases in which the enlargement of the air spaces is accompanied by destruction and to use the term "pulmonary overinflation" if there is dilatation of air spaces without destruction. It is probable, however, that in most (if not all) cases of emphysema, both mechanisms are involved at the same time, with one or the other being predominant. As Heard pointed out, it is difficult to sharply separate pulmonary overinflation from emphysema on this basis, since it is not possible to determine at what point the slightest amount of destruction can be recognized.

The forms of emphysema that will be discussed are centrilobular, panlobular, paraseptal, paracicatricial, variants of panlobular and centrilobular types, and interstitial. The clinical emphysema syndromes that are most frequently encountered in practice usually are related to sufficiently widespread or severe centrilobular and/or panlobular emphysema.

Centrilobular emphysema. Centrilobular emphysema (centriacinar emphysema) is usually a destructive lesion in which destroyed and enlarged respiratory bronchioles tend to become confluent and form emphysematous spaces situated toward the center of the acini. The lesions tend to be most frequent and severe in the upper areas of the lungs. Black pigment is often seen in the walls of the respiratory bronchioles and in the perilobular septa. The so-called focal emphysema of coal workers is a form of centrilobular emphysema.

Panlobular emphysema. Panlobular emphysema (panacinar emphysema) is characterized generally by destruction and fairly uniform dilatation of all air passages distal to the terminal bronchiole, so that the entire acinus is affected. Although it occurs in any part of the lung, it tends to become more severe in lower lobes and anterior zones. Panlobular and centrilobular emphysema may occur together in lungs in varying degree as well as separately.

• • •

Morphologically, early lesions of centrilobular emphysema can be readily differentiated from panlobular emphysema. In the centrilobular (centriacinar) type, the emphysematous spaces (respiratory bronchioles) are surrounded by alveoli that appear normal, whereas in panlobular (panacinar) emphysema, all structures in the acinus are rather uniformly distended. In advanced centrilobular emphysema, the peripheral parenchyma may be compressed and distorted or even destroyed, so that the condition may be indistinguishable from panlobular emphysema. However, the presence of persisting normal alveoli would reveal that it is centrilobular. In severe panlobular emphysema, the alveolar spaces are enlarged and the walls appear stretched, thin, bloodless, and often ruptured. The constriction of vessels in the alveolar walls causes pallor and dryness of the lung tissue.

In patients with clinical symptoms, the type of emphysema observed at autopsy may be centrilobular or panlobular, but in advanced disease both types commonly are present. In such instances, the lungs are voluminous, pale, and dry and of peculiar pillowlike consistency because of loss of normal elasticity. They fail to collapse when the chest is opened. Bullae (localized emphysematous air spaces greater than 1 cm in diameter) and blebs (intrapleural collections of air) may be seen on the surface of the lungs.

Emphysema is associated with an increase in the residual air content of the lungs and a proportionate decrease in vital capacity. It occurs more frequently in men than in women, and the highest incidence is in persons in the sixth decade. The chest tends to be barrel shaped, with a wide costal angle and a low position of the diaphragm. The decreased pulmonary mobility and elasticity and the obliteration of alveolar capillaries tend to cause stagnation in the pulmonary circulation and throw more work on the right side of the heart. There may be hypertrophy of the right side of the heart (cor pulmonale), and eventually there may be failure and passive congestion.

The *etiology* and *pathogenesis* of centrilobular and panlobular emphysema are not clearly understood. However, it appears that cigarette smoking, air pollution, and infection, the same factors that are responsible for chronic bronchitis, play a significant role in many instances. The coexistence of chronic bronchitis and emphysema suggests that chronic bronchitis may predispose to the development of emphysema. Inflammatory damage of the air spaces and airway obstruction may be the initiating factors. It must be noted, however, that emphysema may occur in some patients who have no history of chronic bronchitis. Some investigators have suggested that parenchymal damage precedes airway obstruction, particularly in panlobular emphysema. Factors such as autoimmunity and cigarette smoke have been incriminated as causes of alveolar damage, possibly by inducing obstruction of capillary blood flow. In such instances, airway obstruction may be secondary. The loss of supporting framework usually provided by the alveolar septa to bronchioles results in collapse of the bronchioles during expiration, followed by air trapping and distention of the air spaces.

Constitutional and hereditary factors may play a part in the pathogenesis of emphysema. An acquired tissue weakness associated with aging has been proposed by some. A congenital or inherited constitutional defect has been reported, with or without chronic bronchitis. In some of these familial cases, a deficiency of the serum enzyme alpha$_1$-antitrypsin, a recessive non–sex linked trait, is associated with the development of panlobular emphysema at an early age, usually without chronic bronchitis, although the mechanism of production of emphysema has not been determined. In animals, it has been shown that proteolytic enzymes cause destruction of lung tissue followed by emphysema. Since alpha$_1$-antitrypsin inhibits proteolytic enzymes in leukocytes, it has been postulated that its absence allows digestion of the pulmonary tissue by circulating or local proteolytic enzymes released from leukocytes or alveolar macrophages. Trypsin inhibitor also has been found to have some antibiotic action, so that its absence may accentuate the effects of inflammation in the lungs.

Paraseptal emphysema. Paraseptal (peripheral lobular) emphysema affects the periphery of the lobule adjacent to interlobular septa and appears to be predominantly destructive. The condition may coexist with centrilobular emphysema, even in the same lobule. Its cause is not known but may be related to infection or other injurious agents. Bullae may result from coalescence of distended alveoli, resulting in so-called primary bullous disease (Fig. 15-25). Generally, paraseptal emphysema is well localized and asymptomatic, unless spontaneous pneumothorax results from rupture of a bulla.

Paracicatricial emphysema. Paracicatricial (scar) emphysema is the result of overdistention and destruction of air spaces in relation to scars, which occasionally may lead to bulla formation.

Variants of panlobular and centrilobular emphysema. *Infantile lobar emphysema,* usually discovered shortly after birth, is predominantly a distensive, rather than a destructive, panlobular emphysema ("pulmonary overinflation"). The distention of the involved lobe may be so marked that it may cause compression atelectasis of the adjacent lobes. It is attributed to obstruction of a bronchus and air-

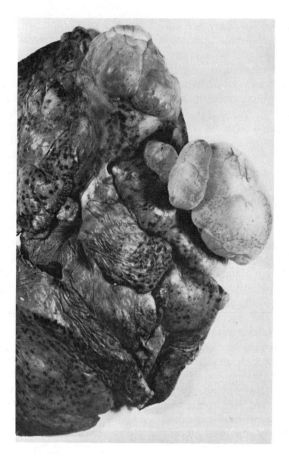

Fig. 15-25. Bullous emphysema of anterior margin of lung. (From Millard, M.: Lung, pleura, and mediastinum. In Anderson, W. A. D., and Kissane, J. M., editors: Pathology, ed. 7, St. Louis, 1977, The C. V. Mosby Co.)

trapping caused by vascular anomalies, collapse of the bronchial wall due to absent or hypoplastic bronchial cartilage, foreign bodies, or infection.

Swyer-James syndrome, MacLeod's syndrome, or *unilateral hyperlucent lung* (the last referring to the typical radiologic appearance) is a form of panlobular emphysema that may be recognized in childhood but may not become manifest until adulthood. It is related apparently to bronchiolitis obliterans of infectious origin.

Compensatory emphysema is a panlobular overinflation of the remaining lung after a portion has been surgically resected or damaged by disease. The *aging lung* is a form of panlobular emphysema in persons past middle age, associated with some loss of elastic tissue and capillaries. The pores of Kohn appear enlarged. The so-called *senile emphysema* is a nondestructive generalized alveolar enlargement produced in association with senile thoracic kyphosis. *Focal emphysema* is considered to be a form of centrilobular emphysema related to pigment deposits surrounding respiratory bronchioles. It is seen particularly in coal workers but may occur in those exposed to other types of dust and also is seen in the general population.

Pulmonary interstitial emphysema. Pulmonary interstitial emphysema is a condition in which air is present in interstitial tissues of the lung rather than in alveolar spaces. Air escapes through ruptured alveolar bases into sheaths of pulmonary vessels precipitated by a pressure gradient of air in alveoli to perivascular sheaths in cases where alveoli are overexpanded or blood vessels are not filled to the normal extent. Predisposing conditions are (1) general overinflation of lung tissue, (2) atelectasis of an area of lung with overinflation of adjacent areas, and (3) decreased blood supply to pulmonary vessels with hyperinflation or increased intra-alveolar pressure.

The air may travel along vascular sheaths to the mediastinum (pneumomediastinum), work upward to the neck, face, and axillae (subcutaneous emphysema), and work downward along the aorta and esophagus into the retroperitoneum. Cyanosis may result from venous stasis because of collapse of pulmonary vessels, and dyspnea may result because of interference with respiratory movement.

Bronchiolar emphysema. "Bronchiolar emphysema" is not a true emphysema but a bronchiolectasis with muscle hypertrophy and fibrosis. It also is called "muscular cirrhosis of the lungs."

Complications. Among the complications of severe pulmonary emphysema are (1) respiratory acidosis, (2) right-sided heart failure (cor pulmonale), (3) erythrocytosis secondary to hypoxemia, (4) peptic ulcers, usually duodenal, and (5) pneumothorax, most often in patients with bullae.

Cardiac disturbance may result from pressure of the distended lungs or pneumomediastinum or from lack of blood because of the venous congestion. Continued accumulation of air in the mediastinum, unless withdrawn, may be fatal from interference with respiration and circulation. Air block in newborn infants may be caused by interstitial emphysema, with pneumothorax resulting from rupture of the pleura.

PNEUMOCONIOSIS

Pneumoconiosis refers to the pulmonary changes caused by the inhalation of dust.

These changes depend on the type and the amount of dust inhaled, the size of the dust particles, the length of time of exposure, and the failure of eliminative mechanisms within the lung, which may be caused by cilia-toxic effects of the dust or to the presence of associated infection. There are several important types:

1 Nonoccupational anthracosis, caused by the inhalation of carbon pigment (i.e., soot particles in the atmosphere), is almost universal in occurrence but, as a rule, is not associated with functional changes and hence is not significant clinically.

2 Silicosis, caused by the inhalation of free silica, is an important occupational disease among miners and others working in rock, sandblasters, metal grinders, and workers engaged in manufacturing products containing silica. It produces a reaction in the lung characterized by the development of nodular areas of hyaline fibrosis. It often is associated with tuberculosis and accelerates this infection. The pulmonary fibrosis predisposes to right-sided heart failure.

3 Coal workers' pneumoconiosis, caused by the inhalation of coal dust and its impurities, occurs in coal miners and others working with coal (e.g., those loading coal into ships).

4 Asbestosis, caused by the inhalation of asbestos fibers, is an important disease. It produces a diffuse fibrosis of the lung. Characteristic asbestos bodies, which are elongated, club-shaped fibers coated with iron pigment, are found in the lung tissue and may appear in the sputum. It causes no particular predisposition to tuberculosis but does predispose to cancer. Right-sided heart failure may result from the pulmonary fibrosis.

5 Silicosiderosis occurs among hematite miners and is characterized by lungs of a bright brick-red color.

6 Pneumoconiosis resulting from inhalation of graphite dust is known to occur among graphite miners. Recently, the disease has been described in a few patients whose occupation was electrotyping.

Also included in this discussion is mention of berylliosis, since lung lesions may be caused by exposure to beryllium dust, but disease also may be induced by breathing beryllium fumes. Other pulmonary diseases caused by inhaling fumes, thus not strictly pneumoconioses, are bauxite lung disease and cadmium pneumonitis. There also are antigenic dusts that may produce pulmonary lesions, but probably by means of hypersensitivity rather than by the nonspecific toxic or mechanical irritant effects that are characteristic of many other dusts.

Nonoccupational anthracosis. A deposit of inhaled carbon pigment is found in some degree in all adult urban dwellers. Whereas the normal color of the lung, as seen in an infant, is grayish pink, the adult lung is flecked by focal and linear deposits of black pigment, evident on both the pleural and cut surfaces. Through function of alveolar phagocytes and lymphatics, the pigment becomes concentrated in the lymphoid tissue of the lungs, peribronchial nodes, and mediastinum. It tends to accumulate particularly in areas in which inflammation or fibrosis has blocked lymphatics. The pigment itself does not stimulate fibrosis. Air spaces are visible in the pigmented areas, and respiratory function is undisturbed. The presence of carbon particles in coal workers is actually a form of anthracosis, but usually it is considered separately as "coal workers' pneumoconiosis" (p. 429).

Silicosis. Silicosis is a most important type of pneumoconiosis because of its frequency as an occupational disease, the severity of the fibrosis, and its promotion of serious tuberculous infection. Inhaled particles of silica (0.5 to 5 μ) become concentrated in the parts of the alveoli that are most fixed (viz., next to vessels, septa, and the pleura), since they are less readily cleared away from these sites by respiratory movements.

The earliest lesions are seen in the walls of the alveoli arising from respiratory bronchioles and alveolar ducts, with formation of reticulin fibers followed by dense collagen. Nodules of hyalinized, collagenous, concentric laminae are formed (Fig. 15-26). Globulins are mixed with the collagen in the nodules. Carbon pigment usually is trapped in the same area, so that some black pigment is evident in the nodules (Fig. 15-27). The particles of silica may be identified by a polarizing microscope. There is evidence that silica can combine with body protein and act as an antigen, so that an antigen-antibody reaction may be a factor in silicosis. Experimentally, the reaction of tissues to silica may be modified by the administration of cortisone.

In early stages, the silicotic nodules are too small to be identified grossly, but ultimately they develop into nodules 3 mm or more in diameter and with sharply defined borders. Islets of this collagenous tissue are scattered throughout the lung, under the pleural surfaces, and in tracheobronchial lymph nodes. Eventually, massive conglomerate areas of fi-

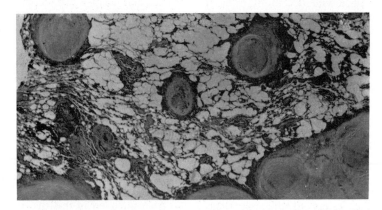

Fig. 15-26. Silicotic nodules in lung as seen in low-power photomicrograph.

brosis may result. Most of the fatal cases terminate with tuberculous infection. Other complications that may develop are cardiac hypertrophy and dilatation, particularly of the right side of the heart, emphysema, and carcinoma of the lung. Obliterative vascular changes appear to be important in the pulmonary hypertension and right-sided cardiac failure. The degree of importance of silicosis in the etiology of pulmonary carcinoma is still undetermined.

A rapidly fatal form of silicosis has been reported that is characterized chiefly by a histologic appearance similar to that of ''pulmonary alveolar proteinosis'' (p. 415) and is called *silicoproteinosis*. In some patients, typical silicotic nodules occur concomitantly.

Coal workers' pneumoconiosis. The lung disease associated with the inhalation of coal dust may appear as a *simple form* or a *complicated form (progressive massive fibrosis)*. Although the term ''anthracosis'' often is applied to the black lungs of coal miners, today there is a tendency to restrict this term to the usually clinically insignificant carbon deposition in lungs of city dwellers referred to previously.

In *simple coal workers' pneumoconiosis,* the coal dust particles (no greater than 5 μ) collect principally in the alveoli arising from respiratory bronchioles, in a manner similar to the silica particles in silicosis, and are usually within macrophages. There is associated reticulin fiber formation, but collagen fibers are not abundant. The respiratory bronchioles undergo compensatory dilatation *(focal emphysema)* due to obliteration of adjacent alveoli, and possibly the dilatation is contributed to by damage to the bronchiolar wall by the dust deposits. Some particles enter lymphatic channels and are taken up by the reticuloendothelial cells in the regional lymph nodes. The changes in this simple form of pneumoconiosis are considered by many investigators to be due to coal dust alone, but there is some debate as to whether the small amount of silica and other impurities in the coal dust may be partly responsible.

In *progressive massive fibrosis* (PMF), large confluent lesions usually are limited to the upper lobes of the lungs. They consist of irregular bundles of dense hyalinized collagenous tissue, with heavy coal dust deposits, and some infiltration by lymphocytes, plasma cells, and macrophages. Obliterative endarteritis of nearby vessels may be present. Some of the nodules may undergo cavitation due to ischemia or superimposed tuberculosis. In advanced disease, pulmonary hypertension and cor pulmonale develop. The silica content in lesions of PMF is usually greater than in simple pneumoconiosis. It is probable that the silica plays a prominent role in the development

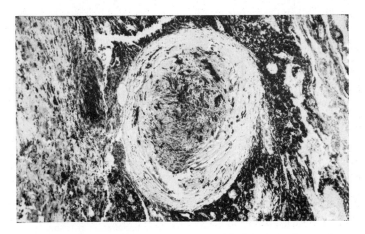

Fig. 15-27. Silicotic nodule of lung. Large amount of black carbon pigment is present also.

of the massive fibrotic nodules, and thus the lesions are often referred to as "anthracosilicosis." Some studies have suggested that the presence of tubercle bacilli is a factor in causing the fibrosis, but this is debatable.

Coal workers afflicted with rheumatoid arthritis may develop nodules rapidly throughout the lungs that resemble rheumatoid granulomas with the addition of concentric bands of coal dust surrounding the central core. This condition is known as *rheumatoid pneumoconiosis* or *Caplan's syndrome*. It may occur in other forms of pneumoconiosis (e.g., silicosis and asbestosis).

Asbestosis. Asbestos is a mineral fibrous structure composed essentially of magnesium silicate. Inhalation of the fibers occurs mainly in the factories during the carding process, in which the fiber is separated from the crushed mineral. It also occurs in a variety of other occupations in which asbestos materials are used. The fibers are deposited in the bronchioles and stimulate fibrosis mechanically rather than by specific chemical action. The lower lobes particularly are affected, and the result is a dif-

fuse rather than a nodular type of interstitial fibrosis. Emphysema, bronchiectasis, and interference with respiratory function may result. Termination is usually by infection or cardiac failure. Tuberculosis occasionally supervenes, but asbestosis does not particularly predispose to tuberculosis. Bronchogenic carcinoma and pleural mesothelioma occur with increased frequency in association with asbestosis. Although there is some controversy as to whether short-fibered asbestos induces tissue reactions, experimental evidence has been presented that suggests that fibers less than 5 μ in length are not pathogenic.

Grossly, the involved lung shows irregular patches and strands of grayish dense scar tissue. Dilated emphysematous air spaces are evident in the involved tissue.

The characteristic asbestos bodies occur singly or in clumps as elongated fibers of variable size and form (up to 140 μ in length). One or both extremities of the fiber are bulbous, and the body is slender and haustrated or segmented (Fig. 15-28). The color is yellowish, greenish yellow, or brown because of the iron

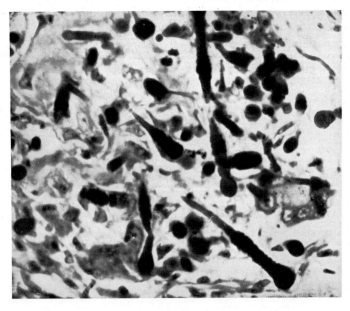

Fig. 15-28. Asbestosis of lung. Note bulbous ends and haustration of asbestos bodies and also giant cells.

pigment deposited on the surface. The bodies stain well with the Prussian blue method for iron. Asbestos bodies may be found in basal lung smears in a considerable proportion of adult urban individuals in the absence of the pulmonary lesions of asbestosis. This may be evidence of exposure of the general public to the many asbestos-containing materials being used today (e.g., home construction materials, brake linings).

The iron-coated asbestos bodies are commonly referred to as "ferruginous bodies." Since inhaled fibers consisting of materials other than asbestos may also be iron-coated and thus become "ferruginous bodies," only those with the central fiber consisting of asbestos are designated "asbestos bodies."

Silicosiderosis. Silicosiderosis is caused by the inhalation of iron-containing hematite by hematite miners. The lungs have a striking brick-red color. Some silica is usually inhaled as well. A diffuse or nodular pulmonary fibrosis may be produced.

Graphite pneumoconiosis. Inhalation of graphite appears to cause a chronic pneumoconiosis with a predilection for the upper portions of the lung. It is characterized by a granulomatous reaction, with areas of fibrosis, necrosis, cavitation, and obliterative changes in blood vessels and bronchi. The lung tissue is black, and the graphite particles are large and cause a giant cell reaction.

Bauxite lung disease. In the manufacture of alumina abrasive powders, exposure to the white fumes evolved from heating a mixture of bauxite, iron, and coke has resulted in a diffuse pulmonary fibrosis with obliterative endarteritis. Amorphous aluminum and silica dust are the prominent constituents of the fumes.

Berylliosis. The inhalation of beryllium fumes or dust may cause either an acute pneumonitis or a granulomatous inflammation with diffuse pulmonary fibrosis (p. 224).

Cadmium pneumonitis. Cadmium inhalation may produce a pneumonitis with interstitial fibrosis in addition to some alveolar exudate.

Antigenic dusts. Dusts from many sources are known to cause respiratory disease. It is possible that nonspecific toxic or mechanical irritant effects may lead to the respiratory disease, but considerable evidence suggests that hypersensitivity plays an important role. Exposure to wood dusts in woodworkers is an example. Inhalation of detergents containing a proteolytic enzyme (derived from *Bacillus subtilis)* used for removal of stains from clothing is another cause of respiratory disease of immunologic nature. Disease caused by inhalation of dust from moldy hay or silage (farmer's lung) and from pigeon droppings (pigeon-breeder's lung) has been mentioned previously (p. 411).

Pleura

Diseases of the pleura are mainly effusions, inflammations, and tumors. With effusions into the pleural cavity, corresponding collapse of lung tissue occurs. The collapse may be limited to one side by immobility of the mediastinum, or it may be locally limited by adhesions.

Hydrothorax. Hydrothorax is the accumulation of edema fluid or transudate in the pleural cavity. It occurs in conditions of generalized edema, as in renal or cardiac disease, or rarely may be caused by local conditions, such as tumor or aneurysm. The fluid is clear, light yellow, of low specific gravity (below 1.015), and low in protein content. In some cases, the fluid is milky because of the fat content (chylous hydrothorax).

Hemothorax. Blood in the pleural cavity may occur in cases of thoracic trauma or from rupture of an aneurysm. A blood-stained pleural fluid is more common than true hemothorax. Its occurence usually is associated with tuberculosis or with malignant tumor of the lung or pleura.

Pneumothorax. Air in the pleural cavity may be introduced from without by wounds or therapeutic procedures, or it may result from a rupture of the lung into the pleural cavity. The most common causes of the latter are tuberculosis and rupture of an emphysematous bleb. In many cases, air in the pleural cavity is associated with a serous or inflammatory exudate.

Pleurisy. Inflammation of the pleura is usually a spread from the lung. Less commonly, it is caused by spread from the abdomen or mediastinum or is blood borne. At times, it appears to be primary in the pleura. Most cases result from infection by bacteria, such as tubercle bacilli, pneumococci, staphylococci, or streptococci. Viral and fungal infections also occur. The apparently primary forms usually are caused by tuberculosis or rheumatic fever. Major causes of pleural exudate are pneumonia, subpleural tuberculosis, carcinoma, pulmonary infarction, acute mediastinitis, subphrenic abscess, and fractured rib.

Pleurisy is classified according to the type of exudate as fibrinous (dry pleurisy), serofibrinous (pleurisy with effusion), and purulent (empyema). The fluid in pleurisy is cloudy or contains flakes of fibrin and has a relatively high specific gravity and high protein content. The exudate containing fibrin and inflammatory cells is evident in sections throughout the inflamed pleura. Pleurisy may resolve and leave little trace, but often organization results in a thickened scarred area of pleura or fibrous adhesions between visceral and parietal layers.

Empyema most commonly is the result of lung infection, but in recent years the number of cases following thoracic surgery has increased. Staphylococci, streptococci, gram-negative bacteria, and pneumococci are the common organisms in empyema cultures, although pneumococci have decreased in predominance compared with earlier years. Organization and formation of adhesions tend to localize the pus in various parts of the pleural cavity. A thick organizing wall of exudate may line the cavity, covering both visceral and parietal surfaces.

Tumors. Most tumors involving the pleura are extensions from malignant tumors in the lung, but primary pleural tumors occur also. Rarely, primary benign tumors arise from subpleural tissues and include fibromas, lipomas, chondromas, and angiomas.

Mesothelioma is an uncommon primary tumor arising from pleural lining cells. A diffuse malignant form occurs as flattened nodular tumor masses on both visceral and parietal layers or spreads diffusely over the pleura, forming a thick layer of tumor tissue. Microscopic characteristics of both epithelial and connective tissue tumors may be present, with a sarcomatous appearance in some areas but also tending to form glandlike spaces or channels. A papillary pattern or some hyaluronic acid may be present. There may be some histologic similarity to synovial tumors (synovioma). Spread may be by invasion of lymphatics and metastasis to mediastinal lymph nodes. Abundant hemorrhagic pleural fluid is a usual accompaniment. A solitary form commonly is fibrous in type but also may contain components of epithelial appearance. It may be benign or malignant.

A frequent association of exposure to asbestos mineral or the finding of asbestos bodies in the lung has been noted in cases of diffuse pleural mesotheliomas. Some association of asbestosis with peritoneal mesothelioma also has been found. Carcinoma of the lung, as noted before, also occurs in patients with asbestosis.

Mediastinum

Tumors. The varied tissue components of the mediastinum may give rise to a great variety of neoplasms, the most frequent being malignant lymphomas, thymomas, teratomas (including dermoid cysts), and neurogenous tumors. Lymphomas and thymomas are discussed in later chapters.

Mediastinal teratomas are generally cystic and are located in the anterior mediastinum. Schlumberger has presented evidence that the origin may be from faulty embryogenesis of the thymus. The majority are benign. In malignant mediastinal teratomas, well-differentiated ectodermal derivatives such as skin or nerve tissue and organoid epithelial structures are absent. Their main complications are mechanical effects on the trachea, great vessels, heart, or lungs.

The mediastinal neurogenous tumors are almost always in the posterior mediastinum. They are of two main types: (1) ganglioneuromas (benign) and neuroblastomas (malignant) arising from cells of the sympathetic nervous system, which occur mainly in children and young individuals, and (2) nerve sheath tumors, including neurilemomas, neurofibromas, and neurogenous sarcomas, found in adults.

Cysts. Mediastinal cysts are mainly of developmental origin. Bronchial cysts are considered developmental reduplication cysts of the respiratory tract. They are lined by ciliated columnar epithelium, and their walls may contain any or all of the tissues normally present in the respiratory tract. They are most common in the posterior part of the superior mediastinum near the bifurcation of the trachea. Esophageal cysts have a muscular wall and a squamous lining. The rare gastroenteric or alimentary cysts have a structure simulating that of stomach or intestine. They are thought to be caused by a pinching off of a diverticulum of the embryonic foregut.

Cystic lymphangioma of the mediastinum, a congenital maldevelopment in a group of lymph vessels, is quite rare. It is a nonencapsulated mass of multiple cystic spaces lined by single layers of endothelium, intimately incorporated with surrounding structures.

Anterior mediastinal cysts may be of thymic or thymopharyngeal duct origin. Pericardial coelomic cysts (pleuropericardial cysts) are discrete and nonadherent, are situated in the anterior inferior mediastinum, and are composed of a fibrous wall lined by a single layer of flat mesotheliallike cells. A rare mediastinal meningocele, usually associated with Recklinghausen's neurofibromatosis, may appear as a cystic structure. The wall is composed of dural and arachnoidal components.

REFERENCES

Abell, M. R.: Arch. Pathol. **61**:360-379, 1956 (mediastinal tumors and cysts).

American Joint Committee for Cancer Staging and End Results Reporting: Clinical staging system for carcinoma of the lung, Chicago, Sept. 1973.

Anderson, W. A. D.: Am. J. Clin. Pathol. **46**:3-26, 1966 (lung cancer).

Arias-Stella, J., and Kruger, H.: Arch. Pathol. **76**:147-157, 1963 (high altitude pulmonary edema).

Auerbach, O., et al.: Cancer **20**:2055-2066, 1967 (bronchial changes in cigarette-smoking dogs).

Auerbach, O., et al.: N. Engl. J. Med. **300**:381-386, 1979 (bronchial epithelial changes in cigarette smokers).

Balows, A., and Fraser, D. W., symposium editors: Ann. Intern. Med. **90**:489-703, 1979 (Legionnaires' disease—symposium).

Beattie, E. J., et al.: The present status of lung cancer; a symposium. In Seventh National Cancer Conference Proceedings, Philadelphia, 1972, J. B. Lippincott Co., pp. 723-728.

Bennett, D. E., et al.: Cancer **23**:431-439, 1969 (adenocarcinoma of lung).

Bensch, K. G., et al.: Cancer **22**:1163-1172, 1968 (oat cell carcinoma of lung: relationship to bronchial carcinoid).

Blackmon, J. A., et al.: Arch. Path. Lab. Med. **102**:337-343, 1978 (pathology of Legionnaires' disease—historical aspects).

Blot, W. J., and Fraumeni, J. F., Jr.: Lancet **2**:142-144, 1975 (arsenic and lung cancer).

Brooks, S. M.: J. Occup. Med **17**:19-26, 1975 (lung cancer—environmental and host factors).

Broome, C. V., et al.: Ann. Intern. Med. **90**:1-4, 1979 (direct immunofluorescent staining for diagnosis of Legionnaires' disease).

Buechner, H. A., and Ansari, A.: Dis. Chest **55**:274-284, 1969 (acute silicoproteinosis).

Carbone, P. P. (moderator): Ann. Intern. Med. **73**:1003-1024, 1970 (prognosis in lung cancer).

Carrington, C. B., et al.: N. Engl. J. Med. **298**:801-809, 1978 (usual and desquamative interstitial pneumonia).

Carroll, R. J.: Pathol. Bacteriol. **83**:293-297, 1962 (lung scars and cancer).

Cassan, S. M., et al.: Am. J. Med. **49**:366-379, 1970 (Wegener's granulomatosis, limited form).

Churg, A., and Warnock, M. L.: Cancer **37**:1469-1477, 1976 (tumorlets—form of peripheral carcinoids).

Cocke, E. W., and Wang, C. C.: CA **26**:194-200, 1976 (cancer of the larynx).

Coombes, R. C., et al.: Br. J. Dis. Chest **72**:263-287, 1978 (biochemical markers in bronchogenic carcinoma).

Crystal, R. G., et al.: Ann. Intern. Med. **85**:769-788, 1976 (idiopathic pulmonary fibrosis).

Dickle, H. A., and Rankin, J.: J.A.M.A. **167**:1069-1076, 1958 (farmer's lung).

Dutz, W.: Pathol. Ann. **5**:309-341, 1970 (*Pneumocystis carinii* pneumonia).

Editorial: Br. Med. J. **1**:571-572, 1974 (types of emphysema).

Editorial: Lancet **2**:506, 1974 (lung tumors in mice exposed to tobacco smoke).

Esterly, J. A., and Warner, N. E.: Arch. Pathol. **80**:433-441, 1965 (pneumocystis pneumonia).

Farrell, P. M., and Avery, M. E.: Am. Rev. Resp. Dis. **111**:657-688, 1975 (hyaline membrane disease).

Fienberg, R.: Am. J. Pathol. **29**:913-931, 1953 (cholesterol pneumonitis).

Figueroa, G. W., et al.: N. Engl. J. Med. **288**:1094-

1096, 1973 (lung cancer in chloromethyl methyl ether workers).

Fishman, A. P.: N. Engl. J. Med. **298**:843-845, 1978 (usual and desquamative interstitial pneumonia).

Fraser, D. W., et al.: N. Engl. J. Med. **297**:1189-1197, 1977 (Legionnaires' disease—description of epidemic).

Gaensler, E. A., et al.: Am. J. Med. **41**:864-882, 1966 (graphite pneumoconiosis of electrotypers).

Gore, I., and Tanaka, K.: Am. J. Med. Sci. **244**:351-361, 1962 (pulmonary embolization).

Gross, P.: Arch. Environ. Health **29**:115-117, 1974 (short-fibered asbestos dust).

Gross, P., and Harley, R. A., Jr.: Arch. Pathol. **96**:245-250, 1973 (asbestos-induced intrathoracic tissue reactions).

Hamman, L., and Rich, A. R.: Bull. Johns Hopkins Hosp. **74**:117-212, 1944 (acute diffuse interstitial fibrosis of the lungs).

Hammond, E. C., et al.: CA **21**:78-94, 1971 (effects of cigarette smoking on dogs).

Hardy, H. L.: Am. J. Med. Sci. **250**:381-389, 1965 (asbestos).

Haugen, R. K.: J.A.M.A. **186**:142-143, 1963 (laryngeal obstruction—"the café coronary").

Heard, B. E.: Pathology of chronic bronchitis and emphysema, Baltimore, 1970, The Williams & Wilkins Co.

Heppleston, A. G.: Am. J. Pathol. **78**:171-174, 1975 (silica-induced alveolar lipoproteinosis).

Herman, D. L., et al.: Cancer **19**:1337-1346, 1966 (giant cell adenocarcinoma).

Hewer, T. F.: J. Pathol. Bacteriol. **81**:323-330, 1961 (pulmonary metastases resembling alveolar carcinoma).

Hoffman, E. O., et al.: Arch. Pathol. **96**:104-107, 1973 (acute silicosis—ultrastructure).

Jick, H., et al.: Arch. Intern. Med. **139**:745-746, 1979 (lung cancer in women).

Johnston, W. W., and Frable, W. J.: Am. J. Pathol. **84**:373-424, 1976 (cytopathology of respiratory tract).

Kent, G., et al.: Arch. Pathol. **60**:556-562, 1955 (pulmonary microlithiasis).

Killburn, K. H., editor: Arch. Intern. Med. **126**:415-511, 1970 (symposium—pulmonary responses to inhaled materials).

Kleinerman, J., et al.: Arch. Pathol. Lab. Med. **103**:375-432, 1979 (coal workers' pneumoconiosis).

Kreyberg, L.: Histological typing of lung tumours, Geneva, 1967, World Health Organization.

Lanza, A. J., editor: The pneumoconioses, New York, 1963, Grune & Stratton, Inc.

Lauweryns, J. M.: Hum. Pathol. **1**:175-204, 1970 (hyaline membrane disease in newborn infants).

Lieberman, J.: N. Engl. J. Med. **281**:279-284, 1969 (alpha-1-antitrypsin deficiency in pulmonary emphysema).

Liebow, A. A.: Tumors of the lower respiratory tract. In Atlas of tumor pathology, Sect. V, Fasc. 17, Washington, D.C., 1952, Armed Forces Institute of Pathology.

Lindsay, M. I., et al.: J.A.M.A. **214**:1825-1832, 1970 (Hong Kong influenza).

Lowell, F. C.: N. Engl. J. Med. **281**:1012-1013, 1969 (editorial—antigenic dusts).

Marinkovich, V. A.: J.A.M.A. **231**:944-947, 1975 (hypersensitivity alveolitis).

McDade, J. E., et al.: N. Engl. J. Med. **297**:1197-1203, 1977 (Legionnaires' disease—isolation of bacterium).

McNary, W. F., Jr., and Gaensler, E. A.: Ann. Intern. Med. **74**:404-407, 1971 (desquamative interstitial pneumonia).

Moran, T. J., and Totten, R. S.: Am. J. Clin. Pathol. **54**:747-756, 1970 (lymphoid interstitial pneumonia).

Moser, K. M., editor: Pulmonary vascular diseases, New York, 1979, Marcel Dekker, Inc.

Naeye, R. L.: Arch. Pathol. Lab. Med. **101**:165-167, 1977 (sudden infant death syndrome).

Nash, G., et al.: N. Engl. J. Med. **276**:368-374, 1967 (pulmonary lesions with oxygen therapy).

Nelson, N.: N. Engl. J. Med. **288**:1123-1124, 1973 (carcinogenicity of halo ethers).

Neubuerger, K. T., et al.: Arch Pathol. **37**:1-15, 1944 (rheumatic pneumonia).

O'Donnell, W. M., et al.: Cancer **19**:1143-1148, 1966 (asbestos and lung cancer).

Patchefsky, A. S., et al.: Ann. Intern. Med. **74**:322-327, 1971 (desquamative interstitial pneumonia).

Perera, D. R., et al.: J.A.M.A. **214**:1074-1078, 1970 (*Pneumocystis carinii* pneumonia).

Pratt, P. C., and Kilburn, K. H.: Hum. Pathol. **1**:443-464, 1970 (pulmonary emphysema).

Reid, L.: The pathology of emphysema, Chicago, 1967, Year Book Medical Publishers, Inc.

Rifkind, D., et al.: Ann. Intern. Med. **65**:943-956, 1966 (pneumocystis pneumonia).

Rodman, T., and Sterling, F. H.: Pulmonary emphysema and related lung diseases, St. Louis, 1969, The C. V. Mosby Co.

Rosen, S. H., Castleman, B., and Liebow, A. A.: N. Engl. J. Med. **258**:1123-1142, 1958 (pulmonary alveolar proteinosis).

Ross, J. M.: Br. Med. J. **1**:79-80, 1941 (blast injury).

Saccomanno, G., et al.: Cancer **27**:515-523, 1971 (histologic types of lung cancer among uranium miners).

Saccomanno, G., et al.: Cancer **33**:256-270, 1974 (carcinoma of lung—cytologic study).

Saltzstein, S. L.: Cancer **16**:928-955, 1963 (lymphomas of lung).

Scarpelli, E. M.: The surfactant system of the lung, Philadelphia, 1968, Lea & Febiger.

Schlumberger, H. C.: Tumors of the mediastinum. In Atlas of tumor pathology, Sect. V. Fasc. 18, Washington, D.C., 1951, Armed Forces Institute of Pathology.

Scoggin, C. H., et al.: N. Engl. J. Med.: **297**:1269-1272, 1977 (high altitude pulmonary edema).

Selikoff, I. J., and Hammond, E. C.: CA **28**:87-99, 1978 (asbestosis in U.S. shipyards).

Shelley, S. A., et al.: N. Engl. J. Med. **300**:112-116, 1979 (surfactant in hyaline membrane disease of newborn).

Spencer, H.: Pathology of the lung, ed. 3, Oxford, 1977, Pergamon Press, Inc. (general reference).

Spencer, H., and Raeburn, C.: J. Pathol. Bacteriol. **71**:145-154, 1956 (bronchiolar carcinoma).

Staub, N. C.: Hum. Pathol. **1:**419-432, 1970 (pathophysiology of pulmonary edema).

Sullivan, K., et al.: Arch. Intern. Med. **131:**521-527, 1973 (empyema thoracis).

Sun, T., et al.: Am. J. Clin. Pathol. **62:**725-731, 1974 (alpha₁-antitrypsin deficiency and pulmonary disease).

Sutherland, T. W., et al.: J. Pathol. Bacteriol. **65:**93-99, 1953 (hamartoma).

Thomson, J. G., and Graves, W. M., Jr.: Arch. Pathol. **81:**458-464, 1966 (asbestos).

Thurlbeck, W. M.: Pathol. Ann. **3:**367-398, 1968 (chronic obstructive lung disease).

Totten, R. S., et al.: Am. J. Med. **25:**803-809, 1958 (farmer's lung).

Valdes-Dapena, M.: In Sommers, S. C., and Rosen, P. P., editors: Pathology annual, part 1, New York, 1977, Appleton-Century-Crofts, pp. 117-145 (sudden unexplained infant death).

Weese, W. C., et al.: Arch. Intern. Med. **131:**516-520, 1973 (empyema of thorax).

Weiss, W., et al.: Cancer **26:**965-970, 1970 (histopathology of bronchogenic carcinoma and prognosis).

Whitcomb, M. E., et al.: Ann. Intern. Med. **73:**761-765, 1970 (*Pneumocystis carinii* pneumonia).

Whitwell, F.: J. Pathol. Bacteriol. **70:**529-541, 1955 (atypical hyperplasia).

Winn, W. C., Jr., et al.: Arch. Pathol. Lab. Med. **102:**344-350, 1978 (pathology of Legionnaires' disease—1977 Vermont outbreak).

Wyatt, J. P.: Am. J. Pathol. **64:**197-216, 1971 (occupational lung disease).

Wyatt, J. P., et al.: Am. Rev. Resp. Dis. **89:**533-560, 721-735, 1964 (pathomorphology of emphysema complex).

16

Liver, gallbladder, and pancreas

Liver

STRUCTURE AND FUNCTION

The liver has a double blood supply, portal and hepatic, but the circulation to the right and left sides of the liver is fairly distinct. This circulatory division of the liver does not correspond with the anatomic lobes, but the right and left halves are divided by a line passing through the middle of the gallbladder fossa to the junction of the hepatic veins with the inferior vena cava. The portal stream from the spleen and stomach goes mainly to the left side of the liver and that from the intestines mainly to the right side.

Microscopically, the liver appears to be divided into lobules. At the center of each is a central (efferent) vein, and arranged around the periphery are portal areas, each containing a bile duct, hepatic artery, and portal vein. The cords of liver cells enclose bile canaliculi and blood sinusoids. The lining of the sinusoids consists of endothelial cells and Kupffer cells. The latter are highly phagocytic and form a part of the reticuloendothelial system.

The liver is the largest organ in the body, and its functions are many and varied. It is concerned with the excretion of bile, but bile pigment is formed only partly in the liver, the other components of the reticuloendothelial system (spleen and bone marrow) playing a major role. The liver forms bile salts and is important in various other biochemical pro-

cesses, such as the formation of plasma proteins, heparin, prothrombin, and fibrinogen, fat metabolism and storage, urea and amino acid formation, and glycogen storage. In the fetus, the liver is a blood-forming organ. A variety of laboratory tests are useful in determining the efficiency of the various hepatic functions and in the clinical evaluation of patients with disease of the liver or jaundice.

An important feature of the liver is a great capacity for regeneration after injury or destruction of its cells, a feature that is important in compensation for effects of injury to liver cells. There is nodular overgrowth of localized regenerating areas (multiple nodular hyperplasia) that at times may be difficult to differentiate morphologically from neoplasia. The compensatory hyperplasia is prevented by deficiency or obstruction in the portal circulation (e.g., in portal cirrhosis) and by confinement and compression caused by fibrosis.

Congenital abnormalities of form are uncommon or unimportant in the liver. *Riedel's lobe* is a downward projection of the right lobe. Acquired changes in form include rib impressions on the surface of a markedly enlarged liver and anteroposterior depressions on the upper surface of the liver caused by the pressure of muscle bundles of the diaphragm.

Congenital biliary atresia is characterized by obstruction of the bile passage, caused by anomalous development of the bile duct. There is severe hepatic fibrosis with distortion of the lobular architecture. Interlobular bile ducts are

436

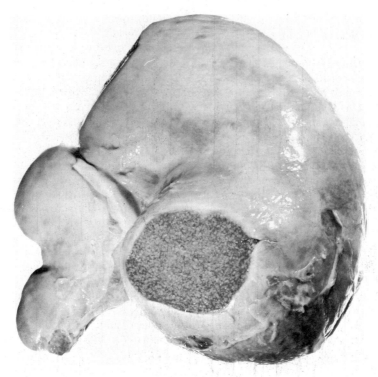

Fig. 16-1. Marked hyalinization of capsule of liver (''sugar-coated'' liver). Small portion of liver has been cut away to expose underlying tissue.

hypoplastic, with ductular proliferation. The hepatic cells show severe degeneration with giant cell change.

POSTMORTEM AUTOLYSIS

Postmortem autolytic changes develop quite rapidly in liver tissue. Bluish black discoloration may occur in the portion of liver adjacent to the transverse colon. Foamy liver results from postmortem infection of the liver by gas-forming organisms (e.g., *Clostridium perfringens*) from the intestinal tract, the bubbles of gas so produced honeycombing the liver tissue.

DEGENERATIONS AND INFILTRATIONS

Cloudy swelling. Cloudy (cellular) swelling is common in the liver as a result of acute infections. The liver is enlarged and has a tense capsule, a softer consistency, and a paler,

more opaque appearance than normal. Microscopically, the liver cells are swollen and have distinct margins and pale granular cytoplasm.

Amyloid infiltration. Amyloid infiltration is common in the liver as well as in the spleen and kidney in patients with tuberculosis and other chronic diseases. The amyloid appears as a hyaline material between the lining cells of the sinusoids and the liver cells. Its continued accumulation causes compression, atrophy, and disappearance of the liver cords (p. 34).

Hyaline substances. Hyaline masses may be found in the cytoplasm of liver cells in portal cirrhosis. They apparently represent an early and specific type of degenerative change in the liver cells (Mallory bodies).

Intracellular hyaline changes also are noted in yellow fever (Councilman bodies) and viral hepatitis (acidophilic bodies). Hyalinization of the hepatic capsule (''sugar-coated'' liver; Fig. 16-1) may occur, e.g., following healing by organization in perihepatitis or associated with long-standing ascites, as in polyserositis (Concato's disease).

Glycogen. Glycogen is normally abundantly present in the cytoplasm of liver cells but in many diseases is much depleted by the wasting that precedes death. Cytoplasmic glycogen is also reduced in diabetes mellitus, although the amount in the liver cell nuclei may be increased and give the nuclei a clear, glassy appearance. Cytoplasmic glycogen is abnormally increased in *von Gierke's glycogen storage disease*. This is a congenital, hereditary defect of glycogen mobilization seen as a rare condition in infants and children. Enlargement because of the accumulation of glycogen may involve the kidneys as well as the liver.

Fatty change. Fatty change in the liver is a common event and may be of very severe degree. Fatty metamorphosis occurs with a variety of infections and intoxications. Prolonged passive congestion tends to cause fatty change in central parts of the lobules. Fatty liver is found in association with obesity, chronic alcoholism, malnutrition and wasting diseases (e.g., tuberculosis and malignant tumors), in some cases of diabetes mellitus, and as a result of certain poisons such as phlorhizin, carbon tetrachloride, chloroform, and ether.

Grossly, the fatty liver, such as that seen in chronic alcoholism, is enlarged and has rounded borders, a tense capsule, yellow or yellowish red color, fairly firm consistency, and some greasiness of the cut surface. Microscopically, the fat is most prominent around the central part of the lobules, but when the fatty change is great, the distribution is diffuse and the fat is in the form of large globules (see Fig. 2-2). The pathogenesis of fatty metamorphosis is discussed on p. 27.

In sudden unexpected death in young adults, prominent fatty change in the liver is frequently the only finding. Unexplained death in chronic alcoholism with severe fatty change in the liver has been caused by massive fat embolism in some cases, but this appears to be an infrequent finding. In a report of idiopathic acute fatty liver in pregnancy, the complication of disseminated intravascular coagulation

was documented and considered a contributory cause of death.

Reye's syndrome. Fatty metamorphosis of the liver is a significant component of Reye's syndrome. This syndrome, which is being recognized with increasing frequency, is characterized by acute encephalopathy along with fatty change in the liver and other organs (e.g., kidneys and heart). It occurs typically in childhood. It may be seen at any age between early infancy and young adulthood but seldom after age 16 years. The syndrome usually begins as a viruslike upper respiratory illness, followed in a few days by vomiting, drowsiness, disorientation, and coma. Mortality is high. A specific cause has not been identified, but viruses and exogenous toxins may play an etiologic role. Reye's syndrome has occurred often in association with virus infections (e.g., influenza, particularly type B, varicella, coxsackie A, and reovirus). In some instances, environmental factors alone or in combination with viral infections have been implicated (e.g., aflatoxins contaminating foods or exposure to pesticides).

The encephalopathy is characterized by cerebral edema without inflammation or demyelination. Swelling of neurons and glial cells and neuronal necrosis may be seen. The fatty change in the liver consists of multiple small lipid deposits throughout the cytoplasm of the hepatocytes. Focal necrosis of hepatocytes and mononuclear inflammatory cell infiltration of liver lobules, particularly in portal areas, may be seen. Ultrastructural changes of mitochondria in the liver and other organs have been described, although such changes have been minimal or absent in some reports. However, there is agreement that functional derangement of mitochondria occurs following injury to the organelles.

According to some investigators, increased serum ammonia concentration is the factor that induces encephalopathy. The hyperammonemia is attributed to disturbed function of the mitochondria in the liver, resulting in a decrease in the activity of the urea-synthesizing enzymes that normally convert ammonia to urea. Others believe that the abnormal mitochondrial function leads to a decrease in fatty acid oxidation that results in fatty acidemia (elevated serum free fatty acids and short-chain fatty acids), which alone or synergistically with hyperammonemia is responsible for the cerebral disorder. A third suggestion is that maintenance of normal water and electrolyte balance in the brain is disturbed because of injured mitochondria so that cerebral edema and coma develop.

Pigmentation. Pigmentation of the liver is common in a number of conditions. The accumulated pigment may be hemosiderin (in congestion, hemolytic conditions, hemosiderosis, and hemochromatosis), malarial pigment (hematin), bile pigment (in obstructive jaundice), or a pigment of uncertain nature (in chronic idiopathic jaundice). In obstructive jaundice, the bile pigment first appears as small plugs in bile canaliculi and later may appear as coarse granules in parenchymal and Kupffer cells.

Chronic idiopathic jaundice. Chronic idiopathic jaundice has been recognized as a distinct condition by Dubin and Johnson and by Sprinz and Nelson. A benign condition easily mistaken for obstructive jaundice, it is characterized by chronic or intermittent jaundice, with abdominal pain, dark urine, pale stools, a high level of direct-reacting bilirubin in the serum, and nonvisualization of the gallbladder on cholecystography. It appears to be a congenital metabolic deficiency in which the liver can conjugate indirect bilirubin with glucuronic acid but has difficulty in excretion, so that the direct-reacting bilirubin accumulates in the serum and is excreted in the urine. The liver is characterized by a heavy accumulation of a dark brown pigment in hepatic cells in the central zones of the lobules. The pigment, formerly considered to be lipofuscin, may be a melanin polymer. Little or no fibrosis or other morphologic change is evident. The liver may be grossly black or greenish black.

CIRCULATORY DISTURBANCES

Chronic passive congestion. Chronic passive congestion is a common and prominent finding in the liver, an organ highly susceptible to circulatory deficiency. Congestive heart failure and inferior vena caval obstruction are among the causes of this disturbance. The effect is particularly in the central parts of the lobules, where stagnation and accumulation of blood dilate the central vein and adjacent portions of the sinusoids (Fig. 16-2). The liver cells, first around the central veins but gradually extending out to the periphery, undergo atrophy resulting from anoxemia and compression. Degenerative changes, particularly of a fatty type, tend to occur. In some severe cases, there may be actual necrosis.

Grossly, the contrasted pattern of red areas (caused by blood-stuffed vessels) and yellowish brown areas (liver cells with fatty degeneration) produces a characteristic "nutmeg" appearance (see Fig. 5-1). Long-standing congestion results in the so-called cardiac cirrhosis (p. 453).

Hemorrhage. Hemorrhage in the liver, which occurs in eclampsia and other conditions, is distinguished from congestion by the finding of red cells outside the sinuses, e.g., between the sinusoidal endothelium and the liver cells.

Edema. Edema in the liver is distinguishable by the presence of a fine web of granular precipitated protein material between the sinus endothelial lining and the liver cell cords (serous hepatitis).

Infarction. Infarction is rare in the liver (Fig. 16-3), presumably because of the abundant and double blood supply. When it does occur, it is most often caused by obstruction of the hepatic artery or its branches (e.g., septic or bland emboli, polyarteritis nodosa, or inadvertent surgical ligation), particularly when there is passive congestion of the liver. Obstruction of the portal vein may cause areas of necrosis in the liver, but usually obstruction of the intrahepatic branches of the portal vein leads to the development of so-called red infarcts of Zahn. These are areas of hyperemia with atrophy of hepatic cells but without actual necrosis.

Thrombosis of hepatic veins. Thrombosis of the hepatic veins occurs in acute and

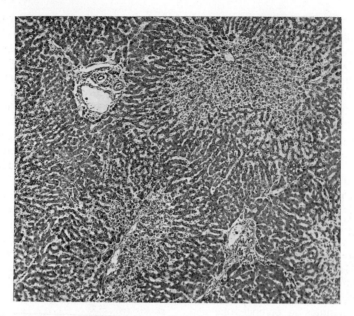

Fig. 16-2. Chronic passive congestion of liver. Central zones of lobules show most severe congestion with centrilobular degeneration and atrophy. ($\times 50$.)

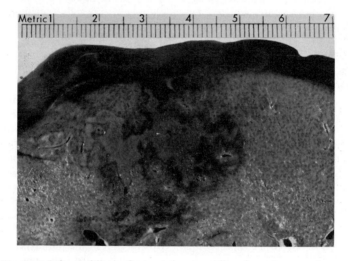

Fig. 16-3. Infarct of liver. Congested zone outlines irregular necrotic area.

chronic forms. It may be caused by a primary hepatic endophlebitis or be secondary to various intrahepatic and extrahepatic conditions that favor thrombosis.

Veno-occlusive disease. Veno-occlusive disease of the liver is a peculiar type of obliterating endophlebitis of the smaller radicals of the hepatic veins that may progress to nonportal cirrhosis. Described in children and young adults in Jamaica, it appears to be associated with toxic substances in "bush teas," made by boiling leaves of plants of the *Senecio* and *Crotalaria* species.

Peliosis hepatis. Peliosis hepatis is a condition in which small blood-containing cystic lesions are distributed throughout the liver. The peliotic cavities may develop as a result of focal parencymal necrosis followed by hemorrhage (parenchymal peliosis hepatis). In some livers, the lesions are believed to represent aneurysmal dilatation of central veins (phlebectatic peliosis hepatis). Most instances of peliosis hepatis have been in patients with tuberculosis. It also has been reported in patients treated with gonadal steroid hormones.

Experimentally, peliosis hepatis has resulted after the transplantation of ovarian or testicular tumors in mice or the inoculation of newborn rats with certain viruses isolated from rat tissues.

NECROSIS

Liver cells undergo necrosis as a result of a variety of poisons of chemical, infectious, and metabolic origin. Adequate stores of glycogen in the liver cells appear to give some protection. The lesions may be classified roughly according to their distribution into the following types:

1 Diffuse necrosis, e.g., "acute red or yellow atrophy"
2 "Focal" necrosis, i.e., small necrotic foci distributed without any constant relationship to particular areas of the liver lobules
3 Zonal necrosis, in which the areas of necrosis are in fairly constant relationship to a particular part of the liver lobules

The zonal necroses may be (1) central, i.e., in the central vein region, (2) midzonal, or (3) peripheral, or in portal areas.

Diffuse necrosis. Diffuse, massive necrosis of the liver has been incorrectly called *acute red* or *yellow atrophy*. It may be caused by a variety of agents, including infections (viral hepatitis) and chemicals or drugs (phosphorus, arsenicals, chloroform, carbon tetrachloride, sulfonamides, and iproniazid). Most cases of diffuse necrosis of the liver, formerly considered idiopathic, now may be accounted for as cases of viral hepatitis. The hepatic changes are essentially the same as those described in fulminating viral hepatitis. The acute form is fatal after a short duration, with fever, gastrointestinal upset, disturbances of hepatic and renal functions, jaundice, crystals of leucine and tyrosine in the urine, and coma.

Except in the most acute cases, the liver is shrunken, often to half its normal size. The capsule is wrinkled, soft, and opaque and mottled patchy yellowish and red in color. In early stages, the yellowish color predominates, but later, when the liver cells have extensively disintegrated, a red color is prominent. Microscopically, one sees a loss of nuclei, granular and fatty degeneration of cytoplasm, and breaking up, disorganization, or complete disappearance of many cells.

In patients with submassive necrosis, the progress of the disease tends to be slower, so that death occurs at a later stage or only after repeated attacks. The lesion is sometimes referred to as *subacute yellow atrophy*. Here, there is an opportunity for removal of the necrotic cells, regenerative hyperplasia from the remaining liver tissue, and development of fibrous tissue. Nodules of hyperplastic liver cells are separated by connective tissue, and bile duct proliferation is in evidence. Complete healing may be achieved, but in some cases the changes are progressive and end in hepatic insufficiency. The healing or healed stage often is referred to as coarsely nodular or postnecrotic cirrhosis.

Focal and zonal necroses. Multiple small areas of necrosis are more frequent in the liver than are diffuse or massive areas of necrosis. Those that have a fairly constant relationship to some part of the liver lobules are referred to as zonal necroses.

Focal necroses, which have no special or constant site in the liver lobules, occur in a variety of severe infections, such as typhoid fever, pneumonia, diphtheria, and tularemia (Fig. 16-4).

Central necrosis is the most common type of zonal necrosis. It occurs with severe chronic passive congestion, particularly if there is

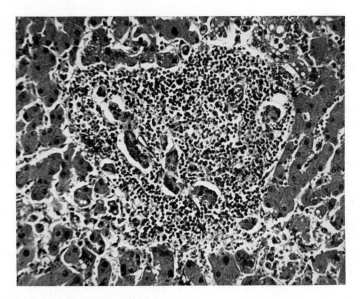

Fig. 16-4. Focal necrosis (and some inflammatory cells) in liver in tularemia.

added infection with streptococci. A variety of poisons, some of industrial importance, such as trinitrotoluene, carbon tetrachloride, and chloroform, produce central necrosis.

Midzonal necrosis occurs in certain infective conditions and is particularly characteristic of yellow fever. In the latter, there are rounded hyaline cytoplasmic masses (Councilman bodies) and sometimes nuclear inclusion bodies in cells of the midzonal region.

Peripheral necrosis often is seen in phosphorus poisoning and in eclampsia, although in the latter condition the necroses are by no means constant in their position but are often focal in distribution and hemorrhagic in character.

Eclampsia. Eclampsia is a toxic complication of the later months of pregnancy (pp. 344 and 663) in which hypertension, albuminuria, edema, and convulsions are prominent features. The lesions in the liver are the most striking, but they cannot be correlated with the severity of the disease and are probably of less importance than the renal changes. Areas of confluent necrosis and associated hemorrhage may be patchily scattered throughout the liver substance, particularly in (but not limited

to) peripheral lobular zones, and irregular areas of hemorrhage beneath the capsule give the liver a grossly mottled appearance.

CHEMICAL AND DRUG INJURY

A number of chemicals or drugs may cause direct toxic injury to the liver, sometimes referred to as "toxic hepatitis." In such instances, the effect is related to dose and usually is manifest shortly after exposure. These direct hepatotoxins (e.g., carbon tetrachloride, chloroform, phosphorus, mushroom [*Amanita phalloides*] toxin) usually produce zonal necrosis and fatty change but may cause massive necrosis of the liver. Repeated exposure to some of these hepatotoxic agents may result in cirrhosis of the liver. Chronic toxic effects, including portal fibrosis and cirrhosis of the liver, have been observed in association with continued long-term use of methotrexate, a folic acid antagonist, for the treatment of cancer and psoriasis. However, several recent reports tend to deemphasize the chronic hepatotoxicity of the drug in patients with psoriasis, suggesting that it alone may not cause severe or irreversible liver changes. Progressive portal fibrosis, focal capsular fibrosis, mild perisinusoidal fibrosis, and focal hypertrophy and hyperplasia of hepatocytes have been observed in patients exposed to vinyl chloride. This chemical is believed to have caused hepatic angiosarcomas in workers exposed to it.

In contrast to the direct hepatotoxins, there are certain drugs that are tolerated by most persons but affect certain susceptible individuals, apparently by hypersensitivity. The liver damage is not dose-related and may be necrosis or cholestasis. For example, iproniazid may produce focal necrosis with inflammation, simulating viral hepatitis. Chlorpromazine causes cholestasis with minimal hepatocellular damage (degenerative changes with little, if any, cellular necrosis). Bile canaliculi contain bile plugs, and the portal areas show an infiltration by mononuclear cells and eosinophils.

Another group of drugs may affect any person who receives them long enough and in sufficient dosage, usually producing cholestasis (jaundice) without hepatocellular damage. Such drugs include the 17-alpha-alkyl-substituted testosterones (e.g., methyltestosterone, norethandrolone, and norethindrone) and oral contraceptive agents. It appears that the cholestatic drugs produce reversible injury to the secretory mechanism, preventing bilirubin glucuronide from entering the canaliculi normally. The bilirubin that does enter the canaliculi is seen microscopically as bile plugs in the centrilobular regions.

In some patients, these cholestatic drugs may produce occasional necrotic liver cells as well as minimal inflammation and, rarely, severe necrosis. In addition, a possible relationship of the gonadal steroid hormones to peliosis hepatis (p. 441) and liver cell tumors (p. 456) has been suggested.

VIRAL HEPATITIS

As noted previously (p. 176), three types of viral hepatitis are recognized. A short incubation type (15 to 50 days), known as hepatitis A, infectious hepatitis, MS-1 type, or epidemic hepatitis, is most commonly seen in children or young adults and usually is transmitted orally but may be acquired by the parenteral route by inoculations. A long incubation type (50 to 160 days), known as hepatitis B, serum hepatitis, or MS-2 type, is a more common type of viral hepatitis in adults, but occurs at any age, and generally is transmitted by injection of human blood products or material contaminated with blood. However, there is evidence that it can be transmitted by other than the parenteral route. The third form of viral hepatitis is referred to as non-A, non-B hepatitis and is usually acquired as a result of the administration of blood or blood products. For discussion of the antigens associated with the various forms of viral hepatitis, see pp. 175 and 176.

Pathologic anatomy. The microscopic features of hepatitis A, hepatitis B, and non-A, non-B hepatitis are similar. Early in the disease, prior to clinical manifestations, biopsy of the liver discloses only occasional cell necrosis, enlargement and increase in number of Kupffer cells, and an increased number of lymphocytes in the sinusoids. At the height of the disease, when symptoms are manifest, there is generalized parenchymal damage with disruption of the normal liver cell cord arrangement. The hepatic cells are swollen and hydropic, particularly in the centrilobular regions. The cytoplasm of many cells shows a "ground glass appearance"; other cells appear markedly vacuolated (ballooning degeneration). Focal necrosis is present. Some of the necrotic cells are shrunken, with the cytoplasm forming a homogeneous, hyaline mass, the "acidophilic body," which may be extruded into a sinusoid. Other necrotic liver cells are absorbed, and a collapsed stroma may be seen in their place. The Kupffer cells are prominent and show proliferation. Lymphocytes and monocytes infiltrate the portal areas and sinusoids throughout the lobules. Occasional plasma cells, eosinophils, and neutrophils may be present. Variable degrees of canalicular cholestasis (bile pigment in canaliculi) are observed. Kupffer cells may contain yellowish pigment. Regeneration of liver cells occurs, and mitotic figures may be seen. Multinucleated liver cells may be present.

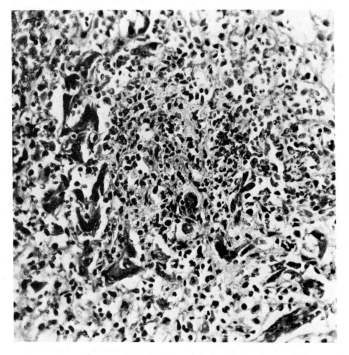

Fig. 16-5. Diffuse necrosis of liver in fulminating viral hepatitis. Loss of liver cells, infiltration by leukocytes, and some proliferation of small bile ducts are evident.

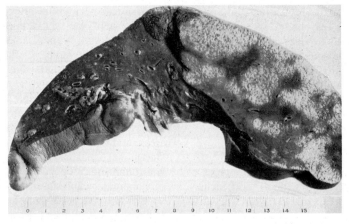

Fig. 16-6. Epidemic hepatitis, nineteenth day. Regenerating tissue evident on right. (From Lucke, B.: Am. J. Pathol. **20:**471-593, 1944.)

With recovery, there is gradual reestablishment of the normal liver cell cord arrangement, although pigmented Kupffer cells and some portal lymphocytic infiltration may remain.

The electron microscopic changes in viral hepatitis are nonspecific and include injured endoplasmic reticulum, detached ribosomes throughout the cytoplasm, and large autophagic vacuoles. Mitochondrial alterations are not prominent in nonnecrotic cells. The acidophilic bodies consist of condensed cytoplasm in which remains of cell organelles are still seen. Viruslike particles have been seen in the liver in some instances of viral hepatitis.

Variants. In most patients with viral hepatitis, there is no recurrence of symptoms following the initial attack. In a small percentage of patients, however, *relapsing hepatitis* occurs within a few months, with clinical and anatomic features similar to the original episode of hepatitis, although usually of milder degree. Other patients may remain almost completely asymptomatic following recovery from the initial attack but show persistent or episodic elevations of transaminase activity for more than a year *(unresolved viral hepatitis or chronic persistent hepatitis)*. Liver biopsy discloses hydropic changes and foci of necrosis of liver cells, which are surrounded by rosettes of lymphocytes. Also, lymphocytes infiltrate the portal areas. The relapsing and unresolved forms of viral hepatitis are nonfatal variants of the disease.

A more serious variant of acute viral hepatitis is that described by some investigators as *progressive viral hepatitis,* which eventually may be fatal. Frequently, the histologic changes in the liver resemble those of the usual form of acute viral hepatitis, as described previously. However, in addition, multiple, larger zones of liver cell necrosis may be seen that are confluent, resulting in bridging bands of collapsed stroma infiltrated by lymphocytes that connect adjacent portal areas or central regions. Such bridging lesions have been called *subacute hepatic necrosis,* and their presence indicates a severe form of the disease that may progress to hepatic failure

and death or to chronic liver disease (cirrhosis). Subacute hepatic necrosis sometimes may be difficult to distinguish from the lesion of "chronic active hepatitis."

Another fatal form of viral hepatitis is *fulminant viral hepatitis*. This infrequent variant is characterized by diffuse, massive necrosis of the liver, which usually becomes moderately reduced in size, is soft in consistency, has a slightly wrinkled capsule, and is dark reddish brown (so-called acute red atrophy). Microscopically, there is massive destruction of hepatic cells, but there is preservation of the architectural framework, sinusoids, and bile ducts (Fig. 16-5). Smaller bile ducts may show proliferative changes. Inflammatory cells may be most numerous about peripheral parts of the lobules. Monocytes, lymphocytes, and plasma cells predominate, with fewer neutrophils and eosinophils. Patients may survive only a few days. If there is less massive (i.e., submassive) necrosis, death may occur after 2 or 3 weeks. In such instances, the stroma is collapsed and the liver is greatly reduced in size. The capsule is markedly wrinkled. The reddish collapsed areas contrast with the masses of persistent, swollen, regenerating hepatic cells that are icteric (yellowish or yellow-green) and form bulging nodular areas (so-called subacute yellow atrophy) (Fig. 16-6).

CHRONIC ACTIVE HEPATITIS

In the literature, chronic active hepatitis is referred to also as "active chronic hepatitis" or "chronic aggressive hepatitis." It is characterized by recurrent attacks resembling mild viral hepatitis and may ultimately result in postnecrotic (coarsely nodular) cirrhosis. The condition frequently is "idiopathic," but in some instances there is suggestion of either an immunologic or viral cause. Hypergammaglobulinemia, with increase in IgG particularly, is often present in patients with chronic active hepatitis. Some patients have positive LE cell preparations, antinuclear antibodies, and anti–smooth muscle antibodies. The disease in these patients is sometimes referred to as "chronic active lupoid hepatitis." In other persons, the lesion is believed to be of viral origin. Australia antigen (HAA) is demonstrated in their sera, but the LE cell preparations are negative and there are no anti–smooth muscle antibodies. There may or may not be a history of a typical acute attack of viral hepatitis as the initial event. The lesion in these patients may be designated "chronic active viral hepatitis."

Microscopically, the liver in chronic active hepatitis may show acute and chronic changes. Usually, there is evidence of hepatic cell damage, inflammation, and fibrosis (Fig. 16-7). The liver cell cord pattern is disturbed. Liver cells are swollen, often with bizarre nuclei. Necrosis of cells, particularly in the periportal zones ("piecemeal necrosis"), is associated with fibrosis, infiltration by mononuclear cells, and ductal proliferation. Fibrous tissue extends from the portal zones and appears between cells or clumps of cells, isolating them sometimes in a rosettelike fashion. Extensive

necrosis with stromal collapse, involving several consecutive lobules, may occur. With progression of the disease, fibrosis becomes more prominent and surrounds regenerative nodules of hepatic cells, leading to postnecrotic (coarsely nodular) cirrhosis.

CIRRHOSIS

Cirrhosis refers to a fibrosis or scarring of the liver that is progressive and not simply the stationary healed end stage of an injury. It is a chronic disease, often accompanied by some degree of liver cell failure and portal hypertension. All parts (although not necessarily each lobule) of the liver are involved with fibrosis. In some cases, there are connective tissue bands disorganizing the lobular architecture and uniting centrilobular zones with portal tracts, accompanied by nodular parenchymal regeneration. Necrosis of hepatic cells is usually present at some stage of the disease.

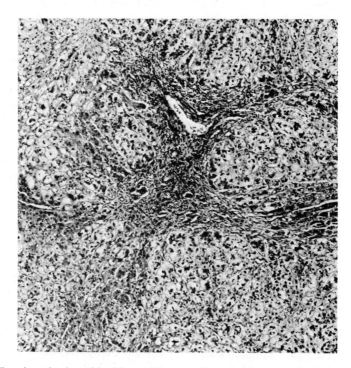

Fig. 16-7. Chronic active hepatitis. Liver cells are swollen, some showing bizarre nuclei. Perilobular necrosis is associated with fibrosis and infiltration by mononuclear cells. Fibrous tissue extends from periphery into lobules, separating cells or clumps of cells.

There are several varieties of cirrhosis, differing in etiology, nature, form, and effects. Numerous classifications are extant, with even more numerous terminologies. Generally agreed to are the three morphologic varieties of portal (Laennec's) cirrhosis, postnecrotic cirrhosis, and biliary cirrhosis. Differentiated among the cases of portal cirrhosis are the fatty cirrhosis of malnutrition or alcoholism and the pigmentary cirrhosis associated with hemochromatosis. Other forms of cirrhosis include cardiac or congestive cirrhosis (the result of a passive congestion of long standing), parasitic cirrhosis (caused by schistosomiasis or clonorchiasis), and syphilitic cirrhosis.

The effects and complications of cirrhosis are mainly obstruction of the portal circulation, gastrointestinal hemorrhage, disturbance of liver function, and development of carcinoma of the liver. In the United States, about 5% of patients with cirrhosis develop primary carcinoma of the liver.

Portal cirrhosis

Portal cirrhosis (Laennec's cirrhosis; fatty nutritional cirrhosis; alcoholic cirrhosis; septal cirrhosis; hobnail liver) occurs at any age but most commonly in middle life and is more frequent in males than in females. A history of chronic alcoholism is present in 50% to 80% or more of the patients, but it also develops in total abstainers. Bouts of jaundice or other evidence of hepatitis occur in some cases. Major clinical signs are ascites, edema, jaundice, enlargement of the liver and spleen, telangiectasis, hematemesis, dermatitis, and disorientation. Ascites is the most constant and striking result. There is obstruction of the portal circulation, and collateral channels of venous return develop. Death may be sudden from the rupture of varices of the esophagus.

The causes of death in portal cirrhosis are mainly acute and chronic infections, hemorrhage from esophageal varices or gastric erosions, hepatic insufficiency, carcinoma of the liver, and cardiac failure. In chronic alcoholics, death may occur from acute hepatic insufficiency before a late stage of hepatic fibrosis and atrophy has developed.

Gross appearance. The disease goes through stages in which both morphologic appearances and associated clinical effects are distinctive. The early stage is an enlarged liver with severe fatty change. In this period there may be few symptoms, but at any time an acute necrosis may develop with sudden hepatic insufficiency. With the progression and development of fibrosis, a fibrofatty stage follows (Fig. 16-8), in which hepatic insufficiency and portal hypertension are clinical manifestations. In the final, late stage of fibrosis and atrophy, portal hypertension and its complications may be dominant clinically. When seen in late stages, the liver is atrophic and smaller than normal (hobnail liver). The general shape is normal, and the color is reddish brown or is yellowish if there is associated fatty change. The whole outer surface is nodular because of rounded, projecting masses of liver cells, 2 to 5 mm in diameter, separated by retracted grayish connective tissue. Consistency of the tissue is much increased. On the cut surface, an interlacing network of gray translucent connective tissue separates prominent nodules of liver cells.

Microscopic appearance. Microscopically, the normal architecture of the liver is completely upset by bands of connective tissue (Fig. 16-9) that redivide the liver into irregular nodules having no constant relationship to central veins or portal regions. Most of the connective tissue is fairly young, only slightly hyalinized, and infiltrated by mononuclear chronic inflammatory cells, mainly lymphocytes and plasma cells. Bile canalicular and pericanalicular changes may be associated with cholestasis and jaundice. Small bile ducts are numerous and prominent in the connective tissue areas. In all stages of the process, degenerative changes and necrosis may be evident in the liver cells. Most characteristically, there is a hyaline accumulation in their cytoplasm, as described by Mallory. The hyaline Mallory bodies, sometimes called "alcoholic hyalin," are differentially stained by chromotrope aniline blue. Although certain electron microscopic studies suggest that the Mallory bodies are related to mitochondrial changes of clump-

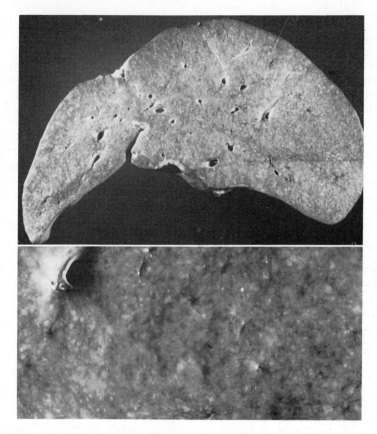

Fig. 16-8. Cirrhosis of liver, fibrofatty stage.

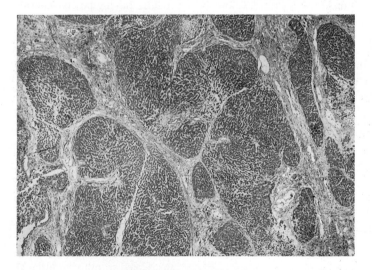

Fig. 16-9. Portal cirrhosis of liver.

ing, enlargement, and bizarre forms or to endoplasmic reticulum, in one investigation they were described as intracytoplasmic meshworks of fibrils with no relationship to any cytoplasmic organelles. They may represent a newly formed protein. In early stages, fatty change is a prominent feature, preceding or associated with the development of fibrosis. Fatty change tends to persist even in late stages (Fig. 16-10), although it may be diminished. Regenerative nodules of liver cells form the bulk of the tissue in advanced cirrhosis and contribute to the distortion of architecture and vascular relationships and to the development of portal hypertension.

In some alcoholics, a clinical state develops, referred to as *alcoholic hepatitis,* that may eventually progress to cirrhosis. It is characterized by fatty metamorphosis, extensive cellular degeneration and necrosis (with intracellular hyaline Mallory bodies), and inflammatory cell infiltration. Electron microscopic changes include enlarged and clumped mitochondria, vesiculation of endoplasmic reticulum, a paucity of rough endoplasmic reticulum, and areas of cytoplasmic degradation.

Etiology. The etiology is still unsettled and much debated. Cirrhosis has been produced experimentally in animals by repeated doses of certain poisons, such as carbon tetrachloride, tars, and combinations of phosphorus and alcohol, manganese chloride and phenylhydrazine, and chloroform with infection. Mallory also found that lead would induce cirrhosis. There has been some controversy as to whether dietary deficiency can lead to cirrhosis. Fatty change in the liver has been observed in children with kwashiorkor, a protein deficiency, but not cirrhosis. However, fatty metamorphosis of the liver that follows intestinal bypass operations for obesity apparently can proceed to cirrhosis. Nutritional cirrhosis in experimental animals has been produced in rats by a diet low in casein but is preventable when methionine or cystine plus choline is added to the diet. The cirrhosis is similar to portal cirrhosis of man except for the presence of a golden brown fluorescent pigment, ceroid. Ceroid is believed to be of lipoidal nature and is developed from liver cells containing fat during the development of cirrhosis.

Clinical experience indicates that alcoholism is a factor in many cases of cirrhosis. It has been suggested that dietary insufficiency in combination with alcoholism results in the liver damage, although there may be a direct metabolic effect of alcohol. The mechanism by which alcohol causes fatty change in the liver is not definitely known. It is probable that any

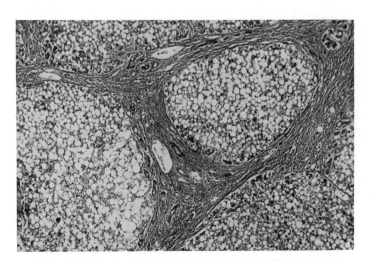

Fig. 16-10. Cirrhosis of liver. Fibrous bands and fatty change.

of the mechanisms resulting in the production of increased cellular triglyceride that are described on p. 27 may be involved. The fatty liver so characteristic of chronic alcoholism may proceed gradually to the development of portal cirrhosis if the individual survives and the insults to the liver continue. Obstruction of lymphatics and sinusoidal blood vessels in the liver by cells swollen from fat or injury may be part of the pathogenetic mechanism. Alcoholism and malnutrition may be associated with an acute type of disease, so-called alcoholic hepatitis (described previously), which may progress to cirrhosis.

Experimentally, fatty change and ultrastructural alterations have been produced in the liver of rats and human volunteers following chronic consumption of alcohol in the presence of an adequate diet. In many investigations, alcohol alone has quite regularly failed to produce hepatic cirrhosis in experimental animals, although it has done so when combined with a high-fat diet in a prolonged experiment. However, recently it was shown by Rubin and Lieber that nonhuman primates (baboons) fed alcohol with a nutritionally adequate diet developed the entire spectrum of liver disease clinically associated with chronic alcoholism in man, i.e., fatty liver, alcoholic hepatitis, and cirrhosis.

Cirrhosis has been observed in patients with alpha$_1$-antitrypsin deficiency, usually but not necessarily with pulmonary emphysema also. Inclusions containing alpha$_1$-antitrypsin have been seen in the cytoplasm of hepatocytes in these cirrhotic livers. It has been suggested that these intracytoplasmic inclusions may interfere with normal hepatic cell function, making the liver more susceptible to injury by some other factor.

Effects. The effects of portal cirrhosis in disturbing the portal circulation are usually more prominent than failure of liver function. Ascites is an outstanding feature and is partly the result of congestion and increased pressure in the portal veins, causing extravasation of fluid along the peritoneal serosa, but reduction of plasma proteins is an important factor contributing to the accumulation of fluid. Additional causative factors are considered to be renal retention of sodium and water (resulting from hyperaldosteronemia and increased secretion of antidiuretic hormone) and increased production of hepatic lymph because of intrahepatic congestion with exudation of lymph through Glisson's capsule. Perfusion experiments have indicated that in some cases portal hypertension may be contributed to by an increased hepatic arterial inflow transmitted to the portal side by abnormal arterioportal anastomoses.

The gradually developing obstruction in the portal circulation permits the development of a collateral venous circulation. The cutaneous vessels over the abdomen and back become distended and prominent. Varices of esophageal veins commonly develop, and the anastomoses with these from the portal circulation are composed of vessels from the coronary veins and from the left gastroepiploic veins and vasa brevia. In the lower third of the esophagus, the rich anastomoses of submucosal veins are poorly supported by connective tissue. Hence, this is a frequent site for varices and venous rupture. Severe hemorrhage complicating cirrhosis also may be from erosive gastritis or peptic ulcers. Varices of hemorrhoidal veins are much less common in association with cirrhosis.

The spleen is enlarged and congested in patients with portal cirrhosis as a result of the obstruction to the portal circulation.

Testicular atrophy is a common accompaniment of the cirrhosis, particularly in patients under 50 years of age. The extensively damaged liver apparently fails to inactivate estrogens, particularly in the absence of sufficient intake of the vitamin B complex. A similar explanation is possible for the occasional occurrence of gynecomastia, palmar erythema, and arterial spider nevi of the skin.

Other evidences of disturbed liver function include hyperbilirubinemia (jaundice), hypoalbuminemia, hypoprothrombinemia, and increased serum transaminases (e.g., SGOT). Derangement of ammonia metabolism may be a factor responsible for the encephalopathy observed in advanced disease, i.e., mental cloudiness, hallucinations, coma, and a peculiar flappy tremor of the hands.

Postnecrotic cirrhosis

Postnecrotic cirrhosis (coarse nodular cirrhosis; toxic cirrhosis) is characterized by irregular involvement of the liver, often with areas of preserved architecture. There may be broad bands of fibrous tissue that follow collapse of the parenchyma. The nodules represent persisting parenchyma. Postnecrotic cirrhosis may result from a variety of causes that produce a massive necrosis of hepatic tissue that is insufficient to cause death but too great to allow structural recovery. The causes include viral hepatitis and hepatotoxic chemicals and drugs. It may directly follow an acute hepatitis or appear after months or years.

The liver is smaller than normal and is characterized by large nodules (1 cm or more in diameter) irregularly distributed in the liver (Fig. 16-11). Thick, dense, grayish septa of fibrous tissue, of varying width, separate the nodules. The nodules are composed of groups of hepatic cells, in which the arrangement may vary from normal to great distortion. Some of the hepatic nodules contain central veins (Fig. 16-12). Bizarre liver cells may be seen, but fatty change usually is not present. The effects are similar to those described for portal cirrhosis.

In *Wilson's disease* (hepatolenticular degeneration), cirrhosis is associated with degenerative changes in basal ganglia of the brain. It appears to be an inherited disturbance of copper metabolism. There is defective synthesis of serum ceruloplasmin and a low serum copper level but increased albumin-bound copper in the serum. Increased accumulation of copper is found in the liver, brain, kidneys, cornea, and other tissues. Clinical symptoms usually arise during adolescence. Symptoms and lesions either of hepatic cirrhosis or of the nervous system may be predominant. Kayser-Fleischer corneal rings, a pigmentation of Descemet's membrane, are characteristic. The cirrhosis is usually the coarse nodular type.

Biliary cirrhosis

Biliary cirrhosis is less common than the portal type. One form is caused by an obstruction in some part of the bile duct system (*secondary biliary cirrhosis*). There may or may not be an associated infection (cholangitis). The obstruction may be intrahepatic or the result of stricture, gallstone, or pancreatic carcinoma interfering with the common bile duct.

The liver is a deep green color (bile stained) and usually is increased in size and weight. Its surface is smooth or only finely granular, and during the early phase the lobular pattern is preserved. The portal areas are lengthened and widened and appear prominent. Hepatic cell degeneration is associated with bile stasis. Intrahepatic bile ducts are dilated and often contain neutrophilic leukocytes. Inspissated masses of bile distend the bile canaliculi. Foci of necrosis, particularly in the periphery of the lobules, may be accompanied by formation of

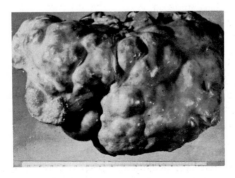

Fig. 16-11. Coarse nodular cirrhosis of liver. (From Anderson, W. A. D.: The liver. In Anderson, W. A. D., editor: Pathology, ed. 3, St. Louis, 1957, The C. V. Mosby Co.)

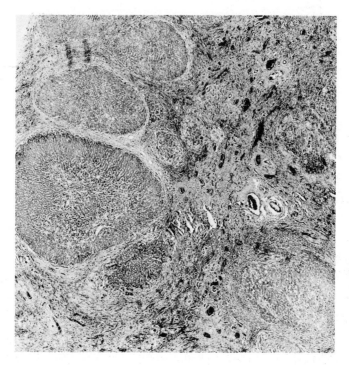

Fig. 16-12. Postnecrotic cirrhosis. Irregular nodules of hepatic tissue are separated by fibrous bands with large scar on right. Central veins are readily apparent in nodule at left center.

"bile lakes." There is increased connective tissue in portal areas and around the periphery of the lobules (Fig. 16-13). Chronic inflammatory cells, mainly lymphocytes and plasma cells, infiltrate this fibrous tissue.

Primary biliary cirrhosis is a disease of unknown cause, occurring most frequently in middle-aged women. It has been called "chronic nonsuppurative destructive cholangitis." There is destruction of cholangioles, infiltration by inflammatory cells (chiefly mononuclear) in the portal areas, and evidence of periportal cholestasis. Occasionally, the disease has followed an episode of "cholangiolitic viral hepatitis." Also, it has been observed in some patients with ulcerative colitis. Drug sensitivity has been suggested as a possible cause. The possibility of an immunologic pathogenetic mechanism is suggested by the demonstration of an antiliver antibody in the sera of patients with primary biliary cirrhosis. The antibody reacts against mitochondrial membranes. Some investigators have identified high serum levels of complement-fixing immune complexes in patients with primary biliary cirrhosis that may be important in the pathogenesis of the disease.

The manifestations of biliary cirrhosis include jaundice, pruritus, hypercholesterolemia, skin xanthomas, and features of the malabsorption syndrome due to impairment in the flow of bile. Evidence of hepatic insufficiency may appear in advanced disease. Portal hypertension does not occur as frequently as in portal or postnecrotic cirrhosis.

Other forms of cirrhosis

Pigment cirrhosis. The liver changes in hemochromatosis may be referred to as pigment cirrhosis. The gross and microscopic features of the liver are those of a portal type of cirrhosis with the addition of large amounts of hemosiderin pigment (p. 48).

Syphilitic cirrhosis. The liver is commonly

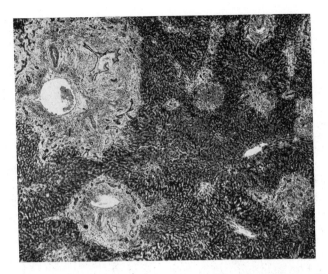

Fig. 16-13. Biliary cirrhosis of liver. (From Edmondson, H. A., and Peters, R. L.: Liver. In Anderson, W. A. D., and Kissane, J. M., editors: Pathology, ed. 7, St. Louis, 1977, The C. V. Mosby Co.)

involved in congenital syphilis, and many spirochetes may be demonstrable in that organ. In some cases, there is a diffuse fibrosis within the lobules. In acquired syphilis, the liver is not so regularly affected, but gummas may occur that heal by fibrous scars and leave a severe distortion of the organ (hepar lobatum).

Cardiac or congestive cirrhosis. Long-continued chronic passive congestion of the liver leads to atrophy of liver cells around the central vein areas, with a relative increase in the connective tissue. There also may be a diffuse fibrosis and alteration of architecture. It is most commonly associated with constrictive pericarditis and rheumatic heart disease.

Parasitic cirrhosis. As a result of the lodgment of ova in the liver, cirrhosis may be produced by infection with *Schistosoma mansoni* and, less frequently, with *Schistosoma japonicum* and *Schistosoma haematobium*. Dense whitish zones of fibrosis develop about intrahepatic portal branches. The external surface may be nodular and similar in gross appearance to Laennec's cirrhosis. Small fibrous nodules, 1 or 2 mm in diameter, may be scattered throughout the liver. Microscopically, the ova or remains of their shells may be found in the fibrous areas. Brownish pigment granules are held in Kupffer cells. Splenomegaly, ascites, and esophageal varices develop in late stages (p. 216).

The liver fluke, *Clonorchis sinensis,* may produce a biliary type of cirrhosis caused by lodgment in biliary channels. There is fibrous thickening with dilatation of bile ducts, and fibrosis and cellular infiltration develop in the portal spaces. Flukes or their remnants may be found in involved areas. Severe visceral leishmaniasis (kala-azar) also may be complicated by cirrhosis.

WEIL'S DISEASE

Weil's disease, or spirochetal jaundice, is caused by infection with *Leptospira icterohaemorrhagiae* and affects particularly the kidneys, liver, capillaries, and skeletal muscles. The liver usually is enlarged and bile stained. The microscopic features are described on p. 191.

GRANULOMATOUS HEPATITIS

Granulomatous lesions in the liver may be produced by numerous infections, by hypersensitivity, and by various generalized granulomatous diseases. Among the causes are brucellosis, tuberculosis, sarcoidosis, and fungal infections.

ABSCESSES

Abscesses of the liver may be bacterial, amebic, or actinomycotic.

Bacterial abscesses. Abscesses caused by pyogenic bacteria are often referred to as *pyogenic abscesses*. These lesions, commonly caused by *Escherichia coli,* staphylococci, and streptococci, may result from:

1 Extension of organisms to the liver by way of the bile ducts (suppurative cholangitis), secondary to obstruction of the common duct

2 Spread of organisms to the liver by way of the portal vein (pylephlebitis) from the appendix, rectum, or other parts of the bowel

3 Spread to the liver from contiguous infected tissue, e.g., a subphrenic abscess

4 Infection carried to the liver by hepatic arteries in septicopyemia

5 Penetrating traumatic injuries

At present, most bacterial abscesses result from common bile duct obstruction, which leads to dilatation of intrahepatic bile ducts, stagnation of bile, and secondary infection by pyogenic organisms. *Pylephlebitis* with multiple liver abscesses was seen most frequently in the past as an extension from an acute suppurative appendicitis. It may result from septic foci elsewhere in the intestine or other sites drained by the portal vein. The abscesses are more abundant in the right lobe. The areas of necrosis vary from microscopic size to a diameter of several centimeters and, by coalescence, can form large cavities. Necrosis, cellular disintegration, and leukocyte accumulation are found in the areas of abscess. Occasionally, there is the complication of rupture or spread of the infection to adjacent tissues. Bacterial hepatic abscesses resulting from the spread of organisms to the liver by the hepatic arteries are usually only a part of a general septicemia, and abscesses are present in other organs as well.

Amebic abscesses. The amebic abscess (tropical abscess) is caused by the spread of *Entamoeba histolytica* from intestinal lesions by way of the portal vein. The lesion begins in the portal areas, with lysis of tissue and only a little accompanying inflammatory reaction. As noted previously, although the lytic lesion is called an abscess, it is not a true abscess. Adjacent abscesses coalesce to produce lesions of considerable size (Fig. 16-14). The larger abscesses tend to become walled off by connective tissue (p. 206).

Actinomycotic abscesses. Actinomycotic abscesses of the liver are the result of spread from intestinal lesions by way of the portal blood. Multiple small ragged abscess cavities in which the actinomycotic colonies can be found are produced (p. 197).

NONSUPPURATIVE BACTERIAL HEPATITIS—NONSPECIFIC

As already noted, bacteria are capable of producing granulomatous hepatitis, a nonsuppurative form of liver infection, and hepatic abscesses. Usually these lesions are caused by bacteria arising from other sites. On the other hand, an occasional instance of nonspecific nonsuppurative bacterial hepatitis with no demonstrable site of origin of the organisms has been reported. A suggested explanation for this is that during a period when the liver function is temporarily altered, the organ's capacity to eliminate bacteria that reach it in the course of a transient bacteremia is impaired and the organisms are able to set up the intrahepatic infection. This type of disorder may be unrecognized clinically for some time and may be a cause of so-called fever of unknown origin. Biopsy of the liver in such instances may reveal a nonspecific inflammatory reaction consisting of lymphocytes in the portal area with loss of hepatocytes at this site, and bacteria may be cultured from the tissue.

CYSTS

Cysts in the liver are commonly hydatid (echinococcus) cysts, cystic distensions of ducts (hydrohepatosis) and congenital cysts.

Hydatid cysts. Hydatid cysts are caused by the lodging in an organ of the larval form of the dog tapeworm *Echinococcus granulosus* (p. 218). The liver is a commonly involved

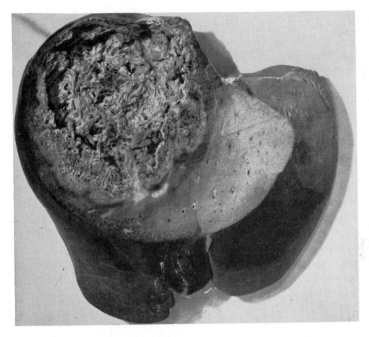

Fig. 16-14. Amebic abscess of liver.

organ. The cyst wall is composed of concentric hyaline laminae, lined by germinal cells from which grow ''daughter'' cysts. Scolices and hooklets of the worm may be identified in the cyst wall or its contents by microscopic examination. Old cysts, in which the parasites are dead, contain a yellowish gray, puttylike material. Alveolar hydatid disease is caused by *Echinococcus multilocularis* (p. 218).

Cystic distention of bile ducts. Cystic distention of the bile ducts, known as hydrohepatosis, is the result of obstruction to bile passages, particularly if such obstruction is intermittent, incomplete, or slow in development.

Congenital cysts. Congenital cysts are uncommon but sometimes are found associated with a congenital cystic condition of the kidneys. They are usually small and cause no disturbance.

TUMORS

Hemangioma. The most common benign tumor of the liver is a cavernous hemangioma (Fig. 16-15) similar to those occurring else-

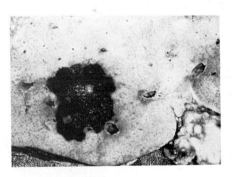

Fig. 16-15. Hemangioma of liver.

where. At autopsy, it often is encountered as an incidental finding. It grows very slowly or remains stationary in size. An unusual tumor is the *hemangioendothelioma of infancy,* which is comparable to the cellular hemangiomas commonly seen in the skin of infants. Frequently, arteriovenous shunts occur within the tumor, causing hypertrophy and dilatation of the heart with resultant congestive heart failure and death.

Adenoma. Benign hepatoma (liver cell adenoma) is relatively infrequent. It is a circumscribed mass of well-formed liver cells that grows expansively, compressing the surrounding liver substance. Bile duct adenoma also occurs and tends to be cystic. Sometimes it is difficult to distinguish morphologically between a liver cell adenoma and focal nodular hyperplasia of the liver. Recently, benign hepatic lesions (reported as "adenomas," "benign hepatomas," "hamartomas," and "focal nodular hyperplasia"), sometimes associated with peliosis hepatis (p. 441), have been described in women taking oral contraceptives. In some patients, regression of their tumors occurred after the use of oral contraceptives was discontinued, suggesting that the hormones played a role in the development of the lesions.

Hamartoma. Hamartoma of the liver is a benign tumorlike malformation of a portion of the liver. It may consist of both proliferating hepatic cells and bile ducts (mixed adenoma of the liver). Most cases occur in infants and children. The lesions are frequently multiple and cystic. A mesenchymal hamartoma occurs in infancy that consists of relatively acellular collagenous connective tissue, remnants of bile ducts, and fluid-filled spaces.

Carcinoma. In the United States, the liver is a very common site for metastatic tumors, whereas *primary carcinoma* occurs less frequently. In the Orient and Africa, primary carcinoma of the liver is much more common. It is a frequent malignant tumor among Japanese males and is very common among black males in some parts of Africa. The high incidence in certain regions appears to result from environmental rather than racial reasons and is associated particularly with nutritional disturbance and cirrhosis or with prevalence of *Clonorchis sinensis* or *Schistosoma* infections. Also, certain substances that may become incorporated in foods may be carcinogenic, e.g., aflatoxins, which are metabolic products of *Aspergillus flavus.* An association between androgenic anabolic steroid therapy and hepatic carcinoma has been reported. An occasional carcinoma has been attributed to other substances, e.g., Thorotrast.

Cancer of the liver occurs at all ages, even in young infants, but the highest incidence is between 50 and 60 years. A considerable proportion of the tumors are associated with cirrhosis in a chronic or late stage. About 75% of patients with cancer of liver cell origin (hepatocarcinoma; Fig. 16-16) and about 25% to

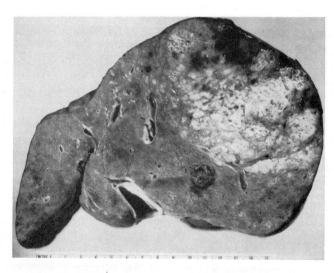

Fig. 16-16. Primary carcinoma of liver (liver cell type).

50% of those with cancer derived from intrahepatic bile ducts (cholangiocarcinoma) have antecedent cirrhosis. In the United States, where the incidence of liver carcinoma is relatively low, about 5% of patients with cirrhosis develop carcinoma of the liver. In some areas (e.g., Africa), where the incidence of carcinoma of the liver is high, about 60% of patients with cirrhosis of the liver develop cancer. In postnecrotic cirrhosis, there appears to be a relatively high incidence of liver cell carcinoma as a late complication. Pigment cirrhosis also is a significant precursor. The incidence of carcinoma is much higher in males than in females.

Grossly, there are three forms: (1) nodular, in which various circumscribed tumor nodules are present throughout the liver, (2) massive, in which a single large tumor occupies one of the lobes, and (3) diffuse, in which the tumor cells are found extensively invading every part of the liver.

Histologically, there are two types—hepatocarcinoma (liver cell carcinoma) and cholangiocarcinoma (bile duct carcinoma)—but some highly undifferentiated tumors are difficult to classify.

Hepatocarcinoma (hepatocellular carcinoma) is more frequent and is composed of cells arranged in columns resembling normal liver cords. These cells are often hyperchromatic and multinucleated or are of giant size. Atypical lobules may be formed, and there is often some bile in or near the tumor cells. A delicate network of capillaries is found in the stroma.

Cholangiocarcinoma is a glandular carcinoma arising from bile ducts. The columnar or cuboidal cells may be in solid clusters or may attempt to form tubules. The connective tissue stroma is dense and shows only a few capillaries. Cholangiocarcinoma has a more rapid course than hepatocarcinoma. Combined liver cell and bile duct carcinomas also occur.

Intrahepatic spread by way of the intrahepatic veins is common, but extrahepatic metastases are not unusual, particularly in regional lymph nodes and lungs. The symptoms are variable, multiple, and often appear unrelated, so that primary liver carcinoma may present diagnostic problems.

Certain *paraneoplastic syndromes*, characterized by metabolic or endocrine abnormalities, have been observed in some patients with hepatocarcinoma, e.g., hypoglycemia (due to excessive intake of glucose by tumor cells or to secretion of insulinlike substance), erythrocythemia (due to secretion of erythropoietin by tumor cells), endocrine changes (gonadotropinlike substance secreted by cancer cells), and hypercalcemia (possibly the result of parathormone-type secretion from cancer cells). *Elevated serum α-fetoprotein* (AFP) levels frequently occur in association with hepatocarcinoma.

Primary carcinomas of the liver in infancy and childhood (hepatoblastomas) are among the most frequent cancers of this age group. They are of the liver cell type, although the cells tend to be smaller, more anaplastic, and more embryonal in appearance than in adults. The condition is to be distinguished from the giant cell transformation of the neonatal liver, which appears to be the response of an immature liver to various injuries or disease processes.

Hepatic sarcoma. *Angiosarcoma* is a highly malignant vascular tumor usually affecting adults. It is reported under various designations, such as "hemangioendothelial sarcoma," "hemangioblastoma," "angioreticular-endothelial sarcoma," and "Kupffer cell sarcoma." Although it is a rare tumor, it has received particular attention recently because of its relatively frequent appearance in workers exposed to vinyl chloride gas in the manufacture of polyvinyl chloride. Hepatic angiosarcomas have been observed also in patients after administration of Thorotrast or after exposure to arsenic.

Embryonal rhabdomyosarcoma, malignant mesenchymoma, and *malignant mixed tumor* occasionally occur in infants and children.

Secondary tumors. Secondary involvement of the liver may occur by direct extension from malignant tumors of the gallbladder, extrahepatic bile ducts, pancreas, and stomach. Distant metastases commonly occur from various carcinomas but particularly from those arising in the gastrointestinal tract, pancreas, kidney, lung, and breast. Metastatic sarcomas also occur, although less frequently.

Gallbladder

The gallbladder is a thin-walled sac in which bile is concentrated by active mucosal absorption of water. The function of the gallbladder is as a reservoir for bile. The chief lesions are inflammation, stone formation, and carcinoma. Inflammation (cholecystitis) causes disturbance of the reabsorptive concentrating activity of the organ. Gallstones (cholelithiasis) result from the precipitation of constituents of bile. They may produce obstruction in the gallbladder, cystic duct, or common duct. Carcinoma is the only common type of tumor of the gallbladder.

JAUNDICE

Jaundice, or icterus, is the condition of hyperbilirubinemia and deposition of bile pigment in the tissues. Bile pigment is formed from the breakdown of hemoglobin by reticuloendothelial cells, particularly in the spleen, liver, and bone marrow.

Prehepatic bilirubin so formed is bound to albumin in the bloodstream and gives an indirect van den Bergh reaction. The indirect-reacting bilirubin is taken up by the parenchymal cells of the liver, where it is conjugated with glucuronides by the enzyme glucuronyl transferase. This conjugated form of bilirubin gives an immediate direct reaction with van den Bergh's reagent and is readily soluble in water. As such, it is excreted in the bile and, if excessive, may be excreted in the urine. Bilirubin excreted with the bile is changed within the bowel to urobilinogen and then to the brown pigment of the stool, urobilin. Urobilinogen may be reabsorbed from the bowel and reexcreted by the liver and kidney. The indirect-reacting (unconjugated) bilirubin is insoluble in water and so is not excreted by the kidneys. For this reason, unconjugated hyperbilirubinemia is often referred to as *acholuric jaundice*.

Jaundice may be classified according to whether the excess bilirubin in the circulation is predominantly unconjugated or conjugated. *Unconjugated hyperbilirubinemia* may result from (1) an overproduction of bilirubin exceeding the capacity of the liver cells to remove it from the bloodstream, (2) a disturbance in hepatocellular uptake and transport to the conjugation site, (3) a disturbance in the conjugation mechanism, or (4) a combination of these factors. *Conjugated hyperbilirubinemia* results from a disturbance in excretion of bilirubin after it is conjugated, involving either defective excretion from the liver cells or interference with excretion along the bile canaliculi or bile ducts, particularly the extrahepatic bile ducts. There is reflux ("regurgitation") of the excess bilirubin into the bloodstream and excretion by way of the kidneys. Bile salts also appear in the urine. The causes of jaundice may be classified as follows.

I Unconjugated hyperbilirubinemia due to
  A Overproduction of bilirubin caused by
    1 Hemolysis of circulating erythrocytes (e.g., hemolytic anemias, drugs, venoms, septicemia, mismatched transfusions)
    2 Destruction of erythrocyte precursors in bone marrow (e.g., thalassemia, pernicious anemia)
    3 Breakdown of masses of extravasated erythrocytes (e.g., massive pulmonary infarcts)
  B Disturbances in hepatic uptake of bilirubin caused by
    1 Certain drugs
    2 Viral hepatitis (recovery phase)
    3 Chronic passive congestion
    4 Idiopathic disease (constitutional hepatic dysfunction or Gilbert's disease)
  C Disturbance in conjugation of bilirubin caused by
    1 Subnormal activity of glucuronyl transferase in newborn, especially premature, infants
    2 Inhibition of glucuronyl transferase by drugs, hepatic cellular disease, breast milk factor affecting nursing infants, etc.
    3 Congenital deficiency or absence of glucuronyl transferase (Crigler-Najjar syndrome)

II Conjugated hyperbilirubinemia due to
  A Disturbance in excretion of bilirubin by liver cells caused by
    1 Hepatic cellular diseases (e.g., hepatitis and cirrhosis)
    2 Drug-induced cholestasis
    3 Familial or hereditary disorders (e.g., Dubin-Johnson and Rotor syndromes)
  B Interference with flow of bile caused by
    1 Obstruction of bile canaliculi by dissociated, swollen hepatic cells (e.g., hepatitis)
    2 Obstruction of biliary tract by neoplasms, calculi, inflammation, strictures, etc.

It should be noted that in some clinical states there may be an increase in both unconjugated and conjugated bilirubin in the serum, e.g., in hepatic cellular diseases such as hepatitis and cirrhosis. In some of these instances, conjugated hyperbilirubinemia predominates to such a degree that the jaundice resembles that caused by obstruction of the extrahepatic bile ducts.

The effects of jaundice other than pigmentation of tissues may be slight in the pure unconjugated type, unless the hyperbilirubinemia is severe, e.g., *kernicterus,* characterized by serious brain damage, may occur in a jaundiced infant, as in hemolytic disease of the newborn. In conjugated jaundice, the effects are probably largely the result of retention of bile salts and their absence from the intestinal tract. Such effects include pruritus and interference with absorption of fats and fat-soluble vitamins (including vitamin K). The latter may give rise to a bleeding tendency caused by prothrombin deficiency.

CHOLECYSTITIS

Inflammation of the gallbladder may be acute or chronic. Chemical damage to the gallbladder wall because of the action of concentrated bile, promoted by an obstruction of the cystic duct, usually by a stone, is probably the most common cause of cholecystitis. In some cases, bacterial infection supervenes. The presence of stones within the gallbladder also may promote an inflammatory process. In nonobstructive or noncalculous cholecystitis,

primary bacterial infection may be responsible, usually caused by streptococci, colon bacilli, and staphylococci. Infection may reach the gallbladder wall from the bloodstream, by direct spread from adjacent organs, from the liver, from the intestine through lymphatics, or by ascending bile ducts from the duodenum.

Acute cholecystitis. In acute cholecystitis, the gallbladder is enlarged, is gray or reddish, and has a thick edematous wall. The mucosa shows areas of necrosis and ulceration, and leukocytes are present in the wall. Purulent exudate may fill the cavity (empyema of the gallbladder). Calculi often are associated with the inflammation and may obstruct the neck of the gallbladder, or they may erode through the softened and necrotic wall.

Chronic cholecystitis. Chronic cholecystitis, commonly associated with gallstones, may be catarrhal, with merely slight thickening, lymphocyte infiltration, and congestion of mucosal folds. In other cases, the changes are greater, with areas of destruction of the mucosa, fibrous thickening of the wall, and a more diffuse infiltration of lymphocytes. Rarely, lymphoid follicles with germinal centers are prominent ("cholecystitis lymphofollicularis"). Occasionally, calcium is deposited in the wall.

In some instances, there is proliferation of the mucosal epithelium with formation of glandlike spaces in the wall of the gallbladder ("cholecystitis glandularis"). The glandlike spaces may represent an increase in the number of epithelium-lined spaces that sometimes are seen in normal gallbladders. The most common type is formed by outpouchings of the mucosa or sinuses, which communicate with the lumen of the gallbladder (Aschoff-Rokitansky sinuses). They may become dilated to form diverticula or cysts, and sometimes calculi are formed within them. The lining epithelium is similar to that of the mucosa of the gallbladder or bowel. A second type of epithelium-lined space in the gallbladder is formed by aberrant bile ducts that communicate with intrahepatic ducts but not with the gallbladder (Luschka ducts). Their lining epi-

Table 16-1. Classification of gallstones

Type	Composition	Appearance	Factors in origin	Changes in gallbladder
Pure gallstones (10%)	Cholesterol (crystalline)	Solitary; crystalline surface	Increased cholesterol content in bile	Cholesterolosis
	Calcium bilirubinate	Multiple; jet black; crystalline or amorphous	Increased pigment content in bile	No change
	Calcium carbonate	Grayish white; amorphous	Unknown	No change
Mixed gallstones (80%)	Cholesterol and calcium bilirubinate	Multiple, faceted or lobulated, laminated, and crystalline on cut surfaces; hue depends on content: cholesterol, yellow; calcium bilirubinate, black; calcium carbonate, white	Chronic cholecystitis plus increased content in bile of cholesterol, calcium bilirubinate, or calcium carbonate	Chronic cholecystitis
	Cholesterol and calcium carbonate			
	Calcium bilirubinate and calcium carbonate			
	Cholesterol, calcium bilirubinate, and calcium carbonate			
Combined gallstones (10%)	Pure gallstone nucleus with mixed gallstone shell	Largest of gallstones, when single; hue depends on composition of shell	As in pure gallstones, followed by chronic cholecystitis	Chronic cholecystitis
	Mixed gallstone nucleus with pure gallstone shell		As in mixed gallstones, followed by increased content in bile of cholesterol, calcium bilirubinate, or calcium carbonate	Chronic cholecystitis

From Halpert, B.: Gallbladder and biliary ducts. In Anderson, W. A. D., and Kissane, J. M., editors: Pathology, ed. 7, St. Louis, 1977, The C. V. Mosby Co.

thelium is similar to that of the intrahepatic bile ducts. In addition to these epithelium-lined spaces, there may be subperitoneal glandlike spaces lined by flattened or cuboidal cells that are apparently of mesothelial origin.

In some instances, features of an acute cholecystitis may be superimposed on the chronic process.

CHOLESTEROLOSIS

In cholesterolosis (strawberry gallbladder), multiple, tiny, yellowish deposits of cholesterol are present in mucosal folds. These yellow areas on the reddish background of a congested mucosa suggest the appearance of a ripe strawberry. There is usually an associated increase of cholesterol in the bile.

Cholesterolosis is often of little significance, but it may be associated with chronic inflammation in the gallbladder wall. Pedunculated mucosal folds containing cholesterol sometimes are pinched off and form the nuclei of stones.

CHOLELITHIASIS

Important factors in the formation of gallstones are disturbances of cholesterol metabolism, infection, and stasis. The incidence increases with age, is greater in women than in men, and is greater in whites than in blacks. The stones may be in any part of the biliary tract, but they are most common in the gallbladder.

Types of gallstones. Three normal constituents of bile—cholesterol, calcium bilirubinate, and calcium carbonate—are the main substances composing gallstones. *Pure gallstones,* which constitute about 10%, are composed almost entirely of one of these substances. *Mixed gallstones,* which are the most frequent type and account for about 80%, contain a mixture of the three substances in varying proportions. *Combined gallstones* are those in which one type of gallstone forms the nucleus and another type forms the outer shell (Table 16-1).

Pure gallstones form when the bile contains an excess of the stone-forming substance, which usually is caused by disturbances of metabolism or of liver function rather than by a local inflammatory reaction. Cholesterol stones are the most frequent, calcium bilirubinate (pigment) stones are secondary in frequency, and calcium carbonate stones are the rarest of the pure gallstones.

The *cholesterol stone* is usually single. It is a crystalline calculus, light in weight and soft, and has a radiate structure evident on its cut surface. It occurs in the absence of infection and is probably of metabolic origin. The gallbladder may show cholesterolosis. The formation of a cholesterol stone appears to be influenced by a metabolic disturbance causing an increased cholesterol content of the bile. The solitary large cholesterol stone may give rise to few or no symptoms and is usually too large to enter and obstruct ducts. It is nonopaque to roentgen rays.

Calcium bilirubinate (pigment) stones are multiple, small, dark brown or black, hard, and brittle. Formed by precipitation of bile pigment in an uninfected gallbladder, they are associated with conditions having increased bilirubin concentration of the bile, such as hemolytic jaundice or pernicious anemia. Stasis favors their formation.

Calcium carbonate stones are rare, soft, white stones, usually formed only when there is complete obstruction of the cystic duct. Stasis may be a factor in deposition of bile pigment and calcium. The more complete the obstruction, the greater the proportion of calcium, which is deposited from the gallbladder wall.

Mixed gallstones are the most common variety (accounting for about 80%). They are composed of varying mixtures of cholesterol, calcium bilirubinate, calcium carbonate, and some organic material. They form in gallbladders in which function is altered, so that the solvents, bile acids, are resorbed faster than the stone-forming substances they hold in solution. The exact mechanism of their formation is uncertain. Chronic cholecystitis usually is associated, although how much this may be the cause or the effect often cannot be determined. The association with cholecystitis has led to the term *infective stones* for this type, although association with a specific bacterial infection is not usually evident.

Mixed stones are usually multiple and sometimes are present in huge numbers. They vary from 0.1 to 2 cm in diameter, are often hard, rough-surfaced stones, and are of varying color and structure according to their composition. Adjacent surfaces may be faceted. They often seem to be composed of concentric laminae laid down over a small nucleus. Some have a lobulated surface with the contour of a mulberry. The mulberry stones appear to form around polypoid projections of the mucosa that contain lipoidal material and when small may remain attached to the mucosa.

Combined gallstones constitute about 10% of gallstones. They occur most often as a solitary stone with a cholesterol nucleus and an outer shell similar to a mixed gallstone. Less often, the nucleus is a mixed stone, and the outer shell is of cholesterol or calcium bilirubinate. The gallbladder containing combined gallstones usually shows chronic cholecystitis.

Effects of gallstones. Biliary calculi do not of themselves produce symptoms, but they may produce injury in three ways:

1 Their presence may induce inflammation (acute or chronic cholecystitis).
2 The chronic irritation of calculi may be a factor in the development of carcinoma of the gallbladder.
3 Stones may cause obstruction at the neck of the gallbladder or in the bile ducts.

The effects of obstruction of bile passages depend on the site and completeness of the obstruction. Large stones such as the solitary cholesterol calculus are often too large to get into bile ducts, although they may obstruct the neck of the gallbladder. Passage of a small calculus, distending biliary ducts, elicits the severe pain of biliary colic.

Complete obstruction of the neck of the gallbladder or the cystic duct leads to hydrops or mucocele of the gallbladder, in which condition the pigmented bile has been absorbed and replaced by a mucoid secretion from the lining of the gallbladder. In some instances, empyema of the gallbladder may develop following bacterial invasion. Obstruction by a stone in the common duct results in only a lit-

tle distention of the gallbladder if the wall has been thickened by inflammation, although bile passages themselves are usually visibly dilated above the obstruction. *Courvoisier's law* states that obstruction of the common bile duct by pressure from the outside, as by a carcinoma of the pancreas, produces a distended gallbladder, whereas obstruction by a stone produces little or no distention of the gallbladder. The usual explanation is that in the latter instance, the gallbladder wall is thickened and contracted as a result of inflammation.

If biliary obstruction is present for a considerable time, the bilirubin excretory function of the liver may become suppressed, and a watery or mucoid fluid, the so-called white bile, is found in bile ducts. Other complications include ascending cholangitis and biliary cirrhosis of the liver.

The pancreas may be affected when a stone is impacted in the ampulla of Vater, which acts as a common opening of pancreatic and bile ducts. In such a case, reflux of irritating bile into the pancreatic duct may give rise to acute pancreatitis (p. 464).

In rare cases, perforation of a gallbladder into a viscus may release a gallstone, which produces intestinal obstruction (gallstone ileus). Inflammatory reaction and adhesions after perforation of the gallbladder also may result in obstruction of the bowel.

CARCINOMA

The only important tumor of the gallbladder is carcinoma. About 75% of cases occur in women, commonly between 50 and 70 years of age. From 65% to 90% of carcinomas of the gallbladder are associated with calculi, which often are thought to have some causative role, probably by mechanical irritation. Among patients in whom gallstones are present at necropsy, about 3% have a carcinoma of the gallbladder. Papillomas and adenomas of the gallbladder occur, but it is uncertain how frequently these precede development of carcinoma. Many so-called papillomas appear to be nonneoplastic cholesterol polyps, and most lesions appearing as polyps by cholecystography are not true adenomas.

Cancer of the gallbladder is an adenocarcinoma in more than 90% of cases but occasionally is of squamous or mixed cell type. Adenocarcinoma may be subdivided into infiltrating scirrhous, papillary, and mucous types.

The *infiltrating scirrhous type* is most common (65%). It forms a firm tumor that spreads widely through the gallbladder wall, causing it to be greatly thickened. The lumen is narrowed and eventually obliterated. Microscopically, it is an infiltrating adenocarcinoma, often with abundant dense fibrous stroma.

The *papillary adenocarcinoma* (22%) forms a friable fungating tumor that grows into the lumen of the gallbladder (Fig. 16-17). Micro-

scopically, it presents stalks of connective tissue stroma covered by atypical columnar epithelium and infiltrated by glandular acini. The papillary type is less malignant and slower in its growth and spread than is the infiltrating adenocarcinomatous variety.

The *mucoid adenocarcinoma* (7%) forms a bulky gelatinous mass in which the tumor cells are distended with mucoid material and may have a signet-ring form.

Squamous cell carcinoma (4%) of the gallbladder is a variety assumed to arise on the basis of metaplasia of the epithelial lining.

Spread of cancer of the gallbladder is usually by direct extension to the liver and metas-

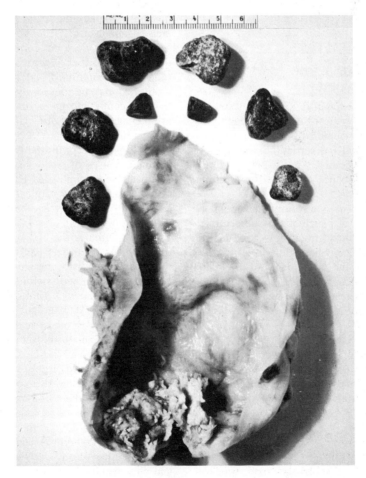

Fig. 16-17. Carcinoma of gallbladder. Papillary adenocarcinoma of fundus and cholelithiasis.

tasis to regional lymph nodes. Further spread may occur by lymphatic and bloodstream metastasis.

Carcinoma may arise in the extrahepatic bile ducts, but much less frequently than in the gallbladder. It occurs usually in the sixth or seventh decade and is slightly more common in men than in women. The cancer, with few exceptions, is adenocarcinoma, and it is commonly associated with extensive fibrosis, often causing thickening of the ducts with subsequent obstruction. Carcinoma in the region of the ampulla of Vater (i.e., the vaterian system) may originate from the common bile duct in some instances. Others may arise from the pancreatic duct or duodenal mucosa.

Pancreas

HETEROTOPIA AND MALFORMATIONS

Heterotopic pancreatic tissue is found at about 14% of autopsies. Such misplaced tissue occurs in the duodenum (80%), stomach, jejunum, or Meckel's diverticulum. It is most commonly asymptomatic, but it may give rise to digestive disturbance or be the site of tumor growth.

Annular pancreas is a rare maldevelopment in which a band of pancreatic tissue encircles and may narrow or obstruct the second part of the duodenum. The pancreatic tissue often intermingles with the muscularis of the duodenum, so that simple resection or division of the ring of pancreatic tissue may be insufficient.

FATTY INFILTRATION

Fatty infiltration of the pancreas is quite common in obesity and may be of severe degree (lipomatous pseudohypertrophy). A minor amount of fatty replacement of atrophic pancreatic tissue is common.

ACUTE PANCREATITIS

Acute pancreatitis is characterized by edema, necrosis, hemorrhage, and suppuration in varying degrees of predominance. The effects are caused by the escape of active lytic pancreatic enzymes, which act on the parenchyma of the gland, blood vessels, and fatty tissue. The condition appears to be brought about by increased pancreatic secretion with partial or complete obstruction of outflow and raised intraductal pressure. It may occur suddenly with severe abdominal pain. If extensive, it may be accompanied by peripheral vascular collapse or shock, and it frequently is fatal. Occurring almost entirely in adult life, it is more common after 40 years of age, and 60% of the cases are in women.

Acute pancreatitis is accompanied by leukocytosis, increased serum amylase in early stages (although it may later return to normal), increased serum lipase, and increased amylase in the urine. The increase of serum amylase does not correlate reliably with the severity of the pancreatitis. Hypocalcemia (due to precipitation of calcium in foci of necrotic fat) may be present in severe cases, and hyperglycemia and glycosuria (due to secondary damage to islets) are found in a small proportion of cases.

Etiology and pathogenesis. Two of the common causes of acute pancreatitis are cholelithiasis and alcoholism. The lesion may also occur as a result of surgical trauma (particularly involving pancreas, biliary tract, stomach, or duodenum) and less frequently after external trauma to the abdomen. A number of other causes have been considered, including hyperparathyroidism, certain drugs (e.g., opiates, thiazides, and steroids), vascular disease, and infections. Although the characteristic destructive damage and reaction in acute pancreatitis are brought about by release of pancreatic enzymes, the mechanism has been a matter of theory and debate. A variety of factors may be responsible and have variable relative importance in different cases.

According to the "common channel" theory, derived from a case described by Opie, an obstruction of the common opening into the duodenum of the biliary and pancreatic ducts causes a reflux of bile into the pancreatic duct, and this results in activation and release of pancreatic enzymes. However, some investigators do not accept the view that reflux of bile is the important factor, although it may occur in some instances. Instead, it is suggested that increased pressure within the pancreatic duct, with rupture and release of enzymes, is the pathogenetic mechanism in acute pancreatitis. The increased intraductal pressure may be brought about by two factors that often act in combination: (1) obstruction of the pancreatic duct caused by a stone or ductal lesion, by spasm of the sphincter of Oddi, or by edema of the duodenal mucosa and papilla of Vater due to surgical trauma or irritants such as alcohol, drugs, or hydrochloric acid, and (2) increased secretion into the pancreatic duct induced by various stimuli, including a heavy meal, alcohol, certain drugs, or the presence of hydrochloric acid in the duodenum.

Another opinion is that reflux of bile-free duodenal secretions is important in the pathogenesis of acute pancreatitis. The lesion has been induced experimentally in animals by creating a closed duodenal loop with the common bile duct ligated, and it was prevented by ligation of the pancreatic duct. Furthermore, intraductal administration of enterokinase (EK), a component of duodenal secretions, has produced acute hemorrhagic pancreatitis in animals. EK converts trypsinogen to trypsin, which in turn may activate other proteolytic enzymes.

Infection, when it occurs, appears to be a later or secondary complication rather than a primary cause of the pancreatic necrosis. However, various bacterial and viral infections may cause pancreatitis of a different nature, as in the case of scarlet fever, typhoid fever, mumps, and coxsackievirus infection. Vascular disease also may cause focal areas of pancreatitis with necrosis. Pancreatic vessels occasionally are involved in the severe arteriolar degeneration and necrosis of malignant hypertension, but a resulting pancreatic necrosis is usually small and overshadowed by the severe renal involvement.

The possibility that nutritional factors may play a role in the development of acute pancreatitis is suggested by experiments on mice in which a choline-deficient diet together with ethionine, which is known to exert a toxic effect on the pancreatic acini as well as on the liver in experimental animals, seemed to potentiate the action of ethionine and caused severe acute hemorrhagic pancreatitis. It is not certain whether nutritional deficiency is a factor in the production of pancreatitis in alcoholics. Terminal acute pancreatitis is an occasionaly incidental finding at autopsy in a variety of conditions, but especially with circulatory failure. More rarely, acute pancreatic necrosis is found as a cause of sudden death, particularly in alcoholics.

Pathologic appearance. The pancreas is enlarged and firm with softer friable areas of necrosis. Various degrees of hemorrhagic and gangrenous changes may involve portions of or the entire pancreas. The gangrenous changes progress rapidly after death. Areas of fat necrosis affect the fat of the pancreas (Fig. 16-18), mesentery, and omentum. These appear as firm, dry, opaque yellow or gray nodules (Fig. 16-19). The necrotic areas of fatty tissue may contain calcium deposits and are surrounded by a zone of hyperemia and leukocytes. Rarely, disseminated foci of fat necrosis occur (e.g., in the skin, pleura, mediastinum, and bone marrow), presumably as a result of liberation of lipolytic enzymes into the lymphatics or bloodstream.

The pancreatic tissue is edematous but is infiltrated by relatively few leukocytes. Blood vessels may have necrosis of their walls and thrombi in their lumina. Inspissated secretion may be found in pancreatic ducts, and metaplasia of duct epithelium with associated acinar dilatation is present in about 50% of the cases. Complications include the development of multiple suppurative abscesses or sinus tracts and pseudocysts. The peritoneal cavity may contain a turbid yellowish or brownish fluid in which globules of fat and an increased concentration of amylase may be present. Pancreatic abscesses complicating pancreatitis, if untreated, can lead to serious consequences and frequently are fatal.

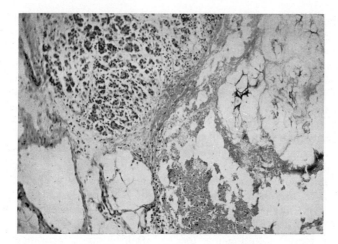

Fig. 16-18. Fat necrosis of pancreas.

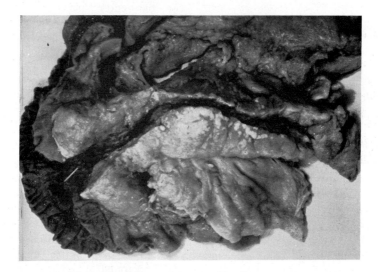

Fig. 16-19. Fat necrosis and acute pancreatitis. White opaque areas represent fat necrosis. Small white rod is in duct opening into duodenum.

CHRONIC (RELAPSING) PANCREATITIS

Chronic pancreatitis is essentially a relapsing pancreatitis resulting from repeated attacks of acute pancreatitis. Frequently, the recurrent episodes are mild and may be undiagnosed clinically. Chronic pancreatitis is manifested by perilobular and interacinar fibrosis, often with increased firmness of the organ. A variable degree of acinar and islet atrophy may be present. The latter type may be associated with diabetes. Dilatation of acini with appearance of a central space or channel suggests some duct obstruction, as does the presence of inspissated material in the lumina of ducts. Dilatation of ducts, hyperplasia of duct epithelium, and lymphocytic infiltration also may be present. Precipitation of calcium salts, mainly calcium carbonate, in pancreatic ducts may form single or multiple calculi. As with acute pancreatitis, there is frequent association with alcoholism or biliary tract disease.

There appears to be a definite relationship of pancreatic fibrosis and insufficiency to the development of fatty change and cirrhosis in the liver, and both commonly are associated with chronic alcoholism.

CYSTS

True cysts in the pancreas may be congenital or caused by duct obstruction. Pseudocysts, which do not have an epithelial lining, result from pancreatitis with degeneration and softening of tissue or from hematomas. Some pancreatic tumors are cystic.

Dilatation of pancreatic acini with inspissation of secretion is seen quite commonly in adults in association with uremia, gastric cancer, small intestinal obstruction, and ulcerative colitis. The genesis and significance of the lesion are unknown.

CYSTIC FIBROSIS

This inherited genetic disorder, which is characterized by an abnormality of secretion by exocrine glands in various organs, including the pancreas, is discussed on p. 17.

DIABETES MELLITUS

Diabetes mellitus is a disease caused by an absolute or relative deficiency of the hormone insulin, which is produced by the islets of Langerhans of the pancreas. This, in turn, gives rise to a disturbance in carbohydrate metabolism, with inability to store glycogen in the liver, excessive accumulation of glucose in the blood (hyperglycemia), and excretion of the excessive sugar in the urine (glycosuria). Fat metabolism also is upset. The fats cannot be completely oxidized, ketone bodies accumulate, and acidosis results. In addition, there is disturbance in protein metabolism. Clinical features are excessive appetite, thirst, and urination.

In a few instances, a demonstrable cause for diabetes exists, e.g., destruction of pancreatic islets by inflammation (acute or chronic pancreatitis) or carcinoma, surgical extirpation of the pancreas, and endocrine disorders (such as Cushing's syndrome or acromegaly). Hemochromatosis may be associated with diabetes, the latter being caused apparently by deposits of iron in the pancreatic islets, although some investigators do not believe that the presence of iron is responsible for the development of the diabetic state. Experimentally, diabetes may be induced in animals by the administration of alloxan, which causes selective necrosis of the beta cells in the islets of Langerhans. Also, pancreatic changes associated with diabeteslike manifestations have been induced by certain viruses in experimental animals. This is of interest in view of the suggestion by some epidemiologists that there is a link between viral infections and the onset of diabetes in human subjects, particularly juvenile-onset diabetes.

In the vast majority of patients, there is no recognizable cause of the disease, but it is generally agreed that heredity plays a major role in the etiology. The mode of inheritance, however, has not been definitely settled. Various precipitating factors may unmask diabetes or aggravate it if it is already manifest, e.g., obesity, stressful situations (such as infection or surgical trauma), and hyperfunction of the thyroid gland, pituitary gland, or adrenal glands. Two distinct clinical types are juvenile diabetes, which has a relatively acute onset, usually before the age of 15 years, and maturity-onset diabetes, which develops gradually and usually after 40 years of age. The typical juvenile diabetic has a low insulin reserve in the pancreas and is more difficult to control, requiring insulin therapy (insulin-dependent diabetes). The mature-onset diabetic usually has a relatively normal insulin reserve in the pancreas, so that diet or use of oral drugs to stimulate release of insulin may control the disease (insulin-independent diabetes). A significant association between the histocompatibility antigens HLA-B8 and Bw15 and juvenile (insulin-dependent) diabetes was reported previously, and more recently a strong association of the disease with the antigens Dw3 and Dw4 has been established. The inherited susceptibility to juvenile diabetes is believed to be related in some way to the HLA antigens. Some evidence suggests that autoimmune factors directed against the pancreatic islets may exist in the juvenile diabetic. The view that viruses may sometimes be a cause of juvenile diabetes was strengthened by the recent report of isolation of a virus from the pancreas of a child who died of diabetic ketoacidosis. It was then shown that this virus could produce diabetes in mice.

In addition to the fully manifest disease (*overt* or *clinical diabetes*), there is a state characterized by an abnormal glucose tolerance, without signs or symptoms of the disease *(chemical diabetes)*. Also, it is now established that there is a *prediabetic state* that eventually may progress to chemical or overt diabetes. Although prediabetics have no demonstrable abnormalities of carbohydrate metabolism, there may be evidence of structural change in the small vessels (microangiopathy) as seen in biopsies of various tissues (p. 471). The person who is suspected of being a prediabetic is one whose mother and father have diabetes, one who has an identical twin with diabetes, or a woman who has a tendency to have large babies and/or to have frequent complications during pregnancies.

The anatomic changes in diabetes mellitus to be considered are the lesions in the pancreas and the lesions in other organs, some of which result from the disturbed metabolism.

Lesions in pancreas

Pathologic changes in the pancreas in diabetes mellitus are concerned with the islets of Langerhans. In about 20% of the cases, no anatomic pancreatic change is demonstrable by the usual histologic methods. Frequently, the changes in the islets are slight and cannot be closely correlated with the clinical severity of the disease.

Gross changes in the pancreas in diabetes are uncommon. Occasionally, the pancreas may be small, under 35 g. Gross fibrosis may be related, but lipomatosis is not significant. Pancreatic lithiasis may or may not be associated with diabetes. In hemochromatosis associated with diabetes, the pancreas is a rusty brown color because of the deposition of hemosiderin. If more than five sixths of the pancreas has been destroyed by other disease processes, such as carcinoma or pancreatitis, diabetes may be produced. However, the bulk of the islets of Langerhans is situated in the tail of the pancreas, and consequently extensive destruction of other portions of the gland will do relatively little harm to them. Since the islets have a structure and blood supply independent of the acini, there is frequently little disturbance of the islets even in advanced involvement of the pancreas by carcinoma or other destructive processes.

The islets comprise 1% to 3% of the weight of the pancreas. There is a wide range of normal variation in the numbers of islets, with estimates ranging from 750,000 to 3,750,000. Sometimes there is a distinct quantitative reduction. It is possible that this quantitative variation may be a factor in hereditary aspects of diabetes.

Histologically, three different types of cells can be identified within the islets: alpha cells, beta cells, and delta (undifferentiated) cells. The beta cells, which are the insulin-producing cells, constitute 60% to 70% of islet cells. They can be specifically stained with aldehyde fuchsin, which gives a purple color to the secretory granules. The alpha cells, which constitute 20% to 30% of islet cells, and the delta cells, 2% to 8%, also can be differentially stained. With fluorescent antibody techniques, it has been demonstrated that beta cells contain insulin and alpha cells contain glucagon. The exact role of the delta cells is not certain, but there is evidence suggesting that they contain both gastrin and somatostatin.

By electron microscopy, the alpha, beta, and delta cells can be differentiated on the basis of their ultrastructure. The secretory granules of the *alpha* cells appear as round, highly electron-dense structures separated from the limiting membrane by a halo. The secretory granules of *beta* cells, by contrast, show great variation in ultrastructure within a single cell and may appear round but often are angular with a crystallinelike structure of the core, and they are surrounded by smooth membranous sacs. In the *delta* cell, the secretory granules appear smudged and less dense, with close approximation of the limiting membrane to the core.

Electron microscopic studies on beta cell granules show their formation in the ergastoplasm, appearing first as an amorphous substance between the two membranous components of the lamellar ergastoplasm and subsequently within sacs that pinch off from the ergastoplasm. Ribonucleoprotein granules attached to the outer surface of the ergastoplasmic sacs disappear, and the beta granule condenses into a dense structure surrounded by a smooth membranous sac. When the beta cell is stimulated to secrete insulin, the granules within their encasing sacs move to the surface of the cell, where the membranous sac fuses with the plasma membrane. It then ruptures, and the granule is liberated into the extracellular space, where it undergoes dissolution. This mechanism of secretion is called emiocytosis. Before the insulin of the liberated granules can enter the bloodstream, it must traverse a basement membrane associated with the beta cell, a space, and finally the capillary endothelium. Theoretically, blockage or impairment of the rate of transfer through any one of these steps in insulin secretion could result in production of a diabetic state.

Pathology of islets. Distinct differences occur in the pathologic changes in classic juvenile diabetes and maturity-onset diabetes. In the juvenile diabetic patient, the number of islets is usually reduced. Degranulation of beta cells and fibrosis of the islets may be present, and, in occasional instances, lymphocytic infiltration is observed. In the maturity-onset diabetic patient, the number of islets is usually normal, the degree of beta granulation may be normal or moderately reduced, and hyaline deposition may be observed within the islets.

In approximately 20% of patients with maturity-onset diabetes, no distinct pathologic changes can be found in the islets.

Amyloidosis is the most common change observed in the islets of patients with maturity-onset diabetes. The amyloid deposits, formerly referred to as "hyalinization" of the islets, appear as an eosinophilic amorphous material deposited around the capillaries of the islets, compressing and displacing the islet cells. By electron microscopy, the hyaline material appears as a fibrillar protein interposed between the basement membrane of the capillary and the basement membrane of the islet cells, similar to amyloid in other situations. The amyloid encases the sinusoids, rarely occluding them, but it ultimately replaces nearly all the epithelial cells of the islets. Sometimes the peripheral cells of the islets attempt to proliferate and the hyaline masses continue to encroach upon the new cells, so that masses of hyaline material much larger than the original islet may be produced (Fig. 16-20). In 97% of cases with amyloidosis of the islets, the patients are over 40 years of age. A similar deposition in the islets is also seen, to a minor degree, in about 2% of nondiabetic persons over the age of 40 years.

Vacuolization (glycogenosis) of beta cells occasionally is seen in untreated, inadequately treated, or comatose diabetic patients. In patients adequately treated with insulin, it is almost never seen. The cytoplasm of the beta cells first becomes vacuolated and later disappears, leaving nuclei and cell membrane alone visible. This change was formerly referred to as "hydropic degeneration," but histochemical studies show that the vacuoles contain glycogen. Electron microscopic studies show that the glycogen accumulates first as small focal masses within the cytoplasm of the beta cell and that, as the hyperglycemic state becomes more severe, the masses increase in size and displace the normal intracellular organelles. Since insulin is formed within the ergastoplasm, obviously the accumulations of glycogen would interfere with insulin synthesis, thus resulting in a further increase in the severity of the diabetic state. Glycogen accumu-

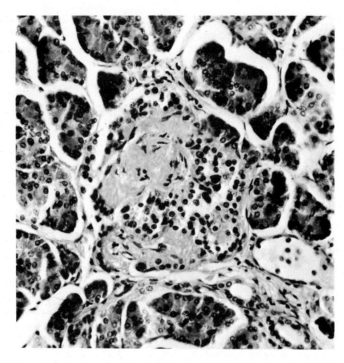

Fig. 16-20. Amyloidosis (so-called hyalinization) of islet of pancreas in diabetes mellitus.

lation in the beta cell is a reversible change and is removed after treatment with insulin and return of the blood sugar level to normal.

Lymphocytic infiltration of the islets may be observed in juvenile diabetic patients. It is particularly evident in those patients who come to autopsy within days or weeks after the onset of diabetes. Its significance is unknown. In involved islets, there may be complete or extensive disappearance of epithelial cells, with scattered lymphocytes replacing them. Some investigators have considered that lymphocytic infiltration may be a transient lesion in the interval between necrosis in the islets and the development of fibrosis. An immunologic (possibly autoimmune) mechanism has been suggested as an explanation for the lymphocytic infiltration. A similar infiltration of islets has been observed in cattle and rabbits receiving repeated administrations of beef insulin. A viral cause for the islet cell damage and lymphocytic infiltration has also been considered.

Fibrosis of islets may develop after "hy-dropic degeneration" or necrosis of the insular epithelium as well as after lymphocytic infiltration. It varies from a slight change to an almost complete replacement of the islet by dense collagen. Even in advanced examples, there is little extension of fibrosis into adjacent acinar tissue. Fibrosis may occur either alone or in combination with other types of pancreatic lesions, such as chronic pancreatitis.

Eosinophilic infiltration sometimes may be observed in and around the islets in children of diabetic mothers and invariably is associated with *islet hypertrophy* and *hyperplasia*. These changes are diagnostic of diabetes mellitus in the mother. That the infiltration of eosinophils in the islets of these infants may represent an antigen-antibody response is suggested by the observation of a similar change in the islets of rats injected with anti-insulin serum.

Hemosiderin may accumulate within beta cells of the islets as well as within acinar cells in *hemochromatosis*. Alpha cells do not contain hemosiderin but tend to be reduced in number. Atrophy of acinar cells and interstitial fibrosis are usually present.

Infants born of diabetic mothers are large and often stillborn and may show severe hypertrophy of their pancreatic islets. It appears that infants born of women with a latent diabetic tendency but without clinical diabetes may sometimes show similar effects.

Lesions in other organs

Lesions occur in organs other than the pancreas, some of which depend on the disturbed metabolism, e.g., changes in the distribution and amount of glycogen in certain tissues. Such changes will not be present in patients in whom the metabolic disturbance is controlled by adequate treatment. Glycogen may be demonstrated in tissues by prompt fixation in alcohol followed by staining with Best's carmine. The glycogen appears as a bright red intracellular material.

The kidney contains excessive glycogen in the epithelium of the terminal straight portions of the proximal convoluted tubules and sometimes the contiguous thin limbs of Henle's loops so that the cells have a water-clear cytoplasm or hydropic appearance (Armanni-Ebstein lesion). This change may be associated with glycosuria from any cause. Nodular glomerulosclerosis (Kimmelstiel-Wilson lesion) is a specific renal lesion frequently associated with diabetes mellitus (p. 351). Diffuse glomerulosclerosis also occurs. Pyelonephritis is another common lesion in diabetes and may be complicated by papillary necrosis (p. 357).

The liver has decreased glycogen storage within the cytoplasm of the liver cells, although the nuclei of the liver cells may have increased glycogen content and appear clear and glassy. The skin, voluntary muscle, and heart also may show some changes in glycogen content.

Vascular lesions involving small blood vessels (diabetic microangiopathy) are widespread in diabetes mellitus. The changes include thickening of basement membranes and accumulation of material resembling basement membrane in the walls of capillaries and arte-rioles. An increase in thickness of the basement membrane of capillaries in biopsies of skeletal muscle, skin, and kidneys has been demonstrated in prediabetic individuals.

Atherosclerotic lesions of medium-sized and larger arteries also are likely to develop in diabetic patients at an earlier age and with enhanced severity. Two important sites of involvement are the coronary arteries, which may result in myocardial infarction, and the vessels of the legs, which subsequently may cause gangrene of the toes. The small-vessel lesions, described previously, may play a role in the vascular insufficiency leading to gangrene.

Peripheral neuropathy tends to occur in older diabetic patients. Areas of demyelination are observed in the peripheral nerves. The lesion may be caused by ischemia resulting from involvement of the small vessels supplying the nerves (the vasa nervorum), or the disturbed carbohydrate metabolism in these patients may have a direct effect on the nerves, causing the degenerative changes.

Proliferative retinopathy appears to be a specific diabetic lesion and is found particularly in patients with severe diabetes of long duration (average, about 17 years). Retinal neovascularization and microaneurysms of capillaries are the characteristic changes. Blindness results in about 25% of cases. There is frequent association of diabetic retinopathy and diabetic renal lesions. Cataracts also may be a complication of diabetes.

Lesions of the skin, in addition to diabetic microangiopathy, include xanthoma diabeticorum, necrobiosis lipoidica, pruritus vulvae, and skin infections.

TUMORS

Primary tumors of the pancreas may be carcinoma arising from ductal or acinar tissue, cystadenoma, or tumors arising from cells of the islets of Langerhans.

Cystadenomas of the pancreas are uncommon. They occur mainly in women, in middle age periods, and most often in the tail of the pancreas. They are rounded, coarsely lobulated cystic tumors (Fig. 16-21) that grow

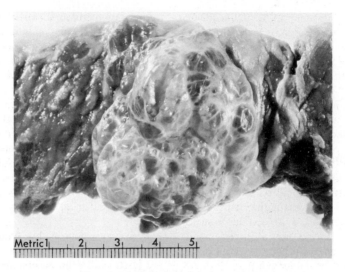

Fig. 16-21. Cystadenoma of pancreas.

slowly and by expansion. The cystic spaces are lined by flattened or cuboidal epithelium, occasionally with papillary infolding. A malignant counterpart, cystadenocarcinoma, also occurs.

Carcinoma. Pancreatic carcinoma occurs more often in men than in women, most frequently in the sixth and seventh decades. It is increasing in frequency and represents the fourth leading cause of cancer deaths in men in the United States. The majority of the carcinomas arise in the head of the pancreas, where early in their course they cause obstruction of the common bile duct. The obstruction produces dilatation of the bile ducts and gallbladder and clinically gives rise to ever-deepening jaundice, often with pain. Spread to neighboring tissue and by metastasis is a late feature. In the less common tumors arising in the body or tail, earlier and more widespread extension and metastasis result in a greater variety of clinical symptoms, and multiple and sometimes widespread venous thrombosis (Trousseau's syndrome) is a frequent complication. A large proportion metastasize to the lung and thoracic lymph nodes and may lead to mistaken diagnosis of primary lung cancer. The prognosis of pancreatic carcinoma is

poor—the 5-year survival rate is less than 2%. In the untreated cases, death usually occurs within a year after the diagnosis is made.

The tumor forms a hard nodular mass within the pancreatic tissue, often fibrous or scirrhous in character, and it is difficult to distinguish grossly from chronic pancreatitis. Microscopically, it may be a cylindrical cell adenocarcinoma originating from the pancreatic duct system or, less frequently, an acinar cell type resembling the parenchyma of the pancreas.

Islet cell tumor. Tumors composed of islet cell tissue occasionally occur in the pancreas, most frequently in the body and tail of the organ. They are usually small, less than 2 cm in diameter, and only rare examples have measured up to 6 cm in diameter. They usually appear well circumscribed, and some have a fibrous capsule. Their increased consistency may make them palpable, and their homogeneous color in contrast with the surrounding lobulated yellowish pancreatic tissue may make them visible. About 80% are single, and about 90% are benign. The majority are insulin-producing (beta cell) tumors. Others are of the nonbeta cell type.

The benign insulin-producing islet cell adenomas *(insulinomas* or *nesidioblastomas)* usually are circumscribed or encapsulated. In some cases, there seems to be microscopic evidence of invasion, but no metastases are present, and there is a clinically benign course. The carcinomas of islet tissue tend to be larger and more infiltrative, but metastasis is often the only good evidence of malignancy. Some metastasizing islet cell carcinomas are well differentiated microscopically.

Microscopically, the insulin-producing islet cell tumors usually are composed of well-differentiated tissue, often with the characteristics and architecture of normal islet tissue, and appear simply as a gigantic islet. The cells, which often seem comparable to beta cells of normal islets, tend to occur in ribbons or cords, with only occasional solid masses or glandular structures. Degenerative changes such as fibrosis, hyalinization, or calcification may be present. The appearance may simulate that of carcinoid tumors or some bronchial adenomas. It is probable that these tumors may arise from ductal tissue as well as from preexisting islet tissue.

Functioning islet cell tumors may give rise to episodes of severe hypoglycemia, often precipitated by fasting or exercise. Nervous system manifestations and even loss of consciousness may occur. The attacks are relieved by the administration of glucose. Multiple petechial hemorrhages and acute degeneration of nerve cells and astrocytes have been described in the central nervous system. The severity of the clinical episodes does not correlate with the size of the islet cell tumor.

Nonbeta islet cell tumors are sometimes associated with gastric hypersecretion and the development of severe and intractable or recurrent peptic ulcers *(Zollinger-Ellison syndrome)*. The ulcers may be atypically located, characteristically resist therapy, and frequently are fatal. Diarrhea and malabsorption occur in some patients, sometimes as the predominant manifestations.

The type of islet cell in the ulcerogenic syndrome has not been definitely settled. In some investigations the neoplastic cells were said to be similar to delta cells. This view is supported by a study of normal pancreatic islets, using an immunofluorescent method, in which gastrin was identified in delta cells. However, in other reports the islet cells of ulcerogenic tumors were described with features resembling alpha cells.

The *ulcerogenic tumors* are sometimes multiple and often malignant. A gastrinlike hormone has been demonstrated in these tumors. Multiple adenomas involving the pituitary, adrenal, and parathyroid glands, as well as the pancreatic islets, sometimes are found in this syndrome. Recently, there have been reports of occasional instances of the Zollinger-Ellison syndrome occurring in association with tumors or hyperplasias of endocrine cells in the stomach or duodenum.

Nonbeta islet cell tumors of the pancreas may be associated with another syndrome characterized by profuse watery diarrhea, hypokalemia, and achlorhydria without gastric hypersecretion or peptic ulceration *(diarrheogenic tumors)*. There is evidence that a secretinlike hormone is responsible for the diarrheal syndrome. The islet cell type in the neoplasms has not been clearly identified. Hypercalcemia is seen in many of the patients, and some investigators believe it may be due to elaboration of parathormone stimulated by low serum magnesium, although parathormonelike secretion from the neoplastic islet cells is a possibility.

An uncommon nonbeta islet cell tumor, consisting of alpha cells, that contains glucagon has been described *(glucagonoma)*. Hyperglycemia occurs with this tumor. Another nonbeta islet cell tumor that may be associated with hyperglycemia contains somatostatin *(somatostatinoma)*. The cells in this tumor resemble delta cells.

In one study, multiple hormones (ACTH, MSH, and gastrin) were found in a single ulcerogenic tumor. Other substances (e.g., serotonin and dopamine) have been identified in islet cell tumors.

REFERENCES

Adam, Y. G., et al.: Ann. Surg. **175**:375-383, 1972 (malignant vascular tumors of liver).

Ahmed, M. N., et al.: Arch. Pathol. **92:**66-72, 1971 (Australia antigen and hepatitis).

Alpert, M. E., and Davidson, C. S.: Am. J. Med. **46:**325-329, 1969 (mycotoxins and hepatic carcinoma).

Al-Sarraf, M., et al.: Cancer **33:**574-582, 1974 (primary liver cancer).

Bagheri, S. A., and Boyer, J. L.: Ann. Intern. Med. **81:**610-618, 1974 (peliosis hepatis and steroid therapy).

Baker, H. de C., et al.: J. Pathol. Bacteriol. **72:**173-182, 1956 (Kupffer cell sarcoma).

Bearn, A. G.: Am. J. Med. **22:**747-757, 1957 (Wilson's disease).

Becker, F. F.: Am. J. Pathol. **74:**179-210, 1974 (hepatoma—a review).

Bergs, V. V., and Scotti, T. M.: Science **158:**377-378, 1967 (peliosis hepatis).

Bhagavan, B. S., et al.: Arch. Pathol. **98:**217-222, 1974 (Zollinger-Ellison syndrome associated with endocrine tumorlets or hyperplasias in gastric antrum).

Bianchi, L., et al.: Lancet **1:**333-337, 1971 (morphologic criteria in viral hepatitis).

Bigelow, N. H., and Wright, A. W.: Cancer **6:**170-178, 1953 (hepatic tumors in children).

Bismuth, H., and Malt, R. A.: N. Engl J. Med. **301:**704-706, 1979 (carcinoma of biliary tract).

Bordi, C.: Arch. Pathol. **98:**274-278, 1974 (Zollinger-Ellison syndrome associated with endocrine cell proliferation in nonantral gastric mucosa).

Boyer, J. L., and Klatskin, G.: N. Engl. J. Med. **283:**1063-1071, 1970 (subacute hepatic necrosis in viral hepatitis).

Brown, C. H., and Crile, G., Jr.: J.A.M.A. **109:**30-34, 1964 (pancreatic adenoma with diarrhea and hypokalemia).

Brown, J., and Straatsma, B. R. (moderators): Ann. Intern. Med. **68:**634-661, 1968 (diabetes mellitus).

Cameron, R., and Heu, P. C.: Biliary cirrhosis, Springfield, Ill., 1962, Charles C Thomas, Publisher.

Cano, R. I. et al.: J.A.M.A. **231:**159-161, 1975 (acute fatty liver in pregnancy with DIC).

Cegrell, L.: Acta Pathol. Microbiol. Scand. (A) **78:**734, 1970 (dopamine in islet cell tumor).

Chang, L. W., et al.: Arch. Pathol. **96:**127-132, 1973 (Reye's syndrome—electron microscopy).

Craighead, J. E.: N. Engl. J. Med. **299:**1439-1445, 1978 (etiology of insulin-dependent diabetes mellitus).

Crocker, J. F. S., et al.: Lancet **2:**22-24, 1974 (fatty viscera and encephalopathy—insecticide and viral interaction).

Cubilla, A. L., and Hajdu, S. I.: Arch. Pathol. **99:**204-207, 1975 (islet cell carcinoma of the pancreas).

Cudworth, A. G., and Woodrow, J. C.: Br. Med. J. **3:**133-135, 1975 (HLA-linked genes in juvenile diabetes).

Cunningham, J. A., and Hardenbergh, F. E.: Arch. Intern. Med. **97:**68-72, 1956 (incidence of gallstones).

Dowdy, G. S., Jr.: The biliary tract, Philadelphia, 1969, Lea & Febiger.

Dubin, I. N.: Am. J. Med. **24:**268-292, 1958 (chronic idiopathic jaundice).

Dubin, I. N., and Johnson, F. B.: Medicine (Baltimore) **33:**155-197, 1954 (chronic idiopathic jaundice).

Editorial: Lancet **2:**1481, 1973 (liver tumors and steroid hormones).

Edmondson, H. A.: Tumors of the liver and intrahepatic bile ducts. In Atlas of tumor pathology, Sect. VII, Fasc. 25, Washington, D.C., 1958, Armed Forces Institute of Pathology.

Edmondson, H. A., and Peters, R. L.: In Anderson, W. A. D., and Kissane, J. M., editors: Pathology, ed. 7, St. Louis, 1977, The C. V. Mosby Co. (liver diseases).

Edmondson, H. A., et al.: Am. J. Pathol. **25:**1227-1247, 1949 (pancreatitis).

Edmondson, H. A., et al.: Am. J. Pathol. **26:**37-55, 1950 (pancreatitis).

Gambill, E. E., editor: Pancreatitis, St. Louis, 1973, The C. V. Mosby Co.

Ganda, O. P., and Soeldner, S. S.: Arch. Intern. Med. **137:**461-469, 1977 (factors in etiology of diabetes mellitus).

Ganda, O. P., et al.: N. Engl. J. Med. **296:**963-967, 1977 (somatostatinoma).

Gibson, J. B.: J. Pathol. Bacteriol. **79:**381-401, 1960 (Chiari's disease).

Greenwald, A. J., et al.: J.A.M.A. **231:**273-276, 1975 (alpha$_1$-antitrypsin and cirrhosis of liver).

Greider, M. H., and Elliott, D. W.: Am. J. Pathol. **44:**663-678, 1964 (electron microscopy of islet cell tumors).

Greider, M. H., et al.: J.A.M.A. **186:**566-569, 1963 (islet cell adenomas).

Greider, M. H., et al.: Lab. Invest. **22:**344-354, 1970 (features of islet cells).

Greider, M. H., et al.: Cancer **33:**1423-1443, 1974 (pancreatic islet cell, ulcerogenic and diarrheogenic tumors).

Haverback, B. J.: J.A.M.A. **193:**279-283, 1965 (exocrine function of pancreas).

Huttenlocher, P. R., and Trauner, D. A.: In Vinken, P. J., and Bruyn, G. W., editors: Handbook of clinical neurology, vol. 29, Amsterdam, 1977, Elsevier/North Holland Biomedical Press, pp. 331-344 (Reye's syndrome).

Johnson, J. D.: N. Engl. J. Med. **292:**194-197, 1975 (neonatal nonhemolytic jaundice).

Kraft, A. R., et al.: Am. J. Surg. **119:**163-170, 1970 (diarrheal syndrome with nonbeta islet cell tumors).

Krementz, E. T., and Becker, M. L.: Adv. Surg. **6:**205-236, 1972 (cancer of the pancreas—a review).

Lacy, P. E.: N. Engl. J. Med. **276:**187-195, 1967 (pancreatic beta cell).

Lacy, P. E., and Kissane, J. M.: Pancreas and diabetes mellitus. In Anderson, W. A. D., and Kissane, J. M., editors: Pathology, ed. 7, St. Louis, 1977, The C. V. Mosby Co.

Lieber, C. S.: J.A.M.A. **233:**1077-1082, 1975 (alcohol, malnutrition, and liver disease).

Lieber, C. S., and Rubin, E.: N. Engl. J. Med. **280:**705-708, 1969 (alcoholic liver).

Lisa, J. R., et al.: Cancer **17:**395-401, 1964 (carcinoma of pancreas).

Lombardi, B., et al.: Am. J. Pathol. **79**:465-480, 1975 (acute pancreatitis in mice fed choline-deficient diet with ethionine).

Lomsky, R., et al.: Nature (Lond.) **223**:618-619, 1969 (immunochemical demonstration of gastrin in islet cells).

Lough, J., and Wiglesworth, F. W.: Arch. Pathol. Lab. Med. **100**:659-663, 1976 (Wilson's disease—EM study).

MacDonald, R. A., and Mallory, G. K.: Am. J. Med. **24**:334-357, 1958 (postnecrotic cirrhosis).

Mann, S. K., and Mann, N. S.: Arch. Pathol. Lab. Med. **103**:79-81, 1979 (enterokinase in experimental acute pancreatitis).

Margolis, G., et al.: Exp. Mol. Pathol. **8**:1-20, 1968 (peliosis hepatitis caused by rat virus).

Maugh, T. H. II: Science **188**:347-351, 436-438, 1975 (viruses and diabetes mellitus).

Mays, E. T., et al.: Am. J. Clin. Pathol. **61**:735-746, 1974 (focal nodular hyperplasia of liver and oral contraceptives).

McGavran, M. H., et al.: N. Engl. J. Med. **274**:1408-1413, 1966 (glucagon-secreting alpha cell carcinoma of pancreatic islets).

Mosely, R. V.: Surgery **61**:674-686, 1967 (primary malignant tumors of liver).

Music, S. I., et al.: J. Fla. Med. Assoc. **60**:25-26, 1973 (Reye's syndrome).

Nadell, J., and Kosek, J.: Arch. Pathol. Lab. Med. **101**:405-410, 1977 (peliosis hepatis).

Nerup, J., et al.: Lancet **2**:864-866, 1974 (HLA antigens in diabetes mellitus).

Nisman, R. M., et al.: Arch. Intern. Med. **139**:1289-1291, 1979 (bridging hepatic necrosis in viral hepatitis).

Nolan, J. P.: N. Engl. J. Med. **299**:1069-1071, 1978 (bacteria in the liver).

O'Sullivan, J. P., and Wilding, R. P.: Br. Med. J. **3**:7-10, 1974 (liver hamartomas and oral contraceptives).

Patek, A. J., et al.: Arch. Intern. Med. **135**:1053-1057, 1975 (alcohol and dietary factors in cirrhosis).

Patton, R. B., and Horn, R. C., Jr.: Cancer **17**:757-768, 1964 (carcinoma of liver).

Popper, H.: N. Engl. J. Med. **290**:159-160, 1974 (editorial—alcoholic hepatitis and cirrhosis).

Rubin, E., and Lieber, C. S.: N. Engl. J. Med. **290**:128-135, 1974 (fatty liver, alcholic hepatitis, and cirrhosis produced by alcohol in nonhuman primates).

Schaffner, F.: Am. J. Med. **49**:658-668, 1970 (electron microscopy in viral hepatitis).

Schaffner, F., et al.: J.A.M.A. **183**:343-346, 1963 (alcoholic hepatitis).

Sherlock, S.: Diseases of the liver and biliary system, ed. 5, Oxford, 1975, Blackwell Scientific Publications Ltd.

Sherlock, S., and Scheuer, P. J.: N. Engl. J. Med. **289**:674-678, 1973 (biliary cirrhosis).

Smith, A. L.: N. Engl. J. Med. **294**:897-898, 1976 (Reye's syndrome).

Smuckler, E. A.: Am. J. Clin. Pathol. **49**:790-797, 1968 (ultrastructure of alcoholic hyalin).

Sprinz, H., and Nelson, R. S.: Ann. Intern. Med. **41**:952-962, 1954 (chronic idiopathic jaundice).

Stary, H. C.: Am. J. Med. Sci. **252**:357-374, 1966 (blood vessels in diabetes).

Suckow, E. E., et al.: Am. J. Pathol. **38**:663-678, 1961 (Thorotrast-induced liver tumors).

Thomas, L. B., et al.: N. Engl. J. Med. **292**:17-22, 1975 (vinyl chloride–induced liver disease).

Unger, R. H.: N. Engl. J. Med. **296**:998-1000, 1977 (somatostatinoma).

Vana, J., et al.: J.A.M.A. **238**:2154-2158, 1977 (liver tumors and oral contraceptives—results of a survey).

Walters, M. N.-I.: J. Pathol. Bacteriol. **92**:547-557, 1966 (adipose atrophy of pancreas).

Wands, J. R., et al.: N. Engl. J. Med. **298**:233-237, 1978 (complement-fixing immune complexes in primary biliary cirrhosis).

Warren, S., LeCompte, P. M., and Legg, M. A.: The pathology of diabetes mellitus, ed. 4, Philadelphia, 1966, Lea & Febiger.

Warshaw, A. L.: N. Engl. J. Med. **287**:1234-1236, 1972 (pancreatic abscesses).

Weinstein, G. D., et al.: Arch. Dermatol. **102**:613-618, 1970 (possible hepatotoxic effects of methotrexate in psoriasis).

Weinstein, L.: N. Engl. J. Med. **299**:1052-1054, 1978 (bacterial hepatitis).

Yanoff, M., and Rawson, A. J.: Arch. Pathol. **77**:159-165, 1964 (peliosis hepatis).

Yoon, J.-W., et al.: N. Engl. J. Med. **300**:1173-1179, 1979 (virus-induced diabetes mellitus).

Zachariae, H., and Schiødt, T.: Acta Derm. Venereol. (Stockh.) **51**:215-220, 1971 (liver biopsy in methotrexate treatment).

Zollinger, R. M., and Grant, G. N.: J.A.M.A. **190**:181-184, 1964 (ulcerogenic tumor of pancreas).

Zollinger, R. M., et al.: Ann. Surg. **168**:502-521, 1960 (secretion-producing nonbeta islet cell tumors).

Zollinger, R. M., et al.: In Tenth Clinical Conference on Cancer, Anderson Hospital and Tumor Institute: Cancer of the gastrointestinal tract, Chicago, 1967, Year Book Medical Publishers, Inc., p. 73 (ulcerogenic tumors of pancreas).

17

Reticuloendothelial system, spleen, and lymph nodes

Reticuloendothelial system

The reticuloendothelial system is composed of widespread cells having the essential and common ability to phagocytose particulate foreign material, such as injected vital dyes or India ink. Some of these phagocytic cells are endothelial cells lining the blood sinuses of the spleen, liver, and bone marrow and the lymph sinuses of lymph nodes. Also, all connective tissues contain elements (undifferentiated mesenchymal cells) that are capable of assuming mobility and phagocytic function. These cells are called histiocytes, clasmatocytes, polyblasts, resting wandering cells, adventitial cells, etc. Both the endothelial cells and the undifferentiated mesenchymal cells are capable of becoming macrophages.

The concept of the reticuloendothelial system has been furthered by Maximow, who pointed out that in the spleen, bone marrow, and lymphatic tissue generally, there exists an undifferentiated mesenchyme, called reticulum, in the form of a nucleated syncytium with an abundant meshwork of fibrils. These fibrils (reticulin) are not seen well in ordinary sections stained by hematoxylin and eosin. However, reticulin fibers are argyrophilic and are stained black by silver salts, which are converted to the black oxide. This syncytium or reticulum is not in itself phagocytic, but under the stimulus of an injury or inflammation, there differentiates from it the mobile phagocytic macrophage. Since the undifferentiated mesenchyme is widespread throughout the body, macrophages likewise have diverse origin. Microglial cells are the corresponding phagocytic cells in the nervous system.

The monocytes of the circulating blood also give rise to phagocytic macrophages. The prevalent view is that the major source of monocytes is the bone marrow and that most of the macrophages at the site of an inflammatory response are derived from blood monocytes. The ordinary lining endothelium of blood vessels and lymphatics, other than in the spleen, lymph nodes, liver, bone marrow, adrenal cortex, and hypophysis, is not actively phagocytic.

Reticuloendothelial cells are important in the normal breakdown of hemoglobin and formation of bile pigment, in fat metabolism, and in defense of the body. The blood is cleared of particulate matter, foreign material, and bacteria in its filtration through the liver, spleen, and bone marrow. The phagocytic cells ingest and remove dead tissue fragments, pigments, bacteria, fungi, and protozoa. For larger masses of particulate matter, they fuse and form foreign body giant cells. The osteoclast of bone is a particular type of such a giant cell. The role of the macrophage in immune responses is referred to in Chapter 4.

Diseases of the reticuloendothelial system fall into three main groups:

1 Infections and inflammations, in which proliferation and phagocytosis by reticuloendothelial cells are prominent, of which histoplasmosis and malaria are excellent examples

2 Lipidoses, or lipid storage diseases, in which, because of disturbed metabolism, fatty substances accumulate in reticuloendothelial cells; the fatty material may be kerasin (Gaucher's disease), sphingomyelin (Niemann-Pick disease), or cholesterol (Schüller-Christian disease and xanthomas)

3 Tumors and tumorlike conditions, which form a large and confusing group of conditions and include monocytic leukemia, Hodgkin's disease, histiocytic lymphoma (reticulum cell sarcoma), and reticuloendotheliosis

Since the large storehouse of reticuloendothelial cells is in the spleen, lymph nodes, bone marrow, and liver, the reticuloendothelial involvement is considered in conjunction with diseases affecting these organs.

Spleen

The average normal adult spleen weighs 150 to 170 g, but the size and weight vary widely. Many of the diseases of the spleen bring about an enormous increase in its size and weight, sometimes 2,000 g or more. The adult spleen is usually not clinically palpable unless it weighs more than 300 g. The cut surface of the normal spleen is moderately firm and light red. The malpighian corpuscles are just visible as small grayish white areas. Small accessory spleens are not uncommon. An accessory spleen is present in about 10% of persons. The tail of the pancreas is a frequent site.

Microscopically, the discernible structures are (1) the white pulp with periarterial lymphoid sheaths and lymphoid follicles (malpighian corpuscles), (2) the red pulp, consisting of sinusoids and cords with erythrocytes and phagocytic histiocytes, and (3) trabeculae or fibromuscular bands, which connect with the splenic capsule.

The spleen is not essential to life, but it has important functions, particularly as the main component of the reticuloendothelial system. Thus, it is important (1) in the breakdown of hemoglobin and formation of bile pigment, (2) in the filtration of organisms or other foreign material from the bloodstream, (3) in the formation of antibodies and immunity, (4) as the reservoir for blood, and (5) for blood formation in the fetus or when there is severe anemia.

Functioning of the spleen in the storage and breakdown of blood elements may get out of balance or equilibrium because of primary (idiopathic or hereditary) factors, or the imbalance may be secondarily caused by various disease processes, mainly of the reticuloendothelial system. The resulting hypersplenism may destroy excessive numbers of circulating red blood cells (as in congenital hemolytic anemia), platelets (as in thrombocytopenic purpura), or neutrophilic leukocytes (splenic neutropenia). All three elements may be excessively destroyed (panhematopenia). Surgical removal of the spleen and accessory splenic tissue is effective in such cases when clinical study has established that bone marrow function is normal and is not a contributing factor.

In primary hypersplenism, there is a diffuse or nodular hyperplasia of the reticulum cells of the spleen proportional to the severity of the disease. In acute stages of hemocytopenia, there is also sequestration in the red pulp and splenic sinusoids of the decreased formed elements of the blood. In secondary hypersplenism, small hemolytic or cytolytic foci may be found in the spleen.

Splenectomy may be beneficial in rupture of the spleen, congenital hemolytic anemia, thrombocytopenic purpura, hypersplenism or primary splenic neutropenia, and thrombosis or anomalous obstruction of the splenic vein.

RETROGRADE CONDITIONS

Atrophy. Reduction in size of the spleen may occur in old age, usually in association with severe arteriosclerosis of splenic vessels. Extreme atrophy may be present in late stages of sickle cell anemia.

Arteriosclerosis. Hyaline sclerosis of small arteries and arterioles in the spleen is very common, its frequency and severity increasing with age. Although more pronounced when there is hypertension and when arteriosclerosis is present elsewhere, the vascular change may be present in the spleen alone. When severe, it may cause multiple small infarcts or necroses in the spleen.

Amyloid. The spleen is a common site for amyloid deposit (p. 34).

Pigmentation. Pigment deposits in the spleen follow excessive breakdown of hemoglobin, such as occurs in chronic hemolytic anemias, multiple blood transfusions, malaria, or chronic congestion. Some brownish hemosiderin pigment in the spleen is a normal finding. In malaria, pigmentation may be excessive, so that the enlarged organ grossly exhibits a slate gray color (p. 208). In sickle cell anemia and chronic congestive splenomegaly, curious areas of fibrosis and pigmentation occur in the spleen (siderofibrotic nodules and Gandy-Gamna bodies, pp. 102 and 500).

Multiple necroses (Fleckmilz). Speckling of the spleen may be caused by widespread and irregular areas of necrosis as the result of confluence of many minute infarcts. The splenic arterioles commonly show marked degenerative changes with frequent thromboses. Most cases are associated with renal disease and uremia.

CIRCULATORY DISTURBANCES

Infarction. Infarction in the spleen is common and frequently is the result of arterial embolism (pp. 111 and 117).

Congestion. Chronic passive congestion in the spleen may be present in conditions of circulatory failure. The spleen is moderately enlarged and firm. Microscopically, the sinusoids appear dilated. Fibrosis occurs if the process continues for a long period.

Chronic congestion also is associated with obstruction of the portal circulation (e.g., from cirrhosis of the liver and portal vein thrombosis). Severe congestion of the spleen is a feature of sickle cell anemia in its earlier phases and of congenital hemolytic anemia. In the long-standing, chronic congestion related to portal hypertension (including Banti's syndrome) and in the late stage of sickle cell anemia, foci of fibrosis with deposits of iron and calcium may be seen (Gandy-Gamna bodies).

Banti's syndrome. Banti's syndrome is a symptom complex dominated by splenic enlargement, nonhemolytic anemia, and leukopenia. The splenomegaly is characterized by congestion and fibrosis. It is accompanied by portal hypertension and often is complicated in later stages by ascites, hematemesis, portal cirrhosis of the liver, and thrombosis of splenic and portal veins. There is a tendency today to discard the term Banti's disease and to consider the condition simply a chronic congestive splenomegaly related to portal hypertension, with the added feature of splenic hyperactivity (hypersplenism). Hypersplenism is evidenced by the anemia and leukopenia.

Recently, the view has been expressed that splenomegaly with portal hypertension associated with slight hepatic fibrosis (i.e., Banti's syndrome) may be the result of exposure to known or unknown chemical agents. This condition has been described in patients who were known to have had chronic exposure to vinyl chloride or arsenicals.

Rupture. Rupture of the spleen is usually the result of direct trauma over the splenic area. Occasionally, there is delayed splenic rupture, with a latent period following the traumatic injury. Splenic rupture also may complicate malaria, infectious mononucleosis, primary splenic tumors, and other conditions on rare occasions. Unless there is prompt operation, fatal intra-abdominal hemorrhage usually results. Autotransplantation of fragments of splenic tissue on peritoneal surfaces throughout the abdominal cavity (i.e., *splenosis*) may complicate splenic rupture. The usually widespread distribution of these implants is in contrast to that of the single or multiple congenital accessory spleens, which are most often found in the region of the spleen or in nearby sites (e.g., in the omentum or on or in the tail of the pancreas).

Partial return of splenic activity, as evidenced by certain hematologic findings, has been reported in children who had an emergency splenectomy because of trauma to the spleen and who subsequently developed splenosis. This return of function resulting from the transplanted fragments of splenic tissue may account, in part, for the low frequency of serious bacterial infection observed in these patients compared with children who had elective splenectomy for hematologic disorders.

INFLAMMATIONS

Acute splenitis (acute splenic "tumor"). Splenic reaction with moderate enlargement accompanies acute systemic infections, particularly bacteremias or septicemias. In such cases, the causative organisms are usually obtainable in cultures from the spleen. Acute splenic "tumor" appears to be a reaction to the presence of foreign protein, whether bacterial or nonbacterial. The term *acute splenic hyperplasia* is sometimes used for the enlarged spleen.

Microscopically, the changes in acute splenitis are congestion and cellular accumulation in the pulp. In some cases, many of the cells are neutrophilic leukocytes, but commonly they are large basophilic mononuclear cells that are lymphoid in character. Phagocytic mononuclear cells containing ingested erythrocytes, bacteria, or necrotic debris may be seen. The lymphoid follicles may be hyperplastic with reactive centers but in some instances are not conspicuous.

Tuberculosis. The spleen usually is involved in generalized miliary tuberculosis. In rare cases, a large localized tuberculous lesion develops in the spleen while the original focus remains quiescent or heals. Small, rounded, hyalinized fibrous nodules, 1 to 3 mm in diameter, are a frequent finding in the spleen and in most cases represent healed tubercles.

Malaria. The spleen is enlarged and heavily pigmented in malaria (p. 208).

Histoplasmosis. The spleen often is greatly enlarged in histoplasmosis because of marked proliferation of reticuloendothelial cells. The small organism can be seen in the cytoplasm of these phagocytic cells (p. 199). Similar splenic lesions occur in kala-azar.

CYSTS AND TUMORS

Cystic cavities in the spleen are rare. Most are pseudocysts resulting from encapsulation of an area of hemorrhage or degeneration in the pulp. Neoplastic cysts (Fig. 17-1) and parasitic (hydatid) cysts are rare occurrences.

Tumors of the spleen, either primary or metastatic, are rather uncommon. Heman-

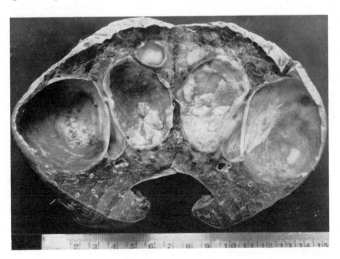

Fig. 17-1. Multiple cysts of spleen.

gioma, although rare, is the most frequent primary benign tumor. Hamartomas and sarcomas, including the malignant lymphomas, also occur. The reason for the relative infrequency of metastatic tumors in the spleen is not known, but it may result from the inequality of exposure to metastasizing tumor cells or from lesser susceptibility than other tissues.

Lymph nodes

The lymph nodes are focal collections of lymphoid and reticuloendothelial cells. Lymphoid tissue is widely distributed in other tissues as well, such as the alimentary canal and spleen. The main elements in lymph nodes are (1) lymph follicles (germinal centers) in the cortex, (2) lymph sinuses, lined by endothelium, and (3) the medulla or pulp, consisting of lymphocytes and reticulum cells in a delicate meshwork of reticulin fibers. As noted previously, cells of the B series (including the antibody-producing cells) are found in the cortical lymphoid follicles and medullary cords; the T cells are in the deep perinodular cortical area.

The lymph nodes are an integral part of the reticuloendothelial system and participate in its diseases. In agammaglobulinemia, they may show an absence of germinal centers and of plasma cells, even after injection of an antigen. Lymphoid aggregations in the spleen and elsewhere may be similarly nonreactive. In deficiencies of the thymus (e.g., thymic aplasia), there is depletion of lymphocytes in the deep perinodular cortical areas of the nodes as well as in the periarterial lymphatic sheaths of the spleen ("thymic-dependent" areas). The main lesions of lymph nodes are inflammations (lymphadenitis) and tumors (primary and metastatic).

Lymphadenitis. Acute lymphadenitis occurs in lymph nodes draining an area of acute inflammation, e.g., in cervical lymph nodes in acute infections of the throat or in axillary lymph nodes in infections of the hand or arm. The lymph nodes are swollen and tender, and, in pyogenic infections, suppuration may occur. Microscopically, the sinuses of the lymph nodes are found filled by neutrophilic leukocytes and some mononuclear cells. In certain infections, the lesions in the lymph nodes are of a characteristic nature (e.g., in tularemia, lymphogranuloma venereum, and tuberculosis). In systemic lupus erythematosus, the lymph nodes are enlarged in 66% of cases, showing edema, engorgement, and sometimes necrosis.

Chronic lymphadenitis, which may be found in nodes draining an area of low-grade inflammation, shows proliferation of mononuclear cells, which fill the sinuses (Fig. 17-2). Fibrosis usually does not occur. The lymphoid follicles may be enlarged and hyperplastic.

Chronic dermatitis with pruritus may have an associated enlargement of lymph nodes. The nodes show reticular hyperplasia, melanin pigment, intracellular fat, and a few eosinophils (lipomelanotic reticular hyperplasia and dermatopathic lymphadenitis).

Infectious mononucleosis. Infectious mononucleosis occurs most frequently in children and young adults. It is characterized by slight enlargement of the superficial lymph nodes, splenomegaly, sore throat, and an increase of mononuclear cells (atypical lymphoid cells) in the blood. Actually, a great variety of tissues may be involved, so that the clinical manifestations are protean. The mortality is almost nil, but fatality has occurred as a result of rupture of the spleen, central respiratory paralysis, and myocarditis. The evidence suggests that the Epstein-Barr virus (EBV) is the etiologic agent. This virus was originally isolated from cell lines derived from Burkitt's lymphoma. EBVs in throat washings and high EBV antibody titers have been demonstrated in patients with infectious mononucleosis.

The large abnormal lymphocyte found in the blood is characterized by a large, eccentric, indented nucleus with a sievelike, coarse network of chromatin. The cytoplasm is basophilic and vacuolated. Occasionally, more immature types may be present. The cell is not pathognomonic, and similar cells may be seen in various viral infections and allergic states. However, the presence of such cells account-

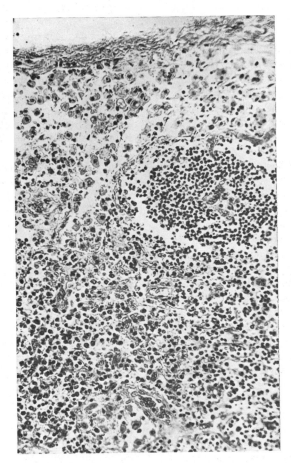

Fig. 17-2. Chronic lymphadenitis. Many large mononuclear cells may be seen in dilated peripheral lymph sinus. (From Richter, M. N.: Spleen, lymph nodes, and reticuloendothelial system. In Anderson, W. A. D., editor: Pathology, ed. 5, St. Louis, 1966, The C. V. Mosby Co.)

ing for more than 10% of white blood cells is very suggestive of infectious mononucleosis. Absence of anemia in uncomplicated cases assists in differentiation from leukemia.

Of diagnostic importance is the Paul-Bunnell test showing heterophil antibodies in the serum, which agglutinate sheep red cells in high dilutions (a titer of 1:160 or more). The highest titers are usually found in the second or third week, and the reaction sometimes persists for several months. However, several other conditions, including viral hepatitis, viral pneumonitis, undulant fever, and serum sickness, may be associated with heterophil

antibodies in the serum. The Davidsohn exclusion test is useful in the presence of relatively low titers. It is based on the fact that the heterophil antibodies of infectious mononucleosis are not absorbed by guinea pig kidney tissue as are the heterophil antibodies of serum sickness and of normal serum. Beef erythrocytes will absorb the heterophil antibodies of both infectious mononucleosis and serum sickness but not of normal serum.

The lymph nodes show a maintenance of architecture (albeit distorted) with distinguishable lymph sinuses and germinal centers. Throughout the pulp, in the sinuses, and on the edges of the germinal centers are large numbers of the specific large mononuclear cells, identical with those characteristic in the blood. Much proliferative activity is evident in the pulp.

The spleen, other lymphoid tissues, and bone marrow show similar changes, with an accumulation of the characteristic cells. Focal areas of mononuclear cell infiltration and necrosis occur in the liver, kidneys, nervous system, heart, and lungs. Involvement of the nervous system may give variable clinical manifestations, and fatalities have resulted from acute polyradiculitis with respiratory paralysis (Guillain-Barré syndrome). Hepatitis similar to that of nonfatal viral or epidemic hepatitis is common, and evidence of hepatic dysfunction or jaundice may be present. The liver shows lymphoid accumulations about portal areas, degeneration and regeneration of hepatic cells, and activity of the Kupffer cells. In rare cases, the hepatic damage is severe, and viral hepatitis may be simulated clinically.

Recent immunologic studies have shown that the vast majority of atypical lymphocytes in acute infectious mononucleosis have surface markers that are characteristic of T lymphocytes. However, the presumed cause of this disease, EBV, has been shown to infect only B lymphocytes. An explanation given for this apparent contradiction is that the uninfected T cells play a part in the immune response to EBV.

Acute infectious lymphocytosis. Under the term *acute infectious lymphocytosis* there has been described an infectious condition in children that is characterized by a relative and absolute lymphocytosis of small lymphocytes of normal appearance. Biopsied lymph nodes show a great proliferation of the reticuloendothelium of the sinuses and hyaline degenerative changes in the lymph follicles. Acute infectious lymphocytosis is differentiated from leukemia and infectious mononucleosis by the normal appearance of the predominating small lymphocytes and the negative heterophil agglutination reaction. The cause is not known.

Kawasaki disease. Often referred to as *mucocutaneous lymph node syndrome,* Kawasaki disease is an acute febrile disease of unknown cause that occurs most frequently in young children and infants. It was first recognized in Japan but is now observed in the United States and in other countries. The disease is characterized by fever; congestion of the conjunctivae, lips, and oral mucosa; erythema and edema of the hands and feet with maculopapular rash and desquamation of the skin; and nonpurulent, tender, swollen cervical lymph nodes. Usually, thrombocytosis, leukocytosis, and elevated sedimentation rate are present. Associated findings may be myocarditis or pericarditis, diarrhea, proteinuria, sterile pyuria, mild jaundice or elevated liver enzymes, and occasionally meningitis and arthritis or arthralgia. Throat culture, antistreptolysin-O titers, streptozyme test, and culture and serologic tests for rubeola, rubella, and other infectious agents are negative. Certain investigators have reported rickettsialike bodies in some patients, but the evidence for rickettsial origin is inconclusive. When the lymph nodes have been examined microscopically, usually in biopsied tissue, nonspecific lymphoid hyperplasia has been observed. Although this is usually a self-limited disease with a favorable outcome, fatalities have been reported in a small percentage of patients.

Death may result from myocarditis or from myocardial infarction caused by coronary thrombosis associated with coronary arteritis. The coronary artery disease with aneurysm and thrombosis that accompanies Kawasaki disease may occur during the first few months of life and is usually fatal. It is possible that infantile polyarteritis nodosa with coronary involvement, which has been recognized in the United States for many years, may be the same disease as fatal Kawasaki disease.

Immunoblastic lymphadenopathy. A new disease with a lymphomalike clinical presentation has been described that is characterized by generalized lymphadenopathy, often with hepatosplenomegaly, and immunologic abnormalities, such as dysgammaglobulinemia or hemolytic anemia. It has been referred to as "immunoblastic lymphadenopathy," "chronic pluripotential immunoproliferative syndrome,'' ''diffuse plasmacytic sarcomatosis,'' and ''angioimmunoblastic lymphadenopathy.'' Microscopically, the appearance of the lymph nodes resembles a malignant lymphoma, particularly Hodgkin's disease, but there are no diagnostic Sternberg-Reed cells. There is a nonneoplastic proliferation of immunoblasts, plasmacytoid immunoblasts, plasma cells, and small lymphocytes. An increase in the number of vessels with endothelial hyperplasia and walls thickened by PAS-positive material is also noted. The disease may be an abnormal immunologic disorder of the B and T cell systems. Occasionally, the disease has evolved into a malignant lymphoma (called immunoblastic lymphoma or immunoblastic sarcoma).

Metastatic tumors. Carcinomas particularly tend to metastasize to regional lymph nodes. The tumor cells are first seen in the sinuses of the periphery or pulp, but lymphoid tissue eventually is replaced by tumor, and invasion occurs through the capsule.

Primary tumors. Primary neoplasms of the lymph nodes are in almost all instances malignant lymphomas, which are discussed in the next section. Rarely do other primary tumors arise in the lymph nodes.

Tumors of reticuloendothelial and lymphoid tissues

Apart from the infections in which proliferation of reticuloendothelial cells is a distinctive feature (malaria, histoplasmosis, and kala-azar) and the lipid storage diseases (Gaucher's disease, etc.), there occurs a variety of tumors and tumorlike conditions involving lymphoid and reticuloendothelial structures. Since they are of obscure causation, etiologic classification fails. The following simplified morphologic classification should be viewed with the realization that gradations and overlappings preclude sharp lines of distinction. The cellular structure of the lymphatic tumors is very labile, and since they are all derived from the same mesenchymal stem cells,

transitions are sometimes observed from one type to another.

Reticuloendotheliosis
Malignant lymphoma
   Non-Hodgkin's types
      Nodular (follicular) type
      Diffuse type
         Lymphocytic type
         Histiocytic type (reticulum cell sarcoma)
         Mixed lymphocytic-histiocytic type
         Undifferentiated (Burkitt) type
         Undifferentiated (non-Burkitt) type
   Hodgkin's disease
   Mycosis fungoides
Leukemia (discussed in Chapter 18)

RETICULOENDOTHELIOSIS

Nonlipid reticuloendotheliosis. Nonlipid reticuloendotheliosis (Letterer-Siwe disease; malignant reticuloblastomatosis; aleukemic reticulosis) is a rare condition in which there is diffuse hyperplasia of the reticuloendothelial system to the point of replacement of normal structures. It may occur at any age but is more frequent in infants and young children. The characteristics include splenomegaly, hepatomegaly, anemia, purpura, and bony changes such as areas of rarefaction and cyst formation. A fatal ending is reached in 2 weeks to 2 years, usually from acute infection. The disease has been termed nonlipid reticuloendotheliosis to distinguish it from the lipid storage diseases, and it is also called *Letterer-Siwe disease,* after Letterer and Siwe, who described cases in 1924 and 1933.

The greatest changes are found in the spleen, lymph nodes, liver, and bone marrow. The enlarged spleen shows scattered, indefinite grayish yellow nodules on the cut surface, and similar nodules may be seen in the liver. In addition, there may be diffuse or nodular lesions of the lungs and involvement of the intestinal lymphoid tissue. Microscopically, there is a great proliferation of large mononuclear cells in organs of the reticuloendothelial system, with distortion of normal structure. These cells are rounded or polyhedral, and some may be very large (up to 50 μ). Multinucleated giant cells may be seen. Occasional mitoses are present. Silver staining shows a proliferation of reticulin fibers in contact with the atypical cells. In some cases, there may be a few neutrophilic or eosinophilic leukocytes.

Leukemic reticuloendotheliosis. This disease is also known as *hairy cell leukemia,* so called because abnormal mononuclear cells with exaggerated, "hairlike" cytoplasmic projections (best seen with phase microscopy and electron microscopy) are present in the peripheral blood. The cells are identified cytochemically by positive staining reaction for tartrate-resistant acid phosphatase. Frequent findings are pancytopenia (anemia, leukopenia, and particularly thrombocytopenia) and splenomegaly, which is sometimes massive. Hepatomegaly occurs in some patients, but enlargement of lymph nodes is seldom observed. Although pancytopenia is the usual finding, some patients may have normal or elevated white blood cell counts with the "hairy" cells. Another characteristic of the disease is that attempts to aspirate bone marrow are frequently unsuccessful, resulting in "dry" taps. Bone marrow biopsy reveals a probable reason for this, namely, an increase in reticulin fibers associated with infiltration of the neoplastic mononuclear cells. The origin of the neoplastic cells has not been definitely established. In various studies, features of both B lymphocytes and monocytes have been described in the same or different patients.

MALIGNANT LYMPHOMA

Malignant lymphoma is a malignant tumor that can arise from any aggregate of lymphoid tissue. It is more frequent in males than females. It may occur at any period of life, but the different types of lymphoma tend to occur in different age groups, e.g., Hodgkin's disease between 20 and 40 years of age, follicular lymphoma usually in older age groups, diffuse lymphocytic and histiocytic types principally in middle and older age groups, and Burkitt's lymphoma commonly in childhood but sometimes in adults.

Constitutional symptoms and blood changes are lacking in early stages. External lymph node enlargement is the most frequent beginning, and the cervical nodes are affected most often. However, enlargement of other nodes may be observed first, e.g., mediastinal lymph nodes in a chest x-ray film. The gastrointestinal tract, nasopharynx, spleen, skin, liver, and other tissues frequently are involved. Direct invasion and extension to contiguous lymph nodes occur early. Later, widespread extension, probably by the bloodstream, often results in involvement of many tissues. Lymphomas are usually radiosensitive.

Etiology. Although the cause of malignant lymphomas in man has not been established, there is evidence that lymphomas, as well as leukemias, in certain animals are caused by viruses, usually RNA viruses with C-type characteristics. Also, some investigators have detected the presence of RNA in human malignant lymphomas that is related to the RNA of the Rauscher (murine) leukemia virus, suggesting involvement of a viral agent in these diseases.

In a central zone of Africa through the equatorial region, lymphoma occurs with high incidence in children between 2 and 14 years of age, with a peak incidence at 5 years of age *(Burkitt's lymphoma).* Most of the cases involve the jaw or abdomen. The distribution is geographic rather than racial, suggesting an infective spread by an insect vector. This and additional immunologic evidence suggest that a viral agent contributes to the pathogenesis of this lymphoma. A virus of the herpes group (EBV) has been isolated from Burkitt's lymphoma cells in tissue culture, and patients with this disease often have a high titer of antibodies for EBV. A reovirus type 3 also has been isolated from Burkitt's tumor tissue by some investigations. Most reports seem to favor the view that EBV, a DNA virus, is the most likely etiologic agent of Burkitt's lymphoma, although this has not been proved. It is therefore of interest that in recent studies the presence of RNA similar to that of a murine leukemia virus has been detected in this as well as in other types of lymphoma. The relationship of this viral-related RNA to EBV has not been established.

Among children, lymphoma resembling the Burkitt's tumor has only recently been described in the United States. Among American patients, the disease appears most frequently in young children, but it also occurs in older children and young adults, the median age being somewhat older than in African patients. In contrast to the latter, a greater frequency of initial involvement in abdominal sites rather than in the jaw is noted in American patients.

Malignant lymphomas have been noted to occur during anticonvulsant therapy, particularly with use of hydantoin derivatives. Also, pseudolymphomatous reactions in lymph nodes have been reported in patients receiving anticonvulsants. Some investigators suggest that the lymphomalike reaction seen in immunoblastic lymphadenopathy (p. 482) may be triggered by a hypersensitivity reaction to therapeutic agents. A higher incidence of malignant lymphomas has been observed in immunosuppressed patients receiving kidney transplants, in certain primary immunologic deficiency syndromes (e.g., ataxia-telangiectasia), and in patients with certain autoimmune diseases (e.g., Sjögren's syndrome). The relationship of the immune system to malignant lymphomas is discussed on p. 491.

Classification. Traditionally, malignant lymphomas have been classified chiefly on the basis of the histologic appearance and degree of differentiation of the neoplasms. In recent years, however, a new approach to the study of malignant lymphomas has been proposed that utilizes immunologic concepts together with morphologic studies in order to derive a more functional classification of these lesions. First, malignant lymphomas will be discussed according to the traditional approach, and then a consideration of some of the current immunologic aspects of these tumors will follow.

Various classifications of malignant lymphoma have been suggested, among which is the following:

Non-Hodgkin's lymphoma
  Nodular (follicular) lymphoma
  Diffuse lymphoma
    Lymphocytic lymphoma (well, intermediate, and poorly differentiated types)
    Histiocytic lymphoma (reticulum cell sarcoma)
    Mixed lymphocytic-histiocytic lymphoma
    Undifferentiated (Burkitt's type) lymphoma
    Undifferentiated (non–Burkitt's type) lymphoma
Hodgkin's disease
Special types of lymphoma (e.g., mycosis fungoides)

Non-Hodgkin's lymphoma. The non-Hodgkin's lymphomas consist of two general groups, nodular and diffuse lymphomas.

Nodular (follicular) lymphoma was formerly regarded as a distinct clinical and pathologic entity, commonly referred to as *Brill-Symmers disease* or *giant follicular lymphoma*. It has been shown, however, that nodular lymphomas can be subdivided into cytologic types similar to certain variants of the diffuse lymphomas. There are three subtypes: poorly differentiated lymphocytic, histiocytic, and mixed lymphocytic-histiocytic types of nodular lymphoma. Throughout the lymph node, the proliferating neoplastic cells form nodules that compress the intervening parenchyma. Some pathologists are of the opinion that the nodules bear no relationship to the normal follicles (germinal centers), but others have presented evidence to support the view that the nodules represent neoplastic transformation of the cells within the normal germinal centers. There is a tendency for the nodular lymphomas to progress into the diffuse form, usually of similar cellular composition, but this does not necessarily occur in all instances. An important problem is the histologic differentiation of nodular lymphoma from inflammatory (reactive) follicular hyperplasia of lymph nodes. Differentiating features are listed in Table 17-1.

In the **diffuse lymphomas,** the growth of the neoplastic cells lacks a follicular pattern. Instead, the cells are distributed diffusely throughout the lymph node, causing a disruption and obliteration of the architecture of the lymphoid tissue (Figs. 17-3 and 17-4). Also, infiltration of the lymph node capsule by the neoplastic cells and extension of the cells into the surrounding adipose tissue are commonly seen (Fig. 17-3). The foregoing features are

Table 17-1. Histologic differences between nodular (follicular) lymphoma and reactive hyperplasia

	Nodular (follicular) lymphoma	Follicular hyperplasia of inflammatory or toxic origin
Follicles	Loss of normal architecture of node	Preservation of nodal architecture
	Closely packed	Scattered
	Diffuse throughout node	More prominent in cortical portion of node
	Slight variation in size and shape of follicles	Great variation in size and shape of follicles
	Fade into surrounding tissue without sharp demarcation	Sharply demarcated reaction centers
	Composed of neoplastic cells usually of one type (or two in mixed form) with lack of phagocytosis	Composed of usual nonneoplastic cells with macrophages containing cellular debris (active phagocytosis)
	Few mitoses, with no significant difference in number inside and outside follicles	Typical mitoses often frequent in reaction centers, with few outside follicles
Interfollicular tissue	Cells densely packed	Cells scattered
	Condensation of reticulum fibers at periphery of follicles	Little alteration of reticulum framework
	Similarity of cell type inside and outside follicles	Lymphocytes at margin of reaction centers, small, mature, and uniform
	Extensive infiltration of capsule and pericapsular fat, sometimes with follicles outside capsule	No or slight infiltration of capsule and pericapsular fat

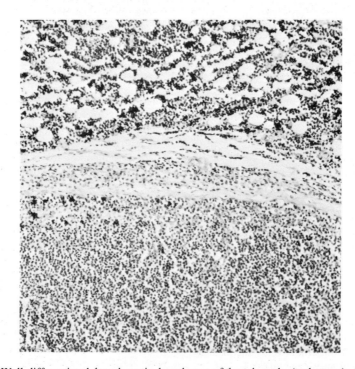

Fig. 17-3. Well-differentiated lymphocytic lymphoma of lymph node (at bottom). Invasion of capsule (center) and extension into adipose tissue adjacent to lymph node (top) are evident. Lymph node architecture is obliterated by lymphoma.

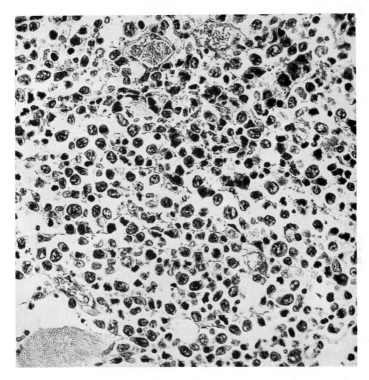

Fig. 17-4. Reticulum cell sarcoma. Highly pleomorphic cellular neoplasm is without organized arrangement. (From Haukohl, R. S., and Anderson, W. A. D., editors: Pathology seminars, St. Louis, 1955, The C. V. Mosby Co.)

among the criteria that distinguish malignant lymphomas from benign reactive hyperplastic lymphadenitis.

In the various forms of diffuse non-Hodgkin's lymphoma, there is a dominance of one cell type in accordance with the above classification, with the exception of the mixed lymphocytic-histiocytic form, which, as the name implies, consists of a mixture of two principal cell types. *Most of the diffuse lymphomas are composed of lymphoid cells,* the size of which may be small, intermediate, or large (corresponding to the well, intermediate, and poorly differentiated lymphocytic types, respectively).

Malignant lymphomas of the histiocytic type consist of larger cells than those in lymphocytic and undifferentiated lymphomas. The individual tumors may be composed of rela-tively uniform cells or of pleomorphic cells. The latter are sometimes atypical and may be in the form of multinucleated giant cells resembling the Sternberg-Reed cells observed in Hodgkin's disease. Silver stains may show fine reticulin fibers surrounding individual cells. Tumors of histiocytic type have been diagnosed as *reticulum cell sarcoma* (Fig. 17-4), but some pathologists do not use this term today. Evidence from recent investigations has led to the suggestion that diffuse histiocytic lymphomas may be derived from transformed lymphocytes (B, T, and null cells) as well as from true histiocytes and that true histiocytic lymphomas are not common.

Burkitt's lymphoma (p. 484) has been considered by some investigators to consist of cells similar to those in the lymphomas of poorly differentiated lymphocytic type. However, others have shown that the cells more closely resemble those in the lymphomas of undifferentiated type. The neoplastic cells in Burkitt's tumor are uniform. Scattered throughout the tumor is a characteristic, but not specific, feature; i.e., the presence of nonneoplastic histiocytes containing ingested pyknotic nuclei and cellular debris, giving a "starry-sky" appearance. In untreated patients, Burkitt's tumors grow relentlessly and rapidly. Young children usually die within 6 months after onset of symptoms. The life expectancy is longer in older children. Regression of the tumors following chemotherapy has been reported.

In contrast to Burkitt's lymphoma with its uniform cell type, the *undifferentiated (non-Burkitt's) lymphoma* is a pleomorphic tumor with considerable variation in size of cells and shape of nuclei. The undifferentiated and histiocytic forms of lymphoma are sometimes classified as *large-cell lymphomas*.

The *prognosis of non-Hodgkin's lymphomas* is correlated with the cytologic type. In several series of cases, the 5-year survival rates were: diffuse lymphocytic lymphoma (all types), 15.9% to 27% (in one series, the well-differentiated cell type was 25% and the poorly differentiated cell type, 3%); diffuse undifferentiated cell lymphoma and reticulum cell sarcoma combined, 12.3% to 21.4%; and follicular lymphoma (all types), 53% to 73%. A system of clinical staging according to the anatomic extent of the disease, similar to that used for Hodgkin's disease (p. 489), also is useful in assessing the prognosis. For example, in one study of patients with non-Hodgkin's lymphomas of all types, the 5-year survival rate was as follows: 55% in stage I, 25% in stage II, and less than 10% in stages III and IV. Patients with follicular lymphoma in stages I and II had a better survival rate than those with diffuse lymphomas in stages I and II, but this favorable difference was not observed in stages III and IV. It has also been shown that the presence of sclerosis in non-Hodgkin's lymphomas is associated with a better prognosis when compared with nonsclerosing tumors of similar histologic type.

Hodgkin's disease. Hodgkin's disease involves lymph nodes or lymphoid tissue elsewhere, as in the alimentary tract, spleen, and often bone marrow. It is sometimes called a lymphogranulomatous type of malignant lymphoma. The etiology is unknown, and its nature has been a matter of debate. The most popular concepts have been that it is (1) a chronic infective granuloma, (2) a viral infection, or (3) a true neoplasm of lymphoid or reticuloendothelial origin. At least one form or stage, often termed Hodgkin's sarcoma, has the characteristics of a malignant tumor. The belief that it is an atypical form of tuberculosis has been almost abandoned. Organisms of the *Brucella* group have been considered, but an etiologic relationship has not been established. There is an immunologic defect in Hodgkin's disease, with an inability to develop delayed hypersensitivity and delayed homograft rejection. The most widely held opinion is that Hodgkin's disease is a form of malignant lymphoma, and it is so considered here.

The beginning is usually a painless enlargement of a group of lymph nodes, most frequently in the neck. Itching is often an accompaniment. Blood changes are inconstant, but there may be a moderate neutrophilic leukocytosis with lymphopenia, and eosinophilia is occasionally present. Anemia develops in later stages. The disease progresses by further involvement of lymphoid tissue, as in other groups of nodes, spleen, etc. In late stages, various viscera become involved. Almost any tissue eventually may be affected, although the nervous system is seldom involved except by Hodgkin's sarcoma.

The enlarged involved lymph nodes are at first discrete but in late stages become matted together. The cut surface of the Hodgkin's tissue has a grayish, translucent, "fish flesh" appearance. Diagnosis is usually made by biopsy of a lymph node. The whole of an enlarged node should be resected for such a purpose.

The microscopic picture of Hodgkin's disease is more complex than that of the other malignant lymphomas and consists of various types. In all types, however, the distinctive Sternberg-Reed cells are present. These are atypical histiocytes (15 to 45 μ) that are irregular in shape and have lobulated or multilobulated nuclei. Often they are binucleated or multinucleated. The nuclei contain prominent, large, usually eosinophilic nucleoli with a clear zone around each nucleolus. The cytoplasm is abundant and usually amphophilic or basophilic but may be eosinophilic.

Attempts have been made to subdivide Hodgkin's disease into histologic groups with prognostic differences. A classification that has been used for years is the one proposed by Jackson and Parker:

1 *Hodgkin's paragranuloma* (10% to 15%), the most limited form with a relatively good prognosis, consisting mainly of lymphocytes and Sternberg-Reed cells

2 *Hodgkin's granuloma,* the most frequent type (80% to 90%), which presents a pleomorphic cellular picture (lymphocytes, plasma cells, neutrophils, eosinophils, reticulum cells, Sternberg-Reed cells), necrosis, and fibrosis; widespread involvement is frequent

3 *Hodgkin's sarcoma,* the least frequent (1% to 5%) but highly malignant type, consisting chiefly of atypical reticulum cells and scattered Sternberg-Reed cells

The usefulness of this classification appears to be limited since the more predictable forms (paragranuloma and sarcoma) constitute only a small group, and the largest group (granuloma) shows a widely variable pattern of behavior.

A more recent classification was proposed at the Conference on Hodgkin's Disease held in 1965 at Rye, N.Y., based on the work of Lukes and associates, and is commonly used at present:

1 *Lymphocytic predominance type* (5%) has a variable histiocytic component (sometimes more than lymphocytes) and may be diffuse or nodular. There are few Sternberg-Reed cells. When lymphocytes predominate, it corresponds to the paragranuloma type.

2 *Nodular sclerosis type* (52%) consists of nodules of abnormal lymphoid tissue separated by orderly bands of collagenous fi-

brous tissue. Few typical Sternberg-Reed cells are seen, but an unusually large variant of Sternberg-Reed cells is more characteristic.

3 *Mixed cellularity type* (37%) consists of eosinophils, plasma cells, neutrophils, lymphocytes, histiocytes, and Sternberg-Reed cells and a variable but not severe degree of irregular fibrosis (Figs. 17-5 and 17-6).

4 *Lymphocytic depletion type* (6%) shows depletion of all cell types, except Sternberg-Reed cells, and involves especially the lymphocytes. It may be associated with diffuse disorderly fibrosis and focal necrosis ("diffuse fibrosis" variant), or it may be characterized by a marked prominence of Sternberg-Reed cells ("reticular" variant), the latter sometimes being pleomorphic and atypical, corresponding to the Hodgkin's sarcoma type.

On the basis of several series of cases as reported in the literature, the 5-year survival rates as correlated with the 1965 Conference classification are presented in Table 17-2.

Prognosis also may be assessed by some system of clinical staging. At a Conference on Staging in Hodgkin's Disease, held at Ann Arbor, Michigan in April 1971, the Staging Classification Committee recommended a combination of clinical staging (CS) and pathologic staging (PS). Clinical staging is determined by history, physical examination, x-ray studies, isotope scans, laboratory tests of blood and urine, and initial biopsy results. Pathologic staging is based on all extra pathologic data obtained as a result of laparotomy, splenectomy, additional lymph node examination, liver biopsy, etc. The pathologic staging is subscripted by symbols indicating the tissue sampled, and the result of histopathologic examination is indicated by + when positive for Hodgkin's disease or − when negative. Liver involvement is always considered to be diffuse and thus stage IV of the disease. The recommended staging classification is as follows:

Stage I Involvement of a single lymph node region (I) or of a single extralymphatic organ or site (I_E).

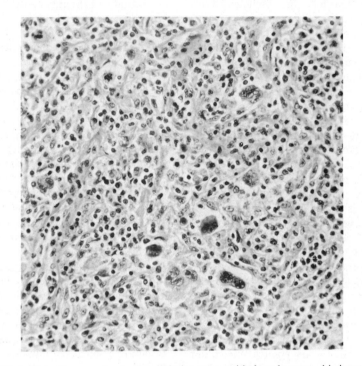

Fig. 17-5. Hodgkin's disease of mixed cellularity type, with lymphocytes, histiocytes, plasma cells, eosinophils, and multinucleated Sternberg-Reed cells.

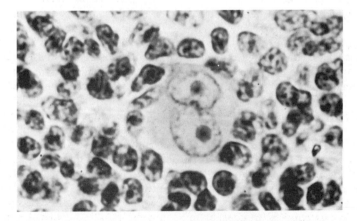

Fig. 17-6. Hodgkin's disease showing Sternberg-Reed cell with two nuclei containing prominent (eosinophilic) nucleoli.

Table 17-2. Reported 5-year survival rates (as to histologic types) in Hodgkin's disease

Lymphocytic predominance	50%-88%
Nodular sclerosis	44%-72%
Mixed cellularity	3%-58%
Lymphocytic depletion	0%-38%
All cases	26%-67%

Stage II Involvement of two or more lymph node regions on the same side of the diaphragm (II) or localized involvement of extralymphatic organ or site and of one or more lymph node regions on the same side of the diaphragm (II_E). An optional recommendation is that the numbers of node regions involved be indicated by a subscript (e.g., II_3).

Stage III Involvement of lymph node regions on both sides of the diaphragm (III), which may be accompanied by localized involvement of extralymphatic organ or site (III_E) or by involvement of the spleen (III_S), or both (III_{SE}).

Stage IV Diffuse or disseminated involvement of one or more extralymphatic organs or tissues with or without associated lymph node enlargement. The reason for classifying the patient as stage IV should be identified further by defining site by symbols.

(Each stage is subdivided into A or B category to indicate absence or presence of general symptoms.)

Examples of the combined staging classification are as follows:

$CSII^A_{(3)}PSIII_{S+N+H-M-}$ means clinical stage II^A with involvement of three node regions and PSIII with spleen positive, abdominal lymph node positive, liver biopsy negative, and bone marrow biopsy negative.

$CSIV^B_{LH}PSIV_{H+M-}$ means clinical stage IV^B with gross evidence of lung and hepar (liver) involvement and PSIV with liver biopsy positive and bone marrow biopsy negative.

Microscopic evidence of vascular invasion in Hodgkin's disease may be another feature used in assessing prognosis. This finding in patients with Hodgkin's disease, regardless of histologic type, appears to be associated with an increased incidence of the disease in non-adjacent lymph nodes and extranodal sites.

Immunologic aspects of malignant lymphoma. Numerous reports have appeared recently that emphasize the relationship of the immune system to malignant lymphomas. As already noted, there is an increased incidence of these neoplasms in patients receiving renal transplants and in those with certain immunologic disorders. Some investigators have suggested that long-lasting immune responses to certain antigens (whether microbial, foreign tissue [transplant], or self-antigens) may lead to the development of the tumors, perhaps by activating a latent oncogenic virus. Various immunologic and cytochemical techniques for identifying surface cell markers or biochemical markers of T and B cells, as well as certain morphologic techniques such as scanning electron microscopy, are being utilized to develop a more functional classification of malignant lymphomas that may lead to a better understanding of the clinical course, prognosis, and therapy of these lesions.

As a result of these studies, it appears that most of the lymphocytic and mixed lymphomas, especially those with a follicular (nodular) pattern, are derived from the B cells. Relatively few lymphomas have been identified as the T cell type. In a significant number of patients with Burkitt's lymphoma, the tumor cells had B cell characteristics. Furthermore, it has been suggested that lymphomas of histiocytes or identifiable reticulum cells may be rare and that most of those lesions previously classified under these designations may be derived from transformed lymphocytes.

In Hodgkin's disease, a T cell abnormality is suspected since patients with this disease show evidence of deficient cell-mediated immune responses, e.g., reduced capacity for graft rejection and depressed antimicrobial cellular immunity, particularly involving certain viral and fungal infections. Some investigators suggest that a defective T cell surveillance system in Hodgkin's disease allows the development of the characteristic Sternberg-Reed cells from the reticulum cells. Others propose that the Sternberg-Reed cells may represent a polyploid expression of transformed lymphocytes or immunoblasts rather than atypical or malignant histiocytes (reticulum cells).

On the basis of their morphologic studies,

Lukes and Collins have recently characterized the cells of the follicle centers according to their degree of cleavage and size, i.e., "small cleaved," "large cleaved," "small noncleaved," and "large noncleaved." They suggest that the follicular center is the site of normal transformation in the B cell system and that the small lymphocyte changes through a cleaved cell phase to the large noncleaved cell. Cells with the morphologic features of these follicular center cell types have been found to make up the majority of nodular and diffuse forms of non-Hodgkin's lymphoma. These authors also report a lymphoma in which the cells are described as "convoluted lymphocytes," i.e., noncohesive lymphocytes with nuclei that have a convoluted-appearing surface. These cells are probably of the T cell type. This lymphoma presents as a mediastinal mass, particularly in adolescent patients, and eventually enters a leukemic phase. The same authors propose the term *immunoblastic sarcoma* for a group of lymphomas that tend to occur in patients with chronic diseases of probable autoimmune nature, such as severe rheumatoid arthritis and systemic lupus erythematosus, and in older patients without immunologic disorders. The tumors are made up of cells that are indistinguishable from large transformed lymphocytes. The lymphomas reported as reticulum cell sarcomas in Sjögren's syndrome, in primary immunodeficiencies, and in graft recipients during immunosuppressive therapy may be of this type.

In 1974, Lukes and Collins proposed a functional classification of malignant lymphomas that relates the cytologic types to immunologic surface markers. The authors concluded that malignant lymphomas are neoplasms of the immune system, including principally the B and T cell systems and rarely histiocytes. In a later report, Lukes and his associates presented results of their surface marker studies of a large group of cases with non-Hodgkin's lymphomas and leukemias (including the lesions reported previously by Lukes and Collins) in which the diagnosis was initially established on a purely morphologic basis. The cases were grouped in accordance with the Lukes-Collins classification (see below). The B cell group constituted most of the cases, and of these the majority were follicular center cell lymphomas. In the T cell group, the most common types were convoluted lymphocytic lymphomas and immunoblastic sarcomas. Most of the lesions composed of small lymphocytes were classified as B cell type and relatively few as T cell type.

1 *B cell type:* Cases with small B lymphocytes, those with plasmacytoid lymphocytes, and those with follicular center cell types (small cleaved, large cleaved, small noncleaved, and large noncleaved); also immunoblastic sarcoma (B cell type) and hairy cell leukemia

2 *T cell type:* Cases with small T lymphocytes and those with convoluted lymphocytes; also mycosis fungoides, Sézary syndrome, immunoblastic sarcoma (T cell type), and Lennert's lymphoepithelial cell lymphoma

3 *Histiocytic type:* Only rarely observed

4 *U cell (undefined) type:* Cases with primitive-type cells not readily classified and without detectable discriminating markers (primarily acute lymphocytic leukemias of childhood)

Mycosis fungoides. Mycosis fungoides, a special type of malignant lymphoma with lesions primarily in the skin, is discussed on p. 694. The *Sézary syndrome* (chronic generalized erythrodermia and lymph node enlargement) may be a form of mycosis fungoides, since similar cells have been identified in each condition. The typical Sézary cell, which appears in the peripheral blood and tissue infiltrates, is large and has a characteristic cerebriform nuclear structure. Studies have shown that Sézary cells have T lymphocyte markers.

LIPIDOSES

The lipidoses (lipid storage diseases) are a group of conditions in which an abnormal accumulation of fatty substance occurs within reticulum cells or tissue histiocytes. Often congenital or familial, they are the result of an abnormality of fat metabolism. It has been debated whether the large fat-holding cells are

Table 17-3. Lipidoses

Disease	Lipid substance	Organs and tissues involved
Gaucher's disease	Cerebroside (kerasin)	Spleen, liver, bone marrow, skin, brain (infantile or acute neurologic form)
Niemann-Pick disease	Phospholipid (sphingomyelin principally)	Generalized—reticuloendothelial, epithelial, and connective tissue cells
Amaurotic family idiocy (Tay-Sachs disease)	Ganglioside	Central nervous system—glial and ganglion cells
Xanthomatoses		
Hand-Schüller-Christian disease	Cholesterol ester	Multiple involvement of skeletal system—bone marrow of skull and femur particularly; lung sometimes involved
Xanthoma palpebrarum	Cholesterol	Skin, particularly of upper eyelids
Xanthoma tuberosum multiplex	Cholesterol	Skin, tendons and tendon sheaths, and periarticular tissues

active participants in the disturbed metabolism or if they simply passively accumulate the lipids in abnormal amount. The main types of lipidoses and the fatty materials involved are outlined in Table 17-3.

Gaucher's disease. Gaucher's disease (cerebroside lipidosis) is a chronic familial disease in which a cerebroside (kerasin) accumulates in reticulum cells of the spleen, liver, lymph nodes, and bone marrow. Rare cases in infancy may have an acute course with early death. Beginning in childhood, it extends into adult life, and the course of the disease may last 20 years or more. The spleen increases progressively in size to reach a weight of 2,000 to 3,000 g. The liver and lymph nodes are enlarged to lesser degrees. Hemosiderosis, pigmentation of skin and conjunctiva, mild anemia, and leukopenia are usually present. An acute infantile form of the disease in which neurologic manifestations are prominent also occurs.

The hypertrophied spleen is firm, reddish brown, and studded with grayish white translucent masses. The liver also is pigmented and shows discrete whitish nodules, and similar masses involve lymph nodes and bone marrow. Microscopically, the distinctive feature consists of the large pale Gaucher cells, which compose the grayish translucent areas (Fig. 17-7). These cells measure 20 to 40 μ or more

in diameter and have a small eccentric nucleus and abundant pale cytoplasm containing fine striations or threads. Multinucleated forms occur. The intracytoplasmic lipid does not stain with the ordinary fat stains. Electron microscopic examination has disclosed that the cellular striations correspond to round, ovoid, or irregular cytoplasmic bodies, which appear related to mitochondria. It has been suggested that the mitochondria are pathogenetically important in the intracellular defect.

Niemann-Pick disease. In Niemann-Pick disease (phosphatide lipidosis), sphingomyelin (a phospholipid), usually with some cholesterol, accumulates in cells of the reticuloendothelial system and in histiocytes in many organs and tissues. Young infants are affected, and death usually occurs before the age of 2 years. The neutral fat, fatty acid, and cholesterol of the blood are increased.

The spleen, liver, lymph nodes, lungs, and bone marrow are most involved, but the lipid-containing cells may be found in any organ. The characteristic cells are smaller than Gaucher cells and have a foamy appearance, caused by many fine vacuoles of lipid in the cytoplasm. There is no hemosiderosis. Lesions that occur in the central nervous system resemble, in some respects, those of the infantile form of amaurotic familial idiocy (Tay-Sachs disease), in which a ganglioside is present in

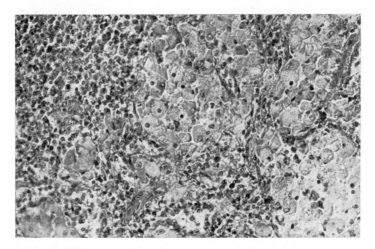

Fig. 17-7. Gaucher's disease of spleen. Note masses of large lipid-filled cells.

the glial and ganglion cells of the nervous system (p. 748).

Xanthomatosis. *Xanthomas* are localized accumulations of cells containing lipid (mainly cholesterol). Grossly, the lesions are yellow. Microscopically, they are made up of large cells filled with doubly refracting lipids. In some cases they are primary or idiopathic, and in other instances they are secondary to disturbances of lipid metabolism, as in primary biliary cirrhosis and diabetes mellitus. The most common sites are in the skin or about tendons. The xanthoma cells are large and rounded and have a vacuolated cytoplasm. Unlike the other lipidoses, the cells of a xanthoma tend to break down and release their fat, so that a granulomatous reaction and fibrosis may be elements in the lesion.

The *Hand-Schüller-Christian syndrome* is an osseous type of xanthomatosis in which the skull particularly is affected. It may occur in childhood or adult life. There is often a characteristic triad of symptoms: defects of membranous bones, exophthalmos, and diabetes insipidus. Blood cholesterol is not increased. The defects in bones are filled by yellow granulomatous material, with many xanthoma cells containing cholesterol. Similar deposits in the pituitary region cause diabetes insipidus and in the orbit lead to exophthalmos. The

lung may be involved and become diffusely fibrosed. There is not much generalized storage in the reticuloendothelial system. It is probable that Letterer-Siwe disease (p. 483) and eosinophilic granuloma (p. 710) are variants of this disease or related conditions. Because the pathologic lesions caused by Hand-Schüller-Christian disease, eosinophilic granuloma, and Letterer-Siwe disease have certain common features, the generic term *histiocytosis X* is sometimes used for this group of disorders.

REFERENCES

Ainsberg, A. C.: N. Engl. J. Med. **288**:883-890, 935-941, 1973 (malignant lymphoma).

Arseneau, J. C., et al.: Am. J. Med. **58**:314-321, 1975 (American Burkitt's lymphoma—clinical aspects).

Banks, P. M., et al.: Am. J. Med. **58**:322-329, 1975 (American Burkitt's lymphoma—pathologic correlations).

Bennett, M. H.: Br. J. Cancer **31**(Suppl. 2):44-52, 1975 (sclerosis in non-Hodgkin's lymphomas).

Braylan, R. C., et al.: In Sommers, S. C., editor: Pathology annual, vol. 10, New York, 1975, Appleton-Century-Crofts, pp. 213-270 (malignant lymphomas—current classification and new observations).

Burkitt, D.: Br. J. Cancer **16**:379-386, 1962 (lymphomas of African children).

Burkitt, D. P., and Wright, D. H.: Burkitt's lymphoma, Edinburgh, 1970, E. & S. Livingstone.

Butler, J. J.: Cancer Res. **31**:1770-1775, 1971 (Hodgkin's disease—prognosis as to histologic types).

Carbone, P. P.: Cancer Res. **31**:1860-1861, 1971 (staging classification for Hodgkin's disease).

Craver, L. F., and Miller, D. G.: The malignant lymphoma, New York, 1966, American Cancer Society.

Fisher, E. R., and Reidbord, H.: Am. J. Pathol. **41:**679-692, 1962 (Gaucher's disease).

Flad, H.-D.: Recent Results Cancer Res. **46:**48-54, 1974 (immunology and immune reactions in malignant lymphomas).

Frizzera, G., et al.: Lancet **1:**1070-1073, 1974 (angioimmunoblastic lymphadenopathy with dysproteinemia).

Golomb, H. M.: Cancer **42:**946-956, 1978 (hairy cell leukemia).

Gough, J.: Int. J. Cancer **5:**273-281, 1970 (Hodgkin's disease—correlation of histopathology with survival).

Gowing, N. F. C.: In Sommers, S. C., editor: Pathology annual, vol. 10, New York, 1975, Appleton-Century-Crofts, pp. 1-20 (infectious mononucleosis).

Kawasaki, T., et al.: Pediatrics **54:**271-275, 1974 (mucocutaneous lymph node syndrome).

Keller, A. R., et al.: Cancer **22:**487-499, 1968 (Hodgkin's disease—correlation of histopathology with prognosis).

Landing, B. H., and Larson, E. J.: Pediatrics **59:**651-662, 1977 (infantile periarteritis nodosa with coronary artery involvement and fatal mucocutaneous lymph node syndrome).

Lee, R. E., et al.: In Sommers, S. C., and Rosen, P. P., editors: Pathology annual, part 2, vol. 12, New York, 1977, Appleton-Century-Crofts, pp. 309-339 (Gaucher's disease).

Lukes, R. J. (chairman): Cancer Res. **26:**1311, 1966 (histologic types of Hodgkin's disease).

Lukes, R. J., and Butler, J. J.: Cancer Res. **26:**1063-1083, 1966 (Hodgkin's disease).

Lukes, R. J., and Collins, R. D.: Cancer **34:**1488-1503, 1974 (immunologic characterization of human malignant lymphomas).

Lukes, R. J., and Collins, R. D.: Recent Results Cancer Res. **46:**18-30, 1974 (functional approach to classification of malignant lymphomas).

Lukes, R. J., and Tindle, B. H.: N. Engl. J. Med. **292:**1-8, 1975 (immunoblastic lymphadenopathy resembling Hodgkin's disease).

Lukes, R. J., et al.: Cancer **19:**317-344, 1966 (Hodgkin's disease).

Lukes, R. J., et al.: Am. J. Pathol. **90:**461-486, 1978. (non-Hodgkin's lymphomas—morphology and surface markers).

Mann, R. B., et al.: Am. J. Med. **58:**307-313, 1975 (immunologic and morphologic studies of T cell lymphoma).

Mann, R. B., et al.: Am. J. Pathol. **94:**103-176, 1979 (malignant lymphoma—a review).

Morens, D. M., and O'Brien, R. J.: J. Infect. Dis. **137:**91-93, 1978 (Kawasaki disease in the United States).

Movat, H. Z., and Fernando, N. V. P.: Exp. Mol. Pathol. **4:**155-188, 1965 (fine structure of lymphoid tissue).

Nathwani, B. N., et al.: Cancer **41:**578-606, 1978 (malignant lymphoma arising in angioimmunoblastic lymphadenopathy).

Pattengale, P. K., et al.: N. Engl. J. Med. **291:**1145-1148, 1974 (atypical lymphocytes in infectious mononucleosis).

Pearson, H. A., et al.: N. Engl. J. Med. **298:**1389-1392, 1978 (splenosis following splenic trauma).

Rappaport, H.: Tumors of the hematopoietic system. In Atlas of Tumor Pathology, Sect. 3, Fasc. 8, Washington, D.C., 1966, Armed Forces Institute of Pathology.

Rappaport, H., et al.: Cancer **9:**792-821, 1956 (follicular lymphoma).

Rappaport, H., et al.: Cancer Res. **31:**1794-1798, 1971 (vascular invasion in Hodgkin's disease).

Rosenberg, S. A.: Cancer Res. **26:**1310, 1966 (staging of Hodgkin's disease).

Roulet, F. C., editor: The lymphoreticular tumours in Africa, Basel, 1964, S. Karger.

Schulz, D. R., and Yunis, A. A.: N. Engl. J. Med. **292:**8-12, 1975 (immunoblastic lymphadenopathy with mixed cryoglobulinemia).

Siegal, F. P., et al.: Am. J. Pathol. **90:**451-460, 1978 (surface markers in leukemias and lymphomas).

Spiegelman, S., et al.: Cancer Res. **33:**1515-1526, 1973 (RNA tumor viruses and malignant lymphomas).

Strauchen, J. A., et al.: N. Engl. J. Med. **299:**1382-1387, 1978 (diffuse histiocytic lymphoma).

Thomas, L. B., et al.: N. Engl. J. Med. **292:**17-22, 1975 (vinyl-chloride liver disease and Banti's syndrome).

van Unnik, J. A. M., et al.: Br. J. Cancer **31:**(Suppl. 2):201,207, 1975 (non-Hodgkin's lymphoma—clinical staging and survival).

18

Blood and blood-forming organs

The conditions in which alteration in the constituents of the blood is the prominent feature are primarily diseases of blood-forming tissue, especially of bone marrow. The changes in the blood, which are most easily studied clinically, are reflections of the basic defect in hematopoietic structure and function. The following is a simplified classification:

Diseases involving red blood cells
  Deficiency of red blood cells and hemoglobin—anemia
  Excess of red blood cells—polycythemia
Diseases involving white blood cells
  Deficiency of white blood cells—leukopenia and agranulocytosis
  Excess of white blood cells—leukocytosis and leukemia
Hemorrhagic diseases

Diseases involving red blood cells

ANEMIA

In anemia, there is a quantitative deficiency of hemoglobin, and usually it is accompanied by a corresponding decrease in number of red blood cells. Different types of anemia show varying degrees of dissociation between the reduction of hemoglobin and of red cells.

General features. Although anemias of particular types have certain pathologic changes that are more or less characteristic, there are also features common to all severe anemias. These include pallor of skin, mucous membranes, fat, and muscle and fatty change in the heart and liver. In severe anemias, fatty degeneration of the myocardium is often of extreme degree and is especially prominent on the endocardial surface, where thrush-breast markings may be seen (p. 27). Atrophic changes frequently affect the mucosa of the alimentary canal. Small hemorrhages of the skin and of the mucosal and serous surfaces are common terminally. Red blood cells may show variations in size (anisocytosis), shape (poikilocytosis), and staining properties (polychromasia).

Classification. An etiologic classification of the anemias is, in many cases, readily correlated with morphologic and other changes in the red blood cells that can be determined by laboratory tests. It is also helpful as a guide to rational therapy. It is recognized, however, that as yet not all anemias are readily classifiable on this basis.

Anemias resulting from defective erythrocyte formation caused by
  Deficiency
    Deficiency of iron (microcytic and hypochromic anemia)
      Inadequate iron intake or absorption
      Excessive iron loss, as in chronic bleeding
      Chlorosis
      Idiopathic hypochromic anemia
    Deficiency of specific hematopoietic principle (macrocytic anemia)

496

Pernicious anemia (vitamin B_{12} deficiency)
Folic acid–deficiency anemia
Megaloblastic anemias of pregnancy, etc.
Other factors
Aplastic anemia
Anemia of nephritis
Anemias resulting from carcinomatosis of bone and osteosclerosis (myelophthisic anemia)
Anemias of thyroid deficiency (myxedema) and scurvy
Anemias resulting from decreased erythrocyte survival (hemolytic diseases)
Hemoglobinopathies (e.g., sickle cell anemia)
Hemolytic disease of newborn infants (erythroblastosis fetalis)
Other hemolytic anemias—congenital and acquired
Anemias resulting from loss of blood
Acute posthemorrhagic anemia
Chronic posthemorrhagic anemia (leads to iron deficiency)

Iron-deficiency anemia. When there is deficiency of iron supply, hemoglobin cannot be formed in sufficient quantity. Hence, the red blood cells are hypochromic, or have a low concentration of hemoglobin, and tend to be of smaller size (microcytosis). Insufficient dietary intake of iron may be responsible for this type of anemia, but other factors such as failure of absorption or faulty metabolism of the iron may be at fault. Blood loss, particularly chronic bleeding, is a significant cause of iron-deficiency anemia.

Chlorosis is an anemia characterized by a faintly greenish pallor of the skin, and it responds remarkably to iron therapy. Rarely encountered now, it is said formerly to have been very common among young women.

Idiopathic hypochromic anemia occurs frequently among middle-aged women. There may be soreness and atrophy of the mucosa of the tongue, and achlorhydria is often present. Dysphagia is a peculiar complication in some patients *(Plummer-Vinson syndrome)*. Iron therapy is effective.

Pernicious anemia. Pernicious anemia (Addison's anemia) was formerly referred to as a primary anemia. It is caused by a deficiency of vitamin B_{12}, which results from a lack of secretion of gastric *intrinsic factor*. The latter is needed for absorption of vitamin B_{12} by the intestinal mucosa. The vitamin deficiency apparently causes defective DNA synthesis in the proliferating cells in the bone marrow without impairing RNA synthesis. This leads to a decrease in the rate of cell division but an increase in intracellular components, so that the cells become enlarged. The result is a megaloblastic anemia with enlarged red cells in the blood (macrocytic anemia). Granulocytes are affected also, so that hypersegmented polymorphonuclear leukocytes appear in the blood. The large red blood cells are well filled with hemoglobin. Intramarrow hemolytic activity (increased destruction of the defective red blood cells) is also present, as is evident from an abundant hemosiderin deposition in the liver, spleen, and bone marrow.

Pernicious anemia occurs most frequently in adults, its highest incidence being in middle-aged and older persons. The adult disease is associated with a gastric disorder. This is usually in the form of mucosal atrophy of the stomach, particularly in the proximal two thirds, with disappearance of oxyntic and peptic cells and replacement of the fundic type of glands by less differentiated abnormal glands (Fig. 18-1). The inflammatory infiltrate in the atrophic mucosa includes lymphocytes and some plasma cells. The pyloric portion is not altered in most cases (p. 530). Antibodies to intrinsic factor and to parietal cells of the gastric mucosa have been identified in some patients, suggesting the role of autoimmunity in pernicious anemia. Certain studies also suggest that cell-mediated response against intrinsic factor may play a role in the pathogenesis. In some patients, the gastric lesion may be related to hereditary predisposition and advancing age.

Other features include soreness of the tongue, atrophy of the epithelium of the tongue, achlorhydria, and gastrointestinal disturbances. A few cases are complicated by degenerative lesions in the dorsal and lateral columns of the spinal cord (subacute combined degeneration, p. 758). In fatal cases, in addition to the gastric and tongue lesions one may see a lemon yellow tinge in the skin and fat,

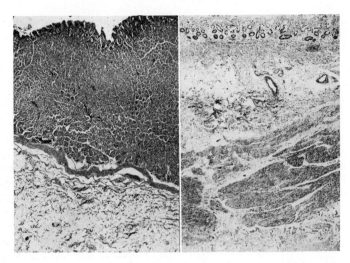

Fig. 18-1. Atrophic gastric mucosa (right) of pernicious anemia contrasted with normal gastric mucosa (left). (×23.)

fatty degeneration in the heart and possibly also in the liver and kidneys, and excessive deposition of hemosiderin in the liver and spleen. The hematopoietic tissue of the bones is hyperplastic, and a deep red marrow is found in the long bones, which normally harbor a yellow fatty marrow. The hyperactive marrow is composed almost entirely of erythroblastic tissue.

Other gastric disorders that may be associated with the adult form of pernicious anemia include gastrectomy and destructive mucosal lesions (e.g., those caused by ingestion of corrosives). A congenital form of pernicious anemia exists that usually becomes manifest in early childhood. In this form, intrinsic factor is lacking, but other constituents of the gastric secretion are normal, and there is no structural defect in the stomach.

Folic acid–deficiency anemia. Megaloblastic anemia may be caused by folic acid deficiency, which, like vitamin B_{12} deficiency, results in intracellular defective DNA synthesis. Folic acid deficiency may occur in certain intestinal disorders accompanied by malabsorption (e.g., *tropical sprue* and the *gluten-sensitive enteropathies,* which include *nontropical sprue* and *celiac disease*). Coincident malabsorption of vitamin B_{12} may also be present, particularly in tropical sprue. A defect in folic acid absorption with resultant megaloblastic anemia has been reported as a complication of ingestion of anticonvulsant drugs and, rarely, in women using oral contraceptives. Folic acid deficiency may be observed also in chronic alcoholics, partly because of inadequate ingestion of folic acid resulting from poor diet and partly because alcohol interferes with the intermediate metabolism of folic acid.

Occasionally, megaloblastic anemia caused by deficiency of folic acid may be seen in pregnancy. However, anemia in pregnancy is most often of the iron-deficiency type.

Aplastic anemia. In aplastic anemia, there is a failure of maturation of blood-forming cells at an early undifferentiated stage. An extreme degree of anemia results, in which evidence of regenerative activity of the blood is lacking and the red blood cells present are of approximately normal size, shape, and staining (normocytic and normochromic). Leukocytes also are depressed. The condition is rapidly progressive and fatal, with hemorrhagic and purpuric phenomena prominent in late stages. The cause is usually unknown, but in some cases it is due to chemical poisons (e.g., benzene and trinitrotoluene), anticancer chemotherapeutic agents (nitrogen mustard, cytoxan, antimetabolites, etc.), antimicrobial agents (chloramphenicol, sulfonamides, etc.), other drugs, and ionizing radiation. A familial form of aplastic anemia occurs in the Fanconi syndrome.

The postmortem findings are those of a severe anemia, such as fatty change of the heart and petechial hemorrhages of serous surfaces. The changes actually found in the bone marrow are variable. The normally red marrow may be aplastic, appearing yellow and fatty. In other cases, however, the marrow is active or even hyperplastic, but it exhibits failure of maturation of the hematopoietic cells at an early stage.

Anemia of nephritis. A hypochromic anemia is a common accompaniment of nephritis, sepsis, and other infective conditions. It apparently results from some toxic effect on the bone marrow and responds poorly to treatment unless the causative factor is removed.

Myelophthisic anemia. Myelophthisic anemia is caused by the replacement of the blood-forming tissue of the bone marrow. Widespread tumor growth replacing marrow tissue may act in this way as a result of multiple myeloma (p. 718) or metastatic carcinoma from the breast, thyroid gland, prostate gland, kidney, etc. A similar effect is observed in osteosclerotic bone disease, in which overgrowth of dense bone encroaches on the marrow (p. 702). Some cases of aleukemic myelosis (myeloid metaplasia) may be associated with marrow fibrosis (p. 507).

Anemia of myxedema and scurvy. The anemia in myxedema and scurvy is not infrequently hypochromic and microcytic. In women with myxedema, menorrhagia is common, and this results in iron deficiency. In scurvy, other nutritional deficiencies are often associated. However, in both of these conditions macrocytic anemia may also occur. In myxedema, this develops because of vitamin B_{12} deficiency that results from a lack of intrinsic factor, and in scurvy, folic acid deficiency may be associated with vitamin C deficiency.

Sickle cell anemia. An inherited disorder of red blood cells in heterozygous form is found in about 8% of black persons. This peculiarity, referred to as sicklemia or sickle cell trait, is the tendency of the cells to assume bizarre shapes when exposed to low oxygen tension, many becoming elongated, pointed, and sickle shaped. The sickling can be observed in blood preserved in sealed moist slide preparations or in tissues fixed in formalin or Zenker's solution (Fig. 18-2).

Sickle cells are found in high percentages in the venous circulation in sickle cell anemia but not in the peripheral circulation of persons who have only the sickle cell trait. The anemia is at least partially hemolytic in type, for the sickled red cells have greater mechanical fragility, and there are signs of red cell destruction as well as of increased regenerative activity on the part of the bone marrow.

Studies have demonstrated chemical differences in hemoglobins, and several varieties are distinguishable by electrophoresis. Sickling or distortion of red blood cells is caused by the presence of hemoglobin S, which, in the absence of oxygen, is no longer soluble and forms crystals and "tactoids." Hemoglobin S is inherited, wholly or in part. A heterozygous person with a mixture of normal adult hemoglobin and hemoglobin S has the sickle cell trait, and sickling may not occur in the bloodstream, although it may be produced in vitro by deprivation of oxygen. A homozygous person with only hemoglobin S may have a sickle cell anemia, for many of the red cells undergo sickling in the peripheral circulation at venous oxygen tensions.

The broader term *sickle cell disease* has been used to include all the hereditary and hematologic conditions in which the sickle cell hemoglobin (Hb S) is present, including sickle cell trait (Hb A-S), sickle cell anemia (Hb S-S), and various combinations of hemoglobin S with other abnormal hemoglobins (e.g., C, D, and E) and with other hereditary diseases such as thalassemia and spherocytosis.

A milder form of sickle cell anemia has been found in persons with a mixture of hemoglobin S and hemoglobin C (sickle cell–Hb

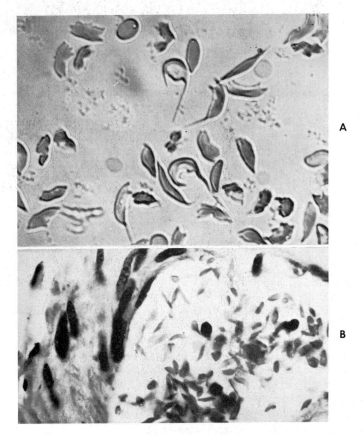

Fig. 18-2. Sickled red blood cells in moist preparation, **A,** and in lumen of blood vessel, **B.**

C disease). Vascular occlusions and hemolytic phenomena similar to those of other sickle cell anemias may be present, sickling occurs in the peripheral blood, and stained smears of the blood show a prominent proportion of target cells.

Pathologic features of sickle cell anemia include the sickled erythrocytes and vascular occlusions, consisting chiefly of masses or aggregates of the sickled red blood cells in the small vessels, although thrombi may occur subsequently. The resultant tissue hypoxia may result in focal hemorrhages (Fig. 18-3) and small or large infarcts. Hemosiderin deposits are found in the spleen, liver, bone marrow, lymph nodes, and kidney. The bone marrow is hyperplastic, and its activity is evident from the regenerative blood picture. The splenic changes in sickle cell anemia are particularly noteworthy. In early stages, the spleen is enlarged, and extreme congestion or hemorrhage is noted around the malpighian corpuscles. Later, fibrosis develops, with noticeable pigment deposits and the formation of siderofibrotic nodules (Gandy-Gamna bodies, p. 478). Fibrotic atrophy of the spleen may progress to an extreme degree (Fig. 18-4).

Sickle cell crises (acute episodes of pain and fever) may occur at intervals in individuals with sickle cell disease. The crises may be precipitated by infection, exposure to cold, or other factors, but at times the cause is not evident. They apparently result from vascular occlusions in various areas, but there may also

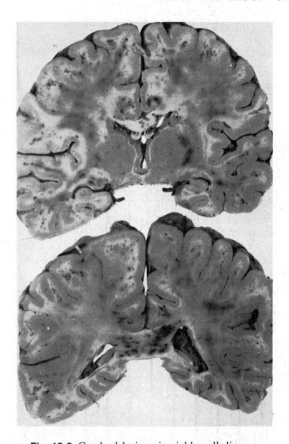

Fig. 18-3. Cerebral lesions in sickle cell disease.

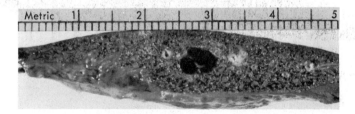

Fig. 18-4. Atrophic and fibrotic spleen of sickle cell anemia.

be hematologic crises of aplastic or hemolytic type. Persons with sickle cell disease have developed symptoms and lesions when exposed to low oxygen tensions during airplane flights and at high altitudes in mountains. Necrosis in the spleen is particularly common, but infarcts also have been observed in the kidneys, brain, and adrenal glands.

In addition to hematuria and infarcts of the kidney, various other renal abnormalities may be observed in patients with sickle cell anemia, including renal vein thrombosis and the nephrotic syndrome. Also, in an occasional patient an autologous immune-complex membranoproliferative glomerulonephritis has been reported. This lesion is believed to have resulted from renal tubular epithelial antigen, released possibly after renal ischemia or some other phenomenon, causing renal tubular damage.

Erythroblastosis fetalis. Erythroblastosis (hemolytic disease of newborn infants) is a congenital disturbance in which immature red blood cells are present in the circulation in excessive number. There is an accompanying excessive hemolysis, and extramedullary hematopoiesis (particularly in spleen and liver) is often present (Fig. 18-5). Some infants have severe edema and ascites (hydrops fetalis), whereas intense and persistent jaundice is prominent in others (icterus gravis neonatorum). The basal ganglia of the brain may show bile pigmentation (kernicterus). Fatty change or even more severe degeneration is sometimes present in the liver. In instances in which edema is severe, the placenta is usually enlarged and thick, with an increase in size of the villi.

The Rh factor is important in the pathogenesis of erythroblastosis. About 15% of persons are said to lack the Rh factor in their blood. The child of an Rh-negative mother and an Rh-positive father tends to inherit the dominant Rh factor. In this case, the fetus may cause the production of anti-Rh agglutinins in the maternal blood, which, in turn, penetrate the placental barrier and cause destruction of fetal red cells.

For a similar reason, Rh-negative mothers are likely to suffer serious hemolytic reactions if transfused with Rh-positive blood.

Hemolytic disease of the newborn infant is caused even more commonly by ABO incompatibility (usually in Group A or Group B children of Group O mothers), but the disease is usually less serious than that caused by Rh incompatibility.

Other hemolytic anemias. In addition to sickle cell and erythroblastic anemias, there are other forms of hemolytic anemia, congenital and acquired. Among these is *hereditary spherocytosis (congenital hemolytic anemia)*. It is a familial disorder that may become manifest at any age but usually is first detected in childhood. The red blood cells are rounded, forming biconvex disks (spherocytes), and are excessively fragile. Their fragility is demonstrated by their decreased resistance to hypotonic saline solutions. In such solutions, laking begins at a concentration of about 0.7%

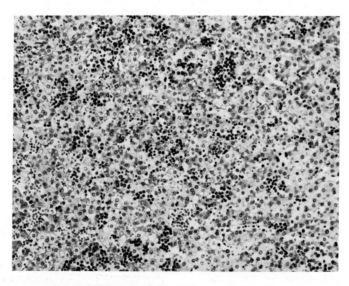

Fig. 18-5. Extramedullary hematopoiesis in liver.

and is complete at 0.46% (corresponding normal figures are 0.44% and 0.35%). The spherocytosis is regarded as a congenital abnormality in the form of the red blood cells that renders them less resistant. It is to be noted, however, that spherocytosis (an increased fragility) may be present in acquired hemolytic anemias also, the changed form resulting from the action of a lytic agent on mature red blood cells. Jaundice results from the excessive bilirubin production, and when the hemolytic action is violent, there may be hemoglobinuria also. Pigment stones often form in the gallbladder. Extreme normoblastic hyperplasia of the bone marrow occurs in an attempt to replace the destroyed red blood cells, and numerous reticulocytes in the circulating blood reflect this regenerative activity.

The spleen shows the changes of greatest interest, being very much enlarged, with distention and congestion of the pulp sinuses. Excess pigment deposit and even siderofibrotic nodules may be present. Histiocytic proliferation, with phagocytosis of red blood cells and giant cell formation, is observed in certain cases. Multiple areas of thrombosis and infarction also may be present. Splenectomy usually is followed by prompt clinical recovery. This is apparently caused by removal of the major mechanism of destruction of the fragile red blood cells, although the fragility of the red cells is not corrected.

Hemolytic anemias of acquired nature may be caused by the direct action of a variety of infectious, physical, and chemical agents. In addition, however, immunologic factors may play a role, as in certain drug-induced hemolytic anemias. Some drugs may form a complex with the antidrug antibody, and the immune complex attaches to red blood cells, usually fixing complement and causing acute intravascular hemolysis. Other drugs, when given in large doses, coat the normal red blood cells and stimulate production of antibody, which reacts with the antigen on the coated cells, resulting in hemolysis. Also, normally occurring protein in the red blood cells may cross-react with antibodies formed against a drug.

Immune hemolytic anemia may occur in association with other systemic diseases, e.g., Hodgkin's disease, other malignant lymphomas, leukemias, sarcoidosis, and systemic lupus erythematosus, or it may occur in the absence of any associated disease *(idiopathic autoimmune hemolytic anemia).*

Anemias caused by hemorrhage. Loss of blood is one of the most common causes of anemia. The loss may be acute and severe, or there may be repeated mild hemorrhages. The anemia is hypochromic in type and may be of severe grade.

POLYCYTHEMIA

Polycythemia is an increase in number of red blood cells. Counts of 7,000,000 to 10,000,000 red cells per cubic millimeter of blood may occur. The cases can be divided into two groups:

1 *Erythrocytosis,* which is a mild type secondary to or compensatory for various conditions in which there is poor oxygenation, as in congenital heart disease of certain types, chronic pulmonary diseases, pulmonary arteriosclerosis, and high altitudes. A form of erythrocytosis has been reported to occur secondary to certain tumors that apparently produce an erythropoietinlike substance.

2 *Erythema (polycythemia rubra; Vaquez-Osler disease),* in which the polycythemia is more pronounced and of unknown etiology or not obviously secondary to a condition of poor oxygenation or an erythropoietin-producing tumor.

Polycythemia rubra usually appears in middle life. It is frequently considered a neoplastic change of erythropoietic cells, comparable to a leukemia. Some investigators have suggested that it may be caused by local anoxemia in the bone marrow itself as a result of arteriosclerotic or inflammatory changes in skeletal vessels, with excessive erythrogenesis as misdirected overcompensation, but this concept is not acceptable to many investigators. The increase of red blood cells is caused by overproduction rather than by any greater longevity or decreased destruction of the cells. Leukopoietic overactivity also develops in some cases, and there may be termination with leukemia or a myelofibrotic syndrome.

The main pathologic finding is engorgement and hyperplasia of bone marrow. The liver and spleen are enlarged and hyperemic. Engorgement of vessels is widespread. Hemorrhages and thromboses are common.

Diseases involving white blood cells

AGRANULOCYTOSIS

Agranulocytosis is a depression of granulocytic (chiefly neutrophilic) leukocyte formation with an extreme decrease in the number of white cells in the blood. It frequently is accompanied by severe infection and ulcerations of the mucosa of the mouth and pharynx (agranulocytic angina). The absence of severe anemia distinguishes agranulocytosis from aplastic anemia, and the absence of thrombocytopenia distinguishes it from aleukemia. Most cases are caused by hypersensitivity to certain drugs, aminopyrine being a frequent and serious offender. Other cases are caused by dinitrophenol, chloropromazine, thiouracil, the sulfonamides, etc. The findings in the bone marrow are variable. Although usually aplastic, in some cases the marrow appears normal or even hyperplastic.

Primary splenic panhematopenia. A condition in which there appears to be excessive destruction of neutrophilic leukocytes and other blood elements by the spleen has been termed primary splenic panhematopenia, or *primary hypersplenism*. In addition to the decrease of granular leukocytes, platelets, and red cells in the peripheral blood, there is splenomegaly and hyperplasia of the bone marrow. Splenectomy often is curative, but unremoved accessory spleens may cause recurrence. Examination of the spleen shows enlargement and increase of reticuloendothelial cells throughout the pulp, with stagnation or sequestration of blood elements in the pulp and sinusoids. It is uncertain whether the

mechanism is simply phagocytic destruction of blood elements or the operation of humoral factors (p. 477).

LEUKEMIA

Leukemia is a condition of lawless overgrowth of white blood cells and proceeds to a fatal ending, although therapy may favorably affect the clinical course in some patients. It is probably best regarded as a neoplastic change in blood-forming tissue, in most cases accompanied by flooding of the blood and tissues with the excess of white cells, many of which are immature or abnormal forms. In some patients, the white blood cell count may be normal or below normal. In such instances, the patient is said to have subleukemic leukemia (subleukemia) or aleukemic leukemia (aleukemia), depending on whether abnormal leukocytes are identified or not identified in the peripheral blood.

Etiology. In most instances, the cause of human leukemia is not known, although much effort has been directed in the search for a specific agent. Ionizing radiation as a cause of human leukemia has been long suspected and has been confirmed by studies on atomic bomb victims in Hiroshima and Nagasaki. The incidence of acute leukemias and chronic granulocytic leukemia was increased in the irradiated population. Exposure to ionizing radiation during fetal life and childhood appears to have a more dangerous leukemogenic effect than in adult life.

Among chemical poisons, benzene appears to have the best established leukemogenic activity.

A possible viral etiology of leukemia has had much recent study. Although viral agents have been accepted as a cause of leukemia in mice, the evidence in human leukemia for a viral etiology is still incomplete. Outbreaks of leukemia cases in "clusters" have suggested an infective agent. Electron microscopy has revealed the presence of particles resembling RNA-type C virus in human leukemic cells. Also, an RNA-directed DNA polymerase (reverse transcriptase) with the biochemical characteristics of the enzyme related to RNA tumor viruses has been isolated from the cytoplasm of human leukemic cells. Recently, it has been reported that the reverse transcriptase identified in leukemic cells from a patient with myelogenous leukemia was identical to that of viruses known to be oncogenic in nonhuman primates.

Most patients with chronic myelocytic leukemia have shown an abnormal chromosome, the Ph[1], or Philadelphia, chromosome, and other chromosomal abnormalities have been observed with less regularity in various leukemias. Patients with Down's syndrome (trisomy of chromosome 21) develop acute leukemia much more frequently than normal children. Genetic damage and somatic mutation may be a possible mechanism of neoplastic transformation in leukemogenesis.

Types. According to the type of white blood cell involved, the leukemias are classed as myelocytic (granulocytic), lymphocytic, and monocytic. Each of these may be acute or chronic, but the acute types are difficult to distinguish from each other. In the lymphocytic leukemias, the lymphatics of the spleen are involved with leukemic cells, but they are not appreciably affected in myelocytic leukemia. In the liver, portal area lymphatic spaces are particularly affected in lymphocytic leukemia, whereas in myelocytic leukemia, the hemic vascular system of the liver and spleen is involved. There is a different age incidence for the various types. Acute lymphocytic (lymphoblastic) leukemia has its maximum incidence in the first decade. Acute myelocytic (myeloblastic) leukemia is unusual in childhood, the incidence being highest after 55 years of age. Chronic myelocytic leukemia occurs between the ages of 25 and 45 years and chronic lymphocytic leukemia between 45 and 60 years. The monocytic type tends to occur more frequently in middle or older age periods. There is evidence that the occurrence of leukemia in persons over 50 years of age is increasing.

Acute leukemia. Acute leukemia may begin suddenly, and it runs a rapid course of a few weeks or months. Early stages may be aleukemic, but later the white blood cell count becomes very high, although less than the extreme figures of chronic leukemia. Anemia and thrombocytopenia are often severe. The majority of white cells in the blood are myeloblasts or lymphoblasts, the distinction between these primitive cells being difficult in some cases. At autopsy, the bone marrow everywhere is hyperplastic and packed with the same primitive white cells. The spleen, lymph nodes, and tonsils usually are moderately enlarged, and their sinuses are filled by the leukemic cells. These cells may also be found infiltrating the liver, heart, kidneys, and other viscera.

Some chronic forms of leukemia may suddenly develop a "blast crisis," during which large numbers of immature blast cells appear in the peripheral blood, as in acute leukemia.

Chronic myelocytic (granulocytic) leukemia. In the myelocytic type of leukemia, there is a great increase in granular leukocytes in the blood, and many immature cells (myelocytes and myeloblasts) are recognizable in blood smears. The total white blood cell count may become very high, reaching 500,000 or more per cubic millimeter in some cases. Platelets also may be increased, but red blood cells progressively diminish in number. The course of the disease may extend over several years before the inevitably fatal end.

The essential lesion is a myeloid hyperplasia throughout the bone marrow, including the marrow of long bones, which normally is yellow and fatty. The marrow tissue is grayish brown and fairly firm. Myelocytes are predominant microscopically, but granular leukocytes in all stages of development are present. The spleen becomes enormously enlarged, dark red, and firm. Masses of granulocytic cells infiltrate the splenic cords and sinuses and obscure the usual splenic architecture. The liver is also considerably enlarged and is infiltrated by granulocytes, the sinusoids being particularly affected. Similar but milder granulocytic infiltration is found in the kidneys, heart, and other viscera. The unusual number of leukocytes in the lumina of blood vessels may be noted in any organ or tissue. Lymph nodes are only slightly enlarged. Infarcts occur commonly in the spleen, more so than in chronic lymphocytic leukemia.

Chronic lymphocytic leukemia. The white blood cell count is lower in lymphocytic leukemia than in the myelocytic type. It is usually below 100,000, and often 90% or more are lymphocytes. Red blood cell reduction and anemia occur in late stages, but to a lesser degree than in myelocytic leukemia.

The lymph nodes all over the body are enlarged (Fig. 18-6), and their normal microscopic architecture is replaced by a diffuse mass of lymphoid cells. The histologic appearance is similar to that observed in diffuse lymphocytic lymphoma, well-differentiated type.

Other lymphoid tissue, as in the tonsils, thymus, and intestine, is similarly affected. The spleen is moderately enlarged by lymphoid hyperplasia, but not to the extreme degree characteristic of myelocytic leukemia. The lymphocytic proliferation involves principally the lymph follicles, although the splenic cords may be infiltrated. Lymphocytic accumulation is found also in the liver, kidneys, skin, etc. The bone marrow is hyperplastic throughout, firm, grayish red, and similar grossly to the marrow of myelocytic leukemia. Except in early stages, the hyperplastic marrow is composed largely of lymphocytes.

Monocytic leukemia. The leukemias in

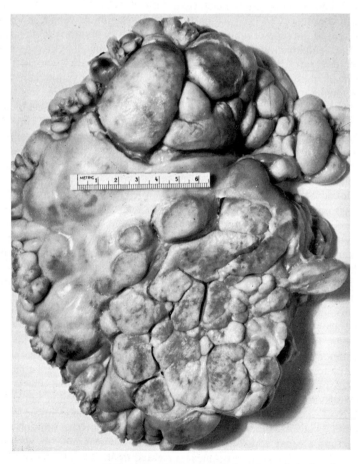

Fig. 18-6. Mesenteric lymph nodes in chronic lymphocytic leukemia.

which mature and immature monocytes are prominent in the blood are referred to as monocytic. Two varieties often are included. The *Naegeli type* is characterized by immature cells intermediate between myeloblasts and monocytes and is probably a variety of myelocytic leukemia. In the *Schilling type,* the immature cells resemble monocytes and histiocytes.

Monocytic leukemia tends to run a rather acute course, often with swelling and hemorrhages of the oral mucosa. Skin lesions are more frequent than in the other types of leukemia.

Leukosarcoma. A localized malignant lymphoma with development of a leukemic blood picture is referred to as a leukosarcoma.

Chloroma. In rare cases of myelocytic leukemia of rather acute type in children or young adults, there are associated tumor masses of a pale greenish color, referred to as chloroma. The greenish color, which may be related to the myeloperoxidase content of the lysosomes in the cells, fades rapidly on exposure to air. The tumor masses are found in close relationship to the periosteum of the bones of the face, ribs, sternum, or vertebrae and, less commonly, in viscera. Microscopically, chloroma is composed of myeloblastic cells.

Primary myelofibrosis. A condition variously termed primary myelofibrosis, myelosclerosis with myeloid metaplasia, aleukemic myelosis, agnogenic myeloid metaplasia, and leukoerythroblastic anemia is considered by some to be a variant form of myelocytic leukemia and by others to be a nonspecific response of potential hematopoietic cells of the spleen and liver to a wide variety of stimuli and of a fundamentally different nature from leukemia.

The disease is characterized by a slowly progressive splenomegaly, with diffuse myeloid metaplasia in a person of middle age or beyond, sometimes with some enlargement of the liver. The liver, and sometimes lymph nodes, also show foci of proliferating myeloid cells and of giant cells of the megakaryocytic type. Usually, there is no significant peripheral lymph node enlargement. Occasionally,

tumorlike masses of extramedullary myeloid tissue are found. The peripheral blood picture is variable, but there may be anemia with the presence of immature red blood cells and leukocytosis with or without leukemoid features. Sometimes, there is an antecedent history of polycythemia rubra vera. The bone marrow is usually fibrotic, although in some instances the marrow may appear normocellular or even hyperplastic. The clinical course often is prolonged but slowly progressive and irreversible. Splenomegaly may be massive in some patients and contributes to the morbidity. Myelofibrosis, sometimes associated with metastatic cancer, malignant lymphomas, or nonneoplastic disease, may produce a similar picture *(secondary myelofibrosis)*.

Cell markers in leukemia. Currently, there is interest in identifying B cell or T cell markers in leukemias as well as in other lymphoproliferative diseases. This approach may lead to a more functional classification of leukemias. However, more investigation is necessary to determine whether these markers have a diagnostic or prognostic significance. In certain studies, most of the patients with chronic lymphocytic leukemia (CLL) were found to have leukemic cells with surface immunoglobulins that were characteristic of B lymphocytes. Only rarely were the leukemic cells in CLL found to be T cell type. Recent studies of the blast cells in acute lymphoblastic leukemia (ALL) reveal heterogeneity in this disease. ALL cells have been identified with either B or T cell markers or with neither B nor T cell markers, which have been referred to by some investigators as "undefined" cells. In certain studies, the "non-B, non-T" cells were the predominant type found in ALL patients. It is of interest that certain characteristics have been noted in the T derived ALL cells that suggest that they are more similar to normal thymocytes than to peripheral T lymphocytes. They were found to contain antigenic determinants shared by thymocytes and not by peripheral T cells, and they were detected by antisera to normal thymocytes. In addition, a thymic-specific enzyme (a type of DNA polymerase known as terminal deoxynucleotidyl transferase or TdT) was detected in circulating blast cells in patients with ALL. This enzyme is lost as cells mature to become peripheral T lymphocytes. An interesting observation was the presence of TdT activity in the cells of some patients with chronic myelocytic leukemia (CML) in blast crisis, suggesting that some patients with CML may undergo a lymphoblastic rather than a myeloblastic crisis.

Hemorrhagic diseases

The oversimplified classic theory of blood coagulation has been expressed as two equations:

$$\text{Prothrombin} + \text{Thromboplastin} + \text{Calcium} = \text{Thrombin}$$

$$\text{Fibrinogen} + \text{Thrombin} = \text{Fibrin}$$

It has been shown that the chemistry of blood coagulation is much more involved and complicated than depicted in the foregoing equations and that numerous factors that have been given various names play some role in the process. A schematic representation of the role of the various factors in blood coagulation is shown in Fig. 18-7. The more common hemorrhagic disorders may be classified in this fashion.

Diminished prothrombin caused by
    Lack of vitamin K
        Dietary origin
            Hemorrhagic disease of newborn infants
        Faulty absorption
            Lack of bile salts
            Obstructive jaundice
            Biliary fistula
            Sprue
    Liver damage
        Faulty utilization of vitamin K

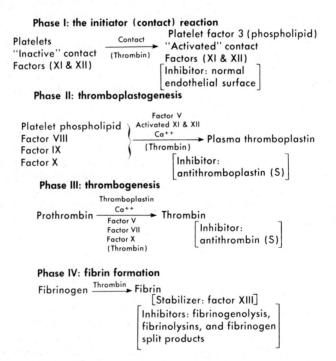

Fig. 18-7. Schematic representation of blood coagulation. (From Miale, J. B.: Normal and abnormal hemostasis. In Anderson, W. A. D., and Kissane, J. M., editors: Pathology, ed. 7, St. Louis, 1977, The C. V. Mosby Co.)

Severe hepatocellular disease (various causes)

Deficiency of platelets or thromboplastin generation

  Abnormality in number or function of platelets

    Thrombocytopenic purpura

    Thrombocytopathic purpura

    Thrombocythemic purpura

  Deficiency of antihemophilic factor (VIII)

    Hemophilia

  Deficiency of factors IX, X, etc.

    Hemophilialike disorders

Decreased fibrinogen

  Acquired

    Nutritional deficiencies

    Diseases of blood-forming organs

    Severe liver damage

    Defibrination (also reduces platelets and other clotting factors), as in

      Amniotic fluid embolism

      Visceral carcinomas

    Excess fibrinolytic activity, as in

      Severe burns

  Congenital

Anticoagulants in blood

  Circulating anticoagulants

    During or following pregnancy

    In leukemia and other neoplasias

    In systemic lupus erythematosus

  Excessive anticoagulant therapy

Primary vascular defects

  Hereditary

    Hereditary hemorrhagic telangiectasia

  Acquired

    Vitamin C deficiency

    Allergic purpura

PURPURA

Purpura is the condition of petechial and ecchymotic hemorrhages in the skin and mucous membranes. Symptomatic purpura occurs in various conditions, such as leukemia, severe anemia, and severe infections such as smallpox and streptococcal septicemia. Certain forms of purpura, however, appear to be entities of themselves. They are associated with a decrease in the number of blood platelets (thrombocytopenia), a normal platelet count but abnormalities of the platelets (thrombocytopathia), or an increase in the number of platelets (thrombocythemia).

Thrombocytopenic purpura. In thrombocytopenic purpura (purpura hemorrhagica;

Werlhof's disease), there is not only a deficiency of platelets but also some weakness or dysfunction of the walls of small blood vessels. Spontaneous hemorrhages occur into the skin, mucous membranes, joints, and intestinal tract. The condition occurs chiefly in children and young adults.

The bone marrow is of normal appearance and contains a normal proportion of megakaryocytes. It has been suggested that the platelet deficiency is caused by thrombocytolysis rather than by deficient formation. Megakaryocytes may be found in the sinuses of the spleen and liver. The spleen also shows enlarged and hyperactive germinal centers. The finding of antiplatelet antibody in patients with this disease suggests that an autoimmune mechanism may play a role in the pathogenesis.

In addition to this primary (immunologic) form of thrombocytopenic purpura, a secondary thrombocytopenia may occur in a variety of known disorders, e.g., aplastic anemia, leukemia, malignant lymphoma, myelofibrosis, and chronic infections, and also as a result of exposure to certain drugs and chemicals and ionizing radiation.

Thrombotic thrombocytopenic purpura. Thrombotic thrombocytopenic purpura (diffuse platelet thrombosis; thrombocytopenic verrucal angionecrosis) appears to be a disseminated disease of the capillaries and arterioles, characterized by diffuse hyaline thrombi. The arterioles and capillaries are partially or completely occluded by a hyaline or finely granular eosinophilic material that may be covered by an endothelial lining. A degenerative process in the vascular walls may be the primary process. The myocardium, renal cortex, capsular zone of the adrenal gland, and brain are mainly involved, but other organs also may show the lesions.

The clinical syndrome is characterized by acute onset with fever, hemolytic anemia, thrombocytopenic purpura, and sometimes bizarre neurologic manifestations (*Moschcowitz's syndrome*). The disease is fatal within a few weeks. The etiology is unknown, but some evidence suggests that hypersensitivity may be concerned, and there may be similarities to some of the so-called collagen diseases (p. 684).

Thrombocytopathic purpura (thrombasthenia). Purpura may be due to morphologic and functional abnormalities (thrombocytopathic) in the presence of a normal number of platelets, although the clinical features simulate those of thrombocytopenic purpura.

Thrombocythemic purpura. An excessive number of circulating platelets (thrombocytosis or thrombocythemia) may be associated with a defect in thromboplastin generation and a hemorrhagic tendency, usually when the count is 1 million or more per cubic millimeter. In some instances, there may also be formation of thrombi.

HEMOPHILIA

Hemophilia is an inherited abnormality of the blood, transmitted as a sex-linked recessive mendelian factor and appearing only in males. The coagulation time of the blood is prolonged, but the bleeding time, clot retraction, prothrombin time, platelet count, and tourniquet test are normal. Severe and prolonged hemorrhages follow trivial injuries. The classical hemophilia (or hemophilia A), which is referred to here, is caused by a deficiency of factor VIII (antihemophilic factor). Certain hemophilialike disorders exist in which other factors are deficient (factor IX [Christmas factor], factor X, etc.).

DEFIBRINATION SYNDROME

A variety of conditions are characterized by an intravascular coagulation with widespread deposition of fibrin in minute vessels but without the formation of large thrombi. During this process, there is a reduction of fibrinogen, as well as of platelets and other coagulation factors, followed by a hemorrhagic tendency.

This syndrome, also referred to as *disseminated intravascular coagulation* and *consumption coagulopathy,* is observed in certain disorders of pregnancy (such as abruptio placentae, prolonged retention of a dead fetus, or amniotic fluid embolism), in association with certain visceral carcinomas, and after tissue trauma, e.g., excessive manipulation of the lung during surgery. In these conditions, the initiating cause of the intravascular coagulation appears to be the release of thromboplastin into the circulation from the placenta, the tumor, or the lung. Increased activity of fibrinolysin in response to the intravascular coagulation may contribute to the hemorrhagic tendency.

REFERENCES

Ainsberg, A. C., and Bloch, K. J.: N. Engl. J. Med. **287:**272-274, 1972 (immunoglobulins on neoplastic lymphocytes).

Brouet, J. C., and Seligmann, M.: Cancer **42:**817-827, 1978 (cell markers in acute lymphoblastic leukemia).

Bryan, W. R., et al.: In Brown, E. B., and Moore, C. V., editors: Progress in hematology, vol. 5, New York, 1966, Grune & Stratton, Inc., pp. 137-179 (viruses in leukemia and lymphomas).

Chanarin, I., and James, D.: Lancet **1:**1078-1080, 1974 (pernicious anemia—autoimmune factors).

Dean, J., and Schechter, A. N.: N. Engl. J. Med. **299:**752-763, 804-811, 863-870, 1978 (sickle cell anemia—molecular and cellular aspects).

Deykin, D.: N. Engl. J. Med. **283:**636-644, 1970 (disseminated intravascular coagulation).

Diggs, L. W.: Am. J. Clin. Pathol. **44:**1-19, 1965 (sickle cell crises).

Gallo, R. C.: Am. J. Pathol. **60:**80-87, 1973 (RNA tumor viruses and leukemia).

Garratty, G., and Petz, L. D.: Am. J. Med. **58:**398-407, 1975 (drug-induced immune hemolytic anemia).

Koneman, E. W., et al.: Am. J. Clin. Pathol. **40:**1-20, 1963 (sickle cell–thalassemia).

Lieberman, P. H., et al.: Cancer **18:**727-736, 1965 (myelofibrosis).

McCaffrey, R., et al.: N. Engl. J. Med. **292:**775-780, 1975 (terminal deoxynucleotidyl transferase in leukemia).

McKay, D. B.: Disseminated intravascular coagulation—an intermediary mechanism of disease, New York, 1965, Harper & Row, Publishers, Inc.

McPhedran, P., and Heath, C. W., Jr.: J.A.M.A. **209:**2021-2025, 1969 (multiple cases of leukemia associated with one house).

Medical News: J.A.M.A. **231:**335-336, 1975 (link between leukemia and RNA tumor viruses).

Miale, J. B.: Laboratory medicine—hematology, ed. 5, St. Louis, 1977, The C. V. Mosby Co. (general reference).

Moloney, W. C.: Cancer **42:**865-873, 1978 (chronic myelogenous leukemia).

Nakai, G. S., et al.: Ann. Intern. Med. **57:**419-440, 1962 (myeloid metaplasia).

Nowell, P. C., and Hungerford, D. A.: Semin. Hematol. **3:**114-121, 1966 (etiology of leukemia).

Quick, A. J.: Hemorrhagic diseases and thrombosis, ed. 2, Philadelphia, 1966, Lea & Febiger.

Rundles, R. W., and Moore, J. O.: Cancer **42:**941-945, 1978 (chronic lymphocytic leukemia).

Sandberg. A. A.: CA **15:**2-13, 1965 (chromosomes and leukemia).

Sandberg, A. A.: The chromosomes in human cancer and leukemia, New York, 1980, Elsevier North-Holland, Inc.

Seligmann, M.: N. Engl. J. Med. **290:**1483-1484, 1974 (B cell and T cell markers in lymphoid proliferations).

Strauss, J., et al.: Am. J. Med. **58:**382-387, 1975 (nephropathy in sickle cell anemia—immune-complex nephritis).

Videback, A.: Acta Haematol. (Basel) **36:**183-197, 1966 (pathogenesis of human leukemia).

Wintrobe, M. M., et al.: Clinical hematology, ed. 7, Philadelphia, 1974, Lea & Febiger (general reference).

19

Mouth, jaws, throat, and neck

The skin of the face and neck is subject to most of the diseases that involve skin elsewhere on the body (Chapter 24). The face is a common site for carcinoma. Carcinomas of the upper half of the face are usually of the basal cell type, whereas squamous carcinoma is more likely to be found on the lower part of the face. The face and neck are common sites for malignant melanoma, sometimes as a transformation of a benign nevus.

Mouth

DEVELOPMENTAL DEFECTS

The most important developmental abnormalities are cleft of the upper lip (harelip) and cleft palate. Clefts occur at places where embryonic processes that should join have failed to unite during embryonic development. In cleft lip, there is a failure of fusion of the processus globularis and the maxillary process on one or both sides, the cleft being slightly to one side of the midline. Cleft palate may be present with or without associated harelip. Hereditary influence is important.

Developmental disturbances also may affect the jaws, teeth, and tongue. Examples are an overgrowth of bone *(exostosis)* that protrudes into the oral cavity and arises in the hard palate *(torus palatinus)* or mandible *(torus mandibularis),* an abnormally small mandible *(micrognathia),* hypoplasia or aplasia of the tooth enamel, fusion of teeth, unusually large or

small teeth, abnormalities in shape or number of teeth, abnormal attachment of the lingual frenulum close to the tip of the tongue ("tongue-tie"), prominently fissured tongue ("scrotal tongue"), cleft or bifid tongue, and so-called *median rhomboid glossitis.* The last-named lesion is incorrectly named since it is not an inflammatory process. This developmental defect involves the dorsum of the tongue posteriorly and is characterized by a smooth, irregularly oval or diamond-shaped depressed or raised area devoid of papillae. It may be mistaken for cancer.

INFLAMMATIONS

Inflammation in the mouth may be a local condition or part of a generalized disease. The two most common oral diseases are *periodontal disease* (gingivitis and periodontitis) and *dental caries* (tooth decay). Although dental caries is not an inflammatory lesion initially, it frequently is accompanied or followed by inflammation of the dental pulp, sometimes with extension to periodontal tissues.

Gingivitis. *Acute* or *chronic gingivitis* (inflammation of the gums) is often the result of local factors, such as impacted food particles, dental plaques, and deposits of calculus. Dental plaques are soft masses adherent to the teeth, consisting of proliferating bacteria and some cellular debris in a sticky polysaccharide-protein matrix. Calcification of some of these plaques results in calculus formation. The calculus, in turn, serves as a site for more plaque formation. Apparently, the superimposed bacterial plaque is the main factor responsible for the irritating effect of calculus. The local factors are more aggravating in patients with systemic conditions that lower the resistance of the gingiva (e.g., diabetes mellitus, hypovitaminosis, drug intoxications, pregnancy, and leukemia).

A severe form of gingival inflammation is *acute necrotizing ulcerative gingivitis* (trench mouth or Vincent's angina), in which *Fusobacterium fusiforme* and *Borrelia vincentii* are the predominant microorganisms. The necrosis and ulceration may extend beyond the gums to other areas of the oral mucosa *(gingivostomatitis)* or to the tonsils and pharynx. Cervical lymphadenitis may occur.

Periodontitis. Periodontal disease includes that which is confined to the gums *(gingivitis)* and that affecting the underlying supporting periodontal tissues, referred to as *periodontitis*. Periodontitis begins as gingivitis. However, not all instances of gingivitis result in periodontitis. Inflammation of the gingiva spreads to the alveolar bone, causing destruction and resorption of the bone, and there is loss of the periodontal ligaments that join the teeth to the bone. With separation of the soft tissues from the bone, "pockets" form about the teeth from which pus may exude *(pyorrhea)*. As the disease progresses, prominent gingival recession, bleeding of the gums, and loosening of the teeth occur. Periodontitis is the major cause of tooth loss in adults beyond the age of 35 years.

Dental caries. *Dental caries* (tooth decay) is characterized by destruction of enamel and dentin initiated by acids formed by the interaction of food debris and bacteria. If the disease is untreated, microorganisms invade the pulp, causing an *acute pulpitis*. Suppuration may occur. Extension to the periapical region frequently is followed by a *periapical* or *dentoalveolar abscess,* which may drain into the oral cavity or the maxillary sinus or to the surface of the skin of the face or neck. More serious complications include *osteomyelitis, cellulitis,* or *septicopyemia.* In patients who develop a more chronic type of infection, the

lesions that may be present are *chronic pulpitis, periapical granuloma* (a localized periapical chronic inflammatory nodule), or a *periapical cyst.* Dental decay is the principal cause of tooth loss up to the age of 35 years.

Recurrent herpes labialis. A common lesion caused by herpes simplex virus consists of vesicles most frequently on the mucocutaneous junction of the lips *(fever blisters* or *cold sores).* These vesicles rupture, forming a crust, and may become secondarily infected. They tend to recur at the same site, being induced by such factors, as trauma, sunshine, febrile illness, and menstruation.

Acute herpetic gingivostomatitis. Another manifestation of herpes simplex virus infection is the appearance of multiple vesicular lesions of the lips and oral mucosa, particularly in children. The vesicles rupture and form ulcers. The gingiva is red, swollen, and tender and bleeds easily. Cervical lymphadenitis occurs.

Herpangina. Herpangina is a self-limited, febrile disease caused by coxsackieviruses and characterized by small vesicles or ulcers of the soft palate, tonsils, or pharynx.

Aphthous stomatitis. Aphthous stomatitis is characterized by painful, recurrent, erosive oral ulcerations, covered by a gray membrane and surrounded by a thin erythematous ring. The primary cause is unknown. The lesions, known as "canker sores," resemble those of recurrent herpes but apparently are not caused by the herpes simplex virus.

Measles. In measles, Koplik's spots are an early sign. They are small yellowish spots on a red background, seen on the mucosal surface of the cheeks in the upper molar region.

Mercurial or arsenical compounds. Mercurial or arsenical compounds may cause ulcerative stomatitis.

Agranulocytosis. Severe ulcerative inflammations of the mouth or pharynx often complicate agranulocytosis.

Leukemias. In leukemias, infiltration of the gingiva is common, with hemorrhage and ulceration.

Thrush. Debilitated infants and children particularly are subject to thrush, a local membranous lesion of the mouth caused by *Candida albicans*.

Noma. Noma is a progressive gangrenous ulcerative condition that may lead to perforation of the cheeks.

Syphilis. Syphilis may be represented by lesions of the lips or mouth in either primary or secondary stages (p. 181).

Tuberculosis. Tuberculous lesions of the mouth are uncommon.

TUMORS

The lesions to be discussed are hyperkeratosis (which may be precancerous), carcinoma, and epulis. Cancer of the mouth is, in most cases, squamous cell carcinoma. It may arise from the lip or any area of the oral mucosa, but in more than one half of the intraoral cases it involves the tongue.

Hyperkeratosis. Hyperkeratosis of the mouth appears as irregular, white, thickened areas on the mucosa of the lips, cheeks, tongue, or elsewhere in the oral cavity. The term *leukoplakia* (''white patch'') is commonly used as a synonym, but this term sometimes is applied to any white patch that may be caused by a variety of diseases. Another term for hyperkeratosis is *leukokeratosis*. Oral cancer frequently is preceded by hyperkeratosis and begins as carcinoma in situ, so that hyperkeratosis probably corresponds to the precancerous keratoses of the skin. The squamous epithelium is thickened, with acanthosis or thickening of the prickle cell layer and chronic inflammatory cells in the subepithelial layers. As transformation occurs, the rete pegs become more irregular and prolonged, and there is intraepithelial development of cells of malignant appearance (epithelial dysplasia). Later, infiltration or invasion may occur.

Hyperkeratosis may be caused by chronic irritation induced by ill-fitting dentures, jagged teeth, alcohol, heavy smoking (especially of pipes and cigars), actinic radiation (lower lip), and chewing tobacco. Syphilis may be a cause. Hyperkeratosis appears to be associated with about 20% of oral cancers. Oral carcinoma is frequently multiple or appears to arise in a multicentric or multifocal manner.

A verrucose, well-differentiated squamous cell carcinoma, of a low degree of malignancy, sometimes develops in hyperkeratosis of the gingivobuccal groove in ''snuff dippers,'' who leave tobacco snuff in this location for extended periods.

Carcinoma of lip. Cancer of the lip is common, particularly in males. About 95% occur on the lower lip at the mucocutaneous junction, and almost all are of the squamous cell type. The infrequent carcinomas of the upper lip are more often of the basal cell type and show little difference in sex incidence. Trauma and chronic irritation resulting from jagged or carious teeth, pipe smoking, actinic radiation, etc. are believed to be contributing causes. Certain types of lesions such as hyperkeratosis and chronic fissures may precede the development of actual cancer. The greatest incidence is in the sixth through eighth decades of life.

The early cancer may be a small nodule, warty excrescence, or chronic fissure. It develops into a painless ulcer, which grows slowly. It is to be distinguished from a syphilitic chancre of the lip, which is less well defined and shows evidence of inflammation.

Metastasis occurs to lymph nodes of the submental and submaxillary groups and, from there, to the jugular chain of lymph nodes. More distant metastasis is rare. Extension to lymph nodes occurs earlier in the forms with microscopic evidence of high malignancy.

Carcinoma of tongue. Cancer of the tongue is more common in men than in women and has its greatest incidence in the sixth through eighth decades. However, it is not rare in women, and those with *Plummer-Vinson syndrome* (iron-deficiency anemia, dysphagia, and atrophy of mucosa of the tongue [p. 497]) are prone to develop it. Its most frequent sites are the lateral borders and undersurfaces of the anterior two thirds of the tongue. Chronic irritations and hyperkeratosis may be contributing etiologic factors, as in other cancers of the mouth. The most usual form is a small ulcer or fissure, but papillary or fungating lesions also occur. The tumors are squamous cell carcinomas of varying grades of differentiation.

Metastasis occurs most frequently to upper deep cervical lymph nodes adjacent to the bifurcation of the common carotid artery. Extension to other groups of nodes and metastasis to other tissues tend to be more widespread than in carcinoma of the lip. Cure rates are higher for cancer of the dorsum and the anterior one third of the tongue than for the posterior one third. In general, carcinoma of the tongue has a poorer prognosis than carcinoma of the lip.

Epulis. The term *epulis* is rather loosely used to indicate any benign growth of the gums, usually of connective tissue type. Most often it is applied to nonneoplastic lesions. There are two main histologic forms: (1) giant cell epulis, in which giant cells and blood vessels are prominent, and (2) fibromatous epulis, in which connective tissue is predominant. The giant cell form is similar histologically to the benign giant cell tumors found elsewhere (p. 715). The variable histologic forms may simply represent stages in the development of an epulis. These lesions often are preceded by local mechanical injury to the place of origin, or they may grow in the socket of an extracted tooth. They are actually reparative growths rather than true neoplasms, and although their clinical behavior is benign, they may recur if incompletely removed.

The focal form of gingivitis gravidarum, or "pregnancy tumor," may simulate an epulis. Developing during the first 2 or 3 months of pregnancy, it appears to be on a hormonal basis. A rare congenital epulis occurs mainly in the incisor region of the maxilla in females. It is histologically distinct and probably is a hamartoma of a tooth bud. It consists of granular cells resembling those of a granular cell "myoblastoma."

There is another hamartomatous growth that is often referred to as an epulis. The so-called congenital pigmented epulis of infancy also has been called melanotic adamantinoma, retinal anlage tumor, etc. It is a rare benign lesion of the maxilla of infants, probably of neural crest origin. The growth has an abundant connective tissue stroma, with tubular or gland spaces lined by cuboidal cells with abundant pigment granules.

Jaws

Developmental abnormalities of the jaws and teeth and dental caries have been referred to previously.

TUMORS

Some of the tumors that occur in other bones also may be found in the bones of the jaws (p. 711). In addition, a group of tumors arise from epithelial or mesoblastic tissues of developing teeth. A simple classification of these includes (1) odontogenic cysts and (2) odontogenic tumors (epithelial and mesodermal).

Odontogenic cysts. *Dentigerous cysts* are benign cystic structures in the jaws that are are lined by epithelium and contain one or more imperfectly developed teeth. Trauma may be important in the development of a cyst about an unerupted tooth. Transformation to ameloblastoma within dentigerous cysts has been reported. *Radicular cysts,* formed by chronic inflammation at the opening of the pulp canal, are lined by a squamous epithelium derived from epithelial rests of Malassez in the periodontal membrane.

Odontogenic tumors. Tumors of odontogenic origin are infrequent but of considerable variety and complexity. They may be grouped into epithelial and mesodermal types. The epithelial odontogenic tumors include a variety of ameloblastic tumors, dentinomas, and various odontomas.

Odontomas are the result of disturbances of tooth development that may lead to an atypical growth of enamel, dentin, cementum, or all three hard substances. Odontomas grow slowly and are surrounded by a capsule. The rare soft odontoma is formed from either the dentinal papilla or periodontal membrane.

Ameloblastomas (adamantinomas; Fig. 19-1) are epithelial tumors arising from cells with a potentiality for forming the enamel organ. Their histologic structure resembles certain developmental stages of the enamel organ, but origin as a downgrowth from oral epithelium also has been considered. They are composed of irregular masses of epithelial cells divided

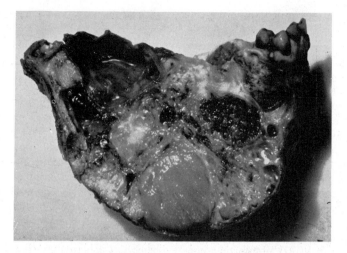

Fig. 19-1. Adamantinoma of jaw.

by a connective tissue stroma. The epithelial masses are outlined by a palisade of dark-staining columnar epithelial cells (Fig. 19-2). In rare instances, some keratinization occurs. Cyst formation is common within the epithelial masses, so that solid, cystic, and combined forms occur.

The tumor is most common in the mandible and usually appears in persons before the age of 35 years. Although it ordinarily does not metastasize, irregular local extension occurs, and the tumor will recur unless removal is complete. A few malignant forms with metastasis have been reported.

Tumors histologically similar to those of the mandible arise in the pituitary region (craniopharyngioma, p. 581) and in the tibia (p. 719).

Mesodermal odontogenic tumors include odontogenic fibromyxomas and cementifying fibromas.

Pharynx

INFLAMMATIONS

Pharyngitis is commonly caused by streptoccal infection, although diphtheria, viruses, and Vincent's organisms also cause characteristic pharyngeal inflammations. The tonsils are most frequently involved and are swollen and reddened with exudate on the surface and in tonsillar crypts. When the crypts are prominently distended with pus, it is often termed follicular tonsillitis. Epidemic tonsillitis is sometimes a milk-borne streptococcal infection. *Quinsy* is a peritonsillar abscess that may complicate acute tonsillitis. *Ludwig's angina* is a diffuse cellulitis or spread of the infection to involve structures of the neck.

TUMORS

Highly malignant tumors occur in the pharynx, arising most commonly from the posterior wall of the nasopharynx or from the tonsil. They are characterized by an earlier age incidence than that of cancers in general, by predominance in the male, and by a tendency to early metastasis to the lymph nodes of the neck or invasion of the base of the skull. Metastasis may appear before the primary growth is noted. As a group, they are highly radiosensitive tumors. This factor, plus their surgical inaccessibility, makes radiation the usual form of treatment. As noted previously, nasopharyngeal carcinoma is one of the lesions linked with the Epstein-Barr virus (p. 258).

Most of these tumors can be classified as (1) squamous cell carcinoma, (2) transitional cell carcinoma, (3) lymphoepithelioma, and (4)

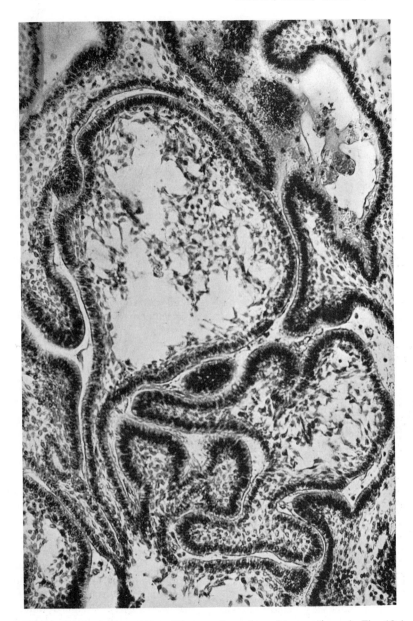

Fig. 19-2. Adamantinoma of jaw. Microscopic section of tumor shown in Fig. 19-1.

malignant lymphoma. Teratomas of the pharynx and solitary myelomas (plasmacytomas) also occur.

Squamous cell carcinoma. Squamous cell carcinoma forms a coarsely granular elevated tumor with an indurated border and ulcerated surface. Its histologic appearance is similar to that of squamous carcinoma elsewhere, with evidence of keratinization.

Transitional cell carcinoma. Transitional cell carcinoma is a type of cancer in which keratinization is absent. It forms a smaller, flatter lesion than does the squamous type, with a finely granular surface. Histologically, the tumor is composed of small uniform cells having large hyperchromatic nuclei and scanty cytoplasm. The cells are more undifferentiated than those of the squamous variety.

Lymphoepithelioma. Lymphoepithelioma, described by Regaud and Schmincke, is a tumor in which wide sheets and cords of undifferentiated malignant epithelial cells are intimately associated with lymphoid tissue or infiltrated with lymphocytes. Many believe that this is not a distinct type of tumor but that its representatives are more properly classified as transitional cell carcinomas, although electron microscopic studies suggest that many of the undifferentiated tumors are squamous cell carcinomas.

Malignant lymphoma. Malignant lymphoma may occur in a localized form or as part of a generalized lymphomatosis.

Nasopharyngeal fibroma. Nasopharyngeal fibroma is an uncommon tumor developing mainly in boys at or near the age of puberty and tending to undergo spontaneous regression by about 25 years of age. It has been considered to arise from periosteum of bone of the vault or posterior wall of the nasopharynx, but a vascular or angiomatous origin with sex-endocrine relationships also has been proposed. The hard tumor is composed of dense but highly vascular connective tissue. It is essentially benign but may be serious because of its progressive growth before sexual maturity and its tendency to profuse hemorrhage.

Salivary glands

Disturbances of the salivary glands include inflammations, duct obstruction (usually caused by calculi), and tumors.

INFLAMMATIONS

Acute parotitis. Acute parotitis occurs in the epidemic virus disease *mumps* (p. 174), but it also may be caused by other microorganisms, particularly *Staphylococcus aureus,*

which involve the gland by way of Stensen's duct when salivary flow is reduced.

Sjögren's syndrome. Sjögren's syndrome occurs mainly in women of menopausal or postmenopausal age. It is generally regarded as an autoimmune disorder and is characterized by dry eyes (keratoconjunctivitis sicca), dry mouth (xerostomia), and dryness of the nose, pharynx, and larynx (nasopharyngolaryngitis sicca), along with inflammation of the salivary glands (sialoadenitis) and, in many cases, rheumatoid arthritis. Lack of secretion of the lacrimal and salivary glands and the submucous glands of the upper respiratory tract is responsible for the characteristic dryness in this condition. In some patients, features of other collagen (autoimmune) diseases, in addition to rheumatoid arthritis, may appear, e.g., systemic lupus erythematosus, polyarteritis, polymyositis, and dermatomyositis. Hypergammaglobulinemia occurs in most cases, and often the rheumatoid factor, antinuclear and antithyroglobulin antibodies, and other autoantibodies may be detected. An increased incidence of malignant lymphomas is observed in patients with Sjögren's syndrome.

The involved salivary glands, which may be enlarged, microscopically show prominent mononuclear cell (chiefly lymphocytic) infiltration. The infiltrating cells cause atrophy of the adjacent acini and may eventually replace a considerable amount of the parenchyma. Small islands of epithelium resulting from ductal proliferation may be seen throughout the glands. Similar microscopic changes may be seen in the lacrimal glands and in the labial and palatal minor salivary glands.

When these changes are found in the salivary glands without the other manifestations of Sjögren's syndrome, the term *Mikulicz's disease* or *benign lymphoepithelial lesion* is sometimes used. The designation *Mikulicz's syndrome* is applied to enlargement of salivary and lacrimal glands resulting from any of a variety of conditions (e.g., sarcoidosis, tuberculosis, Sjögren's syndrome, leukemia, Hodgkin's disease).

Ranula. Ranula is a cystic lesion in the floor of the mouth that may arise from a sublingual gland, a mucous gland, or the submaxillary duct.

Mucocele. A mucocele consists of a localized pool of mucus in a cavity within the connective tissue about a minor salivary gland. Spillage of the mucus is caused by rupture of ducts following obstruction or mechanical trauma. The cavity in which the mucus lies is surrounded by granulation tissue and contains mucus-laden macrophages in addition to the fluid.

Uveoparotid fever. Uveoparotid fever (Heerfordt's syndrome) is a granulomatous involvement of the parotid glands and uveal tract (iris and ciliary body). It appears to be a form of sarcoidosis (p. 149).

TUMORS

A variety of tumors occur in the salivary glands, including both the major salivary glands and the minor foci of salivary gland tissue of the palate and other areas of oral mucosa. However, a very large proportion of salivary gland tumors occur in the parotid gland, are benign, and are "mixed tumors." The submaxillary glands are involved with some frequency. The sublingual gland is involved only rarely.

Benign mixed tumor. Benign "mixed" tumors, commonly referred to as *pleomorphic adenomas,* may develop at any age, but the highest incidence is in early or middle adult life. About 90% occur in the parotid gland, and about 60% occur in females. There are various theories of origin, but most evidence suggests that the neoplasms arise from intercalated ducts and that both epithelial and myoepithelial cells participate in formation of the lesions. Theories of origin from embryonal rests or branchial cleft tissue have little supporting evidence. "Mixed" tumors are solitary, irregularly round or oval, often lobulated, and usually 2 to 5 cm in diameter, although occasional examples may be much larger. The tumors have a capsule of varying thickness, often with defective areas through which neoplastic tissue extends into the surrounding salivary gland. Complete removal is difficult, and recurrence after excision is not infrequent, the incidence of recurrence being estimated to vary from 5% to 45%. Recurrent tumor masses are often multiple separate nodules. One of the serious complications of the removal of a parotid tumor is injury to the facial nerve.

The histologic picture is complex and variable (Fig. 19-3). The neoplastic cells are both epithelial and myoepithelial ("basket") cells in

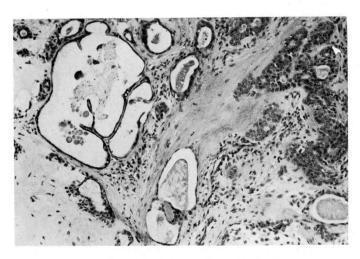

Fig. 19-3. Mixed tumor of parotid gland.

the midst of a stroma that may be composed of fibrous, myxomatous, myxochondroid, chondroid, or even osseous tissues. The neoplastic cells form a variety of patterns. They may be abundant and closely packed, producing a densely cellular appearance, or they may be sparse and widely separated by the stroma. In some areas, the neoplastic cells are in a stellate or spindle pattern and blend imperceptibly with a myxomatous or myxochondroid matrix. The epithelial cells may form an adenomatous, ductal, or cylindromatous pattern. Occasionally, metaplastic squamous epithelium may be present. It has been suggested that the mucoid material in the myxomatous stroma is a product of myoepithelial cells and that the characteristic cartilagelike areas seen in "mixed" tumors develop by transformation of this mucoid material. However, it is also possible that areas of true cartilage and even bone may be formed by metaplasia from fibroblastic stroma.

Mixed tumors often grow very slowly and may be present for years with few symptoms. Rapid enlargement in a tumor that has been present for years and stationary or only slowly growing suggests a malignant change in the tumor. Some investigators doubt that benign mixed tumors transform to the malignant variety and consider the latter to be malignant mixed tumors from the outset.

In a few pleomorphic adenomas, tyrosine or calcium oxalate crystals have been described, being present usually in the myxomatous or chondroid areas. The significance of these crystals is not known. Of these two, the tyrosine crystals have been observed more frequently. They are recognized as rosettelike or petallike structures in the tissues. In one report, foci of calcification were noted in several malignant mixed tumors, particularly in those that metastasized. Among the illustrations of the calcific foci in this report was one depicting "flower petallike" structures that resembled the tyrosine crystals described and illustrated by other investigators.

Oncocytoma. Oncocytoma (oxyphil cell adenoma) is a rare, benign, encapsulated salivary gland tumor composed of cells with eosinophilic granular cytoplasm and small dark nuclei. These cells are oncocytes (oxyphil granular cells), which contain a large number of closely packed mitochondria that fill the entire cytoplasmic compartment.

Papillary cystadenoma lymphomatosum. Papillary cystadenoma lymphomatosum (adenolymphoma; *Warthin's tumor*) is a benign, encapsulated cystic tumor occurring in or at-

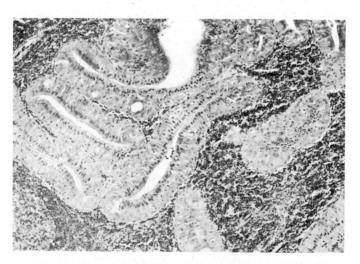

Fig. 19-4. Adenolymphoma (Warthin's tumor) of salivary gland.

tached to the parotid gland. It is rounded, soft, and 2 to 6 cm in diameter. Microscopically, it is composed of papillary, tubular, or cystic epithelial structures having a double layer of deeply eosinophilic cells and set in a lymphoid tissue (Fig. 19-4). The tumor occurs predominantly in males. Athough the origin is debatable, most evidence suggests that the lesion arises from salivary gland or duct tissue inclusions in lymph node tissue either in the parotid gland or adjacent to the gland. It has been shown that the characteristic lymphoid component of this tumor consists predominantly of B lymphocytes.

Malignant mixed tumor. Malignant mixed tumors of salivary gland tissue probably arise most often as a malignant change in a previously existent benign tumor and at a later average age (about 10 years) than benign mixed tumors. However, as mentioned earlier, some investigators have expressed the view that they are malignant from the outset. The malignant mixed tumors are usually larger than benign tumors and tend to be fixed to underlying tissues or to the skin, which may be ulcerated. Regional lymph nodes may be enlarged by metastasis. Although the gross appearance may be similar to that of the benign mixed tumors, there is a greater tendency to areas of softening, necrosis, hemorrhage, or cyst formation. Histologically (Fig. 19-5), the pattern of the tumor cells may be predominantly glandular, basaloid, spindle, squamous, or undifferentiated, but usually areas having the appearance of "benign" mixed tumor are also seen.

Mucoepidermoid carcinoma. Mucoepidermoid carcinomas of salivary tissue are of ductal origin and contain both mucus-secreting and epidermoid cells (Fig. 19-6). They vary greatly in degree of malignancy. About 90% occur in the parotid gland, and the remainder occur in the submaxillary glands. Rare examples have been reported within the mandible. Those of low-grade malignancy occur more frequently in females in the fourth to fifth decades and seldom involve the facial nerve. Those of higher grade malignancy tend to be larger, occur with equal frequency in males and females, occur at a slightly later average age, and are more likely to produce pain or to be associated with facial nerve paralysis. Encapsulation of the tumor is usually incomplete or lacking, and a cystic structure is common. Rare squamous cell carcinomas without a mucus-secreting element also occur.

Adenocarcinoma. Adenocarcinoma (adenoid cystic carcinoma; cylindroma) is a rela-

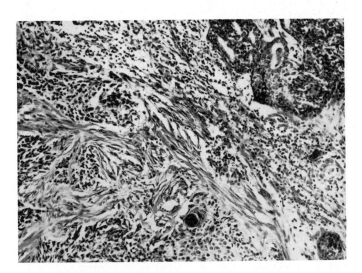

Fig. 19-5. Malignant mixed tumor of parotid gland.

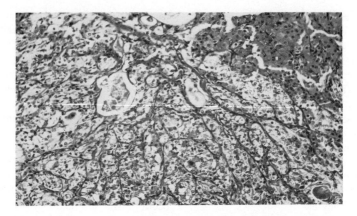

Fig. 19-6. Mucoepidermoid tumor of parotid gland.

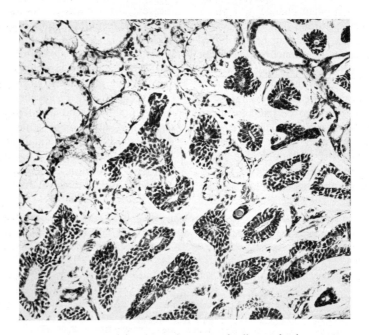

Fig. 19-7. Adenoid cystic tumor of salivary gland.

tively infrequent salivary gland tumor arising with about equal frequency in parotid and submaxillary glands. It tends to be of relatively slow growth and low-grade malignancy. The tumor cells are small and dark staining, with relatively abundant cytoplasm, and they grow in solid masses, in anastomosing cords, or with an adenoid cystic pattern (Fig. 19-7).

Acellular areas between strands of tumor cells contain mucoid material and tend to undergo hyalinization.

Perineural lymphatic extension of the tumor is common. Adenocarcinomas of various other patterns or of anaplastic appearance also occur but are infrequent.

Acinic cell adenocarcinoma. Acinic cell

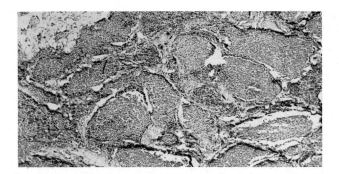

Fig. 19-8. Carotid body tumor. Tendency to rounded masses of tumor cells is evident.

adenocarcinoma is an uncommon malignant tumor that chiefly affects the parotid gland. Most of the tumors are composed of round or polyhedral cells with slightly granular cytoplasm and small, dark, eccentric nuclei. The tumor cells resemble the serous cells of the salivary gland acini. Some tumors consist of clear cells and resemble "hypernephroma."

Neck

CAROTID BODY TUMORS

The rare tumors of the carotid body are found at the upper end of the common carotid artery in close relationship to the point of bifurcation. They are generally benign, slowly growing tumors that tend to be encapsulated. A few reported cases have metastasized.

Microscopically, the tumors are composed of rounded groups of large polyhedral epithelial cells with small uniform nuclei and poorly defined boundaries (Fig. 19-8). The cells have a tendency to an alveolar arrrangement and are closely associated with a vascular fibrous stroma. Spindle cells are prominent in some tumors. An abundant innervation, as well as cells containing argentaffin granules, has been demonstrated.

Rare tumors of the middle ear arise from the glomus jugularis of the temporal bone and have a similar character and histologic appearance *(glomus jugularis tumors)*. Similar tumors also may arise from other so-called paraganglionic glomera in relation to various vessels and nerves in the neck and upper mediastinum. Tumors composed of the chemoreceptor cells associated with parasympathetic nerves have been called *chemodectomas*.

CYSTS

Cysts of the neck, arising from vestigial rests, may be of thyroglossal duct origin (midline) or branchiogenic origin (lateral). Lymphatic vessels also may give rise to cysts.

Thyroglossal cysts. A thyroglossal cyst may occur anywhere between the base of the tongue and the thyroid gland. The lesions are smooth-walled cysts lined by columnar or flattened epithelium.

Branchial cleft cyst. The branchial cleft cyst most frequently appears near the angle of the jaw. The cyst lining is squamous epithelium, and lymphoid tissue is abundant in the wall.

Cystic hygroma. The cystic hygroma is a lymphangiomatous cyst of the neck, usually of congenital origin (p. 296 and Fig. 13-13).

REFERENCES

Albers, G. D.: J.A.M.A. **183:**399-409, 1963 (branchial anomalies).
Azzopardi, J. G., and Smith, O. D.: J. Pathol. Bacteriol. **77:**131-140, 1959 (salivary gland tumors).
Baden, E.: In Sommers, S. C., editor: Pathology annual, vol. 6, New York, 1971, Appleton-Century-Crofts, pp. 475-568 (odontogenic tumors).
Chaudhry, A. P., and Gorlin, R. J.: Am. J. Surg. **95:**923-931, 1958 (papillary cystadenoma lymphomatosum).
Collins, N. P., and Edgerton, M. T.: Cancer **12:**235-239, 1959 (branchiogenic carcinoma).

Cossman, J., et al.: Arch. Pathol. Lab. Med. **101**:354-356, 1977 (Warthin's tumor).

Costero, I., and Barroso-Moguel, R.: Am. J. Pathol. **38**:127-141, 1961 (carotid body tumor).

Dietert, S. E.: Am. J. Clin. Pathol. **63**:866-875, 1975 (Warthin's tumor).

Dyke, P. C., et al.: Arch. Pathol. **91**:89-92, 1971 (calcium oxalate crystals in mixed tumor of parotid gland).

Evans, R. W., and Cruikshank, A. H.: Epithelial tumors of the salivary glands, Philadelphia, 1970, W. B. Saunders Co.

Foote, F. W., Jr., and Frazell, E. L.: Tumors of the major salivary glands. In Atlas of tumor pathology, Sect. 4, Fasc. 11, Washington, D.C., 1954, Armed Forces Institute of Pathology.

Gerughty, R. M., et al.: Cancer **24**:471-486, 1969 (malignant mixed tumors of salivary glands—calcific deposits).

Glickman, I.: N. Engl. J. Med. **284**:1071-1077, 1971 (periodontal disease).

Godwin, J. T., et al.: Am. J. Pathol. **30**:465-477, 1954 (acinic adenocarcinoma).

Gorlin, R. J., et al.: Cancer **14**:73-101, 1961 (odontogenic tumors).

Micheau, C.: Ann. Anat. Pathol. (Paris) **18**:469-476, 1973 (tyrosine crystals in mixed tumor of parotid gland).

Nochomovitz, L. E., and Kahn, L. B.: Arch. Pathol. **97**:141-142, 1974 (tyrosine crystals in pleomorphic adenomas of salivary glands).

Page, R. C., et al.: J.A.M.A. **240**:545-550, 1978 (periodontal disease).

Schermer, K. L., et al.: Cancer **19**:1273-1280, 1966 (glomus jugulare tumors).

Schneider, M.: Am. J. Med. Sci. **244**:628-645, 1962 (oral cancer).

Scopp, I. W.: Oral medicine, ed. 2, St. Louis, 1973, The C. V. Mosby Co.

Spiro, R. H., et al.: Cancer **41**:924-935, 1978 (acinic cell carcinoma of salivary glands).

Stecker, R. H., et al.: J.A.M.A. **189**:838-840, 1964 (snuff-dipper's carcinoma).

Sun, C. N., et al.: Arch. Pathol. **99**:208-214, 1975 (oncocytoma of parotid gland—EM study).

Svoboda, D., et al.: Exp. Mol. Pathol. **4**:189-204, 1965 (nasopharyngeal carcinoma).

Vickers, R. A., and Gorlin, R. J.: Cancer **26**:699-710, 1970 (ameloblastoma—histopathology).

20

Alimentary tract

Although divided into various anatomic regions, all portions of the alimentary canal consist of a hollow tube lined by a mucous membrane and having a muscular wall with peristaltic or sphincteric actions controlled by nerve influences. The same types of disease processes occur in each and follow the same general rules, but they vary in their relative frequency and importance in the different portions. These types are (1) congenital malformations, (2) diverticula, (3) inflammations and ulcerations, (4) obstructions of the lumen, acute and chronic, and (5) tumors. The main lesions of the alimentary canal are outlined in Table 20-1.

Esophagus

Congenital atresia. Congenital atresia of the esophagus is the only developmental abnormality that is common. In most cases, there is an associated tracheoesophageal fistula.

Diverticula. Diverticula may be of the *pulsion* type, with pressure within the esophagus forcing the wall outward at a weak point, or they may be the result of *traction* caused by inflammatory adhesions to surrounding structures. The pulsion type is more common and usually involves the posterior wall at the upper end of the esophagus. The traction type is usually anterior and at about the level of the tracheal bifurcation. Adhesions to tuberculous

mediastinal lymph nodes are the usual initiating factor.

Esophagitis. Esophagitis resulting from infection is not a common lesion, although fungal (e.g., candidal) esophagitis may occur in debilitated patients (see Fig. 10-1). Acute and subacute erosive esophagitis occurs near the lower end of the esophagus, especially as a terminal event in elderly or debilitated patients. The inflammatory process appears to begin or to localize largely in the lamina propria of the mucosa, and the erosive action of regurgitated gastric juice appears to play a role. Acid peptic erosion (peptic esophagitis) may occur in association with other conditions. For example, involvement of the esophagus in progressive systemic sclerosis (scleroderma) results in a thickening and rigidity of the wall that permits regurgitation of gastric contents followed by inflammation and ulceration. Peptic esophagitis also occurs in patients with hiatus hernia.

Various forms of chronic irritation may result in the formation of white plaques (*leukoplakia*) in the esophageal mucosa (Fig. 20-1).

Gastroesophageal lacerations. Gastroesophageal lacerations at the cardiac orifice of the stomach (*Mallory-Weiss syndrome*) are an infrequent cause of gastric hemorrhage. Longitudinal lacerations through the cardioesophageal junction have occurred commonly in patients with a history of alcohol abuse. Vomiting and retching often precede hematemesis, and gastritis and hiatus hernia are pres-

525

Table 20-1. Lesions of gastrointestinal tract

Disease process	Esophagus	Stomach	Duodenum
Congenital malformations	Atresia; tracheoesophageal fistula	Pyloric stenosis caused by hypertrophy and spasm of muscle of pylorus	Rare
Diverticula	*Pulsion type*—pressure from within, bulging at weak point, at upper end; *traction type*—caused by pull of inflammatory adhesions, usually at level of tracheal bifurcation	Uncommon	Fairly common
Inflammations and ulcerations	Relatively unimportant; follow swallowing of corrosive chemicals; varices at lower end in obstructions of portal circulation (cirrhosis of liver) sometimes associated with overlying inflammation and/or ulceration	Gastritis resulting from various poisons and irritants; chronic peptic ulcer very frequent and important; acute ulcers may accompany severe burns and acute central nervous system lesions	Chronic ulcer (peptic) very common in first portion; acute ulceration may accompany severe burns
Obstructions	Congenital; fibrosis following ingestion of corrosives; tumors; cardiospasm and functional strictures of lower end; pressure from without	Usually at pylorus; may be congenital (infancy), scar of healed ulcer, carcinoma, bezoars or concretions (masses of indigestible material)	Uncommon, except at pylorus
Tumors	Benign—uncommon; carcinoma—prognosis extremely poor; squamous cell type common; adenocarcinoma rare (occurs at lower end)	Benign—uncommon; malignant—carcinoma common and important; types: polypoid, ulcerating, and scirrhous or infiltrating; sarcoma uncommon	Rare

ent in many cases. Complete rupture of the esophagus *(Boerhaave syndrome)* is a more serious surgical emergency, with a high mortality from chemical mediastinitis.

Stenosis. Stenosis of the esophagus may be caused by the swallowing of corrosive chemicals such as lye. The resulting dense fibrous tissue repair causes such stricture of the lumen that the swallowing of solids and eventually even liquids is impossible. Tumors of the esophagus also obstruct the lumen and give rise to dysphagia. Pressure on the esophagus from without, as by a mediastinal or pulmonary tumor, enlarged lymph nodes, or aortic

Small intestine	Appendix	Colon	Rectum and anus
Uncommon, except for abnormalities of mesenteric attachment and rotation and Meckel's diverticulum	Rare	Congenital dilatation (megacolon—Hirschsprung's disease)	Atresia
Meckel's—persistence of omphalomesenteric duct, 1-3 ft proximal to ileocecal junction; other types uncommon	In rare cases, may follow appendicitis	Common in descending and sigmoid regions—often become inflamed (diverticulitis)	Uncommon
Typhoid—ulcerations of lymphoid areas of ileum; regional ileitis—chronic inflammation of terminal ileum; tuberculosis—chronic ulcerations of lower ileum; chemical poisons and uremia—may cause ulcerations of ileum; lesions of jejunum rare	Acute appendicitis common; complicated by perforation, abscess formation, peritonitis, and pylephlebitis	Bacillary dysentery; amebic dysentery; chronic ulcerative colitis; cholera; tuberculosis—may involve cecal region; actinomycosis—in cecal region; uremia; mercury	Nonspecific chronic inflammation with sinus or fistula formation common; involvement in lymphogranuloma venereum
Paralytic—e.g., in mesenteric thrombosis; mechanical—blockage of lumen; strangulation—obstruction and interference with blood supply; biochemical disturbance, with dehydration and electrolyte loss resulting	Commonly caused by fecalith or fibrosis; important in pathogenesis of appendicitis	Acute obstruction as in small bowel; chronic obstructions from tumors and inflammatory fibrosis	Acute obstruction uncommon; chronic obstruction from tumors, impacted feces, and in lymphogranuloma venereum
Rare; carcinoids similar to those of appendix occur, but less often; may metastasize to liver and produce carcinoid syndrome (serotonin production)	Carcinoid—a small yellow argentaffin tumor that histologically may resemble carcinoma; true carcinoma rare	Benign—polyps and adenomas common; carcinoma—common, particularly in distal portions of colon and rectum; gross types: (1) annular constricting and ulcerating and (2) papillary; histologic varieties: (1) adenocarcinoma, (2) mucoid, and (3) scirrhous	

aneurysm, produces variable degrees of esophageal obstruction.

Cardiospasm. Cardiospasm (*achalasia*) or functional stricture of the lower end of the esophagus is caused by spasm of the cardiac sphincter. It appears to result from neurogenic imbalance of sphincteric action. Degenerative changes have been found in afferent vagal fibers. As in other types of obstruction, the esophagus above the stricture becomes dilated. Idiopathic muscular hypertrophy of the lower esophagus is a rare condition sometimes associated with spasm.

Varices. Varices at the lower end of the

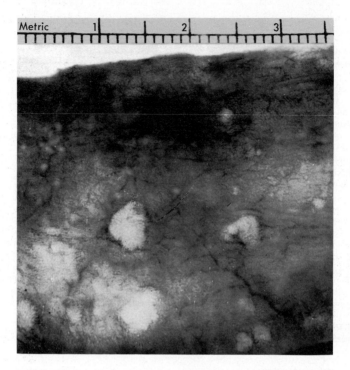

Fig. 20-1. Leukoplakia of esophagus. Irregular white areas are prominent on mucosal surface.

esophagus occur in chronic portal hypertension usually secondary to cirrhosis of the liver. Hemorrhage from the varices is influenced both by the increased hydrostatic pressure and by mucosal ulceration.

Benign tumors. Benign tumors are uncommon. Fibrous polyps, polypoid lipomas, and leiomyomas may project into the lumen and occur mainly at the level of the cricoid cartilage. Intramural leiomyomas may be found at any level.

Congenital cysts. Cysts containing derivatives of the primitive foregut occur in the middle and lower thirds of the esophagus.

Carcinoma. Carcinoma is the only type of tumor common in the esophagus. It occurs more frequently in persons after the age of 50 years, and more than 80% occur in men. The three esophageal sites at which carcinoma commonly develops are (1) the lower third, at about the level of the diaphragm, (2) the middle third, at the level of the tracheal bifurca-

tion, and (3) the upper third, at the level of the cricoid cartilage. Most carcinomas occur in the middle third, although the lower third also is a frequent site. They occur less commonly in the upper third. Of interest is the fact that carcinoma in the postcricoid segment occurs in a high percentage of women with the Plummer-Vinson syndrome (sideropenic dysphagia) (p. 497).

The *gross types* are (1) an infiltrating or scirrhous form, which grows around the esophagus and soon produces stenosis and obstruction of the lumen, (2) a medullary type, which is a soft, bulky, ulcerating tumor, and (3) a polypoid form, which is least common.

These tumors are *squamous cell carcinomas* of varying degree of differentiation. In rare instances, an *adenocarcinoma* may be present at the lower end of the esophagus. It may arise from ectopic gastric mucosa or may be an upward extension of an adenocarcinoma of the cardiac end of the stomach. Carcinoma with both squamous and glandular patterns (adeno-acanthoma) also occurs in the cardioesophageal region.

Metastasis is more widespread in the highly undifferentiated tumors, with the liver, lungs, and lymph nodes draining the area being most frequently involved. The outlook in carcinoma of the esophagus is usually extremely poor.

Stomach and duodenum

CONGENITAL PYLORIC STENOSIS

Great hypertrophy of the circular muscle fibers of the pylorus is characteristic of congenital pyloric stenosis. Usually accompanied by spasm, it produces stenosis and obstruction of the pyloric orifice. Symptoms begin shortly after the first week of life, with vomiting, visible gastric peristalsis, and often a palpable hardened pylorus. Symptoms may subside in a few weeks or continue for months. Recovery results after surgical splitting of the circular muscle fibers of the pylorus.

Although the condition is congenital, its pathogenesis is unknown, and the relative importance of spasm and muscle hypertrophy in the production of symptoms is a debatable point. Myenteric ganglion cells and nerve fiber tracts have been shown to be fewer in number in the hypertrophied pyloric region, and the ganglion cells show degenerative changes. The condition occurs predominantly in males.

Duodenal obstruction in infancy also may be caused by an *annular pancreas,* a malformation in which a band of pancreatic tissue is wrapped around the duodenum.

POISONS

Various ingested corrosives leave their mark on the stomach as well as on the mouth, pharynx, and esophagus. The effects vary with the type and strength of the poison. Certain powerful poisons, such as phenol and related compounds, may cause immediate fixation and death of gastric mucosa. The fixed tissue is firm and grayish white or brownish. Microscopically, the cells appear well preserved.

Sloughing of the dead tissue occurs in patients who survive for some time.

Strong acids, such as hydrochloric and sulfuric, burn the tissues, which then appear yellowish or brown, necrotic, and hemorrhagic. Action on the blood in contact with the acid results in dark brown pigmentation because of hematin formation. Microscopically, the tissue appears massively necrotic and disintegrated. The degree of inflammatory reaction depends on the period of survival after ingestion of the poison.

Strong alkalies, such as lye, also produce necrosis with softening and discoloration, although the pigmentation may be less distinct.

Various weaker corrosive poisons result in lesser degrees of the same type of change, with more opportunity for the development of severe inflammatory reaction.

GASTRITIS

Acute gastritis. Acute gastritis may be caused by various irritant foods, alcoholic drinks, aspirin, other drugs, and poisons.

Chronic gastritis. Chronic gastritis occurs in hypertrophic and atrophic forms.

Chronic hypertrophic gastritis is characterized by thickening of the mucosa and submucosa. The lining of the stomach is excessively rugose or even polypoid. There is a hyperplasia of the mucosal epithelium, and in the submucosa there is an increase in connective tissue, with infiltration of chronic inflammatory cells. Multiple polyps may develop. The condition is rather rare but clinically may be difficult to differentiate from a cancer. Chronic gastritis with hypertrophy of the rugae is sometimes associated with loss of protein into the lumen *(Menetrier's disease).*

Chronic atrophic gastritis is a nonspecific change that becomes more frequent with advancing age. It may be particularly prominent in persons with chronic alcoholism, chronic pellagra, and pernicious anemia. The normal rugae of the stomach are less prominent. Hypochlorhydria or achlorhydria is a common accompaniment.

Microscopically, the mucosa is atrophic, with a scarcity of mucosal glands. There may be an increase of leukocytic infiltration and lymphoid aggregation in the mucosa and submucosa. The mucosa of the pylorus and corpus may be metaplastic and transformed to an intestinal type, and there may be a change of parts of the mucosa of the corpus to a pyloric type (pseudopyloric metaplasia). There is an increase of mucus-producing gland cells at the expense of the chief and parietal cells. Small cysts may be present in deeper parts of the mucosa. The interglandular connective tissue and the muscularis mucosae are thickened.

The importance of chronic gastritis with metaplasia in predisposing to carcinoma of the stomach is debatable, but the two conditions are commonly associated.

In pernicious anemia, there is an extreme atrophy involving all coats of the stomach wall. This change is localized in the upper two thirds of the stomach and does not affect the pyloric antrum or duodenum. In the involved area, the stomach wall is extremely thin, but there is an abrupt transition to normal thickness at the junction with the pyloric mucosa. Only a few scattered glands remain in the involved area, the specialized oxyntic and peptic cells having entirely disappeared (see Fig. 18-1). The inflammatory cell infiltrate may be minimal, particularly if the atrophy is severe. These changes appear to be the morphologic basis of the achylia gastrica present in pernicious anemia.

Carcinoma of the stomach is at least three times more common in persons with pernicious anemia. The possibility that atrophic gastritis and pernicious anemia are autoimmune disorders has been considered. Patients with both of these conditions frequently have serum antiparietal cell and anti-intrinsic factor antibodies.

Specific gastritis. Rarely, local granulomatous or ulcerative lesions may occur in syphilis, tuberculosis, and the mycoses. In some instances, as in syphilis, a diffusely infiltrative lesion occurs that may be of the leatherbottle (linitis plastica) type and is grossly indistinguishable from scirrhous carcinoma.

On occasion, sarcoidosis, eosinophilic granuloma, and xanthomatosis produce lesions in the stomach.

BEZOARS

Bezoar is a term applied to an accumulation of foreign material in the stomach and intestine. There are four varieties: (1) trichobezoar, or hair ball, (2) phytobezoar, or food ball, (3) trichophytobezoar, or combined hair and food ball, and (4) shellac bezoar, or concretion.

PYLORIC OBSTRUCTION

In adults, stenosis and obstruction at the pylorus may result from the contracting scar of an ulcer or from carcinoma. The stomach becomes greatly dilated and filled by stagnant food and fluid. Persistent vomiting results in loss of chlorides and acid and the production of so-called gastric tetany (i.e., alkalosis and a chloride insufficiency occur). An increase in nonprotein nitrogen of the blood and evidence of renal insufficiency may be present. The kidneys show significant tubular degeneration and often calcium deposits in the degenerated tissue. Other obstructions high in the intestinal tract produce a similar result.

ULCERS

The term *peptic ulcer* refers to ulceration in areas that may be acted upon by acid gastric juice, i.e., the stomach, the first portion of the duodenum, and, after gastrojejunostomy, the jejunum. *Acute ulcerations* or *erosions* are superficial and often hemorrhagic areas of mucosal loss. These common acute ulcers heal easily and give rise to little trouble. It is believed, however, that they may form the starting point for chronic peptic ulcers. *Chronic peptic ulcers* are more serious than the acute ulcers because of their persistence, annoying symptoms, and the complications of hemorrhage, perforation, stenosis, and malignant change. The term *peptic ulcer,* when unqualified, usually refers to this serious chronic type.

Acute ulcer

Acute ulcers or erosions are quite common and may be produced by a variety of injuries, such as coarse or excessively hot foods, septicemias, and burns of the skin. The variety complicating extensive superficial burns is known as *Curling's ulcers*. Found in only a small proportion of fatal burns, they usually occur in the duodenum and stomach, but they also have been seen in the intestine.

Acute hemorrhagic ulcerations of the stomach or duodenum occasionally occur in patients with acute lesions of the central nervous system (Fig. 20-2), especially of the hypothalamus *(Cushing's ulcers),* with other types of stress, or with shock or in those who have been treated by adrenal steroid hormones. Acute ulcers are usually small, involve only the mucosa and superficial layers of submu-

cosa, and are often hemorrhagic. They usually heal readily but in certain areas and circumstances may become chronic. Acute ulcers are more frequent in the stomach than in the duodenum. Serious upper gastrointestinal bleeding may occur in some patients with acute hemorrhagic ulcers.

Chronic peptic ulcer

Etiology. The etiology of chronic peptic ulcer is not thoroughly understood. The one factor of established importance is the *action of acid-pepsin gastric content*. Chronic peptic ul-

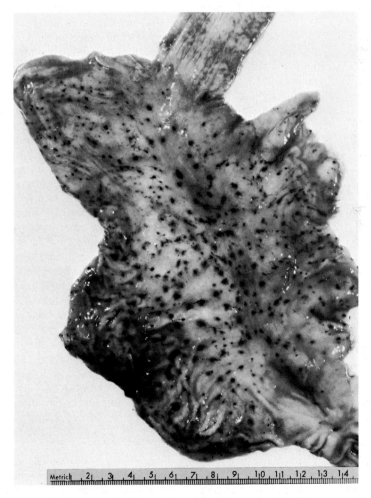

Fig. 20-2. Multiple acute hemorrhagic erosions (ulcers) associated with acute central nervous system lesion (cerebral infarct).

cers develop only in areas exposed to acid-pepsin secretion: the duodenum, stomach, lower part of the esophagus, jejunum at the site of a gastrojejunostomy, and Meckel's diverticulum containing gastric mucosa. In the rare Zollinger-Ellison syndrome (hypersecretion of gastric acid associated with pancreatic adenoma), peptic ulceration occurs in the jejunum as well as in the duodenum. Ulceration does not occur in acid-pepsin–secreting mucosa but in adjacent areas.

Although chronic ulcers in the duodenum and stomach, the two common sites, have certain features in common, there are obvious differences that have led some investigators to consider them different disease entities.

Duodenal ulcers are much more common than gastric ulcers and occur most often in males, usually between 20 and 50 years of age. Individuals with Group O blood and those unable to secrete A, B, and H substances in the saliva and gastric secretions are more susceptible to duodenal ulceration. It is the duodenal ulcer that tends to occur in the professional or executive person who is hard driving and under mental stress. Most patients with duodenal ulcers secrete a greater than normal amount of gastric acid and have a greater than normal number of parietal (acid-secreting) cells in the stomach.

On the other hand, chronic gastric ulcers are not characterized by the great preponderance in males as are the duodenal ulcers, tend to occur in an older age group, and are associated with a normal or low amount of gastric secretion with no increase in the number of parietal cells.

Despite these differences, it can be said that the peptic ulcers in both sites are caused by too much gastric acid secretion with respect to the degree of protection provided for the mucosa.

The factors that normally protect the gastroduodenal mucosa against digestion by gastric secretions include (1) a layer of mucus, (2) dilution or buffering of gastric juices by swallowed food and saliva and by the alkaline small intestinal juices, and (3) an adequate blood supply. Although it has been suggested that decreased resistance of the mucosa plays a role in the development of peptic ulcers, there is no general agreement on this point. Significant changes of the aforementioned protective factors have not been demonstrated conclusively in ulcer subjects. Impaired tissue resistance is considered by some investigators to be more important in the pathogenesis of gastric ulcers than duodenal ulcers. Chronic gastritis is frequently but not always associated with chronic gastric ulcers. The possible relationship of these ulcers to local trauma such as that caused by the passage of coarse, indigestible foods has been noted. Localized mucosal damage caused by changes in vascular supply (e.g., vasospasm, thrombosis, embolism) or by bacterial infection has been thought by some to be responsible for ulcer formation, but such a mechanism is not regarded by many writers today to be of major significance. Smoking may favor ulcer production or interfere with healing of one already present.

The influence of the nervous system has long been considered a factor in the cause of peptic ulcers. A hypersecretion of gastric acid may be mediated through the vagus nerve and possibly through adrenal cortical steroids as a result of hypothalamic–anterior pituitary stimulus brought about by anxiety, other emotional states, or other types of stress.

A familial history is present in many patients with peptic ulcers, suggesting a hereditary predisposition in certain instances. Of interest is the observation of an increased incidence of peptic ulcers in patients with chronic lung diseases such as pulmonary emphysema associated with CO_2 retention, with hyperparathyroidism, with rheumatoid arthritis, or with polycythemia vera. Most frequently, the ulcers are of the duodenal type.

Various factors have been thought to prevent healing once the ulcer is established. These include hyperacidity and stasis, the traumatic effects of food, tobacco smoking, and the pull of muscle about the ulcer. The rather constant location of gastric ulcers on the lesser curvature has caused emphasis on functional and anatomic factors. Contraction of oblique muscle fibers forms a groove (magenstrasse) along the distal part of the lesser curvature, along which food or liquid may be forced without mixing with the rest of the gastric content. Usually, gastric ulcers are located in or near the magenstrasse. This region, in comparison with other parts of the gastric mucosa, is exposed to more trauma, lacks protective mucin production, and is subjected to greater muscle traction.

Gross appearance. Peptic ulcers are highly constant in location, being found in the pyloric portion of the stomach, most commonly on the posterior wall near the lesser curvature, and in the first portion of the duodenum proximal to the ampulla. Gastric ulcers are usually situated a few centimeters proximal to the pyloric ring. Ulcers right at the pylorus are more commonly carcinomatous. Duodenal ulcers occur in the first portion (duodenal bulb) on the anterior or posterior wall. Peptic ulcers are usually single but may be multiple.

The ulcers vary in size from a few millimeters to 3 cm in diameter. They usually do not extend and become very large. Large ulcers of

the stomach are usually carcinomas rather than chronic peptic ulcers. An ulcer in the duodenum is almost never a carcinoma.

The chronic ulcers appear as indurated, deep, punched-out or funnel-shaped areas (Fig. 20-3). The proximal or cardiac side of the gastric ulcer is usually steep with overhanging edges, whereas the distal or pyloric side tends to be sloping or terraced. The base of the ulcer is covered by roughened, grayish, necrotic material or may contain granular or blood-tinged exudate. Hyperemia or some fibrous thickening may be present around the edge of the ulcer. Variable degrees of fibrosis and distortion of the organ develop. When marked fibrosis spreads around the stomach, contraction tends to produce an hourglass deformity. Fibrous adhesion to adjacent organs, such as the pancreas or liver, may be present. Fibrosis about a duodenal ulcer shortens the distance between the pyloric ring and the opening of the ampulla.

Microscopic appearance. At the edge of the ulcer, the mucosal and muscle layers end rather abruptly, although there may be some

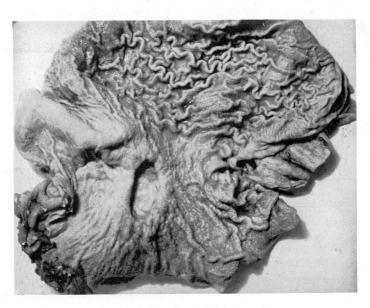

Fig. 20-3. Chronic ulcer of stomach.

overhanging of the epithelium. Occasionally, there is some downward proliferation of the marginal epithelium, producing an appearance that should not be confused with malignancy.

The whole thickness of the base of the ulcer is composed of fibrous scar tissue, the muscle layers usually being completely gone. Over this fibrous base are successive layers of granulation tissue, necrotic and hyalinized materials, and exudate. Inflammatory cells may be found not only in this layer of exudate on the surface but also in the granulation tissue and about the edges. Blood vessels in the base often show inflammation in early ulcers and later show intimal thickening with narrowing or even obliteration of the lumen.

When healing occurs, it is by organization and fibrosis, with the mucosa from the edges growing inward to cover the area. Contraction of the scar tissue sometimes produces pyloric stenosis.

Complications. The complications and sequelae of peptic ulcer include hemorrhage, perforation, malignant change, and scar contraction with pyloric stenosis or deformity of the stomach.

Small hemorrhages commonly accompany peptic ulcers. Repeated small hemorrhages produce secondary anemia. A severe or even fatal hemorrhage may follow erosion of a larger vessel. Endarterial changes in the vessels of the base protect against this to some extent. On the other hand, the vessel walls, being held in rigid scar tissue, may be unable to retract after erosion. Alimentary azotemia may occur after massive hemorrhage from a peptic ulcer, apparently because of absorption of breakdown products of the digested blood.

Perforation results when the ulcer continues to penetrate deeply. Perforation into the peritoneal cavity produces shock and soon results in peritonitis. This is likely to occur in ulcers of the anterior wall of the stomach or duodenum. In other older ulcers of the posterior wall, adherent to some surrounding structure, perforation may occur into the adherent organ (e.g., the pancreas).

Relationship to carcinoma. The relationship of carcinoma to peptic ulcers is controversial. However, one cannot exclude the possibility that carcinoma may arise from a chronic gastric ulcer in a very small percentage of patients, although it is highly unlikely that malignant change ever develops in a duodenal ulcer.

Evidence that an ulcerating gastric cancer arose from a previously benign chronic ulcer is given by:

1 Complete destruction of the muscle layers of the stomach in the base of the ulcer
2 Fusion of the muscularis mucosae and muscle wall at the margin of the ulcer
3 Intimal thickening of blood vessels
4 The presence of carcinoma in only one part of the wall and its absence in the base of the ulcer and in other portions of the wall

Criteria used in the distinction of benign and malignant gastric ulcers are presented in Table 20-2. A malignant ulcer tends to be bowl shaped, with an edge that is raised and nodular but does not overhang the crater and with a smoothing out of the mucosal folds around the margin. Benign ulcers occur less frequently than malignant ulcers on the greater curvature and in the region of the cardia. In

Table 20-2. Comparison of benign and malignant gastric ulcers

	Ulcerating carcinoma	Chronic ulcer
Duration	Less than 2 yr	Often more than 2 yr
Age (yr)	More frequently past 40	Frequently begins under 40
Size of ulcer (diameter)	Usually over 2.5 cm	Usually less than 4 cm; commonly 1 to 2.5 cm
Position	Usually at or very near pylorus	Commonly 2 to 3 inches from pylorus
Edge of ulcer	Raised; rounded	Sharp; punched-out; terraced on pyloric side

the presence of hypochlorhydria or achlorhydria, a gastric ulcer is more likely to be malignant rather than a simple peptic ulcer. The reverse is true if there is severe hyperchlorhydria.

None of the criteria for the distinction of benign and malignant gastric ulcers is uniformly reliable. Sometimes, the distinction is impossible without microscopic examination and application of the usual histologic criteria of malignancy.

TUMORS
Benign tumors of stomach

Benign tumors of the stomach are uncommon compared with carcinoma and are of little clinical significance unless they obstruct the pylorus. Leiomyoma (Fig. 20-4) and adenoma are the most frequent types. The mucosa may be involved by a polypoid adenoma or by multiple polyps (Fig. 20-5). Regenerative polyps, usually less than 2 cm in diameter, are more common than neoplastic true adenomatous polyps and have not been shown to become malignant. Adenomatous polyps may undergo malignant change but account for few gastric cancers since they are uncommon. Some of the fibroid polyps appear to be of inflammatory origin. Fibroma and lipoma also occur.

Carcinoma of stomach

Malignant tumors of the stomach cause about 5% of all cancer deaths in the United States. The death rate from cancer of the stomach has been steadily declining, the reason for which is unknown. Carcinoma of the stomach is more common in males than in females (in proportion of almost 2:1). More than 90% occur in persons past 50 years of age.

Differences in racial or geographic incidence are striking, carcinoma being much more common in areas such as Japan, Chile, Iceland, Austria, and central Europe than in the United States. In Japan, the high incidence has been related to the frequent consumption of pickled vegetables, dried salted fish, and possibly rice coated with asbestos-contaminated talc (used to improve appearance and taste of the rice). The high incidence in Iceland may be related to dietary intake of carcinogens, particularly in smoked meat and fish.

Hereditary susceptibility appears to be of some importance, and numerous studies have indicated a relatively high incidence in certain families or among relatives. The high incidence in the Napoleon Bonaparte family is of historic interest. Studies on correlation of the incidence of certain blood group factors and gastric cancer have confirmed the importance of a genetic basis of susceptibility.

Conditions that may be associated with, and sometimes precede or predispose to, carcinoma of the stomach are chronic gastritis, chronic gastric ulcer, and adenomatous polyps. The proved frequency of these conditions progressing to carcinoma is not sufficient to

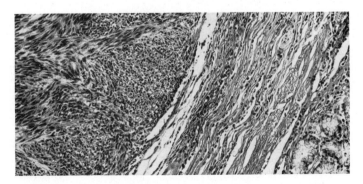

Fig. 20-4. Leiomyoma of stomach. Margin of tumor is shown in center, with tumor at left and normal mucosal glands at right.

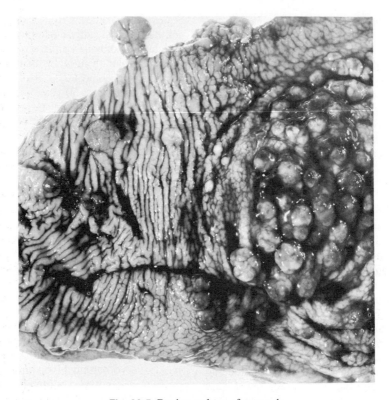

Fig. 20-5. Benign polyps of stomach.

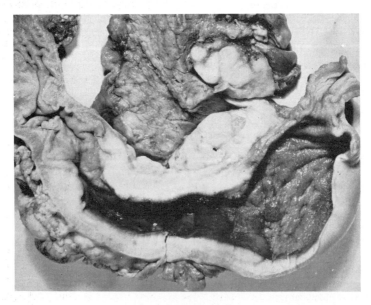

Fig. 20-6. Diffuse scirrhous carcinoma of stomach (linitis plastica). Note considerable diffuse thickening and contraction of wall.

account for more than a small proportion of gastric cancers.

Carcinoma may occur anywhere in the stomach, but the majority develop from mucus-secreting cells of the antrum and pylorus and more particularly along the lesser curvature. A few are found on the greater curvature and about 10% in the fundus or in the region of the cardia. Although the relative proportions vary in the different sites, as compared with benign ulcers, there is much overlapping.

Types. *Gross pathologic classification* of carcinoma of the stomach appears of greater practical usefulness than does microscopic classification. The following gross forms are recognized: polypoid or fungating, ulcerative or penetrating, diffuse spreading or infiltrating (scirrhous), and superficial spreading.

The *polypoid* or *fungating* carcinoma is a soft bulky tumor that projects into the cavity of the stomach. The tumor may be large before many symptoms are produced. The surface tends to become ulcerated and infected, and it bleeds easily. Eventually, the tumor infiltrates and penetrates the muscle wall, but the course may be relatively slow. This fungating form constitutes up to 25% of gastric cancers and is a relatively favorable form for surgical removal.

The *ulcerative* or *penetrating* carcinoma is the most frequent form of gastric cancer, con- stituting up to 30%. The growth is primarily away from the lumen, and ulceration is early and prominent. The ulcer tends to be shallow and bowl shaped, with an edge that is raised and nodular but does not overhang the crater. The mucosal folds around the ulcer's margin tend to be smoothed out. Despite the described differences, a gross distinction from a benign ulcer is sometimes difficult. If the diameter of the ulcer is more than 4 cm, it is usually an indication of malignancy, but size alone is not a reliable criterion.

The *diffuse spreading* or *infiltrating (scirrhous)* carcinoma constitutes about 10% of gastric cancers. The growth extends in the wall of the stomach without producing either a localized tumor mass or a prominent ulcer. Abundant fibrous stroma forms, so that the involved portion of the stomach becomes contracted, thick walled, and firm. It may begin at the pylorus, encircling this region and producing obstruction. The proximal extension may be only a short distance, or the whole stomach may be involved. The diffuse infiltrating type *(linitis plastica;* Fig. 20-6) results in a small, very thick-walled stomach (leather-bottle stomach). Histologically, malignant cells are sometimes quite scarce in the midst of the abundant connective tissue stroma and may be difficult to find (Fig. 20-7). The outlook is poor, and cure is rare. Extensive intra-

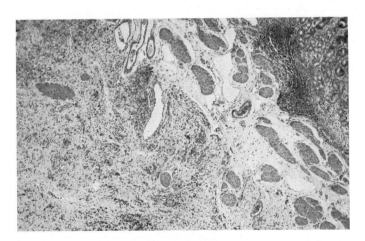

Fig. 20-7. Linitis plastica (sclerosing carcinoma) of stomach. Mucosa at right.

mural (tubal) spread along the alimentary tract sometimes occurs.

Superficial spreading carcinoma, an infrequent and relatively favorable type, extends into the mucosa (Fig. 20-8) and submucosa. It is found mainly in the antrum and pylorus. The mucosa and submucosa may be thickened by the tumor, but abundant fibrous stroma is lacking. Subsequent deeper penetration and metastasis may occur.

A considerable number of late extensive cancers of the stomach cannot be classed into the gross types because their distinctive features have been lost.

Microscopic classification is relatively unimportant from a practical standpoint. Carcinomas of the stomach are adenocarcinomas, derived from mucus-secreting and glandular cells, with varying degrees of differentiation (Fig. 20-9). Mucus production may occur in any of the varieties of gastric carcinoma, either in small localized areas or involving the whole tumor. Large mucoid areas grossly appear translucent and gelatinous. Accumulation of mucus in the cytoplasm of the tumor cells displaces and flattens the nucleus at one side of the cell, giving it a signet-ring appearance (Fig. 20-10). Also, there may be areas of extracellular mucus. Other microscopic varieties may show a predominance of gland formation or papillary structure, infiltrating spheroidal cells, or highly anaplastic undifferentiated cells. A metaplastic squamous cell component (adenoacanthoma) or squamous cell carcinoma rarely occurs in the pyloric area.

Grading of gastric carcinomas has been done on a histologic basis (Broders' system), and staging has been done according to the degree of spread. Prognosis appears to be related to the degree of penetration of the cancer into or through the wall of the stomach and to the presence or absence of lymph node or distant metastases, which are features on which staging systems of cancer are based. Also, some investigators have correlated structural features in the tumor and regional lymph nodes with survival. For example, lymphocytic reaction in the stroma of the tumor and follicular hyperplasia and sinus histiocytosis in regional lymph nodes have been considered to indicate a better prognosis.

Spread and metastases. Carcinoma of the

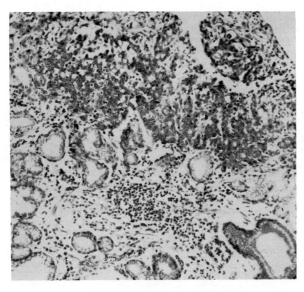

Fig. 20-8. Superficial spreading carcinoma of stomach. Only gastric mucosa is shown, and neoplastic cells are in upper half of photomicrograph.

stomach spreads by direct growth and invasion, by lymphatics, through the peritoneal cavity, and by the bloodstream.

Direct spread in the stomach wall is very important in prognosis. Diffusely infiltrative tumors of the linitis plastica type have the poorest outlook, but the degree of intramural spread in other types is also important. Intramural extension that is rapid or extensive, or spread beyond the limits of visibility or palpability, is associated with poor chances of survival, whereas sharp circumscription of the tumor is an important feature suggesting a good prognosis. Direct spread also may extend intramurally into the esophagus, the first portion of the duodenum, the gastrohepatic and gastrocolic omenta, and adjacent areas of the pancreas, spleen, transverse colon, liver, and diaphragm. When the peritoneal surface is reached, peritoneal dissemination may occur, with numerous peritoneal deposits or ovarian metastases. The ovaries may be involved by bilateral (Krukenberg) tumors.

Metastasis to perigastric regional lymph nodes is one of the main factors affecting prognosis in resectable tumors. From tumors

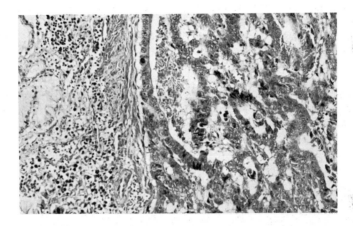

Fig. 20-9. Adenocarcinoma of stomach. A few normal mucosal glands are at left.

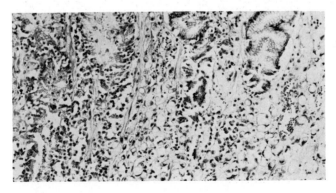

Fig. 20-10. Adenocarcinoma of stomach. Mucin-containing tumor cells of signet-ring type are infiltrating gastric mucosa.

in the distal portions of the stomach, metastases are found in the inferior gastric, subpyloric, and superior gastric nodes. From cancers in the proximal portion of the stomach, the pancreaticolineal group of nodes is most often involved. Further spread by lymphatics occurs to the celiac, lumbar, mesenteric, pelvic, and mediastinal nodes and to the thoracic duct. By way of the thoracic duct, miliary carcinomas of the lungs may develop, as well as involvement of the left supraclavicular lymph node (Virchow's node).

Bloodstream metastasis most frequently involves the liver, lungs, and bones.

Cytologic diagnosis. Cytologic study for diagnosis has not been readily applied to gastric cancer because of the difficulty of getting exfoliated malignant cells for study, the hazard of cellular digestion by gastric enzymes that destroys cytologic features, and difficulties in interpretation of morphology of some types of gastric tumor cells. Tumor cells have been more readily obtained by use of an abrasive gastric balloon and by lavage with mucolytic agents such as chymotrypsin or papain. Proper preparation by first controlling food intake and gastric lavage keeps digestive effects on the exfoliated tumor cells to a minimum. By proper technique and careful interpretation of the nuclear characteristics of enlargement,

variation in size, increase in chromatin, irregular borders, large nucleoli, and mitoses, gastric cancer cells can be recognized with dependable frequency.

Fiberoptic endoscopes are available today not only for inspection and biopsy of suspicious lesions but also for obtaining cytologic specimens by different techniques (e.g., use of a brush or sponge, or washing and aspiration).

Sarcoma of stomach

Sarcoma constitutes about 2% of cancers of the stomach. The varieties include leiomyosarcoma (Fig. 20-11), fibrosarcoma, and malignant lymphoma. Some of the so-called round cell sarcomas probably are highly anaplastic carcinomas. Malignant lymphoma is the most common variety. It forms an intramural tumor, is similar to malignant lymphoma elsewhere, and is highly radiosensitive. It may be primary in the stomach or be only part of a more generalized involvement. The mucosa may be greatly thickened, with giant rugae, multiple nodules, or a single bulky polypoid growth. Ulceration occurs in late stages. The pylorus is not often involved, and obstruction is unusual. Histologic varieties include Hodgkin's disease, small lymphocyte type, mixed lymphocytic-histiocytic type, and histiocytic

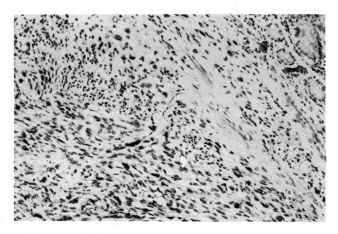

Fig. 20-11. Leiomyosarcoma of stomach. Mucosal glands are at upper right.

(reticulum cell) type (most frequent). The last variety may be difficult to differentiate from anaplastic carcinoma.

Carcinoma of duodenum

The duodenum is a rare site for cancer, even as a malignant change in a chronic duodenal ulcer. Most carcinomas of the duodenum arise at or about the ampulla of Vater and hence usually obstruct the bile and pancreatic ducts, with the early appearance of jaundice. Some probably originate from bile duct epithelium rather than from duodenal mucosa, and others originate from aberrant pancreatic tissue. Cysts of the duodenum are rare. They may be cysts of Brunner's glands or enterogenous cysts.

Intestinal tract

The main types of diseases of the small and large bowel are (1) inflammatory and infective conditions, including inflammations of diverticula and of the peritoneum, (2) diverticula, (3) obstructions, and (4) tumors. Other lesions and syndromes also will be considered herein (e.g., Whipple's disease, malabsorption syndromes, protein-losing enteropathies, melanosis coli, pneumatosis cystoides intestinalis, and pilonidal sinus).

INFLAMMATIONS

Inflammations may involve large portions of the tract, but often one region is affected exclusively or more prominently, so that the terms *enteritis* (small intestine), *ileitis, appendicitis, colitis, sigmoiditis,* and *proctitis* (rectum) may be used to indicate inflammation of the particular region. The causes are classified in three main groups:

1 Poisons, either endogenous (e.g., in uremia) or exogenous (mercury poisoning, botulinum food poisoning)
2 Infections (typhoid, dysentery, cholera, tuberculosis, etc.)
3 Undetermined causes (ulcerative colitis, regional ileitis, etc.)

In the last group, certain lesions may be related to immunologic factors (e.g., ulcerative colitis).

The inflammation may be of the following types:

1 Catarrhal, i.e., a superficial inflammation involving the mucosa accompanied by abundant secretion of mucus
2 Follicular, in which, in addition to catarrhal inflammation, there is a severe hyperplasia of the lymph follicles
3 Pseudomembranous or membranous, characterized by the formation of a false membrane composed of necrotic mucosa and a fibrinous exudate (sometimes called diphtheritic)
4 Ulcerative, in which sloughing of necrotic areas and ulceration are often of distinctive nature
5 Others are hemorrhagic, necrotizing, suppurative, granulomatous, etc.

Some types of infection of the bowel may be catarrhal, pseudomembranous, or ulcerative, depending on their stage or degree of severity. Various inflammations and ulcerations of the intestinal tract are listed in Table 20-3.

Intestinal inflammations caused by poisons

Endogenous inflammations. *Uremia* is accompanied by intestinal lesions in about 20% of the cases. The earliest changes in the mucosa are areas of hyperemia and edema, followed by hemorrhage, necrosis, pseudomembranous change, sloughing, and ulceration. Uremic ulcers are most common in the lower ileum, cecum, and ascending colon, but they also occur in other parts. The change is probably caused by localized interference with circulation to the involved area of bowel, and sclerotic or necrotic changes in blood vessels are often evident in the affected region. Irritation from excessive ammonia in the intestinal content, because of excretion of excess urea, also has been suggested as a causative factor.

Exogenous inflammations. Poisoning by heavy metals, such as mercury bichloride, and other corrosives, may produce an intense hemorrhagic and pseudomembranous inflammation of the bowel. The ileum and colon are

Table 20-3. Inflammations and ulcerations of intestinal tract

	Etiology and pathogenesis	Region of bowel involved predominantly	Nature of lesion
Chemical poisons	Corrosive action of ingested salts of mercury and other heavy metals	Ileum and colon	Hemorrhagic and pseudomembranous
Uremia	Localized blood vessel changes; (?) ammonia poisoning	Lower ileum, cecum, and ascending colon	Hemorrhagic, pseudomembranous, and ulcerative lesions
Burns	In 1% to 6% of fatal burns; possible relation to adrenal damage	First part of duodenum, stomach, and small intestine—in order of frequency	Acute; ulcerative
Typhoid and paratyphoid	Organisms ingested in contaminated water and food; generalized infection	Ileum—Peyer's patches and solitary lymph follicles	Hyperplastic and necrotic; involvement of lymphoid tissue
Bacillary dysentery	Ingested dysentery bacilli produce localized infection of intestine	Large intestine, especially distal portion	Pseudomembranous inflammation with widespread necrosis and abundant exudate
Amebic dysentery	Ingested *Entamoeba histolytica* locally affects intestine	Large intestine	Local invasion and tissue lysis by parasite
Ulcerative colitis	Etiology uncertain	Large intestine, especially distal portion	Chronic ulcerative inflammation
Cholera	Ingested cholera vibrios of Koch produce infection of intestine	Entire intestinal tract, but particularly colon	Acute catarrhal inflammation; reddening of mucosa; sometimes hemorrhages
Regional enteritis	Etiology uncertain	Ileocecal region with or without involvement of colon	Great thickening of segment of ileum
Tuberculosis	Usually secondary to pulmonary lesion, caused by swallowing sputum; occasionally primary from infected milk or food	Ileocecal region—starts in lymphoid tissue	Tubercle formation in lymphoid tissue of bowel; sometimes hyperplastic with thickening of bowel wall
Actinomycosis	Ingested ray fungus	Ileocecal region and appendix	Suppurative and ulcerative, with thickening of bowel wall
Lympho-granuloma venereum	Chlamydiae; Frei reaction positive	Rectum	Chronic suppurative and granulomatous

most greatly involved (Chapter 11). Ulcerations may occur.

Enteric-coated tablets containing potassium chloride appear to have been responsible for ulcerative lesions of the small intestine. They were administered to relieve potassium deficiency in patients receiving thiazide diuretics.

A small proportion of users have developed serious circumferential lesions, which appear to be hemorrhagic infarcts. Rapid release and absorption of the potassium chloride in a short segment of intestine appears to initiate the vascular stasis leading to infarction and ulceration.

Character of ulcers	Microscopic appearance	Complications
Ragged, small, and superficial; may be coalescing and extensive		
No specific form, hemorrhagic, multiple, sometimes extensive	Hyaline thickening, inflammation, and necrosis of small arteries in affected area	
Acute, usually single; may be long and narrow		Hemorrhage; perforation
Ulcers involve Peyer's patches; oval; in long axis of bowel	Proliferation of large mononuclear phagocytic cells	Perforation; hemorrhage
Shallow, ragged, very numerous, and coalescent; not undermined	Superficial fibrinopurulent exudate	Dehydration; stenosis may follow healing
Undermined edges; flask-shaped on section	Amebae in tissues; leukocytic infiltration when secondarily infected	Perforation; liver abscess
Extensive, ragged, chronic, coalescing ulcerations surrounding islands of hyperplastic mucosa	Nonspecific inflammation of mucosa and submucosa; crypt abscesses	Severe hemorrhage; sometimes malignant change in polypoid mucosal islands
No ulcers but superficial desquamation of surface epithelium	Loss of epithelium from mucosa	Extreme dehydration
Not specific	Extreme thickening of entire wall; sarcoidlike aggregates of epithelioid and giant cells	Obstruction of bowel; mesenteric lymph nodes affected; perforation; fistula
Affect lymphoid tissue but tend to encircle bowel	Caseous necrosis; epithelioid, giant, and lymphoid cells	Stenosis of gut; perforation and peritonitis
Not specific	Suppuration; characteristic ray fungus in lesions	Pylephlebitis; chronic draining sinus or fistula
Not specific	Often not characteristic; focal abscesses	Obstruction of lumen (rectal stricture)

Intestinal inflammations caused by infection

Among the most important intestinal infections are those caused by the coli-typhoid-dysentery group of organisms. This group consists of aerobic gram-negative bacilli. One division of the group, distinguished by the inability to ferment lactose, consists of highly pathogenic organisms, such as those of typhoid, paratyphoid, and dysentery. A second division, composed of lactose fermenters, includes the colon bacillus and closely related organisms. They are of very low pathogenicity.

Typhoid fever. Infection with *Salmonella*

typhosa is characterized by involvement of lymphoid and reticuloendothelial tissues, with hyperplasia of large mononuclear phagocytic cells. It is a generalized infection in all cases, but involvement of the lymphoid tissue of the intestine (Peyer's patches and solitary lymph follicles) is usually the most prominent feature, and ulceration there gives rise to the most dangerous complications of perforation and hemorrhage.

The typhoid bacilli are ingested with water, milk, or food that has been contaminated, usually by chronic carriers. The febrile illness often includes severe mental clouding and toxic symptoms in addition to intestinal disturbances, and it lasts for about 4 weeks. The blood culture is usually positive during the first week but is less regularly so later. The stool culture is more frequently positive during the second and third weeks. Urine culture is positive in about 20% of cases in the third and fourth weeks. The Widal reaction, which is the demonstration of specific agglutinins in the patient's serum, is usually positive after the first week. This test may be invalidated as a diagnostic procedure if the patient has had a recent inoculation with typhoid vaccine, which may produce a positive reaction. At autopsy, the organisms are most easily isolated from the spleen or gallbladder. The leukopenia that occurs, with a decrease in the number of granulocytes and relative increase in nongranular white blood cells, is in accordance with the body's reaction to the organism (i.e., proliferation of mononuclear cells rather than exudation of polymorphonuclear leukocytes).

Intestinal lesions. The lower ileum and cecum, where lymphoid tissue is most abundant, are involved earliest and most severely. The more proximal parts of the small intestine and the more distal parts of the large intestine show a later and less severe reaction. In early cases, Goodpasture has demonstrated the growth of a small gram-negative form of the organism in young plasma cells of the lymphoid follicles. The early changes in Peyer's patches and lymphoid follicles are congestion and edema, followed soon by a great proliferation of large mononuclear leukocytes, the

characteristic cells of typhoid fever. These involved lymphoid regions stand out as prominent irregular projecting areas on the mucosal surface. The large mononuclear cells in the lesions are actively phagocytic, and in their cytoplasm can be seen remnants of ingested lymphocytes, plasma cells, and sometimes the large gram-negative typhoid bacilli.

At about the seventh to tenth day, necrosis begins in the affected patches. Tiny necrotic areas slough off, leaving small ulcers that, by their coalescence, form rounded or oval areas of ulceration having the size, shape, and situation of Peyer's patches. The long axis of these ulcers is in the direction of the long axis of the bowel, in contradistinction to tuberculous ulcers, which tend to encircle the gut.

This process of ulceration, particularly if rapid, may result in hemorrhage. The ulcers usually involve only the mucosa and submucosa, but deeper extension and perforation may occur, particularly as the result of secondary infection. Perforation is most likely to occur in the lower ileum, where the lesions are earliest and most severe. Generalized peritonitis follows, except in cases of slower perforating processes, which allow a walling off and localization of the peritonitis.

On recovery, surface epithelium grows over the ulcerated area, but there is little regeneration of the glandular epithelium or lymphoid tissue. There is no scar formation or contraction of the bowel.

Lesions in other organs. Although intestinal lesions are usually primary and predominant in typhoid fever, the infection is a generalized one, and various other organs, such as the spleen, liver, lymph nodes, bone marrow, and gallbladder, are rather constantly involved. The reaction tends to be similar everywhere, with proliferation of large mononuclear cells and foci of necrosis. The necrotic lesions are mainly caused by the endotoxins of *Salmonella typhosa,* but vascular blockage by accumulated mononuclear cells is a contributing factor. Exaggerated vascular hyperreactivity to catecholamines (due to endotoxemia [?] or serotonin release [?]) may be a factor contributing to focal necrotic lesions.

The *spleen* is enlarged up to 400 or 500 g. It is red and soft and exceedingly engorged with blood. In addition to this extreme congestion, collections of large mononuclear cells are seen microscopically. Small focal areas of necrosis may be present.

The *liver* likewise shows small focal necrotic lesions, irregularly distributed in the lobules.

Mesenteric *lymph nodes* also show microscopic necrotic foci and great accumulation of large mononuclear cells. Similar changes may be found in *bone marrow,* where the formation of granulocytes is in abeyance.

The *gallbladder* is usually infected, and the organisms can be cultivated from the bile. Morphologic change in the gallbladder usually is slight, but acute cholecystitis may accompany or follow typhoid fever. A focus of infection may remain here, however, and excretion of organisms by way of the bile and intestinal tract results in a chronic carrier of the disease.

Cloudy swelling and even fatty degeneration affect the heart, liver, and kidneys in typhoid fever as in other acute infections. Zenker's degeneration of voluntary muscle is not uncommon. Rarer complications of typhoid fever include meningitis, suppurative periostitis or osteomyelitis, hemorrhagic pneumonia, and thrombosis of the veins of the legs.

Paratyphoid fever. The illness of paratyphoid infection is similar to that of typhoid fever, although it is of shorter duration, is less severe, and has a lower mortality. The lesions produced are essentially similar but of less severe degree. The organisms that usually produce this disease are *Salmonella paratyphi* A, *Salmonella paratyphi* B, and *Salmonella choleraesuis.*

• • •

In addition to typhoid fever and paratyphoid fever, *Salmonella* organisms are responsible for an important form of *food poisoning* in which acute gastroenteritis is produced. The organisms usually are less virulent types of salmonellae, the most common of which in the United States is *Salmonella typhimurium.*

Dysentery. Dysentery is a term loosely used to indicate diarrhea with pus, blood, or mucus in the stools. Several unrelated conditions may thus be included under this term. The important types of dysentery are caused by *Shigella dysenteriae* and by *Entamoeba histolytica.*

Bacillary dysentery. There are several varieties of dysentery bacilli, which may be distinguished by fermentative and antigenic reactions. They produce an endotoxin that has a local effect on the intestinal mucosa, and some also produce an exotoxin that may affect the nervous system.

The dysentery organisms reach the intestinal tract by means of contaminated food and drink. Dysentery is endemic but also tends to break out in epidemics, particularly in hot weather and when many persons live together under crowded and unhygienic conditions. An acute febrile illness lasting 6 to 8 weeks results, but the infection is localized in the bowel, and positive cultures are rarely obtained from the blood. Repeated flare-ups or even a chronic condition may occur.

The large intestine is involved almost exclusively, specific lesions being rare in other organs. The distal parts of the colon are more severely affected. Occasionally, the terminal ileum becomes involved. The lesion is of a diphtheritic or pseudomembranous type, with necrosis and desquamation of surface layers and abundant fibrinopurulent exudate (Fig. 20-12). In some very acute cases, death occurs from toxemia before any severe lesions have developed in the bowel. In most cases, however, there are widespread necrotic areas in the mucosa of the large intestine and abundant exudate. Sloughing of necrotic areas leaves an extremely ragged ulceration of the colon. The ulcers are usually shallow, are not undermined, and vary a great deal in size and shape. Their coalescence denudes large areas, leaving only occasional islands of intact mucosa. Severe diarrhea, excessive fluid loss, dehydration, and exhaustion accompany this condition of the bowel. Severe hemorrhage is uncommon. Perforation also is unusual and usually results in localized rather than generalized peritonitis.

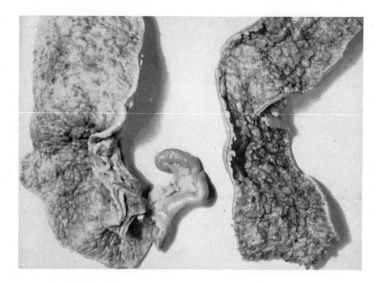

Fig. 20-12. Bacillary dysentery in large intestine.

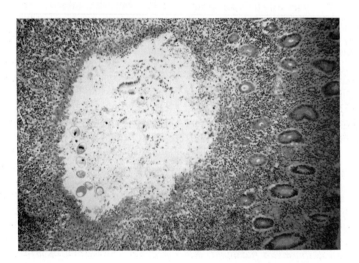

Fig. 20-13. *Balantidium coli* infection of bowel. (AFIP.)

Microscopic study shows the necrosis or ulceration of the mucosa with exudate on the surface. All layers of the bowel wall are edematous and infiltrated by neutrophilic leukocytes, but the submucosa is most greatly involved. Recovery is accompanied by healing of the ulcers and sometimes by scar formation and stenosis of the bowel. In healing, small mucosa-lined cysts may be formed that continue to harbor the organisms.

Amebic dysentery. Entamoeba histolytica infection of the large intestine produces large, undermined, and flask-shaped ulcerations. The amebae can be identified microscopically in the adjacent tissues. Leukocytes are present when there is secondary infection. Occasionally, a localized amebic granuloma may clinically simulate other inflammations or tumors of the colon. For detailed consideration, see p. 206.

Balantidial dysentery. A rare ulcerative dysentery is caused by the ciliated protozoan parasite *Balantidium coli,* the natural host of which is the pig. The parasites invade the mucosa of the large intestine and may produce chronic ulcers, sometimes deep and undermined. Lymphocytes, eosinophils, and neutrophils may form a mild inflammatory exudate. The parasites are easily recognized in the lesions by their large size (50 to 100 μ) and the large, dark elongate nucleus (Fig. 20-13).

Cholera. Cholera is an Asiatic and tropical disease caused by the *Vibrio cholerae* or *comma* bacillus. It spreads in epidemic fashion, particularly by contamination of water and food. The infection is almost always limited to the intestinal tract, where there is an acute catarrhal inflammation and distinct reddening of the mucosa. Profuse diarrhea, with flakes of whitish material in the watery stools (rice water stools), is characteristic and results in profound dehydration. Cholera bacilli produce their damage chiefly by the action of powerful toxins, altering the permeability of the epithelium, without penetration by organisms. This is in contrast to organisms such as *Shigella,* which invade and multiply in lining cells, causing necrosis and intense inflammation, or typhoid bacilli, which penetrate the intestinal epithelium without significant change initially but multiply in the lymphoid tissue of the intestine and lymph nodes.

Pseudomembranous enterocolitis. Pseudomembranous enterocolitis is a serious form of intestinal inflammation that appears to be increasing in frequency. There is extensive denudation of the intestinal mucosa with variable degrees of pseudomembrane formation and great exudation of fluid into the lumen of the bowel. The clinical features are profuse diarrhea, dehydration, shock, and a fulminant course to a usually fatal outcome. The lesion is associated with a variety of conditions, but a clearly defined etiologic mechanism has not been established. Formerly, it was commonly

observed as a complication of abdominal surgery, particularly gastrointestinal operations. However, it also occurs in association with nonsurgical illnesses, such as myocardial infarction and other cardiovascular disorders, hematologic diseases (e.g., leukemia, aplastic anemia, carcinomatosis, chronic liver disease, and septicemia. Of importance is the fact that many patients develop pseudomembranous enterocolitis while receiving antibiotics. In some of these patients, antibiotic-resistant staphylococci have been found that sometimes seem to have followed alteration in the bacterial flora of the intestine as a result of the use of antibiotics. In recent studies, resistant toxin-producing clostridia, which proliferate in the intestine during antibiotic therapy, have been implicated as a cause of antibiotic-associated pseudomembranous enterocolitis.

Tuberculosis. Tuberculous infection of the intestine may be primary, the organisms being ingested with milk or other food. More commonly, it is secondary to a pulmonary lesion as a result of the swallowing of infected sputum. A considerable proportion of fatal cases of pulmonary tuberculosis show intestinal lesions.

The lesions begin and are most common in the lower ileum but from there extend upward and downward to involve the small intestine and colon. The lymphoid tissue of the bowel is affected, and yellowish areas of caseous necrosis develop in the mucosa and submucosa. Ragged ulcers result from sloughing of this necrotic material. The lesions extend by lymphatics, which run laterally, encircling the gut. Hence, the ulcerative lesions tend to be elliptical, extending laterally and partially encircling the bowel (Fig. 20-14). When such an ulcer is deep and extensive, its healing may produce significant contraction and stenosis of the bowel.

The microscopic appearance is similar to that of tuberculosis elsewhere, with caseous necrosis and lymphoid, epithelioid, and giant cells. Perforation of a tuberculous ulcer is uncommon and usually results only in a localized peritonitis or abscess formation, since peritoneal reaction has walled off the area. Severe

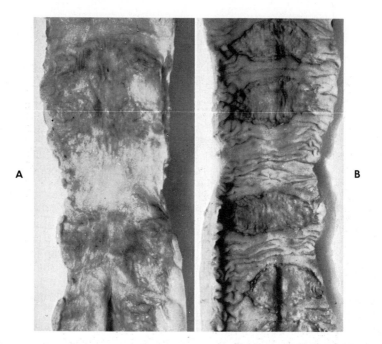

Fig. 20-14. Tuberculous enteritis. Note oval ulcers tending to encircle bowel. Change in serosal surface may be seen in **A.**

hemorrhage rarely occurs, because blood vessels in the lesions are involved by periarteritic and endarteritic changes as they are in tuberculous pulmonary cavities. Occasionally, a hyperplastic form of tuberculosis occurs around the ileocecal region, with great thickening of the bowel wall. Such lesions may be difficult to distinguish grossly from regional enteritis and tumors.

Actinomycosis. The ileocecal region or appendix is one of the common sites for actinomycosis. Characteristic features are thickening of the bowel wall, ulceration, and suppurative areas containing the ray fungus. Pylephlebitic spread to the liver is a frequent complication. Appendectomy is likely to be followed by a chronic sinus or fistula if the appendiceal infection was actinomycotic.

Lymphogranuloma venereum. Lymphogranuloma venereum may cause inflammation (proctitis) and stricture of the rectum. This lesion occurs particularly in women and generally represents a complication of the primary lesion on the genitalia (p. 194).

Intestinal inflammations of undetermined cause

Ulcerative colitis. Ulcerative colitis (proctocolitis) is of debatable etiology but usually is considered as a specific entity. Among suggested causes are infection, immunologic derangement, lack of protective enzymes in the bowel wall, neurogenic and psychogenic disturbances, mucolytic and proteolytic enzymes acting on the mucosa, and alterations in the ground substance of the connective tissue. In some patients, a family history of the disease is obtained in a proportion much higher than would be expected by chance.

Interest in immunologic factors has increased over the years. Sensitivity to food (particularly milk) and autoimmunity have been considered to be possible mechanisms in the pathogenesis of ulcerative colitis, based on some suggestive, but not conclusive, evidence. For example, a greater tendency to form antibodies against milk proteins has been noted among colitis patients compared with normal subjects, autoantibodies to colonic tis-

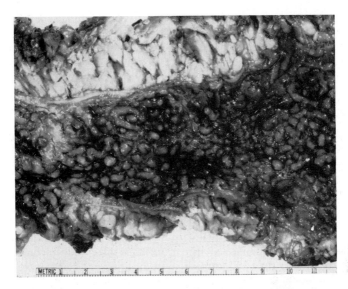

Fig. 20-15. Chronic ulcerative colitis with polypoid regeneration of mucosa.

sue have been identified in patients with colitis, and lymphocytes obtained from patients with this disease tend to be cytotoxic for fetal colon cells in vitro. Bacteria, such as *Escherichia coli,* are possible sources of antigen that may produce antibodies that cross-react with colonic tissue.

Most cases of colitis occur in early or middle adult life. The course frequently extends over years, with remissions and relapses. The large intestine is involved, the rectum and sigmoid being affected earliest, and spread occurs proximally. The disease may be restricted to the rectum (proctitis). Occasionally, extension to the distal ileum may occur. Hyperemia and edema of the mucosa are followed by the appearance of small areas of necrosis and ulceration. Initially, there is infiltration of the mucosa and submucosa by leukocytes (lymphocytes, plasma cells, neutrophils, and eosinophils) as well as mast cells. This is accompanied or followed by changes in the crypts of Lieberkühn, viz., diminished mucus content of the crypt epithelium, segmental dilatation of crypts with degeneration and thinning of epithelial cells, and accumulation of neutrophils around and within the affected crypts ("crypt abscesses"), often followed by undermining of adjacent mucosa, which sheds and thus

leads to ulcer formation. It is also possible that ulcers may form as a result of direct damage to the mucosal epithelium and lamina propria. Richly vascular granulation tissue appears in the base of the ulcers. Strips and tags of mucosa surrounded by the ulcerations become edematous and hyperplastic, projecting as inflamed polypoid masses, so-called pseudopolyps (Fig. 20-15).

Typically, ulcerative colitis is primarily a mucosal disease. Although the submucosa is affected, there usually is no involvement of the muscularis or serosa, except in the fulminating case. This is in contrast to Crohn's disease, which involves all layers of the bowel wall. Fibrosis occurs in ulcerative colitis, but stenosis is not as likely to develop as it does in Crohn's disease. Perforation with peritonitis is a possible complication. This is likely to occur in a fulminating form of the disease that is characterized by acute toxic dilatation of the colon *(toxic megacolon).* Another serious complication is severe hemorrhage.

Malignant change not infrequently occurs in the polypoid mucosa and may be highly malignant with early metastasis. The frequency of death from cancer of the colon in patients with ulcerative colitis is six to eight times that in others of the same age and sex. The cancer is more likely to occur 10 years or more after the onset of the colitis. It appears at an earlier average age, may arise from multiple sites, and tends to be less well circumscribed and to have a very fibrous stroma. Cancers occurring with ulcerative colitis are more evenly distributed throughout the colon. Other complications may include renal tubular degeneration, particularly of a hydropic or vacuolar type (p. 355), fatty liver, chronic active hepatitis, cirrhosis of the liver, interstitial pancreatitis, fluid and electrolyte disturbances, protein loss, arthritis, erythema nodosum, conjunctivitis, uveitis, venous thrombosis, and amyloidosis.

It should be noted that some reports suggest that when the disease remains limited to the rectum (ulcerative proctitis), the prognosis is better and there are fewer and less serious complications than in diffuse ulcerative colitis.

Regional ileitis (enteritis). Regional ileitis (Crohn's disease) is a chronic, often granulomatous, inflammation affecting distal portions of the ileum. It is characterized grossly by considerable regional thickening of the bowel wall with corresponding stenosis of the lumen, mucosal ulceration, and enlargement of regional mesenteric lymph nodes (Fig. 20-16). Histologically, its unique feature consists of focal masses of epithelioid and giant cells in the involved intestine and in mesenteric lymph nodes. These lesions may occur in small numbers or even be entirely absent. Important clinical features are a palpable mass in the abdomen, signs of chronic obstruction, abdominal pain, and loss of weight.

The etiology of regional ileitis is unknown, although various infectious agents (bacterial and viral) and hypersensitivity have been considered as possible causes. Histologic similarity has suggested a possible relationship to Boeck's sarcoid, and there appears to be a disturbed lipid absorption metabolism. It is to be distinguished from the granulomatous lesions of tuberculosis and actinomycosis, which also commonly involve the ileocecal region, by the different histologic picture and demonstration of the specific causative organisms of the latter conditions. Lymphogranuloma inguinale may involve the bowel and is differentiated by the presence of a positive Frei reaction, its microscopic appearance (p. 194), and its usual involvement of the rectum rather than the ileum. There are instances, however, in which Crohn's disease may affect the colon, with or without involvement of the ileum. Any portion of the colon may be involved (*regional colitis, granulomatous colitis,* or *Crohn's disease of the colon*). Involvement of the anus may occur also.

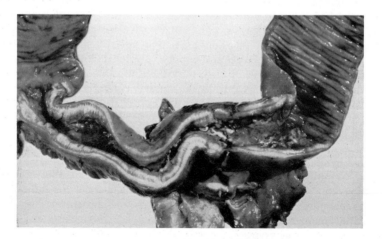

Fig. 20-16. Regional ileitis (enteritis).

Regional ileitis appears grossly as a garden-hose thickening of a segment of ileum, either at or within a few feet of its termination. In its acute stage, the involved area is red and edematous. Later, it tends to be rigid, firm, fibrous, and ulcerative. The bowel is dilated proximal to the constricted lumen of the involved segment. The adjacent mesentery contains enlarged lymph nodes. Perforation may occur, but the effects usually are limited by peritoneal adhesions.

Microscopically, the main feature is extreme thickening of the bowel wall. There is a progressive granulomatous lymphangitis with focal lymphatic obliteration that produces elephantiasis of the intestinal wall, mesentery, and regional lymph nodes. There is also chronic inflammation, often with prominent lymphoid nodules and noncaseating aggregates of epithelioid cells and multinucleated giant cells. Tubercle bacilli cannot be demonstrated in these lesions. Similar sarcoidlike lesions are often present in the enlarged mesenteric nodes. Obstructive lymphedema is constantly present in the thick submucosa. Ulcerations of various depths develop, floored by granulation tissue. Eventually, a diffuse cellular infiltration involves the bowel wall, with thickening of the muscle coat and adhesions of the serosa. In some patients with Crohn's disease, even without colonic lesions, small granulomatous lesions have been identified in biopsy specimens of the sigmoidoscopically normal rectal mucosa.

Complications of regional ileitis include intestinal obstruction, perforation, fistula formation, malabsorption syndrome, fluid and electrolyte disturbances, protein loss, arthritis, and amyloidosis.

Necrotizing enterocolitis. *Idiopathic necrotizing enterocolitis* is a disease that affects premature infants but also may occur in full-term neonates. Although it is referred to as "enterocolitis," there usually is minimal or no inflammatory reaction. The essential features are hemorrhage and necrosis, the latter resembling the ischemic or infarct type. Obstruction of the intestinal tract or major vessels is not evident. Disseminated intravascular coagula-tion may be an associated feature, but it is not certain whether this is secondary or primary. The possibility that this microcirculatory effect may be mediated by a Schwartzmann reaction, an endotoxemia, or other factors has been considered. The mortality among affected infants is high. Recovery may be followed by intestinal stricture resulting from healing of necrotic lesions. Other complications include perforation of the bowel and pneumatosis intestinalis.

Hemorrhagic necrotizing enterocolitis has been described as a fulminating and fatal complication of *leukemia* in adults. In these cases, leukemic infiltration of the intestinal wall was absent or minimal and the mesenteric vessels were patent. Bacterial or fungal invasion of the bowel and bloodstream, acute peritonitis, and shock commonly were present. The pathogenesis of the intestinal lesion was not determined, but possible factors that were considered include prior treatment with broad-spectrum antibiotics, chemotherapeutic agents, severe granulocytopenia, thrombocytopenia, bacteria, and fungi.

Inflammation of appendix

Inflammation in the appendix has the same features and follows the same course as inflammation elsewhere. Its importance is caused by its frequency as a serious surgical condition with significant complications. Obstruction of the appendiceal lumen by fecaliths and interference with vascular supply are important features in its pathogenesis. Spread of the infection beyond the appendix rather than the lesion in the appendix itself is the factor that causes mortality.

Acute appendicitis. The full story of the cause of acute appendicitis is not yet known. The nervous strains and dietary habits of modern life have been vaguely suggested as predisposing factors. The essential factor causing the wall of the appendix to react with inflammation is invasion by bacteria. The common organisms in the inflamed appendix are colon bacilli and varieties of streptococci, organisms commonly found in the intestinal lumen. Obstruction of the lumen and subsequent vascular occlusion brought about by the increasing luminal pressure are considered to be factors of importance in the etiology of appendicitis. They probably act by breaking down the resistance of the wall of the appendix to invasion by the potential pathogens in the lumen.

Morbid anatomy. Acute appendicitis is often classified as (1) catarrhal, (2) suppurative, and (3) gangrenous. In catarrhal appendicitis, the inflammation is limited to the mucosal and submucosal layers. It is usually a mild type or an early stage of the suppurative type. In suppurative appendicitis, the inflammation is usually more diffuse, involving the muscle and serosal layers as well, and the lumen is filled with pus. In gangrenous appendicitis, interference with circulation by the inflammatory exudate leads to areas of necrosis extending through the wall of the appendix.

The beginning of acute appendicitis is usually a superficial ulceration of the mucosa. Spread occurs from the mucosa to the serosa in a wedge-shaped area and then travels rapidly lengthwise in the muscular and serous coats. Grossly, the appendix appears swollen, the serosal vessels are congested, and the surface of the serosa has lost its normal shininess or may be covered by discernible fibrinous or fibrinopurulent exudate. The muscular walls are thick and edematous. The lumen frequently contains pus (Fig. 20-17). The mucosa may show areas of hemorrhage and ulcerations. The causes of luminal obstruction may be swelling of lymphoid tissue, the formation of a calculus or a fecalith (a firm, dried fecal concretion; Fig. 20-18), or marked fibrous thickening of a portion of the appendiceal wall. Over a large fecalith, the wall is likely to be thin and gangrenous. Gangrenous areas show a grayish green or black discoloration, have a thick flaky layer of fibrin on the surface, and often have a small perforation.

Microscopically, the early stage of acute appendicitis is often difficult to discern, particularly if the section is not through exactly the right area. The normal lymphoid cellularity of the mucosa and submucosa may be confusing. Ulceration of the mucosa or a purulent exudate in the lumen may be seen if the section is through the proper area. In most cases of acute appendicitis, the diagnosis is obvious from the infiltration of leukocytes in the muscular and serous layers.

Complications. Many milder cases of acute

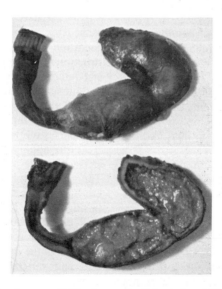

Fig. 20-17. Acute appendicitis. Lumen is distended and filled with pus.

appendicitis subside without surgical interference, but in other cases spread of the infection may occur with serious or fatal results. Such spread is usually to the peritoneum as a result of gangrene or perforation. If there has been opportunity for the walling off and limitation of the infection to the region around the appendix, a localized abscess may result. This localized peritonitis is much less dangerous than the generalized peritoneal spread that quite commonly occurs. In some cases, spread from the appendix is by infection of portal veins draining the inflamed organ (pylephlebitis) and leads to the production of multiple abscesses in the liver. A false diverticulum of the appendix may follow appendicitis.

Chronic appendicitis. Chronic appendicitis has been a subject of controversy because it is often difficult to correlate the clinical symptoms attributed to the appendix with the anatomic findings. In some cases, there is evidence of obstruction from a fecalith or other cause but without any active inflammatory process discernible in the wall of the appendix. Very often, the anatomic finding is a fibrous thickening of the submucosa and mucosa, with atrophy of the mucosal glandular elements and with or without a hyperplasia of the submucosal lymphoid tissue. In its extreme degree, such fibrosis may completely obliterate the lumen. Although this fibrosis may be the end result or healed stage of previous, recurring attacks of acute inflammation in some patients, it may be of noninflammatory origin in others. Masson's studies have indicated that in some cases the thickening of the submucosa and the obliteration of the lumen are largely caused by proliferation of smooth muscle bundles and nervous elements associated with Meissner's plexus, the so-called musculonervous complex of the appendix.

Lesions in measles. In measles, the lymphoid tissue of the appendix, as well as in the throat, spleen, and remainder of the intestinal tract, is distinctly hyperplastic. In early stages, there are characteristic giant cells in the mucosa and lymph follicles (see Fig. 8-9).

Oxyuris vermicularis infection. In children, pinworms commonly infect the appendix, where they may obstruct the lumen. In most instances they cause little damage, but in some cases they may be associated with the clinical picture of acute appendicitis (p. 212).

Mucocele. Complete obstruction of the

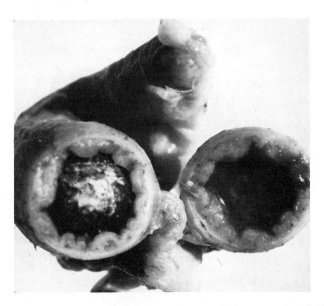

Fig. 20-18. Fecalith obstructing lumen of appendix in acute appendicitis.

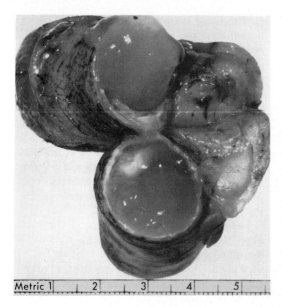

Fig. 20-19. Mucocele of appendix.

proximal portion of the appendix sometimes results in a cystlike dilatation (mucocele) of the distal part (Fig. 20-19). The contents of the dilated sac are a thick mucoid material. Malignant mucoceles are lined by a thick papillary layer of mucus-secreting cells. In some instances, rupture of the mucocele may cause *(pseudo) myxoma peritonei,* although this is more commonly a complication of ovarian mucinous cystadenocarcinoma.

DIVERTICULA OF INTESTINE

A diverticulum of the intestine may be true or false. A true diverticulum has all layers of the bowel in its wall. The common example is the congenital Meckel's diverticulum. False diverticula are acquired herniations of the mucosa through a weak place in the muscularis of the bowel. Their walls contain only mucosal and serosal layers. They occur in both the small and large intestine and are particularly common in the latter.

Meckel's diverticulum. Meckel's diverticulum is caused by the persistence of the proximal portion of the omphalomesenteric duct, which normally atrophies during early fetal life. It is found in 1% to 2% of persons. It varies up to 30 cm in length but is usually about the size of a small finger. It is situated 1 to 3 ft. proximal to the ileocecal junction (averaging 80 cm). Its structure is similar to that of the bowel wall, but heterotropic tissue, such as gastric or duodenal mucosa, or pancreatic tissue may be found in it. Peptic ulcer, subject to the complications of hemorrhage and perforation, has been reported in such tissue.

The most common lesion of Meckel's diverticulum is inflammation. Pathologically, this is similar to appendicitis, which it may mimic clinically. More rarely, it may promote intestinal obstruction by intussusception or adhesions, or it may be the seat of a tumor. Hemorrhage from the bowel is an important complication of the diverticula containing gastric mucosa.

Patent omphalomesenteric (vitelline) duct is comparatively rare. A communication is demonstrable between the umbilicus and the ileum. The intestine may prolapse through the umbilical fistula.

Acquired diverticula. The common sites for diverticula are the esophagus, duodenum, and colon, but they also occur in the small intestine. In these sites, they are commonly false diverticula, although some may have muscle fibers in their walls. In the small intestine they occur along the mesenteric attachment (Fig. 20-20), whereas in the colon they are situated away from the mesenteric attachment between the taeniae or longitudinal muscle bands of the colon (Fig. 20-21). The descending and sigmoid portions of colon have the highest incidence. The protrusion often is into appendices epiploicae, so that the diverticula are readily overlooked. They vary up to several centimeters in diameter. Microscopically, their wall is found to be composed of a thinned mucosa and serosa between which may be a few connective tissue and muscle fibers.

When present without complications, the condition is known as *diverticulosis.* The common complication is inflammation, or *diverticulitis* (Fig. 20-22). This is promoted by the lodging of fecal matter in the sacs. Spread of

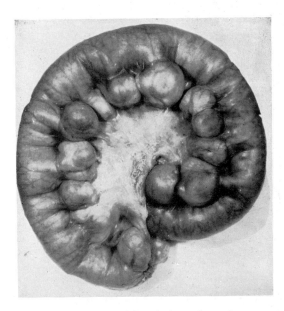

Fig. 20-20. Diverticulosis of small intestine. Diverticula are located at mesenteric border and have large stomas. (Courtesy Dr. J. R. Schenken.)

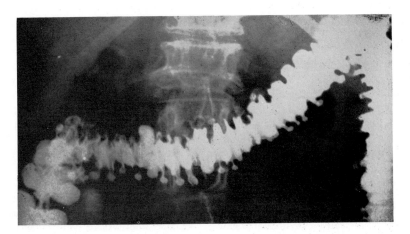

Fig. 20-21. Roentgenogram of diverticulosis of colon. Diverticula are small, and stomas are narrow. (Courtesy Dr. H. Hunt and Dr. R. Moore.)

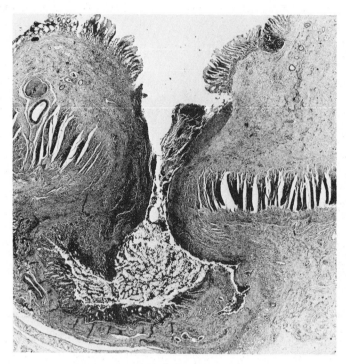

Fig. 20-22. Diverticulum of colon. Lining of diverticulum shows inflammation and necrosis (diverticulitis).

inflammation to surrounding tissue *(peridiverticulitis)* may occur also. The chronic inflammatory process causes thickening of the bowel wall and adjacent tissues with constriction of the lumen of the bowel. The gross appearance may closely simulate that of carcinoma.

INTESTINAL OBSTRUCTION

Complete obstruction to the passage of intestinal contents either by a mechanical obstruction of the lumen or by a paralysis of the bowel wall, particularly when high up in the intestinal tract, may bring about death in a relatively short time unless relieved. Such complete obstructions are usually acute and are distinguished from partial mechanical obstructions of bowel lumen, which are compatible with life for long periods and hence are termed chronic obstructions.

The most common causes of intestinal obstruction, in order of frequency, are hernias, adhesions, and neoplasms. Less frequent causes include volvulus, intussusception, inflammatory lesions, strictures, and foreign objects.

Chronic partial mechanical obstruction of the intestine may be caused by a large variety of conditions, such as tumors in the bowel or pressure on it from the outside, adhesive or fibrous bands (Fig. 20-23), and impacted feces. Perforation of an inflamed gallbladder into the intestinal tract with extrusion of a large gallstone may lead to intermittent upper intestinal obstruction *(gallstone ileus)*. Above a point of chronic partial obstruction, the bowel is distended and there is hypertrophy of the muscle wall. There is, of course, danger that the obstruction may become complete and acute at any time.

An *acute* obstruction may be a simple mechanical obstruction, or there may be an associated interference with the blood and nerve supply of the intestine, in which case it is said to be strangulated. Interference with the blood supply to a segment of intestine, as in thrombosis of mesenteric vessels, results in a paralytic obstruction, although there may be no mechanical blockage. Neurogenic factors may produce an *adynamic (paralytic) ileus,* e.g., after operations or as a result of peritonitis, severe pain (renal colic), or systemic infection. Obstructions with strangulation occur in hernias and as a result of volvulus (twisting) or intussusception. Necrosis or infarction of the bowel wall occurs unless the blood supply is promptly restored. The involved portion of intestine becomes congested, edematous, hemorrhagic, and finally gangrenous. Ulcerations occur in and above obstructed portions of intestine (stercoral ulcers).

The *clinical effects* of intestinal obstruction vary, depending on the site and type of obstruction. For example, vomiting with loss of fluid and electrolytes occurs more rapidly and is more serious in high intestinal obstruction than in low. This results in dehydration and biochemical disturbances, and eventually renal insufficiency, shock, and even death may occur unless proper therapy is instituted early. Contributing to the loss of fluid by vomiting is intraluminal loss of fluid resulting from decreased fluid absorption and increased fluid secretion by the intestinal mucosa, an effect of the increased intraluminal pressure caused by distention of the bowel. In obstruction with strangulation, which results in ischemia of the intestine that in turn may produce infarction, the clinical effects tend to be more severe than in simple obstruction.

Hernia. An abdominal hernia is an abnormal protrusion of abdominal viscera outside the usual confines of the abdominal wall. Such protrusion may be through the inguinal canal, through the femoral canal, at the umbilicus, through a weak scar of an abdominal wound (ventral hernia), or through the diaphragm. Internal hernias are protrusions into intra-abdominal pouches.

A hernia becomes strangulated when there is a tight constriction of the loop of bowel at the neck of the sac. The constriction first compresses veins in which the pressure is low, causing congestion and swelling of the herniated loop. This, in turn, increases the constriction until eventually the arterial supply is cut off as well, and the involved tissue soon becomes gangrenous.

Diaphragmatic hernia. Herniation through the diaphragm may be congenital (i.e., caused by abnormality of development) or may be acquired as a result of trauma or wounds of the diaphragm.

Congenital diaphragmatic hernia is encountered quite frequently in newborn infants or young children (Fig. 20-24). It is about ten times more frequent on the left side than on the right. The hernia may be *true,* with the existence of a hernial sac composed of peritoneum and pleura, or more commonly, it is *false,* with no hernial sac existing, since the pleura and peritoneum are absent over the opening. Congenital false hernia is caused by abnormal persistence of the pleuroperitoneal canal, which connects the primitive pleural region with the abdominal region and normally becomes covered by a membrane about the seventh or eighth week of fetal life. An excessive mobility of the intestinal tract usually is associated because of the abnormal attachment of mesenteries.

Herniation also may occur through the esophageal hiatus.

Internal hernia. Occasionally, intra-abdominal hernias may occur, most commonly in or about the paraduodenal fossae, into the transverse mesocolon, or through the foramen of Winslow.

Adhesions. Congenital peritoneal bands, or more commonly, acquired peritoneal adhesions of inflammatory or postoperative origin may cause kinking or compression of the intestine, particularly the small intestine, with resultant intestinal obstruction. The adhesions and bands may predispose to a volvulus in some instances.

Neoplasms. Intestinal obstruction caused by neoplasms occurs most frequently in the large intestine, a common site for carcinoma in both sexes. The annular stenosing type of carcinoma, which tends to occur particularly in the rectosigmoid region, is the type that causes obstruction most frequently.

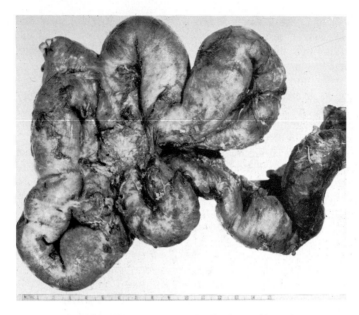

Fig. 20-23. Fibrous peritoneal adhesions of bowel.

Volvulus. Volvulus is a twisting or rotation of a loop of bowel that, by its occlusion of blood vessels, may result in strangulation. The coil of intestine becomes obstructed and gangrenous.

Intussusception. The invagination or passage of one portion of intestine into another segment is known as intussusception. The invaginated part tends to be carried along by peristaltic activity, dragging with it mesentery and blood vessels, which eventually become obstructed, so that congestion, edema, hemorrhage, inflammation, and adhesions occur. These changes may make reduction very difficult. Necrosis of the invaginated segment eventually develops. The condition is more common in young children, usually beginning in the ileocecal region. Sometimes polyps or other tumors of the intestine are dragged along by peristalsis and start an intussusception.

Multiple small intussusceptions of the small bowel may be found incidentally at autopsy. They are caused by irregular intestinal contractions at the time of death and, being without inflammatory changes, are easily reduced.

Congenital megacolon. Congenital megacolon, or Hirschsprung's disease, is a marked dilatation of the large intestine with hypertrophy of the muscle fibers. The basic defect is a lack of ganglion cells in Auerbach's (myenteric) and Meissner's (submucous) plexuses in the narrowed segment distal to the dilated segment of bowel. The aganglionic area usually does not extend higher than the sigmoid colon. The distended bowel produces considerable abdominal enlargement, and fecal evacuations occur after abnormally long intervals.

WHIPPLE'S DISEASE

Whipple's disease, sometimes referred to as *intestinal lipodystrophy,* is a rare and serious disorder. It is characterized by generalized manifestations, including fever, polyserositis, arthralgia and arthritis, diarrhea, intestinal malabsorption, and progressive emaciation, but the predominant lesion is in the small intestine.

The mucosa of the small intestine is thickened, with clubbing of villi, and shows dilated lymphatics and infiltration with large

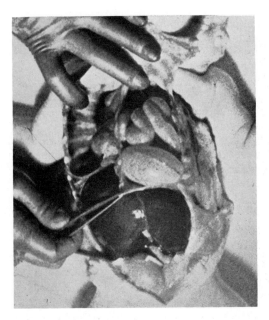

Fig. 20-24. Congenital diaphragmatic hernia. Note stomach and loops of bowel in left thoracic cavity. Diaphragm is held in forceps.

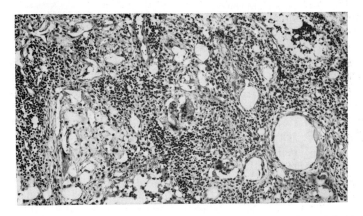

Fig. 20-25. Lymph node in Whipple's disease. Clear areas represent sites of lipid. Large pale histiocytes and some giant cell reaction are shown.

pale histiocytes. Mesenteric lymph nodes are enlarged, have lost their normal architecture, and show dilated spaces and sinuses filled with amorphous fat, large pale histiocytes, and some multinucleated giant cells (Fig. 20-25). The intestinal and lymph node histiocytes contain abundant mucopolysaccharide demonstrable by periodic acid–Schiff staining. Some of the material in the cells is in the form of sickle-shaped particles. Similar PAS-positive histiocytes have been observed in other organs also, e.g., liver and spleen.

Such evidence has suggested that Whipple's disease might be an intracellular defect within histiocytes or reticuloendothelial cells. However, antibiotic-sensitive bacilliform organisms have been demonstrated within and near macrophages, which suggests the possibility of an infectious origin of the disease. Some investigators interpret the previously mentioned sickle-shaped particles as being derived from the cell wall of phagocytized bacteria. Other evidence also suggests that Whipple's disease is a multisystem infection.

MALABSORPTION SYNDROME

The malabsorption syndrome is characterized by impaired absorption of fats, vitamins, proteins, and other nutrients and is manifested by steatorrhea, abdominal distention and pain, vitamin deficiencies, loss of weight, edema, and hematologic disorders (e.g., anemia). The syndrome may be *secondary* to a variety of disorders including:

1 Hepatobiliary and pancreatic diseases, in which lack of bile or pancreatic enzymes causes impairment of digestion or breakdown of fat, which is necessary for absorption

2 Intestinal conditions, such as regional enteritis, surgical resections, bacterial and parasitic infections, Whipple's disease, lymphomas, amyloidosis, and scleroderma, in which disturbances of mucosal absorption occur

The *primary* form of malabsorption syndrome is due to a primary mucosal cell abnormality, as in gluten-sensitive enteropathy and tropical sprue.

Gluten-sensitive enteropathy includes celiac disease in infants and children and nontropical sprue (adult celiac disease). The condition is related to the ingestion of wheat products containing a fraction (gluten) that causes damage to the intestinal mucosa. The mucosal villi become progressively thickened, blunted, and somewhat shortened, so that the surface appears flattened. These changes, which are sometimes referred to as "villous atrophy," are most prominent in the jejunum, which is a usual site for biopsy. Electron microscopic study reveals distortion and decrease in number of microvilli of the mucosal epithelial cells.

A genetic deficiency of an intracellular peptidase in the breakdown of the gluten in wheat had been considered as the basic defect. However, recently there have been investigations that suggest an immunologic basis for the disease, i.e., damage to the intestinal mucosa by an immune reaction induced by gluten antigens. Nevertheless, there may also be a genetic factor that predisposes the individual to hypersensitivity to gluten. Other studies have shown an association between celiac disease and alpha$_1$-antitrypsin deficiency. Many patients with gluten-sensitive enteropathy have histocompatibility antigen HLA-B8.

Tropical sprue is accompanied by pathologic changes similar to, but not as marked as, nontropical sprue. Macrocytic anemia is a common feature. The cause is not known, but infection has been incriminated as a possible cause.

PROTEIN-LOSING ENTEROPATHIES

Protein may be lost in the intestine, resulting in hypoproteinemia and edema. This may be idiopathic but often is associated with intestinal and extraintestinal diseases. Among the gastrointestinal diseases producing this syndrome, some of which also may be associated with malabsorption and steatorrhea, are chronic hypertrophic gastritis (*Menetrier's disease*), regional enteritis, ulcerative colitis, other inflammations, and lymphangiectasia of the small intestine. Chronic constrictive pericarditis may cause the syndrome.

MELANOSIS COLI

Melanosis coli is a symptomless condition of brown or black discoloration of the mucosa of the large intestine caused by a melaninlike pigment held in large mononuclear cells. The pigment also may be found in the submucosa and sometimes in mesenteric lymph nodes. The condition may be related to colonic stasis, as in chronic constipation.

PNEUMATOSIS CYSTOIDES INTESTINALIS

Pneumatosis cystoides intestinalis (or pneumatosis intestinalis) is an uncommon disorder characterized by gas-filled cysts in the submucosa and/or subserosa of the small bowel and sometimes of the colon. Occasionally, the esophagus may be involved (pneumatosis cystoides esophagi). Ranging in size up to several centimeters, the cysts may be lined by flattened endotheliumlike cells, forming pseudolymphatic spaces, or, if the cysts have been recently formed, by mononuclear cells and multinucleated giant cells.

The cysts may occur following pulmonary alveolar rupture, as in emphysema of the lungs. Air escapes into the mediastinum and thence to the retroperitoneum, after which it extends along the mesenteric vessels to the intestinal wall. The cysts also may be produced as a result of air entering the intestinal mucosa following trauma (e.g., endoscopic biopsy) or in association with inflammatory lesions, particularly those with ulceration and obstruction.

PILONIDAL SINUS

Pilonidal sinus, or sacrococcygeal sinus, is a very common lesion that, in some cases, may be a remnant of the neurenteric canal or an infolding of the epithelial layer of skin. Commonly, however, it is an acquired condition caused by the penetration of hairs into subcutaneous tissues, with chronic mild infec-tion. It occurs in the midline a few centimeters posterior to the anus, the sinus extending inward toward a cystic cavity in the subcutaneous tissue above the sacrococcygeal vertebrae (Fig. 20-26).

Microscopically, the usual features are hair shafts, multinucleated giant cells of the foreign body type, and abundant lymphocytes and plasma cells (Fig. 20-27).

Troublesome recurrence is likely to follow incomplete removal or infection in adjacent tissue. Cancer in a pilonidal sinus is extremely rare.

TUMORS OF SMALL INTESTINE

Tumors are uncommon in the small intestine. Various benign tumors such as *fibromas, myomas,* and *lipomas* may involve the small bowel, but *carcinoma* is rare. Brunner's gland *adenomas* occur rarely. *Carcinoid tumors* are encountered more often. *Multiple polyposis* of the stomach and small bowel may be associated with focal melanin pigmentation of the lips and mouth *(Peutz-Jeghers syndrome),* inherited as an autosomal dominant trait. Such polyps rarely become malignant. An occasional instance of carcinomatous transformation has been reported. The polyps in Peutz-Jeghers syndrome contain more than one type of cell (e.g., columnar cells and goblet cells), and the possibility that they are hamartomas has been considered. *Malignant lymphomas* of various types may involve the ileum as well as

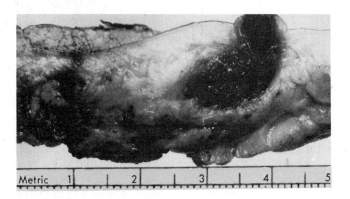

Fig. 20-26. Pilonidal sinus.

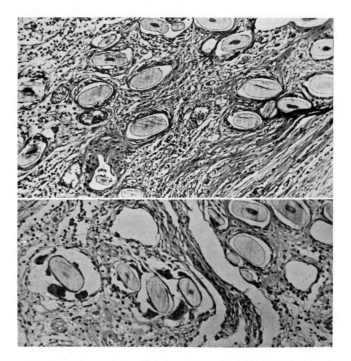

Fig. 20-27. Pilonidal sinus. Note shafts of hairs, some of which have foreign body giant cells around them, and infiltration of chronic inflammatory cells.

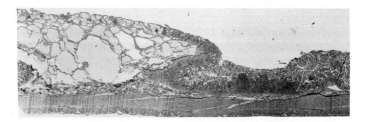

Fig. 20-28. Angioma of intestinal mucosa.

the region of the cecum or ascending colon. In some cases, a malignant lymphoma of the small bowel is focal in nature and may be cured by complete excision. *Angiomatous lesions* (Fig. 20-28) of the alimentary tract are rare except in association with vascular lesions elsewhere as part of one of the hereditary vascular dysplasias.

CARCINOID TUMORS

Carcinoid tumors (argentaffinomas) are distinctive neoplasms that have infiltrative and metastasizing potentialities but are of a low grade of malignancy. The tumor cells are believed to arise from Kultschitsky cells, i.e., argentaffin and chromaffin cells found at the base of Lieberkühn's glands, which produce

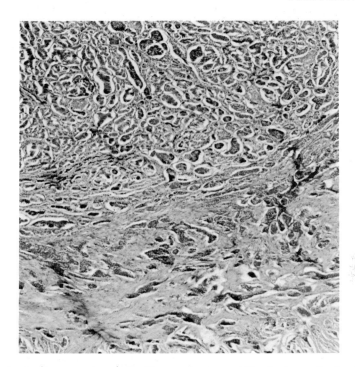

Fig. 20-29. Carcinoid tumor of appendix. Tumor of mucosa obliterates lumen (top) and infiltrates wall of appendix (bottom).

serotonin (enteramine; 5-hydroxytryptamine). A small proportion of carcinoid tumors may have liver metastases that produce excess serotonin and a distinctive clinical syndrome (the carcinoid syndrome). Other substances, such as bradykinin, have been identified that may contribute to the symptoms of this syndrome.

About 60% of carcinoid tumors occur in the appendix and most often near the tip, where they may form a yellowish annular thickening that encircles the lumen (Fig. 20-29). In the appendix, carcinoid tumors have a biologically benign course. They are not circumscribed, may infiltrate the muscularis, and in rare cases metastasize to lymph nodes, but distant metastases do not occur. Carcinoid tumors of the appendix do not give rise to the clinical carcinoid syndrome.

About 40% of carcinoid tumors arise from the remainder of the gastrointestinal tract, any part of which may be involved, although the ileum is the most frequent site (Fig. 20-30).

They most often occur as small yellowish or grayish submucosal masses with intact overlying mucosa and only uncommonly form large ulcerating or fungating masses. They are often multiple (25%). Infiltration of the muscularis and spread to lymph nodes are common, and about 15% metastasize to the liver. In all cases, the degree of malignancy is low, and the natural course of the disease tends to be long and slow. Carcinoid tumors also have been reported to occur in the bronchus, gallbladder, pancreas, Meckel's diverticulum, and ovarian dermoid cysts.

The cells composing a carcinoid tumor are remarkably uniform, and only very rarely are there mitoses or cells of polymorphous or giant form. The compact uniform cells have distinct nuclei but ill-defined borders and occur in solid clusters, sheets, islands, or cords with a variable but usually scanty stroma. Distinct gland formation is not commonly seen. Chrome and silver salts stain granules in the

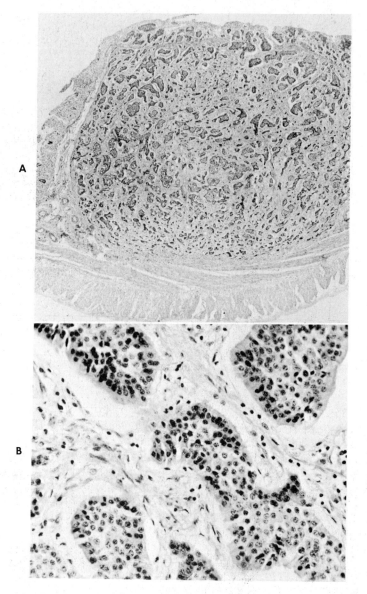

Fig. 20-30. Carcinoid tumor of ileum, producing nodule in mucosa. **A,** Overlying epithelium partly denuded. **B,** High-power view to show cellular details.

cytoplasm. A small proportion of carcinoid tumors, particularly those of the rectum and colon, fail to stain with silver and are considered to arise from preenterochrome cells.

The *carcinoid syndrome* occurs in some of the cases in which there are metastases in the liver, presumably caused by the production of large amounts of serotonin as well as other vasoactive substances, such as bradykinin. It is characterized by episodic flushing of the skin (beginning in the face and spreading over the trunk and extremities), a plethoric coloration or cyanosis, intestinal hyperperistalsis with diarrhea, asthmalike bronchoconstrictive attacks, and cardiac symptoms resulting from tricuspid and pulmonary valve involvement. In late stages, there may be much wasting, weight loss, and cutaneous telangiectases or pellagralike lesions.

The cardiac lesions are a fibrous thickening of the tricuspid and pulmonary valves, usually with tricuspid insufficiency and pulmonic stenosis. The thickening appears to be caused by a fibrous tissue growth without elastic fibrils superimposed on an intact valve cusp. It has been postulated that these changes are caused by exposure to large quantities of serotonin from the hepatic carcinoid metastases but that this substance tends to be destroyed in the lungs so that the left side of the heart is usually not similarly exposed. However, instances of left-sided heart involvement have been described.

Serotonin (5-hydroxytryptamine; enteramine) is derived from tryptophan and is a smooth muscle–stimulating and vasoconstrictive substance carried normally by the blood platelets. The large amount of serotonin produced by a functioning carcinoid tumor results in an excess of 5-hydroxy-3-indole acetic acid in the urine, a valuable laboratory diagnostic test.

Some of the manifestations may be attributed to the excess serotonin, such as those related to hypermotility of the intestines and endocardial lesions of the heart. Also, because of excess production of serotonin from dietary tryptophan, less of the latter is converted to nicotinic acid and protein, so that pellagralike changes are produced. The cause of the typical flushing is probably not the serotonin but possibly bradykinin or some other vasoactive substance.

Although the carcinoid syndrome is produced most often from an intestinal carcinoid tumor that has metastasized to the liver, it appears that the carcinoid type of bronchial adenoma may have a similar effect.

In rare examples, a functioning carcinoid tumor, composed of nongranular argyrophil cells, appears to produce 5-hydroxytryptophan, a precursor of serotonin.

CARCINOMA OF APPENDIX

Apart from carcinoid tumors, the appendix is rarely a site of primary carcinoma. Malignant mucocele of the appendix is a type of carcinoma in which the dilated appendix is filled with gelatinous material, and the mucosa has prominent papillary folds of mucus-secreting epithelium. Peritoneal spread with production of (pseudo) myxoma peritonei may result from rupture or spillage at the time of surgical excision. A colonic type of carcinoma, similar in structure to tumors of the large bowel, is the rarest variety of carcinoma of the appendix.

Carcinoid tumors of the appendix must be distinguished from the rare true adenocarcinoma of the appendix by (1) situation in the distal rather than the proximal part of the appendix, (2) the distinct yellow color, (3) argentaffin and chromaffin granules in the cytoplasm, (4) lack or paucity of metastases, and (5) absence of glandular arrangement.

TUMORS OF COLON AND RECTUM

Unlike the small bowel, the colon and rectum are common and important sites of *carcinoma*. The incidence is greatest in the rectum (50%), followed by the sigmoid (20%), the cecum and ascending colon (16%), the transverse colon and splenic flexure (8%), and the descending colon (6%). The tumors may begin as polypoid, sessile, or ulcerated neoplasms. The infiltrating ulcerative type may spread to lymph nodes while at an early and small stage. The tumors vary in rate of growth and degree of malignancy, but in some cases metastatic spread is late and cure is possible by excision. Grading by Dukes' method based on degree of spread is helpful in prognosis. The age of greatest incidence is after 50 years, but younger ages are not exempt.

Carcinoma of the colon is significantly (six to eight times) more common in patients with chronic ulcerative colitis than in the general population and occurs at a younger average age (p. 549). Carcinoma of the rectum and colon affects both sexes about equally. Although in men it occurs less frequently than lung carcinoma and in women it occurs less often than breast cancer, considering both sexes together it is almost equal in frequency to lung cancer. The possibility that the diet is etiologically related to colorectal cancer has been discussed previously (p. 263).

Other tumors that occur commonly in the rectum and colon are the *neoplastic polyps* (adenomatous polyps and villous adenomas). *Carcinoids* are less frequent tumors of the rectum and colon and may metastasize. Other uncommon rectal or anal tumors are *benign lymphoma (benign lymphoid polyp), basaloid carcinomas, mucoepidermoid tumors,* and *malignant melanoma* of the anorectal region.

Adenoma and polyposis

Neoplastic polyps of the colon and rectum are common. They occur in any portion of the large bowel but most frequently (60% or more) in the sigmoid and rectum, i.e., the same areas in which carcinoma is most frequent. The polyps are true adenomatous tumors and are to be distinguished from the inflammatory and hyperplastic areas of mucosa that simulate them in chronic dysentery and ulcerative colitis.

There are two types of neoplastic polypoid disease of the intestine: (1) diffuse polyposis, in which large numbers of polyps involve the colon and rectum, and (2) localized or solitary polyposis, in which there is only one or a few polyps present.

Familial polyposis coli (see Fig. 12-13) is hereditarily transmitted as an autosomal, non–sex linked dominant trait. This diffuse multiple polyposis is present in early life and often is complicated by carcinoma at an early age. The term *Gardner's syndrome* is applied to those instances of familial polyposis coli in which there are multiple tumors or tumorlike lesions elsewhere (skin, subcutaneous tissues, and bones), such as epidermal cysts, fibromas, lipomas, and osteomas (particularly of the skull and mandible). In contrast to familial polyposis of the large bowel, the polyps in the Peutz-Jeghers syndrome (p. 561) occur less frequently in the colon and rectum and rarely undergo malignant change.

Some of the confusion regarding the malignant potentialities of polypoid tumors results from the failure to differentiate clearly different types of polypoid lesions of the bowel. The term *polyp* simply refers to an outgrowth from a mucous membrane.

Adenomatous polyps are characterized by a relatively normal covering epithelium over a mass of elongated, bizarre-shaped mucosal glands, often with goblet cells. These lesions usually have a stalk (i.e., are pedunculated; Fig. 20-31). They are very common, and estimates of their incidence in adults have ranged from 10% to 50%. Apart from diffuse multiple polyposis, the importance of the ordinary adenomatous polyp as a precursor of carcinoma is debatable. Arising as a local hyperplasia of mucosal glands, it often shows focal areas of atypical cells, but carcinoma arising in such lesions is probably infrequent.

Villous polyps, also called *papillary adenomas, villous adenomas,* and *villous papillomas,* are composed of branching, fingerlike processes of surface origin. They usually are broad based or sessile rather than pedunculated, and the villi have cores of vascularized connective tissue. They may be multiple but also occur in solitary fashion in the rectum of older adults. They are distinguished by their broad attachment to the bowel wall, a villous architecture resulting from a disproportionate growth of surface epithelium, and a great tendency to recur after local removal. They are potentially malignant, and carcinomatous change may develop in any part. *Mucus-secreting villous adenomas* occasionally cause hypokalemia, hyponatremia, and dehydration due to profuse secretion from the mucosa of the tumor. The electrolyte imbalance may be severe, with sudden collapse and death.

Juvenile or *childhood polyps* are characterized by a prominent stromal growth and eosinophilic cell exudate. The surface may be ulcerated and covered by granulation tissue. The glands in the polyp show cystic dilatation with intraluminal epithelial projections. Juvenile polyps remain benign.

Differentiation of benign polyps from those that have become malignant or from small polypoid carcinomas may be difficult. Tendency to ulceration is greater in the malignant polyps. Since malignant change can occur in any

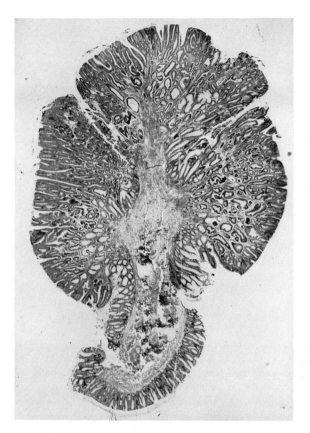

Fig. 20-31. Pedunculated benign polyp of large bowel. (From del Regato, J. A., and Spjut, H. J.: Ackerman and del Regato's Cancer, ed. 5, St. Louis, 1977, The C. V. Mosby Co.)

part of a polyp, sections from various portions must be examined before cancer can be ruled out. Sections from the base and from the tip are particularly likely to show malignancy. The important criteria of malignancy are (1) invasion of underlying tissue (muscularis mucosae) or of lymphatics or blood vessels, (2) anaplasia of the epithelial cells, and (3) disorderly arrangement of glands.

Less common benign tumors of the large intestine are *lipomas* and *leiomyomas*. *Lymphoid polyps* occur in the rectum and are benign.

Carcinoma

Gross features. The two main gross types of carcinoma of the colon and rectum are (1) annular constricting and (2) papillary. The *annular constricting* type is often ulcerative.

This type is seen especially in the rectosigmoid region (Fig. 20-32). It grows around the bowel, thickening and contracting the wall and narrowing and obstructing the lumen. The *papillary* variety grows as a bulky mass projecting into the bowel lumen, a type found particularly in the right half of the colon (Fig. 20-33). Necrosis and infection of the tumor mass and inflammatory lymphadenitis are common with this type. Bleeding and anemia also occur.

Histologic features. Histologically, the tumors nearly always show some tendency to gland formation and hence may be termed adenocarcinoma (Fig. 20-34). When this tendency is slight, the tumor cells form solid masses with scanty alveolar formation, and hence the tumor is of a medullary type. Stroma

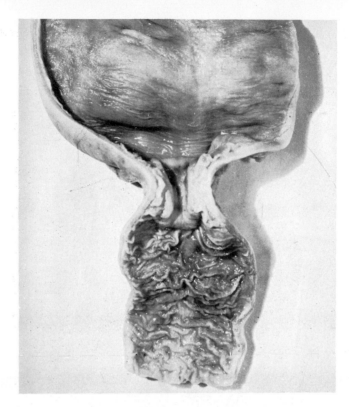

Fig. 20-32. Adenocarcinoma of sigmoid colon. Tumor encircles bowel and constricts lumen. Note dilatation of colon proximal to region of chronic obstruction.

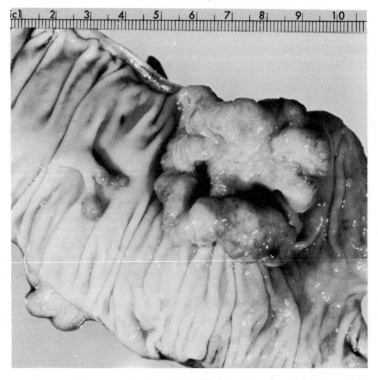

Fig. 20-33. Carcinoma of colon with adjacent benign pedunculated polyps.

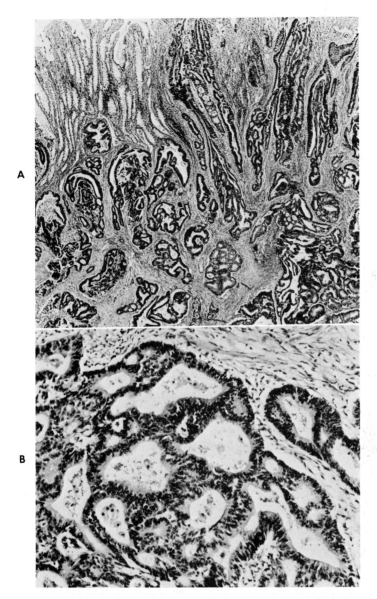

Fig. 20-34. Adenocarcinoma of colon. **A,** Note portion of normal mucosa at top left. Neoplasm replaces mucosa at top right and infiltrates wall of colon. **B,** High-power view showing adenocarcinoma infiltrating wall of colon, associated with proliferating fibrous stroma.

is often scanty or moderate in amount, but it may be so abundant that the tumor is scirrhous. Mucin production is prominent in about 5%. There may be an accumulation of mucin in individual cells so that they have a signet-ring appearance, or the mucoid material may be formed by the tumor alveoli, with mucinous deposition in a considerable area in which only a few tumor cells are evident.

Grading and staging. Classification according to degree of malignancy is important for prognostic and therapeutic purposes. There are two main methods, histologic grading and clinical staging, and these methods can be combined for greatest effectiveness.

The histologic method is based on the criteria of invasiveness, glandular arrangement, nuclear polarity, and frequency of mitosis and indicates rate of growth of the tumor. Grade I tumors are characterized by a well-differentiated, compact glandular structure, nuclei of the cells close to the basal portion, little tendency to invasion of surrounding tissue, and infrequent mitoses. These tumors most nearly resemble adenomas and are sometimes termed "malignant adenomas." In grade II tumors, the glandular arrangement is preserved but irregular, the nuclei are in variable positions, there is a greater invasive tendency, and there are more frequent mitoses. In grade III tumors, the glandular structure is almost completely gone, cells grow in solid masses, the cell polarity is lost, invasion is irregular, and mitoses are numerous. The practical value of this system of grading, if used alone, has been questioned.

The mucoid carcinoma of the signet-ring type tends to be of high malignancy, grade II or III, whereas carcinomas not of the signet-ring type are often of lower malignancy, grade I or II.

Dukes' method of classification is based on the degree of spread and appears to be more valuable for prognostic purposes. In group A are placed the carcinomas that have not spread through the bowel wall; in group B, those that have penetrated the bowel wall but have not invaded the adjacent lymphatics; and in group C, those that have invaded the local lymphatics. A TNM clinical stage classification also has been proposed.

The determination of *carcinoembryonic antigen* (CEA) serum values has been suggested as a technique for assessing the prognosis and management of patients with colorectal carcinoma, particularly in monitoring for tumor recurrence following resection (p. 255).

Spread and metastasis. Spread tends to be earlier in the flat, sessile growths than in the papillary type. It occurs by growth laterally around the bowel and outward through the wall. Local lymphatics then become affected. From a rectal cancer, this lymphatic involvement may be downward, lateralward, or frequently upward along the superior hemorrhoidal vessels by way of the retrorectal lymph nodes to the nodes of the pelvic mesocolon. Spread by the bloodstream most commonly produces metastasis in the liver. Next to the liver and regional lymph nodes, the peritoneum and lungs are the most frequent sites of metastasis.

Effects. The disturbances produced by carcinoma in the colon and rectum depend on the type and location of the growth. Because the symptoms are often slight until a late stage, the condition must be kept in mind and investigation made on the least suspicion. Ulceration usually is accompanied by slight bleeding, so that blood is detectable in the stools. Chronic obstruction is often a late development, usually in the annular stenosing type of carcinoma. The bowel above the obstruction is dilated.

Lymphoma

Benign lymphoma of the rectum (lymphoid polyp) is more frequent than primary malignant lymphoma of the rectum, which is rare. Most occur in the lower rectum or anal region. Lymphoid tumors of the large intestine proximal to the rectum are more likely to be malignant than benign.

A form of malignant lymphoma occuring throughout the gastrointestinal tract, *multiple lymphomatous polyposis,* must be differentiated from *nodular lymphoid hyperplasia,* which occurs chiefly in the small intestine and may be associated with hypogammaglobulinemia. Smaller foci of lymphoid hyperplasia may be seen throughout the intestinal tract in association with a variety of conditions and are sometimes referred to as *enterocolitis lymphofollicularis.*

Malignant melanoma

Melanoma of the rectum occurs predominantly at the anorectal junction or in the anus itself. It is often polypoid or pedunculated. The tumor is highly malignant, and the prognosis is poor.

Peritoneum

The peritoneum is a closed sac in the male, but in the female it communicates with the genital tract by openings at the ends of the fallopian tubes. The smooth, shiny peritoneal lining is composed of flattened mesothelial cells, beneath which are a basement membrane and a small amount of connective tissue containing abundant blood vessels and lymphatics. The total surface area is very large, and through the peritoneum there is ready absorption with equal facility in all parts. The omentum actively functions to wall off inflamed areas and to retard the spread of peritonitis.

Inflammation is the most important lesion of the peritoneum. Ascites is the accumulation of excessive fluid in the peritoneal cavity. Primary tumor *(mesothelioma)* of the peritoneum is rare, but metastatic growths involving peritoneum are common. Mesotheliomas may have epitheliumlike structures that do not secrete mucin, although hyaluronic acid may be present. Primary *retroperitoneal tumors* are of various histologic types, and some may arise from remnants of the urogenital fold. Most of the tumors are sarcomas, but epithelial cysts, lipomas, and other benign tumors also occur. Fibromatous and other solid tumors occur uncommonly in mesentery and omentum.

PERITONITIS

Infection of the peritoneum may result by spread (1) from a ruptured viscus (e.g., perforated peptic ulcer or gangrenous appendix), (2) through an inflamed but unruptured bowel wall (e.g., gangrenous infarct of the bowel), (3) from or by way of the internal genitalia (e.g., in puerperal endometritis and bacterial salpingitis), or (4) rarely, through the bloodstream. The peritoneal infection may be walled off so as to be limited to a localized area, as in periappendiceal abscess or subphrenic abscess, or there may be generalized involvement. Death may be caused by the absorption of toxins or by paralytic obstruction of a portion of intestine. Sterile inflammation of the peritoneum may be caused by the presence of a noninfective substance in the peritoneal cavity (e.g., blood resulting from hemorrhage, bile leaking from a perforation in the biliary system, or talc introduced during surgery).

Acute peritonitis has been described as occurring in hyperemic, exudative, and plastic stages. These changes may be found locally or diffusely. In the hyperemic stage, one sees great dilatation and congestion of peritoneal vessels, which gives the peritoneal surfaces a pinkish blue color. This stage occurs early, e.g., probably within an hour after the perforation of an ulcer. It is rapidly followed by the exudative stage, in which the exudate may be serous, fibrinous, purulent, or hemorrhagic, or any of these combined. In the plastic stage, the exudate forms adhesions that wall off the affected region or join peritoneal surfaces. Organization or fibrosis may occur.

Coliform bacterial peritonitis. Coliform bacteria, especially *Escherichia coli,* are common causative organisms in peritonitis. There is usually an abundant purulent exudate, which may have a fecal odor.

Streptococcal peritonitis. Streptococcal peritonitis is often a fulminating infection, in which only a thin, serous exudate is found. It is one of the most serious types of puerperal infection.

Gonococcal peritonitis. Gonococcal peritonitis is usually localized to the pelvis and originates from an infected fallopian tube. It tends to become chronic and forms fibrous adhesions.

Pneumococcal peritonitis. Pneumococcal peritonitis may be primary in female children, the organisms reaching the peritoneum through the fallopian tubes, or it may be secondary to pneumococcal infection in the lung or elsewhere. It used to be a common complication of the nephrotic syndrome in children but seldom is seen today.

Biliary peritonitis. Biliary peritonitis is

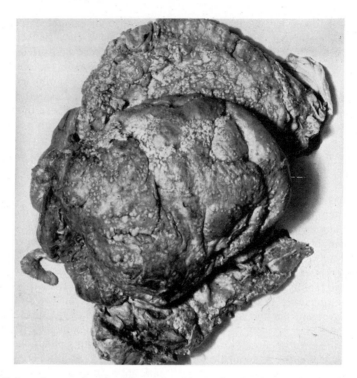

Fig. 20-35. Tuberculous peritonitis. Viscera bound together by dense tuberculous exudate and granulation tissue.

caused by chemical irritation of the peritoneum by bile, most often as a result of rupture of a common bile duct after a surgical procedure involving the gallbladder or biliary tract. In some cases, the bile is infected, and bacterial irritation is added.

Tuberculous peritonitis. Tuberculous peritonitis commonly results from local spread of the infection from a fallopian tube, the intestine, or a mesenteric lymph node, but hematogenous infection from distant sources may occur. Tiny tubercles may fleck all peritoneal surfaces. They appear as yellowish opaque spots surrounded by a reddish zone. The exudate may be very abundant and serous so that a large amount of fluid accumulates in the peritoneal cavity. This is the moist form. A dry or plastic type also occurs that is characterized by the matting together of abdominal viscera by firm adhesions or by a dense granulomatous tissue (Fig. 20-35).

• • •

Various rare types of peritonitis, such as the *rheumatic* and *actinomycotic* forms, also occur. *Periodic peritonitis* is a peculiar hereditary disorder that occurs in repetitive episodes among persons of Armenian, Arabic, or Jewish extraction. Recurring attacks of fever and nonspecific acute peritonitis of unknown cause, sometimes accompanied by signs of pleuritis and arthritis, are characteristic of this disease, which is also known as *familial Mediterranean fever*.

ASCITES

In ascites (edema of the peritoneal cavity), very large amounts of transudate may accumulate. This is seen in conditions in which edema is generalized, such as in congestive heart failure, nutritional edema, and nephrotic syndrome, and also occurs as a result of obstructions to the portal circulation as in cirrhosis of the liver. The watery fluid has a low specific gravity (usually less than 1.015) and a low protein content (less than 2% or 3%).

Fluid accumulation in the abdomen also may be an exudate resulting from inflammation, as in the moist form of tuberculous peritonitis. In such cases, the fluid has a higher cellular and protein content and a higher specific gravity.

Tumor metastasis to the peritoneum also may be associated with abundant fluid, particularly with ovarian cystadenocarcinomas. It is often possible to identify tumor cells in the centrifuged sediment of such fluid.

REFERENCES

Altshuler, J. H., and Shaka, J. A.: Cancer **19**:831-838, 1966 (squamous carcinoma of stomach).

American Joint Committee for Cancer Staging and End Results Reporting: Staging system for carcinoma of the stomach, Chicago, June 1971.

American Joint Committee for Cancer Staging and End Results Reporting: Clinical staging system for carcinoma of the esophagus, Chicago, October 1973.

Anderson, W. A. D.: Cancer **34**:909-911, 1974 (stage classification of cancer of colon and rectum).

Asman, H. B., and Pierce, E. R.: Cancer **25**:972-981, 1970 (familial multiple polyposis).

Ballard, J., and Shiner, M.: Lancet **1**:1014-1017, 1974 (ulcerative colitis—immunofluorescent studies).

Bartlett, J. G., et al.: N. Engl. J. Med. **298**:531-534, 1978 (toxin-producing clostridia and pseudomembranous colitis).

Bayless, T. M., and Knox, D. L.: N. Engl. J. Med. **300**:920-921, 1979 (Whipple's disease—a multisystem infection).

Becker, F. F., et al.: J.A.M.A. **194**:559-561, 1965 (Whipple's disease).

Black, M. M., et al.: Cancer **27**:703-711, 1971 (prognosis in gastric carcinoma).

Boley, S. J., et al.: J.A.M.A. **192**:763-768, 1965 (potassium and small intestinal ulcers).

Boley, S. J., et al.: J.A.M.A. **193**:997-1000, 1965 (potassium and small intestinal ulcers).

Brooks, F. P., editor: Gastrointestinal pathophysiology, ed. 2, New York, 1978, Oxford University Press (general reference).

Burdick, D., et al.: Cancer **16**:854-861, 1963 (Peutz-Jeghers syndrome).

Burkitt, D. P.: Cancer **28**:3-13, 1971 (epidemiology of colorectal cancer).

Callaghan, P. J., and Del Beccaro, E. J.: J.A.M.A. **180**:333-334, 1962 (carcinoma of appendix).

Cammerer, R. C., et al.: J.A.M.A. **235**:2502-2505, 1976 (pseudomembranous colitis).

Cassella, R. R., et al.: J.A.M.A. **191**:379-382, 1965 (spasm of esophagus).

Castleman, B., and Krickstein, H.: Gastroenterology **51**:108-112, 1966 (polyps and carcinoma).

Crowder, B. L., et al.: CA **18**:212-218, 1968 (gastrointestinal carcinoids).

De Dombal, F. T.: Br. Med. J. **1**:649-650, 1971 (ulcerative colitis).

Devroede, G. J., et al.: N. Engl. J. Med. **285**:17-21, 1971 (cancer, life expectancy, and ulcerative colitis).

Dungal, N.: J.A.M.A. **178**:789-798, 1961 (gastric cancer).

Editorial: J.A.M.A. **187**:57, 1964 (Boerhaave syndrome).

Editorial: Lancet **2**:501-502, 1974 (immunologic aspects of celiac disease).

Elliott, G. B., and Elliott, K. A.: Am. J. Roentgenol. Radium Ther. Nucl. Med. **89**:720-729, 1963 (pneumatosis intestinalis).

Fisher, E. R.: J.A.M.A. **181**:396-403, 1962 (Whipple's disease).

Folley, J. H.: N. Engl. J. Med. **282**:1362-1364, 1970 (ulcerative proctitis).

Foltz, E. L.: J.A.M.A. **187**:413-417, 1964 (peptic ulcer).

Goldgraber, M. B., and Kirsner, J. B.: Cancer **17**:657-665, 1964 (carcinoma and ulcerative colitis).

Goldgraber, M. B., et al.: Gastroenterology **34**:809-839, 840-846, 1958 (carcinoma and ulcerative colitis).

Goligher, J. C.: Br. Med. J. **1**:653-655, 1971 (ulcerative colitis).

Greenwald, A. J., et al.: J.A.M.A. **231**:273-276, 1975 (celiaclike disease and alpha$_1$-antitrypsin).

Halsted, J. A., and Zimmerman, H., editors: Med. Clin. North Am. **52**:1275-1501, 1968 (symposium on gastrointestinal and liver diseases).

Helwig, E. B., and Hansen, J.: Surg. Gynecol. Obstet. **92**:233-243, 1951 (lymphoma of rectum).

Horn, R. C., Jr., et al.: Arch. Pathol. **76**:29-37, 1963 (malignancy in Peutz-Jeghers syndrome).

Hornick, R. B., et al.: N. Engl. J. Med. **288**:686-691, 739-746, 1970 (typhoid fever).

Ingelfinger, F. J.: Nutr. Today **3**(3):2-10, 1968 (gluten-induced enteropathy).

Kennedy, B. J.: Cancer **26**:971-983, 1970 (TNM classification for stomach cancer).

Kraft, S. C., and Kirsner, J. B.: Gastroenterology **60**:922-951, 1971 (immunology and inflammatory bowel disease).

Kyriakos, M.: J.A.M.A. **229**:700-702, 1974 (malignant tumors of the small intestine).

Lane, N., and Lev, R.: Cancer **16**:751-764, 1963 (familial polyposis).

Lewin, K. J., et al.: Cancer **42**:693-707, 1978 (lymphomas of the gastrointestinal tract).

Lightdale, C. J., et al.: J.A.M.A. **226**:139-141, 1973 (causes of upper gastrointestinal tract bleeding).

Lim, F. E., et al.: Cancer **39**:1715-1720, 1977 (gastric lymphoma).

Little, J. M., et al.: Lancet **2**:659-663, 1969 (pseudomyxoma peritonei).

MacGregor, I. L.: J.A.M.A. **227**:911-915, 1974 (carcinoma of colon and stomach—causes).

Marks, C.: Carcinoid tumors, Boston, 1979, G. K. Hall & Co.

Matsudo, H., et al.: Arch. Pathol. **97**:366-372, 1974 (Japanese gastric cancer).

McGovern, V. J.: In Sommers, S. C., editor: Pathology

annual, vol. 4, New York, 1969, Appleton-Century-Crofts, p. 127 (differential diagnosis of colitis).

Ming, S. C., and Goldman, H.: Cancer **18**:721-726, 1965 (gastric polyps).

Morson, B. C., and Dawson, I. M. P.: Gastrointestinal pathology, ed. 2, Oxford, 1979, Blackwell Scientific Publications Ltd.

Otto, H. F., and Begemann, F.: Virchows Arch. [Pathol. Anat.] **350**:368-388, 1970 (Whipple's disease).

Pettet, J. D., et al.: Surg. Gynecol. Obstet. **98**:546-552, 1954 (pseudomembranous enterocolitis).

Reid, J. D.: J.A.M.A. **229**:833-834, 1974 (intestinal carcinoma in Peutz-Jeghers syndrome).

Robinson, M. J., et al.: Arch. Pathol. **96**:311-315, 1973 (enterocolitis lymphofollicularis).

Rodin, A. E., et al.: Arch. Pathol. **96**:335-338, 1973 (necrotizing enterocolitis).

Rotterdam, H., et al.: Am. J. Clin. Pathol. **67**:550-554, 1977 (microgranulomas in sigmoidoscopically normal rectal mucosa in Crohn's disease).

Sheahan, D. G., et al.: Cancer **28**:408-425, 1971 (multiple lymphomatous polyposis of the gastrointestinal tract).

Shiffman, M. A.: J.A.M.A. **179**:514-522, 1962 (familial multiple polyposis).

Shiner, M.: J.A.M.A. **188**:45-48, 1964 (sprue).

Silverberg, E.: CA **30**:23-38, 1980 (cancer statistics).

Sorokin, J. J., et al.: J.A.M.A. **228**:49-53, 1974 (carcinoembryonic antigen assays).

Spratt, J. S., Jr., and Ackerman, L. V.: J.A.M.A. **179**:337-346, 1962 (adenocarcinoma of colon).

Steinberg, D., et al.: Arch. Intern. Med. **131**:538-544, 1973 (necrotizing enterocolitis in leukemia).

Truelove, S. C.: Br. Med. J. **1**:651-653, 1971 (ulcerative colitis).

Valdes-Dapena, A. M., and Stein, G. N.: Morphologic pathology of the alimentary canal, New York, 1970, W. B. Saunders Co.

Valtonen, E. J.: Gastroenterologia (Basel) **104**:309-320, 1965 (bezoars).

Vanasin, B., et al.: J.A.M.A. **217**:76-77, 1971 (pneumatosis cystoides esophagi).

Walker-Smith, J., and Andrews, J.: Lancet **2**:883-884, 1972 (celiac disease and alpha$_1$-antitrypsin).

Watts, H. D., and Admirand, W. H.: J.A.M.A. **230**:1674-1675, 1974 (Mallory-Weiss syndrome).

Waxler, B., et al.: Cancer **44**:221-227, 1979 (hyaluronic acid in mesotheliomas).

Wynder, E. L., and Reddy, B. S.: Cancer **34**:801-806, 1974 (epidemiology of colorectal cancer).

21

Endocrine glands

Pituitary gland (hypophysis)

STRUCTURE AND FUNCTION

The pituitary gland is a small endocrine structure (0.5 to 0.9 g) situated in the sella turcica. Its main divisions are anterior and posterior lobes. At the posterior part of the anterior lobe is the pars intermedia, although in man this has no distinct histologic separation from the anterior lobe.

The important anterior lobe arises from Rathke's pouch (craniopharyngeal duct), an evagination of the roof of the posterior nasopharynx. From there, the cells migrate upward to reach their final position in the sella turcica. Small portions of pituitary tissue may be left along this course and give rise to epithelial tumors (Rathke's pouch tumors) or simply remain as small remnants of pituitary tissue (Fig. 21-1). Such ectopic nests of pituitary tissue most often are found in the pharyngeal mucosa (pharyngeal pituitary gland) or in the body of the sphenoid bone. Cells of the anterior lobe extend upward over the stalk toward the base of the brain as the pars tuberalis.

The posterior lobe develops as a downgrowth from the floor of the third ventricle and hence is of nerve origin. It becomes enveloped anteriorly by the anterior lobe. It is directly continuous with the neural tissues of the pituitary stalk, which carries the supraopticohypophyseal tract of nerve fibers. These fibers from the supraoptic and paraventricular nuclei ramify throughout the posterior lobe (Fig. 21-2).

The blood supply of the anterior lobe is by a portal system of large thin-walled vessels. This vascular link with the nervous system may convey trophic substances from the hypothalamic area, providing a neurohumoral mechanism regulating anterior lobe hormones.

The *anterior lobe* contains three main types of cells distinguishable by the ordinary hematoxylin and eosin tissue stains. Although proportions vary slightly with age and sex, about 50% are *chromophobe* cells, which have a cytoplasm devoid of specific granulation. The chromophobes probably give rise to the other two types, *acidophils* (40%) and *basophils* (10%), by the accumulation of specific cytoplasmic granules, which respectively stain red with acid dyes and blue with basic dyes. Histochemical staining methods, such as the periodic acid–Schiff (PAS) stain with orange G, methyl blue, or alcian blue, the aldehyde thionine–PAS–orange G stain, and an aldehyde-fuchsin method, enable the three main varieties to be further subdivided. Such methods give promise of better correlation between categories of cells and the hormones they produce, although there is some confusion because of varying terminologies and interpretations. The percentages of the cells, as reported by various authors using different histochemi-

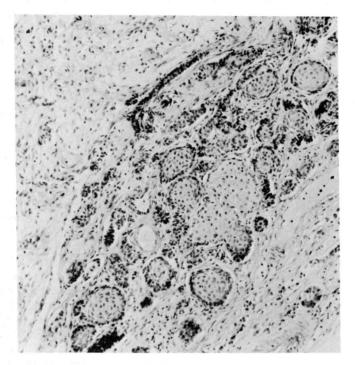

Fig. 21-1. Epithelial remnants of Rathke's pouch in pituitary gland.

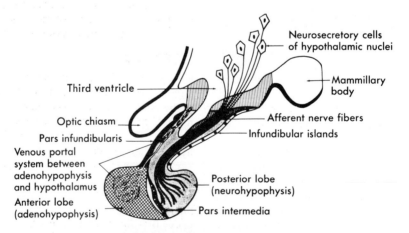

Fig. 21-2. Diagrammatic representation of pituitary gland showing neural and vascular relationships.

cal techniques, are markedly varied and unlike the proportions noted in the routine hematoxylin-eosin–stained sections. Electron microscopy is useful in the identification of the cell types, particularly in tumors in which the usual staining reactions are atypical. Certain immunohistologic techniques also are available (e.g., fluorescent antibody demonstration of ACTH in cells).

The anterior lobe elaborates a number of hormones. These may be listed as a growth-promoting (somatotropic) hormone (STH), a lactogenic (luteotropic) hormone (LTH or prolactin), a thyrotropic hormone (TSH), an adrenocorticotropic hormone (ACTH), and gonadotropic hormones (GTH), which are follicle-stimulating (FSH) or luteinizing (LH), the latter also referred to as interstitial cell–stimulating hormone (ICSH). In human beings, the anterior lobe apparently also elaborates a melanocyte-stimulating hormone (MSH or intermedin).

Although future studies may determine differently, the results of investigations already completed suggest that the hormones are secreted by the following cells (names in parentheses are synonyms for the cells):

STH—acidophil (alpha cell)
LTH—acidophil (epsilon-eta cell)
TSH—basophil (theta cell; blue beta cell; beta 2 cell; S_2 cell)
GTH—basophil (delta cell; S_1 cell)
MSH—basophil (zeta cell; purple beta cell; beta 1 cell; R cell)
ACTH—basophil (zeta type) and also large chromophobe (hypertrophic amphophil cell; gamma cell)

It is of interest that some chromophobes are now considered a possible source of hormones, although formerly all chromophobes were regarded as nonsecretory cells. The gonadotropic hormones generally are considered to be associated with one type of basophil, but certain investigators believe that FSH and LH (ICSH) may be secreted by different cells, perhaps subtypes of the delta basophil.

The *posterior lobe* is composed of neuroglial cells (pituicytes), nerve fibers, and some hyaline bodies. This portion of the pituitary gland is connected by nerve tracts with supraoptic and paraventricular nuclei of the floor of the third ventricle, forming an important endocrine unit, the neurohypophysis.

Hormones of the posterior lobe are vasopressin (antidiuretic hormone [ADH]) and oxytocin. *Vasopressin* is responsible for pressor and antidiuretic activities. The pressor effect is peripheral vasoconstriction and rise in blood pressure. The antidiuretic action controls resorption of water by the renal tubules. *Oxytocin* stimulates uterine contractions. These hormones appear to be formed by neurons of the hypothalamic nuclei. The neurosecretory material reaches the posterior lobe by the supraopticohypophyseal tract, where it is stored as an extracellular deposit demonstrable by aldehyde-fuchsin and other stains.

The indistinct *pars intermedia* contains the same cells as the anterior lobe, although basophils are more numerous. A few small cystic spaces containing pink-staining colloidlike material are usually present at the junction with the posterior lobe. A few basophils are sometimes found in the adjacent posterior lobe, especially in males over 50 years of age. In animals with a pars intermedia that is more distinct than in man, this area is considered to be the site of formation of MSH. In man, the site of origin of this hormone is not definitely known, although it is suggested that it is the anterior lobe. Basophils of the pars intermedia type are found in the anterior lobe.

DISEASES

Pathologic changes in the pituitary gland may be (1) adenomas or hyperplasias, which may result in pituitary hyperfunction, pressure effects, or both, and (2) destructive lesions resulting from inflammation, thrombosis, embolism, atrophy, or pressure from adjacent tumors, which are associated with hypofunction of the gland.

Adenomas

Tumors developing from cells of the anterior lobe of the pituitary gland are usually benign adenomas. Some, however, develop local invasion characteristics consistent with malignancy and have considerable nuclear variability and mitoses. Carcinomas with distant metastases rarely develop from pituitary cells. Other rare pituitary tumors are teratomas, including those called ''ectopic pinealomas,'' which resemble tumors arising in the pineal body.

The pituitary adenomas are usually classified as *chromophobe, acidophil,* and *basophil adenomas,* in accordance with the staining characteristics of their cells. They are so designated in the present discussion. However, certain investigators prefer to classify the tumors in accordance with electron microscopic and immunocytologic findings, taking into consideration the cell type from which the tumors arise and the endocrine function of the component cells. Accordingly, the different types include *growth hormone, prolactin, corticotroph, TSH,* and *gonadotroph cell adenomas* as well as *acidophil stem cell adenoma* and *undifferentiated cell adenoma (oncocytic* or *nononcocytic.)*

Chromophobe adenoma. Chromophobe adenoma is the most common type of pituitary tumor (Fig. 21-3). It varies from less than a millimeter to several centimeters in diameter. Generally, the chromophobes elaborate no specific hormone, and the effects are simply

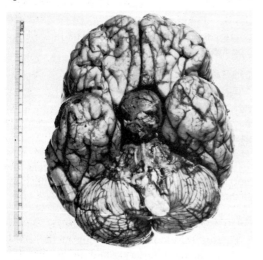

Fig. 21-3. Chromophobe adenoma of pituitary gland.

caused by pressure of the expanding growth. Such pressure effects are on the surrounding glandular tissue of the pituitary gland, the bony and membranous walls of the sella turcica, and the optic chiasm. Pressure on the surrounding normal glandular tissue may produce various symptoms of hypopituitarism.

The tumor tissue is soft, grayish white, and susceptible to hemorrhage, degeneration, necrosis, and cyst formation. Occasional chromophobe adenomas may involve the nasopharynx, and rarely invasion of the nasal cavity occurs. Some pituitary tumors in patients with Cushing's syndrome consist of chromophobes or chromophobes mixed with basophils.

In rare cases, adenomas of parathyroid and pancreatic islet cells have been associated with pituitary chromophobe or acidophil adenomas (pluriglandular or polyendocrine adenomatosis).

Acidophil adenoma. Tumors composed predominantly of acidophils cause clinical syndromes prominently featured by overproduction of growth hormone. If the adenoma develops within the growing period before ossification is complete, *gigantism* results; if it develops after bone growth is completed, *acromegaly* is produced. Acromegaly is characterized by overgrowth and thickening of bones, conspicuous in the skull, face, mandible, and peripheral portions of the extremities. Overgrowth of the heart, tongue, and viscera and fibrous hyperplasia of the skin and subcutaneous tissue also occur. Other disturbances usually present are sexual disorders of impotence or amenorrhea and glycosuria.

Eventually, pressure effects result from continued growth of the adenoma, although these tumors tend to be smaller than chromophobe adenomas and frequently are confined to the sella. The pressure first may be on other portions of the gland, giving rise to evidence of hypopituitarism, and then on suprasellar regions, where pressure on the optic chiasm or optic nerves produces visual disturbances.

Microscopic foci of hyperplasia of acidophils without tumor formation are quite common and usually are not associated with hormonal disturbances.

Basophil adenoma. The least common type of pituitary adenoma is composed of basophilic cells. The basophil adenoma is usually the smallest of the functioning pituitary tumors. It is sometimes found associated with the clinical condition of *Cushing's syndrome,* the clinical features of which are obesity (confined to the face, neck, and trunk), hypertension, polycythemia, a dusky cyanotic tinge of the skin, purplish striae on the breast and abdomen, hirsutism, and sexual disturbances. As noted previously, pituitary adenomas consisting of chromophobes or chromophobes mixed with basophils may also be associated with this syndrome. Hypersecretion of ACTH by the pituitary neoplasms stimulates the adrenal glands to produce excess cortisol (hypercortisolism), which is responsible for the clinical features of Cushing's syndrome. In recent years, microadenomas of the pituitary have been diagnosed more frequently by improved radiologic techniques and, even in the absence of radiologic evidence of the tumor, by means of transsphenoidal microsurgical exploration of the pituitary in patients with Cushing's syndrome. Selective removal of the microadenomas usually corrected the hypercortisolism.

Other varieties of Cushing's syndrome not associated with pituitary tumors are discussed on p. 613. It should be noted that some writers refer to the variety associated with pituitary tumors as *Cushing's disease,* since Harvey Cushing first described this relationship in 1932; nevertheless, it is quite appropriate to refer to all varieties as *Cushing's syndrome.* In some patients with this syndrome, bilateral adrenalectomy has later been followed by a clinically manifest ACTH- (and MSH-) secreting pituitary adenoma and progressive hyperpigmentation *(Nelson's syndrome).* The adenoma in Nelson's syndrome has a tendency to undergo spontaneous infarction. It is not certain whether the removal of the adrenal glands is responsible for inducing a new tumor or stimulating a preexisting microscopic tumor. The latter is most probable in view of the frequent demonstration recently of pituitary microadenomas in patients with Cushing's syndrome.

A constant change in nonneoplastic pituitary basophils that occurs in Cushing's syndrome with or without pituitary adenomas is replacement of the cytoplasmic substance by a hyaline material *(Crooke's hyaline change).* The change is caused by the excess cortisol. A similar change has been described after use of large doses of adrenal corticosteroids.

Hypopituitarism

Injuries or destructive lesions of the pituitary gland are not frequent. Pressure effects may be produced by tumors in or around the sella. Syphilis may cause a diffuse fibrosis of the pituitary gland. Tuberculosis, sarcoidosis, and other granulomas sometimes involve the gland, as may amyloid deposits in amyloidosis. The anterior pituitary cells contain mucopolysaccharide in gargoylism (Hurler's disease). In xanthomatosis of the Hand-Schüller-Christian type, the neurohypophysis is commonly involved. Lymphomas and metastatic carcinomas sometimes involve the gland. Diabetic patients who develop destructive lesions of the pituitary gland may show the Houssay phenomenon (hypoglycemia and an increase in sensitivity to insulin). Septicemia and embolism occasionally affect the hypophysis.

The most common type of severe injury is a necrosis that occurs after childbirth, particularly in those cases in which there has been severe postpartum hemorrhage and shock. The necrotic area undergoes fibrosis, and if extensive, hypopituitarism results.

Simmonds' disease. Simmonds' disease is the result of severe hypopituitarism in the adult. It is uncommon in men, for most cases appear to be the late effects of a postpartum necrosis of the pituitary gland. The condition is characterized by loss of sexual function, low metabolic rate, weakness, cachexia, loss of hair, loss of pigmentation of the skin, and premature senility. Not only is there atrophy or destruction of the anterior lobe of the pituitary gland, but there is also fibrosis or atrophy of the thyroid gland, parathyroid glands, adrenal glands, ovaries, and endometrium. Low blood pressure, hypoglycemia, and evidence of myxedema are usually present. Cachexia is not invariably present and is not a necessary feature of hypopituitarism. The cachexia is dependent mainly on loss of appetite and subsequent undernutrition. An unrelated condition, *anorexia nervosa,* is characterized by severe cachexia resulting from undernutrition. It has some of the clinical features of Simmonds' disease, but changes in the pituitary gland and other endocrine glands are lacking.

Sheehan has emphasized the danger and frequency of postpartum ischemic necrosis of the pituitary gland in women who suffer hemorrhage and circulatory collapse at the time of parturition. The anterior lobe of the pituitary gland normally hypertrophies during pregnancy and involutes rapidly during the puerperium. A sudden reduction of blood flow to the gland results from hemorrhage at the time of delivery, and if, in addition, there is severe general circulatory collapse, the blood flow to the gland may be reduced sufficiently to cause focal ischemic necrosis. The diminished circulation has been attributed to several mechanisms (e.g., vascular spasm and disseminated intravascular coagulation). The type of hypopituitarism that subsequently develops is often called *Sheehan's syndrome.* It varies in severity with the amount of pituitary tissue that has been destroyed by infarction. Atrophy of the supraoptic and paraventicular nuclei may be found when there is atrophy of the posterior lobe, and in severe cases there is loss of nerve fibers in the stalk.

Diabetes insipidus. Diabetes insipidus is characterized by an excessive output of urine that is of low specific gravity and without sugar. Excessive thirst and intake of fluid accompany the condition. Secretion of antidiuretic hormone is apparently by the cells of the hypothalamic nuclei, with storage in the posterior lobe of the pituitary gland. The antidiuretic hormone conserves water by increasing reabsorption of water by the renal tubules, particularly by the distal convoluted and collecting tubules. Interruption of the supraopticohypophyseal tract anywhere from the nuclei in the floor of the third ventricle downward to the posterior lobe may produce a deficiency of ADH, which results in diabetes insipidus. Known causes include trauma, neoplasms, granulomatous inflammations (e.g., sarcoidosis), eosinophilic granuloma, xanthomatous lesions of Hand-Schüller-Christian disease, and local infections.

Either hypothalamic or pituitary injury may result in diabetes insipidus, although injury of the posterior lobe alone may not do so. The anterior lobe must be functioning for development of diabetes insipidus, although the relationship is obscure. Idiopathic diabetes insipidus also occurs. In addition, a rare familial form exists.

Progeria. Progeria (Hutchinson-Gilford syndrome) is a condition of dwarfism and premature senility. A decreased number of acidophils in the anterior lobe of the pituitary gland has been described, but the primary cause is unknown.

Other pituitary syndromes. Various other clinical syndromes are related to disturbances of pituitary function. They are less clear-cut, and their pathologic basis is less definite. *Dystrophia adiposogenitalis* (Fröhlich's syndrome) is characterized by adiposity of the trunk and a feminine configuration. It is probably a hypopituitarism and often is related to pressure on the pituitary gland by tumors. *Dwarfism* of the Lorain-Levi syndrome may be attributable to hypopituitarism. Failure of sexual development is a common accompaniment.

Conditions in which a pathogenetic relationship to the pituitary gland is rather questionable include the Laurence-Moon-Biedl syndrome, mongolism, and Morgagni's syndrome. The *Laurence-Moon-Biedl syndrome* is characterized by obesity, hypogenitalism, polydactylism, pigmentary retinal changes, and failure of proper mental development. There is a genetic basis, and although there is no demonstrable pituitary or hypothalamic lesion, a functional hypothalamic-pituitary disturbance cannot be excluded. *Mongolism,* a prenatal developmental disorder caused by the presence of an additional small acrocentric chromosome, also shows evidence of pituitary involvement, with secondary changes in the thyroid gland, adrenal glands, and gonads.

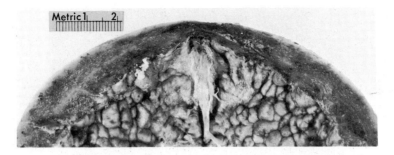

Fig. 21-4. Skull in hyperostosis frontalis interna. Note multiple bony projections toward cranial cavity.

Morgagni's syndrome is an endocrine disturbance occurring mainly in women after menopause. It is characterized by *hyperostosis frontalis interna* (Fig. 21-4), virilism with hirsutism, and obesity. The underlying endocrine changes are imperfectly known. It has been suggested that displacement of the brain by the bony thickening strains the pituitary stalk, providing a basis for the various changes that could be of pituitary or hypothalamic origin, although there may be no demonstrable lesion of the pituitary gland.

Craniopharyngioma

Remnants of Rathke's pouch (craniopharyngeal duct) give rise to cystic or solid tumors (craniopharyngiomas [Fig. 21-5], pituitary adamantinomas, and suprasellar cysts). Composed of epithelium derived from the mouth cavity, the tumors consist of a squamous type of epithelium. This epithelium resembles the ameloblasts of the developing enamel organ, and consequently the tumors are sometimes similar in microscopic appearance to the adamantinoma (ameloblastoma) (Fig. 21-6), which arises in the jaw (p. 515). A few cystic tumors of the pituitary gland have been lined by ciliated epithelium. Calcification is common in craniopharyngiomas and may be sufficient to be of value in radiologic diagnosis.

Many of the craniopharyngeal tumors develop from the region of the hypophyseal stalk, are cystic, and lie above the diaphragm of the sella (hence the commonly used term *suprasellar cyst),* although a few are intrasel-

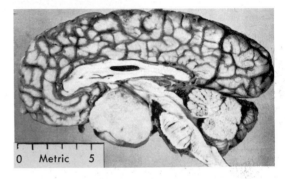

Fig. 21-5. Craniopharyngioma.

lar. The tumors constitute about 3% of intracranial neoplasms. Being of congenital origin, they may be found in early age periods, often before 15 years of age. They are benign growths, their serious effects being caused by pressure. Various types of hypopituitarism and stunting of growth may result, including Fröhlich's syndrome, dwarfism, and diabetes insipidus.

Tumors of neurohypophysis

Tumors of the neurohypophysis are very uncommon. Atypical teratomas ("ectopic pinealomas"), lymphomas, and gliomas are all quite rare. In the posterior lobe of the pituitary gland and stalk, small masses of rounded cells with granular cytoplasm have been termed *choristomas.* They appear to be of glial origin and without known significance.

Infundibuloma is a term used for a rare tu-

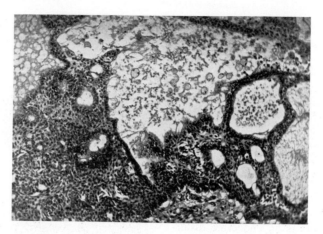

Fig. 21-6. Cystic craniopharyngioma (adamantinoma of hypophyseal duct).

mor that appears to be of neurohypophyseal derivation and that simulates the structural pattern of the infundibulum. Occurring in children, it grows slowly in the floor of the third ventricle, causing pressure effects on neighboring structures. The cells resemble pituicytes, and the tumor has a distinctive vascular pattern.

Thyroid gland

STRUCTURE AND FUNCTION

The thyroid gland develops as a downgrowth from the region of the primitive pharynx. A mass forms at the base of the tongue and extends downward as a long tube, the thyroglossal duct, its final position being in front of the trachea and thyroid cartilage. The upper end of the thyroglossal duct is marked by a small depression at the root of the tongue, the foramen cecum. Normally, the duct is obliterated during fetal life. Failure of the complete downgrowth and disappearance of this tissue leaves aberrant thyroid tissue at the base of the tongue (lingual thyroid) or in the neck anywhere along the course of the thyroglossal duct. These nests of thyroid tissue may give rise to midline (thyroglossal duct) cysts, which must be distinguished from the lateral (branchial cleft) cysts of the neck.

The units of thyroid tissue are glandular follicles or acini. They are lined by a layer of epithelial cells, the luminal borders of which have many microvilli that are apparently related to the secretory and resorptive function of these cells. The lumina of the follicles contain colloid consisting of several proteins, predominantly thyroglobulin. The latter is synthesized in the follicle cells and secreted in an apical direction into the intraluminal colloid. The thyroid cells actively take up plasma iodide along their outer (basal) borders (''active transport'' or iodide ''trapping'' mechanism). It is believed that the iodide is incorporated into the thyroglobulin molecules at the cell-colloid interface, initiating the synthesis of the thyroid hormones, thyroxine (T_4) and triiodothyronine (T_3). T_4 and T_3 are stored in the thyroglobulin of the follicular colloid. The exact site and mechanism of release of the thyroid hormones are not certain, but the following has been suggested. As necessary, the colloid is resorbed by the cells through the process of pinocytosis, the droplets fuse with lysosomes, T_4 and T_3 are released from thyroglobulin following protease hydrolysis of the latter, and the hormones are secreted into the plasma. Certain ions (e.g., nitrate, thiocyanate, and perchlorate) interfere with the active transport of iodide from the plasma. The thiouracil compounds interfere with the synthesis of hormones in the thyroid gland, apparently by inhibiting the oxidation of iodide to iodine and blocking the coupling of iodotyrosines to form the active hormones.

Factors that influence the activity of the thyroid gland include the amount of iodide available for synthesis and the thyrotropic-stimulating hormone (TSH) of the pituitary gland. A deficiency of iodine from any cause promotes hyperplasia and enlargement of the thyroid gland. TSH secretion from the pituitary gland is regulated by the level of thyroid hormones in the plasma. When the thyroid hormone level is decreased, the output of TSH is increased, and this, in turn, stimulates hyperplasia and increased secretion of the thyroid gland. An excess of plasma thyroid hormones depresses TSH output, causing a reduction in size and secretion of the thyroid gland. It is possible that some conditions increase TSH output by direct stimulation of the hypothalamus, inducing the latter to secrete a thyrotropic-releasing factor (TRF).

The thyroid gland controls the rate of general body metabolism. Its proper secretion is necessary for normal physical, sexual, and mental development and function. Abnormalities of thyroid function may be in the direction of deficiency (hypothyroidism) or excess (hyperthyroidism). Hypothyroidism gives rise to cretinism in infants and children and myxedema in adults. Hyperthyroidism may occur in severe form with a diffuse enlargement of the thyroid gland (Graves' disease; exophthalmic goiter) or in a milder form in which the thyroid enlargement is nodular (toxic nodular goiter). The thyroid hormone acts to accelerate oxidation or rate of metabolism of cells or of the whole organism. The protein-bound iodine of the blood is an index of the amount of circulating thyroid hormone and closely correlates with thyroid function in hyperthyroidism or hypothyroidism.

Since the histologic structure of the thyroid gland reflects its functional activity, a condition of underactivity or overactivity sometimes may be judged by microscopic examination. It must be borne in mind, however, that the activity of the normal thyroid tissue is cyclic and that in diseased thyroid glands different portions of the gland may show different stages or degrees of activity.

The type of epithelium lining the follicles is the most important criterion of thyroid activity. The height of acinar epithelium acts as an index of functional activity and probably also of the action of thyrotropic hormone of the pituitary gland. Secretory activity is characterized by cellular hypertrophy with a change of resting low cuboidal epithelium to a columnar type. When activity becomes excessive, epithelial proliferation (hyperplasia) also occurs. Infoldings of the follicle wall result from the cellular increase and may be simply slight elevations or definite lacelike papillae. Increase in thyroid activity also is accompanied by changes in the mitochondria, membrane permeability, and enzyme activities. The nature of the colloid content of the follicles also may indicate the degree of activity. Under conditions of glandular activity and active resorption into the circulation, the colloid is very pale staining and vacuolated, particularly about its periphery. Apparently, this represents the transformation of the intrafollicular colloid into a thinner, more soluble form. Continued preponderance of resorptive activity over colloid formation eventually produces exhaustion of the gland. When iodine is administered to an individual with a hyperactive thyroid gland, colloid storage is promoted and for a time may predominate over resorption, with resulting clinical improvement. The improvement, however, is only temporary, since the tendency to excessive resorptive activity still exists, and more colloid has been made available.

In addition to the thyroid hormones T_4 and T_3, another hormone has been demonstrated in thyroid extracts of various animals. This hormone, *thyrocalcitonin,* is produced by parafollicular "C" cells, which have a different embryologic origin than the follicular cells, arising from the ultimobranchial cleft, which initially originated from the neural crest. Thyrocalcitonin lowers the serum calcium level, presumably by decreasing resorption of calcium from bones and possibly enhancing incorporation of calcium in bones. The hormone is also known as *calcitonin*.

DISEASES

The term *goiter,* or struma, refers to an enlargement of the thyroid gland. Such enlargement may be related to several different etiologic factors, it may be diffuse or nodular (adenomatous), and it may be associated with a deficient, normal, or excessive production of hormone. A large variety of classifications of goiter have served to confuse the subject unnecessarily. Five main types may be recognized. It is to be noted that the term *goiter* is used here in a broad sense to include all thyroid enlargements, whereas some writers restrict the term to the nonneoplastic enlargements.

Simple (colloid) goiter, which is endemic to certain regions and usually has its origin in iodine deficiency

Diffuse goiter with hyperthyroidism (exophthalmic goiter; Graves' disease; Basedow's disease)

Nodular (adenomatous) goiter
  With hyperthyroidism (toxic nodular goiter)
  With hypothyroidism (cretinism; myxedema)

Inflammatory goiter
  Subacute (granulomatous) thyroiditis
  Hashimoto's disease (lymphadenoid goiter; struma lymphomatosa)
  Riedel's struma (struma fibrosa; woody thyroiditis; invasive fibrous thyroiditis)
  Lymphocytic (lymphoid) thyroiditis

Neoplastic goiter
  Benign (adenoma)
  Malignant (carcinoma)

Simple (colloid) goiter

In certain regions of the world, goiter is endemic and occurs with great frequency *(endemic goiter).* Such regions occur particularly about great mountain ranges, but in North America a goiter belt also occurs around the Great Lakes and St. Lawrence Valley. The thyroid enlargement is a response to insufficient iodine intake resulting from a deficiency of iodine in the soil and water in these regions. Bacterial contamination of water supplies may interfere with availability or absorption of iodine and give rise to goiter. Endemic goiter

may be prevented by the addition to the diet of minute amounts of iodine, as by the use of iodized salt. The condition occurs more commonly in females and is particularly likely to develop at a time when the thyroid gland is subjected to extra functional stress, as in adolescence or pregnancy. Simple goiter also may occur sporadically in women because the extra functional stress of adolescence and pregnancy results in a relative deficiency of iodine.

Deficiency of iodine apparently leads to diminished production of thyroid hormone, which, in turn, causes increased output of TSH from the pituitary gland, followed by growth of the thyroid gland. In relatively few patients other factors, besides iodine deficiency, cause colloid goiter. The ingestion of certain plant foods containing goitrogenic substances (thiocyanates or thiouracil-related compounds) that interfere with formation of thyroid hormone may be responsible.

Gross examination of simple goiters shows great variation in size. There may be diffuse involvement of the entire gland, or involvement may be nodular, with patchy "adenomatous" areas. The enlargement is probably always diffuse in the beginning, but successive cycles of uneven hyperplasia and involution give rise to the nodularity. The cut surface of the gland has a highly translucent appearance because of the abundant colloid. Degenerative changes are often evident, particularly in the nodular type, and there may be hemorrhage, cyst formation, and calcification. Coarse, irregular connective tissue trabeculae separate the adenomatous nodules.

Microscopically, the goiter may be composed of large distended follicles filled with abundant, deeply staining colloid and lined by a low cubical or flattened inactive type of epithelium (Fig. 21-7). Such a "colloid goiter" is in an involutional phase and has been preceded by a stage of hyperplasia in response to the iodine deficiency. Subsequent flare-ups of hyperplasia, followed by involution and colloid accumulation, produce a nodular colloid goiter.

In some cases of simple goiter, the thyroid gland is composed of small inactive follicles

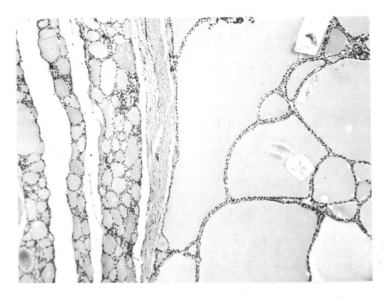

Fig. 21-7. Nodular colloid goiter. Note flat epithelium, abundant colloid, and fibrous band separating nodule. (×85; courtesy Dr. S. E. Gould; from Sommers, S. C.: Thyroid gland. In Anderson, W. A. D., and Kissane, J. M., editors: Pathology, ed. 7, St. Louis, 1977, The C. V. Mosby Co.)

without excess colloid accumulation. This variety is termed by some the parenchymatous or microfollicular type.

Hyperthyroidism

Hyperthyroidism is the result of a hyperplastic, overactive thyroid gland that secretes an excess of hormone into the circulation. Hyperthyroidism may be of all grades of severity, with that associated with diffuse thyroid hypertrophy and hyperplasia (exophthalmic goiter) being more serious, in general, than that with nodular goiter. There appears to be no fundamental difference between the diffuse and the nodular hyperplastic goiters as far as the thyroid factor itself is concerned. Histologic changes of hypertrophy and hyperplasia within the thyroid gland indicate excessive secretory activity. The quantitative concept must be borne in mind, however, in any attempt at functional interpretation from a tissue section. In the diffuse goiter of Graves' disease, such functional interpretation may be fairly accurate. In nodular goiter, there is great variation in activity in different portions of the gland and hence also in the microscopic picture. This precludes accuracy in any attempted estimation of function.

Laboratory determinations that may be helpful in the diagnosis of hyperthyroidism include (1) the basal metabolic rate, (2) the protein-bound iodine level of the serum, (3) the uptake of radioactive iodine by the thyroid gland, and (4) the rate of conversion of radioactive iodine into iodine bound by protein.

Diffuse goiter with hyperthyroidism. Diffuse goiter with hyperthyroidism (exophthalmic goiter; Graves' disease) is the most acute and severe type of hyperthyroidism. It occurs particularly in young and middle-aged adults. The incidence is sporadic and not limited to the goiter belts.

The actual stimulus for the hyperactivity of the thyroid gland was thought to be an excess of the pituitary thyrotropic hormone, although there is evidence that TSH does not have a primary pathogenetic role. It has been suggested that autonomous thyroid hyperactivity or a thyroid stimulator of nonpituitary origin may be involved. In favor of the latter concept is the finding of a gamma globulin in the serum of many patients with Graves' disease that stimulates release of hormone from the thyroid and induces hyperplasia of the gland. This globulin, referred to as *long-acting thyroid stimulator* (LATS), is believed to be an autoantibody to some cellular component of the thyroid gland. It is possible that the globulin (which apparently is IgG produced by lymphocytes) acts against the normal inhibitor of mitosis in the thyroid gland. Thus, the removal of mitotic inhibition could lead to hyperplasia, followed by hyperfunction. LATS and other thyroid autoantibodies have been demonstrated in the serum of relatives of patients with Graves' disease, Hashimoto's disease, and myxedema.

LATS is not found in all patients with Graves' disease, and recently some doubt has been raised as to its role. Other immune factors have been implicated in the origin of the disease. In certain studies, several immunoglobulins (IgE, IgM, and IgG) as well as complements C1q and C3 have been demonstrated within the follicular basement membrane and stroma of the thyroid glands in patients with Graves' disease, but not in normal thyroid glands or in those with toxic or nontoxic adenomas. The multiplicity of antibodies found in the glands suggests that LATS may not be the only initiator of Graves' disease. The possibility that a cell-mediated mechanism may be involved has been considered.

Although thyroid enlargement is usually associated with Graves' disease, it is often slight and does not necessarily parallel the severity of the clinical symptoms. Exophthalmos, or protrusion of the eyes, is an inconstant feature. It is apparently not a direct result of hyperthyroidism and cannot be reproduced by thyroid extract. TSH is not regarded as the cause, but the possibility that another factor of pituitary origin is responsible has been considered, viz., an exophthalmos-producing substance (EPS). It has been suggested that EPS may be a component of TSH. Some investigators implicate LATS as the cause of exophthalmos, but not all are in agreement with this view. Increased metabolic rate, tachycardia, and nervous excitability are prominent features more closely related to the thyroid hyperfunction. A negative iodine balance is present. Cardiac damage may occur, often marked by disturbances of rhythm, such as atrial fibrillation. Hyperthyroidism may develop slowly or suddenly and proceed through a course that may be rapid or may be prolonged by a series of exacerbations and remissions. The result may be an exhausted condition of the gland, with actual hypothyroidism.

The gross appearance of the thyroid gland is similar in all parts. Although it may not be much enlarged, it is highly vascular and has a characteristic meaty and firm consistency. The cut surface has a solid, firmly lobulated appearance, without the translucence imparted by a rich colloid content. By the promotion of colloid accumulation, a preoperative iodine administration may change the aspect to a glistening translucence not unlike that of the normal gland.

Microscopically, characteristic features of thyroid hyperactivity are evident throughout the gland (Fig. 21-8). The epithelial cells of the follicles are tall and columnar, and their nuclei are closely packed and basal in position. Papillary epithelial proliferation with lacelike projections into follicle lumina is often considerable. New follicles with small lumina may be formed. The colloid is decreased in amount, thin, pale, and vacuolated or scalloped around the edges. Accumulations of lymphocytes, often with distinct germinal centers, are frequently prominent. By itself, the lymphoid hyperplasia is not good evidence of thyroid hyperfunction. Ultrastructural changes that reflect the activity of the cells have been described—viz., increase in number and length of apical microvilli, prominence of endoplasmic reticulum with increase of ribosomes, increase in number of mitochondria, hypertrophy of the Golgi apparatus, large number of apical vesicles, formation of colloid droplets, and fusion of the latter with lysosomes.

The preoperative administration of iodine

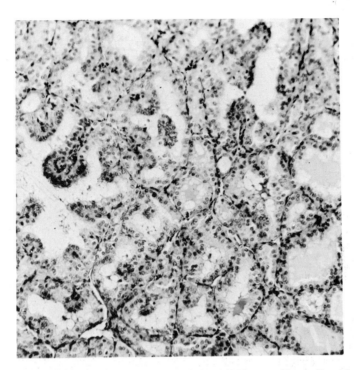

Fig. 21-8. Diffuse hyperplasia of thyroid gland in Graves' disease. Note tall epithelium lining follicles, papillary projections of epithelium into follicle lumina, and vacuolization and scantiness of colloid.

usually causes a change in this picture before it is seen in the laboratory. The epithelium is changed to a cuboidal form, the acini becoming larger, with less infolding of epithelium and containing a more deeply stained colloid. This involutional change is not diffuse, and patchy areas still exhibit a hyperplastic character. The lymphoid accumulations are not influenced by the iodine medication.

Thiouracil and other thiourea derivatives have been found to be therapeutically effective in relieving hyperthyroidism. However, there may be an increase in size of the thyroid gland, which microscopically may show a very great degree of hyperplasia and little colloid content. The effect in this case does not appear to be preventable by iodine. It is postulated that thiouracil prevents oxidation of iodide to iodine and coupling of iodotyrosines. Meanwhile, the thyroid gland itself is increasingly stimulated to hyperplasia by the unopposed pituitary thyrotropic hormone because of the decreased synthesis of thyroid hormones. The extreme degrees of hyperplasia of thyroid tissue that may be seen as a result of thiouracil or thiocyanate therapy must be distinguished with care from neoplastic lesions of the thyroid gland. In children, cobalt compounds used in the treatment of anemia have produced goiters that are characterized by severe hyperplasia but depressed function.

Exophthalmos associated with goiter appears to result mainly from swelling and edema of the orbital contents. There is an increase of fat in the orbits and eyelids, and the fatty tissue becomes swollen and edematous. The extrinsic muscles of the eye also may be swollen. Compression of orbital veins by increased contraction of ocular muscles may be a factor in the increased accumulation of fluid. The severity of the exophthalmos is not correlated with the degree of hyperthyroidism. Secondary ulceration of the cornea may complicate severe exophthalmos.

Various other organs may show changes in severe hyperthyroidism. Lymphoid hyperplasia is generalized, not simply in the thyroid gland itself. The thymus often is enlarged, and even the blood may show a relative lymphocytosis. The heart shows few changes, despite the frequent occurrence of cardiac complications. There may be cardiac hypertrophy and some myocardial degeneration and fibrosis. Voluntary muscles, such as the quadriceps, also may show degenerative changes. Some skeletal osteoporosis is common. The liver is affected by hyperthyroidism and, in severe cases, may show fatty degeneration and necrosis. The adrenal glands also may be involved by degenerative and atrophic changes.

Nodular goiter with hyperthyroidism. Hyperthyroidism with a nodular goiter is probably fundamentally the same condition as Graves' disease. The nodularity is the result of recurring cycles of hypertrophy and hyperplasia affecting the gland in irregular fashion. Because the hyperactivity may appear in a previously existent simple goiter, it is sometimes termed *secondary Graves' disease*. The condition tends to occur in later life, the degree

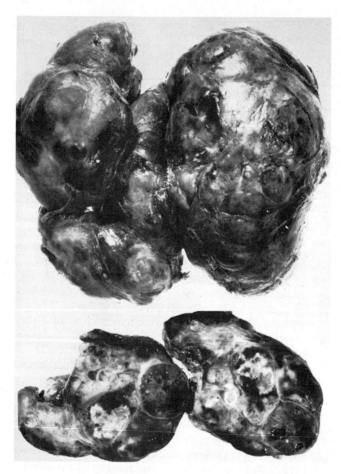

Fig. 21-9. Nodular goiter, with fibrosis, hemorrhage, and necrosis evident on cut surface.

of hyperthyroidism is milder, and exophthalmos is usually absent. Large nodular goiters may cause disturbance by pressure on surrounding structures (e.g., the trachea).

Both the gross and microscopic appearance is extremely variable. The enlargement of the thyroid gland may be great and irregular. Areas of degeneration are often present (Fig. 21-9). Nodular or adenomatous areas of varying size may show fibrosis around them. Their cut surface may be meaty and firm, indicating hyperplasia, or it may be soft and translucent because of colloid storage. The appearance is often quite variable in different portions of the gland, both grossly and microscopically. Hence, there is difficulty of evaluation in terms of function, which evidently depends on the total balance of hyperplasia and involution.

Hypothyroidism

Insufficient function of the thyroid gland produces the condition of cretinism in early life and myxedema in the adult. Although fundamentally the same, the clinical syndromes differ because of the retardation and distortion of physical, sexual, and mental development in the childhood form. Skeletal growth is stunted and distorted, the skin is thick and coarse, hair is scanty, metabolism is depressed, and both sexual and mental development are of low degree.

Cretinism. Cretinism is a congenital deficiency of thyroid function. It may occur as a nongoitrous sporadic form, caused by failure of proper development of the thyroid gland, in which the gland is absent or hypoplastic (athyreotic cretinism). Goitrous cretinism also exists, either in regions in which goiter is endemic (goitrous endemic cretinism) or as a sporadic form (goitrous sporadic cretinism).

In goitrous sporadic cretinism, there is evidence of a genetic basis for a biochemical abnormality with a defect in the synthesis of thyroid hormone. The goitrous glands in these cases show severe epithelial hyperplasia, with irregular and pleomorphic epithelial cells and adenomalike nodules (Fig. 21-10).

Myxedema. Myxedema is the antithesis of Graves' disease. The general metabolism is low, heat tolerance is increased, and physical and mental activities are retarded. The skin becomes dry, coarse, and thickened by subcutaneous accumulation of a mucoid material. This results in the appearance of a nonpitting edema, particularly prominent on the face, neck, and hands, which feature has given origin to the term *myxedema*. Specific cytologic changes may be found in the exocrine sweat glands, with PAS-positive granules in the large pale cells of the secretory coil. The hair tends to become coarse and scanty. Loss of sexual desire and impotence or amenorrhea are common. The condition responds readily and effectively to thyroid administration.

Mild degrees of myxedema may follow operative removal of most of the thyroid gland or result from exhaustion of the gland after severe hyperthyroidism. Pituitary deficiency may be associated with a secondary thyroid deficiency caused by a lack of thyrotropic hormone. Prolonged ingestion of iodides as medication has been known to produce goiter and myxedema.

Most cases of primary myxedema are of unknown etiology. Circulating antibodies to thyroglobulin are demonstrable in the sera of about 80% of patients with primary myxedema. This and the histologic appearance suggest that the condition may be a late stage of chronic diffuse (Hashimoto's) thyroiditis. The thyroid tissue is atrophic and inactive, often displaying severe fibrosis, and lymphocytic infiltration is present, often of marked degree (Fig. 21-11). Vacuolization and mucoid degeneration of skeletal muscle fibers have been noted. A similar degeneration in the media of the aorta, leading to dissecting aneurysm and fatal rupture, has been described in induced hypothyroidism. The heart is dilated, there is a loss of muscle tone, and interstitial edema and some scarring may be present. Mucoid (basophilic) degeneration has been observed in myocardial fibers. Atherosclerosis of advanced degree may be present in young adults with myxedema.

Inflammation

Since the thyroid gland appears quite resistant to most infections, inflammatory pro-

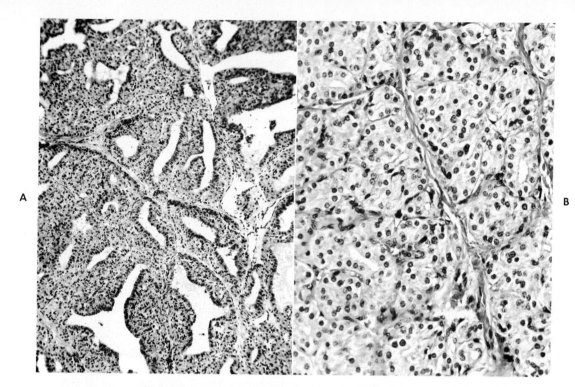

Fig. 21-10. A, Congenital goiter with hyperplastic appearance. **B,** Goiter from cretin with pale and notably hyperplastic epithelium. (**A,** ×85; **B,** ×240; courtesy Dr. S. E. Gould; from Sommers, S. C.: Thyroid gland. In Anderson, W. A. D., editor: Pathology, ed. 6, St. Louis, 1971, The C. V. Mosby Co.)

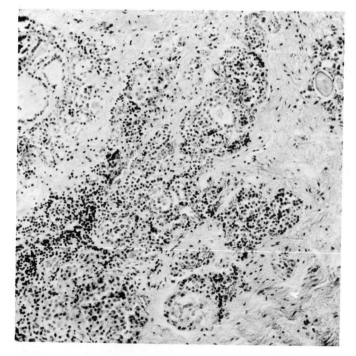

Fig. 21-11. Thyroid gland in myxedema showing atrophy, fibrosis, and lymphocytic infiltration.

cesses in the gland are uncommon. Direct spread may occur from neighboring tissues. Also, thyroiditis may be produced by trauma or radiation. However, distinctive types of supposedly inflammatory conditions are termed subacute (granulomatous) thyroiditis, Hashimoto's disease, Riedel's struma, and lymphocytic (lymphoid) thyroiditis.

Subacute (granulomatous) thyroiditis. Subacute (de Quervain's) thyroiditis occurs predominantly in female adults. The clinical onset may be acute, with sore throat, pain or swallowing, pain and tenderness in the thyroid gland, and some fever. The effects are often mild, and local pressure symptoms are not prominent. The sedimentation rate is elevated. The serum protein-bound iodine level is near the upper limit of normal or is elevated, but the uptake of radioiodine by the gland is depressed. The alpha$_2$ globulin fraction of the serum may be elevated, probably because of colloid entering the bloodstream from destruction of follicles.

The thyroid gland is slightly to moderately enlarged, and involved areas are firm and yellowish white. Some degree of perithyroiditis is frequent. The microscopic changes are focal, with degeneration of follicles, infiltration of leukocytes (lymphocytes and plasma cells), and a variable amount of fibrosis (Fig. 21-12). Groups of histiocytes and giant cells produce a tuberculoid appearance, but caseous necrosis is not present. The giant cell formation often appears to be a reaction to altered colloid, and some giant cells seem to be formed by fusion of follicle cells around colloid masses.

The cause is obscure, but a viral infection has been suggested. Some cases have shown evidence of a relation to the virus of mumps. In other instances, antibodies against

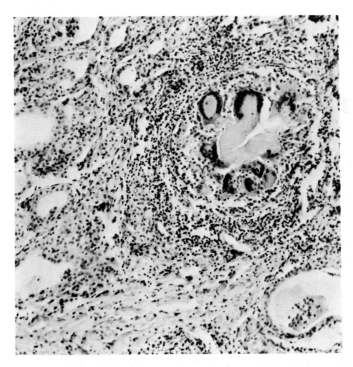

Fig. 21-12. Subacute (granulomatous) thyroiditis. There are multinucleated giant cells, lymphocytes, fibrosis, and few thyroid follicles.

other viruses have been demonstrated (e.g., echovirus, coxsackievirus, and adenovirus). Subacute thyroiditis is usually a self-limited disease, commonly persisting for 1 to 3 months.

Hashimoto's disease. Hashimoto's disease, or *struma lymphomatosa*, is a condition in which excessive lymphoid tissue develops in the thyroid gland, often with prominent lymphoid follicles and a crowding out and replacement of thyroid acini. A characteristic feature is alteration of thyroid epithelium with enlargement, an abundant oxyphilic cytoplasm (Fig. 21-13), and nuclei that may be hyperchromatic and of variable size and shape. The altered follicle cells are called Hürthle or Askanazy cells. The associated change of thyroid parenchyma is accompanied by a varying degree of interstitial fibrosis. The thyroid tissue is usually diffusely and symmetrically enlarged, with uniformly firm rubbery consistency and a white to yellowish brown color (Fig. 21-14). The condition may occur at any age, but most cases seem to be in women over 40 years of age. Moderate diffuse enlargement of the thyroid gland is usual. Functional disturbance is usually not a prominent feature, but hypothyroidism (myxedema) may be present in later stages.

As to the origin of this disease, the prevalent view is that *autoimmunity* plays a significant role. In most of the patients with Hashimoto's thyroiditis, autoantibodies against thyroglobulins are identified, and in some patients autoantibodies against thyroid cytoplasmic components and against colloid antigens other than thyroglobulins also are found. Lesions similar to thyroiditis in man have been produced experimentally following injection of thyroid extract into animals immunized against the extract. Whether the antibodies produce damage to the thyroid gland is not certain, but there is some evidence that a cell-mediated mechanism may play a role in causing the thyroiditis (p. 88).

The lesser degree of lymphoid infiltration in other thyroid lesions also may represent a localized immune response. Antithyroid antibodies have been demonstrated in Graves' disease and in primary myxedema, as well as in Hashimoto's disease. Some investigators believe that these three disorders are interrelated and may be variants of the same process.

Riedel's struma. Riedel's struma (struma fi-

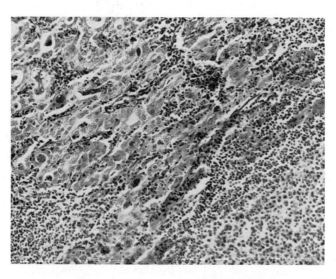

Fig. 21-13. Hashimoto's thyroiditis. In addition to lymphoid infiltrate, altered follicle cells show granular oxyphilia. (From Sommers, S. C.: Thyroid gland. In Anderson, W. A. D., and Kissane, J. M., editors: Pathology, ed. 7, St. Louis, 1977, The C. V. Mosby Co.)

brosa; woody thyroiditis; invasive fibrous thyroiditis) is a rare condition characterized by a thyroid gland of very firm consistency. Its essence is a slow progressive replacement of thyroid tissue by dense scar tissue (Fig. 21-15) and extension of the fibrous tissue to involve surrounding structures. Sometimes, only a portion of the gland is affected. It occurs at any age, but usually in adults, and almost as frequently in men as in women. It may be as-

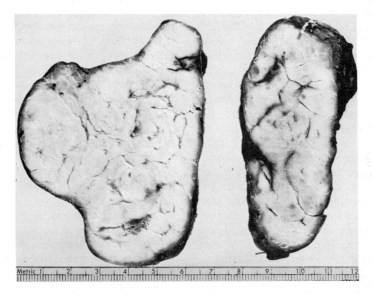

Fig. 21-14. Thyroid gland in Hashimoto's disease.

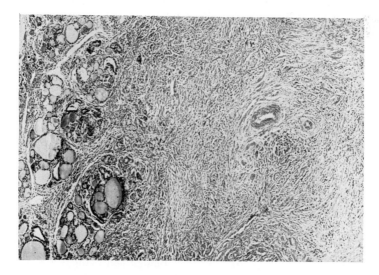

Fig. 21-15. Riedel's struma. Dense but irregular fibrosis involves thyroid tissue. (From Anderson, W. A. D., and Winship, T.: Thyroid gland. In Anderson, W. A. D., editor: Pathology, ed. 5, St. Louis, 1966, The C. V. Mosby Co.)

sociated with mild hypothyroidism and is easily confused clinically with carcinoma. Clinical manifestations are mainly severe pressure symptoms.

Although extensive fibrosis is the essential microscopic feature, lymphoid accumulation is frequently prominent, and forms occur that have suggested a transition from Hashimoto's disease to Riedel's struma. The fibrous thyroid tissue is hard, gritty, and white and often without any gross resemblance to normal thyroid tissue. Capsular involvement is an important and distinctive feature. Extensive involvement of adjacent structures of the neck by the dense fibrous tissue makes surgical resection difficult.

Lymphocytic (lymphoid) thyroiditis. Sporadic cases of goiter in children and young women have been characterized by extensive lymphocytic infiltration but without the oxyphilic changes in follicular epithelium that occur in Hashimoto's struma. However, this is considered by some to be an early phase or a form of Hashimoto's disease. The thyroid gland is diffusely enlarged, and there is an intact capsule. The cut surface of the tissue is grayish white or yellowish white. Clinical evidence of mild hypothyroidism is present in some cases. Serum protein-bound iodine levels are variable but sometimes elevated. Radioiodine uptake shows no significant change.

Tumors

The common neoplasms of the thyroid gland are adenomas and carcinomas. Some carcinomas of the gland are believed to originate in a benign adenoma. Atypical adenomas and adenomas with atypical foci are probably precancerous lesions. In reported cases, from 6% to 20% of solitary thyroid nodules have been found to be carcinomatous.

Adenoma

The so-called adenomas of nodular goiters are not true tumors but are localized areas of hyperplasia or involution. The criteria for true thyroid adenomas are as follows:

1 Complete encapsulation
2 Homogeneous texture throughout, although degenerative changes may be present
3 Definite variation of the tissue of the adenoma from that outside the capsule
4 Evidence of compression of adjacent thyroid tissue

Papillary adenoma is a variety composed of papillary or cystadenomatous structures. Active or cellular papillary adenomas are difficult to distinguish from papillary carcinomas unless invasion is seen. Some believe that it is not possible to classify papillary thyroid tumors into benign and malignant tumors on histologic grounds.

The more common type of benign tumor is *follicular adenoma*. Follicular adenomas may consist of colloid-containing follicles resembling the normal thyroid, either small *(microfollicular)* or large *(macrofollicular),* or both. Those composed of large follicles containing abundant colloid often are referred to as *colloid adenomas.*

Other variants described are *embryonal, fetal,* and *Hürthle cell adenomas.*

Embryonal and *fetal adenomas* are so called because of resemblances to embryonic or fetal thyroid tissue. The embryonal type is composed of cords and trabeculae of cells, with little tendency to gland formation. The fetal adenoma consists of small follicles lined by epithelium and often separated by abundant hyaline colloidlike material or abundant and edematous stroma.

Hürthle cell tumors are composed of large, polyhedral cells, with prominent granular nuclei and abundant pale eosinophilic cytoplasm (Fig. 21-16). The cells are arranged in solid-looking masses and clumps, but with formation of small alveoli. Stroma is usually small in amount. The origin of the distinctive cells is uncertain. They formerly were considered to be retrogressive variants of thyroid follicle cells, but they are rich in mitochondria and oxidative enzymes, suggesting that they are hyperplastic or metaplastic.

Benign and malignant forms of Hürthle cell tumors occur. Criteria for malignancy are the same as those in other thyroid tumors, vascular invasion being most important. In general,

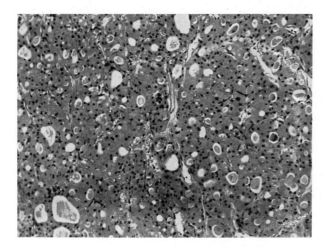

Fig. 21-16. Hürthle cell tumor of thyroid gland.

the Hürthle cell change tends to be associated with a decreased growth capacity and a more favorable prognosis.

Hürthle cells frequently are seen in thyroid glands, apart from tumors, apparently as an alteration occurring in thyroid cells as a result of injury (e.g., by radiation) or exhaustion after overstimulation. Various thyroid tumors may show a Hürthle cell change in focal areas.

Carcinoma

It is said that carcinoma of the thyroid gland may arise from a benign adenoma, but how often this occurs, if at all, has not been determined accurately. A carcinoma may be well differentiated histologically, resembling an adenoma, so that diagnosis and prognosis are often very difficult. Invasion, particularly capsular and vascular invasion, may be the only evidence of malignancy. Some of the well-differentiated tumors that invade blood vessels and produce secondary growths in other organs have been given the anomalous name of "benign metastasizing struma." Although invasion of blood vessels, lymphatics, or capsule is the most reliable microscopic evidence of malignancy, in many cases cellular anaplasia is present, and the usual histologic criteria of malignancy can be applied. Hyperfunction is rarely an accompaniment of thyroid cancer,

even though well-differentiated cancer cells may show evidence of function and take up radioactive iodine.

Malignant tumors of the thyroid gland are, with rare exception, of epithelial nature (carcinomas). Fibrosarcoma and lymphosarcoma are relatively uncommon. Carcinoma of the thyroid gland occurs in all age periods, but the highly malignant undifferentiated carcinomas almost all occur after the age of 40 years. Thyroid carcinomas occurring in childhood have often been in children who have received irradiation to the area during infancy, usually for an enlarged thymus.

The different histologic varieties of thyroid carcinoma show extreme variation in their natural history. Some papillary carcinomas may exist over a period of several decades, whereas many undifferentiated carcinomas may cause death within 6 months or a year. Between the extremes are follicular cancers of varying degrees of differentiation and malignancy. Mixed papillary and follicular carcinomas are common.

Papillary carcinoma. Papillary carcinoma, the most common form of thyroid carcinoma, generally occurs in a younger age group than the other types. The tumor epithelium is arranged on fibrovascular stalks projecting into cystic spaces (Fig. 21-17). Metastatic deposits

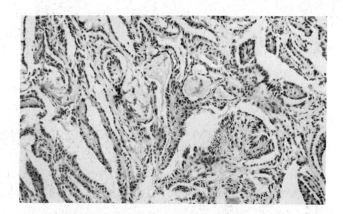

Fig. 21-17. Papillary carcinoma of thyroid gland.

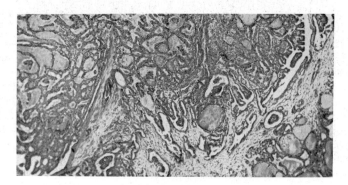

Fig. 21-18. Follicular carcinoma of thyroid gland.

show a similar architectural pattern. Psammoma bodies may develop from the hyalinized stroma of the papillae. The presence of psammoma bodies may be considered evidence of malignancy. Areas of squamous metaplasia are often present, but squamous metaplasia in the thyroid gland is not ordinarily a precancerous lesion.

Papillary carcinomas of the thyroid gland are usually of a low grade of malignancy, grow slowly, and may exist over many years. They have a tendency to local infiltration and spread to cervical lymph nodes, but distant metastasis tends to be uncommon or late. Metastases in the cervical lymph nodes may be mistaken for "lateral aberrant thyroid." Lym-

phatic invasion, rather than blood vessel invasion, is characteristic of this form of cancer, although both do occur.

Follicular carcinoma. Follicular carcinomas of the thyroid gland are of varying degrees of undifferentiation and malignancy (Fig. 21-18). Many of them appear as encapsulated adenomalike tumors, are distinguishable only by vascular or capsular invasion, and have a relatively good outlook. Some follicular carcinomas show a Hürthle cell change, in some parts or as a whole, which is usually an indication of slow growth. The more undifferentiated follicular carcinomas may show solid masses of cells, with relatively little formation of distinct follicular lumina, great cellular and nu-

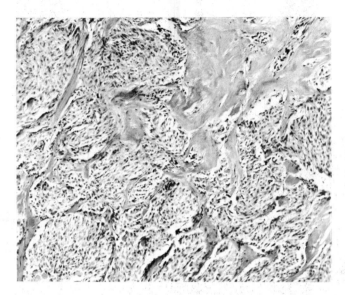

Fig. 21-19. Medullary carcinoma of thyroid gland. Stroma of tumor contains amyloid. (From Sommers, S. C.: Thyroid gland. In Anderson, W. A. D., and Kissane, J. M., editors: Pathology, ed. 7, St. Louis, 1977, The C. V. Mosby Co.)

clear variability, and numerous mitoses. Such tumors are of a relatively higher grade of malignancy.

Metastases occur in the cervical lymph nodes, the lungs, and bones. This tumor has a greater predilection for bones than any other thyroid cancer. The well-differentiated metastatic tumors take up radioactive iodine.

Medullary (solid) carcinoma. Medullary carcinoma, arising from parafollicular "C" cells, consists of solid sheets and trabecular masses of pleomorphic cells separated by a fibrous stroma in which usually are found deposits of amyloid (Fig. 21-19). This tumor occurs in patients at an average age of about 50 years and, like the follicular carcinoma, metastasizes by way of the lymphatics and blood vessels. Although it is an undifferentiated neoplasm histologically, it does not show the features of the anaplastic tumors.

Calcitonin may be demonstrated in the tumor tissue, and high concentrations of the hormone in the plasma may be detected or may be stimulated by infusions of calcium in patients with medullary carcinoma. Occasion-ally, hypocalcemia has been reported in association with the tumor. Also, high histaminase activity and prostaglandins have been demonstrated in the tumors. In some instances, medullary carcinoma may be the site of ectopic hormone production, e.g., ACTH or serotonin, causing endocrine disorders such as Cushing's syndrome and the carcinoid syndrome.

Association with pheochromocytomas, parathyroid adenomas, and neurofibromas has been reported, sometimes with evidence of a familial pattern.

Anaplastic carcinoma. Anaplastic carcinomas may be of small cell, spindle cell, giant cell (Fig. 21-20), or epidermoid varieties. They are of high malignancy. The highly anaplastic carcinomas may arise from a change in malignant character occurring in papillary or follicular carcinomas.

Anaplastic carcinomas occur in the older age group. They tend to invade locally and spread widely by way of the bloodstream. They are rapidly fatal, with death usually occurring within 1 year.

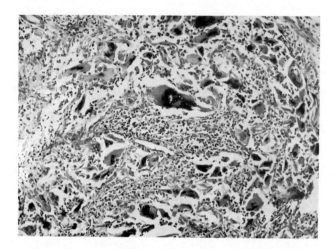

Fig. 21-20. Anaplastic giant cell carcinoma of thyroid gland.

Nonencapsulated sclerosing carcinoma. An incidental microscopic finding in a thyroid gland removed surgically for another lesion is a minute papillary or follicular carcinoma within a small scar that invades the adjacent tissue (nonencapsulated) (Fig. 21-21). The prognosis is excellent in such cases.

Struma ovarii

Struma ovarii is a teratoma of the ovary in which thyroid tissue is the sole or chief constituent. Malignancy and metastasis may occur rarely. Functional activity of the tissue seldom is sufficient to produce clinical hyperthyroidism.

Parathyroid glands

STRUCTURE AND FUNCTION

The parathyroid glands are usually four in number and are situated on the posterior surface of the thyroid gland or are embedded in the thyroid tissue but separated from it by a connective tissue capsule. There is considerable variation in their position, particularly in the site of the lower pair of glands, which are derived from the third branchial pouch in close association with portions of the thymus. One or both of the lower parathyroid glands may be found in the mediastinum in or near the thymus.

Histologically, the basic cell type in normal parathyroid glands is the *chief cell,* which is responsible for synthesis and secretion of parathyroid hormone and consists of two types: light (resting) and dark (active) chief cells. The light cells have abundant glycogen; scant granular endoplasmic reticulum; small Golgi complexes; few vacuoles, vesicles, and secretory granules; and large amounts of lipid. The dark cells have sparse glycogen; prominent granular endoplasmic reticulum; prominent Golgi complexes; numerous vesicles, vacuoles, and secretory granules; and few fat droplets. In man, the chief cell is the only cell present in normal parathyroid glands before puberty. Just before puberty, the *oxyphil cells* appear and increase in number with age. Their nuclei are smaller than those of chief cells, and the cytoplasm is filled with numerous mitochondria but does not contain secretory granules. The oxyphil cell is derived from the chief cell through a transitional or intermediate form. In normal glands, oxyphil cells do not appear to have the ability to synthesize and secrete hormone, but in neoplasms and in primary hyperplasia, they have the organelles re-

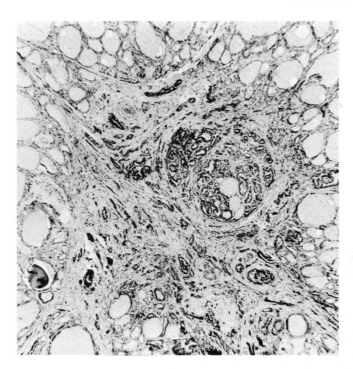

Fig. 21-21. Small follicular thyroid carcinoma in midst of dense fibrous tissue (nonencapsulated sclerosing carcinoma).

quired for synthesis, secretion, and storage of hormone. Another type of cell derived from the chief cell is the *water-clear cell,* which is the prominent cell type in primary water-clear cell hyperplasia of the parathyroid glands. It has been shown in recent studies that the cells in this form of hyperplasia represent a distinct cell type that is not present in the normal glands. Electron microscopically, the cytoplasm contains characteristic vacuoles not seen in other parathyroid cells. Certain chief cells seen in normal, hyperplastic, or neoplastic parathyroid glands may have a cytoplasm that appears clear because of the removal of intracellular glycogen during preparation of the tissue section for light microscopy, and they have been referred to as "water-clear" cells. However, some investigators propose that the term *water-clear cell* be used only for the cells in primary water-clear cell hyperplasia. The cellular elements in the normal gland may be diffuse or compact, but usually they have a definite arrangement in irregular strands or trabeculae. There may be occasional acinar arrangement. Fat cells are often quite abundant between the parenchymal cells.

The parathyroid glands are important in the regulation of calcium and phosphorus metabolism. Parathyroid regulation maintains the diffusible ionized portion of serum calcium (i.e., the portion of serum calcium not bound to protein) within a narrow normal quantitative range. The mechanism of regulation appears to be by promotion of renal phosphate excretion and through mobilization of calcium from bones by stimulation of osteoclasts. It is thus evident that disturbances of parathyroid hormone production may be expected to produce changes in calcium and phosphate regulation, with lesions not only in the parathyroid glands themselves but also in bones and kidneys. Hypoparathyroidism, or insufficient hormone production, is associated with tetany (neuromuscular irritability). Hyperparathyroidism, in which there is excessive hormone, may result in the skeletal changes of osteitis fibrosa cystica, calcium deposits in soft tissue (metastatic calcification), and renal calculi. Hypercalcemic crises (calcium intoxication) may occur in hyperparathyroidism and be rapidly fatal unless recognized and treated.

As noted previously, thyrocalcitonin (calcitonin), produced by thyroid parafollicular cells, is also important in controlling calcium and bone metabolism. Its hypocalcemic effect (e.g., decreasing resorption of calcium from bones) partly counters the action of parathyroid hormone.

Dietary hypercalcemia, known as the *Burnett* or *milk-alkali syndrome,* may simulate primary hyperparathyroidism with secondary renal damage. It usually is caused by prolonged excessive intake of milk and absorbable alkalies. There is hypercalcemia without hypercalciuria, ocular calcinosis known as "band keratopathy," pruritus, azotemia, and mild alkalosis.

DISEASES
Hyperparathyroidism

Hyperparathyroidism may be primary or secondary. The primary form originates in the parathyroid glands, most often as a tumor (adenoma) of one gland or, rarely, as an idiopathic hypertrophy and hyperplasia of all glands. In secondary hyperparathyroidism, there is diffuse hyperplasia of all glands. A mild degree of such secondary parathyroid hyperplasia occurs in chronic renal disease, osteomalacia, and rickets and may be produced experimentally by phosphate injections. Long-standing chronic renal insufficiency may produce pronounced parathyroid hyperplasia and skeletal changes (p. 360). Pancreatitis is an occasional complication of hyperparathyroidism.

Hyperparathyroidism is characterized clinically by weakness, polyuria, pain in the bones, skeletal changes, increased serum calcium and phosphatase levels, and decreased serum phosphate level. The bony changes seen on x-ray film may appear first as subperiosteal

bone resorption, followed by generalized loss of bone density and later cyst formation. Renal or skeletal disease is usually prominent. Renal disease in association with hyperparathyroidism is discussed on p. 361 and the hyperparathyroid skeletal disease, osteitis fibrosa cystica, on p. 705.

Parathyroid adenoma. Parathyroid adenoma is a benign tumor involving a single gland or portion of a gland. Occasionally, two glands may be involved. Adenomas are most commonly composed of chief cells, but in many cases there is a mixture of this type with oxyphil cells, transitional oxyphil cells, and cells resembling "water-clear" cells on light microscopy. The last-named cells have been identified as glycogen-filled chief cells that do not contain the characteristic vacuoles of the distinct type of cell seen in primary water-clear cell hyperplasia. In some patients, the adenomas may be composed mainly of oxyphils (Fig. 21-22) or of cells resembling the "water-clear" type. Although many adenomas are functional, oxyphil cell adenomas often do not cause hyperparathyroidism. The individual cells in the adenomas, as well as their nuclei, may be increased in size. Cells with multiple nuclei may be seen, but mitotic figures are not usually present. In some adenomas, annulate lamellae have been identified in chief cells by electron microscopy, a feature that is not observed in normal chief cells. Commonly, the cellular elements of the adenomas are compactly arranged, with loss of the normal pattern of cells and a decrease in fat and connective tissue. However, variability of cellular arrangement exists, so that trabecular, pseudoglandular, or follicular patterns may be seen.

Parathyroid carcinoma. Parathyroid carcinomas are rare, but functioning metastases have been reported.

Primary hyperplasia. In primary hyperplasia, all the parathyroid glands are enlarged. Originally, only hyperplasia of the water-clear cells was described, the cells being enlarged (hypertrophied) as well as increased in number. There is now recognized, however, a primary hyperplasia of chief cells, which, ac-

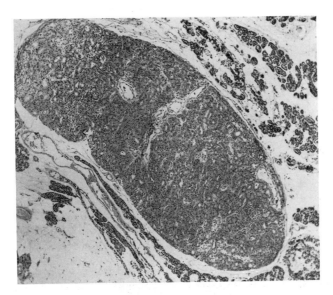

Fig. 21-22. Small oxyphil adenoma of parathyroid gland.

cording to recent studies, occurs more commonly than primary water-clear cell hyperplasia. In *primary chief-cell hyperplasia,* the chief cells are similar to those seen in adenomas of the parathyroid glands. It is difficult to distinguish the cells in these two conditions, even by electron microscopy. Not infrequently, the cells in primary hyperplasia may consist of a mixture of chief cells, oxyphil cells, and transitional oxyphil cells.

In *primary water-clear cell hyperplasia,* the cells are large and have clear cytoplasm and basally oriented nuclei. The cells usually are arranged in cords or sheets but sometimes form acini. The cytoplasm of the cells contains characteristic spherical vacuoles that are ultrastructurally distinct from the secretory granules in the chief cells present in normal, hyperplastic, or neoplastic parathyroid glands.

Secondary hyperparathyroidism. Secondary hyperparathyroidism is characterized by enlargement of all the glands (Fig. 21-23), usually because of increased numbers of chief cells. Some of the chief cells have small cytoplasmic vesicles and swollen mitochondria in a clear cytoplasm, but the vesicles are not as large or as distinctive as the vacuoles in the

water-clear cells seen in the less common form of primary parathyroid hyperplasia. Mature oxyphil cells and transitional oxyphil cells may also be increased in secondary hyperparathyroidism. The various glands are not necessarily enlarged to the same degree, but all show a decrease of interstitial fat.

Hypoparathyroidism

Manifested clinically by tetany, hypoparathyroidism is most commonly seen after operations on the thyroid gland in which the parathyroid glands were accidentally removed or had their blood supply disturbed. Idiopathic cases also occur.

Tetany. Tetany is a manifestation of neuromuscular hyperirritability caused by low blood and tissue calcium. It occurs also in conditions other than hypoparathyroidism, such as rickets, osteomalacia, and hyperventilation.

Pseudohypoparathyroidism is a rare genetic disorder characterized by short stature, mental retardation, hypocalcemic tetany unresponsive to parathyroid extract, and osseous abnormalities (Albright's hereditary osteodystrophy). There is a normal secretion of hormone from the parathyroid glands. It has been suggested

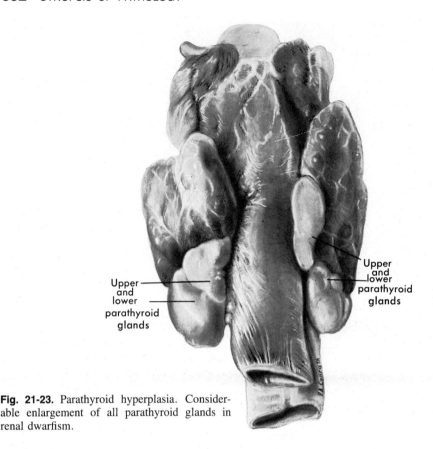

Fig. 21-23. Parathyroid hyperplasia. Considerable enlargement of all parathyroid glands in renal dwarfism.

that the target tissues, bones and kidneys, are unresponsive to parathyroid hormone because of the genetic defect. An increased secretion of thyrocalcitonin is considered by some investigators to play a role.

Polyendocrine disease

Several syndromes that have a strong familial incidence are characterized by functioning adenomas in more than one endocrine gland. Pancreatic islets, parathyroid glands, the anterior lobe of the pituitary gland, adrenal glands, and the thyroid gland may be involved with varying frequency and combinations. Peptic ulcer is a frequent manifestation. Some cases of the Zollinger-Ellison syndrome (p. 473) may have a polyendocrine background.

The familial disease characterized by adenomas of several endocrine glands, frequently associated with the Zollinger-Ellison syndrome, is variously known as *polyendocrine* or *multiple endocrine adenomatosis, Wermer's syndrome,* and *multiple endocrine neoplasia, type 1.* Polyendocrine disease characterized by pheochromocytoma, medullary thyroid carcinoma, and sometimes hyperparathyroidism is referred to as *multiple endocrine neoplasia, type 2,* or *Sipple's syndrome.*

Thymus

STRUCTURE AND FUNCTION

The thymus is an epithelial and lymphoid structure prominent during childhood. Its relative size is greatest at birth, when it weighs about 13 g, and its absolute size is greatest at puberty, when the average weight is about 30 g. In adult life, it undergoes atrophy and replacement by fatty tissue.

The epithelial elements are derived from the third branchial cleft, and the lymphoid structures develop later in fetal life. The epithelial cells form concentric collections known as Hassall's corpuscles.

The thymus is an important source of T lymphocytes. In addition to this lymphopoietic function, it also appears to have erythropoietic and myelopoietic activity, at least during fetal life. Its important function is related to immune mechanisms (p. 81).

PATHOLOGIC CHANGES

Pathologic changes in the thymus consist of developmental defects (absence, aplasia, hypoplasia), atrophy, hyperplasia, and cyst and tumor formation.

Developmental defects, atrophy, and hyperplasia

In some patients, there may be a congenital developmental defect of the third and fourth pharyngeal pouches, resulting in total absence of the thymus or a very small thymus that is inadequate for proper immunologic function (*DiGeorge's syndrome* or *III-IV pharyngeal pouch syndrome*). In this syndrome, there is also a lack of development of the parathyroid glands. Anomalies of the aortic arch may be present as well. In these patients, the cell-mediated immune responses are depressed. Although immunoglobulin production is usually normal, there may be a deficiency of humoral response to certain antigens.

In *severe combined immunodeficiency disease (Swiss-type lymphocytopenic agammaglobulinemia)*, hypoplasia of the thymus and a deficiency of antibody formation coexist, so that there is a depression of both cell-mediated and humoral immune responses. A hypoplastic thymus consists of a small number of poorly developed lobules separated by fibrous septa, lacking in small lymphocytes and Hassall's corpuscles (Fig. 21-24).

In addition to the physiologic thymic atro-

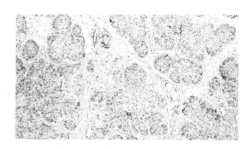

Fig. 21-24. Hypoplasia of thymus gland.

phy that occurs after puberty, atrophy may develop in most serious illnesses or infections of childhood.

Hyperplasia of the thymus occurs in hyperthyroidism (Graves' disease), in acromegaly, in some cases of Addison's disease, and in eunuchs. It also is observed in some patients with myasthenia gravis.

The concept of *status thymicolymphaticus* is that of a constitutional abnormality in certain persons characterized by an enlarged thymus, generalized lymphoid hyperplasia, hypoplasia of the aorta, atrophy of the adrenal glands, and underdevelopment of the testes or ovaries. Such persons are supposedly subject to sudden death as a result of relatively trivial stimuli (e.g., mild trauma, anesthesia). It is probable that the thymus plays no role in the condition other than being part of the generalized lymphoid hyperplasia. That such a condition actually exists is often doubted.

Cysts

Cysts of the thymus may be congenital or acquired, but they seldom are large enough to produce symptoms. So-called *Dubois' abscess* is a rare thymic cyst caused by persistence of the embryonic duct, giving rise to epithelial structures. It may be associated with congenital syphilis. Cystic change in Hassall's corpuscles may occur in infections and during physiologic involution of the thymus. In the anterior mediastinal fat pads of older adults, small cysts may be found that have atrophic thymic tissue in their wall, thus probably representing thymic cysts.

Tumors

Tumors of the thymus are uncommon, but they represent one of the important types of anterior mediastinal neoplasms. Although their histologic pattern varies considerably, they are collectively termed *thymomas* (Fig. 21-25). Some are well encapsulated, but others are nonencapsulated or incompletely encapsulated and extend or infiltrate locally, although distant metastasis is not frequent.

Commonly, the thymomas are classified according to the predominant cell type: (1) epithelial, (2) spindle, (3) lymphocytic, and (4) mixed (lymphoepithelial). The spindle-cell type is apparently a variant of epithelial thymomas. One form of thymic tumor has been described as "granulomatous thymoma," consisting of a combination of epithelial cell masses and a granulomatous component resembling the nodular sclerosing form of Hodgkin's disease. Some investigators believe that such a tumor should be regarded as Hodgkin's disease arising in the thymus rather than a true thymoma. Another tumor that occasionally involves the thymus resembles the testicular seminoma or ovarian dysgerminoma. The origin of this tumor, which is sometimes referred to as "seminomalike thymoma," is not known. Lipomas of the thymus occur rarely but may be large. Another rare tumor is a malignant thymoma consisting of epithelial cells with areas of rhabdomyosarcomatous differentiation that presumably originate from thymic "myoid" cells.

It should be noted that certain authors contend that the lymphocytes in "lymphocytic" or "lymphoepithelial" thymomas are not neoplastic and that these tumors are simply epithelial thymomas with an associated lymphocytic component of varying degrees. Malignant lymphomas of the lymphocytic type involving the thymus must be differentiated from the thymomas that have a lymphocytic component.

Tumors of the thymus may be asymptomatic, but in some patients they produce symptoms caused by compression or infiltration of adjacent mediastinal structures. About 35% to 50% of patients with thymomas have been reported to have symptoms of myasthenia gravis, although the incidence in individual series is sometimes reported as being much higher. At times, a paraneoplastic syndrome may be associated with a thymoma (e.g., Cushing's syndrome, aregenerative anemia, or pancytopenia).

A poorer prognosis is associated with thymomas that are nonencapsulated or incompletely encapsulated and invasive than with those that are well encapsulated and show no evidence of capsular invasion. Also, the prognosis is less favorable in patients with thymomas complicated by myasthenia gravis.

Thymus in myasthenia gravis

Myasthenia gravis is characterized by weakness or abnormal fatigability of voluntary muscles that is believed to be caused by interference with transmission of impulses across the myoneural junction. This condition, which is simulated by curare poisoning, is temporarily overcome by administration of cholinergic drugs (e.g., neostigmine). Foci of lymphocytes (lymphorrhages) are found in the affected muscles. Lymphocytic infiltration has also been described in the thyroid gland and other organs. Foci of degeneration and necrosis in the myocardium and myocarditis have been observed in some myasthenic patients, especially those with an associated thymoma.

Most of the patients with myasthenia gravis have an associated thymic lesion, but the exact nature of this association has not been clearly established. In the majority of instances, the thymic lesion consists of lymphoid hyperplasia with formation of germinal centers, and in the others it is a thymoma. In some thymomas, there may be lymphoid hyperplasia with germinal centers in the remaining thymic tissue about the tumor. Some myasthenic patients have been reported to be improved by thymectomy, particularly female patients whose thymus glands showed lymphoid hyperplasia with germinal centers.

It has been postulated that autoimmunity plays a role in the pathogenesis of myasthenia gravis. In addition to the presence of abnormalities of the thymus gland in most of the patients with this disease and the relief of

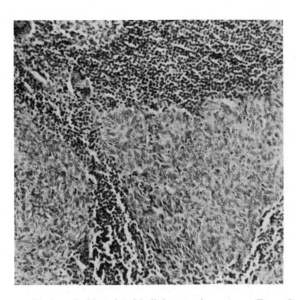

Fig. 21-25. Thymoma with lymphoid and epithelial-appearing areas. (From Smith, S. B.: Thymus. In Anderson, W. A. D., and Kissane, J. M., editors: Pathology, ed. 7, St. Louis, 1977, The C. V. Mosby Co.)

symptoms as a result of thymectomy in some of them, there is other evidence suggesting a relationship with autoimmunity. Myasthenia gravis is sometimes associated with other diseases of probable autoimmune origin (e.g., rheumatoid arthritis and systemic lupus erythematosus). Cross-reactions have been demonstrated between antimuscle antibodies in the sera of myasthenic individuals and certain cells of the thymus. The reactive elements in the thymus that may be the source of antigen are believed to be the thymic myoid cells. Antinuclear and antithyroid autoantibodies have been detected in some myasthenic patients. In one study, in vitro immunologic reactivity was demonstrated between thymocytes of patients with myasthenia gravis associated with thymic hyperplasia and their own peripheral blood lymphocytes, but not in patients with myasthenia associated with thymomas or in control patients. In addition, there was evidence of an increased percentage of B lymphocytes with IgM receptors in the thymus glands of myasthenic patients as compared with the control group. It has been shown that the his-

tocompatibility antigen HLA-B8 is significantly associated with myasthenia gravis in young females with thymic lymphoid hyperplasia, but it is uncommon in older myasthenic patients and those with thymomas.

Experimental "autoimmune thymitis," characterized by a dense lymphocytic infiltration around Hassall's corpuscles, was induced by immunizing animals with thymic antigens in Freund's complete adjuvant. This condition was associated with a neuromuscular block similar to that occurring in myasthenia gravis, and there was evidence that this block was caused by a humoral substance released from the damaged thymus. Subsequently, a polypeptide, "thymopoietin" (formerly known as "thymin"), was isolated from bovine thymus and was shown to depress neuromuscular transmission. This substance was also found to have a specific lymphopoietic effect in that it induced differentiation of T cells (not B cells) in vitro. In contrast to the concept that an anticholinergic thymus hormone is responsible for the neuromuscular block is the view that antibodies may be directed against the neuromuscular junction. Certain investigators have demonstrated serum globulins in some myasthenic patients that appear to have an inhibitory effect on muscle acetylcholine receptors by interacting with them. In electron microscopic studies, significant ultrastructural alterations have been observed in the postsynaptic membrane at the motor endplates in myasthenic patients.

The possibility has also been considered that a viral infection of the thymus may be the cause of the thymic abnormalities and the resultant myasthenia gravis.

Pineal body

STRUCTURE AND FUNCTION

The function of the pineal body is yet unknown. There is some evidence that it has a secretory function, although it is not essential to life, pregnancy, or parturition. Several neurohumoral substances (e.g., serotonin and histamine) as well as a skin-lightening agent (melatonin), which appears to be an antagonist of the pituitary melanocyte-stimulating hormone, have been reported in bovine pineal tissue. It has been suggested that the pineal body secretes an adrenotropic hormone affecting aldosterone secretion, but this has not been proved.

At about the time of puberty, regressive structural changes are initiated in the pineal body. There is an increase in interstitial connective tissue, which accentuates fibrous trabeculae and gives the gland a lobulated appearance in microscopic section. Calcareous concretions (acervuli) also begin to form about puberty and are almost constant after the sixteenth year. In adult life, they are sometimes sufficiently dense to be evident on x-ray film.

Areas of neuroglial hyperplasia, often with irregularly cavitated centers, are quite commonly present in the pineal body. True cysts also occur, usually lined by ependymal cells.

TUMORS

Tumors of the pineal body constitute its only important lesion. Pineal tumors are of three types: (1) pinealomas, (2) teratomas, and (3) gliomas.

Pinealomas are tumors composed of pineal parenchymal cells and have a microscopic appearance similar to that of some stage of embryonic development of the pineal body (Fig. 21-26). Two types of cells are usually present: large pale cells with prominent rounded nuclei and indefinite cytoplasm, resembling cells of the adult period, and fewer small, round, dark cells, resembling lymphocytes. The tumors are locally invasive and malignant. Pinealomas also may have a structure resembling the adult pineal body.

Athough some evidence has suggested that the usual pinealoma is really an atypical teratoma, there are also *teratomas* of the pineal body that are similar to teratomas elsewhere in the body and contain bone, teeth, cartilage, epithelium, hair, etc.

Gliomas of the pineal body usually closely resemble the ependymomas that arise in other areas of the brain, but spongioblastic pineal tumors also occur.

Because of their situaiton, pineal tumors soon obstruct the aqueduct of Sylvius, producing internal hydrocephalus and considerable increase of intracranial pressure. Certain pineal tumors in preadolescent boys have been associated with precocious sexual development (pubertas praecox or macrogenitosomia praecox). A similar condition of hypergenitalism has been associated with midbrain lesions or tumors as well as with various endocrine disturbances.

Adrenal glands

STRUCTURE AND FUNCTION

The adrenal glands consist of two distinct glands, cortex and medulla, which have different origins and functions. The cortex is of mesodermal origin from the urogenital ridge and is thus closely related to gonads and other urogenital organs. The medulla originates from the neural crest in common with sympathetic nerve cells. Although anatomically as-

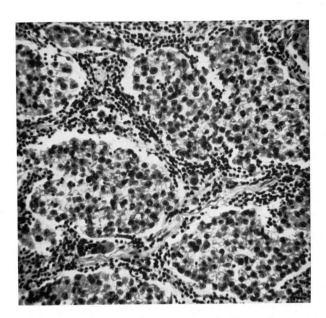

Fig. 21-26. Pinealoma showing two types of cells usually present.

sociated in man, the cortex and medulla are quite separate in their function and pathology and are best considered as separate glands. The cortex, which is essential for life, is associated with salt and water (electrolyte) metabolism, protein and carbohydrate metabolism, and development and maintenance of secondary sexual characteristics (androgen production). The adrenal glands are essential for adjustment to changes in internal and external environment. The adrenal medulla secretes epinephrine, the effects of which simulate sympathetic stimulation. Survival is possible in the absence of the medulla. Accessory adrenal tissue may be found between the origins of the celiac and superior mesenteric arteries, in or on the kidneys, and attached to the genital tract.

The adrenal glands are relatively largest at the time of birth, when they are usually one-third the size of the kidney. The large size results from a highly vascular inner cortical tissue that degenerates soon after birth and disappears almost entirely during the first year of life. In adult life, the adrenal glands are about one-thirtieth the size of the kidney.

ADRENAL CORTEX
Structure and function

Although numerous steroids have been isolated from adrenal tissue, three are recognized as principal cortical hormones in man: cortisol, corticosterone, and aldosterone. The first two, which have an effect on carbohydrate metabolism, are called glucocorticoids. Aldosterone has its main effect on salt and water metabolism and is termed a mineralocorticoid.

The adrenal cortex is divided into zones descriptively named, from without inward, zona glomerulosa, zona fasciculata, and zona reticularis. Internal to these, the highly vascular zone that exists at birth is replaced by a thin juxtamedullary zone. Some brownish pigment, of no known significance, is often present in the inner part of the cortex.

The outer zone, the zona glomerulosa, is composed of rounded clusters of cells. It appears to be the zone mainly concerned with the group of adrenal steroids termed mineralocorticoids and is concerned principally with control of water and electrolyte metabolism. The naturally occurring hormone is aldosterone, and its synthetic relative is called deoxycorticosterone. These hormones bring about reabsorption of sodium and chloride by the renal distal convoluted tubules, with a corresponding loss of potassium, and provide the mechanism by which sodium, potassium, and extracellular fluid are maintained in normal osmotic balance. Output of aldosterone appears to be regulated by changes in the relations of sodium, potassium, and extracellular fluid and is not under control of the anterior pituitary gland. Aldosterone also antagonizes the activity of hydrocortisone (cortisol), which inhibits inflammatory reactions and produces a decrease of circulating eosinophils. Urinary excretion of aldosterone provides an index of the amount of circulating hormone. The electrolyte composition of sweat serves as an index of the effect of the mineralocorticoid on the sodium content of the tissues. An increase of the hormone (secondary hyperaldosteronism) may be brought about by a prolonged low sodium intake, and it also occurs in conditions of generalized edema or persistent hypertension. Primary hyperaldosteronism occurs from the activity of certain adrenal cortical tumors and hyperplasias. Selective hypoaldosteronism appears to be rare.

The thick middle zone of the cortex, the zona fasciculata, is composed of parallel cords of cells that are rich in lipids and appear pale or vacuolated. It is a site of formation of the glucocorticoids, which influence intermediate carbohydrate metabolism. The production of the glucocorticoids is under the control of the anterior pituitary adrenocorticotropic hormone (ACTH), and, in turn, the glucocorticoid level controls the adrenocorticotropic activity of the anterior pituitary gland. The main glucocorticoids are cortisol (compound F) and corticosterone. Synthetic derivatives used therapeutically are prednisone and prednisolone. The glucocorticoids cause acceleration of gluconeogenesis from protein and deposition of liver glycogen, with related effects on the metabolism of carbohydrates, protein, and fat. They suppress inflammatory response (antiphlogistic activity) and cause eosinopenia, lysis of lymphoid cells, and atrophy of lymphoid tissues. The glucocorticoids are important in resistance to nonspecific stress. They

are not without some mineralocorticoid activity, just as aldosterone has some weaker glucocorticoid action. Prolonged medication with cortisone or its relatives may produce the phenomena seen in Cushing's syndrome.

The inner zone, the zona reticularis, is usually narrow and made up of an interlacing network of "compact" cells, which are eosinophilic and contain abundant phosphatase and ribonucleic acid. It appears to be the site principally concerned with the androgenic sex hormones (nitrogen hormones). These hormones are involved in masculinization (androgenic function) and also are anabolic, increasing the synthesis of amino acids and protein from nitrogen. Their amount is reflected in the urinary excretion of 17-ketosteroids. Some estrogen production also may occur. According to some views, the zona reticularis is also the ordinary site of formation of glucocorticoids, with additional formation in the zona fasciculata when there is unusual stimulation.

The assignment of separate functions to the different zones is provisional, and it is uncertain as to how distinct the functional separation may be. Ascorbic acid is stored in the zona reticularis and inner part of the zona fasciculata, and its concentration parallels the lipid content of the cortex. Lipid material is present throughout the cortex but is most abundant in the zona fasciculata. The shift of lipid patterns gives some indication of adrenal cortical activity caused by pituitary adrenotropic hormone. When ACTH is administered, the cells of the inner part of the zona fasciculata have a decrease of their lipid and become similar to the "compact" cells of the zona reticularis. Increasing the amount of ACTH stimulation extends this change outward in the zona fasciculata. The lipids in adrenocortical cells consist of doubly refractile cholesterol, anisotropic neutral lipids, and steroids. The lipids tend to be depleted as the gland becomes exhausted.

Lesions

Lesions in the adrenal cortex may be grouped roughly as regressive and destructive changes and hyperplasia and tumors.

Regressive and destructive lesions

Adrenal cortical tissue is most commonly injured or destroyed by hemorrhage, infarction, metastatic tumors, infections, and amyloid deposits.

Hemorrhage and necrosis. Extensive hemorrhage into the adrenal glands or thrombosis of adrenal vessels may produce acute adrenal insufficiency. Hemorrhage is particularly common in newborn infants, in some cases from trauma incident to birth. Adrenal hemorrhage or focal necrosis also may occur with extensive burns or in various infections. Small areas of hemorrhagic necrosis may occur in eclampsia. In newborn infants, the highly vascular inner zone of the cortex may be mistaken for hemorrhage unless carefully examined.

Various acute infections may severely damage the adrenal cortex, the necrosis of cells transforming the solid cords of cells of the zona fasciculata into apparent tubular structures containing inflammatory exudate. The adrenal damage may bear some relation to the circulatory collapse that occurs in some of the patients. Small focal areas of inflammation or necrosis are common wth generalized infections or toxemias. Histoplasmosis and blastomycosis quite commonly involve the adrenal glands.

Massive bilateral hemorrhages of the adrenal glands may occur in cases of fulminating meningococcemia, in which rapid death occurs, often before there is any great involvement of the meninges *(Waterhouse-Friderichsen syndrome).* The fatal outcome appears to result from the overwhelming meningococcemia, with acute adrenal insufficiency having only a minor role. The hemorrhages in the adrenal glands, skin, and elsewhere appear to be the result of toxic injury of capillary endothelium. Only about 2% to 4% of meningococcal infections have the complication of the Waterhouse-Friderichsen syndrome. Overwhelming septicemia due to other organisms (e.g., *Haemophilus influenzae,* staphylococci, or pneumococci) may be associated with this syndrome.

Atrophy of the adrenal cortex may be produced by the continued administration of cortisone. Loss of lipid occurs first, particularly in the zona fasciculata, and the adrenal glands decrease in weight and show narrowing in the cortex and loss of color. The changes seem to be reversible in most instances and appear to be caused by suppressed endogenous production of corticotropin by the pituitary gland. Basophils of the anterior pituitary gland may show loss of granularity of their cytoplasm.

Addison's disease. Chronic adrenal cortical insufficiency produces the clinical condition of Addison's disease. Symptoms appear when about 80% of adrenal cortical tissue has been destroyed. In about 70% of cases, the bilateral destruction of the adrenal glands formerly was caused by tuberculosis. In most of the remaining cases, there was atrophy or destruction from unknown causes, thought by some to result from unsuspected chemical or drug poisoning. In the United States, cortical necrosis or atrophy (Fig. 21-27) now appears to account for about two thirds of the cases.

The pathogenesis of the cortical necrosis or atrophy usually is unknown. Thus, the disorder is commonly referred to as "idiopathic Addison's disease." Autoimmunity, however, has been suggested as a possible mechanism, since in many of the patients, autoantibodies to adrenal tissue have been demonstrated. In some of the patients, there are associated diseases of autoimmune nature, particularly of other endocrine organs. The adrenal medulla usually is unaffected in idiopathic Addison's disease. The incidence of tuberculosis as a cause of Addison's disease is decreasing. In the case of the tuberculous lesions, both cortex and medulla of the adrenal glands usually are destroyed. Active tuberculous lesions usually are found elsewhere. Amyloidosis, inflammatory changes, fibrosis, histoplasmosis, and torulosis of the cortex sometimes cause Addison's disease, but bilateral metastatic tumors or gummas only rarely are a cause.

Addison's disease is characterized by extreme weakness, low blood pressure, and pigmentation of the skin. The pigmentation is caused by excessive melanin, presumably from the increased secretion of the melanocyte-stimulating hormone of the pituitary gland, which results from lack of inhibition by

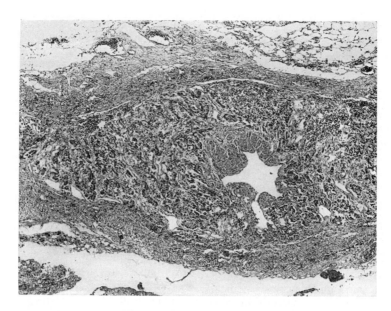

Fig. 21-27. Adrenal gland in Addison's disease showing cortical loss. Only medulla is seen, which is focally infiltrated with lymphocytes. (From Anderson, W. A. D., and Cleveland, W. W.: Adrenal glands. In Anderson, W. A. D., editor: Pathology, ed. 5, St. Louis, 1966, The C. V. Mosby Co.)

the adrenal cortical hormones. It may be irregular in distribution and often is best seen in the mucous membranes of the lips or mouth or in scars. Urinary excretion of ketosteroids is decreased to a low level. Salt metabolism is disturbed, there being excessive loss of sodium salt in the urine with low sodium and chloride levels and a rise in potassium in the plasma. High sodium and low potassium intake relieves many of the symptoms. Adrenal cortical extracts successfully replace the hormonal deficiency.

Schmidt's syndrome is the combination of idiopathic Addison's disease with chronic lymphocytic thyroiditis. It is found mainly in females, and generally the adrenal insufficiency precedes recognizable thyroid disease. Circulating antibodies against thyroid tissue and also against adrenal tissue may be present. Some patients also have diabetes mellitus, and it has been suggested that such cases may be a polyendocrinopathy and that the basis may be immunologic.

Anencephaly. The adrenal glands frequently have been reported as defective or absent in anencephalic monsters. Usually they are present but atrophic and, histologically, are of the adult rather than the infantile type. The adrenal atrophy is believed to be secondary to pituitary changes.

Hyperplasia and tumors

Hyperplasia of the adrenal cortex may be nodular or diffuse and is usually bilateral. It may be observed as a nonspecific finding in some patients with acromegaly, hyperthyroidism, cancer, hypertension, or diabetes mellitus. Specific clinical endocrine syndromes with which adrenocortical hyperplasia may be associated include Cushing's syndrome, adrenogenital syndrome, and primary hyperaldosteronism. These conditions are discussed below. Adrenocortical hyperplasia also occurs following adminstration of ACTH.

Adrenocortical nodules are small circumscribed growths that are not true neoplasms

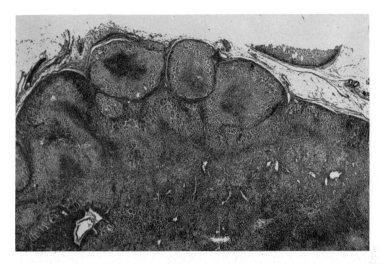

Fig. 21-28. Adrenal cortex (low power) showing multiple adrenocortical nodules with varying degrees of encapsulation.

and are not associated with an endocrine syndrome. They are found in a considerable proportion of autopsies on adults, particularly in older persons and in those who died of hypertension or cardiovascular diseases. The functional significance of the nodules is not known. It has been suggested that they represent a regenerative process following ischemic focal cortical atrophy resulting from local vascular disease (Fig.21-28).

True adenoma occurs as a yellowish mass that is usually 1 or 2 cm in diameter but may grow to considerable size. It is usually single and unilateral. Although it is well circumscribed and has a definite capsule, it may press upon and deform the remainder of the gland. *Carcinomas* are similar to the adenomas but contain areas of atypical and malignant-looking cells. Invasion of veins or the capsule may be seen, and metastasis occurs readily to distant organs and to the opposite adrenal gland. *Myelolipoma* is a tumorlike nodule of adipose and hematopoietic tissue, resembling bone marrow (Fig. 21-29). It may be an incidental finding in the adrenal glands of adults. Occasionally, certain benign mesenchymal tumors occur in the adrenal gland,

e.g., neurilemoma, neurofibroma, leiomyoma, angioma, and lipoma (Fig. 21-30).

In persons having a functioning adrenal cortical adenoma or carcinoma, the opposite adrenal gland may be atrophic and insufficient to meet sudden functional demands. Consequently, an acute adrenal insufficiency may develop after surgical removal of the tumor.

Adrenal cortical hyperfunction

Hyperplasias, adenomas, or carcinomas of the adrenal cortex may be associated with excessive hormonal production and clinical effects, although not infrequently these lesions are encountered without apparent hormonal effects. Those that are associated with excess hormone production may result either in a clinical syndrome in which the effects of one type of adrenal cortical hormone are dominant or in a mixed picture in which the effects of excess of more than one hormonal principle are evident. Although the varying excesses of the different hormones produce gradations in the clinical features, cases may be grouped into three classes, with some exceptions: the adrenogenital syndrome, Cushing's syndrome, and primary aldosteronism.

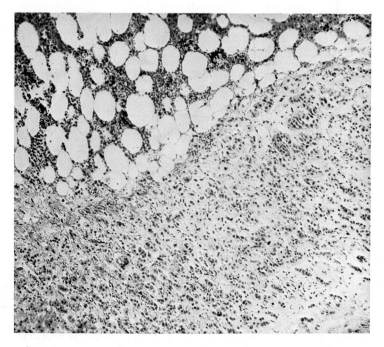

Fig. 21-29. Myelolipoma of adrenal gland. Fatty and myeloid tissue, resembling bone marrow, have formed a tumorlike nodule enclosed by adrenal cortical tissue.

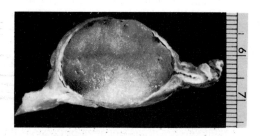

Fig. 21-30. Lipoma of adrenal gland.

Adrenogenital syndrome. The adrenogenital syndrome is an adrenal virilism in which an excess of androgenic hormones produces the dominant effects. Overgrowth of cortical tissue that produces male hormone causes a variety of sexual disturbances, depending on the age at which it occurs. *Congenital virilism* appears to be an inborn metabolic fault in which incompletely oxygenated steroids instead of cortisol are secreted into the bloodstream. The

resulting lack stimulates excess production of pituitary corticotropin, which, in turn, causes hyperplasia of the adrenal cortex and a large output of androgens.

The most common form of congenital virilism results from 21-hydroxylase deficiency. In some patients, aldosterone as well as cortisol formation is decreased, so that salt loss is added to the clinical features. An 11-hydroxylase deficiency is characterized by virilism with hypertension. The affected female infant or child with congenital virilism has hypertrophy of the clitoris and labial fusion that resembles a scrotum but has normal internal genitalia (i.e., pseudohermaphroditism). In the male infant or child, the phallus may be enlarged (macrogenitosomia). In both sexes, accelerated skeletal growth occurs, with early closure of the epiphyses. The hyperplastic adrenal gland in this condition consists of "compact" cortical cells extending from the corticomedullary junction up to the zona glomerulosa.

Adrenal virilism in older children and adults may also be caused by adrenal cortical hyperplasia but is more likely produced by an adrenal cortical tumor (adenoma or carcinoma). In boys, it is characterized by precocious sexual and muscle development, with genitalia of adult size and secondary sexual characteristics. In girls, pseudosexual precocity with masculinity occurs, with the appearance of pubic hair and hypertrophy of the clitoris. Adult females become masculinized, the change being characterized by hirsutism, enlarged clitoris, atrophy of the breasts, amenorrhea, deepening of the voice, and various masculine characteristics. Urinary excretion of 17-ketosteroids is excessive. The virilization must be distinguished from that produced by certain ovarian tumors. Rarely, an adrenal carcinoma may produce excess estrogen and cause feminization of males or precocity in young females.

Cushing's syndrome. Cushing's syndrome is produced by excessive secretion of cortisol and is most commonly caused by adrenal cortical hyperplasia involving the zona fasciculata and in some instances the zona reticularis as well. Cushing's syndrome is more common in women than in men (3:1 or 4:1). Clinical characteristics are obesity of the face, neck, and trunk, polycythemia and a dusky color of the skin, purplish striae of the skin of the abdomen, buttocks, and flanks, hypertension, osteoporosis, a tendency to diabetes mellitus, weakness and fatigue, and sexual impotence or amenorrhea.

Most of the clinical effects can be reproduced by the administration of an excess of glucocorticoids. In the common variety of spontaneously occurring Cushing's syndrome, anterior pituitary gland secretes an overproduction of ACTH, which stimulates the adrenal cortex. The source of the ACTH secretion may be a pituitary tumor (basophil or chromophobe adenoma), but in some patients no pituitary tumor is demonstrated, suggesting the possibility that a functional hypothalamic-pituitary disturbance may be operative (i.e., over-stimulation of the pituitary by hypothalamic corticotropin-releasing factor). Until recently, relatively few patients with Cushing's syndrome had demonstrable pituitary tumors, but with improved radiologic techniques and the use of transsphenoidal microsurgical exploration of the pituitary, microadenomas have been identified frequently in patients with the syndrome, suggesting that the association of pituitary adenomas with Cushing's syndrome may be more common than previous reports have indicated. A fairly constant associated change in patients with Cushing's syndrome is hyalinization of pituitary basophils (Crooke's hyaline change).

Less commonly, Cushing's syndrome is caused by an adrenal cortical adenoma or carcinoma (Fig. 21-31). An increasing number of instances are being observed in association with neoplasms of nonendocrine tissues that secrete ACTH, especially oat cell carcinoma of the lung. In addition to lung cancers, other nonpituitary tumors of nonendocrine or endocrine origin that are known to secrete ACTH include thymomas, pancreatic islet cell tumors, thyroid medullary carcinoma, neuroblastoma, and ovarian tumors. They are referred to as *ectopic ACTH-secreting tumors.*

Primary aldosteronism. Primary aldosteronism *(Conn's syndrome)* results from excess mineralocorticoid, which is caused usually by an adenoma of the adrenal cortex and much less frequently by adrenal cortical carcinoma or hyperplasia. The tumors are 1 to 5 cm in diameter, bright yellow in color, and composed of large, clear, lipid-containing cells (Fig. 21-32). The cells resemble those of the zona fasciculata. Smaller zona glomerulosa–like cells also may be present or may even be the predominant cell type. In hyperplasia, the zona glomerulosa is involved.

Aldosteronism is characterized clinically by periodic severe muscle weakness, intermittent tetany and paresthesia, polyuria, polydipsia, and hypertension. Edema is not present. There is excessive loss of potassium in the urine, and the blood levels of potassium are low. Alkalosis is present, manifested by the elevation of pH and carbon dioxide content. The urinary

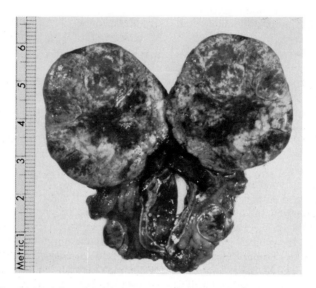

Fig. 21-31. Adrenal carcinoma associated with Cushing's syndrome.

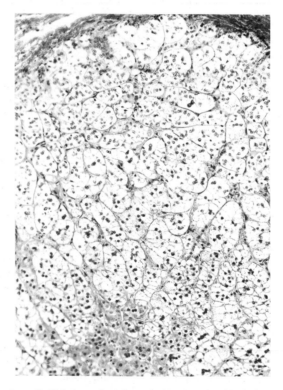

Fig. 21-32. Large, clear, lipid-laden adrenal cortical cells associated with hyperaldosteronism. (×125; courtesy Dr. S. E. Gould; from Anderson, W. A. D., and Cleveland, W. W.: Adrenal glands. In Anderson, W. A. D., editor: Pathology, ed. 5, St. Louis, 1966, The C. V. Mosby Co.)

aldosterone level is high. Before recognition of their true nature, some of these cases have been called ''potassium-losing nephritis.'' Conn has noted that in certain cases of primary aldosteronism, the potassium level in the blood may be normal, at least initially.

Some of the cases of normokalemic primary hyperaldosteronism may masquerade as essential hypertension but have as their basis aldosterone-secreting adrenal cortical adenomas. Overproduction of aldosterone and suppression of plasma renin activity are diagnostic of an aldosterone-secreting adrenal cortical tumor.

Increased aldosterone secretion is frequently present in advanced stages of hypertensive disease and in malignant hypertension. The increased rate of aldosterone secretion appears to be secondary to and to correlate with increased plasma renin levels. Secondary aldosteronism as part of a syndrome associated with renin-producing tumors of the kidney was referred to on p. 349.

Adrenal cortex in eclampsia. The adrenal cortex may have a role in the toxemias of pregnancy, although specific changes may not be present. A hyperadrenalism involving mineralocorticoids and glucocorticoids appears to produce some of the features accompanying pregnancy, but enzymes of the placenta normally suppress or inactivate certain of the effects of the adrenal hormones. Ischemic placental lesions may interfere with this mechanism and result in preeclampsia or eclampsia with convulsions.

ADRENAL MEDULLA
Structure and function

The medulla of the adrenal gland has its origin from ectoderm, in common with sympathetic nerve tissue. The cells of the medulla stain with chrome salts, as do certain other tissues, such as abdominal paraganglia and the carotid body. Their function, production of epinephrine and norepinephrine, is not essential for life. Epinephrine causes contraction of some vessels and dilatation of others (e.g., the coronary arteries), tachycardia, and increased cardiac output. Norepinephrine constricts vessels and causes increased peripheral resistance.

Epinephrine has a greater effect on oxygen consumption and glycogenolysis.

Lesions

Functional disturbances caused by destructive lesions of the medulla may be overshadowed by the associated involvement of the cortex, as in the tuberculous type of Addison's disease. The only lesions of the adrenal medulla that are of practical importance are tumors.

Tumors

Tumors of the adrenal medulla or other parts of the sympathetic nervous system are composed of immature or mature cell types comparable to those that occur in embryonic development of medullary and sympathetic nerve tissue. The most immature form, the precursor of the other types, is the sympathogonia, a small, dark, lymphocytelike cell that differentiates into neuroblasts (sympathoblasts and pheochromoblasts). The sympathoblasts mature as ganglion cells, and the pheochromoblasts develop into pheochromocytes, the mature cells of the adrenal medulla. Tumors composed of the immature forms (sympathogonioma and neuroblastoma) are highly malignant, whereas those composed of mature forms (ganglioneuroma and pheochromocytoma) are usually benign.

Sympathogonioma. Sympathogoniomas usually develop during intrauterine life or in early infancy, are highly malignant and invasive, and metastasize early. They are composed of small dark cells resembling lymphocytes, some of which group to form rosettes. No neurofibrils are formed.

Neuroblastoma. Characteristically, neuroblastoma (sympathoblastoma) is a highly malignant tumor that occurs almost exclusively in infants and young children. It arises either in the adrenal medulla or in sympathetic ganglia. Microscopically, it is extremely cellular, is composed of small, rounded, dark cells resembling lymphocytes, and has the characteristic feature of rosette formation (circular grouping around a fine fibrillar network) (Fig. 21-33).

Usually, the neuroblastoma differs from the

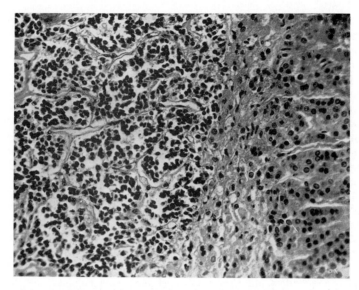

Fig. 21-33. Adrenal neuroblastoma in newborn infant. (From Anderson, W. A. D., and Cleveland, W. W.: Adrenal glands. In Anderson, W. A. D., editor: Pathology, ed. 5, St. Louis, 1966, The C. V. Mosby Co.)

sympathogonioma only in its somewhat greater maturity, and some differentiated ganglion or pheochrome cells may be present. The cells tend to be larger and irregular or oval in shape, and they may have elongated cytoplasmic processes. Tumors having similar histologic structure are the medulloblastoma of the midbrain and the retinoblastoma of the eye. They also arise from undifferentiated neural elements and occur in childhood.

Rare examples of neuroblastoma have given evidence of secretion of epinephrine or norepinephrine. However, there usually is evidence of abnormalities of tyrosine metabolism, with formation of excessive 3,4-dihydroxyphenylalanine (dopa). The excess dopa is metabolized through dopamine to homovanillic acid (HVA) or through dopamine and norepinephrine to vanillylmandelic acid (VMA). The urinary excretion of these terminal metabolites may be detected and measured, providing an effective method for diagnosis and for following results of treatment. VMA is the metabolite that is usually measured. Increase of these urinary metabolites also has been reported with ganglioneuromas and ganglioneuroblastomas.

Adrenal neuroblastoma spreads early and widely by the lymphatics and bloodstream. Sites commonly involved are retroperitoneal lymph nodes, bones, liver, and lungs. In rare instances, the tumor cells of a neuroblastoma mature to ganglion cells, producing a benign ganglioneuroma.

Ganglioneuroma. The ganglioneuroma is a benign tumor composed of large differentiated sympathetic ganglion cells and often a few nerve fibers (Fig. 21-34). It may occur in either a child or an adult. Although the common origin is from the adrenal medulla, it may arise in any part of the abdominal sympathetic system or, very rarely, in the central nervous system. It produces symptoms only by virtue of the large size to which it may grow. A form also occurs in which undifferentiated or incompletely differentiated cells are mixed with some ganglion cells and nerve fibers (ganglioneuroblastoma).

Pheochromocytoma. Chromaffinoma (pheochromocytoma) is a rare tumor composed of a differentiated mature type of cell resembling those cells that normally compose the adrenal medulla. About 90% of these tumors

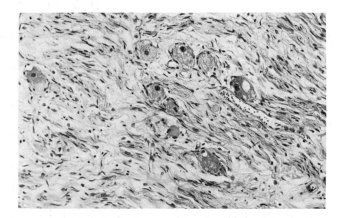

Fig. 21-34. Ganglioneuroma. Tumor composed of irregular jumble of nerve cells and fibers.

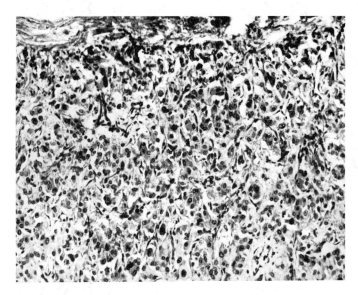

Fig. 21-35. Pheochromocytoma of adrenal gland.

arise in the adrenal gland, somewhat more frequently on the right, and about 10% of those of adrenal origin are bilateral. Some 10% or less arise in extra-adrenal sites, usually near the kidneys, adrenal glands, aortic bodies, or organs of Zuckerkandl, or, rarely, in the urinary bladder. Those arising from extra-adrenal chromaffin tissue have been called paragangliomas.

The tumors are usually less than 10 cm in diameter, circumscribed, and yellowish brown, frequently with cystic, necrotic, or hemorrhagic areas. The tumor cells are large and irregular or polyhedral and occur in groups surrounded by a vascular fine connective tissue stroma (Fig. 21-35). Mitoses are absent. Some of the cells are stained brown by fixation in bichromate. Most pheochromocytomas are benign, and malignancy should not be considered in the absence of invasion or metastasis. The rare malignant pheochromocytomas tend to have a spindle cell growth pattern predominating.

The tumor affects adults more frequently than children. In some cases, there is evidence of familial occurrence, and association with thyroid carcinoma of the medullary type and hyperparathyroidism due to parathyroid hyperplasia or adenoma has been noted (multiple endocrine neoplasia, type 2). It occurs also with somewhat greater than usual frequency in patients with multiple neurofibromatosis.

Although some pheochromocytomas are clinically asymptomatic, many produce symptoms as a result of catecholamine content (epinephrine and norepinephrine). Paroxysmal attacks characterized by hypertension, tachycardia, hyperglycemia, sweating, and trembling are most characteristic and are particularly epinephrine effects. Tumors in which persistent secretion of norepinephrine predominates may give rise to persistent hypertension. Extra-adrenal pheochromocytomas may secrete only norepinephrine. Catecholamines or their metabolites may be demonstrated in urine or blood as a diagnostic procedure. Catecholamines may be assayed also in the fresh tumor tissue. Surgical resection of a functioning tumor may be followed by hypotension and shock.

Glomic tissue tumors (chemodectomas or nonchromaffin paragangliomas). Glomic tissue tumors may arise in the carotid and aortic bodies, the glomus jugulare, and retroperitoneal space. Some examples have been found to secrete norepinephrine (p. 523).

Apudomas (neuroendocrine tumors). Some of the tumors described in this chapter and elsewhere in the book have recently been grouped together as *apudomas,* tumors composed of APUD cells. They have also been designated as *neuroendocrine tumors.* Included in this group are intestinal carcinoid, bronchial carcinoid and oat cell carcinoma, chemodectoma, pheochromocytoma, melanoma, neuroblastoma, pancreatic islet tumor, pituitary adenoma, pinealoma, and medullary carcinoma of the thyroid. The APUD cells are endocrine cells that, although located in different regions of the body, have common properties, i.e., the ability to synthesize peptide or amine hormones and the ability to take up, decarboxylate, and store amine precursors such as 5-hydroxytryptophan and dopa. They also have high levels of nonspecific esterases or cholinesterases and α-glycerophosphate dehydrogenase. It has been suggested that the cells also have a common origin, the neuroectoderm; thus, they have been referred to also as *neuroendocrine cells.* The term ''APUD'' is an acronym derived from following characteristics of the cells: *a*mine content, amine *p*recursor *u*ptake, and *d*ecarboxylation.

REFERENCES

Abdow, N. I., et al.: N. Engl. J. Med. **291**:1271-1275, 1974 (thymus in myasthenia gravis).

Almon, R. R., et al.: Science **186**:55-57, 1974 (serum globulin in myasthenia gravis).

Anderson, D. R.: Am. J. Ophthalmol. **68**:46-57, 1969 (LATS and endocrine exophthalmos).

Batsakis, J. G., et al.: Am. J. Clin. Pathol. **39**:241-251, 1963 (sporadic goiter).

Baylin, S. B., et al.: Am. J. Med. **53**:723-733, 1972 (histaminase activity in medullary carcinoma of the thyroid).

Bieger, R. C., and McAdams, A. J.: Arch. Pathol. **82**:535-541, 1966 (thymic cysts).

Black, W. C., and Haff, R. C.: Am. J. Clin. Pathol. **53**:565-579, 1970 (parathyroid chief cell hyperplasia).

Bloodworth, J. M. B.: Endocrine pathology, Baltimore, 1968, The Williams and Wilkins Co.

Brewer, D. B.: J. Pathol. Bacteriol. **77**:149-162, 1959 (papillary carcinoma of the thyroid gland).

Browne, F. J.: Lancet **1**:115-119, 1958 (adrenal gland and eclampsia).

Carpenter, C. C. J., et al.: Medicine (Baltimore) **43**:153-180, 1964 (Schmidt's syndrome).

Carpenter, W. B., and Kernohan, J. W.: Cancer **16**:788-797, 1963 (retroperitoneal ganglioneuroma).

Castleman, B., et al.: Cancer **38**:1668-1675, 1976 (primary parathyroid hyperplasia).

Catt, K. J.: Lancet **2**:1383-1389, 1970 (thyroid gland).

Chatten, J.: Am. J. Med. Sci. **248**:715-727, 1964 (thymus in systemic disease).

Cohen, K. L.: Arch. Intern. Med. **138**:575-579, 1978 (pituitary tumors following adrenalectomy).

Cohen, R. A., et al.: Ann. Intern. Med. **61**:1144-1161, 1964 (pineal gland).

Cohen, R. B.: Cancer **19**:552-556, 1966 (adrenal cortical nodules).

Conn, J. W.: J.A.M.A. **183**:775-781, 871-878, 1963 (hyperaldosteronism).

Conn, J. W., et al.: J.A.M.A. **193:**200-206, 1965 (aldosteronism in hypertensive disease).

Conn, J. W., et al.: J.A.M.A. **195:**21-26, 1966 (aldosteronism in hypertensive disease).

Conomy, J. P.: Arch. Intern. Med. **138:**691-692, 1978 (Nelson's syndrome).

Cope, O.: N. Engl. J. Med. **274:**1174-1182, 1966 (hyperparathyroidism).

Cope, O., et al.: Ann. Surg. **148:**375-388, 1958 (primary chief cell hyperplasia of parathyroid glands).

Craven, D. E., et al.: Arch. Intern. Med. **129:**567-569, 1972 (familial multiple adenomatosis).

Currie, A. R., Symington, T., and Grant, J. K., editors: The human adrenal cortex, London, 1962, E. & S. Livingstone, Ltd.

Datta, S. K., and Schwartz, R. S.: N. Engl. J. Med. **291:**1304-1305, 1974 (infectious [?] myasthenia).

Daughaday, W. H.: N. Engl. J. Med. **298:**783-794, 1978 (Cushing's disease and basophilic microadenomas).

Delta, B. G., et al.: J.A.M.A. **194:**507-511, 1965 (thymus and agammaglobulinemia).

Drachman, D. B.: N. Engl. J. Med. **298:**136-142, 186-193, 1978 (myasthenia gravis).

Eylan, E., and Zmucky, R.: Lancet **1:**1062-1063, 1957 (thyroiditis and mumps virus).

Forcier, R. J.: Arch. Intern. Med. **129:**638-641, 1972 (autoimmunity and multiple endocrine abnormalities).

Fox, F., et al.: Cancer **12:**108-116, 1959 (maturation of neuroblastoma to ganglioneuroma).

Gaillard, P. J., Talmage, R. V., and Budy, A. M., editors: The parathyroid glands, Chicago, 1965, University of Chicago Press.

Garry, R., and Hall, R.: Lancet **1:**693-695, 1970 (mitosis in thyroid gland and LATS).

Giarman, N. J., et al.: Fed. Proc. **18:**394, 1959 (neurohumoral content of pineal body).

Goldstein, G.: Ann. N.Y. Acad. Sci. **249:**177-185, 1975 (isolation of thymopoietin).

Goldstein, G., and Mackay, I. R.: The human thymus, St. Louis, 1969, Warren H. Green, Inc.

Good, R. A., and Gabrielson, A. E., editors: The thymus in immunobiology, New York, 1964, Harper & Row, Publishers, Inc.

Gordon, P. R., et al.: Cancer **31:**915-924, 1973 (medullary carcinoma of the thyroid gland).

Graze, K., et al.: N. Engl. J. Med. **299:**980-985, 1978 (familial medullary thyroid carcinoma).

Hale, J. F., and Scowen, E. F.: Thymic tumors—their association with myasthenia gravis and their treatment by radiotherapy, London, 1967, Lloyd-Luke (Medical Books) Ltd.

Hazard, J. B.: Am. J. Clin. Pathol. **25:**289-298, 399-426, 1955 (thyroiditis).

Hazard, J. B.: Am. J. Pathol. **88:**213-249, 1977 (thyroid C cells and medullary carcinoma—a review).

Hazard, J. B., et al.: J. Clin. Endocrinol. Metab. **19:**152-161, 1959 (medullary carcinoma of the thyroid gland).

Ibanez, M. L., et al.: Cancer **19:**1039-1052, 1966 (thyroid carcinoma).

Irvine, J.: Hosp. Tribune, June 14, 1971, p. 16 (Addison's disease).

Irvine, W. J., editor: Thyrotoxicosis, Baltimore, 1967, The Williams & Wilkins Co. (Proceedings of an International Symposium, Edinburgh, May 1967).

James, V. H., editor: The adrenal gland, New York, 1979, Raven Press.

Jordan, R. M., et al.: Arch. Intern. Med. **139:**340-342, 1979 (pituitary tumor infarction in Nelson's syndrome).

Kernohan, J. W., and Sayre, G. P.: Tumors of the pituitary gland and infundibulum. In Atlas of tumor pathology, Sect. 10, Fasc. 36, Washington, D.C., 1956, Armed Forces Institute of Pathology.

Keynes, W. M., and Till, A. S.: Q. J. Med. **40:**443-456, 1971 (medullary carcinoma of the thyroid gland).

Kitay, J. I., and Altschule, M. D.: The pineal gland, Cambridge, Mass., 1954, Harvard University Press.

Kleinfeld, G.: Cancer **12:**902-911, 1959 (functioning tumors of parathyroid glands).

Klinck, G. H., and Winship, T.: Cancer **8:**701-706, 1955 (occult sclerosing carcinoma of the thyroid gland).

Kovacs, K., et al.: In Sommers, S. C., and Rosen, P. P., editors: Pathology annual, part 2, vol. 12, New York, 1977, Appleton-Century-Crofts, pp. 341-382 (pituitary adenoma—new classification).

Laragh, J. H.: N. Engl. J. Med. **289:**745-746, 1973 (control of aldosterone secretion).

Laragh, J. H., et al.: Circ. Res. **18**(Suppl. I):158-174, 1966 (aldosterone in hypertension).

Lathem, J. E., and Hunt, L. D.: J.A.M.A. **197:**558-590, 1966 (pheochromocytoma of urinary bladder).

Levine, G. P., and Rosai, J.: Hum. Pathol. **9:**495-515, 1978 (thymic hyperplasia and neoplasia).

Lindsay, S., and Chaikoff, I. L.: Cancer Res. **24:**1099-1107, 1964 (effects of radiation on the thyroid gland).

Lindstrom, J.: Fed. Proc. **37:**2828-2831, 1978 (autoimmune response, acetylcholine receptors, and myasthenia gravis).

Lischner, H. W., and DeGeorge, A. M.: Lancet **2:**1044-1049, 1969 (role of the thymus in humoral immunity).

McDermott, F. T., and Hart, J. A. L.: Br. J. Surg. **57:**657-661, 1970 (medullary carcinoma of the thyroid gland with hypocalcemia).

McGowan, G. K., and Sandlor, M., editors: J. Clin. Pathol. **20**(Suppl. 1):309-414, 1967 (symposium on the thyroid gland).

Meachim, G., and Young, M. H.: J. Clin. Pathol. **16:**189-199, 1963 (granulomatous thyroiditis).

Meissner, W. A., and Warren, S.: Tumors of the thyroid gland. In Atlas of tumor pathology, Fasc. 4, Series 2, Washington, D.C., 1969, Armed Forces Institute of Pathology.

Meyer, P. C.: Br. J. Cancer **16:**16-26, 1962 (nodular goiter and carcinoma of the thyroid gland).

Moon, H. D., editor: The adrenal cortex, New York, 1961, Harper & Row, Publishers, Inc.

Nichols, J., and Delp, M.: J.A.M.A. **185:**643-646, 1963 (craniopharyngeal pituitary gland).

Pearse, A. G. E.: In Friesen, S. R., editor: Surgical endocrinology; clinical syndromes, Philadelphia, 1978, J. B. Lippincott Co., pp. 18-34 (APUD concept).

Purves, H. D.: In Harris, G. W., and Donovan, B. T., editors: The pituitary gland, vol. 1, London, 1966, Butterworth & Co. (Publishers) Ltd., p. 147 (cytology of adenohypophysis).

Roediger, W. E. W.: Cancer **36:**1758-1770, 1975 (cells of the thyroid gland).

Rosai, J., and Levine, G. D.: Tumors of the thymus. In Atlas of tumor pathology, Fasc. 13, Series 2, Washington, D.C., 1976, Armed Forces Institute of Pathology.

Rose, E., and Royster, H. P.: J.A.M.A. **176:**224-226, 1961 (Riedel's struma).

Roth, S. I.: Am. J. Pathol. **61:**233-248, 1970 (water-clear cell hyperplasia of parathyroid glands).

Roth, S. I., and Capen, C. C.: Int. Rev. Exp. Pathol. **13:**161-221, 1974 (parathyroid gland—EM and functional correlations).

Russell, W. O., et al.: Cancer **16:**1425-1460, 1963 (thyroid carcinoma).

Schantz, A., and Castleman, B.: Cancer **31:**600-605, 1973 (parathyroid carcinoma).

Schimke, R. N., and Hartmann, W. H.: Ann. Intern. Med. **63:**1027-1039, 1965 (familial pheochromocytoma).

Sclare, G.: J. Pathol. Bacteriol. **85:**263-278, 1963 (thyroid gland in myxedema).

Sheehan, H. L.: Q. J. Med. **8:**277-309, 1939 (postpartum necrosis of the pituitary gland).

Sheehan, H. L.: Am. J. Obstet. Gynecol. **68:**202-223, 1954 (postpartum necrosis of the pituitary gland).

Sherwin, R. P.: Cancer **12:**861-877, 1959 (pheochromocytoma).

Stowens, D.: Arch. Pathol. **63:**451-459, 1957 (neuroblastoma).

Symington, T.: Functional pathology of the human adrenal gland, Baltimore, 1969, The Williams & Wilkins Co.

Thomison, J. B., and Shapiro, J. L.: Arch. Pathol. **63:**527-531, 1958 (adrenal lesions in meningococcemia).

Tischler, A. S., et al.: N. Engl. J. Med. **296:**919-925, 1977 (neuroendocrine neoplasms).

Tyrrell, J. B.: N. Engl. J. Med. **298:**753-758, 1978 (pituitary microadenomas in Cushing's disease).

Volpe, R.: N. Engl. J. Med. **287:**463-464, 1972 (immunologic basis of Graves' disease).

Warren, S., and Meissner, W. A.: Tumors of the thyroid gland. In Atlas of tumor pathology, Sect. 4, Washington, D.C., 1953, Armed Forces Institute of Pathology.

Werner, S. C., et al.: N. Engl. J. Med. **287:**421-425, 1972 (immunoglobulins and complement in Graves' disease).

Whitehead, R.: J. Pathol. Bacteriol. **86:**55-67, 1963 (hypothalamus in hypopituitarism).

Williams, C. M., and Greer, M.: J.A.M.A. **183:**836-840, 1963 (neuroblastoma).

Williams, E. D.: In Symmers, W. S. C., editor: Systemie pathology, ed. 2, vol. 4, London, 1978, Churchill Livingstone, pp. 2040-2066 (parathyroid glands).

Williams, E. D., et al.: J. Clin. Pathol. **19:**103-113, 1966 (medullary carcinoma of thyroid gland).

Wilton, A., et al.: J. Pathol. Bacteriol. **67:**65-68, 1954 (Crooke's change).

Wolman, L.: J. Pathol. Bacteriol. **72:**575-586, 1956 (pituitary necrosis).

Wolman, L.: J. Pathol. Bacteriol. **77:**283-296, 1959 (infundibuloma).

Wolstenholme, G. E. W., and Porter, R., editors: The thymus; experimental and clinical studies, Boston, 1966, Little, Brown & Co.

22

Female genitalia

The important pathologic conditions of the female genitalia are inflammations, endocrine disturbances, tumors, and cysts. Many gynecologic diseases are closely related in both functional and morphologic aspects to hormonal imbalance. The endocrine factors important in gynecologic pathology are the pituitary gonadotropic hormones and the ovarian and placental hormones.

HORMONAL RELATIONSHIPS

Pituitary gonadotropic hormones. The two pituitary gonadotropic hormones that act on the ovaries are the follicle-stimulating hormone (FSH) and the luteinizing hormone (LH). FSH stimulates growth of the ovarian follicle, but full development of the follicle, ovulation, and secretion of estrogen are dependent on the addition of LH. Estrogen enhances the effect of FSH and LH in regard to the follicle growth and also plays a role later in maintenance of the corpus luteum. LH is required for luteinization of the follicle and thus formation of the corpus luteum, from which both estrogen and progesterone are secreted.

In animals, luteotropic hormone (LTH) is necessary for maintenance of the corpus luteum and its progesterone secretion, but this role in man is uncertain.

Ovarian hormones. The two ovarian hormones that normally are controlled by the pituitary gland are of known chemical nature and structure, and they exert pronounced effects on the endometrium, vagina, and other tissues. Menstrual changes and periodicity are dependent on these hormones.

Maturing ovarian follicles produce estrogen. This hormone has been isolated in a number of closely related forms, all characterized by the ability to produce estrus (heat) in castrated animals. The names given to these estrogens are estradiol, estrone, and estriol. Certain estrogenic substances can be derived synthetically (e.g., stilbestrol). The basic chemical structure of estrogens is the phenanthrene ring system. Thus, there is a chemical structural resemblance to certain naturally occurring sterols and to some potent carcinogenic materials, a relationship that has caused much interesting speculation.

Estrogen, formed by the mature ovarian follicle, is a sexual growth-stimulating substance that acts especially on the uterus and vagina. It brings about the proliferative endometrial growth characteristic of the first half of the menstrual cycle (p. 642). In addition, it controls the rhythmic activity of the uterine musculature and causes cornification of the vaginal epithelium and growth of the duct system of the breast. At puberty, estrogen is responsible for the appearance of the various secondary sexual characteristics.

The ovarian follicle ruptures at about the middle of the menstrual cycle and then forms the corpus luteum. This luteinized follicle produces not only estrogen but also a new and characteristic hormone called progesterone.

This latter substance also is a sterol, of known chemical formula, and has been isolated, crystallized, and synthesized. It has a close structural relationship to the male sex hormone testosterone.

Progesterone also affects the endometrium, vagina, and breast. In the endometrium, it brings about a secretory phase (p. 642). The endometrium remains hypertrophied, but the glands become very irregular in outline and secretory in function. The stromal cells of the endometrium begin a decidualike change. The endometrial changes occur in preparation for the receipt of a fertilized ovum. If conception does not occur, the corpus luteum atrophies, the endometrium breaks down, and menstruation occurs. However, if pregnancy occurs, the corpus luteum continues to develop and produces progesterone, its effects being important in the maintenance of the pregnancy in its early phases.

In addition to its effect on the endometrium, progesterone inhibits contractility of the uterus, suppresses ovulation and menstruation, and causes a mucus-secreting phase in vaginal epithelium and a lobular proliferation of the breast.

Hormones of pregnancy. During pregnancy, human chorionic gonadotropin (HCG) is produced and is found in the urine. The biologic pregnancy tests (Aschheim-Zondek; Friedman) are based on the demonstration of this hormone in the urine. This substance is anterior pituitary–like (APL) in its action. Another placental gonadotropin has been discovered, known as human placental lactogen (HPL). Although HPL is luteotropic in the rat, it is not certain yet whether it maintains corpora lutea in man. The placenta also seems capable of producing progesterone, an action important in the maintenance of later stages of pregnancy.

Ovaries

DEVELOPMENT AND STRUCTURE

The ovaries, as well as the testes, first appear as *genital ridges* (thickenings of celomic epithelium and underlying mesenchyme) on the medial side of the mesonephros. Soon, primordial cells migrate from the yolk sac into the genital ridges. In this indifferent stage, it is not possible to make a distinction between the ovaries and the testes. Enormous numbers of primitive follicles develop as the ovary differentiates. The cortex of the ovary is composed of these primitive graafian follicles and a dense connective tissue stroma. The so-called epithelial cells of the follicles (i.e., granulosa cells) and the stromal cells (including theca cells, which are specialized stromal cells around follicles) have a common mesenchymal origin. Their close relationship is evident in certain tumors (e.g., granulosa–theca cell tumors). The primordial follicles consist of a central ovum surrounded by a layer of low cuboidal epithelium, the granulosal membrane. As the follicle matures and enlarges under the influence of the pituitary hormones, the granulosa becomes more cuboidal and several layers thick. A central cavity appears, the ovum being at one pole surrounded by a mass of granulosa cells, the discus proligerus. Around the follicle is a specialized layer of connective tissue cells, the theca interna. *Call-Exner bodies* are small, rounded, clear, glandlike areas found in the granulosa layer, and similar structures appear in tumors composed of granulosa cells. About the middle of the menstrual cycle, the follicle ruptures and the ovum is extruded. The ruptured follicle develops into a *corpus luteum* under the influence of LH of the pituitary gland.

At the time the follicle ruptures, many other follicles are approaching maturity. Their further development is stopped after ovulation of the one follicle, and they undergo regression. These atretic follicles form cysts that, in some cases, reach considerable size. Usually, the cystic stage is promptly followed by fibrosis, forming a small hyalinized area, the *corpus fibrosum*.

In the development of the corpus luteum after follicular rupture, the granulosa is vascularized, and the cells become large and polyhedral with abundant vacuolated cytoplasm. They are then called lutein cells and form a bright yellow zone. Hemorrhage into the follicular lumen usually occurs, and in some cases this is abundant. The mature corpus luteum is much larger than the follicle, measuring up to 10 or 15 mm in diameter.

If fertilization does not occur, regression of the corpus luteum begins shortly before menstruation. Fatty change of the lutein cells is followed by atrophy, fibrosis, and hyalinization. This results in a convoluted hyalinized mass, the *corpus albicans,* which slowly regresses further and disappears. Occasionally, the corpus luteum fails to regress but develops into a cyst *(corpus luteum cyst).* Also, if pregnancy occurs, the corpus luteum does not regress but becomes even larger and more prominent.

INFLAMMATION (OOPHORITIS)

Inflammation of the ovary is secondary to inflammation elsewhere, most commonly spreading from the tube. Oophoritis secondary to tubal infection is usually caused by the gonococcus, streptococcus, or *Bacteroides* species. Acute and chronic abscesses may occur. An abscess often involves a corpus luteum, the organisms apparently gaining entrance to the ovary through a ruptured follicle. Oophoritis is followed by fibrosis and adhesions to surrounding structures. Occasionally, there is hematogenous infection of the ovary, as in mumps. Inflammatory reactions in the ovary are similar to those elsewhere.

Tuberculous oophoritis is almost always secondary to tubal tuberculosis. Tuberculous peritonitis is usually present as well. The microscopic picture is the same as in tuberculosis elsewhere in the body.

CYSTS

Cysts of the ovary are of two main groups: nonneoplastic cysts and neoplastic cysts (i.e., cystic tumors). The latter will be considered with other ovarian tumors. Several types of cysts are noted in Fig. 22-1.

Ovarian cysts sometimes rupture and cause intraperitoneal hemorrhage. The clinical aspects depend on the amount of intraperitoneal hemorrhage, which, in rare cases, may be quite massive. Clinical differentiation of such cases from other acute abdominal conditions may be difficult. Nonneoplastic cysts are of four main types: follicular, luteal, theca-lutein, and endometrial.

Follicular cyst. A follicular cyst is caused by the distention of an unruptured, graafian follicle. It is extremely common and usually remains small but occasionally reaches several centimeters in diameter. Lining granulosa cells are evident in the smaller cysts, but the larger cysts may be lined by a single layer of low cuboidal epithelium. Hemorrhage into the cyst occasionally occurs.

Luteal cyst. A luteal cyst is the result of dilatation of a corpus luteum. It occurs less frequently than the follicular type and must be distinguished from the normal corpus luteum hematoma, the large corpus luteum of pregnancy, and the hemorrhagic cysts of endometriosis. Luteal cysts are recognized microscopically by remnants of granulosa-lutein cells found in the wall.

Theca-lutein cyst. Theca-lutein cysts are found in the ovaries in association with choriocarcinoma and hydatidiform mole (p. 654). These cysts are multiple and bilateral and are lined by theca-lutein cells, i.e., the lutein cells lining the cyst are believed to arise from the theca interna rather than the granulosa.

Endometrial cyst. Endometrial cysts, or chocolate cysts of the ovary, are caused by endometriosis. They may reach a size of several centimeters, are often bilateral, and may be associated with endometriosis elsewhere (p. 646). Hemorrhage into the cyst cavity results in a thick chocolatelike content. This is not a distinctive feature, however, for a similar content may be found in hemorrhagic cysts of other types. Identification is by finding endometrial glands in some part of the cyst wall. Beneath the lining, there is often a layer of swollen mononuclear phagocytic cells that contain blood pigment and are easily confused with luteal cells.

Stein-Leventhal syndrome. Multiple bilateral cystic follicles with hyperplasia of the theca interna cells may be associated with the Stein-Leventhal syndrome (Fig. 22-2). This is

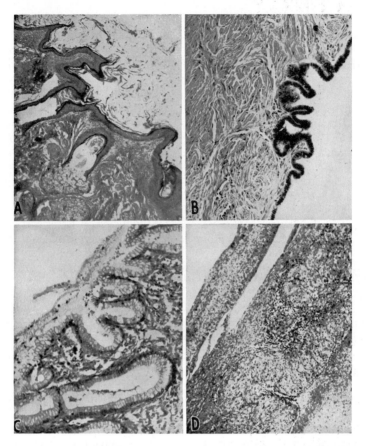

Fig. 22-1. Ovarian cysts showing characteristic linings. **A,** Dermoid cyst, with keratinizing squamous epithelium and sebaceous glands. **B,** Serous cystadenoma, lined by dark-staining cuboidal cells. **C,** Mucinous cystadenoma, lined by pale columnar cells with basal nuclei. **D,** Corpus luteum cyst, lined by thick layer of large luteal cells. (From Berman, J. K.: Synopsis of the principles of surgery, St. Louis, 1940, The C. V. Mosby Co.)

a clinical syndrome characterized by sterility, hirsutism, and menstrual irregularities that may progress to oligomenorrhea or amenorrhea. The ovaries have thickening of the tunica albuginea in addition to the cysts. Although androgenic activity is evident, various hormonal patterns are found. However, the normal cyclical fluctuations of hormonal levels are lacking. Endometrial hyperplasia may be present, and endometrial carcinoma occurs with increased frequency in association with this syndrome.

Hyperthecosis (thecomatosis), a condition characterized by nests of lipid-containing lutein cells in the ovarian stroma, which is often hyperplastic and dense, may clinically resemble the polycystic (Stein-Leventhal) syndrome. Usually, however, in addition to hirsutism, women with hyperthecosis often develop overt virilism and, in some instances, also hypertension, obesity, and a disturbance in glucose tolerance.

TUMORS

Various classifications of ovarian tumors have been proposed. The tumors may be clas-

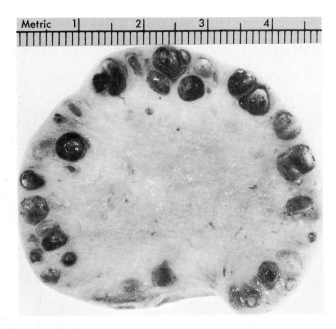

Fig. 22-2. Polycystic ovary in Stein-Leventhal syndrome.

sified as to whether they are cystic or solid, benign or malignant, or functioning (endocrine-producing) or nonfunctioning. The following classification is based on the origin and histopathologic features of the tumors. It should be noted that the origin of certain tumors (e.g., Brenner tumor, mesonephroid or clear cell tumor, and lipoid cell tumor) is debatable.

1 Tumors of surface epithelial origin
  a Serous cystomas
    (1) Serous benign cystadenoma
    (2) Serous cystadenoma of low potential malignancy*
    (3) Serous cystadenocarcinoma
  b Mucinous cystomas
    (1) Mucinous benign cystadenoma
    (2) Mucinous cystadenoma of low potential malignancy*
    (3) Mucinous cystadenocarcinoma
  c Endometrioid tumors
    (1) Endometrioid benign tumor
    (2) Endometrioid tumor of low potential malignancy*
    (3) Endometrioid carcinoma
  d Cystadenofibroma—benign and malignant
  e Clear cell (mesonephroid) tumors
    (1) Benign
    (2) Of low potential malignancy*
    (3) Malignant
  f Brenner tumors
    (1) Benign
    (2) Intermediate proliferative type
    (3) Malignant
2 Germ cell tumors
  a Dysgerminoma
  b Cystic teratoma (dermoid cyst)
  c Solid teratoma
    (1) Well-differentiated (adult) teratoma
    (2) Immature (embryonal) teratoma
  d Embryonal carcinoma
  e Endodermal sinus tumor
  f Choriocarcinoma
3 Sex cord stromal tumors
  a Granulosa-theca cell tumors

---

*These are epithelial tumors with proliferating activity of epithelial cells and nuclear abnormalities but with no infiltrative, destructive growth; also called ''borderline'' lesions.

---

*These are epithelial tumors with proliferating activity of epithelial cells and nuclear abnormalities but with no infiltrative, destructive growth; also called ''borderline'' lesions.

b Arrhenoblastoma (androblastoma; Sertoli-Leydig cell tumor)
  c Gynandroblastoma
4 Lipoid cell tumors
5 Collagen-producing stromal tumors
  a Fibroma
  b Fibrosarcoma
  c Sclerosing stromal tumor
6 Primary carcinoma—undifferentiated; unclassified
7 Metastatic tumors—various types including Krukenberg tumor

As with other malignant tumors within the female pelvis, a clinical stage classification of ovarian cancers is helpful in evaluating the prognosis, i.e., a four-stage classification (stages I through IV) based on the extent of the disease.

Most of the ovarian tumors are of the cystic variety. For example, the combined incidence of serous and mucinous cystomas (benign and malignant) is more than 50% of all ovarian neoplasms, the cystic teratoma (dermoid cyst) varies from 15% to 25% of ovarian tumors, and a number of other neoplasms are also cystic. The less common solid tumors are of wide variety, some forms being quite rare. Tumors with endocrine function usually are found among the solid tumors. Endocrine syndromes may be produced by ovarian neoplasms as well as by certain nonneoplastic lesions.

Tumors of surface epithelial origin

These tumors consist of one or more types of epithelium and stroma of variable degree and originate from the surface epithelium (celomic mesothelium) that covers the ovary.

Serous tumor. The serous tumors are characteristically cystic (cystomas) and constitute about 30% of ovarian tumors. In 30% to 50% of cases, the tumors are bilateral, particularly the borderline and malignant types.

Serous cystadenomas may be unilocular or multilocular and sometimes reach enormous size. The cyst cavity contains a clear fluid with a rich content of serum proteins. There may be a smooth lining of epithelial cells (simple type), but frequently there are papillary projections into the cavities. This papillary growth may be so great that the tumor in some of the loculi appears almost solid. The lining cells of the cyst are cuboidal or columnar epithelium and sometimes are ciliated. Calcium deposits are common in the papillary masses. The papillary tendency, sometimes with extension through the capsule so as to form papillary excrescences on the serosal surface, is more characteristic of the lesions of low potential malignancy (''borderline'') and of the serous cystadenocarcinomas. However, small surface excrescences may occur occasionally in the benign cystomas.

Serous cystadenocarcinoma is the most common type of ovarian cancer (Fig. 22-3). It usually is characterized by a papillary architecture, often with a surface papillary component. Some of these tumors have a tubal type of epithelium, often showing cilia, are sometimes termed endosalpingomas, and have a low degree of malignancy. Others have a greater degree of anaplasia and are often seen only in later stages of disease when extension has occurred and operability is poor, and so the prognosis is poor. Psammoma bodies may be present.

Mucinous tumor. Mucinous cystomas generally occur less frequently than the serous type, forming about 20% of ovarian tumors. These cystomas are usually unilateral, being bilateral in only 5% to 15% of cases. Most of the bilateral tumors are malignant.

Mucinous cystadenomas contain a mucoid material. They are thin walled and multilocular and have a smooth lining usually without papillary growth. The cysts are lined by a single layer of tall columnar epithelial cells with basal nuclei and a clear secretory cytoplasm resembling those in the endocervical mucosa. Intracystic papillary processes may be present, but less commonly than in serous cystadenomas. They are usually regarded as evidence of potential malignancy. Papillary projections occur more frequently in the malignant tumors *(mucinous cystadenocarcinomas)*. Mucinous cystadenomas do not become malignant as commonly as do the serous cystadenomas, but occasionally a proliferative adenocarcinomatous change occurs. Mucinous cystadenocarcinomas make up about 5% of ovarian cancers.

Rupture of a mucinous cystoma, usually the

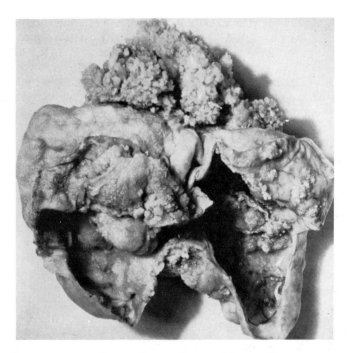

Fig. 22-3. Papillary serous cystadenocarcinoma of ovary. Note papillary masses growing on external surface of cyst.

malignant form, implants the secretory epithelium over the peritoneal cavity. Continued secretory function of the implants causes an accumulation of large quantities of gelatinous material in the abdomen, a condition called *(pseudo) myxoma peritonei*. It may be difficult to find the epithelial elements on biopsy of the peritoneal tissue.

Some investigators have suggested that the mucinous tumors are of germ cell origin (teratomatous), since in occasional instances a nodule of dermoid cyst may be found in the wall of a mucinous cyst and in some cases the lining epithelium contains cells resembling the "goblet cells" of intestinal epithelium or argentaffin cells. Occasionally, a nodule of Brenner tumor may appear in the cyst wall.

Endometrioid tumor. Endometrioid tumors are characterized by the presence of tubular glands resembling benign or malignant glands of the uterine endometrium. The benign and potentially malignant ("borderline") forms are not common. Most of the lesions are malignant, constituting 15% to 20% of ovarian cancers. These are *adenocarcinomas* and are often confused with serous or mucinous adenocarcinomas. Squamous differentiation of the neoplastic cells is common, and, when present, the lesion may be designated *adenoacanthoma*. Often an endometrioid carcinoma of the ovary is associated with a carcinoma of the endometrium in the same patient. Usually, they are both primary tumors, although it sometimes may be difficult to exclude metastasis from one site to the other.

An endometrioid tumor of the ovary may be cystic or solid. The cysts have a relatively smooth lining, but their lining may be papillary, and they contain a chocolate-colored fluid. It is to be noted that endometriosis involving the ovary also may consist of a cyst containing similar fluid; however, this lesion lacks features of a neoplasm. It is discussed with the other nonneoplastic cysts of the ovary (p. 623).

Cystadenofibroma. Cystadenofibroma is a benign variant of a cystadenoma, consisting of abundant fibrous stroma with tubular structures and small cysts. Grossly, it may resemble a fibroma. The epithelial component usually resembles that of a serous cystadenoma, although it may be mucinous or endometrioid in appearance. Malignant change in a cystadenofibroma is uncommon.

Clear cell (mesonephroid) tumor. The tumors of this group are composed of clear cells and/or hobnail-shaped cells arranged in tubules, cysts, and solid masses in a dense fibrous stroma. The clear cells contain glycogen and resemble those of a clear cell (hypernephroid) carcinoma of the kidney. The tumors may be benign or of low potential malignancy ("borderline") but usually are malignant. The clear cell carcinomas constitute about 5% of the ovarian cancers. Grossly, they may appear solid or microcystic or may occasionally have larger cysts containing hemorrhagic (chocolate-colored) fluid with polypoid masses protruding into the cavity. They are bilateral in about 10% of cases.

It is commonly held that the clear cell tumor arises from the pluripotential surface epithelium of the ovary. Some of the clear cell carcinomas include a mixture of elements resembling other ovarian tumors arising from the surface epithelium, e.g., endometrioid, serous, or mucinous carcinoma. The term "mesonephroid" for this group of tumors has been used because they bear a certain resemblance to an ovarian tumor described by Schiller that he considered to originate from mesonephric elements or remnants. According to Teilum, the tumor originally described by Schiller as a "mesonephroma ovarii" may be a variant of a germ cell tumor, one that recapitulates stages in the phylogenetic development of extraembryonic structures, such as the allantois and yolk sac (i.e., endodermal sinus tumor).

Brenner tumor. Brenner tumors are uncommon benign tumors usually found after the age of 50 years and are almost always unilateral. As a rule, they are without hormonal function, but a few have been accompanied by hyperestrinism similar to that of granulosa cell tumors. They are small, firm, circumscribed tumors that occur alone or in the wall of a mucinous cystadenoma. Grossly, they resemble a fibroma. Microscopically, they are characterized by islands or strands of epithelial cells of transitional or uroepithelial type set in a dense fibrous stroma (Fig. 22-4). Frequently, the nuclei of the epithelial cells have a characteristic longitudinal grooving or folding. Similar infolding may be evident in the nuclei of Walthard's cell islets, giving them an appearance reminiscent of puffed wheat. Some of the epithelial islets may have cystic centers, which are sometimes lined by columnar mucus-producing cells.

The origin of Brenner tumors is debatable. Various theories have suggested that they arise from the undifferentiated cells in Walthard's islets, from displaced urogenital epithelium similar to that of the renal pelvis or ureter, or from follicular granulosa cells or that they are of teratomatous origin. The prevalent view is that they originate from the pluripotential surface epithelium of the ovary by a process of metaplasia.

Walthard's islets occur most frequently on the posterior aspect of the lateral portion of the fallopian tube, less frequently in the mesosalpinx, and still less commonly in the ovary. These small nests of cells are regarded as focal areas of metaplasia of the celomic epithelium (pelvic peritoneum) and, by central degeneration, may form small cysts. Similar nests are sometimes found in the serosa near the appendix, and they have been described in men in the epididymis, testis, and spermatic cord. There has been an occasional report of a Brenner or Brenner-like tumor in the testis.

Rare malignant Brenner tumors are described. An intermediate proliferative variety has been reported also that appears to have a favorable prognosis in contrast to the frankly malignant type.

Germ cell tumors

In this category are tumors of undifferentiated types, those with predominantly extraembryonic structures, and others with mature or immature structures derived from any or all of the three embryonic layers.

Dysgerminoma. Dysgerminoma (seminoma) is believed to arise from the primordial

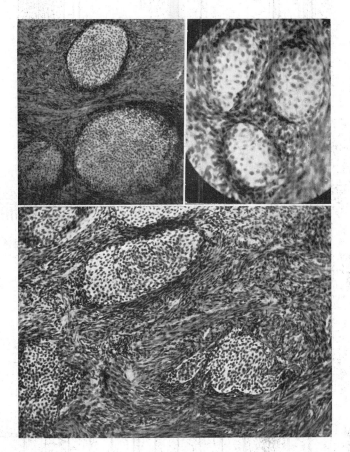

Fig. 22-4. Brenner tumor of ovary. Small islands of tumor cells are present in fibrous stroma.

germ cells of the sexually indifferent embryonic gonad. An entirely similar tumor (seminoma) occurs in the testis. It has no hormonal effects, but it often is associated with congenital hypoplasia of the internal genitalia or with pseudohermaphroditism. Such associated changes are not caused by the tumor and remain after its removal. Occasionally, a positive Aschheim-Zondek test has been reported, but this was due to a coexistent choriocarcinoma or an associated pregnancy.

Most dysgerminomas occur before the age of 35 years and sometimes are found during childhood. The degree of malignancy is variable. They form fairly large encapsulated or nodular tumors of rubbery consistency, grayish pink color, and friable cut surface. About 15% are bilateral.

Microscopically, they are composed of cords and nests of cells with round hyperchromatic nuclei and a small amount of indistinct pale cytoplasm (Fig. 22-5). The cell cords are separated by loose fibrous trabeculae infiltrated with lymphocytes. Giant cells of the Langhans' type may be present. Mitoses are often numerous. Occasional cases may be combined with choriocarcinoma or teratomatous tissues.

Dermoid cyst. Cystic teratomas constitute about 15% to 25% of ovarian tumors. They are rounded masses of any size up to that of a grapefruit, with an opaque grayish wall. The

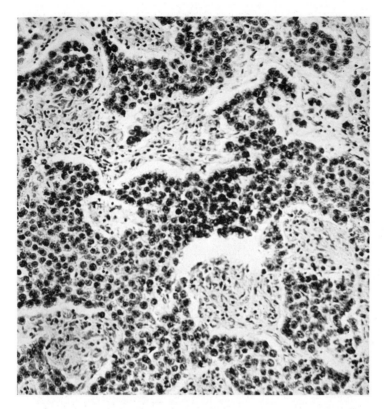

Fig. 22-5. Dysgerminoma of ovary. Note rounded hyperchromatic nuclei, scanty and indistinct cytoplasm, and lymphocytes infiltrating stroma.

cyst content is a greasy, grayish yellow sebaceous material mixed with a variable amount of hair (Fig. 22-6). The cyst lining tends to be rough or granular, and at one point is a small raised or thickened area from which the hair arises. Section through this dermoid tubercle shows skin tissue and appendages, which give rise to the cyst contents. In addition to squamous epithelium, sebaceous glands, and hair follicles, a variety of other tissues may be found, such as cartilage, bone, teeth (Fig. 22-7), thyroid tissue, respiratory tract epithelium, and intestinal tissue. Occasionally, the tumor consists almost completely of thyroid tissue *(struma ovarii)*, and in a few instances it may be functional, producing hyperthyroidism. Also, a *carcinoid* tumor may rarely arise in a dermoid cyst.

Dermoid cysts of the ovary are benign tumors, but in about 2% one element may become malignant. This is most frequently the squamous epithelium. Other complications are torsion with hemorrhagic infarction and, infrequently, a granulomatous peritonitis resulting from a leakage of cyst contents. The most popular theory of their origin is that they represent spontaneous growth of a totipotential ovum, i.e., it seems to be an attempt of a germ cell to form a new individual under unfavorable circumstances.

Solid teratoma. Occurring much less frequently than the benign cystic teratoma (dermoid cyst) is the solid teratoma, which usually is malignant. A "benign" form of solid teratoma has been described, consisting of well-differentiated structures derived from all three germ layers, but it is frequently associated with peritoneal implants *(mature or adult*

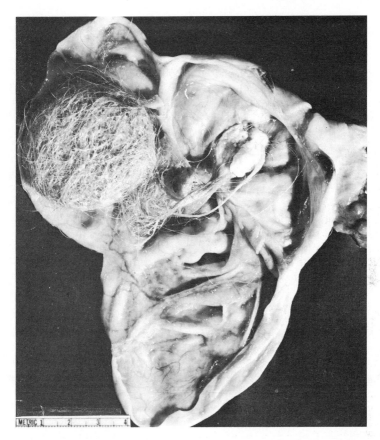

Fig. 22-6. Dermoid cyst of ovary showing hair and dermoid tubercle. (Courtesy Dr. J. F. Kuzma.)

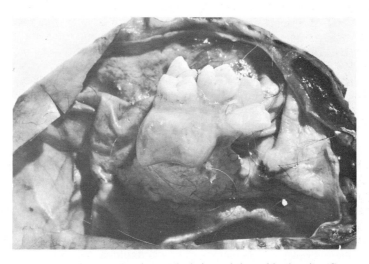

Fig. 22-7. Dermoid cyst of ovary showing teeth, hair, and dermoid tubercle. (Courtesy Dr. J. F. Kuzma.)

teratoma). A solid, malignant teratoma that metastasizes is known to occur in children and young women *(embryonal teratoma).* The various elements of the tumor are usually undifferentiated, often resembling embryonic tissues, but foci of recognizable tissue may be seen (e.g., cartilage, bone, lymphoid tissue, and muscle). Areas suggestive of carcinoma or sarcoma may be present. A teratoma consisting of predominantly undifferentiated carcinoma is often referred to as "teratocarcinoma." Neuroectodermal elements are frequent.

Embryonal carcinoma. Embryonal carcinoma is a rare, highly malignant ovarian tumor of germ cell origin that is analogous to embryonal carcinoma of the adult testis. It is characterized by masses of large primitive pleomorphic cells forming solid sheets or nests, with occasional formation of papillary processes and glandlike clefts. Mitotic figures, frequently atypical, are numerous. Isolated multinuclear giant cells resembling syncytiotrophoblasts are present. Intracellular and extracellular hyaline droplets, similar to those seen in endodermal sinus tumors, may be present focally. Two tumor-associated antigens have been identified in embryonal carcinoma, i.e., human chorionic gonadotropin in the syncytiotrophoblastlike cells and α-fetoprotein in the mononuclear embryonal cells. In a recently reported series, the tumors occurred in patients ranging from 4 to 28 years of age. Frequently, signs and symptoms of hormonal stimulation were observed clinically, i.e., precocious puberty, amenorrhea, irregular vaginal bleeding, or mild hirsutism.

Endodermal sinus tumor. The endodermal sinus tumor was so named by Teilum, who presented evidence of its origin from extraembryonic mesoblast and yolk sac endoderm. Occurring in children and young adults, it is more common than embryonal carcinoma of the ovary, and it resembles somewhat infantile embryonal carcinoma of the testis. Histologically, it usually exhibits a reticular pattern, characteristic papillary formations that simulate endodermal sinuses of the rat placenta (Schiller-Duval bodies), and intracellular and extracellular hyaline droplets. α-Fetoprotein

may be identified in the hyaline droplets, cell cytoplasm, and intercellular spaces. A polyvesicular vitelline pattern (multiple spaces resembling yolk sac vesicles) may be seen in some tumors. Unlike embryonal carcinoma of the ovary, endodermal sinus tumors are rarely associated with endocrine manifestations.

Choriocarcinoma. *Primary ovarian choriocarcinoma,* composed of cytotrophoblastic and syncytiotrophoblastic elements, is rare and probably arises from primordial germ cells but also may develop from an ovarian pregnancy. *Metastatic choriocarcinoma* from the uterus is also uncommon but more frequent than the primary ovarian form. Other elements (e.g., teratomatous or dysgerminomatous) may be present in the primary type. Choriocarcinoma usually produces chorionic gonadotropin.

Sex cord stromal tumors

These tumors are believed to originate from the gonadal stroma and constitute most of the endocrine-producing tumors, which are either estrogenic or androgenic in their effects. The most common endocrine tumors of the ovary are those that produce excess female sex hormones (estrogen). There are two such tumors, the granulosa cell and the theca cell types. Other ovarian endocrine tumors produce masculinizing hormones. These latter tumors include the arrhenoblastoma and lipoid cell tumor.

It should be noted that occasionally a tumor may show an opposite hormonal effect to what is usually expected based on its histologic appearance. For example, instances of thecoma with masculinizing effects and of arrhenoblastoma with feminizing (estrogenic) effects have been reported.

In addition to the aforementioned neoplasms, a small group of primary and metastatic tumors of the ovary, which usually are not hormonally active, may be associated with the production of estrogens or androgens. Other rare types of ovarian tumors that arise from germ cells (e.g., choriocarcinoma and struma ovarii) may produce hormones other than estrogens and androgens.

Granulosa cell tumor. The granulosa cell

tumor is the most common ovarian endocrine neoplasm and is estimated to make up 5% to 10% of ovarian carcinomas. Occurring at any age, it is characterized by production of excessive estrogenic hormone. In the child, this causes precocious sexual changes, with the development of the breasts and onset of menstruation. These changes of precocious puberty disappear after removal of the tumor. During the reproductive period, the tumor may cause either excessive menstrual bleeding or periods of amenorrhea. After menopause, the hyperestrinism causes resumption of menstrual bleeding. Endometrial hyperplasia is present in these cases as a result of the excessive estrogen. Granulosa cell tumors and thecomas are described as separate tumors here, but often elements of both are present in individual tumors, so that frequently they are considered as *granulosa–theca cell tumors.*

Since many granulosa cell tumors are relatively benign or of very low grade malignancy, complete removal results in cure. Ten percent or more are obviously malignant and form metastases. The origin of these tumors is believed to be either from ovarian mesenchyme, perhaps containing embryonal rests of granulosa cells (progranulosa cells of ovarian mesenchyme), or from persistent granulosa cells of atretic follicles.

Granulosa cell tumors are unilateral circumscribed tumors that have a smooth or slightly nodular surface and are a few millimeters to 30 cm in diameter. The cut surface shows a fleshy, pale yellow or grayish tissue, sometimes with cystic areas. Gross features alone are not characteristic enough for diagnosis.

Histologic structure is widely variable, both in different specimens and in the same tumor. The main types are folliculoid, cylindromatous, and diffuse. In the *folliculoid type,* there is formation of folliclelike structures, sometimes with surrounding stroma (Fig. 22-8). Call-Exner bodies (p. 622) may be seen. The *cylindromatous type* has solid cords and strands of tumor cells separated by a small amount of fibrous stroma (Fig. 22-9). In the *diffuse type,* there may be solid, sarcomalike, patternless masses of tumor cells. Areas of luteinization are not uncommon, and when this

is predominant, the designation "luteoma" has sometimes been used. Lipid-containing fibromatous areas like those that characterize theca cell tumor also may occur, indicating their close relationship.

Adenocarcinoma of the uterus has been observed to be quite frequent in association with granulosa cell and theca cell tumors of the ovary. This suggests hyperestrinism as a possible contributing etiologic factor in endometrial carcinoma.

Theca cell tumor (thecoma). Theca cell tumors often are considered a type of granulosa cell tumor, but they usually present distinctive morphologic features that warrant separate consideration. Rarer than granulosal tumors, these fibromatous neoplasms occur at a later age and are characterized by a content of doubly refractive lipid (cholesterol). Excess production of estrogenic hormone results in irregular uterine bleeding with endometrial hyperplasia. Generally, the thecoma is benign. In rare instances, it is malignant and has the characteristics of a spindle cell sarcoma. There is evidence that the theca cell tumors have their origin in cortical stromal hyperplasia of the ovary.

Grossly, these tumors are unilateral, solid, encapsulated tumors of firm consistency and, in general, quite like the more common ovarian fibroma. The cut surface shows a yellowish fibrous tissue structure. Histologically of fibromatous appearance, they have bundles of broad spindle cells that irregularly interlace. Doubly refractive lipid within tumor cells and in surrounding connective tissue is the diagnostic feature.

Arrhenoblastoma. Arrhenoblastoma (androblastoma; Sertoli-Leydig cell tumor) is an uncommon solid ovarian tumor that, by hormone production, causes loss of feminine characteristics followed by masculinization. It is thought to arise from rests of male-directed cells persisting from early stages of gonadal development. Most of these tumors occur at about 20 to 40 years of age, and about 20% are clinically malignant. Defeminizing changes of amenorrhea, sterility, and atrophy of the breasts are followed by development of the masculine characteristics of hirsutism, deep-

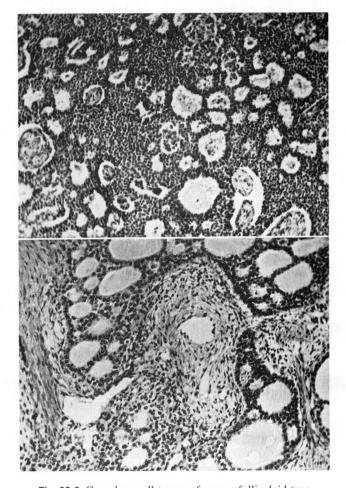

Fig. 22-8. Granulosa cell tumor of ovary, folliculoid type.

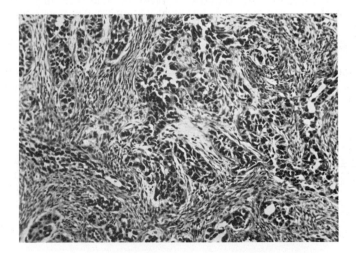

Fig. 22-9. Granulosa cell tumor of ovary, cylindromatous type.

ening of the voice, and enlargement of the clitoris. Clinical differentiation must be from other causes of masculinization, such as adrenal cortical tumors. Arrhenoblastomas vary greatly in their degree of hormonal activity.

Grossly, the tumors are small or of moderate size, gray or yellowish, firm, and unilateral. Microscopically, there is wide variation in appearance, with highly undifferentiated, intermediate, and undifferentiated varieties. The more undifferentiated types have the greatest clinical masculinization. The most differentiated type (testicular tubular adenoma) shows a pronounced tubular arrangement closely imitating the testis. The undifferentiated type consists of sheets and masses of cells having a sarcomatous appearance. In the intermediate grades, there are varying degrees of imperfect attempted tubule formation. An arrangement resembling sex cords and areas having cells similar to the interstitial (Leydig) cells of the testis may be present. Crystalloids of Reinke may be found in the Leydig cells. The tumor usually contains considerable lipid.

Gynandroblastoma. Ovarian tumors have been described that give rise both to masculinization and to evidences of hyperestrinism. The secondary sexual characteristics change in a male direction but with continuation of cycle menstrual bleeding. The microscopic pattern in such cases is not constant but usually presents combinations of the features found in arrhenoblastomas and granulosa cell tumors. It has been suggested that gynandroblastomas are of teratomatous nature.

Lipoid cell tumor

Lipoid cell tumor (hilus cell tumor; Leydig cell tumor; adrenal rest tumor; luteoma) is a rare tumor that produces masculinization with clinical effects similar to those of the arrhenoblastoma. Some patients with this tumor may manifest certain features of Cushing's syndrome. The exact origin and proper terminology of the lipoid tumor are still debated. Origins suggested are (1) from luteal cells, (2) from Leydig cells, (3) from rests of adrenal cortical tissue in the ovary, or (4) that it is a lipid form of arrhenoblastoma.

The lipoid cell tumor is usually benign, unilateral, of small or moderate size, and orange-yellow and has a high fat content. Microscopically, it is composed of large pale cells resembling steroid hormone–producing cells (i.e., lutein, Leydig, and adrenal cortical cells), but the specific identity of these cells is not certain. Some tumor cells contain crystalloids of Reinke in their cytoplasm, similar to Leydig cells. Clinically, malignant behavior of lipoid cell tumors has been observed in some instances.

Collagen-producing stromal tumors

These tumors arise from the ovarian stroma or possibly from the nonspecific connective tissue in the capsule or about blood vessels.

Fibroma. Fibroma is a firm, whitish, usually unilateral, circumscribed tumor that may reach a considerable size. The cut surface is firm and may be homogeneous or trabeculated. Microscopically, it is composed of well-differentiated, regular connective tissue, is of uniform pattern, and shows little evidence of active growth.

Ascites is sometimes associated with ovarian fibroma, particularly when it is prominently edematous, and hydrothorax may be present as well (*Meigs' syndrome*). Both disappear after removal of the tumor. Other solid ovarian tumors (theca cell, granulosa cell, and Brenner tumors) also may have an associated ascites and hydrothorax. The fluid is a transudate, apparently originates in the peritoneal space, and reaches the pleural space by transdiaphragmatic passage.

Fibromas must be distinguished from theca cell tumors, which have an endocrine function. Although similar in many respects to fibromas, theca cell tumors have a more yellowish color grossly, and microscopically they exhibit a high fat content.

Fibrosarcoma. The malignant counterpart of the fibroma (fibrosarcoma) is a rare tumor.

Sclerosing stromal tumor. Another tumor derived from the ovarian stroma, which has collagen as a major component, has been reported recently as a "sclerosing stromal tumor." It has been separated from the fibromas because of certain characteristic clinicopathologic features, among which are the tendency of cellular areas to undergo collagenous sclerosis (not hyalinized plaques as in fibromas and thecomas), prominent vascularity, focal (not diffuse) edema, and occurrence at a much earlier age than the fibromas or thecomas. The tumor appears to be benign and hormonally inactive.

Primary carcinoma (undifferentiated; unclassified)

Certain primary carcinomas are so poorly differentiated that their origin cannot be determined. These tumors tend to be solid and are less common than the cystic types discussed previously. They are frequently bilateral, are variable in size, shape, and consistency, and often have areas of necrosis. Microscopically, malignant epithelial cells may form well-defined glands (adenocarcinoma) but more commonly form solid sheets of cells (medullary form). Spread occurs to the peritoneum, by the lymphatics to lumbar and other lymph nodes, and occasionally by the bloodstream to involve distant organs.

Metastatic tumors

Metastatic tumors of the ovaries may arise from various sites in the body but most frequently from carcinomas of the gastrointestinal tract, the genital tract, and the breast. Leukemia and malignant lymphomas also may spread to the ovaries.

Krukenberg tumor. Krukenberg tumors are a particular type of metastatic ovarian cancer, usually bilateral, in which the tumor cells are mucous producing. The distended cytoplasm and flattened nuclei of individual cells produce a signet-ring appearance. The primary tumor is usually in the stomach (80%), intestinal tract, or gallbladder and often is inconspicuous. The possible modes of spread to the ovaries are by retrograde metastasis along the lymphatics and by peritoneal implantation. In rare instances, a strikingly similar or identical Krukenberg type of tumor has been reported to be primary in the ovary.

Grossly, Krukenberg tumors are firm, solid, lobulated growths of moderate size and have a variegated appearance on the cut surface. Microscopically, there are mucoid epithelial cells having a signet-ring appearance and arranged in solid masses or small clusters (Fig. 22-10). Occasionally there is a tendency to gland formation. The stroma may be abundant and cellular. Since the tumor is usually the result of metastatic spread, the prognosis is often poor.

Endocrine tumors

Throughout the foregoing discussion of ovarian tumors, it was noted that some of them produce hormones. Most of these functioning tumors are of sex cord stromal origin. Less commonly, however, other types of ovarian tumors may produce endocrines, e.g., certain tumors of germ cell origin and, interestingly, a group of tumors that usually are considered to be hormonally inactive.

Functioning sex cord stromal tumors. These tumors, which usually produce feminizing or masculinizing effects or occasionally both, include granulosa–thecal cell tumors, arrhenoblastoma, Leydig cell tumors (lipoid cell tumors), and gynandroblastoma. They are discussed on pp. 632-635.

Tumors with functioning stroma. Certain usually hormonally inactive ovarian tumors occasionally are associated with feminizing effects and, less commonly, virilizing manifestations. The hormone is produced not by the epithelial component but by its stroma. The relatively few such tumors that have been reported include Brenner tumors, cystadenomas, cystadenocarcinomas, cystadenofibromas, and Krukenberg tumors.

Functioning germ cell tumors. Occasionally, a *cystic teratoma* (dermoid cyst) may have prominent thyroid gland component (struma ovarii) or carcinoid component and, in rare instances, may be associated with hyperthyroidism or the carcinoid syndrome, respectively. *Choriocarcinoma* of the ovary usually produces chorionic gonadotropin.

Fallopian tubes

The fallopian tubes have a muscular wall covered on the outer surface by peritoneum and lined by a mucosa that is thrown up into

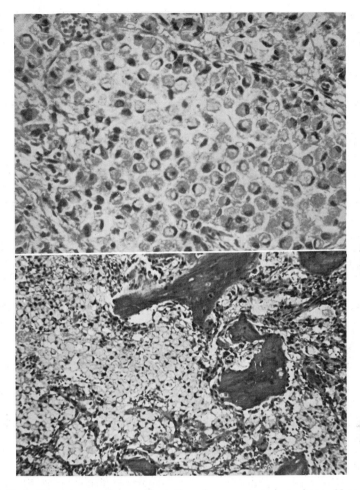

Fig. 22-10. Krukenberg tumor. Lower illustration shows metastasis to bone. Note signet-ring cells.

intricate papillary arborescent folds. Some of the cells lining the mucosa are ciliated, whereas others are nonciliated and appear to have a secretory function. The tubal epithelium undergoes some cyclic changes with the menstrual cycle.

In the mesosalpinx between the fallopian tube and ovary, there are vestigial structures (Fig. 22-11). From some of these structures, cysts may develop that frequently are small but at times are quite large *(parovarian cysts)*.

SALPINGITIS

Inflammation is the most common tubal lesion. Salpingitis may be caused by gonococcal infection or by other bacteria. The latter include streptococci, staphylococci, *Escherichia coli,* and *Bacteroides* species. The gonococcus reaches the tubes from an infection of the cervix and spreads by way of the endometrium. Nongonococcal infection of the tube is commonly the result of postabortal or postpartum spread from an infected uterus.

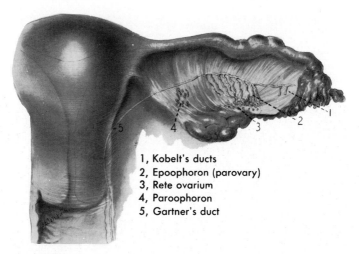

1, Kobelt's ducts
2, Epoophoron (parovary)
3, Rete ovarium
4, Paroophoron
5, Gartner's duct

Fig. 22-11. Vestigial structures of broad ligament. (Redrawn after Schiller, W.: The female genitalia. In Anderson, W. A. D., editor: Pathology, ed. 2, St. Louis, 1953, The C. V. Mosby Co.)

Less than 5% of cases of salpingitis are tuberculous.

Acute salpingitis. In acute salpingitis, the tube is swollen and reddened and has a purulent exudate in the lumen. Microscopically, the mucosal folds are enlarged, edematous, and diffusely infiltrated by neutrophilic leukocytes. Later, this inflammatory exudate also involves the muscularis and serosa of the tube. The fimbriated extremity may become adherent to the ovary, and extension of the infection to the ovary by way of a ruptured follicle produces a tubo-ovarian abscess. With subsidence of the inflammation to a subacute phase, a greater proportion of lymphocytes and plasma cells compose the exudate.

In nongonorrheal acute salpingitis, there is greater enlargement of the tube, and the inflammatory infiltration is proportionately greater in muscular and serosal layers.

Chronic salpingitis. In chronic salpingitis, the thickened mucosal folds are infiltrated by lymphocytes and plasma cells, and the muscularis and serosa may be similarly involved. Adhesions may be present between mucosal folds and, when great, result in a glandlike or follicular pattern (follicular salpingitis) (Fig. 22-12). The lumen often becomes blocked by

adhesions. The purulent exudate may accumulate and greatly distend the blocked tube into a large retort-shaped mass (pyosalpinx). Resorption of the exudate ultimately leaves the cavity filled with a watery fluid (hydrosalpinx) (Fig. 22-13). The mucosal folds may be very atrophic and flattened (hydrosalpinx simplex), or, because of adhesions, the folds may form a number of distended compartments (hydrosalpinx follicularis).

Salpingitis isthmica nodosa. Salpingitis isthmica nodosa may be a form of chronic salpingitis in which the medial portion of the tube is nodular. Microscopically, one sees considerable thickening of the wall, because of increase of muscle, and a number of small irregular lumina lined by mucosal epithelium that probably represent outpocketings of the tubal lumen. These epithelium-lined spaces must be distinguished from endometriosis and from tumor. A noninflammatory and even congenital origin has been suggested by some authors.

Tuberculous salpingitis. Tuberculous salpingitis is secondary to tuberculosis elsewhere, usually in the lungs, but is the primary site of tuberculosis in the female genitalia. From the tube, spread often occurs to the endometrium and peritoneum. The microscopic

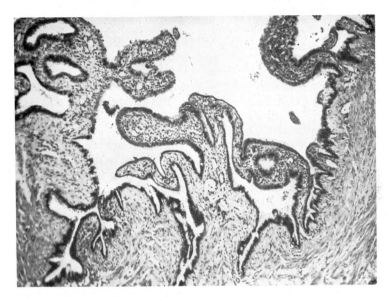

Fig. 22-12. Chronic salpingitis. Adherent mucosal folds give appearance of glandlike follicles. (From Faulkner, R. L., and Douglass, M.: Essentials of obstetrical and gynecological pathology, ed. 2, St. Louis, 1949, The C. V. Mosby Co.)

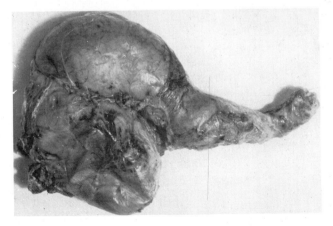

Fig. 22-13. Hydrosalpinx. Note retort-shaped deformity of fallopian tube.

appearance is similar to that of tuberculosis elsewhere in the body, with epithelioid and giant cells and caseation.

TUMORS

Primary carcinoma of the tube is a rare lesion. The tube is greatly enlarged and sausage shaped. Microscopically, it is usually a papillary carcinoma. Metastatic carcinoma of the tube is more frequent than the primary form and is usually from the ovary or uterus.

Rare small benign tumors of distinctive appearance, which have been termed *adenomatoid tumors,* may be found in relationship to the fallopian tube or to the testicular tunic or epididymis in the male. They are composed of large and small acini lined by flattened or cuboidal cells. Their genesis is obscure, and their mesothelial, epithelial, or lymphangiomatous origin is a matter of debate (p. 382 and Fig. 14-41).

TUBAL PREGNANCY

Ectopic pregnancy results when a fertilized ovum becomes implanted in any site other than the endometrium. In most cases, the ectopic site is in a fallopian tube (Fig. 22-14). An important factor causing tubal pregnancy is the effect of chronic salpingitis, which prevents passage of the fertilized ovum into the uterus or delays it until the trophoblast is developed sufficiently for successful implantation. Chorionic villi penetrate the tubal wall. A decidua forms in the endometrium similar to that which would form if the implantation were in the uterus. In addition, atypical changes known as the *Arias-Stella reaction* may be seen in the endometrial glands in some women with ectopic pregnancy. This reaction, consisting of marked cellular atypism and mitotic activity together with pronounced glandular proliferation, may be mistaken for adenocarcinoma. It may also occur in association

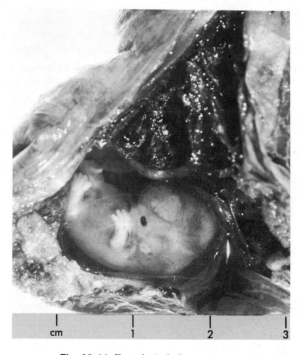

Fig. 22-14. Ectopic (tubal) pregnancy.

with intrauterine pregnancy and trophoblastic disease (hydatiform mole and choriocarcinoma).

In most cases of tubal pregnancy, death of the ovum occurs in a few weeks. Tubal rupture is common. This may be internal bleeding into the tube (hematosalpinx) or external bleeding into the abdominal cavity. In the latter case, bleeding is usually profuse and sometimes fatal. Tubal abortion occurs when the ovum breaks away and is expelled from the tubal orifice. This usually causes hematosalpinx and often profuse bleeding into the abdominal cavity. Tubal pregnancy is the most common cause of hematosalpinx. When the ovum dies, the uterine decidua may be discharged as a thick cast. In rare instances, the abdominal cavity or the ovary may be the site of an ectopic pregnancy.

Uterus

The uterus has a thick muscular wall, the myometrium, and a lining layer, the endometrium, composed of glands set in a connective tissue stroma. The main portion is the corpus, or body of the uterus, and the smaller lower part, the neck or cervix of the uterus, protrudes into the upper part of the vagina. The cervical lining also contains glands, although distinctive from those of the body of the uterus, and surrounds a narrow canal. The portion of cervix that protrudes into the vagina is covered by squamous epithelium.

The uterus undergoes remarkable hypertrophic changes during pregnancy, followed after delivery by normal regressive or involutional changes. One of the serious complications of this process is infection, i.e., a puerperal endometritis and myometritis, which in severe cases may spread widely by the lymphatics and veins.

The endometrium undergoes cyclic changes under the influence of ovarian hormones. These changes are in preparation for implantation of a fertilized ovum and, failing this, culminate in menstruation. Ovarian endocrine imbalance may disturb the endometrial cycles,

so that pathologic hyperplasia or other abnormalities result. Tumors arising from the endometrium are most commonly adenocarcinomas. Endometritis is most often caused by abnormal retention of placental tissue, but tuberculous endometritis not uncommonly follows tuberculous salpingitis. Ectopic endometrial tissue (endometriosis) is quite frequent in various situations in the pelvis. Most commonly, the misplaced islands of endometrium are in the muscular wall of the uterus, the condition here being termed *adenomyosis*.

The chief lesion of the myometrium is a benign tumor of smooth muscle, termed a *leiomyoma*, but because it often has abundant fibrous stroma, it is sometimes referred to as a fibromyoma or fibroid. These tumors are extremely common, particularly among blacks, are often multiple, and reach large sizes. A small proportion undergo sarcomatous change.

Fibrosis uteri is a frequently misused term for a diffuse hypertrophy of the uterus accompanied by abnormal bleeding, usually affecting multiparous women between the ages of 40 and 50 years. The symmetrically enlarged uterus is thick walled, smooth, and freely movable, but fibrosis is often not greater than can be accounted for by physiologic aging. Endocrine imbalance, parity changes with deficient involution, and chronic inflammation are probable causal factors.

ENDOMETRIUM

Pathologic disturbances of the endometrium include abnormalities of the cyclic hormonal changes, inflammation, tumors, and ectopic endometrium (endometriosis).

Cyclic changes. The cyclic changes are controlled by the ovarian hormones of the maturing follicle (estrogen) and the corpus luteum (progesterone). The estrogenic effect is essentially to stimulate proliferation of endometrial glands. Progesterone promotes a secretory activity of the glands and a decidualike change in the stromal cells. If pregnancy fails to occur, the corpus luteum degenerates, and there is a breakdown of the endometrium with hemorrhage and sloughing of all except the most basal layer (menstruation). Thus, there are three main phases in the menstrual cycle: (1) menstrual (first to fourth day), (2) proliferative (fifth to fourteenth day of cycle), which is controlled by estrogen, and (3) secretory (fifteenth to twenty-eighth day), in which progesterone as well as estrogen influences the endometrium. The beginning of the cycle is counted from the first day of menstruation, since that is a point most easily determined. Ovulation usually occurs near the middle of the cycle (fourteenth day) and is followed shortly by corpus luteum formation and a progesterone effect on the endometrium. The histologic changes are summarized in Table 22-1.

During the *menstrual phase* (first to fourth day), there is denudation and breakdown of the endometrium, with thrombosis of blood vessels and infiltration of leukocytes. Except for a basal layer, the endometrium is desquamated. From the remaining basal tissue, there is rapid regeneration. The basal layer does not participate in the histologic changes of the cycle.

The *proliferative phase* (fifth to fourteenth day) extends from the end of menstruation to ovulation and is controlled by estrogen from the developing ovarian follicle. It is characterized by active proliferation of cells and formation of straight tubular glands (Fig. 22-15). At first, the endometrium is 1 to 2 mm in thickness and contains three or four glands per low-power field, set in a loose stroma. The lining epithelial cells are columnar, have nuclei at all levels and are crowded together or "piled up." In the latter part of this stage, mitoses may be numerous in the glands. The glands in this phase appear very regular in outline and either elongated or round, depending on the direction in which they have been sectioned. Toward the end of this phase, the nuclei of the glandular cells are basal in position, and the cells become longer. The average number of glands now may be six or seven in a low-power field, and the endometrium is 2 to 2.5 mm in thickness. The stromal cells are elongated and spindly and have scanty cytoplasm.

The *secretory* (differentiative or progestational) *phase* (fifteenth to twenty-eighth day) extends from ovulation to the beginning of menstruation. Its characteristic features are the effect of progesterone produced by the corpus

Table 22-1. Histology of menstrual cycle

Day of cycle	Ovary	Endometrial phase	Endometrial histology
1 to 4	Degenerating corpus luteum	Menstrual	Infiltration of leukocytes; degeneration and breakdown of endometrium; hemorrhage and sloughing of endometrium
5 to 12	Developing follicle / Mature follicle	Proliferative (estrogen)	Regeneration of endometrium from basalis; glands rounded, regular, with piled-up cells; mitoses; stromal cells elongated and spindly with scanty cytoplasm
13 to 15	Ovulation		
16 to 28	Corpus luteum	Secretory (estrogen + progesterone)	Glandular epithelium lines up in single layer; subnuclear vacuolization, followed soon by peripheral vacuolization of glandular epithelium with basal nuclei; glands tortuous, saw-toothed; stroma edematous in early stages; later, stromal cells swollen, rounded, finally decidualike; congestion of blood vessels and infiltration of polymorphonuclears and lymphocytes in final stages

luteum. Hence, when these changes are present, ovulation may be assumed to have occurred. The main features are tortuosity of the glands, evidence of secretory activity, and, in later days of the phase, a swelling and rounding up of the stromal cells so that they resemble decidual cells.

Early in the secretory phase, the columnar glandular cells become more regularly arranged into line, no longer appearing "piled up." Clear vacuoles of glycogen appear at the base of the cells, pushing the nuclei into a more central position (Fig. 22-16). This subnuclear vacuolization is one of the important early indications of this phase. It is soon followed by vacuolization of peripheral parts of the cells and sinking of the nuclei to a basal position. The glands become twisted and have

a very irregular, saw-tooth appearance (Fig. 22-17). In the early days of this phase, the stroma is loose and very edematous, particularly in its central portions, so that a spongy layer may be distinguishable between a lining compact layer and the basal portion. Late in the phase, the stromal cells become swollen and rounded, possess abundant cytoplasm, and are young decidual cells. The endometrium at this time may be 4 to 7 mm in thickness. The blood vessels are more prominent, particularly the spiral arterioles. The vessels are congested, and there may be small hemorrhages. At the end of this phase, there is an infiltration of polymorphonuclear leukocytes and lymphocytes in the stroma.

Hyperplasia. *Cystic glandular hyperplasia* of the endometrium is an exaggeration of the

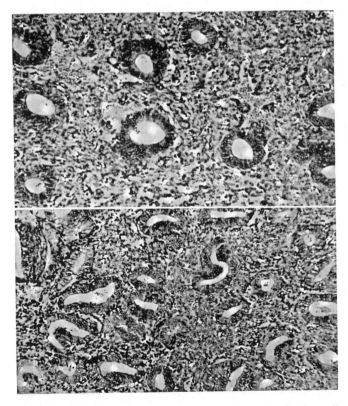

Fig. 22-15. Endometrium in proliferative phase. Rounded and regular glands are lined by several layers of cells.

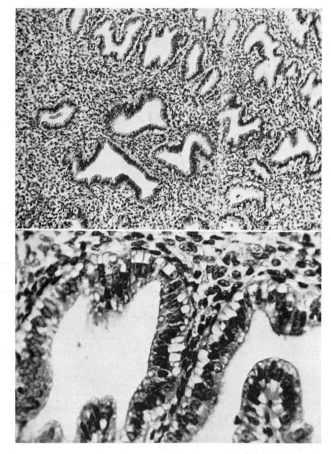

Fig. 22-16. Endometrium in early secretory phase. Subnuclear vacuolization is characteristic feature.

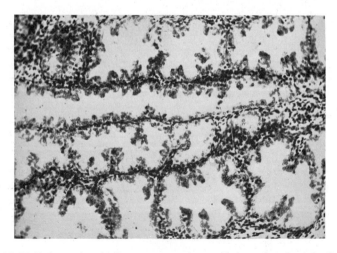

Fig. 22-17. Endometrium in late secretory phase with irregular glandular lining.

changes of the proliferation phase of the menstrual cycle. It may be caused by excessive estrogen production, either absolute or relative, because of failure of ovulation and corpus luteum formation. Follicular retention cysts are usually present in the ovaries. Most cases of endometrial hyperplasia occur after the age of 35 years, and it is most common around the menopausal period. Its chief symptom is irregular and persistent bleeding (functional uterine bleeding). The bleeding is believed to occur when there is a sharp drop or withdrawal of estrogenic hormone, and hence it is not correlated with the degree of hyperplasia, nor is it a regular and invariable accompaniment. Endometrial hyperplasia also accompanies tumors having excess estrogenic hormone production, such as granulosa cell and theca cell tumors. During the reproductive years, it is a benign lesion, but after menopause, endometrial hyperplasia may predispose to adenocarcinoma.

The hyperplastic endometrium is thickened, velvety, and often roughened by folds or irregular polypoid projections. Curettage produces abundant endometrial fragments that are firm, smooth, intact, nonnecrotic, and nonfriable and hence usually distinguishable grossly from the abundant but friable and necrotic masses obtained when there is carcinoma of the uterus.

Microscopically, the endometrium has the features of proliferative endometrium, with the addition of much irregularity in the size of the glands. Some glands are small, some are medium sized, and others show cystic enlargement. When the last are abundant, the endometrium has a characteristic "Swiss cheese" appearance (Fig. 22-18). Proliferative activity

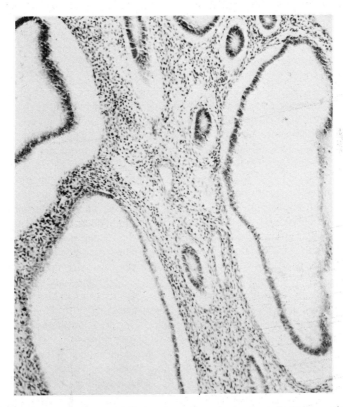

Fig. 22-18. Endometrial hyperplasia. "Swiss cheese" appearance results from cystic dilatation of endometrial glands.

(mitoses) is sometimes evident in the stroma as well as in the glandular epithelium. The endometrium appears similar at all levels, without layering. Small focal areas of degeneration and necrosis with thrombosis of small vessels are sometimes present.

Occasionally, a *focal hyperplasia* of the endometrium occurs. Microscopically, the lesion may appear benign or it may be very proliferative ("adenomatous" or "atypical" hyperplasia), so that it may be difficult to differentiate from carcinoma in situ or minimal carcinoma.

Polyp. Endometrial polyps are localized areas of benign overgrowth of endometrium, attached by a narrowed pedicle or base. Endometrial hyperplasia may be polypoid in form, but polyps also occur singly and without generalized endometrial change. They may undergo cyclic changes with the rest of the endometrium, but often they show a proliferative type of change only, with cystic glandular dilatation and a picture similar to that of endometrial hyperplasia. Large polyps often ulcerate and bleed or show considerable inflammation. Malignant change in a polyp is uncommon.

Endometritis. Inflammation of the endometrium is not a common clinical condition but may result from puerperal infection (streptococcal, staphylococcal, etc.), gonorrhea, or tuberculosis. The most severe form is the acute puerperal infection, which is often associated with myometritis, infective thrombophlebitis, and lymphangitis. Hence, the infection may spread throughout the pelvis and to other parts of the body. Gonococcal endometritis is usually less important than gonococcal tubal and cervical inflammation. Tuberculous endometritis is secondary to tuberculosis of the fallopian tube and shows the usual microscopic picture of epithelioid and giant cells. Postabortive endometritis is commonly seen in curettings sent to the laboratory and is identified by finding remnants of retained chorionic villi.

Pyometra refers to pus in the uterine cavity associated with inflammation of the endometrium. It is frequently, but not always, accompanied by cervical stenosis, the most common cause of which is a malignant tumor, usually cervical carcinoma. Anaerobic microorganisms, alone or in combination with aerobic microbes, are most often the causative agents.

Endometriosis. Endometriosis refers to the condition of ectopic endometrium—endometrial tissue in an abnormal position. The most common abnormal site is the muscular wall of the uterus, the lesion being due to benign invasion by endometrium. Here, the condition is termed *adenomyosis* or internal endometriosis. Other common sites are the ovary, fallopian tube, or peritoneal surfaces any place in the pelvis (Fig. 22-19). Occasionally, the condition involves laparotomy scars or the umbilicus. It also occurs infrequently in the cervix uteri, vagina, vulva, urinary bladder, and rectum. Rarely, distant sites are involved. Endometriosis in any situation is found only in the female and during the period of ovarian activity.

There are two main theories regarding extrauterine endometriosis, neither of which satisfactorily explains all cases. Sampson presented evidence that it is caused by retrograde menstruation, i.e., viable fragments of endometrium that pass through the fallopian tube at the time of menstruation and implant on serosal surfaces. The second theory is that it is caused by celomic metaplasia, i.e., an abnormal differentiation of certain areas of celomic epithelium. The serosal cells of the peritoneum and the mucosa of the uterus, tubes, and vagina have a common origin, and some hormonal factor may stimulate the metaplasia in extrauterine sites. Spread of endometrial fragments by the lymphatics and blood vessels also has been suggested, especially for distant foci of endometriosis. Adenomyosis appears to be the best understood as an exaggerated invasiveness of the endometrium. There is usually a direct continuation of the uterine mucosa with the endometrial areas in the myometrium. Adenocarcinoma only rarely develops in adenomyosis.

The extrauterine endometrial masses are usually small cysts, often only a few millimeters in diameter, containing a thick, chocolatelike fluid and possessing a hemorrhagic lin-

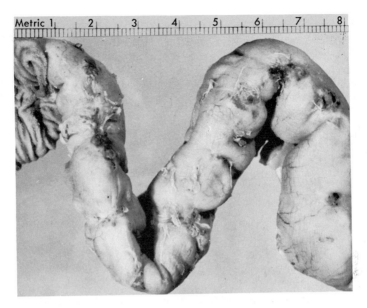

Fig. 22-19. Endometriosis of ileum.

ing. In the ovary, these chocolate cysts may be several centimeters in diameter but in rare cases are very large. They are easily confused with hemorrhagic corpus luteum cysts. When endometrial implants of pelvic peritoneum are numerous, they cause considerable irritation and development of pelvic adhesions. The aberrant endometrial tissue may respond to ovarian hormonal stimuli with periodic "menstrual" bleeding—hence, the cystic dilatation by accumulation of chocolate-colored hemorrhagic material. Rupture of cysts causes peritoneal irritation, fibrosis, and adhesions. Very rarely, malignant change may supervene in ovarian endometriosis, resulting in adenocarcinoma or in adenoacanthoma if there is also squamous metaplasia.

Identification of endometriosis depends on microscopic recognition of endometrial glands and stroma (Fig. 22-20). In the larger endometrial cysts, as in the ovary, this may be difficult because of atrophy of much of the endometrial lining of the cysts. The symptoms caused by endometriosis are often those of chronic pelvic inflammation, although dysmenorrhea may be prominent.

TUMORS OF CORPUS UTERI

Tumors arising from the body of the uterus include the following:

Leiomyomas (fibroids), which arise from myometrium and occasionally, by malignant change, result in sarcoma

Adenocarcinoma, which arises from endometrial glands, and its variant, adenoacanthoma

Sarcoma, which is derived from endometrial stroma or myometrium

Mixed tumors of mesodermal origin

Hydatidiform mole and choriocarcinoma, which, respectively, are caused by cystic degeneration and malignant change in chorionic villi

Rare tumors of the uterus include hemangioma, lipoma, and rhabdomyosarcoma. Hemangiomas of the endometrium or myometrium may be a source of vaginal bleeding. Hemangiopericytomas of the uterus also occur and have been confused with stromal myosis.

Leiomyoma (myoma; fibroid)

The most common tumor of the uterus is a benign smooth muscle growth of the muscular wall. Some evidence has suggested that it may arise from the smooth muscle of blood vessel

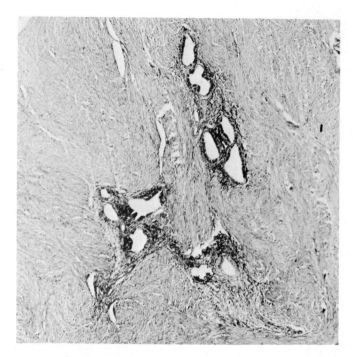

Fig. 22-20. Adenomyosis (endometriosis) of uterus. Islands of endometrial glands and stroma are surrounded by myometrium.

walls rather than from uterine muscle fibers. It occurs during the reproductive age and tends to regress after menopause, even if the latter is induced. It is said to occur in 20% of women over 35 years of age and has a much higher incidence in black women. The tumors are frequently multiple, grow to large size, and are subject to degenerative changes because of their poor blood supply. They distort the uterus, have secondary effects on the endometrium, and interfere with pregnancy and delivery. A small proportion become malignant. A variant form of myoma of the uterus may be very vascular and is sometimes termed *angiomyoma.*

Etiology. The cause of uterine myomas is unknown, although a relationship to hyperestrinism has been postulated. Evidence for this is incomplete. Sterility is quite common with leiomyomas, probably as an effect rather than a cause.

Gross appearance. Most leiomyomas in-

volve the body of the uterus (Fig. 22-21), but a troublesome small proportion are in the cervix. The tumors begin in the myometrium as *intramural* (or "interstitial") growths. With continued expansive growth, they may take up a position beneath the peritoneum (*subserous* fibroids) or the endometrium (*submucous* fibroids). In either case, they can become pedunculated and attached by a narrow pedicle or neck that carries their blood supply and that is easily twisted. *Intraligamentous* fibroids are those that extend out between layers of the broad ligament. In rare cases, the omentum becomes adherent to a pedunculated fibroid and provides a new blood supply. The uterine attachment may be lost, and it becomes a *wandering,* or *parasitic,* fibroid. The tumors are always well circumscribed and easily shelled out from their surrounding pseudocapsule. They are usually multiple (Fig. 22-22) and vary in size from a few millimeters to enormous growths many centimeters in diam-

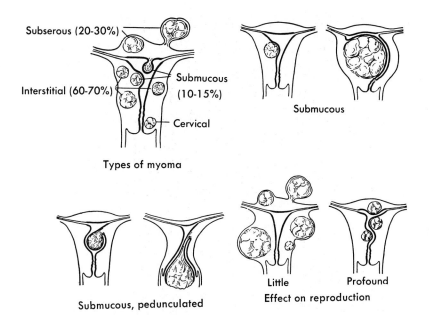

Subserous (20-30%)

Submucous (10-15%)

Interstitial (60-70%)

Cervical

Types of myoma

Submucous

Submucous, pedunculated

Little

Profound

Effect on reproduction

Fig. 22-21. Types of myomas of uterus. Submucous myomas cause enlargement of surface area of endometrium, which tends to bleed. Myomas disturb pregnancy when they distort and encroach upon endometrium and uterine cavity. (From Mengert, W. F.: J. Mich. Med. Soc. **49:**1302-1307, 1950.)

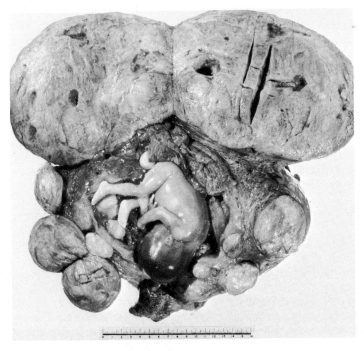

Fig. 22-22. Gravid uterus with multiple, varying-sized leiomyomas.

eter, and weights up to 100 lb have been reported. On being cut, a fibroid tends to bulge outward as a result of retraction of surrounding myometrial tissue. The cut surface is firm and has a characteristic whorled, trabeculated appearance because of interlacing bundles of muscle fibers.

Microscopic appearance. Microscopically, the bundles of smooth muscle cells can be seen running in all directions and producing the whorled pattern. When they are cut longitudinally, the muscle cells are spindle shaped with elongated rodlike nuclei. When they are cut across, the cells appear rounded with central round nuclei. The fibrous stroma may be slight but is variable in amount. The prominent fibrous component in some of these tumors is responsible for the popular designation "fibroid." Mitoses are rare, and there is little variation in the size, shape, and staining properties of the cells. A rare clear cell leiomyoma as well as other atypical smooth muscle tumors of the uterus have been described.

Secondary changes. Degenerative changes in fibroids are very common, mainly because of their poor blood supply. These secondary changes include hyaline degeneration (most common), necrosis and red degeneration, calcification, and cystic degeneration. Telangiectatic and fatty changes occur but are unusual. Infection of a fibroid is most common in the submucous type. Sarcomatous change affects only a small proportion of fibroids (probably less than 2%) and often may be suspected grossly when the cut surface of the tumor is soft, white, and brainlike in consistency and appearance. Rare cases of uterine leiomyomas, which appear benign microscopically, metastasize and appear to be low-grade myosarcomas.

Effects. The more important effects on the uterus are caused by the interstitial and submucous fibroids. They may result in great distortion of the uterus and its cavity, so that growth and accommodation of a fetus or its delivery may be impossible. With submucous fibroids, the overlying endometrium becomes thin and atrophic. Infection, endometrial inflammation, and sometimes bleeding result from submucous growths. Associated with large myomas, a few cases of polycythemia have been reported, the erythrocytosis disappearing on removal of the tumor. The erythrocytosis is due to secretion of erythropoietin or similar substance by the large tumors.

Adenocarcinoma

Carcinoma of the body of the uterus is an adenocarcinoma arising from endometrial glands. Although it is less common than carcinoma of the cervix, recent reports suggest that the incidence of endometrial carcinoma is increasing. Its peak incidence is after menopause at about 55 years of age. It appears to have a greater frequency in infertile women and to have some genetic and endocrine dysfunctional basis.

Ovarian - stromal hyperplasia, presumably associated with increased estrogen production, is found with abnormal frequency in women with endometrial carcinoma. The chief symptom is postmenopausal bleeding, the diagnosis being made, except in advanced cases, by curettage and microscopic examination of tissue fragments. Postmenopausal hyperplasia of the endometrium appears to have some relationship to the development of adenocarcinoma. There is evidence that carcinoma of the endometrium is often preceded by hyperplasia, which may appear atypical or adenomatous. Some of the focal or polypoid atypical hyperplasias may be considered as carcinoma in situ. Recent reports have indicated that menopausal and postmenopausal women who take estrogens have an increased risk of endometrial carcinoma. It has also been suggested that the prolonged use of sequential oral contraceptives may play a role in the development of endometrial hyperplasia and carcinoma. The association of adenocarcinoma of the uterus with feminizing (e.g., granulosa-theca cell) tumors of the ovary has already been mentioned.

Gross appearance. The cancer may involve the endometrium diffusely, making it thick, rough, and polypoid, before there is much myometrial invasion. The tumor tissue tends to be bulky and friable and often has areas of

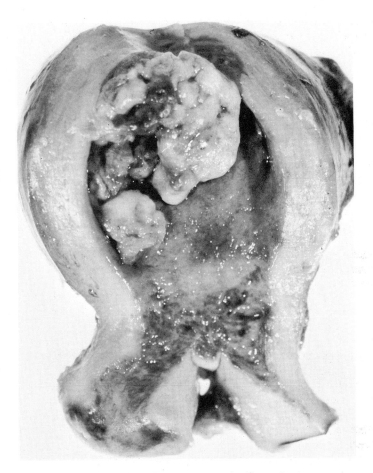

Fig. 22-23. Polypoid carcinoma of endometrium.

necrosis. In other cases, the tumor tissue is localized to one part of the fundus and may be polypoid in form (Fig. 22-23).

Microscopic appearance. Microscopically, there is usually a well-differentiated glandular structure but with considerable irregularity and lawlessness of pattern (Fig. 22-24). Often, the glands are closely and irregularly placed, with little stroma between them. Actual invasion through basement membranes may not be seen except in the more malignant examples. The cells show varying degrees of differentiation. There may be great variation in size, shape, and staining of cells and many typical and atypical mitoses in the highly malignant types. Histologic grading, on the basis of the propor-

tion of differentiated and undifferentiated cells, gives some indication of prognosis.

Spread. Spread of adenocarcinoma of the uterus is chiefly by the lymphatics to involve the lumbar glands at the lower end of the aorta and sometimes the inguinal glands. There is a variable degree of direct invasion of the myometrium, and extension to the cervix occurs readily. In some cases, there is implantation on the tubes, ovaries, or peritoneum. Blood vessel spread is a late event.

Adenoacanthoma. Adenoacanthoma of the uterus is a type of adenocarcinoma in which there are areas of squamous epithelium among the gland-forming tumor cells (Fig. 22-25). The squamous metaplasia is from certain "in-

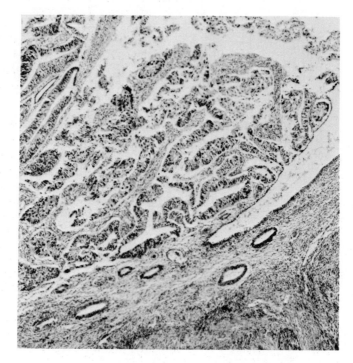

Fig. 22-24. Adenocarcinoma of endometrium. Adjacent nonneoplastic endometrium appears atrophic.

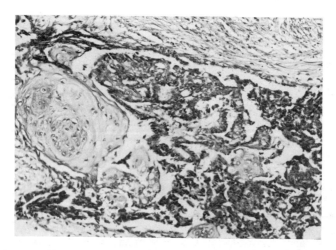

Fig. 22-25. Adenoacanthoma of endometrium. Areas of glandular and squamous epithelium are intermixed.

different'' cells beneath the columnar epithelium that possesses the ability to form squamous epithelium.

Sarcoma

Sarcoma of the uterus is relatively uncommon, constituting about 3% of uterine cancers. It is most common during the fourth and fifth decades. Sarcoma may arise from leiomyomas or de novo from muscle or connective tissue elements of the uterus. Its symptoms do not easily distinguish it from other uterine malignancies. Rhabdomyosarcomas rarely occur in the uterus in pure form but sometimes occur as part of a mixed mesodermal tumor.

The gross appearance may suggest the diagnosis but often is not distinctive. In leiomyosarcoma, the firm consistency and whorled appearance of fibroids are lacking, and the tissue is soft, rubbery, and fleshy.

Microscopically, the tumor may be of spindle cell, round cell, or mixed type. The degree of malignancy rather accurately parallels the number of mitoses. Spread beyond the uterus occurs by direct extension, by the bloodstream to the lungs and liver, and to a lesser extent by the lymphatics.

Endometrial stromal sarcoma is often polypoid. It is relatively rare and often of complex composition. Spread of the tumor is similar to that of leiomyosarcoma. In addition to frank endometrial sarcoma, there occurs a lesion suggestive of endometriosis but composed only of stromal cells. Such lesions, called *stromal endometriosis* or *endolymphatic stromal myosis* because of their tendency to permeate lymphatics or blood vessels, also have been considered neoplastic, either lowgrade stromal sarcomas or hemangiopericytomas.

Mesodermal mixed tumor

The mixed tumors of the uterus are probably caused by inclusion and persistence in the müllerian organs of mesenchymal cells, which have the capacity for differentiation into various mesodermal tissues. Most cases arise in the body of the uterus and occur about the fifth decade. Those arising in the cervix occur at an earlier age. The mesodermal mixed tumors are highly malignant and have a poor prognosis.

The growth begins in the mucosal layer and assumes a polypoid form. Although not distinctive clinically, it is very constantly manifested by a sanguineous discharge from the vagina. Portions of the tumor are sometimes passed per vaginam.

Various types of tissue occur in these tumors, but myxomatous tissue and cartilage are most constant (Fig. 22-26). Striated muscle fi-

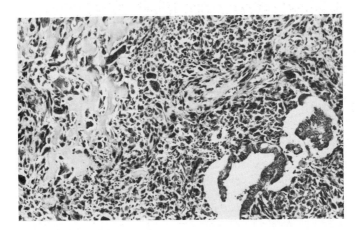

Fig. 22-26. Mesodermal mixed tumor of uterus. Glandular, cartilaginous, and undifferentiated areas are evident.

bers are frequent constituents. Myxosarcomatous and undifferentiated sarcomatous elements also are common. The solitary uterine tumors with intermingled carcinomatous and nonspecific sarcomatous components often are designated carcinosarcoma. Homologous carcinosarcomas, not of the mesodermal mixed tumor type, are rare.

Sarcoma botryoides is frequently classified with mixed tumors of the uterus, although it appears to be a distinct entity. Grossly, it is a nodular (grapelike) growth, most often involving the upper vagina and occurring almost exclusively in infancy or early childhood. Some consider it a form of embryonal myosarcoma originating in the subepithelial tissues. Fusiform cells, striated cells, and tumor giant cells commonly compose the tumor. Nodular protruding growths in the vagina and vulva are characteristic, but spread may occur also to the cervix and pelvic organs, with eventual widespread metastases.

Hydatidiform mole and choriocarcinoma

Hydatidiform mole and choriocarcinoma arise from fetal membranes rather than from the tissues of the mother, but they have the ability to invade and destroy maternal tissues extensively. Determination of the degree of malignancy and prognosis from microscopic examination is a difficult procedure with many pitfalls. The term *trophoblastic disease* is commonly applied to these lesions.

The normal chorionic villus is covered by two layers of trophoblastic cells. The inner layer of Langhans' cells is composed of cuboidal cells with a pale nucleus and cytoplasm. The outer, or syncytial, layer consists of masses of cytoplasm having multiple very dark nuclei. These trophoblastic cells are normally invasive and even in normal pregnancy may be found invading the myometrium and even blood vessels. Some trophoblastic cells may be carried to the lungs but always regress and disappear. This normal event may cause confusion in diagnosis, being mistaken for malignant invasion. The benign invasion (infiltration with syncytium only) is sometimes called

syncytial endometritis, or *syncytioma.* Occasionally, a part of the placenta fails to be detached after abortion or delivery and remains implanted in the endometrium. Such a *placental polyp* may be a cause of abnormal bleeding.

Park* has outlined a concept of degrees of primary trophoblastic abnormality that enables a classification according to varying severity.

1 *Simple dysfunction* causing death of the embryo but with no histologic change in the villi
2 *Dysfunction causing oversecretion of fluid* into the villous stroma, with death of the embryo (hydropic abortion)
3 *Benign neoplasia with oversecretion of fluid*—hydatidiform mole
4 *Locally malignant neoplasia with oversecretion of fluid*—chorioadenoma destruens
5 *Metastatically malignant neoplasia with oversecretion of fluid*—choriocarcinoma that follows a hydatidiform mole
6 *Metastatically malignant neoplasia without villous disturbance*—choriocarcinoma that follows an abortion or term pregnancy

Hydatidiform mole is a hydropic degeneration of chorionic villi, which become enlarged into clusters of grapelike vesicles. Blood vessels are scanty, and there is some proliferation of trophoblastic cells. This abnormality occurs about once in every 2,000 pregnancies, and although it is benign, the patient must be carefully followed, since some cases (1.25% to 2.5%) progress to malignant choriocarcinoma. Various gradations occur between the benign hydatidiform mole and the malignant choriocarcinoma. Greater degrees of trophoblastic proliferation in moles appear to indicate a correspondingly greater risk of development of choriocarcinoma.

Some degree of hydatidiform degeneration of chorionic villi is found in two thirds of spontaneously aborted pathologic ova, apparently caused by the absence or defectiveness of fetal circulation. The typical hydatidiform mole appears to be derived from a pathologic

---

*Adapted from Park, W. W.: In Collins, D. H.: Modern trends in pathology, New York, 1959, Harper & Row, Publishers, Inc., p. 191.

ovum in which the embryo was absent or defective but that failed to abort at the usual time. In a recent cytogenetic study, the karyotype of hydatidiform moles was predominantly 46XX, and only paternal chromosomes were found to be transmitted to the moles, suggesting that the moles were androgenetic in origin.

Chorioadenoma destruens (Fig. 22-27) is a highly proliferative variant of hydatidiform mole that usually follows delivery of a hydatidiform mole. It tends to run a benign course but may penetrate the serosa and lead to hemorrhage or infection and, rarely, may spread to pelvic structures.

Choriocarcinoma is a very malignant and rare tumor. It most frequently follows a hydatidiform mole (1 in 50 instances) but may develop after an abortion (1 in 15,000 instances) or after a term pregnancy (1 in 160,000 instances). Considering all types of pregnancy, it occurs in about 1 of 40,000 consecutive pregnancies.

There is massive overgrowth of both Langhans' and syncytial cells, which exhibit many of the atypical features of malignant cells elsewhere. The arrangement of the cells may suggest primordial placental villi, but fully developed chorionic villi are not formed. Nevertheless, histologic interpretation or diagnosis is frequently difficult or unreliable. Invasion occurs freely in the pelvis, and spread by the bloodstream occurs to the lungs, brain, and other organs. The ovaries are involved by multiple lutein cysts that reach a large size.

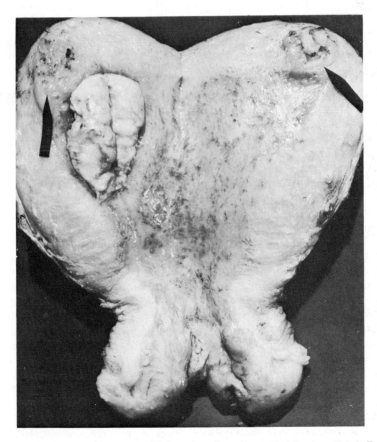

Fig. 22-27. Chorioadenoma destruens, with invasion of uterine wall. (Courtesy Dr. J. F. Kuzma.)

Chorionic gonadotropin may be demonstrated in blood and urine when living trophoblastic tissue is present in the body and hence is often important in the diagnosis and management of hydatidiform mole and choriocarcinoma. Quantitative tests are even more useful than the ordinary qualitative procedures. It has been noted that spinal fluid gives a positive qualitative test in the presence of mole or choriocarcinoma but not in normal pregnancy. Spontaneous regression of metastases has been noted in rare cases. Chemotherapy with folic acid antagonists (methotrexate) has produced significant regression of metastases and good results in some cases.

Choriocarcinoma occurs also in the ovary (rare) and, in the male, as a form of germ cell (teratoid) tumor of the testis. Its microscopic features and malignancy in such cases are similar, and the hormone titers are also elevated.

Benign placental tumors are rare, and almost all are hemangiomas *(chorangiomas)*. They are usually a vascular nodule, 2 or 3 cm in diameter, with varying proportions of capillary proliferation and stromal cells. In some cases, there is a clinical association of hydramnios and prematurity.

Cervix uteri

The cervix, or neck of the uterus, connects the vagina with the uterine cavity. It has an internal os, a canal lined with mucosa having high columnar epithelium and racemose glands, an external os, and a vaginal portion. At the external os there is a rather sharp line dividing columnar epithelium of the endocervix from the squamous epithelium that covers the portion that protrudes into the vagina.

The main lesions of the cervix are inflammation (cervicitis), polyp formation, and carcinoma. Carcinoma of the cervix is a frequent and highly important tumor. In most cases, it is a squamous cell carcinoma arising from epithelium of the vaginal portion. Adenocarcinoma of the endocervix is uncommon, and when it does occur, it is often difficult to be sure that its origin has not been from endometrium.

CERVICITIS

Acute cervicitis. Acute cervicitis may be the result of gonococcal infection (p. 126), but often it may be caused by other organisms, such as streptococci, staphylococci, and *Escherichia coli*.

Chronic cervicitis. Chronic cervicitis may be due to traumatic or mechanical factors in addition to bacterial causes. It is one of the most common gynecologic lesions and is the usual cause of vaginal discharge or leukorrhea. In chronic cervicitis, the chief microscopic change is an infiltration of plasma cells and lymphocytes. Inflammatory obstruction of the outlets of endocervical glands often results in their cystic dilatation (nabothian cysts).

Erosion. Erosion of the cervix is a lesion in which there is an area of loss of the squamous covering of the cervix and eventual replacement by columnar epithelium of the endocervix. This is to be distinguished from *ectropion,* or eversion of the endocervical mucosa, caused by laceration of the cervix. Cervical erosion is commonly associated with chronic cervicitis, but it may be congenital in nature.

Epidermidization (squamous metaplasia). Epidermidization is a common change in the cervix, particularly in the healing phase of erosions. Squamous epithelium invades beneath the lining of cervical glands, with a gradual lifting up and replacement of the cylindrical epithelium by squamous epithelium (Fig. 22-28). This process is benign and is distinguished from carcinoma by the normal appearance of the squamous epithelial cells, the infrequency of mitoses, and the absence of invasion of interstitial tissues.

Tuberculous cervicitis. Tuberculous cervicitis is rare and usually secondary to tuberculosis in the fallopian tube. Although the gross appearance may simulate carcinoma, the usual picture of tuberculosis is seen microscopically.

CERVICAL POLYP

In benign cervical polyp, there is a localized overgrowth or heaping up of cervical mucosa, which becomes pedunculated and inflamed. It often is associated with inflammation of the cervix. A polyp tends to cause in-

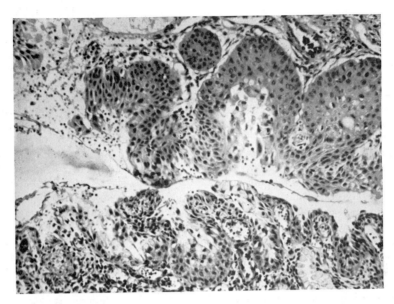

Fig. 22-28. Squamous metaplasia in cervix. Squamous epithelial cells of benign appearance are replacing glandular linings. (From Faulkner, R. L., and Douglass, M.: Essentials of obstetrical and gynecological pathology, ed. 2, St. Louis, 1949, The C. V. Mosby Co.)

termenstrual spotting or bleeding—hence, clinically it must be differentiated from carcinoma. Epidermidization is common in cervical polyps, but carcinomatous change occurs in very few.

CARCINOMA

Carcinoma of the cervix is one of the most important and frequent forms of cancer affecting women. About 95% are squamous cell carcinomas, the remainder being adenocarcinomas arising from the cervical canal or from remnants of Gartner's duct. Mixed squamous cell and adenocarcinoma also may accur. The peak incidence occurs in women between 40 and 50 years of age, but many cases occur in women in their thirties. Clear cell adenocarcinomas of the cervix occurring in young female patients who have had prenatal exposure to stilbestrol have recently been reported (p. 662). The most important factor in prognosis of cervical carcinoma is the degree of extension when treatment is instituted and secondarily, the histologic type of malignancy. Spread is mainly by the lymphatics. In-

volvement of the bladder and ureters frequently occurs, and uremia is a common terminal event.

Since early cases are not distinctive grossly, early diagnosis depends on cytologic study and biopsy of suspicious areas. Colpomicroscopy also may be helpful in diagnosis of incipient lesions. The Papanicolaou smear technique, which is frequently used for the detection of cancer, is referred to on p. 257. The commonly used system of reporting cytologic findings according to a numerical classification indicates the cytopathologist's opinion as to the degree of probability that a particular lesion is cancer. Currently, however, as a result of increased knowledge of cytologic changes in cancer, there is a tendency for cytopathologists to make a cellular diagnosis that approaches the validity of histopathologic examination. Cytology is also important in the diagnosis of cancer of the body of the uterus.

Etiology. The cause of cervical carcinoma is not known, but there are certain factors that are possibly significant. The chronic irritation of untreated lacerations from childbirth and other types of chronic cervicitis have been considered predisposing factors, but these have been somewhat discredited. Epidemiologic studies have shown an association with early and frequent coitus, particularly where there is lack of circumcision and poor penile hygiene. The importance of early coitus is alluded to in the hypothesis that in early adolescence, as well as in the first pregnancy, the cervical epithelium undergoes active cellular growth or physiologic metaplasia, making it more susceptible to possible mutagenic factors that may induce atypical changes. In experimental animal studies and in observations of human subjects shortly after coitus, sperm DNA has been detected in close association with the nuclei of cervical epithelial cells, suggesting that sperm may play a role in producing atypical changes that could lead to the development of carcinoma. The role of sperm is considered to be important, not because of an inherent specific mutagenic property, but because of the receptivity of the target tissue to possible mutagens during certain active physiologic growth periods.

Evidence has been presented that the venereally transmitted herpes simplex virus type 2 (HSV-2) may play an etiologic role. Seroepidemiologic studies have shown significantly higher frequencies of HSV-2 antibodies in patients with cervical cancer, both invasive and preinvasive, as compared with control patients. In a prospective study, women with HSV-2 genital infection were found to develop cervical anaplastic changes more frequently than control women. Cervical dysplasia occurred twice as often and carcinoma in situ eight times as often in those with the herpetic infection, suggesting that the viral infection may precede the development of cervical carcinoma. Certain investigators, by means of immunofluorescent techniques, have detected HSV-2 antigens in cells exfoliated from women with preinvasive and invasive cervical carcinoma. Other scientists have isolated from cervical, vaginal, and vulvar cancers of women a soluble membrane antigen that reacted with antiserum prepared in a guinea pig against semipurified HSV-2. Other studies have shown that hamster cells may be trans-

formed by HSV-2 in vitro and that malignant neoplasms may be produced in hamsters by inoculation with these transformed cells.

Carcinoma in situ. Early cases of cervical carcinoma have been recognized that exhibit characteristic cytologic changes of malignancy but without invasion. They have been variously termed intraepithelial carcinoma, preinvasive carcinoma, carcinoma in situ, etc. Squamous cell carcinoma in situ is a lesion in which an area of the squamous epithelial surface is replaced by anaplastic cells similar to those of invasive cancer but with no stromal invasive penetration demonstrable. The entire thickness of the epithelium is more or less involved, with loss of normal stratification (Fig. 22-29). The anaplastic cells show altered polarity, an increased number of mitoses, and relatively large, hyperchromatic, and irregular nuclei. The cytologic features are thus indistinguishable from invasive cancer, but evidence for the presence or absence of invasion sometimes may be inconclusive, and occasionally invasion is shown only by multiple or serial sections. Rounded buds of cells pushing into and displacing the underlying stroma from the basal layer of the surface epithelium do not constitute evidence of invasion. Likewise, extension of the anaplastic cells may occur into the underlying glands, even appearing to replace such glands, but without extension through a basement membrane and so without definite stromal or lymphatic invasion.

The anaplastic or atypical cervical epithelium may involve only the basal part of the surface epithelium or less than the full thickness, without loss of stratification (Fig. 22-30). Such ''dysplasia,'' ''atypical epithelium,'' or ''basal cell hyperplasia'' is to be distinguished from carcinoma in situ. Its significance is uncertain, and although it may sometimes be only a temporary disturbance, there is evidence also that transformation to carcinoma in situ may occur. In such transformation, there may be stages in which distinction between the two lesions is unreliable or a matter of individual judgment. Basal cell hyperactivity or dysplasia is sometimes present on the periphery of areas of carcinoma.

The significance of carcinoma in situ also is

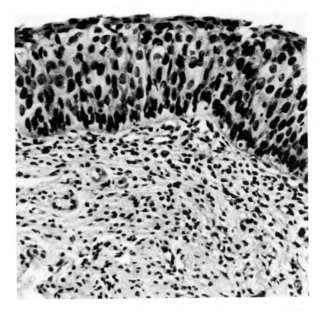

Fig. 22-29. Carcinoma in situ of cervix. Entire thickness of squamous epithelium is replaced by disorderly arranged, atypical cells with large, hyperchromatic nuclei and scanty cytoplasm. Some mitotic figures may be seen. There is no invasion of underlying stroma.

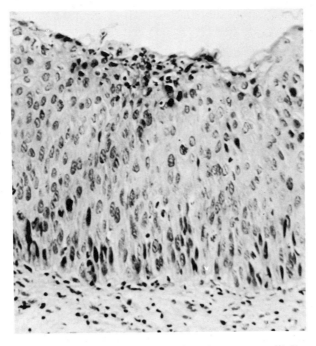

Fig. 22-30. Dysplasia of cervical mucosa. Stratification of squamous epithelium is still evident, but there is proliferation of atypical cells in basal layer and in other areas. Note large, hyperchromatic nuclei and some mitotic figures.

not entirely clarified. The site of the change is most often the squamocolumnar junction of the cervix or the transitional zone. It may arise from subcylindrical reserve cell anaplasia or from anaplastic squamous epithelium that arose from subcylindrical cell anaplasia. Carcinoma in situ appears to develop from a field of abnormal cells rather than from a single cell. A certain proportion of cases progress to invasive cancer after a latent interval of months or years. A microinvasive stage is sometimes recognized. On gross inspection, no characteristic lesion is seen, but there may be changes that may be recognized by colpomicroscopy. The average age of women with carcinoma in situ appears to be about 10 years younger than the average of those with invasive cervical carcinoma.

Invasive carcinoma. The gross appearance of invasive carcinoma of the cervix is not distinctive in early stages. It presents a small, hardened granular or friable area at the margin of the external os. Later, the tumor may grow outward, forming an everting growth of cauliflower appearance, or it may be inverting, extensively invading the cervix and vaginal wall, which are hardened and thickened. The Schiller test is of clinical value in bringing early suspicious areas into prominence when iodine is painted on the cervix. Normal cervical epithelium, because of its glycogen content, stains brown with iodine, whereas carcinomatous cells are deficient in glycogen and remain unstained.

Microscopically, the usual form of cervical carcinoma is composed of squamous epithelial cells showing varying degrees of differentiation and atypicalness in their size, shape, staining reactions, polarity, and pattern. Invasiveness is evident except in the earliest or in situ cases. Some keratin pearl formation may be present in the more highly differentiated examples. In the infrequent form of cervical cancer, adenocarcinoma, the pattern and degree of differentiation vary in individual cases. A mixture of squamous and adenocarcinoma or adenoacanthoma may occur. Clear cell adenocarcinoma of the cervix has recently been observed in young female patients who

have had intrauterine exposure to stilbestrol. A similar type of cancer has also been reported to occur in the vagina under the same circumstances (p. 661).

Grading and prognosis. In the cervix, as elsewhere, the degree of malignancy of a tumor may be estimated from its growth activity and the immaturity or undifferentiation of the cells.

The system of Broders is applicable in other situations as well and has been discussed on p. 246. The tumors are classified into four grades: grade I, less than 25% undifferentiated cells; grade II, 25% to 50% undifferentiated cells; grade III, 50% to 75% undifferentiated cells; and grade IV, more than 75% undifferentiated cells. Grade I and grade II tumors are less malignant and less radiosensitive. Grade III and grade IV tumors are more malignant and more radiosensitive.

Martzloff divided the tumors according to the predominant cell type: (1) spinal cell, (2) transitional cell, (3) spindle cell, and (4) adenocarcinoma.

The Broders and Martzloff systems of grading have not been found to be of very dependable prognostic value. Wentz and Reagan have divided squamous cell carcinoma into three histologic groups: a large cell nonkeratizing type, a keratinizing cancer, and a small cell carcinoma. These types appear to have significant differences of survival time—persons with the large cell nonkeratinizing cancer have a high rate of survival, whereas the small cell carcinoma is associated with the lowest rate of survival.

Histologic grading indicates rate of growth and degree of radiosensitivity but is probably less important in prognosis and as a guide to treatment than is the degree of extension of the tumor at the time examined. Clinical stages of the disease have been designated by the International Federation of Gynecology and Obstetrics (FIGO) and are presented here with the corresponding "T" (primary tumor) designation of the TNM classification in parentheses.

Stage 0 Carcinoma in situ (TIS)

Stage I Carcinoma confined to cervix; extension to corpus disregarded (T1)

Ia: Early stromal invasion; microinvasive carcinoma (T1a)

Ib: All other stage I lesions; occult cancer marked "occ" (T1b)

Stage II Carcinoma extends beyond cervix but not to pelvic wall; involves vagina but not lower third (T2)

IIa: Carcinoma does not infiltrate parametrium (T2a)

IIb: Carcinoma infiltrates parametrium (T2b)

Stage III Carcinoma extends to pelvic wall; involves lower third of vagina; includes cases with hydronephrosis or nonfunctioning kidney not related to other causes (T3)

IIIa: Carcinoma does not extend to pelvic wall (T3a)

IIIb: Carcinoma extends to pelvic wall and/or associated with hydronephrosis or nonfunctioning kidney (T3b)

Stage IV Carcinoma extends beyond true pelvis or clinically involves mucosa of bladder or rectum (T4)

IVa: Carcinoma spreads to adjacent organs (T4a)

IVb: Carcinoma spreads to distant organs (T4b)

A correlation between clinical staging and 5-year survival rates has been noted. It is generally agreed that the 5-year survival rate for adequately treated cervical carcinoma in stage 0 approaches 100%, but the rates for stages I to IV vary considerably in different reports. In a report published under the auspices of FIGO (1976), the rates (based on results from 109 institutions in 27 countries) were as follows: stage I, 79.2%; stage II, 58.1%; stage III, 32.5%; and stage IV, 8.2%. However, rates that are higher and lower for each of these stages have been reported by other investigators.

Combined consideration of the histologic grade or type and the degree of extension leads to the most accurate prognosis.

A diagnosis of cervical or endometrial carcinoma often can be made by expert examination of a cervical or vaginal smear, but it should be confirmed by biopsy or curettage (p. 255).

Extension and metastasis. Direct extension of cervical carcinoma occurs in a radical manner and may massively involve the vagina and body of the uterus. Involvement of the parametrium may be by direct extension or by lymphatic permeation. Lymphatic extension is important, with metastasis developing in the periaortic, iliac, and hypogastric nodes and sometimes in the sacral, obturator, lumbar, and inguinal nodes. In late stages, there may be some spread by the bloodstream. The cause of death is often obstruction in the urinary tract (e.g., blocking of ureters), leading to uremia, or hemorrhage resulting from erosion of a large vessel. Uremia and infection are more often the cause of death than is wide or distant spread of the cancer.

Vagina

Various inflammatory lesions may occur in the vagina. Those that are clinically significant are gonococcal vaginitis (p. 126) and inflammation caused by *Candida albicans* (p. 198) or *Trichomonas vaginalis*. Tumors also occur, the most important of which are carcinoma and sarcoma botryoides, although these are very uncommon in relation to other cancers occurring in female patients. Carcinoma in situ of the vagina has been reported only rarely. Usually, carcinoma is either the squamous cell type or adenocarcinoma.

Squamous cell carcinoma. Squamous cell carcinoma usually occurs in postmenopausal women. It may arise in any part of the vagina, but it most commonly involves the posterior wall. Metastases may occur to inguinal or iliac lymph nodes.

Adenocarcinoma. Until recently, adenocarcinoma was considered a rare form of vaginal carcinoma that occurred more frequently in women of postmenopausal age. However, today an increasing number of these tumors is being reported, particularly *clear cell adenocarcinoma* in young female patients. In 1970, an unusual occurrence of a cluster of seven cases of this neoplasm in young females was reported by Herbst and Scully. Subsequently, the tumors were found to be associated with intrauterine exposure of the patients to diethylstilbestrol (DES), the lesions appearing 14 to 22 years after the mothers had received DES for threatened abortion. Since then, a central registry established for the study of clear cell carcinoma of the genital tract in young females has been conducting an investigation of this lesion, which has been observed in the cervix uteri as well as in the vagina. As of May 1976, 300 cases have been entered in the registry. Of the patients whose maternal history has been investigated, an intrauterine exposure to DES or chemically related nonsteroidal estrogens was documented in about two thirds. The average age of the patients at the time of diagnosis was 17 years, the youngest being 7 years and the oldest 28 years. About two thirds of the tumors were confined to the vagina, and the remainder were in the cervix. Microscopically, the presence of clear cells with distinct cell walls is a characteristic feature of these adenocarcinomas, and the clear cells may appear in the form of nests, cords, or solid masses. *Vaginal adenosis* (noncarcinomatous proliferation of glands) has also been observed commonly in young females exposed to stilbestrol in utero. A chronic inflammatory reaction usually accompanies the adenosis, and in many instances squamous metaplasia involves the glands in this abnormality. In addition, cervical ectropion and vaginal and cervical transverse ridges have been observed frequently in female patients exposed to DES in utero.

Clear cell adenocarcinoma of the vagina and cervix in these young persons is a serious form of cancer. Lymph node metastases have been associated with tumors as small as 1.5 cm and with a significant number of those believed to be confined to the vagina, the cervix, or the cervix and vagina. Recurrence following treatment (particularly of large tumors) has occurred often. The incidence of clinical evidence of metastases to the lungs or supraclavicular lymph nodes in these patients was found to be much higher than in recurrent squamous cell carcinoma of the vagina or cervix. Vaginal cytology in young girls with abnormal bleed-

ing or a history of prenatal exposure to stilbestrol may play an important role in detecting clear cell adenocarcinoma.

Some nonneoplastic abnormalities of the testes, epididymides, and penis in male subjects have been linked to intrauterine DES exposure also.

Other tumors and tumorlike lesions. *Sarcomas* of the vagina are rare. *Fibrosarcomas* and their variants tend to occur in adults but may be seen in children. *Sarcoma botryoides,* a malignant mixed mesodermal tumor, may present as a grapelike, nodular growth in the vagina of infants or children. Mesodermal mixed tumors also occur in women, usually postmenopausally, but in the uterus (p. 653).

Vulva

The vulva, which includes the structures from the pubis to the perineum, is subject to inflammatory lesions, atrophic changes, and tumors. Being covered by skin, the vulva is involved by the same inflammatory and neoplastic lesions that affect skin elsewhere, and many vulvar lesions are such skin conditions. In addition, venereal lesions occur frequently, including gonorrhea, syphilis, chancroid, lymphogranuloma venerum, and granuloma inguinale.

VENEREAL LESIONS

Gonorrheal inflammation. Gonorrhea of the vulva affects particularly the urethra, periurethral Skene's ducts, and Bartholin's glands. The squamous epithelium of adult vulvar and vaginal mucosa is resistant to gonorrheal infection, although the thin mucosa of infants is not. Bartholinitis is most commonly the result of gonorrheal infection, and in acute stages there is much swelling of the gland caused by purulent exudate. In chronic phases, there may be blockage of the duct and cystic distention of the gland. Chronic gonorrheal infection may linger long in Skene's ducts and Bartholin's glands.

Syphilis. The primary chancre of syphilis

may involve the vulva, and in the secondary stage flat condylomas occur there (p. 181).

Granuloma inguinale. Granuloma inguinale is a spreading ulcerative granulomatous lesion affecting the vulvar region. There is a subcutaneous infiltration of neutrophils, plasma cells, and characteristic large, foamy mononuclear cells that contain in their cytoplasm the encapsulated causative organisms, the Donovan bodies (p. 192).

Lymphogranuloma venereum. Lymphogranuloma venereum is caused by the agent of the ornithosis-LGV group (*Chlamydia* or *Bedsonia*). Ulceration and productive lesions (elephantiasis) involve the vulva, and spread occurs to pararectal lymphatics (p. 194).

HYPERPLASTIC VULVITIS

Hyperplastic vulvitis is characterized by hyperplasia of the squamous epithelium, increased keratin on the surface or hyperkeratosis (sometimes hyperparakeratosis), and nonspecific chronic inflammation in the underlying epidermis. Epithelial hyperactivity may be represented by thickening and elongation of the rete ridges and in some instances by dysplastic changes, e.g., cellular atypism with variation in size of cells and nuclei, hyperchromatic nuclei, and mitotic figures. It has been stated that hyperplastic vulvitis has a tendency to develop into epidermoid carcinoma, although the frequency of this development has been debated.

Clinically, hyperplastic vulvitis is a local or diffuse white lesion of the vulva (sometimes with redness superimposed). The term *leukoplakia* ("white patch") has been used commonly by pathologists as a synonym for this lesion. However, it is more appropriate to use the term in a clinical sense rather than as a histopathologic diagnosis, and it can be applied to a variety of distinct conditions of the vulva that produce white lesions, including *kraurosis* (atrophy and shrinkage) and *lichen sclerosus et atrophicus*.

CARCINOMA

The most important tumor of the vulva is epidermoid carcinoma. It occurs in elderly women, usually after 60 years of age, and is frequently associated with hyperplastic vulvitis. The microscopic features are similar to those of epidermoid carcinoma elsewhere on the skin. Spread of the cancer occurs locally and by the lymphatics. At first there is lymphatic extension to the superficial inguinal nodes, and later there is extension to the deep inguinal, hypogastric, and iliac nodes.

In rare instances, adenocarcinoma arises from Bartholin's gland or from the minor vestibular glands. Some of these tumors have a cylindromatous architecture. Epidermoid carcinoma may arise from a duct of Bartholin's gland.

OTHER TUMORS

Hidradenoma of the vulva is an uncommon benign tumor of apocrine sweat gland origin. The epithelium shows papillary and glandular structures. It is easily mistaken for adenocarcinoma (Fig. 22-31). Also rare are *tumors of the clitoris,* which have a more sarcomatous appearance.

Toxemia of pregnancy

The etiology of the toxemias of pregnancy (eclampsia and preeclampsia) is still uncertain. The main theories are that it is (1) a form of hypertensive cardiovascular renal disease, modified and colored by the metabolic disturbances of pregnancy, (2) an endocrine dysfunction, in which the pituitary gland plays the main part, or (3) the result of a toxic material absorbed from the placenta, particularly from areas of infarction caused by ischemia.

One view (Browne) is that the normal protective enzyme (oxidase of trophoblastic origin) of the placenta becomes ineffective when the placenta is rendered ischemic from any cause and its oxygen tension is lowered. The enzyme normally inactivates excess adrenal cortical pressor hormones produced normally in pregnancy by placental corticotropin secretion and by increased pituitary corticotropin secretion. When the placental inactivating enzyme becomes ineffective, hypertension re-

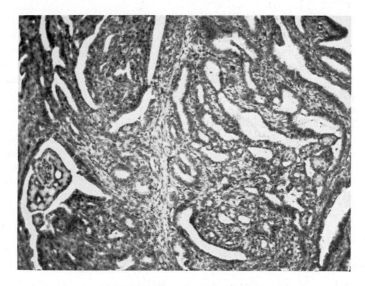

Fig. 22-31. Hidradenoma of vulva.

sults, with the clinical manifestations of pre-eclampsia. Eclampsia, with its characteristic convulsions, appears to be a manifestation of hypertensive encephalopathy.

Lesions are found in the kidneys, liver, placenta, and sometimes other organs. The changes in the kidney have been described (p. 344). Glomerular capillaries frequently show occlusions. Narrowing of capillary loops of glomerular tufts, mainly by subendothelial deposits of electron-dense material of fibrinous nature and swelling of endothelial cells and mesangium, is common. Hyaline droplets may be found in glomerular epithelium. Degenerative changes in convoluted tubules are the usual findings.

The liver may show gross lesions that, although not constantly found, are so characteristic as to be diagnostic. Irregular large and small areas of hemorrhage may be evident on both the capsular and cut surfaces. Areas of hemorrhagic or anemic necrosis are common. Microscopically, there are hemorrhages and necrosis of hepatic cells. These lesions are located particularly in periportal areas, although any part of the liver lobule may be involved. The lesions have been attributed to thrombi in vessels of the portal areas. Diffuse degenera-

tive changes are present in hepatic cells, and sometimes destructive changes are so severe and widespread as to be classed as ''acute yellow atrophy.''

Necrotic and hemorrhagic areas similar to those of the liver are occasionally found in other tissues, such as the adrenal cortex. Areas of infarction very constantly occur in the placenta. The pituitary gland has been described as having increased numbers of basophils that may show hyaline degenerative changes. Basophilic invasion of the posterior lobe of the pituitary gland probably has no significance as far as eclampsia is concerned.

Widespread lesions in the microcirculation may be important in eclampsia, accounting for some of the pathologic changes. Intravascular fibrin deposition in arterioles and capillaries throughout the body (disseminated intravascular coagulation) appears to be responsible for the necrosis and hemorrhages seen in eclampsia and for the uncommon bilateral renal cortical necrosis and pituitary necrosis associated with pregnancy. It has been suggested that the mechanism underlying the fibrin deposition is similar to that in the generalized Schwartzmann reaction.

REFERENCES

Alexander, E. R.: Cancer Res. **33:**1485-1496, 1973 (etiology of cancer of the cervix other than herpesvirus).

American Joint Committee for Cancer Staging and End Results Reporting: Manual for staging of cancer, Chicago, 1977 (cancer of gynecologic sites, pp. 89-100).

Antunes, C. M. F., et al.: N. Engl. J. Med. **300:**9-13, 1979 (endometrial cancer and estrogen use).

Aurelian, L.: Fed. Proc. **31:**1651-1659, 1972 (herpesvirus type 2 and cervical cancer).

Benson, R. C.: Cancer of the female genital tract, ed. 3, 1969, American Cancer Society.

Boivin, Y., and Richart, R. M.: Cancer **18:**231-240, 1965 (hilus cell tumors of ovary).

Bransilver, B. R., et al.: Arch. Pathol. **98:**76-86, 1974 (Brenner tumors and Walthard cell rests).

Browne, F. J.: Lancet **1:**115-119, 1958 (eclampsia).

Caruso, P. A., et al.: Cancer **27:**343-348, 1971 (ovarian teratomas).

Chalvardjian, A., and Scully, R. E.: Cancer **31:**664-670, 1973 (sclerosing stromal tumors of ovary).

Cummings, P. A., and Langley, F. A.: J. Pathol. **110:**167-175, 1973 (nature and origin of Brenner tumor).

Czernobilsky, B.: In Sommers, S. C., and Rosen, P. P., editors: Pathology annual, vol. 12, part 1, New York, 1977, Appleton-Century-Crofts, pp. 201-216 (cystadenofibroma, adenofibroma, and malignant adenofibroma of ovary).

Fine, G. R., et al.: Cancer **31:**398-410, 1973 (mesonephroma of the ovary).

Grady, H. G., and Smith, D. E., editors: The ovary, Baltimore, 1963, The Williams & Wilkins Co.

Gusberg, S. B., and Frick, H. C. III: Corssaden's gynecologic cancer, ed,. 5, Baltimore, 1978, The Williams & Wilkins Co.

Hart, W. R., and Norris, H. J.: Cancer **31:**1031-1045, 1973 (borderline and malignant mucinous tumors of ovary).

Herbst, A. L., et al.: N. Engl. J. Med. **284:**878-881, 1971 (adenocarcinoma of vagina associated with stilbestrol therapy).

Hollingshead, A., et al.: Proc. Soc. Exper. Biol. Med. **141:**688-693, 1972 (reactivity between HSV-2 and cervical tumor cell membrane antigens).

Hurt, W. G., et al.: Am. J. Obstet. Gynecol. **129:**304-315, 1977 (adenocarcinoma of the cervix).

Johnson, L. D., et al.: Cancer **17:**213-229, 1963 (carcinoma in situ of cervix).

Kajii, T., and Ohama, K.: Nature **268:**633-634, 1977 (androgenetic origin of hydatidiform mole).

Kempson, R. L., and Bari, W.: Hum. Pathol. **1:**332-349, 1970 (uterine sarcomas).

Kottmeier, H. L., editor: Annual report on the results of treatment in carcinoma of the uterus and vagina, vol. 16, Stockholm, 1976, International Federation of Gynecology and Obstetrics (staging).

Kreutner, A., Jr., et al.: Fertil. Steril. **27:**905-910, 1976 (endometrium in oral contraceptive users).

Kurman, R. J., and Craig, J. M.: Cancer **29:**1653-1664, 1972 (endometrioid and clear cell carcinoma of the ovary).

Kurman, R. J., and Norris, H. J.: Cancer **37:**1853-1865, 1976 (atypical smooth muscle tumors of the uterus).

Kurman, R. J., and Norris, H. J.: Cancer **38:**2404-2419, 1976 (endodermal sinus tumor of ovary).

Kurman, R. J., and Norris, H. J.: Cancer **38:**2420-2433, 1976 (embryonal carcinoma of ovary).

Lauchlan, S. C.: Cancer **19:**1628-1634, 1966 (Brenner tumors).

Leventhal, M. L.: Am. J. Obstet. Gynecol. **84:**154-164, 1962 (Stein-Leventhal syndrome).

Li, M. C.: Ann. Intern. Med. **74:**102-112, 1971 (trophoblastic disease).

Martzloff, K. H.: Bull. Johns Hopkins Hosp. **34:**141-149, 1923 (carcinoma of cervix uteri).

McAdams, A. J., Jr., and Kistner, R. W.: Cancer **11:**740-747, 1958 (vulva).

Meeker, J. H., et al.: Am. J. Clin. Pathol. **37:**182-195, 1962 (hidradenoma).

Miles, P. A., and Norris, H. J.: Cancer **30:**174-186, 1972 (proliferative and malignant Brenner tumors of the ovary).

Morris, J. L., and Scully, R. E.: Endocrine pathology of the ovary, St. Louis, 1958, The C. V. Mosby Co.

Nahmias, A. J., et al.: Cancer Res. **33:**1491-1497, 1973 (herpesvirus type 2 and cervical anaplasia—prospective study).

Naib, Z. M., et al.: Cancer **23:**940-945, 1969 (genital herpetic infection).

Nelson, J. H.: Recent changes in the international classification of gynecological malignancy. In Seventh National Cancer Conference Proceedings, Philadelphia, 1972, J. B. Lippincott Co., pp. 233-237.

Nelson, J. H., Jr., and Hall, J. E.: CA **20:**150-163, 1970 (dysplasia and early carcinoma of cervix).

Neubecker, R. D., and Breen, J. L.: Cancer **15:**546-556, 1962 (embryonal carcinoma of ovary).

Nogales-Fernandez, F., et al.: Cancer **39:**1462-1474, 1977 (endodermal sinus tumor).

Norris, H. J., and Taylor, H. B.: Cancer **19:**755-766, 1459-1465, 1966 (mesenchymal tumors of uterus).

Norris, H. J., and Taylor H. B.: In Bloodworth, J. M. B.: Endocrine pathology, Baltimore, 1968, The Williams & Wilkins Co., p. 14 (ovaries in endocrine disorders).

Norris, H. J., et al.: Obstet. Gynecol. **28:**57-63, 1966 (mesenchymal tumors of uterus).

Novak, E. R., and Woodruff, J. D.: Gynecologic and obstetric pathology, ed. 8, Philadelphia, 1979, W. B. Saunders Co. (general reference).

Ober, W. B.: In Sommers, C. C., and Rosen, P. P., editors: Pathology annual, vol. 12, part 2, New York, 1977, Appleton-Century-Crofts, pp. 383-410 (experimental toxemia of pregnancy).

Oertel, Y. C.: Arch. Pathol. Lab. Med. **102:**651-654, 1978 (Arias-Stella reaction).

Park, W. W.: In Collins, D. H.: Modern trends in pathology, New York, 1959, Harper & Row, Publishers, Inc., Chap. 10 (disorders of trophoblast).

Rapp, F., and Duff, R.: Cancer Res. **33:**1527-1534, 1973 (transformation of hamster cells by HSV-2).

Reagan, J. W.: Am. J. Clin. Pathol. **62:**150-164, 1974 (cellular pathology and uterine cancer).

Riotton, G., and Christopherson, W. M., in collaboration with Lunt, R.: Cytology of the female genital tract, Geneva, 1973, World Health Organization.

Robboy, S. J., et al.: Cancer **34:**606-614, 1974 (clear cell adenocarcinoma of vagina and cervix in young females).

Robboy, S. J., et al.: Arch. Pathol. Lab. Med. **101:**1-5, 1977 (intrauterine DES exposure—Registry of Clear Cell Adenocarcinoma of Genital Tract).

Roth, L. M., and Hornback, N. B.: Cancer **34:**1761-1768, 1974 (clear cell adenocarcinoma of the cervix in young women).

Rywlin, A. M., et al.: Cancer **17:**100-104, 1964 (clear cell leiomyoma).

Sawin, C. T.: The hormones; endocrine physiology, Boston, 1969, Little, Brown & Co.

Scully, R. E.: Cancer **17:**769-778, 1964 (stromal luteoma of ovary).

Scully, R. E.: Hum. Pathol. **1:**73-98, 1970 (recent progress in ovarian cancer).

Scully, R. E.: Am. J. Pathol. **87:**685-720, 1977 (ovarian tumors—a review).

Semmens, J. P.: Obstet. Gynecol. **19:**328-350, 1962 (congenital anomalies).

Serov, S. F., and Scully, R. E., in collaboration with Sobin, L. H.: Histologic typing of ovarian tumors, Geneva, 1973, World Health Organization.

Silverberg, S. G., et al.: Cancer **39:**592-598, 1977 (endometrial carcinoma in oral contraceptive users and nonusers).

Spiro, R. H., and McPeak, C. J.: Cancer **19:**544-548, 1966 (metastasizing leiomyoma).

Sternberg, W. H., and Roth, L. M.: Cancer **32:**940-951, 1973 (Leydig cell tumors).

Taft, P. D., et al.: Acta Cytol. **18:**279-290, 1974 (cytology of clear cell adenocarcinoma of genital tract).

Teilum, G.: Cancer **11:**769-782, 1958 (testicular and ovarian neoplasms).

Teilum, G.: Cancer **12:**1092-1105, 1959 (mesonephric tumors).

Tweeddale, D. N., and Pederson, B. L.: Am. J. Med. Sci. **249:**701-717, 1965 (serous neoplasms of ovary).

Wentz, W. B., and Reagan, J. W.: Cancer **12:**384-388, 1959 (grading of cervical cancer).

Yoonessi, M., and Hart, W. R.: Cancer 40:898-906, 1977 (endometrial stromal sarcoma).

23

Breast

The breasts have their origin from skin similar to that of other cutaneous glands and are regarded as modified sweat glands. The breast of a woman is composed of multiple subdivisions, or lobes, separated from each other by septa consisting of dense fibrous tissue admixed with adipose tissue. Each lobe is drained by a duct that emerges at the nipple as an independent opening. Each of these ducts branches and rebranches as it extends inwardly. The terminal buddings, which develop into acini during pregnancy and lactation, and their surrounding stroma constitute the lobular subdivisions of the lobes. The specialized connective tissue of the lobules (intralobular stroma) is a loose reticular or myxomatous type and is sharply defined from the more dense collagenous interlobular fibrous tissue that is admixed with adipose tissue. In the terminal branching duct system, there is a layer of flattened cells beneath the lining epithelium, the so-called myoepithelial cells.

During fetal development and until about 4 months after birth, the breast develops a duct system of 15 to 25 branching epithelial channels. Quiescence then follows until puberty, when there is renewed growth of the ducts. This developmental period is transient in males and is followed by quiescence and involution. In females, the ductal development continues during adolescence and is accompanied by increase in the surrounding fibrous and fatty tissue and by development of buds of cells at the ends of the tubules or ducts. Aci-

narlike structures differentiate from these buds under hormonal stimulation as sexual maturity is reached. With the occurrence of pregnancy and lactation, there is maximum acinar development, and the acini show secretory activity. Mild cyclic changes involving hyperplasia followed by involution occur with each menstrual cycle. In the latter part of the cycle, some epithelial hyperplasia is noted, along with an increase in the specialized intralobular stroma that becomes edematous. After the onset of menstruation, these changes regress, and desquamation of epithelial cells and lymphocytic infiltration of the intralobular stroma are seen.

The normal development of the breast at puberty is related to an increase of estrogen in the circulation. Also, during pregnancy, estrogen plays a prominent role in the development of the ductal portion of the glandular tissue, whereas progesterone is chiefly responsible for acinar development. Prolactin (LTH) and/or growth hormone act synergistically with estrogen and progesterone to bring about full development of the breast during pregnancy. Other hormones, such as thyroxine, hydrocortisone, and insulin, appear to be necessary also for full differentiation of the mammary epithelium. Lactation is initiated by prolactin, the secretion of which increases as the circulating levels of placental estrogen and progesterone are diminished following parturition. Hydrocortisone secretion, which is increased at this time, may be contributory. The dense glandular structure (Fig. 23-1) and hy-

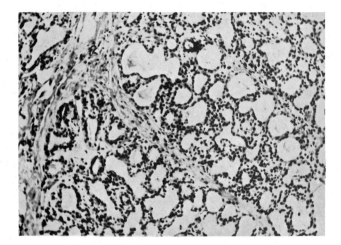

Fig. 23-1. Lactating breast.

peractive epithelium of the breast during pregnancy and lactation are a revelation of the power of physiologic hormonal stimulation. After menopause, involutionary changes occur, with dense connective tissue gradually replacing the glandular tissue and the breasts decreasing in size.

Pathologic changes in the breast consist of disturbances of the cyclic (hormonal) activity, the irritant effects of retained secretions, acute and chronic infections, and tumors.

HYPERTROPHY

Excessive development of the breasts is usually associated with endocrine disturbances. Hypertrophy in the male (gynecomastia), for example, may be associated with some of the tumors of the testis and less often with tumors of the adrenal cortex or pituitary gland. Precocious puberty in female children usually has an associated excessive mammary growth and is found with granulosa cell and theca cell tumors of the ovary, adrenal cortical disturbances, and certain destructive lesions of the hypothalamus. Overgrowth of the breasts during adolescence (virginal hypertrophy) or during pregnancy (gravid hypertrophy) appears to be an excessive response to hormonal stimuli

on the part of abnormally sensitive mammary tissue.

Gynecomastia. Gynecomastia is an enlargement of the breast tissue of males that usually is caused by proliferation of connective tissue and ducts. The lesion may be unilateral or bilateral. Gynecomastia occurs not uncommonly during normal puberty and adolescence without a known cause, but it is usually self-limited and disappears within a few months. Transitory hypertrophy of the breast of unknown cause also appears in old men, although decreased androgenic hormone influence has been considered an etiologic factor. In other instances, gynecomastia is associated with hormone-producing lesions, such as testicular tumors and adrenal cortical hyperplasia and neoplasms. Hepatic disease (cirrhosis), dietary deficiency, and estrogen therapy (e.g., for prostatic carcinoma) may result in gynecomastia. Certain developmental anomalies of the genital tract, as in Klinefelter's syndrome, also may be associated with gynecomastia. Certain drugs, other than hormonal substances, may cause gynecomastia, e.g., digitalis glycosides, spironolactone, and tricyclic compounds (antidepressants). Gynecomastia does not predispose to tumor formation. Pseudogynecomastia is an enlargement of the mammary regions caused by the deposition of fat.

MAMMARY DYSPLASIA

Mammary dysplasia is characterized by varying degrees of proliferative change in the epithelium and connective tissue of the breast, often with cystic dilatation of the ducts. The term *chronic cystic mastitis,* although commonly used, has evident defects in that the condition is not a chronic inflammation in the usual sense and is not always cystic. The following terms referring to various phases or forms of this condition may be encountered: fibrocystic disease, fibrocystic mastitis, cystic hyperplasia, chronic cystic mastopathia, Schimmelbusch's disease, mazoplasia, cystipherous desquamative hyperplasia, cystoplasia, cystic disease of the breast, adenosis of the breast, and adenofibrosis.

Mammary dysplasia appears to result from an imbalance of hormones (estrogen and progesterone) influencing the breasts or an irregular and abnormal response of the breast tissue to those endocrine influences. The irritative effects of retained secretions and desquamated material have been considered another causative factor.

Mild degrees of the conditon are very common, being usually a tender or painful area of breast tissue of increased density. The pain and swelling may be mainly premenstrual and caused by vascular engorgement. In such cases, there may be *lobular fibrosis* and relatively little epithelial activity. In more severe cases, the affected area is diffusely nodular or "shotty." Such nodularity is mainly caused by epithelial hyperplasia, fibrosis, and microscopic cyst formation, and this lesion has been referred to as *adenosis* and *adenofibrosis*. In a more advanced lesion, one or more large cysts may result from secretory changes *(cystic* or *fibrocystic disease)*. Firm, freely movable masses varying in size are sometimes palpable. When the nodularity is not diffuse, the condition must be distinguished from carcinoma. The age of greatest incidence is between 35 and 45 years.

The three forms of mammary dysplasia are described separately, but mixtures of these may occur in a single lesion.

Lobular fibrosis. The form of mammary dysplasia that is associated with a minimal degree of change is lobular fibrosis. It is characterized clinically by periodic swelling, discomfort, and fine nodularity of the breast. Microscopically, there is intralobular fibrosis that merges with the connective tissue stroma of the breast. Lobular ducts may be dilated, but there is no cyst formation. The condition has no etiologic relationship to carcinoma and should be sharply distinguished from cystic (fibrocystic) disease of the breast.

Adenosis. In adenosis, epithelial hyperplasia is a prominent feature. There is proliferation of small ducts, some of which may be dilated and microcystic. Hyperplastic epithelium usually lines the proliferating ductules, forming several layers of cells and sometimes small papillomas. Proliferation of myoepithelial cells may contribute to the epithelial hyperplasia. This type of cell proliferation may also be seen in cases of cystic disease. Intralobular fibrosis frequently occurs in adenosis, causing compression and distortion of the proliferating epithelial masses. Such a lesion, known as *adenofibrosis* or *sclerosing adenosis,* may be misinterpreted as carcinoma. The dominant overgrowth of hyalinizing connective tissue produces variability in the shape and pattern of the epithelial cells by constricting them. Thin isolated epithelial columns result, and microscopically there is a simulation of invasiveness and pleomorphism. However, in this benign lesion, mitoses are absent except in the florid stage, and nuclear staining is regular. Electron microscopic studies in sclerosing adenosis show that the cells resemble those of the normal mammary gland, possessing intact basement membranes, evidence of secretory activity, well-formed mitochondria, etc. On electron microscopy, infiltrating duct carcinoma cells lack intact basement membranes and other structural refinements.

Cystic disease. The gross appearance of this common form of mammary dysplasia is often distinguished by the presence of cysts. Involved areas are grayish, of rubbery consistency, and not sharply outlined. The cysts may be of varying size and number, but they are not always grossly visible. The colorless content of the cysts shining through their tense, translucent walls gives them a bluish color (blue-domed cysts). Occasionally, the contents of the cysts are brown or yellow from altered blood pigment. The cut ends of dilated ducts may release casts of grayish desquamated material.

The microscopic features consist of (1) epithelial changes, (2) cyst formation, (3) fibrous hyperplasia, and (4) lymphocytic infiltration. These features exist in varying combinations and proportions and some may be entirely absent. The cysts, which vary from microscopic size to several centimeters in diameter, are believed to be dilated ducts rather than glands. They are lined by a single layer of flattened or cuboidal epithelium.

Hyperplastic epithelial changes may be present in ducts and glands. Solid buds of epithelial cells may be formed, or localized proliferations of the lining of ducts cause irregular papillary projections into the lumen. Bridges of epithelial cells may unite opposite walls, or the lumen may be completely filled by the proliferative epithelium. Sometimes, the hyperplastic epithelial cells are large, clear, or eosinophilic and of a type suggesting apocrine sweat gland epithelium. Irregular atrophic changes may be present in the epithelium instead of hyperplasia. In those cases in which intraductal proliferation is great and papillary masses fill the lumen (intraductal papillomatosis) or solid epithelial overgrowth occludes ducts, differentiation from carcinoma may be difficult. Such distinction must be based on the histologic character of the cells and the presence or absence of invasion beyond the ductal basal membrane.

Fibrous hyperplasia with increase in connective tissue stroma is usual, and occasionally the stromal overgrowth is great enough to simulate the appearance of a fibroadenoma. Infiltration of lymphocytes in the stroma is a common but inconstant finding. Their presence originally suggested that the condition was of an inflammatory nature, but they are now known to be part of the involutionary phase of cyclic activity.

Relationship to carcinoma. The relationship of cystic or fibrocystic disease to carcinoma has been a greatly debated point and obviously is of importance. That it is not precancerous and that it causes no great likelihood of malignant change has been the view of some investigators. At the other extreme, it is considered that at least 20% of breast carcinomas have passed through a type of chronic cystic mastopathy. Whether or not chronic cystic mastopathy should be considered a truly precancerous lesion, several statistical studies have shown that it is associated with a definitely greater likelihood of development of breast cancer. The incidence of carcinoma in women with cystic disease has been reported to be about three to five times that of the general female population. Some authors report prominent epithelial hyperplasia as a finding that has a significant frequency relationship to subsequent carcinoma of the breast.

GALACTOCELE

Galactocele is a cyst containing milk that results from a duct obstruction during lactation. It is a rare lesion.

FAT NECROSIS

The uncommon condition of fat necrosis in the breast is usually the result of trauma. The necrotic areas are opaque and are grayish yellow or chalky in appearance. The microscopic appearance is characterized by areas of necrosis, leukocytic infiltration, lipid-containing histiocytes, and multinucleated foreign body giant cells. Fibrosis may occur in older lesions, causing a hardness and fixation that may lead clinically to a mistaken diagnosis of cancer.

MASTITIS AND ABSCESS

Acute infection in the breast is most commonly caused by staphylococci or streptococci that gain entrance via a cracked nipple during the period of lactation. By one of the main ducts, spread occurs into the breast substance, where a localized *abscess* forms.

Chronic periductal or *plasma cell mastitis* is an inflammation in and about larger ducts near the nipple, usually found in older women near menopausal age. It may simulate carcinoma on gross examination. The disease is associated with dilatation of ducts filled with inspissated, lipid-containing secretion *(duct ectasia)*. Escape of the contents of the ducts into the periductal tissue is believed to cause the inflammatory response, consisting of many plasma cells, lymphocytes, and macrophages.

Tuberculous mastitis, secondary to tuberculosis elsewhere in the body, is a rare lesion today.

TUMORS

The breast tumors may be classified as follows (the malignant category being modified from Foote and Stewart*):

Benign
Epithelial
  Papilloma
Mixed epithelial and mesenchymal
  Fibroadenoma
    Intracanalicular
    Pericanalicular
    ''Adenoma''
Mesenchymal—breast tumors only by location in mammary gland and in no way distinctive—viz., lipoma, angioma, fibroma, myoma
Malignant
Mammary ducts
  Noninfiltrating tumors
    Papillary carcinoma (intraductal)
    Comedocarcinoma (intraductal)
  Infiltrating carcinoma
    Paget's disease
    Papillary carcinoma
    Comedocarcinoma
    Carcinoma with productive fibrosis (scirrhous, simplex)
    Medullary carcinoma
    Colloid carcinoma
Mammary lobules
  Noninfiltrating—in situ lobular carcinoma
  Infiltrating—lobular adenocarcinoma
Epithelial or mesenchymal origins such as tumors of skin, skin appendages, and supporting tissues

---
*Modified from Foote, F. W., Jr., and Stewart, F. W.: Surgery **19:**74-99, 1946.

of breast; are same as found elsewhere in body—sweat gland tumors, basal or squamous cell carcinoma of skin, liposarcoma, malignant lymphoma, etc.

Benign tumors

Fibroadenoma. Fibroadenomas are compound epithelial and connective tissue tumors in which growth of fibrous tissue is associated with hyperplasia of glandular cells. There are two types: pericanalicular, in which fibrous overgrowth surrounds the glandular spaces, and intracanalicular, in which proliferated connective tissue projects into the ducts as polypoid masses. Fibroadenoma of the breast is not a precancerous lesion. Its occurrence does not increase the chances of carcinoma developing in the breast. Only rarely is carcinoma reported as arising in a fibroadenoma.

The fibroadenomas are firm, lobulated, encapsulated tumors that are easily movable in the breast and usually remain quite small. Microscopically, the pericanalicular form shows great proliferation of connective tissue around the acini, so that each tubule appears to be surrounded by a ring of fibrous tissue. In the intracanalicular form, a more diffuse growth of the connective tissue draws out and distorts the acini, so that polypoid masses of connective tissue covered by a layer of epithelium project into the lumen (Fig. 23-2). If the pedicles of these masses are not included in the section, the duct lumina appear to be filled with rounded masses of connective tissue covered by a layer of epithelium. The connective tissue component of a fibroadenoma is usually loose and myxomatous in appearance. Occasionally, the epithelial component of a fibroadenoma is so prominent that the lesion is regarded as an *adenoma.*

Cystosarcoma phyllodes (giant mammary myxoma) is a very large bulky tumor of slow growth derived from a fibroadenoma. Grossly, it has a cauliflowerlike appearance, with multiple frondlike masses or cystic spaces into which project polypoid masses. Microscopically, myxomatous connective tissue is the predominant feature, forming polypoid masses covered by a layer of epithelium. Although

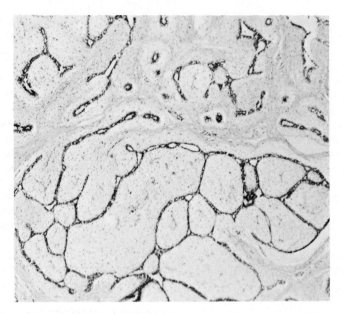

Fig. 23-2. Fibroadenoma of breast showing mainly intracanalicular pattern and areas of pericanalicular pattern.

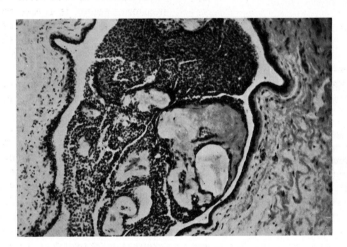

Fig. 23-3. Intraductal papilloma of breast.

generally benign in nature and successfully treated by wide local excision, malignant (sarcomatous) variants have been described. They appear to be sarcomas that develop in the fibroepithelial tumors, but only the mesenchymatous elements appear to be malignant and are found in metastases.

Duct papilloma. Duct papilloma (adenocytoma; intracystic papilloma) is a papillary epithelial tumor that projects into a dilated duct, often quite close to the nipple (Fig. 23-3). It occurs most commonly in the fourth or fifth decade and is often multiple. The tumor may or may not be palpable clinically, but discharge from the nipple, often bloody, is a common symptom. Grossly, the papilloma forms a soft arborescent papillary growth, projecting into a cystic space that contains a clear or hemorrhagic fluid.

Three microscopic forms are sometimes differentiated: fibrous, glandular, and transitional. The fibrous type consists of ramifying stalks of connective tissue covered by epithelium that project into the dilated duct. Fusion of the stalks results in pseudoglandular structures. The glandular type shows hyperplastic or adenomatous acini invaginated into a duct or cyst. The fibrous and glandular types are benign. The transitional cell type resembles in appearance a papilloma of the bladder. Although histologically benign, there is greater danger of carcinoma developing on the basis of this transitional cell type.

Malignancy in an intracystic papillary tumor is suggested by great variation in size, shape, and staining of cells and their nuclei, frequent mitoses, and invasion. Penetration of the basement membrane and invasion of stroma are the most important indications of malignancy (p. 677).

Cancer

The breast is the most common site of carcinoma in women but rare as a site in males. *In women,* carcinoma of the breast may occur at any adult age but is most common between 40 and 60 years of age. As in other carcinomas, the *etiology* is incompletely known. Certain factors, however, have been considered. Among these are hereditary predisposition, hormonal influence, oncogenic viruses, and irradiation. The role of *heredity* is suggested by the observation that breast cancer occurs more frequently in women with a family history of the disease than in the general population. The influence of *hormones* is suggested by other observations: (1) production of mammary cancer in experimental animals by administration of estrogen, (2) tendency for breast cancer to develop in single women, infertile married women, and late married women (possible role of unopposed estrogen activity during a long reproductive life span),

(3) lower risk of breast cancer among fertile women (one suggestion being that multiple pregnancies interrupt the ovarian cycle, causing less exposure to estrogens), (4) association of mammary carcinoma in postmenopausal women with ovarian cortical hyperplasia or endocrine tumors that produce estrogens, and (5) regression of advanced cancer of the breast in some premenopausal women following ovariectomy. The relationship of fibrocystic disease of the breast to cancer has been discussed previously (p. 670). This lesion appears to predispose to carcinoma of the breast, but there is no certain way of determining which case will develop a malignant tumor and which will not.

It has been hypothesized that the urinary estrogen profile in women is the determinant of their breast cancer risk. The estrogens that are measured in the urine are estrone, estradiol, and estriol. According to certain studies, it appears that there is an inverse relationship between the risk of breast cancer and the proportion of *estriol* in the urinary estrogens. Certain studies have shown that Japanese and Chinese women living in the Orient, who have a lower breast cancer risk than North Americans, excrete a much higher proportion of their estrogen as estriol. One may speculate that the lower incidence of breast cancer among Orientals is a result of a protective effect of estriol against neoplastic transformation in the mammary tissue; however, the possible role of other factors (e.g., genetic and environmental) cannot be excluded. The hypothesis regarding the protective effect of a high estriol ratio (i.e., estriol/estrone plus estradiol) was supported, in part, by experimental evidence that estriol did not produce mammary tumors in rodents in contrast to estrone and estradiol, which did. However, this hypothesis has been challenged in other reports, and more recently some investigators have reported that under certain conditions estriol can induce mammary cancer in mice.

Viruses are known to be associated with mammary tumors in animals, but definite evidence of a viral cause in human breast cancer is not available yet, although there are reports of RNA virus–like particles being identified in breast milk and in some tissue specimens of breast cancer in human patients. A possible relationship between *ionizing radiation* and carcinoma of the breast has been suggested (p. 261).

Carcinomas occur most commonly in the upper outer quadrant of the breast and least frequently in the inner lower quadrant. In a relatively small group of patients, carcinoma occurs simultaneously in both breasts. Sometimes, cancer in one breast is followed by cancer in the opposite breast. In the latter instance, it is not always possible to determine whether the second cancer is another primary tumor or a metastatic lesion from the other breast.

Classification of breast carcinoma into the various anatomic and histologic types is a useful procedure, since the morphologic type is one of the factors that is considered in determining prognosis. Such classifications cannot always be strict, however, for different portions of the tumor may show a different condition. Likewise, the degree of differentiation of the tumor cells (in size, shape, arrangement, and staining) also indicates the degree of malignancy. In prognosis, however, such anatomic considerations are only one factor to be considered in conjunction with the size of the tumor, the presence or absence of metastases, the age and condition of the patient, pregnancy, etc. Methods of classification that combine histologic grading and clinical staging (degree of progression or spread) appear most useful for prognosis. The presence of plasma cells and histiocytes in adjacent axillary lymph nodes, considered to be evidence of resistance to spread of the tumor, has been related to better prognosis.

Carcinoma of the male breast accounts for less than 1% of breast cancers. As in women, it is found at an average age of about 56 years, it occasionally is bilateral, and a history of trauma is not usually found. It is most often an infiltrating duct carcinoma. Gynecomastia is not in itself a precursor, but some reported cases of cancer have followed prolonged massive therapy with female hormones, which also may cause the develop-

ment of gynecomastia. Orchiectomy has been effective in some cases in producing remissions, particularly in the presence of bone metastases. The prognosis generally is worse than in carcinoma of the female breast. This is due partly to the fact that the vast majority of lesions in males occur beneath the nipple area, from which there is a greater tendency for metastasis to internal mammary lymph nodes, whereas in women carcinoma tends to occur more frequently in the upper outer quadrant.

Scirrhous carcinoma. Scirrhous carcinoma forms a hard nodule that occurs most frequently in the upper outer quadrant of the breast. The tumor is not encapsulated and soon becomes adherent to skin or deep fascia. The cut surface is composed of a hard, gritty, grayish, translucent tissue, with occasional opaque, yellowish areas of necrosis (Fig. 23-4). There is no definite margin, but irregular lines of fibrous tissue radiate into the surrounding tissue.

Microscopically, there are thin masses and columns of epithelial cells separated by an abundant dense fibrous stroma (Fig. 23-5). The columns may be one cell layer in width ("single filing" phenomenon). Gland formation is slight. Mitoses are infrequent.

Scirrhous carcinoma tends to progress more slowly than the medullary type and has less tendency to ulcerate or form a bulky tumor but has a poorer prognosis. The origin of scirrhous carcinoma generally is believed to be ductal epithelium. In a recent histochemical and electron microscopic study, however, one investigator considers the cell of origin to be myoepithelial, in contrast to the medullary carcinoma, which originates from ductal epithelial cells.

Medullary carcinoma. Medullary carcinoma forms a soft massive tumor of relatively rapid growth that tends to ulcerate and form a fungating mass on the surface (Fig. 23-6). Microscopically, it shows masses of malignant epithelial cells separated by a scanty stroma, which sometimes is infiltrated by lymphocytes. There is often some tendency to gland formation. Medullary carcinoma has a better prognosis than scirrhous carcinoma.

Intraductal carcinoma. Intraductal carci-

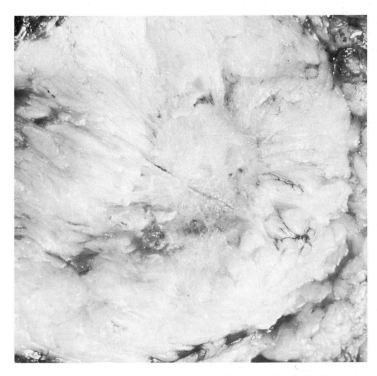

Fig. 23-4. Scirrhous carcinoma of breast. (Courtesy Dr. J. F. Kuzma.)

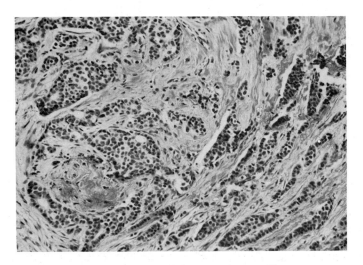

Fig. 23-5. Infiltrating scirrhous carcinoma of breast.

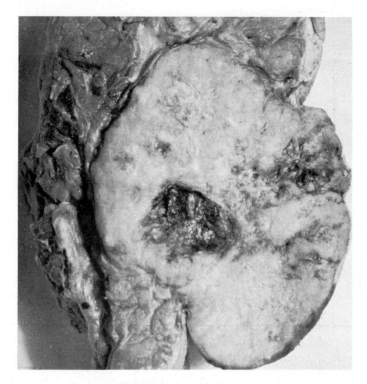

Fig. 23-6. Medullary carcinoma of breast.

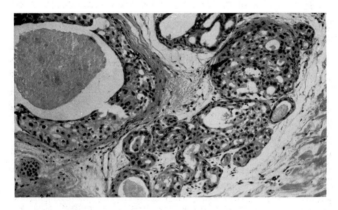

Fig. 23-7. Intraductal carcinoma of breast.

noma includes two types of tumors: (1) *malignant papillary tumors,* arising from ducts and sometimes representing a malignant change in a duct papilloma, and (2) *comedocarcinoma,* so called because on the cut surface, plugs of tumor cells may be expressed from ducts, giving an appearance similar to that when sebum is expressed from a comedo. In comedocarcinoma, dark-staining oval cells proliferate within the ducts, forming neoplastic masses

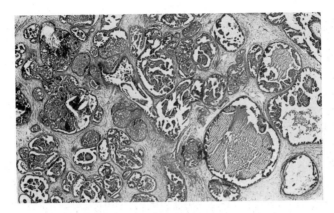

Fig. 23-8. Intraductal papillary carcinoma of breast.

that tend to fill the lumen but often have necrotic centers consisting of granular amorphous debris (Fig. 23-7). The tumor cells grow diffusely along ducts and for a long time remain within the ducts, so that evidence of invasion may be absent. Comedocarcinoma grows slowly, metastasizes late, and has a relatively favorable prognosis.

Papillary carcinomas, particularly if well differentiated, may be difficult to differentiate from benign intraductal papillomas. Features distinguishing a papillary carcinoma are a single type of epithelial cell covering the papillary projections, nuclear hyperchromatism, a cribriform glandular pattern, a delicate or absent connective tissue stroma, epithelial invasion of stroma, intraductal carcinoma in adjacent ducts, and usually absence of sclerosing adenosis in adjacent breast tissue (Fig. 23-8). Subsequently, the intraductal carcinomas invade the stroma of the breast beyond the ducts (infiltrating types).

Mucinous (colloid) carcinoma. Mucin-producing carcinoma of the breast is an infrequent tumor that remains small for a long period, is likely to cause protrusion and enlargement of the nipple, and has a cystic character on palpation. The mucoid nature is evidenced grossly in the tumor by a gray, translucent appearance that may be diffuse throughout or involve only a portion of the tumor. When the gelatinous change occurs in a papillary carci-

noma, the change is likely to be diffuse. Those tumors showing partial mucin-producing change are usually of the scirrhous type. The mucinous material is secreted by the tumor cells, which, by electron micrographic study, show elaborate organelle structure. Microscopically, there are nests of tumor cells surrounded by loose stroma distended with mucoid material (Fig. 23-9). The survival rate of patients with mucin-producing carcinomas is better than that associated with the more common infiltrating duct or scirrhous carcinomas.

Inflammatory carcinoma. In occasional cases, signs of inflammation in the breast (edema, redness, and heat) may arise simultaneously with the development of a breast cancer or after a tumor has been present for some time. The inflammatory signs are caused by lymphatic blockage and congestion caused by cancer cells. The cancer cells grow in lymphatic spaces and veins and disseminate rapidly throughout the breast, and tumor nodules appear in the skin. Such ''inflammatory'' or ''acute'' carcinomas progress rapidly and have a poor prognosis.

Lobular carcinoma. Lobular carcinoma is believed to arise from the epithelium within terminal ramifications of the intralobular ducts. *In situ lobular carcinoma,* a preinvasive form of breast cancer, produces a proliferative pattern in one or more lobules without

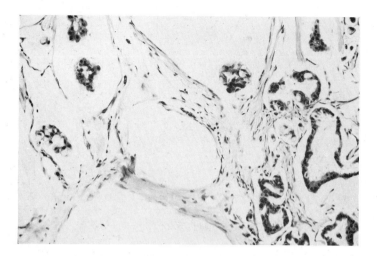

Fig. 23-9. Mucinous (colloid) carcinoma of breast.

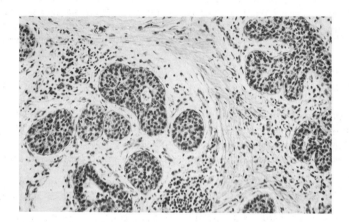

Fig. 23-10. Lobular carcinoma of breast.

forming a distinct tumor mass. The neoplastic epithelial cells fill the lumina of the small terminal ducts and distend them, but the general pattern of the lobule usually is maintained (Fig. 23-10). At times, however, the terminal ductules, filled with tumor cells, are closely packed together with minimal intervening stroma (lobular confluence). The proliferating cells may be fairly regular and normal in appearance, or they may be larger and variable in size and shape, with some hyperchromatism and occasional mitoses. An *infiltrating lobular*

carcinoma also has been described that somewhat resembles carcinoma of the scirrhous type.

Paget's disease of nipple. Paget's disease presents as a chronic eczematous lesion of the nipple, often with extension to adjacent skin of the breast, and is associated with a duct carcinoma in the underlying breast. Section of the involved skin shows characteristic clear, hydropic "Paget" cells in the epidermis. The exact relationship of the epidermal change to the underlying duct cancer has been a matter of debate. The Paget cells have been considered by some as degenerated epidermal cells, possibly melanocytes, and interpreted by others as tumor cells arising from the underlying duct cancer. The latter view seems to be the most prevalent. The carcinoma associated with Paget's disease of the nipple has a relatively higher age incidence than the usual forms of carcinoma of the breast.

A similar epidermal change in other parts of the body (extramammary Paget's disease) occurs in the axillary or anogenital regions, associated with a tumor of an underlying apocrine gland. Paget's disease of the nipple may be simulated clinically in the presence of a benign adenoma of the nipple, which histologically may resemble a sweat gland adenoma.

Sarcoma. Sarcoma is an uncommon tumor of the breast. It may arise from the connective tissue stroma, from a preexisting fibroadenoma, from fat, or from underlying muscle tissue.

Adenofibrosarcoma, which represents a malignant form of adenofibroma, is the most frequent type. The malignant transformation of the connective tissue is accompanied by benign epithelial elements. The tumor tends to remain circumscribed until a considerable size is reached, but there is a distinct tendency to recurrence after local removal. Eventually, it may metastasize. This lesion has also been termed *adenosarcoma* and *malignant cystosarcoma phyllodes* (p. 671).

Primary sarcomas do not originate in fibroadenomas but in the mesenchymal elements of the breast itself. They have no epithelial components. Various types have been described, including fibrosarcoma, myxosarcoma, liposarcoma, myosarcoma, angiosarcoma, osteosarcoma (presumably following metaplasia of fibroblasts), and malignant lymphomas.

Carcinosarcomas are rare cancers of the breast in which both carcinomatous and sarcomatous elements occur. They appear to be carcinomas in which the stroma has undergone sarcomatous change.

Spread. Direct invasion and metastasis by the lymphatics and the bloodstream are all-important in breast cancer. Scirrhous carcinoma particularly tends to invade adjacent tissues and often involves pectoral muscles. Spread by the lymphatics may be by direct growth along the channels (lymphatic permeation) or, more commonly, by tumor emboli. Lymphatic spread to the axillary nodes is most common, but occasionally there is early involvement of the mediastinal nodes. Spread to the supraclavicular nodes is usually a late feature. Spread to the opposite breast may occur. Pleural and lung involvement may be by direct extension through the pectoral fascia to subpleural lymphatics, or it may be from mediastinal nodes. Spread by the bloodstream gives rise to metastases in the lungs, bones, adrenal glands, brain, ovaries, and liver.

Lymphangiosarcoma may complicate chronic edema of an arm after mastectomy for cancer of the breast, although metastases in the edematous tissue from the original carcinoma also may occur and may simulate such tumors.

REFERENCES

Bloom, H. J. G., et al.: Br. Med. J. **2**:213-221, 1962 (breast cancer—natural history).

Buzanowski, K., et al.: Cancer **35**:450-456, 1975 (carcinoma arising in fibroadenoma of breast).

Chrichlow, R. W., et al.: Ann. Surg. **175**:489-494, 1972 (male mammary cancer).

Davis, H. H., et al.: Cancer **17**:957-978, 1964 (cystic disease and cancer).

Dickinson, L. E., et al.: N. Engl. J. Med. **291**:1211-1213, 1974 (estrogen profiles of Oriental and white women).

Fisher, E. R.: Am. J. Clin. Pathol. **66**:291-375, 1976 (ultrastructure of human breast and its disorders).

Fishman, J., et al.: Cancer Res. **38**:4006-4011, 1978 (plasma hormone profiles and breast cancer).

Haagensen, C. D.: Clin. Obstet. Gynecol. **5**:1093-1101, 1962 (lobular carcinoma).

Haagensen, C. D.: Diseases of the breast, ed. 2, Philadelphia, 1971, W. B. Saunders Co.

Halverson, J. D., and Hori-Rubaina, J. M.: Am. Surg. **40**:295-301, 1974 (cystosarcoma phyllodes of the breast).

Handley, R. S., and Thackray, A. C.: Br. J. Cancer **16**:187-194, 1962 (adenoma of nipple).

Hussey, H. H.: J.A.M.A. **228**:1423, 1974 (gynecomastia).

Jenson, E. V.: N. Engl. J. Med. **291**:1252-1254, 1974 (newer endocrine aspects of breast cancer).

Karsner, H. T.: Am. J. Pathol. **22**:235-315, 1946 (gynecomastia).

Kraus, F. T., and Neubecker, R. D.: Cancer **15**:444-455, 1962 (papillary carcinoma).

Leis, H. F.: CA **27**:209-232, 1977 (breast cancer).

Longscope, C., and Pratt, J. H.; Cancer Res. **38**:4025-4028, 1978 (plasma and urine estrogen ratios).

McDivitt, R. W., Stewart, F. W., and Berg, J. W.: Tumors of the breast. In Atlas of Tumor Pathology, Series 2, Fasc. 2, Washington, D.C., 1968, Armed Forces Institute of Pathology.

Morreal, C. E., et al.: J. Natl. Cancer Inst. **63**:1171-1174, 1979 (urinary excretion of estrogens in postmenopausal women with breast cancer).

Murad, T. M.: Cancer **27**:288-299, 1971 (histochemical and electron microscopic classification of breast cancer).

Norris, H. J., and Taylor H. B.: Cancer **23**:1428-1435, 1969 (carcinoma of male breast).

Oberman, H. A.: Cancer **18**:697-710, 1965 (cystosarcoma phyllodes).

Orr, J. W., and Parish, D. J.: J. Pathol. Bacteriol. **84**:201-208, 1962 (Paget's disease).

Report and Commentary: The carcinogenic hazard of radiation to the breasts, CA **20**(1):24-31, 1970.

Richter, G. O., et al.: Cancer **20**:363-370, 1967 (scirrhous carcinoma of breast).

Rudali, G., et al.: Eur. J. Cancer **11**:39-44, 1975 (mammary cancer produced in mice with estriol).

Sandison, A. T.: An autopsy study of the adult human breast, National Cancer Institute Mongraph No. 8, Washington, D.C., 1961, U.S. Health Service.

Schlom, J., and Spiegelman, S.: Am. J. Clin. Pathol. **60**:44-56, 1973 (virus involvement in murine and human mammary carcinoma).

Wellings, S. R., and Roberts, P.: J. Natl. Cancer Inst. **30**:269-287, 1963 (electron microscopy—sclerosing adenosis and duct carcinoma).

Wolff, B.: Br. J. Cancer **20**:36-40, 1966 (histologic grading of carcinoma of breast).

24

Skin

The general principles of inflammations, infections, and neoplasms apply to the skin as elsewhere in the body, modified in some instances by the position and structure of the skin.

STRUCTURE

The skin is composed of two main layers, the epidermis and the dermis (corium). The *epidermis,* or outer portion, has a well-defined basal layer of columnar cells next to the corium that dip down between papillae of the corium to form interpapillary processes. The cells of the basal layer undergo a gradual change to the flattened, resistant, cornified squamous cells found on the surface. In the malpighian layer of the epidermis, the prickle cells have prominent fingerlike process (desmosomes or ''spines'') that adhere to those of adjacent cells, forming the so-called intercellular bridges. The outer cornified layer of epidermis may undergo excessive growth (hyperkeratosis), be imperfectly cornified (parakeratosis), undergo degeneration or abnormal cornification (dyskeratosis), or be atrophic with diminished cornification. Tumors arising from epidermal cells are common. Inflammatory lesions involving epidermis frequently produce vesicles and bullae (edema), pustules, and ulcers.

Small masses of ''sex'' chromatin may be identified in the nuclei of epidermal or buccal epithelial cells—Barr body in females and the Y body in males (p. 5). Sex determination from skin biopsy or buccal smear by this method may be useful in pseudohermaphroditism.

The *corium,* or *dermis,* is the inner layer of the skin beneath the epidermis. It is a fibrous layer, consisting of collagenous, elastic, and reticular fibers, that contains hair follicles, sebaceous glands, blood vessels, lymphatics, and nerve endings. Beneath the dermis is an adipose tissue layer, actually the deeper continuation of the dermis but sometimes described as a third layer of the skin, which is often referred to as the *hypoderm,* or *subcutaneous tissue.* In inflammations of the skin, it is usually in the corium that cellular, vascular, and degenerative changes are most prominent. Hypertrophy, atrophy, and neoplasia are types of pathologic change that affect elements of the corium.

Sebaceous glands are small racemose glands that occur in association with hair follicles. They may undergo hypertrophic, atrophic, cystic, and neoplastic changes. The sweat glands are tubular glands that form a coil. The common type is a small gland that discharges through a spiral duct passing through the epidermis. Larger sweat glands known as apocrine glands open into hair follicles and are found mainly in the axillary and genital regions. Sweat glands may be diminished in number, but functional disorders are more common than anatomic changes. Rarely, tumors may arise from sweat glands (benign tumors and carcinoma). Blood vessels, lymphatics, and nerves of the corium, in addition to being involved in inflammatory processes, may give rise to tumors. Disturbances of a fatty nature in the skin usually take the form of an abnormal deposit of lipid (xanthoma) or a neoplasm of adipose tissue (lipoma and liposarcoma). Degenerative and inflammatory lesions of adipose tissue also occur. Changes in the pigment deposits in the skin occur in a number of local and internal conditions (e.g., Addison's disease), and pigmented cells give rise to tumors (pigmented nevi and malignant melanomas).

INFECTIONS AND INFLAMMATIONS

A variety of inflammatory skin lesions of infectious or noninfectious origin, both nonspecific and granulomatous, have already been considered in previous chapters (e.g., acute bacterial, tuberculous, leprotic, fungal, viral, and rickettsial infections; sarcoidosis; rheumatic nodules; tophus of gout; fat necrosis with foreign body reactions). In this discussion, a few more examples will be considered.

Contact dermatitis. Nonspecific inflammation of the skin may be caused by direct contact with a substance to which the skin is sensitized *(allergic contact dermatitis)* or by exposure to potentially irritating agents *(primary irritant dermatitis)*. The dermatitis may be acute, subacute, or chronic.

Characteristic features of the acute and subacute forms include erythema (hyperemia), intraepidermal edema and vesicle formation, oozing, crust formation, and inflammatory cells in the dermis (lymphocytes, neutrophils, and eosinophils). In chronic contact dermatitis, the epidermis is thickened because of proliferation of the prickle cells (acanthosis), and there are areas of excess keratin on the surface (hyperkeratosis), along with areas of imperfect cornification where nuclei may still be seen in the horny layer (parakeratosis). Lymphocytes, histiocytes, and eosinophils appear in the dermis. Grossly, the skin may appear thickened, with exaggeration of the normal skin markings (lichenification), and scaling may be observed.

Atopic dermatitis. Atopic dermatitis is a hypersensitivity state to which the patient is predisposed by hereditary or constitutional factors rather than an acquired hypersensitivity to specific allergens. The patients have a personal or family history of allergic disorders, such as hay fever or asthma. The skin is dry and itchy, being particularly sensitive to heat, perspiration, and external irritants. The lesions may be multiple, characterized by thickened, excoriated, lichenified patches with histologic features similar to those of chronic contact dermatitis described previously *(generalized neurodermatitis)*.

A localized form of chronic dermatitis occurs in which the lesion resembles that of atopic dermatitis, but allergy is not thought to be causative. In this condition, referred to as *circumscribed neurodermatitis* or *lichen simplex chronicus,* psychogenic factors play a role.

Psoriasis. Psoriasis is a chronic, recurrent disorder of unknown cause, although heredity is a factor. It is characterized by papules and plaques that are dry and usually covered by thin silvery scales. The extensor surfaces of the extremities (e.g., elbows and knees) are common sites of involvement, but the scalp, nails, back, buttocks, and anogenital regions are often affected also.

The microscopic features, which are characteristic, include the following:

1 Acanthosis with regular downward prolongations of the rete ridges that are rounded at the ends
2 Thinning of the suprapapillary portions of the epidermis
3 Prominent parakeratosis
4 Absence of stratum granulosum
5 Nonspecific inflammation with edema of the upper dermis, especially of the papillae, which also contain dilated venules
6 Foci of neutrophils in the epidermis ("Munroe microabscesses")

Patients with psoriasis sometimes develop a form of arthritis similar to rheumatoid arthritis. In psoriatic arthritis, however, serologic tests for the rheumatoid factor are usually negative, and the terminal interphalangeal joints are involved rather than the proximal inter-phalangeal joints as in rheumatoid arthritis. The incidence of diabetes mellitus and a positive family history of this metabolic disorder are said to be higher among those with psoriasis.

Lichen planus. Lichen planus is a chronic, pruritic, nonspecific dermatitis of unknown cause, characterized by discrete, small, shiny, angular, reddish violet, flat-topped papules. The lesions usually are restricted to a few areas but may be generalized. The oral mucosa may be involved. Sometimes, bullous lesions occur.

The microscopic picture is distinctive, with hyperkeratosis, prominence of the stratum granulosum, irregular acanthosis, "saw-tooth" appearance of the rete ridges, degeneration of the basal layer of the epidermis, and a thick bandlike infiltrate of lymphocytes in the dermis immediately adjacent to the epidermis. Macrophages containing melanin from basal cells are seen in the upper dermis. Also, hyaline or colloid bodies, which probably develop from damaged basal cells, may be present in the lower epidermis or subepidermally. The bodies show immunofluorescence for immunoglobulins, complement, and fibrin.

Erythema multiforme. Erythema multiforme is an acute or subacute dermatitis, usually self-limited, which is characterized by macules, papules, vesicles, and bullae. The papules have clearing centers and elevated borders. Mucous membrane lesions may occur in some patients.

The cause of this disorder is unknown, but often it is associated with ingestion of certain drugs, rheumatic fever, streptococcal or other bacterial infections, viral and fungal diseases, and visceral cancer. A severe form of the disease, the *Stevens-Johnson syndrome,* occurs in children and young adults, with sudden febrile onset and predominantly bullous lesions of the skin and mucous membranes.

Pemphigus vulgaris. Pemphigus vulgaris is an uncommon disease that, without corticosteroid therapy, is usually fatal. Bullous lesions appear on the skin and mucous membranes. The bullae form intraepidermally following in-tercellular edema, loss of cohesion between epidermal cells, and separation of the cells (acantholysis). There is minimal inflammation of nonspecific type in the dermis. When death occurs, it is caused by bronchopneumonia, septicemia, or other complications. Malnutrition resulting from inability to eat in the presence of oral lesions may be contributory.

Pemphigus may be an autoimmune disease, since IgG antibodies are usually demonstrated in the serum and in the epithelial intercellular spaces of the skin and oral lesions. Deposits of C3 may also be demonstrated in the lesions. One of the diseases that must be differentiated from pemphigus is **bullous pemphigoid,** which generally has a good prognosis, except in some old, debilitated patients. In bullous pemphigoid, the bullae form just beneath the epidermis, and deposits of IgG and C3 may be identified in the dermal-epidermal junction (basement membrane zone) of the skin and mucous membranes. In both pemphigus and bullous pemphigoid, therefore, the deposits are present at the sites where bullae form. IgG antibodies may also be demonstrated in the serum in bullous pemphigoid.

Granuloma annulare. Granuloma annulare is a chronic dermatitis of unknown cause, consisting of a group of nodules arranged in a ringlike or circinate fashion. There is an intradermal zone of fibrinoid necrosis, surrounded by palisaded epithelioid cells, lymphocytes, and fibroblasts. An occasional giant cell of the foreign body type may be seen. It is similar to rheumatic or rheumatoid nodules, which differ in being subcutaneous. Also, the lesion may be mistaken for necrobiosis lipoidica. Histochemical and electron microscopic studies have suggested that granuloma annulare may result from delayed hypersensitivity.

Necrobiosis lipoidica. Necrobiosis lipoidica consists of one or more demarcated, irregularly circular plaques with yellowish centers and slightly elevated violaceous borders, most frequently present on the anterior aspects of the legs. The centers become depressed and atrophic and may ulcerate.

Microscopically, there is degeneration of the dermal collagen. The collagen fibers are swollen, homogeneous, and partly fragmented. Nearby are foci of lymphocytes and histiocytes and often small granulomas with epithelioid cells and multinucleated giant cells. Lipid may be demonstrated by fat stains in areas of collagen degeneration. Sometimes, endothelial proliferation of vessels and even thrombosis may be observed.

The lesions occur in diabetic patients but also may be observed in persons without diabetes. In some of the latter, diabetes mellitus appears after the onset of the skin lesions.

Erythema nodosum. Erythema nodosum is an inflammation involving chiefly the subcutaneous tissue and is associated with systemic diseases, such as rheumatic fever, streptococcal infections, coccidioidomycosis, and drug reactions. The lesions usually appear on the anterior aspects of the legs in the form of reddish tender nodules raised above the skin, without necrosis or ulceration. Neutrophils, lymphocytes, histiocytes, and occasionally eosinophils are present in the subcutaneous tissue, associated with involvement of vessels, particularly veins (vasculitis).

Weber-Christian disease. Weber-Christian disease (relapsing, febrile, nodular, nonsuppurative panniculitis) is characterized by crops of subcutaneous painful nodules and is accompanied by fever and systemic manifestations. Its cause is unknown. In some cases, lesions in the internal fat areas have been described (e.g., perivisceral and mesenteric).

The characteristic lesion consists of lobules of fat that show degenerative changes, lymphocytic infiltration, and sometimes giant cell granulomas. Neutrophils, according to some authors, may be seen in an early stage of the lesion. Vasculitis also may be noted. Septa between the fatty lobules show relatively little change in early stages. A somewhat similar panniculitis may be seen in erythema nodosum, erythema induratum, and fat necrosis caused by trauma or chemical agents.

Sclerema neonatorum. A generalized form of sclerema neonatorum occurs in the first few weeks of life and is characterized by widespread patchy hardening of subcutaneous tissue. The visceral fat also may be involved. There is a foreign body type of granulomatous inflammatory reaction of the subcutaneous adipose tissue associated with precipitation of fatty acid crystals. Death usually occurs in a few weeks. A localized self-limited form also exists. A deficiency in the composition of the fat and birth trauma are considered to be factors in sclerema neonatorum.

Scleredema. Scleredema is an uncommon benign condition characterized by firm nonpitting edema that may affect the face, neck, thorax, or arms. Effusions into pleural, pericardial, and joint spaces also may occur. Young women are most frequently affected. Recovery may occur spontaneously after a course of several months to years. Persistent scleredema has been observed in some patients with diabetes mellitus. Inflammation in the tissues is not striking, usually evidenced as a slight lymphocytic infiltration.

The disease is not to be confused with *sclerema neonatorum* and must be distinguished from *scleroderma*. The cause of scleredema is unknown, but it often occurs after an upper respiratory tract infection.

IMMUNE DISORDERS OF CONNECTIVE TISSUE (DIFFUSE COLLAGEN DISEASES)

There are various systemic diseases that are characterized as primary disturbances of connective tissues of the body, with certain clinical and morphologic similarities. A grouping together of these conditions as *diffuse collagen diseases* has been popular and productive, although the conditions are not necessarily related to the same cause. They also have been known as "diffuse collagen-vascular diseases," because lesions of blood vessels accompany the connective tissue changes throughout the body. Evidence suggests that hypersensitivity or autoimmunity plays an important role in the pathogenesis of these diseases, and the designation *immune disorders of connective tissue* has been proposed for this group of diseases. Today, these diseases are more commonly referred to as disorders of connective tissue rather than of collagen, since injury is not restricted to collagen nor is the latter necessarily involved first.

Commonly grouped as connective tissue disorders are systemic lupus erythematosus, dermatomyositis, progressive systemic sclerosis (scleroderma), polyarteritis nodosa, thrombotic thrombocytopenic purpura, rheumatic fever, and rheumatoid arthritis. The first three of these diseases are discussed here. The others are considered elsewhere. These diseases, with their widespread connective tissue involvement, are to be distinguished from the localized connective tissue disturbances of the skin, such as keloids, balanitis xerotica obliterans, acrodermatitis chronica atrophicans, granuloma annulare, and necrobiosis lipoidica.

Connective tissue is composed of fibrous connective tissue cells or fibroblasts, intercellular fibers, and an amorphous ground substance that lies between them. The intercellular fibers are of three kinds: collagen, elastic, and reticulin. The collagen fibers are generally most abundant and easily seen, but the elastic and reticulin fibers can be differentially stained, the latter being argyrophilic. The homogeneous, viscid ground substance is composed of mucopolysaccharides and is generally inconspicuous. In the diffuse connective tissue disorders, the ground substance may undergo conspicuous alteration. Among the components of connective tissue, only the fibroblasts are living structures. The inert fibers and ground substance may be acted upon and undergo change but are incapable of active response to injury. The connective tissues show varying combinations of degeneration and fibroblastic proliferation. The most characteristic change is a localized "fibrinoid" degeneration of connective tissue. The ground substance becomes increased in quantity and prominence, the collagen fibers become swollen and fragmented, and the debris becomes fused into a prominently eosinophilic area lacking normal structural detail and taking on staining reactions similar to those of fibrin. The fibrinoid formation has been considered characteristic of an allergic reaction, but it is probably not specific for injury of any particular type (p. 31).

Dermatomyositis. Dermatomyositis is an inflammatory and degenerative condition of the skin, subcutaneous tissue, and striated muscles. Although many features suggest an infective origin, no organism has been found, and the cause is unknown. In some cases (7% to 15%), there is an associated malignant neoplasm somewhere in the body. Occasionally, remission of dermatomyositis follows removal of the tumor, suggesting that tumor antigens may have initiated the lesions of dermatomyositis by stimulating formation of antibodies that cross-react with the patient's tissues. Inflammatory changes in small blood vessels of involved tissues often appear as an important feature. The histologic changes are not specific for dermatomyositis but are similar to those of scleroderma and other conditions. Resemblances to systemic lupus erythematosus have been noted.

The skin shows atrophy of the epidermis, edema, swelling of endothelial lining of small vessels, and perivascular and diffuse infiltration of lymphocytes and plasma cells. Muscle fibers show focal lymphocytic infiltration and degenerative changes varying from swelling and loss of striations to hyaline or vacuolar changes and necrosis. Sarcolemmal nuclei may be increased. Serum creatine phosphokinase and other enzyme levels are elevated because of muscle damage. Vital muscles of deglutition and respiration may be affected and promote terminal pneumonia. Heart muscle as well as skeletal muscle may be involved.

Progressive systemic sclerosis. *Scleroderma* may be circumscribed *(morphea)* or systemic *(progressive systemic sclerosis)*. Although both forms are similar histologically, the systemic disease is more serious. It consists of diffuse thickenings of the skin that often are associated with pigmentation and vascular phenomena similar to those of Raynaud's disease. The pathologic changes are mainly collagenous fibrosis and intimal proliferation of small arterioles leading to narrowing of their lumina. Electron microscopy has revealed changes in the capillaries—viz., thickening and reduplication of the basement membrane and thickening and degeneration of the endothelium. It has been proposed that the vascular disease, particularly at the microvascular level, plays a primary role in the pathogenesis of progressive systemic sclerosis. Inflammatory cell infiltration, chiefly lymphocytic, is usual in the early stages. The vascular and connective tissue changes involve viscera, such as the esophagus, gastrointestinal tract, heart, lungs, and kidneys, as well as skin. Atrophic changes occur in voluntary muscles.

Systemic lupus erythematosus. Systemic lupus erythematosus (SLE) has been recognized to be associated with important systemic and visceral manifestations involving particularly the heart and kidneys. It occurs most commonly in women. The duration may be a few weeks to years, and the prognosis varies, depending on which organs are involved.

Some evidence suggests that systemic lupus erythematosus may be an allergic reaction of tissues, apparently an autoimmune disease. Patients develop autoantibodies to their cells and cell constituents. Hypergammaglobulinemia is frequently present. Interestingly, paramyxoviruslike particles have been identified in tissue biopsies from some patients, and serum antibodies to viral RNA have been demonstrated in others. The question has been raised as to whether viral infection may lead to formation of antibodies that cross-react with the patient's tissues.

The essence of systemic lupus erythematosus has been stated to be a widespread and characteristic alteration or fibrinoid degeneration of connective tissue, with a special predilection for injury to this tissue in the heart, glomeruli, blood vessels, skin, spleen, and retroperitoneal tissues.

In patients with active systemic lupus erythematosus, the LE cell test is usually positive. An LE cell appears to be a mature polymorphonuclear leukocyte that has phagocytized a homogeneous purple-staining mass of chromatin (nuclear) material (Fig. 24-1). A factor (the LE factor) present in the gamma globulin fraction of plasma or serum of patients with systemic lupus erythematosus is capable of reacting with nuclear constituents of normal neutrophils in vitro, transforming the nuclei to homogeneous rounded masses that are rendered susceptible to phagocytosis, usually by granulocytes, forming the LE cells (*LE cell phenomenon*). The LE factor sometimes induces formation of rosettes of clumped leukocytes, which surround the altered nuclear material (*LE rosette phenomenon*). Similar hematoxylin-staining bodies may be seen in sections of various tissues in acute lupus erythematosus. These "hematoxylin bodies" contain partially depolymerized DNA. In addition to the LE factor, a variety of other antinuclear

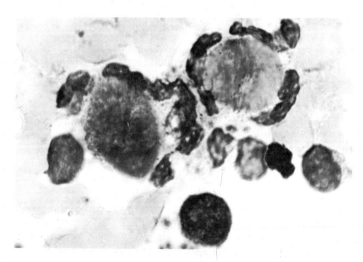

Fig. 24-1. LE cells. Note homogeneous masses of altered nuclear material phagocytized by neutrophils. (Courtesy Dr. J. F. Kuzma.)

autoantibodies, as well as antibodies to cytoplasmic constituents, have been described.

Various cutaneous lesions occur, including erythematous and maculopapular lesions that are frequently symmetrical, involving the face, neck, and extremities. A characteristic "butterfly" malar erythema sometimes is seen. The histologic changes in the skin usually consist of epidermal atrophy, liquefaction degeneration of the basal layer, dermal edema with fibrinoid changes in the connective tissue, which also may affect the walls of small vessels, and mild perivascular leukocytic (chiefly lymphocytic) infiltration. Bullous and ulcerative lesions also may occur. In a small group of patients with systemic lupus erythematosus, subcutaneous nodules that are histologically similar to the rheumatoid nodules in rheumatoid arthritis have been reported. A band of immunoglobulins at the dermal-epidermal junction of the skin may be demonstrated by immunofluorescence in patients with lupus erythematosus *(lupus band test)*.

Nonbacterial atypical verrucous endocarditis, as described by Libman and Sachs, occurs in a considerable proportion of cases (p. 314). Renal changes also are frequent and are described on p. 349. The spleen shows a characteristic periarterial fibrosis of the central arteries, assuming a pattern of thick concentric rings of collagen fibers.

Some patients receiving certain drugs, such as hydrazides, anticonvulsants (Dilantin), and procainamide, develop antinuclear factors and manifestations similar to systemic lupus erythematosus.

TUMORS
Benign tumors and epidermal hyperplasias

Verruca vulgaris. The common wart, or verruca vulgaris, is not a true neoplasm but a hyperplastic lesion of the epidermis that is infective in origin and caused by a filtrable virus. Sometimes, however, it is loosely referred to as a "papilloma." Electron microscopic studies have shown virus particles associated with nucleoli of cells of the stratum spinosum. The virus particles appear related to

basophilic inclusions seen in ordinary sections. Certain investigators have reported seeing also, on occasion, cytoplasmic virus particles in cells containing particles in the nucleus. There is hypertrophy of the outer keratinized layer and proliferation (acanthosis) of the prickle cell layer, and irregular downward prolongations of the rete ridges are seen. There may be some infiltration of mononuclear inflammatory cells about blood vessels of the corium.

The lesion occurs most often in children and appears commonly on the fingers and the hands, although it may occur elsewhere.

Condyloma acuminatum. There are several other forms of verrucae, including the *verruca plana* (flat wart), *verruca plantaris* (plantar wart), and *condyloma acuminatum* (venereal wart), which are caused by the same allied strains of virus as that causing verruca vulgaris. Condyloma acuminatum occurs on the glans penis, on the mucosal surfaces of the vulva, and about the anus. It consists of groups of verrucous nodules that coalesce to form a cauliflowerlike lesion.

Microscopically, there is papillomatosis of severe degree, with acanthosis, slight hyperkeratosis, spotty parakeratosis, and vacuolization of the upper epidermal cells. In the dermis, there are dilated capillaries and inflammatory cell infiltration, usually mononuclears. The lesion must be differentiated from condyloma latum resulting from syphilis.

Acanthosis nigricans. Although acanthosis nigricans is not itself a neoplasm, in adults it frequently is associated with a visceral carcinoma. It is characterized by patchy, warty, pigmented lesions, particularly occurring in the axilla, groin, or mammary region or on the knees or elbows. It is a papillary hyperkeratosis of the skin with underlying acanthosis and considerable melanin pigmentation of the basal layer.

Pigmented papilloma (seborrheic keratosis). Pigmented papilloma, also known as *basal cell papilloma,* occurs most commonly on the trunk and less often on the arms, neck, and face. It is brown or black, has a greasy surface, and appears "stuck on" the skin.

Clinically, it may be mistaken for malignant melanoma.

Microscopically, the lesion consists of thickened epidermis in which there are cystic areas containing keratin. The cells resemble basal cells. Those about the keratin cysts are more mature squamous cells. The cysts appear to form from invaginations of the horny layer. Melanin is usually present in the cells of the tumor. The lower limit of the tumor is on a level with the adjacent normal epidermis, thus accounting for the gross ''stuck on'' appearance. The surface is covered with varying amounts of keratin, which causes the greasy appearance grossly (Fig. 24-2).

Keratoacanthoma. Keratoacanthoma (molluscum sebaceum) is a rapidly growing, keratotic, papular lesion of the skin that undergoes spontaneous resolution. It is most common on the face and probably arises from the pilosebaceous apparatus.

Histologically, the lesion is characterized by a superficial crater containing a keratin mass, surrounded by papillary hyperplastic squamous epithelium. The epithelial cells may suggest the appearance of a low-grade squamous cell carcinoma. Some regular extensions may be seen at the margins, but irregular invasive activity is absent. Similar multiple self-healing keratoses and carcinomalike lesions of the skin have been described.

Tumors of skin appendages. Benign tumors may arise from the sweat glands, sebaceous glands, or hair follicles. Sweat gland tumors (known by various terms, such as spiradenomas, syringomas, cylindromas, and hidradenomas) are somewhat more common than sebaceous adenomas. A verrucous, papillary, and sometimes cystic tumor of sweat gland origin (syringadenoma papilliferum) may grow rapidly and to a considerable size. The majority of such tumors occur on the scalp or face, and a few are associated with basal cell carcinoma.

Hidradenomas arising from the vulva have a distinctive appearance, with narrow, branched, anastomosing papillary fronds (see Fig. 22-31). The lesion arising from hair follicles (trichoepithelioma) consists of single or multiple nodules. The multiple lesions, also known as ''epithelioma adenoides cysticum'' or ''Brooke's tumor,'' consist of strands of cells resembling basal cell carcinoma, but they have cystic spaces filled with hyaline or keratinized material.

Mesenchymal tumors. Fibromas, lipomas, leiomyomas, and neurofibromas may occur. These are discussed in Chapter 12. Hemangiomas, lymphangiomas, and glomus tumors are considered in Chapter 13.

Precancerous lesions

A variety of skin and mucosal conditions, although not themselves neoplastic, give rise to carcinoma so frequently that they may be termed precancerous. These are (1) the keratoses—senile or solar, localized (cutaneous horn), and arsenical, (2) occupational derma-

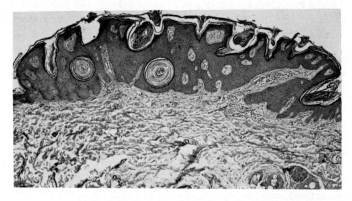

Fig. 24-2. Seborrheic keratotic lesion of skin.

toses (from tar products), (3) x-ray and radium dermatitis, (4) xeroderma pigmentosum, and (5) hyperkeratosis ("leukoplakia") of mucous membranes (p. 514).

Keratoses. The precancerous keratoses are characterized by a hyperkeratosis, or thickening of the outer cornifying layers of epithelium. This may be accompanied by atrophy of remaining portions of the skin. A striking feature is the presence of atypia in the cells of the lower layers of the epidermis (i.e., hyperchromatic nuclei, irregular size and shape of nuclei, loss of polarity, and mitotic activity).

Exposure to sunlight appears to be a causative factor (thus called *actinic,* or *solar, keratosis).* It is also known as *senile keratosis.* However, although it tends to occur in persons past middle age, it is not limited to old age. A localized hyperkeratosis may produce a fingerlike projection, or *cutaneous horn. Arsenical keratosis,* a lesion that is similar to actinic keratosis histologically, develops usually on the palms or soles from continued absorption of arsenicals.

Occupational dermatoses. The occupational dermatoses are chronic inflammatory conditions or hyperkeratoses caused by long-continued irritation by certain chemicals. Tar and mineral oils and their products and derivatives are most important in this respect.

Radiation dermatitis. Dermatitis resulting from overexposure to radium or roentgen rays is particularly likely to occur in certain sensitive skins and often has carcinoma as a late sequel. The carcinomatous change usually is preceded by hyperkeratoses, fissures, ulcers, or scars.

Xeroderma pigmentosum. In xeroderma pigmentosum, there is abnormal sensitivity of the skin to sunlight. Apparently, an inability of cells to repair ultraviolet radiation damage to DNA exists, which may be related to carcinogenesis. The condition usually appears in infancy or early childhood. Exposed areas of skin develop spotty pigmentations, warty hyperkeratoses, atrophy, and telangiectasia, and multiple cancers appear. The disease is a genetic disorder with an autosomal recessive inheritance pattern.

Carcinoma

In the epidermis, the two innermost layers are most active (i.e., the basal layer and the spinous cell layer). The outer layers that undergo physiologic degeneration and death (keratinization) have little or no growth activity. Hence, the main types of carcinoma of the skin arise from or simulate the inner active layers of epithelium and are known as basal cell carcinoma and squamous cell carcinoma (spinous cell carcinoma). There are also mixed forms, in which the fundamental types of basal and squamous cells are present in varying proportion. Finally, there occasionally occurs a carcinoma arising from special structures of the skin, such as hair follicles and sebaceous or sweat glands.

Carcinoma of the skin usually develops in persons after middle age. It occurs particularly on exposed and unprotected parts of the skin (i.e., face, neck, arms, etc.). Injury by excessive exposure to sunlight, heat, wind, roentgen rays, arsenicals, and other chronic irritants seems to be important in causation. The development of actual cancer often is preceded by benign keratoses or other precancerous lesions. Because the lesions are readily accessible, treatment usually results in cure if they are recognized in time. Size when first treated is important in prognosis. The histologic grade of malignancy is next in importance in prognosis.

Basal cell carcinoma (rodent ulcer). Basal cell carcinoma is the most frequent type of skin cancer. It is particularly common on the upper two thirds of the face and about the nose and eyelids. It is a tumor of low-grade malignancy and slow growth. It rarely metastasizes but erodes its way into surrounding tissues with ulceration and much local tissue destruction. This is the "rodent ulcer" form. It also may have a nodular or fungating form. The origin of some of the tumors of basal cell type appears to be from hair follicles or the anlage of hair follicles.

Microscopically, the tumor is composed of cords and masses of cells with deeply basophilic nuclei. Each mass of cells tends to have a definite margin composed of a palisaded row of cells that stain deeply with hematoxylin. Mitotic figures are not abundant. There is ordinarily no keratinization or prickle cell formation. However, in about 10%, there is some prickle cell formation or a few nests of keratinization. Occasionally, the pegs of basal cells tend to form a glandular or adenoid picture. Since excessive pigment is sometimes present, the tumor could be confused with a melanoma on gross examination.

Squamous cell carcinoma. Squamous cell carcinoma occurs not only in the skin but also wherever squamous or transitional epithelium is found. Hence, it may involve the lip, mouth, tongue, larynx, cervix uteri, bladder, and esophagus. It also may arise in other situations (e.g., bronchial mucosa or gallbladder), presumably by a metaplastic change of the lining epithelium.

Squamous cell carcinoma of the skin, like other types, is most common in persons after the fifth decade and frequently is related to some chronic injury or irritation. The tumor may appear as a projecting nodular mass or as an ulcer (Fig. 24-3). Growth is more rapid than in the basal cell type, and metastasis occurs to regional lymph nodes. Distant metastases are less common than with squamous cell carcinoma of mucous membranes.

Microscopically, there is much greater irregularity than in the basal cell type. It is composed of irregular downgrowths and masses of enlarged epithelial cells, which show great variations and irregularities. Mitoses may be numerous and often are atypical. The amount of keratinization is variable. The keratinized cells are seen in concentric nests, or ''pearls'' (Fig. 24-4). The masses of keratin and the presence of prickle cells are the chief differential features for this type of tumor.

The squamous cell carcinoma that arises from the lip, tongue, intraoral mucosa, glans penis, or vulva tends to grow, penetrate, and metastasize more rapidly than the squamous cell carcinoma of the skin.

The lower lip is a particularly common site

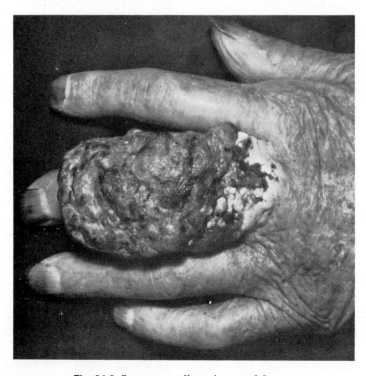

Fig. 24-3. Squamous cell carcinoma of finger.

for carcinoma. The lesions are nearly all of the squamous cell type. The less frequent carcinomas of the upper lip are usually of the basal cell variety. Chronic irritation, as from excessive exposure to sunlight, pipe smoking, or bad oral hygiene, may be a predisposing factor. Hyperkeratosis may precede the formation of a carcinoma. The tumor may be papillary or ulcerative. Metastasis to submental and submaxillary nodes readily occurs (p. 514).

Epidermal hyperplasia, which develops in certain chronic ulcers or chronic inflammatory processes, may imitate the appearance of squamous cell carcinoma (pseudocarcinomatous hyperplasia), and differentiation may be difficult. In this reactive hyperplasia, the epidermal cells usually are limited by a definite basement membrane, and there is less irregularity of cells and architectural arrangement. The clinical features are often an aid in the differentiation.

Basosquamous (metatypical) carcinoma. The mixed cell type of carcinoma of the skin contains prominent features of both basal and squamous carcinoma.

Malignant tumors of skin appendages. Basal cell carcinomas may arise from the epithelium of hair shafts. Sebaceous carcinoma, which is rare, may be confused with basal cell or squamous carcinoma, but it resembles se-

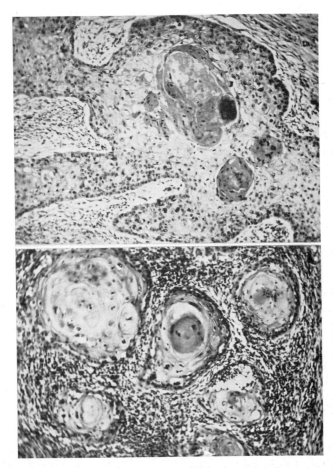

Fig. 24-4. Squamous cell carcinoma. Note rounded masses of keratinized material, so-called keratin pearls or epithelial pearls.

baceous gland tissue in at least some portion. Carcinoma of sweat gland origin is uncommon. Extramammary Paget's disease may be associated with an adenocarcinoma arising in an apocrine gland, as in the vulva. Malignant change rarely occurs in a trichoepithelioma, a tumor arising from hair follicles.

Intraepidermal carcinoma. Intraepidermal carcinoma or carcinoma in situ is limited to the epidermis. One variety is known as Bowen's disease, which involves the skin. A lesion bearing some resemblance to Bowen's disease is erythroplasia of Queyrat, which affects the glans penis (p. 378).

Bowen's disease appears as a dull red patch of skin on the trunk or extremities, often with areas of crusting. Microscopically, all layers of the epidermis show large hyperchromatic nuclei surrounded by halos in the cytoplasm. Mitotic figures are seen in the affected cells. Acanthosis, hyperkeratosis, and parakeratosis are evident. A viruslike particle has been demonstrated microscopically within basal and spinous cells in some instances. Bowen's disease is associated with internal cancer in a significant number of cases. Sometimes, the visceral cancer appears several years after the diagnosis of Bowen's disease has been made.

Although Bowen's disease is described here as a carcinoma in situ, it should be noted that some authors may regard it as a precancerous lesion.

Malignant mesenchymal tumors

Dermatofibrosarcoma protuberans. Dermatofibrosarcoma protuberans may appear as a plaque or protuberant mass that histologically resembles a low-grade fibrosarcoma. It grows slowly and with recurrence unless widely removed, but metastasis is unusual.

Fibrosarcoma. Fibrosarcoma of the skin also may form protuberant masses. It grows more rapidly and has a more serious outlook.

Kaposi's disease. Multiple idiopathic hemorrhagic sarcoma, or Kaposi's disease (sarcoma), is an infrequent condition of unknown origin and of uncertain nature. Its incidence in the black population in Africa is relatively frequent. A large majority of cases occur in men.

The lesions are multiple and variable in form, but usually they are hemorrhagic and pigmented. They tend to involve the extremities, particularly the lower, in symmetric fashion. Mucous membranes also may be affected, and rarely viscera may be involved without external lesions. Temporary spontaneous regressions occur, but eventually lesions may develop in lymph nodes and internal organs, particularly the gastrointestinal tract and lungs. There is a controversy as to whether the lesions in the lymph nodes and viscera represent metastases or multicentric foci of origin. Lymph node involvement is common in the African cases. The histologic appearance of the lesions in lymph nodes and internal organs is similar to that of the skin lesions.

The cutaneous lesions involve the dermis and are characterized by irregular fascicles or bundles of spindle-shaped cells, which intertwine and are irregularly interrupted by vascular slits (Figs. 24-5 and 24-6). The vascular spaces often are congested by red blood cells, but they do not appear to be lined by identifiable endothelium. The spindle-shaped cells are often poorly defined, and their nuclei are fusiform, oval, or round. Varying amounts of focal hemorrhage, deposits of blood pigment, and fibroblastic proliferation may be present. The late stage is characterized by obliteration of the vascular spaces, increased mitoses, and large nuclei, the appearance changing to that of an angiosarcoma, fibrosarcoma, or undifferentiated sarcoma.

It has been debated whether the condition should be classed as a chronic granulomatous inflammation or as a true tumor (angiosarcoma). Current opinion favors regarding Kaposi's disease as a neoplasm of the vascular system with multifocal origin, although evidence also has suggested that it is a disease of the reticuloendothelial system, probably related to the lymphomas.

The occurrence of Kaposi's disease with leukemia or malignant lymphoma (e.g., lymphosarcoma, Hodgkin's disease, and mycosis fungoides) in the same patient has been reported by several investigators. Although malignant lymphoma and Kaposi's disease may

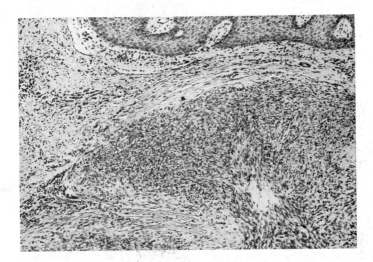

Fig. 24-5. Kaposi's disease. Irregular area of thin spindle cells and small vascular slits occupies dermal tissue.

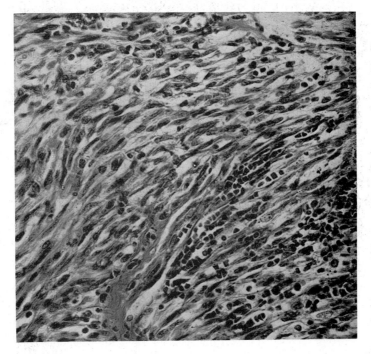

Fig. 24-6. Kaposi's disease. Lesion is disorganized mixture of vascular slits and thin spindle cells. (From Haukohl, R. S., and Anderson, W. A. D., editors: Pathology seminars, St. Louis, 1955, The C. V. Mosby Co.)

occur together, there are some patients without the former disease but with extracutaneous Kaposi's lesions, involving principally lymph nodes, who present a lymphomalike picture clinically. Also, several instances have been reported in which bone marrow plasmacytosis and abnormal serum and urine proteins have been detected in association with Kaposi's sarcoma. Occasionally, multiple myeloma and Kaposi's sarcoma have been observed in the same patient.

Mycosis fungoides (granuloma fungoides). Mycosis fungoides is considered by most authors to be a variant of malignant lymphoma, rather than a granuloma, involving principally and primarily the skin. The term *mycosis* is a misnomer, since the lesion is not a fungal disease. In early stages, there is an eczematoid eruption, followed by a tumor phase in which there may be ulceration. In the tumor stage, there is a dense, massive accumulation of cells in the dermis, with thinning and flattening of the overlying epidermis. In the cellular tumorlike mass, the cells are polymorphic, appearing as mononuclear cells, lymphoblasts, and plasma cells. Some neutrophilic leukocytes, eosinophils, and giant cells may be present. The lesion may closely resemble Hodgkin's disease. Occasionally, there may be an involvement of internal organs, in addition to the skin.

Recent evidence, including clinical, cytologic, and immunologic data, suggests that mycosis fungoides and the Sézary syndrome (p. 492) are closely related and are part of a spectrum of cutaneous lymphomas consisting of thymus-derived T cells.

Pigmented nevi and malignant melanomas

Both benign and malignant tumors may arise from melanocytes (i.e., cells capable of producing melanin pigment). The pigment actually produced in a particular tumor may be either small in amount or abundant. The extremely common benign form is called a pigmented nevus. The relatively rare malignant form is referred to as a melanocarcinoma, or malignant melanoma. Melanomas occur most commonly in the skin but also are found in the mouth, rectum, eye, and meninges and rarely in other sites.

The melanocyte is thought to be a modified basal cell of the epidermis and is capable of producing a pigmented material from 3,4-dihydroxyphenylalanine (dopa) by means of an oxidizing ferment that it contains. Melanin probably is produced by oxidation of some substance closely allied to dopa and to epinephrine.

Concerning the origin of the neval cells in the ordinary pigmented nevi, there are several theories:

1 All neval cells originate from epidermal melanocytes, with "dropping off" into the dermis in the case of intradermal nevi.
2 Neval cells are developed from epidermal melanocytes in junctional nevi or from both the epidermal melanocytes and Schwann cells of dermal nerve sheaths in compound nevi and intradermal nevi.
3 Neval cells originate from a more primitive precursor cell (nevoblast), derived from the neural crest, which can differentiate into a melanoblastic nevoblast that gives rise to epidermal neval cells or into a schwannian nevoblast that develops into intradermal neval cells.

Pigmented nevi. Pigmented nevi are found in almost every person. Commonly, they occur in early years of life, grow to a certain size, and then remain stationary, but some of them may become atrophic and fibrotic. They are flat or raised pigmented lesions, with or without hair. Nevi on the ventral surface of the hands and feet and on the genitalia are usually junctional nevi or nevi with a junctional component. The junctional nevus is the type that may precede malignant change.

The nevi may be grouped as follows:

1 Junctional nevus (dermoepidermal nevus)
2 Intradermal nevus (common mole or neuronevus)
3 Compound nevus
4 Juvenile melanoma
5 Blue nevus (Jadassohn-Tièche nevus)

The *junctional nevus* is characterized by clusters of enlarged, rounded, loosened cells of the basal layer of the epidermis. In the *intradermal nevus,* or common mole, the clusters and cords of the neval cells are found only in the dermis. Histologically, the epidermis is thinner than normal and may be flat or papillary. Beneath the epidermis are nests of rounded or polygonal pale-staining "neval cells" that contain variable amounts of melanin. The cells occur in islands, separated by connective tissue, but there is no sharp line of separation or encapsulation, and the cells may extend somewhat irregularly into subcutaneous tissue. The *compound nevus* is a combination of the junctional and the intradermal nevus.

The *juvenile melanoma,* which occurs in children before puberty, is a special form of compound nevus with distinct histologic features that distinguish it from the malignant melanomas of adults. Juvenile melanomas do not metastasize or run a malignant course.

The *blue nevus* is a benign, bluish black, flat or slightly raised lesion. It is composed of interlacing bundles of elongated or spindle cells that are abundantly pigmented and usually situated quite deep within the dermis, thus differing from the ordinary pigmented nevus. It is believed that blue nevi are derived from dermal melanocytes that failed to disappear during embryonic life, but schwannian cell or epidermal origin of the melanocytes has been considered by some.

Lentigo maligna (circumscribed precancerous melanosis of Dubreilh). Lentigo maligna (also known as *Hutchinson's melanotic freckle*) is a spreading pigmented macule, several centimeters in diameter, occurring on the exposed surfaces of the body, particularly the skin of the temple and malar regions of the face. It develops usually in elderly patients and tends to give rise to malignant melanoma after many years. Sunlight appears to play a role in the development of the lesion and its progression to malignant transformation. The relationship of lentigo maligna to malignant melanoma is similar to that of solar keratosis to squamous cell carcinoma.

The histologic features of lentigo maligna include atrophy of the epidermis with loss of rete ridges, solar degeneration of the dermis, and hyperplasia of the melanocytes in the base of the epidermis, with pleomorphism, atypism, some mitotic figures, and increased pigmentation. The lesion differs from the *benign lentigo* (lentigo senilis, or senile freckle), which consists of multiple dark brown spots on exposed surfaces of middle-aged or older persons and also is related to sunlight. In the senile freckle, there is an increase of melanocytes, but they are not atypical, and the epidermis is not atrophic. In fact, the rete ridges are elongated. The simple *juvenile freckle* (ephelis) consists only of hyperpigmentation of the basal layer of the epidermis, without increase in melanocytes or elongation of rete ridges.

Malignant melanoma. Malignant melanoma *(melanocarcinoma)* frequently arises de novo (i.e., without a preexisting lesion). However, it may arise in a lengito maligna or in a preexisting nevus, either a junctional nevus or the junctional component of a compound nevus. Three main types of malignant melanoma are recognized: (1) malignant melanoma arising in lentigo maligna, (2) superficial spreading malignant melanoma, and (3) nodular (pagetoid) malignant melanoma. The superficial and nodular types occur most commonly in persons between 30 and 60 years of age, the peak incidence being in the fifth decade. The melanoma arising in lentigo maligna has its peak incidence in the eighth decade. Clinical malignancy is rare before puberty. Most reports indicate that malignant melanoma occurs less frequently in black persons.

Microscopically, the *malignant melanoma arising in lentigo maligna* differs from lentigo maligna in that there is an increase in the number of atypical melanocytes followed by invasion of the dermis, at first limited to the papillary dermis but eventually showing the same invasive patterns as any of the melanomas. The invasive tumor frequently is composed of spindle cells.

The *superficial spreading malignant melanoma* is usually smaller than the melanoma arising in lentigo maligna and occurs anywhere on the body surface, although it occurs often on the surfaces exposed to solar radiation. It also may occur in mucosae (e.g., conjunctiva, mouth, genitalia, and anal canal). Microscopically, the abnormal proliferating melanocytes appear in all parts of the junctional zone of the epidermis, are less pleomorphic than in the melanoma arising in lentigo maligna, have an epitheliallike and often pagetoid appearance, and tend to form nests or clusters (Fig. 24-7). Invasion of the dermis tends to occur much earlier than in the melanoma arising in lentigo maligna.

In certain instances, the clinical and histologic features of malignant melanoma arising in lentigo maligna and superficial spreading malignant melanoma overlap. When there is difficulty in distinguishing between the two, it has been suggested that the lesion be diagnosed as "malignant melanoma with an unclassified radial growth phase." As in the first two types, the growth in this lesion initially is characterized by a relatively superficial spread of tumor cells in a radial fashion before the cells penetrate deeper into the dermis.

Nodular malignant melanoma characteristically is invasive and is the most malignant

form. It may occur on exposed and unexposed skin, and most melanomas of the mucosa are of this type. The lesion tends to be more invasive than the other types of melanoma, and the cells usually show more anaplasia. Invasion is associated with junctional activity in the epidermis. The malignant melanocytes at the dermoepidermal junction invade the dermis from the beginning. There is no initial radial type of growth as in the other types of malignant melanoma. The cells in the dermis may be epitheliallike or spindle shaped or both. Bizarre tumor giant cells may be seen.

Malignant melanomas usually are radioresistant. The prognosis for nodular melanoma is worse than for the other types of melanoma. The melanoma arising in lentigo maligna has the best prognosis of the three types. The tumors with the worst prognosis are those with metastases and those exhibiting deep invasion involving the lower dermis and subcutaneous fat, which are more likely to occur in the nodular melanomas. Metastases occur by way of the lymphatics and blood vessels. They usually appear first in the regional lymph nodes

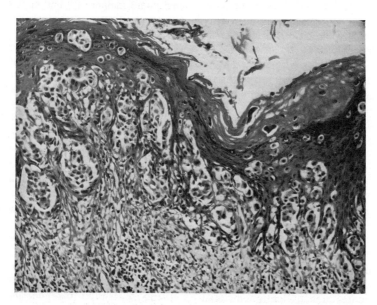

Fig. 24-7. Superficial malignant melanoma showing evidence of epidermal origin. (Courtesy Dr. A. C. Allen.)

but may be noted first in the viscera. Spread by the bloodstream results in widespread metastases, often involving unusual sites. Melanuria may occur with widespread metastases.

• • •

Pigmented papillomas (seborrheic keratoses) of the skin are benign epithelial tumors easily mistaken clinically for pigmented nevi or malignant melanoma, but they contain no neval cells. Sclerosing hemangiomatous tumors may be highly pigmented by hemosiderin and must be distinguished from melanotic tumors. A familial disorder characterized by melanin-pigmented spots of the lips and mouth (and, to a lesser degree, of the skin), associated with intestinal polyposis, is known as the Peutz-Jeghers syndrome (p. 561).

Tumorlike conditions

Keloid. Keloids are fibromalike lesions developing in the dermis, usually as the result of trauma but sometimes spontaneously. They occur in persons having a constitutional factor predisposing to their development and are relatively more common in black persons. Various types of minor or severe traumatism initiate their growth. They are particularly common after burns, are frequently multiple, and may reach a considerable size (Fig. 24-8).

Histologically, keloids are composed of thick, intertwining, hyalinized bands of collagen fibers. Mitoses are unusual except in early stages. Skin appendages are absent, and the overlying epidermis may be thinned out and its processes flattened. An ordinary scar tends to be more cellular and contains thinner collagen fibers.

Xanthoma. Xanthomas are plaquelike or nodular lesions characterized by the presence of lipids in a localized area of the corium. They are usually multiple and occur in various situations and quite commonly on the eyelids (xanthelasma). They may occur in association with hyperlipemia, as in diabetes mellitus, biliary cirrhosis, and idiopathic hypercholesterolemia, but not necessarily so. They should not be considered true neoplasms (p. 494).

Histologically, the characteristic feature of the lesion is the presence in the dermis of lipid-containing histiocytic foam cells and connective tissue proliferation (Fig. 24-9). Lipids can be demonstrated in the xanthoma cells, and crystals of lipid material may lie in the

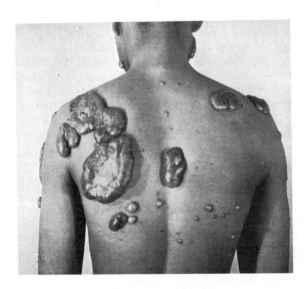

Fig. 24-8. Keloids.

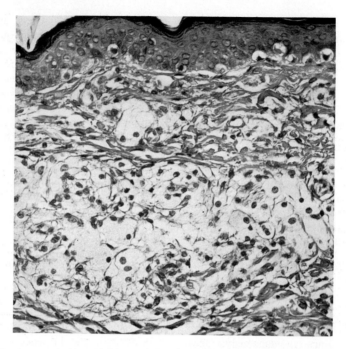

Fig. 24-9. Xanthoma of skin. Lipid-containing foam cells form poorly circumscribed mass in dermis.

tissues. Giant cells are sometimes present. Inflammatory reaction usually is evident in the diabetic xanthomas, particularly about the margins of the nodule.

Pyogenic granuloma. Pyogenic granuloma is an ulcerating, projecting, tumorlike mass of exuberant granulation tissue with abundant, enlarged blood vessels. The lesion resembles a capillary hemangioma and frequently is referred to as ''granuloma telangiectatum.'' The so-called pregnancy tumor, or granuloma gravidarum, arising on the gums during pregnancy, is a similar lesion.

Sebaceous, epidermoid, and dermoid cysts. Certain lesions of epithelial origin are cystic tumorlike formations in the skin, varying in size from a few millimeters to several centimeters. Within the cyst is a cheesy, grayish white substance composed of keratinized material, desquamated partially cornified cells, and granular debris (see Fig. 12-16). The walls are composed of epidermis (epidermoid or epidermal cysts) or may have skin appendages as

well, i.e., sweat glands, sebaceous glands, and hair (dermoid cysts). Epidermoid cysts have a tendency to familial and hereditary occurrence, but some are of traumatic origin as a result of implantation of some surface epithelium in the corium. The dermoid cysts are congenital inclusions of the skin.

The term *sebaceous cyst* is often loosely used to refer to almost any cyst of the skin having soft, semisolid contents. However, true retention cysts of sebaceous glands do occur and have sebaceous gland cells as part of the lining. Sebaceous cysts and epidermal cysts, which may not be distinguishable clinically, are often called *wens*.

REFERENCES

Ackerman, L. V., and Murray, J. F., editors: Symposium on Kaposi's sarcoma, New York, 1963, Hafner Publishing Co., Inc.

Allen, A. C.: The skin, ed. 2, New York, 1967, Grune & Stratton, Inc.

Caplan, R. M., and Curtis, A. C.: J.A.M.A. **176:**859-864, 1961 (xanthoma).

Chapman, G. B., et al.: Am. J. Pathol. **42:**619-642, 1963 (wart—fine structure).

Clark, W. H., Jr., editor: Symposium; cutaneous pathology as related to systemic disease, Hum. Pathol. **4:**153-239, 1973.

Clark, W. H., Jr., and Mihm, M. C., Jr.: Am. J. Pathol. **55:**39-68, 1969 (lentigo maligna and lentigo-maligna melanoma).

Clark, W. H., Jr., et al.: Semin. Oncol. **2:**83-103, 1975 (developmental biology of primary human malignant melanomas).

Cox, F. H., and Helwig, E. B.: Cancer **12:**289-298, 1959 (Kaposi's sarcoma).

Curth, H. O., et al.: Cancer **15:**364-382, 1962 (acanthosis nigricans).

Dubois, E. L., et al.: J.A.M.A. **220:**515-518, 1972 (rheumatoid nodules in systemic lupus erythematosus).

Emmett, E. A.: J. Occup. Med. **17:**44-49, 1975 (occupational skin cancer).

Gardner, D. L.: Pathology of the connective tissue diseases, Baltimore, 1966, The Williams & Wilkins Co.

Graham, J. H., and Helwig, E. B.: Cancer **32:**1396-1414, 1973 (erythroplasia of Queyrat).

Hargraves, M. M.: Mayo Clin. Proc. **44:**579-599, 1969 (symposium on systemic lupus erythematosus).

Jordon, R. E.: J. Invest. Dermatol. **67:**366-371, 1976 (complement activation in pemphigus and bullous pemphigoid).

Lever, W. F., and Schaumburg-Lever, G.: Histopathology of the skin, ed. 5, Philadelphia, 1975, J. B. Lippincott Co.

Lubin, J., and Rywlin, A. M.: Arch. Pathol. **92:**338-341, 1971 (lymphomalike lymph node changes in Kaposi's sarcoma).

Lutzner, M., et al.: Ann. Intern. Med. **83:**534-552, 1975 (mycosis fungoides, Sézary syndrome, and T cell lymphomas).

Mazzaferri, E. L., and Penn, G. M.: Arch. Intern. Med. **122:**521-525, 1968 (Kaposi's sarcoma associated with multiple myeloma).

McGovern, V. J.: Pathology **2:**85-98, 1970 (malignant melanoma).

McGovern, V. J.: Cancer **32:**1446-1457, 1973 (classification of malignant melanoma).

McGovern, V. J.: Malignant melanoma; clinical and histological diagnosis, New York, 1976, John Wiley & Sons, Inc.

Mihm, M. C., et al.: N. Engl. J. Med. **289:**989-996, 1973 (cutaneous malignant melanoma—a color atlas).

Monroe, E. W.: Arch. Dermatol. **113:**830-834, 1977 (lupus band test).

Montgomery, H.: Dermatopathology, New York, 1967, Harper & Row, Publishers, Inc.

Nordquist, R. E., et al.: Cancer Res. **30:**288-293, 1970 (viruslike particles in Bowen's disease).

Norton, W. L., and Nardo, J. M.: Ann. Intern. Med. **73:**317-324, 1970 (vascular disease in scleroderma).

Platt, L. I., and Kailin, E. W.: J.A.M.A. **187:**182-186, 1964 (sex chromatin frequency).

Reed, W. B., et al.: J.A.M.A. **207:**2073-2079, 1969 (xeroderma pigmentosum).

Rywlin, A. K., et al.: Arch. Dermatol. **93:**554-561, 1966 (lymphomalike presentation of Kaposi's sarcoma).

Shur, P. H., and Sandson, J.: N. Engl. J. Med. **278:**533-538, 1968 (systemic lupus erythematosus).

Strukov, A.: Arch. Pathol. **78:**409-420, 1964 (collagen diseases).

Umbert, P., and Winkelmann, R. K.: Arch. Dermatol. **113:**1681-1686, 1977 (granuloma annulare—histochemical and EM study).

Wermuth, B. M., and Fajardo, L. F.: Arch. Pathol. **90:**458-462, 1970 (metastatic basal cell carcinoma).

Yeh, S.: Hum. Pathol. **4:**469-485, 1973 (skin cancer in chronic arsenicism).

Zelickson, A. S., editor: Ultrastructure of normal and abnormal skin, Philadelphia, 1967, Lea & Febiger.

25

Bones, joints, and tendons

Bones

The bones are not inert matter but are active living substance influenced by vascular and biochemical factors, endocrine and nutritional changes, infections, and trauma. The bone marrow has the important function of blood cell formation.

Bone formation occurs by a process of ossification and calcification. In long bones there is ossification in cartilage (endochondral ossification), i.e., there is first a growth of cartilage, which later degenerates and disappears and is replaced by bone formed by osteoblastic activity. In flat bones of the skull, bone is formed in membrane (intramembranous ossification) by differentiation of connective tissue cells into osteoblasts, which progressively lay down bone. A long bone increases in length by progressive ossification on the diaphyseal side of the growing epiphyseal cartilage. Increase in width of a bone occurs by the formation of new bone on the surface under the periosteum. With increase in width, the marrow also increases in size because of resorption of adjacent bone by osteoclasts.

In the formation of bone, a proper supply of calcium and phosphorus is essential. For this, there must be a sufficiency of dietary mineral intake, sufficient vitamin D to promote absorption of calcium, and proper function of the parathyroid glands. The calcium is laid down in bone in the form of a complex calcium phosphate and calcium carbonate compound with the assistance of an enzyme, phosphatase, which hydrolyzes phosphoric esters to form inorganic phosphate. Phosphatase is found in high concentration in growing bone. Vitamin C also is essential for bone formation. Skeletal growth is controlled by the anterior lobe of the hypophysis.

Once deposited in bone, the calcium is not necessarily there permanently but is in a storehouse from which it may be quickly and easily withdrawn. Mobilization of calcium from the bones is brought about by parathyroid hormone. Excess of this hormone will raise the level of calcium in the blood at the expense of the bones. The calcium and phosphate concentration of the blood is very stable and delicately balanced by storage or removal from bones. Bone resorption generally is associated with activity of osteoclasts (bone phagocytes). They may be multinucleated and are similar to foreign body giant cells. The role of calcitonin in calcium and bone metabolism was referred to previously (p. 600).

DEVELOPMENTAL ANOMALIES

The developmental disorders of the skeleton frequently appear at birth (congenital), but in some instances they become manifest some years later. These disturbances are commonly referred to as *skeletal dysplasias*. The term "dysplasia" (literally, bad or disturbed formation) implies altered growth resulting from an intrinsic defect in bone. This is in contrast to the term "dystrophy" (literally, bad or disturbed nutrition), which is applied to skeletal abnormalities related to defective nutrition or metabolism induced by disturbances extrinsic to bone (e.g., vitamin deficiencies and hormonal disorders). Unfortunately, synonyms for some of the dysplastic lesions still include the suffix "dystrophy," which was used at a time when a sharp distinction was not made between dysplasia and dystrophy.

The pathologic processes in the dysplasias may represent hypoplasia (e.g., achondroplasia and osteogenesis imperfecta) or a proliferative reaction (e.g., enchondromatosis), which may originate in one or more of the anatomic zones of the bone (epiphyseal centers, cartilage growth plate, metaphysis, or diaphysis). Some of the skeletal dysplasias are discussed in the following paragraphs.

Achondroplasia. Achondroplasia (chondrodystrophia fetalis) is one of the most frequent forms of dwarfism. The defect is primarily in the growth plate, where there is failure of cartilage proliferation and ossification. There is extreme shortness of the bones of the extremities, whereas the bones of the trunk and head are much less affected. The head may appear larger than it is, but sometimes hydrocephalus is present. Since endochondral growth and ossification have been deficient, the tubular bones are short and seem to be disproportionately thick. The condition is hereditary and often evident at birth. Intelligence is not affected. There is usually autosomal dominant transmission, but some cases occur from spontaneous mutations.

Spondyloepiphyseal dysplasias. Spondyloepiphyseal dysplasias constitute a group in which the disturbances are of the osseous centers of vertebrae, carpal and tarsal bones, and the epiphyses of long bones. The dysplasias occur in various genetic forms. The predominant clinical features are dwarfism and spinal deformities. In the past, *Morquio's disease,* an autosomal recessive condition, was regarded as a form of spondyloepiphyseal dysplasia; however, it is now known to be a disorder of mucopolysaccharide metabolism *(mucopolysaccharidosis, type IV).*

Gargoylism. Gargoylism is characterized by a hereditary abnormal metabolism of mucopolysaccharides. Various forms of the syndrome were described by Hunter (1917) and Hurler (1919). Gargoyle facies and hepatomegaly are the most constant features, followed by mental retardation, flexion contractures, corneal cloudiness, splenomegaly, and lumbar kyphosis. The form known as *Hurler's syndrome (mucopolysaccharidosis, type I-H)* is transmitted as autosomal recessive, whereas the sometimes less severe form, *Hunter's syndrome (mucopolysaccharidosis, type II),* is an X-linked recessive condition. Corneal cloudiness is not a feature in the latter form.

Chondroectodermal dysplasia and dysplasia epiphysealis punctata. Chondroectodermal dysplasia *(Ellis–van Creveld disease)* and dysplasia epiphysealis punctata are relatively rare genetic abnormalities.

Enchondromatosis. Enchondromatosis *(Ollier's disease)* is essentially a hamartomatous growth of cartilage cells within the metaphysis of several bones, causing thinning of the overlying cortices and distortion of growth in length. Considerable growth of the cartilage masses occurs mainly in the hands and feet. The proliferating cartilage cells apparently arise from epiphyseal chondroblasts that fail to mature properly and are left stranded by the advancing epiphyseal line. Transition of enchondromas to a malignant form (chondrosarcoma) has been observed.

Osteochondromatosis. Osteochondromatosis *(hereditary multiple exostoses)* is transmitted as a dominant trait. A disturbance in proliferation and ossification of bone-forming cartilage results in multiple cartilaginous and osteocartilaginous growths, usually benign and often roughly symmetric. Secondary distortions and deformities of the skeleton may occur, such as inequality of length of limbs. Malignant change occurs occasionally. The exostoses occur mainly in the long bones.

Osteogenesis imperfecta. Osteogenesis imperfecta (fragilitas ossium) is a hereditary, autosomal dominant disease in which there is mesenchymal hypoplasia. Although the prominent feature in osteogenesis imperfecta is fragility of bones, other tissues are affected, including sclera, teeth, and skin. Recent biochemical studies have shown that abnormalities of collagen and noncollagenous bone proteins may be present in patients with osteogenesis imperfecta. Blue sclerae are often present, the sclerae being thinner than normal and defective in fibrous tissue so that the underlying pigmented choroid shines through. The basic disturbance in bone is believed to be a deficient osteoid production. The bones have thin cortices with a decrease in the cancellous elements. The trabeculae of the medulla are delicate and widely separated (Fig. 25-1). The delicate bones fracture with extreme ease, and affected infants are often born with multiple fractures. In other cases, fractures and deformity develop later. Healing occurs with abundant callus but poor ossification. There is an increase of the acid mucopolysaccharide content of the cartilage of the epiphyses and the long bones, which may inhibit ossification. There is a characteristic disturbance of dentin, similar to that in the bones. Deafness

caused by otosclerosis develops in many cases. Aminoaciduria and a low blood creatinine level also may be found.

Osteopetrosis. In osteopetrosis (marble bone or *Albers-Schönberg disease*), a rare hereditary and familial dysplasia, great increase occurs in the thickness and density of the bones. The defect appears to be a failure of resorption of calcified chondroid and primitive bone. Two forms are described: an autosomal recessive malignant form and an autosomal dominant benign or tarda form. The former is manifested clinically in infancy, and death, usually occurs before the end of the second decade. Profound anemia (osteosclerotic anemia) develops because of encroachment on the hemopoietic tissue of the marrow. The vertebrae, pelvic bones, base of the skull, proximal ends of the femurs, and distal ends of the tibias are most affected. Pressure on cerebral nerves in narrow foramina of the skull causes optic atrophy, deafness, and facial palsy. Although of increased density, the bones are chalky and tend to fracture more easily than normal.

The dominant benign form may be asymp-

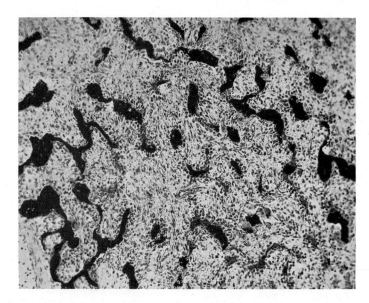

Fig. 25-1. Osteogenesis imperfecta. Note very delicate, well-calcified bone trabeculae within fibrous tissue. Osteoblasts are of irregular shape and arrangement. (Courtesy Dr. W. H. Bauer.)

tomatic for years and is often associated with only radiologic evidence of the disease. However, pathologic fractures as a result of bone fragility, osteomyelitis of the mandible, and facial palsy or deafness caused by compression of cranial nerves by bony overgrowth may occur.

Fibrous dysplasia. Polyostotic fibrous dysplasia of bone (osteitis fibrosa disseminata) appears to be a defect of development involving mainly bone but sometimes extraskeletal tissues as well. Symptoms of pain, disability, and deformity of a limb usually begin in childhood, and the disease runs a slow and protracted course.

The skeletal lesions, usually multiple, are entirely or predominantly unilateral and are most common in the femur and tibia. There is a disturbance in maintenance of cancellous bone. Following physiologic lysis of normal bone, there is replacement by a peculiar fibrous tissue in which abnormal bone forms by metaplasia. The lesions are roentgenologically like those in hyperparathyroidism, but uninvolved skeletal areas show no decalcification. The serum calcium level is normal or only slightly elevated, calcium balance and the serum phosphorus level are normal, and the serum phosphatase level is elevated. In some cases, there are pigmented areas of the skin. In another small group of cases in girls, precocious skeletal and sexual maturation occurs in addition to the cutaneous pigmentation and fibrous dysplasia of bone (*Albright's syndrome*).

A monostotic form of fibrous dysplasia is also described that has none of the clinical or metabolic features of the polyostotic form. Some investigators consider the monostotic form to be an entity distinct from polyostotic fibrous dysplasia.

The lesions show thinning of the cortex of the bone and replacement of the spongiosa and marrow by a rubbery whitish fibrous tissue that is gritty from the presence of spicules of newly formed bone. Cyst formation is absent, although there may be smaller areas of focal cystic degeneration. Microscopically, fibrous tissue replaces the spongiosa, fills the marrow

cavity, and is irregularly traversed by tiny trabeculae of primitive, poorly calcified new bone. Small islands of hyaline cartilage may be present. Malignant transformation of fibrous dysplasia to sarcoma occasionally occurs.

SKELETAL LESIONS IN VITAMIN DEFICIENCIES

Skeletal lesions form a prominent feature in vitamin C deficiency (*scurvy*) and in vitamin D deficiency (*rickets* and *osteomalacia*).

Scurvy. See p. 236.

Rickets. See p. 236.

Osteomalacia. Osteomalacia is the adult counterpart of rickets and is caused by a deficient supply of calcium and vitamin D. It is rare except in countries in which undernutrition is great, occurs almost exclusively in women, and is aggravated by the high calcium demand of pregnancy. The lumbar vertebrae, pelvis (Fig. 25-2), and long bones of the lower limbs are most affected, and severe pelvic deformities may interfere with childbirth. The changes are less limited to growing ends of bones than in rickets. A large proportion of poorly calcified osteoid tissue composes the soft bones, so that they are gradually bent and deformed by muscles and tendons. The bone marrow is fibrous, gelatinous, and sometimes hemorrhagic, and, as in rickets, the parathyroid glands often are found to be enlarged.

OSTEOPOROSIS

Osteoporosis is a reduction in the amount of calcified bone mass per unit volume of skeletal tissue. The most common form, *senile osteoporosis*, occurs in the aged. The spine (Fig. 25-3), pelvis, and peripheral limb bones are affected earliest and most severely. There is increased liability to fractures and deformity. The cause is uncertain. Although lessened physical activity has been considered to play a role, hormonal changes such as diminished estrogen or androgen appear to be more important. Dietary deficiencies may be contributory. Another contributing factor that has been suggested is excessive or unbalanced action of parathyroid hormone. It has been postulated

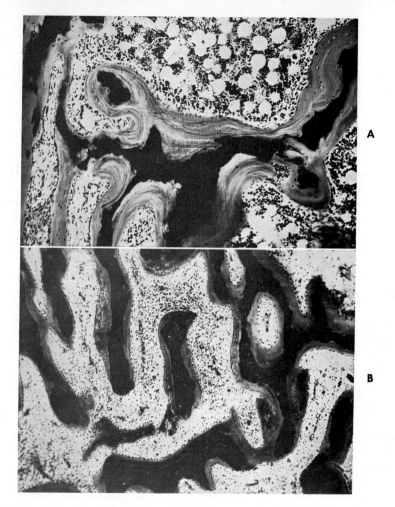

Fig. 25-2. Osteomalacia and rickets. **A,** Osteomalacia (symphysis pubis). Well-calcified remnants of old bone are coated with extremely wide osteoid tissue. **B,** Rickets. Note broad osteoid zones surrounding well-calcified bone trabeculae.

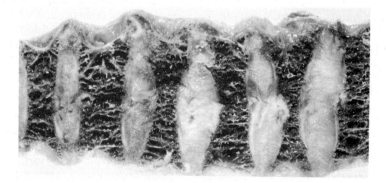

Fig. 25-3. Osteoporosis of vertebrae. Note separation of bone trabeculae, collapse of central portions of vertebral bodies (biconcavity), and resultant expansion of intervertebral discs (biconvexity).

that the normal aging process in the kidneys, resulting in obsolescence of nephrons and decrease in glomerular filtration, may stimulate parathyroid gland hypersecretion.

In the *postmenopausal osteoporosis* of women, hypoestrinism appears to be the cause. A lack of estrogen leads to an inadequate formation of bone matrix because of insufficient stimulation of osteoblasts. Excess of corticosteroids, as in *Cushing's syndrome* or after the administration of *cortisone* or *ACTH,* also leads to inadequate stimulation of osteoblasts. Generalized osteoporosis also is seen in clinical states characterized by decreased formation of matrix because of an insufficient amount of available protein and vitamin C, as in *nutritional deficiency states,* or because of an increased catabolism of protein, as in *hyperthyroidism* and *diabetes mellitus.* A *local osteoporosis* involving individual bones may be seen, e.g., osteoporosis in a single bone after immobilization or localized osteoporosis (atrophy) in an area of a bone being compressed by a tumor or an aneurysm.

SKELETAL LESIONS IN ENDOCRINE DISTURBANCES

In addition to osteoporosis, other skeletal abnormalities may be produced by endocrine disturbances, particularly by pituitary, thyroid, and parathyroid disorders.

Gigantism. Excessive secretion of somatotropic hormone (STH) from an acidophil (or sometimes a chromophobe) adenoma of the pituitary gland causes exaggerated skeletal growth if the disturbance occurs during the period of normal growth, when the ossification centers are still active. There is excessive growth of fibrous tissue also.

Acromegaly. If excessive STH occurs after the period of normal bone growth, when the ossification centers have closed, there is abnormal excessive bone growth due to enchondral bone formation from the deep layers of articular cartilage and intramembranous bone formation from periosteal fibrous tissue. The result is marked thickening of bones without proportional longitudinal growth. Prominence of the bones of the hands, feet, face, and jaw is characteristic.

Generalized osteitis fibrosa (cystica). Osteitis fibrosa (cystica) (Recklinghausen's disease) is caused by hypersecretion of parathyroid hormone, usually the result of an adenoma in one gland. It is characterized by demineralization, bone resorption, and fibrous replacement of the deossified areas (Fig. 25-4). Associated with the disease are decreased neuromuscular sensitivity to galvanic stimulation, hypercalcemia and hypophosphatemia, elevated serum phosphatase level, and often metastatic calcification in other tissues, particularly the kidney.

The essential change in osteitis fibrosa is an osteoclastic resorption of bone and its replacement by connective tissue in which there are abortive attempts at new bone formation. This may be of any degree. When mild, the gross change in the bones is merely a slight porousness and, microscopically, mild generalized osteoporosis and marrow fibrosis. With progression of the condition, there is more and more loss of osseous tissue, which is replaced by connective tissue. Immature, poorly calcified bone develops in the connective tissue. The newly formed bone soon may again undergo resorption. Osteoclasts are abundant. Large fibrous scars develop in the place of the original spongy bone. Some of the lesions are brownish and often are called brown or giant cell tumors, although they are not true neoplasms. The brown tumors are areas of round and spindle cells, fibroblasts, and giant cells. The giant cells show phagocytosis of red cells or hemosiderin, which imparts the brown color to the lesion.

Cysts are not always formed, and the presence of cysts or brown tumors is not necessary for the diagnosis. The cysts may be minute or large and single, multilocular, or multiple. They result from degeneration or hemorrhage and are lined by connective tissue.

When osteitis fibrosa is severe, the involved bones are soft and easily deformed or cut, and the skeletal lesions may be varied, with extreme decalcification, deformities, cysts, and giant cell formation. The long bones and spine are most involved, followed by the pelvis, skull, and jaw. The degree of functional stress and strain apparently is a factor in localization.

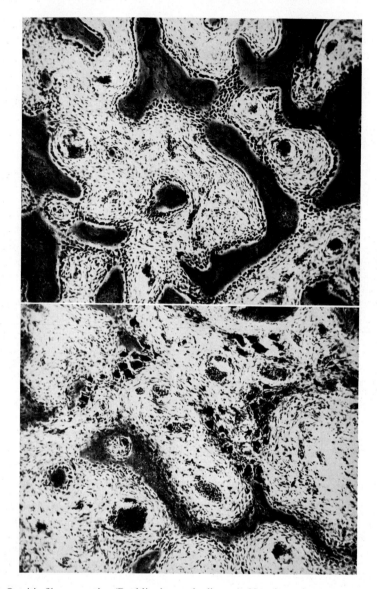

Fig. 25-4. Osteitis fibrosa cystica (Recklinghausen's disease). Note irregular arrangement of newly formed bone trabeculae, which exhibit narrow osteoid zones and osteoclastic resorption. Marrow is fibrous and hyperemic.

HYPERTROPHIC OSTEOARTHROPATHY

In hypertrophic osteoarthropathy, formerly called "hypertrophic pulmonary osteoarthropathy," there is symmetric enlargement (clubbing) of the distal phalanges of the fingers and toes, with swelling of the joints. Subperiosteal deposition of bone is increased, with thickening of connective tissue around the bone and joint. Similar changes also occur in the periosteum of the tubular bones of the extremities. The lesions usually are associated with conditions of chronic anoxemia or with some toxemia. Chronic lung abscess, bronchiectasis, empyema, pulmonary tumors, and congenital cardiac defects are conditions with which hypertrophic osteoarthropathy is often associated.

OSTEITIS DEFORMANS (PAGET'S DISEASE OF BONE)

Paget's disease of bone is a curious condition that usually occurs in persons past 50 years of age. It is characterized by osteoclastic resorption of bone and simultaneous overgrowth of new, poorly calcified, irregular bony spicules. There is also excessive periosteal growth of bone with deficient calcification. The result is an increase in thickness of bones with simultaneous distinct softening, so that severe bowing or other deformities occur. The spine, sacrum, femur, cranium, sternum, pelvis, tibia, and jaws are most commonly involved. The blood phosphatase level is high, but blood calcium and phosphorus concentrations are not changed. The calcium balance is positive, and the parathyroid glands apparently are uninvolved. Sarcoma may be superimposed in some cases and has a very poor prognosis. The sarcoma is usually an osteosarcoma but may be a fibrosarcoma or a chondrosarcoma.

Grossly, the thickened bones are often extremely soft, light, and porous, although in late stages a more hardened state may develop. Microscopically, there is evidence of osteoclastic resorption and formation of new bony trabeculae. Between the new trabeculae, there is an excessive amount of loose connective tissue. Irregularly shaped plates of new and old bone stain with varying degrees of density and are separated by irregular lines of ground substance, a feature that imparts a mosaic appearance to the bony tissue (Fig. 25-5). This mosaic arrangement is the diagnostic characteristic of the microscopic appearance of the bone in fully developed Paget's disease. Increased vascularity often appears in the lesions. Increased blood flow and oxygen tension in the venous blood of the affected limb and increased cardiac output followed by cardiac failure have been observed in patients with Paget's disease of bone. These features have been attributed to the increased vascularity in the bone lesions, which behave in the manner of an arteriovenous fistula, although actual anatomic arteriovenous shunts have not been demonstrated in the lesions.

DISTURBANCES OF CIRCULATION

Like other tissues, bone is dependent on adequate blood supply for preservation of its structure and function. Certain circulatory malformations (e.g., arteriovenous fistula) sometimes affect the circulation of a limb and cause overgrowth of the bone. Necrosis (infarction) occurs in bone when the circulation is seriously reduced. This is commonly a result of trauma, and in fracture some necrosis usually occurs near the ends of the fragments. Fracture or dislocation of the hip may interrupt the blood supply through the ligamentum teres and result in aseptic (avascular) necrosis of the head of the femur. In adults, blockage of circulation in bone may cause infarction.

ASEPTIC (AVASCULAR) NECROSIS

One form of aseptic necrosis of bone is the result of an interruption of the circulation such as occurs at the site of a fracture, as mentioned in the preceding paragraph. A second form is idiopathic aseptic necrosis, which occurs most commonly in the epiphyses of growing children. *Osteochondritis deformans* (Legg-Perthes disease; coxa plana) is a caries and rarefaction of the head of the femur in children 5 to 10 years of age. A similar rarefaction of bone affects the tibial tubercle in *Osgood-Schlatter disease*, the tarsal scaphoid in *Köhler's disease*, and the semilunar bone of the wrist in *Kienböck's disease*.

Osteochondritis dissecans is an aseptic necrosis involving subchondral bone, with secondary changes in adjacent cartilage, which may show softening and degeneration. The involved tissue may be extruded, forming a loose body in the joint. Most cases occur in young adults, the knee being most often in-

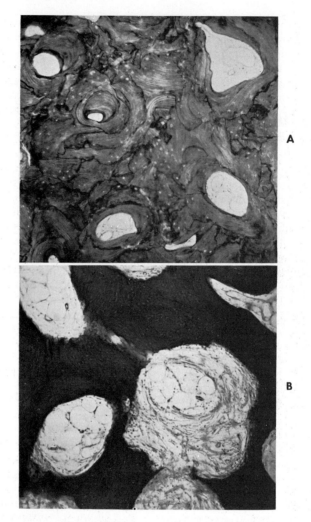

Fig. 25-5. Paget's disease of bone. **A,** Note mosaic structure. **B,** Fibrosis of fatty marrow proceeding from periphery of marrow space.

volved. Trauma usually is considered a causative factor.

INFLAMMATORY LESIONS

The skeletal tissues, like the soft tissues of the body, respond to injuries by a process of inflammation. In many cases, the injurious agent is of bacterial nature, as in osteomyelitis caused by staphylococci, but other inflammatory processes are of more obscure etiology. In

acute inflammation, it is the periosteum, the contents of the haversian canals, and the bone marrow that are mainly involved. In more chronic processes, changes in the osseous portions are also prominent, for in the chronic condition there is time for changes to occur in the hard tissues.

Osteomyelitis. Microorganisms may reach bone directly through a wound (e.g., a compound fracture), may spread to bone from an adjacent tissue (e.g., from a suppurative infection of a tooth or of the middle ear), or may be brought to bone by the bloodstream from a distant focus of infection, which may or may not be clinically apparent. When the inflammation is restricted to periosteum, it is properly called a periostitis, and when it involves bone substance, an osteitis. In most cases, bone and marrow tissue is involved as well as periosteum, and the term *osteomyelitis* is commonly used. Osteomyelitis is usually caused by bacteria and only occasionally by fungi and other nonbacterial organisms. The most common cause by far is the staphylococci, but streptococci, particularly in infants, and gram-negative bacilli also are important causative agents. Interestingly, a relatively high incidence of hematogenous osteomyelitis caused by *Salmonella* is observed among patients with sickle cell anemia.

Since the availability of antimicrobial agents, the incidence and mortality of osteomyelitis have declined considerably. Adequate therapy for the osteomyelitis shortens the course of the disease and tends to limit spread of the infection. In subsequent paragraphs, the features of untreated disease will be considered.

Acute hematogenous osteomyelitis is mainly a disease of childhood and is uncommon after the age of 30 years. It usually is caused by *Staphylococcus aureus* but may be caused by other pyogenic bacteria. The original focus of the organisms is often not discoverable, although sometimes it is obvious, such as a furuncle or carbuncle. At the onset, fever, local pain, and leukocytosis occur. Radiologic changes in the involved bone are not discernible in the early acute stage.

The affected focus is usually in a long bone of an extremity and either is situated close to the end of the diaphysis near the epiphyseal cartilage or is more superficial, lying just beneath periosteum. These are situations in a growing bone that have relatively high vascularity and are subject to trauma. Spread of the infection may be outward to form a subperiosteal abscess and inward to reach the central canal and thence spread widely in the bone. In most cases, the epiphyseal cartilage opposes spread to the epiphysis. Purulent exudate forms and may be seen in the haversian canals and marrow spaces and beneath the periosteum. Fragments of bone become necrotic, influenced by thrombosis of haversian vessels (Fig. 25-6). This dead bone (sequestrum) undergoes digestion and removal only very slowly and with great difficulty. Its continued presence prolongs the inflammation and prevents healing. An irregular casing of new bone (involucrum) may form around the sequestrum. Occasional complications of acute osteomyelitis include extension into a joint, formation of fistulous tracts, and pyemia. Some cases become chronic and persist for years with draining fistulous tracts. The complication of secondary amyloidosis, involving particularly the liver, spleen, and kidneys, may occur in such cases.

Brodie's abscess is a circumscribed focal chronic osteomyelitis. In most cases, the chronic abscess is found in the upper end of the tibia. It may be the sequel of an acute osteomyelitis with organisms of low virulence.

Nonsuppurative nonspecific inflammation. There sometimes occurs a localized condition that is apparently of inflammatory nature in which the specific cause is unknown. *Sclerosing osteitis* (Garré's disease) is an example and is characterized by intense pain in a local area of dense cortical bone.

Syphilis. Syphilis, either congenital or acquired, may produce a chronic osteitis, osteochondritis, or periostitis. In congenital syphilis, osteochondritis of a long bone is particularly characteristic. The epiphyseal line is irregularly widened, opaque, and yellowish gray. Microscopically, there is great irregularity of bone formation in this area, with a chronic inflammatory reaction and severe endarteritis and periarteritis. In acquired syphilis, there may develop an actual gumma or a chronic fibroproliferative periosteal infection of bones with spread into the subjacent bony tissue. Periarteritis and endarteritis are also prominent in the skeletal lesions. The incidence of skeletal involvement in syphilis has

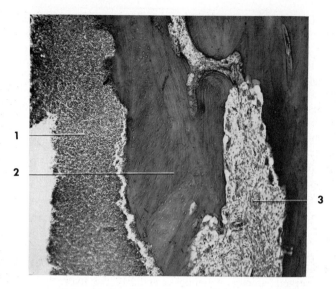

1
2
3

Fig. 25-6. Acute osteomyelitis with formation of a sequestrum. *1,* Pus. *2,* Formation of seques-trum. *3,* Granulation tissue. (From Weinmann, J. P., and Sicher, H.: Bone and bones, ed. 2, St. Louis, 1955, The C. V. Mosby Co.)

been considerably reduced in the United States.

Tuberculosis. A chronic granulomatous form of osteomyelitis is caused by the tubercle bacillus. Children are the victims more fre-quently than adults. The bovine form of the organism accounts for a small proportion of cases. The infection is brought to bone by the bloodstream in most cases, although the pri-mary focus is often insignificant and may be difficult to find. The vertebrae, ends of the long bones of the legs, and bones of the hands and feet are the most frequent sites. Bony tra-beculae are gradually destroyed and replaced by tuberculous granulomas or by caseous and creamy material. In long bones, either the epiphysis or the diaphysis is involved, and spread often occurs to the adjacent joint.

Tuberculosis of vertebrae (Pott's disease of spine). Tuberculosis of the vertebrae usu-ally occurs during childhood. Several verte-brae may be involved. The lesions start in the bodies, produce bony destruction, and spread similarly to destroy adjacent intervertebral discs. Thus weakened, the affected vertebrae

tend to collapse, producing an acute anteflex-ion or angular kyphosis. Complications in-clude compression of the spinal cord and ex-tension of the tuberculous pus to produce a "cold abscess," which may burrow beneath the psoas muscle and appears as a swelling in the inguinal region.

EOSINOPHILIC GRANULOMA

Eosinophilic or solitary granuloma of bone occurs mainly in children and adolescents. Al-though several bones may be affected, more commonly only one is involved. The lesion may be seen in almost any bone except those of the hands or feet and gives rise to local pain and tenderness. Systemic manifestations are usually absent. The blood may show a leuko-cytosis or eosinophilia in some cases.

The involved area of bone shows a soft brownish tissue, which may have yellowish streaks or regions of hemorrhage and cyst for-mation. Microscopically, there are collections of histiocytes, among which are eosinophilic leukocytes and lesser numbers of multinu-cleated giant cells, lymphocytes, and plasma cells. In late stages, the eosinophils may be scarce, the histiocytes have abundant foamy cytoplasm, and fibrosis develops. The prognosis is good when a single lesion is present, since it may be effectively treated by radiation or curettement. It has been suggested that multiple eosinophilic granuloma is a variant of the basic process of *histiocytosis X,* other examples of which are Hand-Schüller-Christian disease and Letterer-Siwe disease (p. 494).

TRAUMATIC INJURY

Minor injuries may cause a localized periostitis. In some cases, this is accompanied by overgrowth of osteoid tissue (callus) in the injured area. More severe injuries may cause *fracture.* In children, relative elasticity of the bone may allow bending without a complete break *(greenstick fracture).* In elderly persons, bones are relatively brittle and fracture with slight trauma. In other cases, very minor trauma may cause a *"spontaneous" fracture* when the bone is weakened by tumor growth or systemic disease. *Compound fractures,* in which there is communication with the exterior, often are complicated by infection. In *comminuted fractures,* the bone is broken into more than two fragments.

Healing of a fracture occurs readily if the broken ends are in apposition and movement is limited. Muscle or other structures between the broken ends may prevent healing, infection retards repair, and excessive movement tends to promote fibrous cartilaginous rather than bony union. When a bone is fractured, hemorrhage and exudation occur between and around the broken ends. The extravasated blood (hematoma) clots and becomes organized by granulation tissue growth. Osteoblastic activity in the periosteum and endosteum produces an overgrowth of osteoid tissue (callus) in the area (Fig. 25-7). Some osteoblasts also may arise from transformed fibroblasts (metaplasia) in the granulation tissue. The osteoid becomes calcified and converted into bone. Some fibroblasts are transformed to chondroblasts that form islands of cartilage that subsequently undergo bone formation. The excess callus in the medullary and exter-

nal parts is gradually removed, and the new bone is knit and shaped by osteoclasts until healing is complete.

TUMORS

Tumors arising in the skeletal tissues are of mesenchymal origin, and hence their malignant representatives are sarcomas. Most bone tumors tend to arise at the ends of bones near epiphyseal lines in areas in which there are complexities of growth and function. Tumors of bone are uncommon. Malignancies of bone probably represent about 1% of all malignant tumors. The tumors may arise (1) from external parts or periosteal tissues (periosteal fibrosarcoma), (2) from the body of the bone (osteogenic, chondrogenic, giant cell, fibrogenic, vascular, and miscellaneous tumors), or (3) from the medulla (myeloma and Ewing's tumor).

From the standpoint of malignancy and prognosis, there are likewise three classes:

1 Benign curable tumors, which include exostosis, osteoma, chondroma of the phalanges, osteoid osteoma, fibroma, bone cyst, and most giant cell tumors

2 Tumors of borderline malignancy and hopeful prognosis, including central chondroma

3 Malignant tumors, usually with poor prognosis, including myeloma, Ewing's tumor, and osteosarcoma

A modification of a commonly used classification that will be used here is as follows:

Periosteal fibrosarcoma
Osteogenic and chondrogenic tumors
    Benign
        Osteochondroma (exostosis)
        Osteoma
        Osteoid osteoma
        Chondroma
        Benign chondroblastoma
    Malignant
        Chondrosarcoma
        Osteosarcoma (osteogenic sarcoma)
Giant cell tumor
    Benign
    Malignant
Fibroma and fibrosarcoma

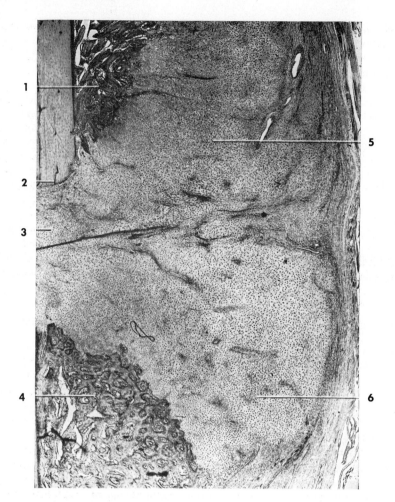

Fig. 25-7. Callus 2 weeks after experimental fracture of tibia of cat. *1* and *4,* Anchoring callus. *2,* Fracture. *3,* Uniting callus. *5* and *6,* Bridging callus. (From Weinmann, J. P., and Sicher, H.: Bone and bones, ed. 2, St. Louis, 1955, The C. V. Mosby Co.)

Vascular tumors
    Benign (angioma)
    Malignant (angiosarcoma)
Ewing's tumor
Multiple myeloma
Other primary tumors
    "Adamantinoma"
    Chordoma
Metastatic tumors
Lesions simulating bone tumors
    Myositis ossificans
    Osteoperiostitis
    Osteitis fibrosa and bone cysts

Periosteal fibrosarcoma. Periosteal fibrosarcoma is a very rare tumor that occurs most frequently in males in early adult life. It arises from the fibrous layer of the periosteum and resembles sarcoma arising from other connective tissue structures. The tumor is single and is found most frequently in long bones, such as the femur and ulna. It forms a fairly large, firm, whitish, circumscribed tumor, and the underlying bone usually shows destructive and sometimes reactive changes. Microscopically, it is similar to fibrosarcoma arising elsewhere.

Osteochondroma (exostosis). Osteochondromas are benign bony or cartilaginous and bony outgrowths from the surface near the end of a long bone. They usually occur in persons between the ages of 10 and 25 years. Microscopically, they show normal laminae of bone beneath a zone of calcifying cartilage, which, in turn, is thinly overlaid by fibrous tissue. To some, the solitary osteochondromas are hamartomas and not true neoplasms.

Hereditary multiple exostoses are a developmental disturbance in which bilateral and symmetric lesions appear in juxtaepiphyseal areas. Transition to chondrosarcoma or osteosarcoma sometimes occurs in one of the exostoses. Malignant transformation rarely occurs in the solitary osteochondromas.

Osteoma. Osteomas are rare benign tumors composed of compact bone. They occur particularly in the skull and facial bones. The term *cancellous osteoma* is sometimes used to refer to the exostosis or osteochondroma. Osteomas are classified by some investigators as hamartomas rather than true neoplasms.

Osteoid osteoma. Osteoid osteoma is a small benign tumor that may be found in almost any bone but is found most frequently in the tibia or femur. It occurs mainly in adolescents or young adults, and pain is the outstanding clinical feature. The tumor consists of a small, well-defined, rounded central nidus that is sharply demarcated from a surrounding zone of bone thickening or sclerosis. The central nidus is only a few millimeters or up to a centimeter in diameter. It consists of a network of osteoid tissue and trabeculae of partly calcified osseous tissue set in a matrix of highly vascular osteogenic connective tissue containing abundant osteoblasts and some osteoclasts. Surgical removal relieves the pain, and there is no recurrence.

It should be noted that some workers have questioned the neoplastic nature of osteoid osteoma, but all agree it is a distinct clinicopathologic entity.

Chondroma. Chondroma (enchondroma) is a benign cartilaginous tumor occurring in the small bones of the hands and feet, ribs, sternum, and spine, usually in persons between the ages of 20 and 30 years. Most frequently found in the phalanges of the hand, it produces a central area of rarefaction. Those chondromas arising in or about the sternum are larger tumors.

Grossly, chondromas are lobulated or trabeculated and pearly gray and may be gelatinous or cystic. Microscopically, they are composed of fairly normal cartilage, the cartilage cells lying in pairs or tetrads in small lacunae. Certain of the cartilaginous tumors that appear to have a benign histologic structure exhibit erratic or malignant behavior and should be considered chondrosarcomas.

Benign chondroblastoma. Benign chondroblastoma is a neoplasm characterized by cartilaginous and giant cell elements that variously has been called a calcifying giant cell tumor and Codman's tumor. It occurs in young persons, most frequently during the second decade, and involves the epiphyseal region of a long bone, principally the humerus, femur, or tibia. Although often very cellular and sometimes causing considerable destruction of bone, it acts in benign fashion and may be satisfactorily treated by curettement or local removal.

Chondrosarcoma. Chondrosarcoma (Fig. 25-8) may be primary or may result from a malignant change occurring in a benign chondroma. The presence of cellular areas consisting of atypical, irregularly arranged cartilage cells with large, sometimes multiple, hyperchromatic nuclei, dispersed throughout a hyaline matrix (Fig. 25-9), differentiates chondrosarcoma from the benign chondroma. Compared with osteosarcomas as a whole, chondrosarcomas occur predominantly in adults between 30 and 50 years of age and have a relatively low degree of malignancy.

Recently described, *mesenchymal chondrosarcoma* is a multicentric tumor composed of an undifferentiated cellular stroma with focal areas of chondroid differentiation. Sometimes, there are zones with a clustering of the small cells about capillary vessels. Because it arises in various bones in young and middle-aged adults, metastases develop in various and sometimes unusual locations. Recurrences are

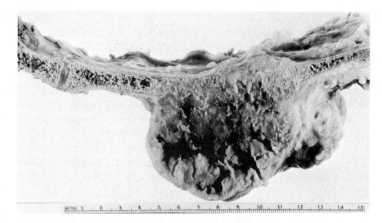

Fig. 25-8. Chondrosarcoma of rib.

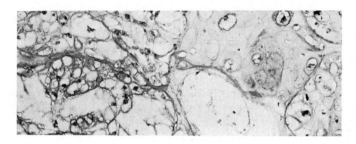

Fig. 25-9. Chondrosarcoma. Neoplastic cartilage cells are very irregular in arrangement, size, shape, and nuclear staining.

common after therapy. Death from the malignant lesion is after variable, but sometimes long, periods.

Osteosarcoma. Osteosarcoma, often referred to as *osteogenic sarcoma,* is composed of osteoblastic (bone-forming) cells that may be derived from the inner layer of periosteum or from the endosteum. Next to multiple myeloma, it is the most frequent malignant tumor of bone. The greatest incidence is in young people between 10 and 30 years of age. In older patients, osteosarcoma may be a complication of Paget's disease of bone. The prognosis of this tumor is extremely poor. The common site is in the shaft of a long bone but near the epiphysis. About 50% occur around

the knee. There is often a history of trauma to the area. Local pain at the site is followed by swelling.

The tumor begins quite superficially but extends both outward and inward, so that subperiosteal and endosteal growth occurs. In late stages, it produces a massive bulbous enlargement of the end of the bone (Fig. 25-10). There may be a bone-destructive (osteolytic) action or a bone-forming (sclerosing or osteoplastic) reaction induced by the tumor. On an x-ray film of the tumor, radiating spicules of newly formed bone may result in a characteristic "sun ray" appearance. Histologically, the picture is extremely variable and complex, and skeletal tissue in all stages of differentia-

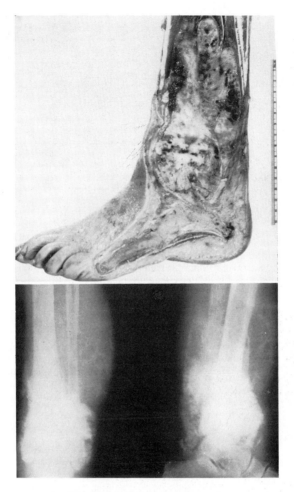

Fig. 25-10. Osteogenic sarcoma.

tion and development may be found (Fig. 25-11). In some cases, marked vascularity, hemorrhage, and necrosis are prominent features (telangiectatic type). The tumor usually spreads by the bloodstream to many organs, especially the lungs, but seldom to other bones.

An uncommon variant of osteosarcoma arising from the external surface of bone is the *parosteal sarcoma* (juxtacortical osteosarcoma). This is a slow-growing tumor that has a better prognosis than the usual central osteosarcoma.

Osteosarcoma develops in extraskeletal soft tissues as a rare event. It must be distinguished from a similar benign lesion that is an atypical form of myositis ossificans. The malignant lesion is distinguished by its cellularity, cellular pleomorphism, mitoses, and atypical osteoid tissue.

In experimental animals, osteosarcomas have been produced by radioactive calcium or strontium deposited in the skeleton.

Giant cell tumor. Giant cell tumor usually involves the epiphyseal region of a long bone. It occurs mostly in early adult life and is rela-

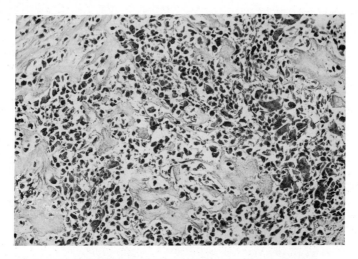

Fig. 25-11. Osteogenic sarcoma. Neoplastic cells are polymorphous with some multinucleated giant cell forms. Irregular areas of osteoid tissue are present.

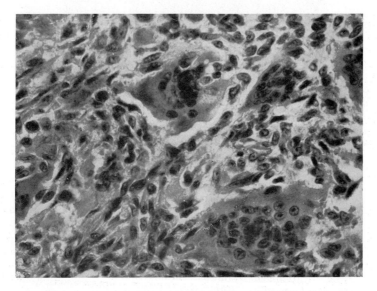

Fig. 25-12. Giant cell tumor of bone. (AFIP 63505; courtesy Dr. G. A. Bennett.)

tively uncommon before the age of 20 years. Pathologic fracture may occur. Grossly, the affected skeletal area is expanded and outlined by a thin shell of bone. The tumor tissue is dark red or reddish brown and of a fleshy or friable consistency. Dark red areas of hemorrhage or yellowish areas of necrosis may be present. Hemorrhage and necrosis sometimes lead to a cystic change. The x-ray film is characteristic, because the tumor produces a rarefied, multilocular cystic or bubblelike appearance. Microscopically, the tumor consists of a highly vascularized stroma composed of spindle-shaped or ovoid cells, with varying numbers of multinucleated giant cells interspersed (Fig. 25-12). The many nuclei of the giant cells tend to accumulate in the center of the cell. In some instances, foci of osteoid formation may be present in the tumors.

There are differing theories of origin of giant cell tumors. It is believed by some that the giant cells represent osteoclasts. Hence, the tumor has been called an *osteoclastoma*. Others have suggested that it arises from undifferentiated supporting connective tissue of the marrow or that it is a tissue reaction to trauma and hemorrhage that may later acquire neoplastic character. Histologically, similar lesions are the giant cell epulis (p. 515), the giant cell tumor of tendon sheaths (p. 727), and the so-called giant cell tumors that occur in osteitis fibrosa cystica (hyperparathyroidism).

Most of the giant cell tumors of bone are benign, but some of them tend to recur after removal. A few are definitely malignant and able to metastasize. The malignant tumors are characterized by abundant compact stromal cells with marked anaplasia, pleomorphism, and a tendency to a whorled arrangement. However, occasional examples of malignant giant cell tumors have not been histologically distinguishable from the ordinary benign giant cell tumors. Because some reported malignant giant cell tumors have contained osteoid tissue, certain investigators have suggested that the lesions are related to osteosarcoma.

In one report, a malignant giant cell tumor and three other instances of neoplasms of bone or soft tissues adjacent to bone (osteosarcoma, fibrosarcoma, and hemangiosarcoma) were described in cats exposed to radiostrontium.

Fibroma and fibrosarcoma. Sharply delimited *fibromas,* without formation of osteoid or bone spicules in the lesions, occur most commonly in the shafts of bones of the lower extremities in children. These *nonossifying fibromas* are benign. A fibroma in which the mesenchymal cells form osteoid or bone spicules has been described (*ossifying fibroma*). Some investigators prefer to call this lesion a *benign osteoblastoma*. The malignant counterpart of a fibroma arising in bone is a *fibrosar-*

coma. It tends to occur in the long bones, especially the femur, particularly in adults. Its occurrence in the periosteal site has already been referred to (p. 712). Fibrosarcoma is not a variant of osteosarcoma and has a better prognosis than the latter.

Vascular tumors. Vascular tumors of bone are uncommon and may be benign or malignant. The benign angioma is similar to angiomatous tumors elsewhere. The malignant angiosarcoma is very uncommon. Rare cases of benign osseous angiomatosis have an associated "massive osteolysis" with progressive localized resorption of bone and resultant deformity.

Ewing's tumor. Ewing's tumor is a malignant neoplasm that occurs in childhood or adolescence and most often involves a long bone. It is accompanied by severe pain, fever, and leukocytosis and hence is easily mistaken for acute osteomyelitis. Its growth in the shaft stimulates reactive formation of multiple new laminae of bone, presenting a layered, onion-like appearance on an x-ray film. The tumor is highly radiosensitive, a characteristic often of diagnostic help, but cure by radiation therapy alone is rare.

The soft, grayish tumor starts in the medulla but rapidly invades and expands the bone. The tibia, femur, humerus, fibula, and clavicle are the most frequent sites. Often, more than one bone is involved. The multiple foci have been regarded as metastases to other bones from the primary site, but some investigators consider them to be multicentric foci of origin. Metastases develop in other organs, including the lungs. Microscopically, Ewing's tumor is composed of small, rounded uniform cells of lymphoblastic appearance arranged in solid sheets and columns or around blood vessels. The lack of stroma is conspicuous, although groups of tumor cells may be bordered by fibrous septa. By silver stains, reticulin can be demonstrated surrounding groups of cells. The tumor cells contain glycogen, a feature that may help to distinguish Ewing's sarcoma from other neoplasms in bone.

The origin of Ewing's tumor was originally believed to be from vascular endothelium (i.e., an endothelial myeloma). It also has been considered to be derived from young reticular cells, although primary reticulum cell sarcoma of bone is said to be distinguishable by reticulin running between individual cells. In a study using tissue culture, histochemical techniques, and electron microscopy, the findings suggested that Ewing's tumor originates from a primitive myeloid cell and that its manner of growth and spread are analogous to plasma cell myeloma.

Multiple myeloma. Multiple myeloma, or generalized myelomatosis, is a fatal disease of later life, with more than 95% of cases occurring in persons past 40 years of age. After diagnosis, the average length of life is $1\frac{1}{2}$ to 2 years. Rarely, persons have survived up to 10 years.

Bone pain, most often in the spine and ribs, is the most frequent beginning. The bone pains are severe, and the bones become weak and brittle, so that fractures occur easily. Roentgenograms may show punched-out osteolytic lesions or generalized resorption of bone or both. Generalized resorption is only recognizable radiologically after 20% to 40% of calcium has disappeared and so is usually evident only in later stages of the disease. Numerous punched-out osteolytic lesions may be seen in the skull ("sieve skull"). Refractory anemia commonly occurs, and there may be some leukopenia. Hypercalcemia and/or hypercalciuria may occur in about 50% of patients with multiple myeloma, but serum alkaline phosphatase is not increased. Renal complications and uremia are frequent. Depositions of amyloid occur in about 10% of cases.

Myelomatosis is a malignant proliferation of immature plasma cells. There is a generalized infiltration of bone marrow by plasmablasts. Localized tumorous overgrowth forms grayish red, soft tumors surrounded by a thin shell of softened bone.

Myelomatosis is to be distinguished from *plasmacytosis*, an increase in the number of normal plasma cells. Bone marrow plasmacytosis occurs in diseases in which serum gamma globulin is increased, such as sarcoidosis, lupus erythematosus, hepatic cirrhosis, kala-azar, and lymphopathia venereum. Increased numbers of mature plasma cells also may occur with some lymphomas, in severe drug reactions, and in cases of agranulocytosis. The immature plasma cells of myelomatosis are more readily differentiated in smears than in decalcified bone marrow sections. The nuclei of the myeloma cells are surrounded by an areola of brightly stained cytoplasm, one or more nucleoli are often seen, and mitoses or multinucleated cells are not infrequent. Hyaline vacuoles may be present in the cytoplasm, may fill the cytoplasm (Mott cells), and may extend to the outer limit of the cytoplasm, which becomes wavy and irregular ("grape cells" of Stich). The grape cells are said to be pathognomonic for multiple myeloma, and the vacuoles, which contain neutral mucoproteins, stain deeply with Giemsa or Wright's stain. The cytoplasm of myeloma cells also may contain fuchsinophilic inclusions (Russell bodies), which consist mainly of gamma globulins rich in glycoproteins.

In multiple myeloma, certain proteins that are practically specific are demonstrable by electrophoretic methods in serum or urine, or both. The proteins, referred to as M-type globulins, are closely related and structurally similar to the normal immunoglobulins. Bence Jones proteins, polypeptide subunits of the M-type globulins, are found in the urine in about 50% of cases of multiple myeloma. Bence Jones demonstrated the proteins as a precipitate in urine made strongly acid and characterized by disappearance of the precipitate on boiling. Trace amounts also may be demonstrable in serum by immunoelectrophoresis.

In about 75% of patients with multiple myeloma, there is hyperglobulinemia, which is mainly an increase of M-type gamma globulins. An antigenic stimulus for the abnormal proliferation of plasma cells and excessive production of the M-type globulins or Bence Jones proteins has not been identified yet. The typical electrophoretic pattern produced by the increased globulin of myeloma is characterized by a steep, high, and narrow-based spike ("church spire peak"). The myeloma globulin in most patients is IgG, and the next most frequent type is IgA. Only a few instances of IgD myeloma and a rare case of IgE myeloma have been reported. Gamma globulins, which react as cryoglobulins, also may be present in myelomatosis. Abnormalities of coagulation (hemorrhagic diathesis) may occur sometimes because of thrombocytopenia and also because of interference with coagulation factors by the M-type proteins. An impaired ability to produce normal antibodies is responsible in part for an increased susceptibility to infections in many patients with myeloma.

In about 10% of patients with multiple myeloma, amyloid may be present, most often deposited in muscle, subcutaneous tissue, lymph nodes, and vessel walls. In viscera, it is mainly in blood vessel walls. The complication of amyloid deposition occurs mainly in patients having Bence Jones protein in the urine but with little or no hyperglobulinemia. Deposition of amyloid in the tongue may produce a striking macroglossia. Skin papules may result from subcutaneous accumulation, hoarseness from involvement of the larynx, and heart failure from myocardial deposition. Amyloid deposition on the synovial membranes of joints is unique to myelomatosis. Amyloid also may appear in the tumor itself.

Renal complications in myeloma patients with Bence Jones proteinuria are mainly caused by tubular obstruction by the precipitated protein. Proximal convoluted tubules, as well as more distant parts of the nephrons, may be obstructed and the tubular lining cells injured. Bence Jones protein casts often elicit a giant cell reaction. Nephrocalcinosis and renal stones also may develop.

Rare cases of *benign plasmacytomas* of bone have been observed, with absence of Bence Jones proteinuria, no hyperglobulinemia, and absence of generalized involvement of bone marrow by plasma cells. Plasmacytomas outside the skeleton may occur, mainly in regions of the upper part of the respiratory tract and oropharynx.

Among the various forms of plasma cell dyscrasia in addition to multiple myeloma is *Waldenström's (primary) macroglobulinemia.*

This condition is generally regarded as a neoplastic proliferation of cells of the lymphocytic-plasmacytic type that normally synthesize IgM macroglobulins. Clinical features include anemia, bleeding manifestations, lymphadenopathy, splenomegaly, hepatomegaly, and lymphocytosis with atypical and plasmacytic forms. The condition may simulate malignant lymphoma or lymphocytic leukemia clinically. Skeletal lesions as seen in multiple myeloma rarely occur. A clinical variant with nervous system involvement (peripheral neuropathy and myelopathy) is known as *Bing-Neel syndrome.*

Adamantinoma. Adamantinoma is an epithelial tumor that usually occurs in the jaw and has a histologic structure resembling the enamel body (p. 515). Rare examples of adamantinoma (so-called) have been found in the tibia or ulna, and although they bear a microscopic resemblance to the lesion in the jaw, it is doubtful that they are of odontogenic origin. The true nature of these tumors is not known. They have been considered by different investigators to be primary bone tumors showing synovial differentiation (synovial sarcoma), malignant angioblastomas, tumors arising from embryonal rests of ectoderm, or tumors arising from implants of epithelial cells of the epidermis or its adnexa resulting from trauma. Electron microscopic studies suggest that the tumors are composed of epithelial cells. Although the "adamantinomas" of long bone grow slowly, they exhibit malignant behavior in that they tend to recur following resection and are capable of metastasizing by the bloodstream or lymphatics.

Chordoma. Chordomas are rare, slowly growing tumors derived from notochordal rests and are found most commonly in the sacrum and in the base of the skull along the clivus. The notochord is the primitive axial skeleton in embryonic life. Notochordal remnants occur in areas other than the sacrum and clivus, e.g., in the nuclei pulposi of intervertebral discs. Grossly, a chordoma is gelatinous or mucinous and tends to compress or invade bone. Microscopically, it is composed of large polyhedral cells disposed in lobules or cords surrounded by a myxomatous matrix. The cytoplasm may contain mucus. Because of inaccessibility, complete removal is difficult, and recurrence is usual.

Metastatic tumors. Certain tumors metastasize to skeletal tissues with particular frequency. These include hypernephroma of the kidney and carcinomas of the prostate gland, lung, ovary, breast, testis, and thyroid gland. A large proportion of metastatic tumors in the skeleton are from bronchogenic carcinomas. Spread is by the bloodstream, and the spine, pelvis, femur, skull, ribs, and humerus are the most frequent sites.

The secondary tumors are often multiple, and pathologic fractures are not uncommon. The metastases are osteolytic, or bone-destroying (Fig. 25-13), except in the case of

carcinoma of the prostate and some well-differentiated mammary carcinomas, which often stimulate an osteosclerotic, or bone-forming, reaction. The undifferentiated bronchogenic tumors may cause little or no bony reaction.

Hypercalcemia is a common accompaniment of metastatic neoplasms in bone, particularly with osteolytic metastases. However, there are some patients who have hypocalcemia in association with skeletal metastases, more so with osteoblastic than osteolytic lesions. The mechanism for development of hypocalcemia is not fully understood.

Lesions simulating bone tumors. The problem concerning clinical differentiation of Ewing's tumor and osteomyelitis has been pointed out. *Myositis ossificans* is a condition

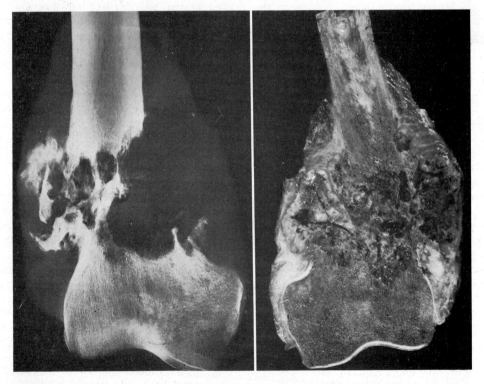

Fig. 25-13. Carcinoma of kidney (hypernephroma) metastasis. Radiologic and gross appearances of slice of femur showing large destructive lesion with pathologic fracture. (From Rosai, J.: Tumors and tumorlike conditions of bone. In Anderson, W. A. D., and Kissane, J. M., editors: Pathology, ed. 7, St. Louis, 1977, The C. V. Mosby Co.)

in which bone develops in muscle tissue. It usually follows trauma and hemorrhage and occurs most frequently in the quadriceps or in muscle about the elbow. The ossification may be extensive and simulate osteogenic sarcoma, and in rare cases there is actual development of malignancy. Parosteal and periosteal forms of posttraumatic ossification also occur. *Osteoperiostitis* is a benign condition in which areas of ossification develop in granulation tissue or hemorrhage beneath a raised periosteum. It is usually of traumatic or syphilitic origin. *Osteitis fibrosa,* in which the lesions microscopically simulate giant cell tumor, is considered on p. 705.

Solitary bone cyst occurs near the end of the shaft of a long bone, most often in the upper part of the shaft of the humerus. Of unknown cause, it is seen most often in childhood or adolescence. The cyst is lined by fibrous tissue. Fracture through the weakened area of bone is a common complication.

Joints

Movable joints have a capsule around cartilage-covered ends of bones and are lined by a synovial membrane, which encloses a cavity containing a small amount of lubricating fluid. The joint is formed of connective tissue derivatives. It functions as an organ of support and passive motion and is affected by mechanical, circulatory, neurologic, and inflammatory changes. Diseases of joints may be classified as (1) specific infectious arthritis, (2) arthritis of rheumatic fever, (3) rheumatoid arthritis, (4) ankylosing spondylitis, (5) rheumatoidlike arthritides, (6) osteoarthritis, (7) traumatic injury, (8) arthritis of gout, (9) arthritis associated with other diseases, and (10) tumors.

The numerically most important diseases of joints are rheumatoid arthritis and osteoarthritis. Being of very common occurrence, they account for a tremendous total of pain, crippling, and disability. Rheumatoid arthritis is essentially an inflammation of synovial membrane, the cause of which is unknown. Os-

teoarthritis is a degenerative change affecting primarily articular cartilage, with secondary hypertrophic changes in the underlying bone. It is often a senescent change and is possibly related to wear and tear and to changes in vascular supply.

ARTHRITIS

Infectious arthritis. Infection of a joint by known organisms is usually the result of hematogenous spread in pyemia or septicemia. Less commonly, the bacteria may reach the joint from an adjacent infection of bone such as osteomyelitis or tuberculosis of bone. Also, there may be introduction from without by penetrating wounds. Any of the pyogenic organisms may thus infect the joints, particularly the staphylococci, streptococci, gonococci, pneumococci, and meningococci. Metastatic infection of joints may occur in gonorrhea, bacterial endocarditis, meningitis, otitis media, pneumonia, typhoid fever, and other infections, although effective antibiotic therapy has decreased the incidence of this complication.

The joint becomes swollen and acutely inflamed. Fluid, at first serous but later purulent, accumulates in the joint cavity. The synovial membrane is greatly congested, swollen, and infiltrated with inflammatory cells. There may be considerable destruction of tissue, so that in healing there is formation of fibrous adhesions (fibrous ankylosis). In some cases, this may be transformed into bone, and a disabling bony ankylosis results.

Gonorrheal arthritis is a complication that usually develops fairly early in an acute gonorrheal infection. Several joints frequently are affected, but only a single joint may be involved.

Tuberculous arthritis is commonly an extension from a tuberculous involvement of bone. It occurs mainly in children and most frequently affects the hip. The synovial membrane is greatly thickened by tuberculous granulation tissue. The inflammation may spread to erode the articular surface. Separation of flakes of cartilage or synovial fringes with adherent fibrin may form small, rounded, firm, loose bodies in the joint (melon seed bodies). Arrest may occur at any stage, or there may be rupture and sinus formation or an end result of fibrous or bony ankylosis.

Arthritis of rheumatic fever. Acute nonsuppurative arthritis is often a prominent feature of rheumatic fever, particularly in the acute cases arising in adolescence or early adult life. Several joints tend to be affected in succession. Acute tenderness and swelling occur, with an excess of turbid fluid in the cavity. The inflammation is predominantly in the synovial membrane, but nodules may develop in subsynovial and periarticular tissues. The histologic character of these may resemble that of the Aschoff bodies of the myocardium or rheumatic nodules elsewhere. The inflammation usually subsides completely without residual disability.

Rheumatoid arthritis. Rheumatoid arthritis is also referred to as atrophic, proliferative, or chronic nonspecific infectious arthritis. It is a very common chronic and disabling disease, with a prevalence in the general population of about 4%. It has its greatest incidence among women of reproductive age and occurs about three times more frequently in women than in men. Although of unknown cause, evidence suggests that it is a chronic inflammation resulting most likely from hypersensitivity or autoimmunity. It usually starts gradually, but it may begin acutely and often is accompanied by general symptoms, fever, leukocytosis, anemia, etc. The small joints of the hands and feet are most frequently affected (Fig. 25-14), and larger joints are involved later. The affected joints show a spindle-shaped swelling, are very painful, and progress to deformity and limitation of movement. Subcutaneous nodules are present in some cases and show a histologic picture somewhat similar to that of rheumatic fever nodules (Fig. 25-15).

Rheumatoid disease is a systemic condition and may include visceral lesions such as granulomas of heart valves, pericardium, myocardium, and pleura. Biopsies of skeletal muscles often show focal accumulations of lymphocytes and macrophages with occasional plasma cells and eosinophils. Secondary amyloidosis is present in some cases. Rheumatoid arthritis may be associated with keratoconjunctivitis and salivary gland swelling as part of Sjögren's syndrome (p. 518). "Rheumatoid fac-

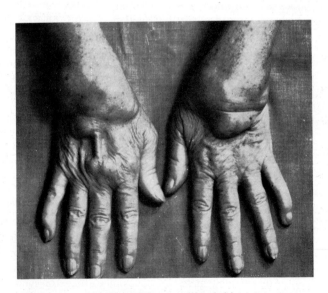

Fig. 25-14. Rheumatoid arthritis.

tor'' is usually present in the serum of patients with rheumatoid disease.

The first and essential change in the joint is in the synovial membrane, which is thickened by a granulation tissue pannus and is infiltrated by many neutrophils, lymphocytes, macrophages, and plasma cells. The cells may be diffusely distributed, but often there are nodular collections, especially of lymphocytes, resembling follicles. By electron microscopy, macrophagelike cells containing numerous lysosomes have been demonstrated (so-called synovial membrane type A cells). The thickened synovial membrane may develop numerous villous processes, in which there may be necrosis, hemorrhage, or fibrosis. Adjacent surfaces form adhesions, so that fibrous ankylosis tends to occur and later may become bony. The joint cartilage is attacked, and there is extension of granulation tissue from the synovial membrane. Inflammatory edema and cellular infiltration also are found in periarticular tissues. An increased effusion

of cloudy and highly cellular fluid is often present in the joint cavity. Vasculitis and perivasculitis are prominent features of both synovial and systemic lesions. It appears that lysosomes released from leukocytes in the synovial fluid, from synovial membrane type A cells, and possibly from chondrocytes play a role in the development of the synovitis and tissue destruction noted in rheumatoid arthritis.

Still's disease is rheumatoid arthritis in children. It is accompanied by fever, leukocytosis, and enlargement of the spleen and lymph nodes. *Felty's syndrome* is a somewhat similar condition in adults, in which chronic arthritis is associated with leukopenia and enlargement of the lymph nodes and spleen.

Ankylosing spondylitis. In ankylosing spondylitis, also known as *Marie-Strümpell spondylitis,* the arthritic changes histologically resemble those seen in rheumatoid arthritis and involve mainly the joints of the spine and the sacroiliac joints. The changes also affect the

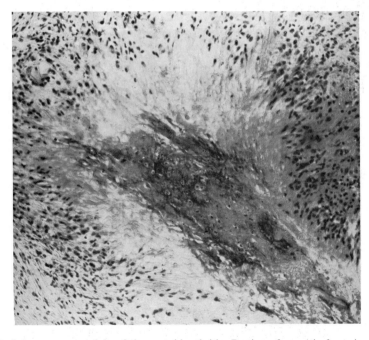

Fig. 25-15. Subcutaneous nodule of rheumatoid arthritis. Portion of necrotic focus is surrounded by palisades of proliferating cells. (AFIP 73941; courtesy Dr. G. A. Bennett.)

intervertebral and costovertebral ligaments. Stiffness and ankylosis of the spine result from ossification of the ligaments and fusion of adjacent vertebrae. Severe kyphosis may be present. Most cases occur in males. Although it was once considered a variant of rheumatoid arthritis, ankylosing spondylitis is now usually regarded as a separate entity because of certain distinctive features:

1 The incidence is very high in men, whereas rheumatoid arthritis occurs mainly in women.

2 It commonly exists without peripheral arthritic manifestations.

3 The serologic reaction for the "rheumatoid factor" is usually negative in the absence of peripheral joint involvement, and even when the latter is present, the incidence of positive tests is low.

4 The cardiovascular disease associated with ankylosing spondylitis is usually an aortitis with aortic valvulitis and insufficiency mimicking syphilitic heart disease, in contrast to the cardiac granulomas of "rheumatoid heart disease."

As pointed out previously (p. 93), some investigators have demonstrated the histocompatibility antigen HLA-B27 in the majority of their patients with ankylosing spondylitis, in contrast to its very low frequency in the general population, suggesting a possible hereditary influence in the origin of the disease.

Rheumatoidlike arthritides. In addition to ankylosing spondylitis, several other forms of arthritis resemble rheumatoid arthritis but lack the rheumatoid factor. Although formerly regarded as variants of rheumatoid arthritis, they usually are classified today as separate entities. These include the forms of arthritis associated with (1) psoriasis (psoriatic arthritis), (2) ulcerative colitis or regional enteritis, and (3) Reiter's syndrome (arthritis, nongonococcal urethritis, and conjunctivitis). Various microorganisms have been suspected but not proved to be the etiologic agents of Reiter's syndrome, including the mycoplasmas and the chlamydiae (bedsoniae).

A new syndrome, called *Lyme arthritis* or *Lyme disease,* has been described recently that must be differentiated from rheumatoid arthritis or one of the rheumatoidlike forms. Its name is derived from the occurrence of an outbreak of the disease in and around Lyme, Connecticut, although it has also been observed elsewhere in the United States. The disease is characterized by recurrent attacks of oligoarticular arthritis affecting particularly the large joints or by migratory polyarthritis in both large and small joints. Usually, the arthritis is preceded by a characteristic annular skin lesion, erythema chronicum migrans, and other clinical manifestations may also occur (e.g., neurologic or cardiac abnormalities). In some patients, chronic arthritis involving one or both knees has been described. Epidemiologic evidence suggests that Lyme disease may be caused by an agent transmitted by a tick vector, a species of *Ixodes*.

Osteoarthritis. Rather than a primary inflammation, osteoarthritis (degenerative, hypertrophic, or senile arthritis) is essentially a degenerative condition of joint cartilage, with reactive and hypertrophic changes in underlying bone. Thus, the term *osteoarthrosis* has been suggested. Affecting the sexes equally, it is a disease of later life, being common in persons past 40 years of age. Large joints, including the hip, tend to be affected, and there is little local inflammation or pain. Although there may be considerable deformity and limitation of movement, complete crippling of a joint is unusual. Trauma and changes resulting from excessive function are most prominent in the causation of osteoarthritis. Other types of injury to the joint, including metabolic and endocrine disturbances, also may be etiologic factors.

Changes begin in the articular cartilage. The cartilage cells degenerate, and the normally smooth surface becomes rigid, frayed, and fibrillated. The elasticity of the cartilage and its cushioning function become reduced. The subchondral bone is thus exposed to excessive functional stresses, and its marrow reacts to this chronic irritation by proliferative changes. Osteoclasts resorb the subchondral bone trabeculae, and blood vessels penetrate into the cartilage. The vascularization of the cartilage is followed by ossification, the bone so formed becoming highly polished (eburnated). Exostoses formed in this fashion at the margins of the joint and periosteal bone formation produce the characteristic bony "lipping" at the edges of the joint. This process occurs prominently in the fingers, forming painless Heberden's nodes. Heberden's nodes are much more common in women than men, and a genetic factor appears to be involved in their pathogenesis. Osteoarthritic changes in the spinal column (spondylitis deformans) may produce kyphosis, extreme rigidity of the back ("pokerback"), and pain caused by the pressure of osteophytic growths on nerve roots. Although bony ankylosis may occur in this type of spondylitis, ankylosis is an uncommon result of osteoarthritis elsewhere.

Traumatic injury. Trauma to a joint may be followed by effusion of fluid into the joint cavity and by acute inflammation of surrounding soft tissues (traumatic arthritis).

Charcot's joint is a condition that occurs in certain cases of tabes dorsalis, neuropathy (e.g., diabetic), and syringomyelia. Destruction of nerve fibers results in loss of sensation in the joint, which is then subjected to unusual trauma. The painless joint is excessively mobile, and destructive changes occur in the joint cartilage and adjacent bone.

Protrusion of an intervertebral disc is a common cause of low back pain and sciatica. The intervertebral discs have a semifluid central matrix (nucleus pulposus) surrounded by circumferentially laminated fibrous tissue and fibrocartilage (annulus fibrosus). Protrusion may involve (1) a bulging disc without detachment from the bone and without a rent in the annulus fibrosus, (2) a herniated disc that extends through a rent in the annulus fibrosus into the spinal cavity, or (3) a slipped disc that has been freed from its anchorage and slipped backward as a result of trauma involving the cartilaginous epiphyseal plate. This sometimes is accompanied by a chip fracture of the vertebral rim. Symptoms are caused by pressure of the protrusion on the spinal cord or one of its branches. Trauma is believed to be the initial cause of herniation or slipping of the disc

rather than primary disease of the disc itself.

Arthritis of gout. Primary gout is a disease of genetic nature that is connected in some fashion with a disturbance of purine (protein) metabolism. The uric acid content of the blood is increased, but this alone does not precipitate an acute arthritic attack. The disease occurs chiefly in middle-aged men. Secondary gout, such as that associated with hematopoietic disorders, also may be accompanied by arthritis (p. 38).

Acute attacks commence suddenly with pain, swelling, and tenderness in a joint (toes, fingers, or knees). There is an effusion into the joint cavity of fluid containing crystals of sodium biurate. The crystals also are present in the synovial membranes and on articular cartilages. Attacks usually recur, so that the arthritis becomes chronic. In addition to synovial inflammation and proliferation, destruction of cartilage and subchondral bone develops. Urate cyrstals apparently produce tissue damage by causing release of lysosomal enzymes from phagocytes, which ingest the crystals (p. 38). Urate crystals also become deposited in surrounding soft tissues, where they elicit some foreign body reaction and chronic inflammation. A tophus is a chalky deposit of the crystals in the subcutaneous tissue, in cartilages of the ear, or occasionally in the eyelids (p. 38 and Fig. 2-13).

Arthritis in other diseases. Systemic diseases, other than those already discussed, in which arthritis frequently occurs include (1) systemic lupus erythematosus, (2) dermatomyositis, (3) serum sickness, (4) polyarteritis nodosa, (5) erythema nodosum, and (6) scleroderma.

TUMORS

Only rarely do tumors arise from joint structures, but chondromas, lipomas, synoviomas, spindle cell sarcomas, and chondrosarcomas have been described.

Synovial sarcoma. Synovial sarcoma is a malignant tumor arising from the lining cells of the synovial membrane of a joint or bursa. Histologically, it shows a distorted picture suggestive of synovia, but the appearance in various examples is far from uniform. A mixed picture of sarcomatous and pseudoepithelial structures is frequently present. There is a groundwork of rounded or spindle cells, with tissue spaces that vary from slitlike clefts to glandlike spaces or pavementlike areas of tissue suggesting low epithelium (Fig. 25-16). Mucinous or serous fluid may be present in glandlike spaces. Papillary villuslike structures or cell tufts are sometimes formed. This tumor is usually regarded as highly malignant. Although some reports indicate that the 5-year survival rate may be as high as 50%, the rate is usually reported to be below that figure. Recurrence often follows local excision of the tumor. Metastases are common in distant organs, such as the lungs, but they may also occur in local lymph nodes.

CYSTS

Various types of synovial or bursal cysts occur. The *popliteal cyst (Baker's cyst)* is one of the most frequent. It may be bursal in origin, or it may be a herniation from the knee joint.

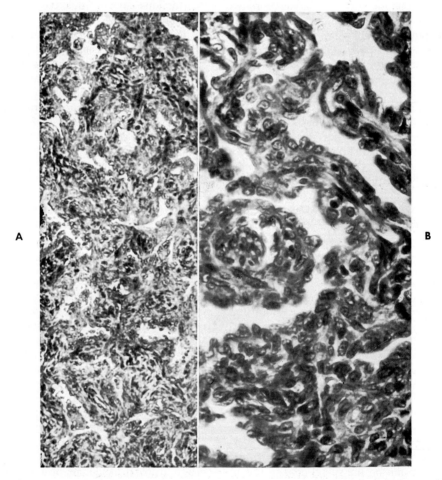

Fig. 25-16. Synovial sarcoma. **A,** Malignant tumor of synovial membrane origin showing characteristic structure. **B,** High-power view of tumor shown in **A.** (AFIP 90623; courtesy Dr. G. A. Bennett.)

The cyst lining may be synovial or may be simply fibrous tissue, with or without an inflammatory exudate.

Tendons

Inflammation. Tenosynovitis is an inflammation of tendon sheaths, usually at the wrist or ankle. It may be traumatic, suppurative, or tuberculous. In the last, with fibrin in the exudate, ovoid melon seed bodies may be formed.

Ganglion. Ganglion is a cystlike swelling arising from a tendon sheath or joint capsule.

It is most common on the back of the hand or wrist. There is proliferation of fibrous tissue of the sheath with mucoid degeneration, producing the cystlike swelling. There is no true lining, and the ganglion does not communicate with the cavity of the tendon sheath.

Tendon sheath tumors. Giant cell tumor (xanthoma) of a tendon sheath is a yellow or yellowish brown tumor that arises near the tendinous insertion, most often in the hand. It has a groundwork of fibrous tissue in which there are scattered giant cells and aggregates of large lipid-containing foam cells (xanthoma cells) (Fig. 25-17). The xanthoma cells are

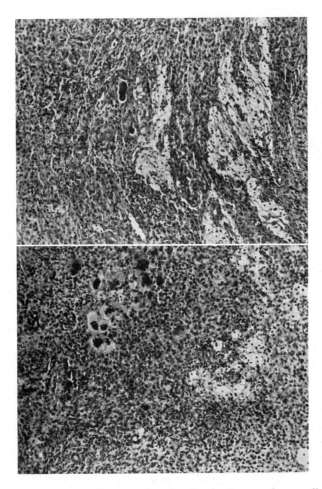

Fig. 25-17. Xanthomatous giant cell tumor of tendon sheath. Note xanthoma cells with distended foamy cytoplasm.

found when there are deposits of iron and cholesterol. Except for this xanthomatous tendency, the tumor is histologically similar to
the giant cell epulis and the benign giant cell
tumor of bone.

**Palmar fibromatosis (Dupuytren's con-
tracture).** Fibrosis of the palmar fascia, with
thickening and shortening, causes flexion of
the fingers, with deformity and inability to
make normal use of the hand. Although the
cause has been considered to be inflammatory,
the condition is characterized mainly by a proliferation of fibrocytes, which may produce
nodular masses and may be mistaken for fibrosarcoma.

Plantar fibromatosis. Plantar fibromatosis
is similar to palmar fibromatosis but does not
ordinarily lead to contractures. Nodular
masses of well-differentiated proliferating fibrocytes arise within the plantar fascia, more
commonly on the medial side. The condition
is benign, and fibrosarcoma arising in this region is very rare. It has been suggested that
the condition is a reactive fibrous hyperplasia
as a result of degeneration of the plantar fascia
that may follow trauma. Complete excision of
the plantar fascia is necessary to prevent recurrence.

REFERENCES

Ackerman, L. V., Spjut, H. J., and Abell, M. K., editors: Bones and joints, Baltimore, 1976, The Williams
& Wilkins Co.
Aegerter, E. E., and Kirkpatrick, J. A.: Orthopedic diseases, ed. 4, Philadelphia, 1975, W. B. Saunders Co.
Albright, F.: J. Clin. Endocrinol. Metab. **7:**307-324,
1947 (fibrous dysplasia of bone).
Beighton, P.: Inherited disorders of the skeleton, Edinburgh, 1978, Churchill Livingstone.
Berlyne, G. M., et al.: J.A.M.A. **229:**1904-1906, 1974
(etiology of osteoporosis—role of parathyroid hor-
mone).
Bland, J. H., editor: Med. Clin. North Am. **52:**447-769,
1968 (symposium on rheumatoid arthritis).
Burkhart, J. M., et al.: Mayo Clin. Proc. **40:**481-499,
1965 (chondrodystrophies).
Caldwell, R. A.: J. Clin. Pathol. **15:**421-431, 1962 (se-
nile osteoporosis).
Collins, D. H.: Pathology of bone, London, 1966, But-
terworth & Co. (Publishers) Ltd.
Coventry, M. B., and Dahlin, D. C.: J. Bone Joint Surg.
[Am.] **39-A:**741-758, 1957 (osteogenic sarcoma).
Coventry, M. B., et al.: J. Bone Joint Surg. [Am.]

27:105-112, 233-247, 460-474, 1945 (intervertebral
discs).
Dahlin, D. C.: Bone tumors, ed. 3, Springfield, Ill.,
1978, Charles C Thomas, Publisher.
Dahlin, D. C., and Henderson, E. D.: Cancer **15:**410-
417, 1962 (mesenchymal chondrosarcoma).
Dahlin, D. C., and Ivins, J. C.: Cancer **30:**401-413,
1972 (benign chondroblastoma).
Dahlin, D. C., et al.: Cancer **25:**1061-1070, 1970 (giant
cell tumors).
Fine, G., and Stout, A. P.: Cancer **9:**1027-1043, 1956
(extraskeletal osteogenic sarcoma).
Gilmer, W. S., Jr., and Anderson, L. D.: South. Med.
J. **52:**1432-1448, 1959 (myositis ossificans).
Hicks, J. D.: J. Pathol. Bacteriol. **67:**151-161, 1954 (sy-
novioma).
Huvos, G., and Higinbotham, N. L.: Cancer **35:**837-
847, 1975 (fibrosarcoma of bone).
Kadin, M. E., and Bensch, K. G.: Cancer **27:**257-273,
1971 (Ewing's tumor).
Kunkel, M. G., et al.: J. Bone Joint Surg. [Am.] **38:**817-
826, 1956 (benign chondroblastoma).
Lichtenstein, L.: Diseases of bone and joints, ed. 2, St.
Louis, 1975, The C. V. Mosby Co.
Lichtenstein, L.: Bone tumors, ed. 5, St. Louis, 1977,
The C. V. Mosby Co.
Llombart-Bosch, A., et al.: Cancer **41:**1362-1373, 1978
(Ewing's sarcoma—EM study).
MacCallium, P., and Hueston, J. T.: Aust. N.Z. J. Surg.
31:241-253, 1962 (Dupuytren's contracture).
Meyer, P. C.: Br. J. Cancer **11:**509-518, 1957 (metastatic
tumors of bone).
Mills, D. M., et al.: J.A.M.A. **231:**268-270, 1975 (HLA
antigens in ankylosing spondylitis).
Osserman, E. F.: In Beeson, P. B., McDermott, W.,
and Wyngaarden, J. B., editors: Cecil textbook of
medicine, ed. 15, Philadelphia, 1979, W. B. Saunders
Co., p. 1852 (plasma cell dyscrasias).
Patterson, C. D., et al.: Ann. Intern. Med. **62:**685-697,
1965 (rheumatoid lung disease).
Pearson, C. M. (moderator): Ann. Intern. Med. **65:**1101-
1130, 1966 (rheumatoid arthritis).
Raskin, P., et al.: Arch. Intern. Med. **132:**539-543, 1973
(hypocalcemia in metastatic bone disease).
Rhodes, B. A., et al.: N. Engl. J. Med. **287:**686-689,
1972 (Paget's disease of bone—absence of anatomic ar-
teriovenous shunts).
Rubin, P.: Dynamic classification of bone dysplasias,
Chicago, 1964, Year Book Medical Publishers, Inc.
Sbarbaro, J. L., Jr., and Francis, K. C.: J.A.M.A.
178:706-710, 1961 (eosinophilic granuloma of bone).
Snapper, I., and Kahn, A.: Myelomatosis, Baltimore,
1971, University Park Press.
Spencer, H., and Whimster, I. W.: J. Pathol. Bacteriol.
62:411-418, 1950 (tumors of tendon sheaths).
Spjut, H. J., Dorfman, H. D., Fechner, R. E., and
Ackerman, L. V.: Tumors of bone and cartilage. In At-
las of tumor pathology, Series 2, Fasc. 5, Washington,
D.C., 1971, Armed Forces Institute of Pathology.

Steere, A. C., et al.: Ann. Intern. Med. **90:**896-901, 1979 (Lyme arthritis—differentiation from rheumatoid arthritis).

Steere, A. C., and Malawista, S. E.: Ann. Intern. Med. **91:**730-733, 1979 (Lyme disease in the United States).

Sykes, B., et al.: N. Engl. J. Med. **296:**1200-1203, 1977 (altered collagen in osteogenesis imperfecta).

Urist, M. R., and Johnson, R. W., Jr.: J. Bone Joint Surg. [Am.] **25:**375-426, 1943 (healing of fractures).

Waldenström, J.: Multiple myeloma, New York, 1970, Grune & Stratton, Inc.

Ward, J. M., et al.: J. Natl. Cancer Inst. **48:**1543-1546, 1972 (bone and soft tissue neoplasms in cats exposed to radiostrontium).

26

Nervous system

STRUCTURE AND REACTION TO INJURY

The nervous system and its supporting structures include a number of basic cells or tissues, each of which exhibits several common types of response to injury. Some of these reactive changes appear to be specific (e.g., the rounding up of microglia to produce fatty granule cells when myelin is destroyed). Many, however, are nonspecific, and the microscopic changes are interpreted with greater difficulty.

Ependyma. The ependymal lining cells of the ventricular system of the brain and the central canal of the spinal cord retain an epithelial character. Very often they are flattened and in some regions may appear in folds or tufts, particularly in the third ventricle. During the developmental period, the ependymal cells are ciliated, and some ciliated ependymal cells may be found in later life. The more common reactions associated with ependymal tissue include proliferation, subependymal gliosis, and inflammation.

Proliferation, manifested by reduplication to several layers of cells, may appear as an aging process. This is common in lower levels of the spinal cord, sometimes to such an extent that the central canal appears obliterated. *Subependymal gliosis* seems to be a response to a chronic toxemia or anoxia, as in alcoholism, the subependymal layer becoming greatly thickened and densely sclerotic. *Inflammation (ependymitis)* is seen in septic conditions of the ventricles and as a result of irritation of the lining cells by other agents, such as *Toxoplasma.* The subependymal layer is swollen and infiltrated with neutrophilic leukocytes, and the lining cells are reduplicated, festooned, and swollen, or they may be eroded.

Neuroglia. The intramedullary supporting glial cells of neuroectodermal origin are astrocytes and oligodendroglia. They are referred to as *macroglia*. The other type of glial cells, *microglia,* is mesodermal in origin and is discussed on p. 734. In sections stained by hematoxylin and eosin, the astrocytes and oligodendroglia must be differentiated by nuclear configuration. The nucleus of the astrocyte is large, oval, pale, and vesicular, with chromatin material deposited in small dustlike particles on a fine linin net. The nuclei of the oligodendroglia are about one-third smaller, are more rounded, and stain darkly, with clumped chromatin masses. Special stains show that the astrocytes possess sucker-foot attachments to blood vessels and a great many fibrillar processes. The oligodendroglia have very few processes. Astrocytes appear in greater number in gray than in white matter. Oligodendroglia are equally numerous in both gray and white matter, forming the "satellite cells" of the neurons and the "interfascicular supporting cells" of the nerve fibers.

Astrocytes may undergo either regressive or reactive changes. Regressive changes are most commonly seen as degenerative processes in tumor cells or in severe toxemia and are manifested by shrinkage and gemistocytosis.

Shrinkage is identified by pyknosis of the nucleus with fragmentation and extrusion. *Clasmatodendrosis* is a regressive change with cytoplasmic swelling, loss of cytoplasmic processes, and nuclear pyknosis. In *gemistocyte formation* or *swelling,* the cells swell and cytoplasm becomes stainable by routine methods. The nuclei are eccentric and may be multiple. These cells often are referred to as "fat astrocytes." Reactive changes in astrocytes are represented by *proliferation,* an increase in the number by amitotic division, and by *gliosis,* a production of glial fibrils forming a dense fibrous network and entering into repair phenomena.

Oligodendroglia may present reactive changes. *Acute swelling* with vacuolation is a nonspecific alteration that may occur as an agonal phenomenon. *Satellitosis* is an apparent increase in the number of oligodendroglia neighboring a nerve cell body and is seen in certain toxic states. It may be seen to occur as incidental to neuronophagia (p. 732).

There are a number of alterations in the nervous system in which the parent reacting element is obscure but glial cells may take part. *Glial nodes* are nests of proliferated glial cells that are prominent in rickettsial and other encephalitides and may be seen near infarcts. Since they are often aggregated close to vessels and house intracellular organisms, the cells may be derived from perithelial cells of vascular adventitia. *Glial plaques* (Alzheimer) are sclerotic nodules representing focal degeneration. They may contain glial fibers and cells with an admixture of fragmented nerve fibers. *Corpora amylacea* are concentric hyaline bodies that, according to electron microscopic evidence, appear to be degenerative bodies in fibrous astrocytes. They are common in persons past 40 years of age and often are conspicuous in premature senility. They stain with iodine but contain neither amyloid nor fat. Histochemically, they appear to contain a complex glucose polymer.

Choroid plexus. The choroid plexus may be regarded as a pia-ependymal membrane invaginated by subarachnoid vasculature. The ependymal epithelium with a thin fibrous substrate is arranged in a foliated or villous pattern with a highly vascular core composed of loose trabecular tissue resembling arachnoid. Alterations in the choroid plexus are common but usually are unimportant. Most often encountered are *cyst formation,* the thin-walled, translucent cysts appearing most frequently at the confluent part of the lateral ventricles; *concretions* (brain sand), amorphous firm bodies that are sometimes quite numerous; and *sclerosis,* a fibrosis of the choroid core.

Neurons. The neurons are the functional units of the nervous system and by their interrelationships provide the physical basis for nervous activity. Each consists of a cell body and its processes. Microscopically, the best criterion for identification is the nucleus. It is large, round, and vesicular and contains a large nucleolus. The nuclear membrane is distinct. The cytoplasm contains varying amounts and patterns of basophilic material known as Nissl substance. Special stains enable identification of neurofibrils, which traverse the cell body and continue into the processes. The shape of the cell body varies greatly. It may be multipolar or unipolar, and the size ranges from a diameter of a few microns to more than 100 μ, depending on location and function.

From the cell bodies arise a varying number of processes. The axon is the process over which a nervous impulse is conveyed to an adjacent neuron or to an end-organ. Those axons (axis-cylinders) attaining a diameter greater than 1.5 μ possess a fatty covering, the myelin sheath. In the central nervous system, this sheath is limited externally by the network of fibrillar processes of supporting cells (oligodendroglia). In peripheral nerves, the myelin is encased in a wrapping supplied by sheath cells (Schwann). Each sheath cell has distinctly marked linear limits that form a constriction (node of Ranvier) around the axis-cylinder, at which point the myelin layer is obliterated. The axis-cylinders terminate in buttonlike knobs (boutons), which provide the contact points at the synapse or in special peripheral structures in muscle or gland.

Changes in body of nerve cells. Changes in the body of nerve cells are difficult to interpret because of the complex nature of the neuron and the distances over which the processes spread. The common reactions of the cell body are shrinkage, swelling, vacuolation, pigment changes, chromatolysis, and neuronophagia.

Shrinkage is indicated by great irregularity in the shape of the cell, pyknosis of the nucleus, clumping and condensation of Nissl substance, and sclerosis or contortion of processes. Shrunken cells are common in senility and other cerebral atrophies and also may appear in chronic infections. Fixation artifacts may mimic shrinkage or sclerosis of cells.

Swelling of nerve cells clouds the irregular surface contour. The cytoplasm stains faintly, the processes fragment, and the cell may be evident in outline only. This change, apparently reversible, occurs in acute toxic states and mild infections. It is the most prominent change in tetanus.

Vacuolation of nerve cells is unusual but occurs in toxic states. It may be seen normally in the hypothalamus, posterior pituitary gland, and peripheral spinal and autonomic ganglion cells.

The appearance of light brown or yellow (lipochrome or lipofuscin) pigment in a perinuclear position or in cytoplasmic blotches is observed commonly in old age and in certain degenerative diseases and is referred to as *pigment degeneration*. This degenerative process should not be confused with the normal (neuromelanin) pigment in cells of certain locations (locus ceruleus and substantia nigra).

In *chromatolysis,* the Nissl substance becomes fine, dispersed, and peripheralized or loses its staining properties altogether. The nucleus of the involved cell is eccentric in position. Because this change is believed to be a specific retrograde response to axon injury, it has been widely used to identify the nuclear or ganglionic origin of damaged fiber bundles in the central and peripheral nervous systems.

Neuronophagia involves reaction of macrophages as well as nerve cells. Phagocytosis of nerve cells is common only in inflammatory diseases and is conspicuous only when the death of the cell is brought about by an intracellular agent. It is a characteristic occurrence in poliomyelitis. A mass of macrophages may be seen occupying the position of, or within, a nerve cell body. The phagocytic cells may be mononuclear cells from the blood or microglia. In satellitosis, on the other hand, the cells are oligodendroglia and are seen around but not within the nerve cell body.

Reactions of axis-cylinder. The reactions of the axis-cylinder to injury include changes in the axon, alterations at the synapse or end-organs, and neuroma formation. By coating the argyrophilic neurofibrillar structure with reduced silver salts, the morphology of the axis-cylinder and its terminal boutons is seen to vary under pathologic influence. The axon may swell in irregular nodules or fragment and become granular. The synaptic change may be a loss of structure, or it may be an accentuation by beading and reduplication of terminal bulbs. Diffuse encephalomyelitis induces the most profound synaptic changes. In peripheral nerves, the end-organs undergo dissolution after severe damage to the nerve.

Neuroma formation occurs as a regrowth reaction to traumatic interruption of nerve fibers. The neuroma is a tangle of regrowing neurofibrils, each spearheaded by a bulbous expansion, the growth cone. Neuromas may develop along the trunk of a nerve at a point of trauma or at the extremity of an amputated limb or stump. The microscopic appearance is complicated by growth of fibrous tissue or by sheath cell proliferation (Fig. 26-1). In a *traumatic neuroma* of some duration, these supporting elements remain, and the argyrophilic substance of the axons disappears. A different type of neuroma *(plantar digital neuroma)* occurs in Morton's metatarsalgia (Morton's toe). This is a tumefacient swelling of a plantar digital nerve, usually the fourth, characterized by degeneration and loss of nerve fibers and fibrosis.

Myelin degeneration. The loss of myelin substance (demyelination) is a prominent pathologic change in both the central and peripheral nervous systems. In considering demyelination as an index of injury, one must remember that some fibers normally possess no myelin. This fatty substance, a complex of

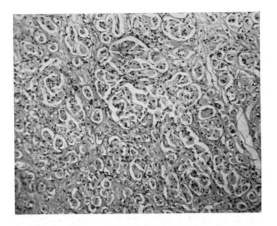

Fig. 26-1. Amputation "neuroma."

at least four lipids, is deposited around fibers of both central and peripheral axons. Injury to the cell body or axis-cylinder causes a degeneration of the myelin, or dissolution of the myelin may occur spontaneously without apparent nerve injury. Demyelination may be recognized in routine hematoxylin- and eosin-stained sections but is best demonstrated by use of special stains, such as the Weigert stain. The Weigert technique stains normal myelin blue or black. Demyelinated areas do not stain and hence are identifiable by contrast. Other techniques are available in which the degenerated or altered myelin is stained but the normal myelin is not.

The demyelinating process and accompanying changes occurring secondary to trauma or interruption of peripheral nerves are called *wallerian degeneration.* This proceeds in both distal and proximal directions from the point of injury. Proximally, the observable alterations in the myelin are usually arrested at the next node of Ranvier. The node probably plays no role in this, since the same limitation of retrograde change is seen in the central nervous system. Proliferation of neurofibrils, proximal to the injury occurs within a few hours. Distally, the axis-cylinders become granular and fragment, and the myelin undergoes dissolution and forms fat droplets. The products of degeneration are removed, mainly by macrophages, in a few weeks.

Simultaneously, regenerative changes occur. The sheath cells (neurilemma; Schwann) proliferate, enlarge, and migrate from both proximal and distal stumps into the defect, bridging it and providing cytoplasmic channels for the regrowing neurofibrils from the proximal stump. The endoneural connective tissue persists, reinforcing the neurilemmal cells. Regrowth may be inhibited by scar tissue and by poor apposition of the stumps. Regrowing neurofibrils will progress at the rate of 0.25 mm per day through the scar and 3 to 4 mm per day through the peripheral stump. Certain of the regrown fibrils slowly enlarge within the Schwann cells and accumulate a myelin sheath. The original status of an individual myelinated peripheral nerve fiber is reestablished in 9 to 12 months. The complete restitution of all fibers of a peripheral nerve probably does not occur.

In the central nervous system, there is a somewhat different process of demyelination. The sheath cells are replaced by oligodendroglia, which lack the remarkable regenerative properties of the former. Central nerve cell processes may be as inherently capable of regrowth as peripheral cells, but only those that possess a neurilemmal sheath can be restored. Consequently, functional repair of interrupted central axons does not occur, although abortive neurofibrillar attempts at regrowth are constantly observed. Hence, disruption of nerve tissue with accompanying demyelination in the central nervous system is an irreversible reaction.

In the area of brain or spinal cord injury or softening, where a large amount of myelin is broken down, the degenerative fatty products are removed by macrophages (microglia). The degeneration of myelin progresses distally from the point of injury. The myelin appears in droplet form and acquires staining reactions, which imply chemical alteration. The droplets will, however, remain in position for months or even years and mark the degenerating tract. Proximally (toward the cell body), the process may progress for a short distance but ordinarily is insignificant.

Demyelination also occurs in association

with certain diseases of the central nervous system (p. 748).

Sheath of Schwann. A membranous covering for peripheral axons is provided by sheath (Schwann) cells. Microscopically, their nuclei appear as elongated structures along peripheral nerves. The sheath cells form a cylindrical tube threaded by an axon and separated from it by a concentric sheath of myelin. When myelin is absent, the axon is covered intimately by the thin-walled sheath cell. Applied to the outside of the Schwann sheath are the collagenous elements of the endoneurium. The reactions to which sheath cells are subject are, principally, hypertrophy and proliferation, and these occur prominently in repair of peripheral nerves.

Nerve cell bodies in peripheral and cranial ganglia are ensheathed by cells commonly referred to as *satellite cells.* Electron microscopy has shown that these cells can perform the function of periaxonal Schwann cells, i.e., the laying down of myelin. Thus, the cells are sometimes termed "satellite Schwann cells."

Meninges. The coverings of the central nervous system include the dura (pachymeninx) and the pia-arachnoid (leptomeninx). The dura is adherent to the cranial periosteum (external layer of dura) but is separated widely from the periosteum of the vertebral canal. The pia follows the surface of the brain closely and is separated from the arachnoid, which is in apposition with the dura, by the subarachnoid space. This space contains cerebrospinal fluid and is bridged by a spongy network of filaments, the arachnoid trabeculae. The principal histologic element of all membranes is collagenous tissue. Elastic fibers appear in the pia-arachnoid and in the innermost layer of the dura. Flattened mesothelial cells (meningothelium) line the subarachnoid and subdural spaces and cover the arachnoid trabeculae. In addition to the lining cells, fibroblasts and fixed histiocytes are identifiable in the membranes. Nests of epitheliallike cells occasionally are encountered buried in the dura. These are arachnoid granulations.

The common reactions of the meninges to injury include the production of macrophages and false dura formation. The macrophages are derived from meningothelium or fixed histiocytes, or both, and appear in greater number in inflammatory conditions. False dura formation amounts to a rapid repair process in which a coagulum forms, later to be invaded by fibroblastic cells. This occurs when dural continuity is interrupted and in walling off of hemorrhage.

Vasculature and related structures. Intimal, medial, and adventitial changes in cerebral vessels are similar to those occurring elsewhere. There are, however, three peculiarities in cerebral vasculature that play prominent roles in reactive phenomena:

1 Vessels less than 70 μ in diameter·contain little or no muscle in the media after 40 years of age.

2 In passing through the subarachnoid space, the vessels acquire a meningothelial sheath and, in penetrating to an intramedullary position, carry a second, outer sheath derived from the pia lining. These concentric wrappings establish a perivascular space (of Virchow-Robin). This space is the morphologic basis for the reaction of perivascular leukocytic infiltration or cuffing. Drainage from the interstitial spaces of the medullary substance passes through the Virchow-Robin channels and, in so doing, may load the space with inflammatory cells or products of degeneration. In addition, exudate reaches the perivascular space through the vessel wall.

3 Vascular adventitial elements provide the parent tissue that reacts to form an abscess wall in response to invasion by certain bacteria.

Vascular disease of the brain is an important cause of morbidity and mortality. Cerebral infarcts (cerebral softening or encephalomalacia) commonly result from vascular obstruction, e.g., thrombosis and embolism (Fig. 26-2).

Microglia (mesoglia). Microglial cells are believed to be mesodermal elements derived from perivascular tissues and are distributed widely throughout the nervous system in postnatal life. Normally, they appear to be at rest (fixed), in which form only the nucleus is evident in ordinary sections.

Compared with the macroglia, the microg-

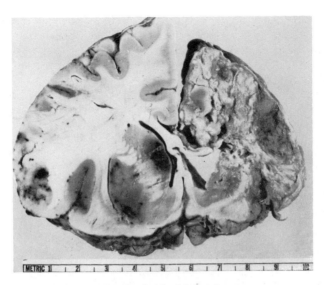

Fig. 26-2. Cerebral infarction.

lial nucleus is small and very compact and may be irregular in shape (round, elongated, or curved). The scanty cytoplasm and thin, branching processes require special staining to be demonstrated. The microglia respond to the products of myelin degeneration *(fatty granule cell reaction)*. In this reaction, the cell processes are pulled in and the nucleus elongates, becoming bipolar. This *rod cell* migrates to the site of injury, where the nucleus becomes rounded and lighter staining. As fat products are engulfed, the cytoplasm becomes globular and the nucleus eccentric. These fat-laden macrophages (fatty granule cells; compound granular corpuscles) often migrate into the perivascular spaces. They are the characteristic cells in an area of cerebral softening (Fig. 26-3).

Cerebrospinal fluid. The cerebrospinal fluid forms a circulatory system peculiar to nervous tissue, perhaps taking the place of the absent lymphatics. The fluid is formed from blood by the choroid plexus of the cerebral ventricles, probably by a process of dialysis, although there may be an active secretory mechanism as well.

Formed mainly in the lateral ventricles, the fluid passes through the interventricular foramina (of Monro) into the third ventricle and through the narrow cerebral aqueduct (of Sylvius) into the fourth ventricle. From the roof and lateral extensions of this ventricle, it escapes through the lateral apertures (of Luschka) and the median aperture (of Magendie) to reach the subarachnoid space. From the large subarachnoid cisterns at the base of the brain, it passes downward into the subarachnoid space of the spinal cord and upward through the narrow aperture of the tentorium cerebelli to bathe the surface of the brain. Most of the fluid is resorbed into the venous bloodstream around the region of the vertex by way of the arachnoid villi, which project into the lumina of the venous sinuses. Some diffusion of fluid probably occurs through the perivascular or Virchow-Robin spaces, by means of which interstitial fluid of the brain tissue is added to the cerebrospinal fluid.

The cerebrospinal fluid reflects by its changes many important disease processes. Normally, the volume is about 125 ml. It is clear and colorless, has a specific gravity of 1.006 to 1.009, and contains fewer than 12 cells (mononuclear) per cubic millimeter in persons past 12 years of age. In disease, there may be color changes caused by fresh hemorrhage or xanthochromia, a yellowish tinge derived from hemoglobin and implying stasis af-

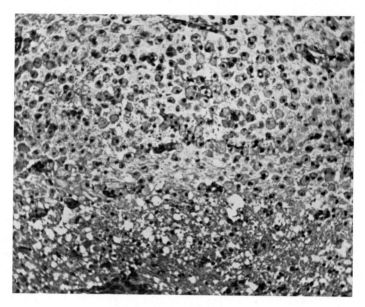

Fig. 26-3. Infarct of brain. Edge is shown, and many compound granular corpuscles (microglia) are evident.

ter hemorrhage. The cell content may be altered in both number and character, and chemical and serologic changes occur that are valuable aids in diagnosis. The most striking change involving cerebrospinal fluid is the mechanical effect resulting from obstruction to its flow (hydrocephalus, p. 747; increased intracranial pressure, p. 762).

TUMORS OF NERVOUS SYSTEM AND RELATED TISSUES

Intracranial tumors as a group have certain peculiarities as a result of their position and the nature of the cells from which they arise. Since they occur within a rigid bony box, their increase of bulk causes damage by increasing intracranial pressure. This is also contributed to by edema of the brain tissue around the growth and often by obstruction to the pathway of cerebrospinal fluid, with some degree of hydrocephalus. A relatively small tumor may press upon or involve vital areas of the nervous system. Most of the intracranial tumors arise from supporting structures (i.e., neuroglia, sheaths of the brain [meninges] or cranial nerves, and blood vessels). Their

greatest incidence is in middle age, but certain types occur mainly in childhood. Most of them do not metastasize, but they may be locally malignant and invasive. Others are quite benign biologically but are serious because of their position. In the relatively few instances of tumors metastasizing beyond the central nervous system (including glioblastomas, medulloblastomas, and ependymomas), the metastases usually occurred after surgical procedures.

In children, the majority of brain tumors are found in the cerebellum, the most frequent being cystic astrocytomas, medulloblastomas, and ependymomas of the fourth ventricle. In adults, brain tumors are found mainly in the cerebrum and are predominantly highly malignant astrocytomas (glioblastoma multiforme).

The tumors of the nervous system and related tissues may be classified as follows:

Primary central neurogenic tumors
  Gliomas (supporting cell tumors)
    Ependymoma
    Oligodendroglioma
    Astrocytoma (grade 1)
    Astroblastoma (astrocytoma grade 2)

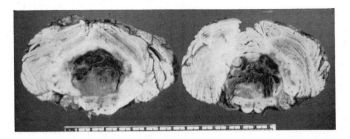

Fig. 26-4. Ependymoma of fourth ventricle.

Glioblastoma multiforme (astrocytoma grades
    3 and 4)
Nerve cell tumors
    Medulloblastoma
    Neurocytoma (ganglioneuroma)
    Neuroblastoma
    Retinoblastoma (neuroepithelioma of retina)
Primary peripheral neurogenic tumors
    Supporting cell tumors
        Schwannoma (neurilemoma)
        Neurofibroma
        Malignant schwannoma
    Nerve cell tumors
        Ganglioneuroma
Tumors of vascular and perivascular structures
    Angiomas
    Sarcoma
    Malignant lymphoma
Meningiomas
Mixed tumors
Hypophyseal tumors
Pineal tumors
Metastatic tumors

Central neurogenic tumors

Tumors of nervous tissue proper include the gliomas and nerve cell tumors. Gliomas constitute almost half of all intracranial tumors, whereas tumors of nerve cells are much less common. Gliomas are less frequent in the spinal cord than in the brain.

Gliomas

Gliomas represent neoplasia of supporting (neuroglial) tissues of the central nervous system.

Kernohan and associates have suggested a simplified classification and grading of the gliomas. This is based on the concept that the more rapidly growing gliomas represent greater degrees of anaplasia or dedifferentiation rather than undifferentiation. Thus, the astrocytoma, astroblastoma, and glioblastoma multiforme are considered to be the same type of neoplasm but of different degrees (or grades) of malignancy. There is a gradual transition between the lowest and highest grades of malignancy. Division into four grades is arbitrary but useful.

The medulloblastoma is commonly classified with the gliomas, but sometimes it is grouped with the nerve cell tumors, as it is here. Perhaps it should be classified separately in a class between gliomas and nerve cell tumors. The tumor apparently arises from immature neural tissue, and the cell of origin is believed to have the ability to differentiate in either a neuronal or a glial direction. However, tissue culture, electron microscopy, and other studies of the tumor cells have not solved this problem yet.

Ependymoma. Ependymomas constitute about 6% of the gliomas. They are derived from ventricular lining cells and appear commonly in the fourth ventricle, along the central canal, and in the filum terminale. They are the most common type of glioma in the spinal cord. Although slow growing, they often interfere with cerebrospinal fluid flow, producing an acute increase of intracranial pressure. Grossly, they are usually distinctly demarcated from the surrounding tissue (Fig. 26-4).

The histology of ependymomas is complex, and they have been classified as follows:

1 Papilloma choroideum, a papillary tumor
    of the choroid plexus, closely simulating

the normal structure but with taller epithelium and often with vacuoles containing mucus—considered by some authors to be a tumor separate from ependymomas

2 Papillary ependymoma, a tumor similar to papilloma choroideum, without mucus in the tumor cells but with abundant myxomatous degeneration in the stroma

3 Epithelial ependymoma, a tumor with many rosettes, i.e., tubular channels resembling the central canal, having cells free of vacuoles and mucus and often containing blepharoplasts (Fig. 26-5)

4 Cellular ependymoma, a highly cellular tumor containing fragments of tissue conforming to the other patterns and often dotted with pseudorosettes

In these ependymomas, mitoses are uncommon. A more undifferentiated form, *ependymoblastoma,* occurs that grows rapidly, is highly malignant, and shows pronounced mitotic activity. *Colloid cyst* of the third ventricle may represent another form of ependymoma, but it has also been suggested that it may arise from paraphyseal tissue. It is benign and grows slowly but causes symptoms by ventricular blockage.

Kernohan and associates have proposed that the ependymomal group of tumors may be graded 1 to 4 according to the degree of anaplasia or dedifferentiation and that such grading of malignancy correlates with the postoperative survival period.

Oligodendroglioma. Oligodendrogliomas grow very slowly and appear most commonly in the cerebral hemispheres of adults. The tumors often contain calcium (roentgenographically visible) and tend to become cystic. Histologically, they are extremely cellular and exhibit very little stroma. The nuclei are small, dark staining, and surrounded by a halo of clear cytoplasm. *Oligodendroblastomas* are rare, highly malignant, rapidly grow-

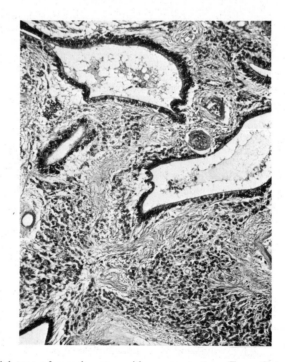

Fig. 26-5. Epithelial type of ependymoma with many rosettes. (From Chason, J. L.: Nervous system. In Anderson, W. A. D., and Kissane, J. M., editors: Pathology, ed. 7, St. Louis, 1977, The C. V. Mosby Co.)

ing variants of this tumor. Cytologic appearance of oligodendrogliomas (i.e., histologic grading) seems to have no good correlation with prognosis.

Astrocytoma. About one half of the gliomas, or one fourth of all intracranial tumors, are astrocytomas. They usually are seen in children and young adults. They occur diffusely throughout the nervous system and are grayish white, fairly firm, and poorly demarcated grossly. They grow slowly and appear benign histologically. The cells are usually uniform, with nuclear structure comparable to that of a normal astrocyte, but the astrocytes appear increased in number (Fig. 26-6). Giant nuclei and mitoses are absent or rare. More cytoplasm is evident than in normal cells, and stroma is densely fibrillated. Very often gem-

istocytes are formed, and occasionally they dominate the histologic picture (gemistocytic astrocytoma; Fig. 26-7).

Astroblastomas are made up of larger cells with short, thick vascular processes and often are arranged in a radial pattern around a blood vessel. They exhibit more rapid growth. The so-called *polar spongioblastomas* also may be considered a variety of astrocytoma. They are dominated microscopically by bipolar or unipolar cells that are thought to be the immediate stem cells from which astroblasts develop. Microscopically, they resemble neurofibromas. The cells and nuclei are regular in size and exhibit no mitoses. They grow slowly.

According to the classification of Kernohan and associates, well-differentiated astrocytoma would be *astrocytoma grade 1,* and as-

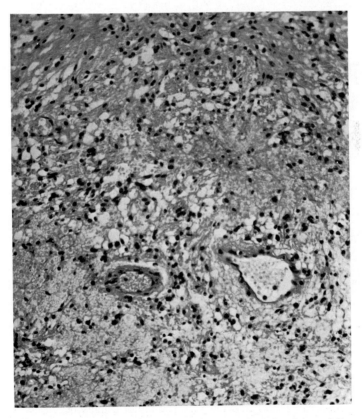

Fig. 26-6. Astrocytoma. Note uniformity of nuclei and abundance of fibers.

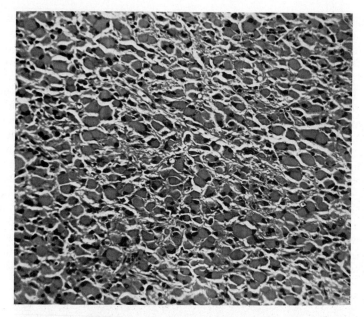

Fig. 26-7. Gemistocytic astrocytoma.

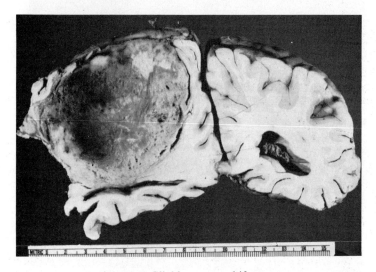

Fig. 26-8. Glioblastoma multiforme.

troblastoma as well as polar spongioblastoma would be *astrocytoma grade 2*.

Glioblastoma multiforme. Glioblastoma multiforme (or *astrocytoma grades 3 and 4*, according to Kernohan and associates) is the second most common of the gliomas. It occurs most frequently in middle-aged adults, somewhat more commonly in men than in women. The tumor usually occurs in the cerebrum and much less frequently in the cerebellum or

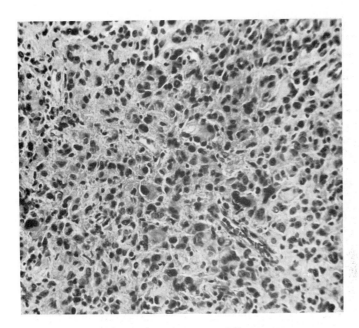

Fig. 26-9. Glioblastoma multiforme.

spinal cord. It usually arises in the white matter and is exceedingly malignant, rapidly expansive, and invasive. It is often grossly hemorrhagic, and its line of demarcation from cerebral tissue is indistinct, although sometimes it appears to be demarcated because of compression of adjacent brain tissues (Fig. 26-8).

Microscopically, the tumors show great variation in size and shape of cells, with giant and multinucleated forms and numerous bizarre mitoses (Fig. 26-9). There is frequently an endothelial hypertrophy and reduplication, imparting the appearance of extremely thick-walled vessels. Patches of necrosis surrounded by radiating clumps of small nuclei are very common. Some of the complex vascular formations appear to be caused by thrombosis and organization.

Syringomyelia. Syringomyelia is a cavitation occurring in the substance of the spinal cord. It appears as a slowly progressive gliosis with subsequent cyst formation. The cavity may be single or multiple, and it varies in form (round, oval, tubular, slitlike, etc.).

The cause is unknown, and although it has been regarded by some as a variety of astrocytoma, its neoplastic character is questionable. Other views are that it may be a congenital lesion or a sequel of a previous inflammation, hemorrhage, or infarct.

Nerve cell tumors

The second group of central neurogenic tumors consists of those stemming from the medulloblast in the direction of the nonsupporting element of the nervous system, the neurocyte. They are often mixed (neuroastrocytoma).

Medulloblastoma. Medulloblastomas are rapidly growing midline cerebellar tumors of children. An occasional instance in adults is reported. The tumors spread by implanting along the ventricles or in the meninges. Microscopically, the cells are small and pear shaped, with a tapered cytoplasmic extremity. They tend to line up in incomplete circles, forming partial pseudorosettes. The tumor cells are radiosensitive, but the response to radiation is temporary.

Neurocytoma (ganglioneuroma). Central neurocytomas are rare tumors characterized by the presence of mature nerve cells in which Nissl substance is demonstrable. They grow very slowly.

Neuroblastoma. Closely related to medulloblastomas, neuroblastomas of the central nervous system are rare tumors composed of neuroblasts, identifiable by large vesicular nuclei in small rounded cells, with little cytoplasm and no Nissl substance. Neuroblasts often can be identified in medulloblastomas.

Retinoblastoma (neuroepithelioma of retina). Occurring in childhood and often familial, retinoblastomas arise from the retinoblast, the counterpart of the neuroblast in the retina. In the familial form, the inheritance pattern is autosomal dominant. Closely related to the medulloblastomas, the retinoblastomas resemble them in behavior, implanting along meningeal spaces. They tend particularly to invade the optic nerve. Microscopically, the cells are small and round, with little cytoplasm, and tend to form rosettes.

Peripheral neurogenic tumors

Neurogenic tumors developing outside the substance of the brain and spinal cord are tumors of peripheral ganglion cells and of the supporting cells of the peripheral nerves. In addition, there are a number of neurogenic tumors arising in the adrenal medulla (p. 615) and chromaffin structures (p. 617). Rarely, neurogenic tumors microscopically resembling neuroblastoma or medulloblastoma may be found in odd sites, such as bone, skin, and muscle, where the stem cell is obscure but is probably related to the migrant cell. Included among the peripheral primary neurogenic tumors are schwannomas (neurilemomas), neurofibromas, and ganglioneuromas.

Supporting cell tumors

Three sources contribute to the morphology of the peripheral nerve: axons of the nerve cells, sheath cells, and fibroblastic tissue from endoneural and perineural supporting structures. The contribution of axons to nerve tumors is insignificant. Tangles of axons appear with their growth cones primarily in reparative processes (amputation neuroma). The relative importance of sheath cells or perineurium in the formation of nerve tumors is a much debated and still unsettled question. These tumors occur along cranial or spinal nerves and at their endings.

Tumors of peripheral nerves (or nerve sheaths) can be classified in three groups. Although there are differences of opinion regarding derivation and terminology, the three types are most commonly called schwannoma (neurilemoma), neurofibroma, and malignant schwannoma.

Schwannoma. Schwannoma (neurilemoma; perineural fibroblastoma) is a solitary encapsulated benign tumor composed of Schwann cells of the nerve sheath. The nerve from which it arises frequently passes to one side or spreads out over the surface of the tumor so that the lesion often can be surgically enucleated with preservation of the parent nerve and without risk of recurrence or malignant change. The larger tumors tend to be cystic. The acoustic nerve is a common site (acoustic

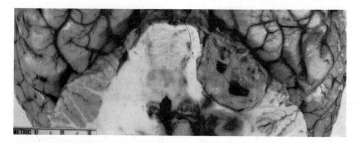

Fig. 26-10. Acoustic neuroma forming tumor at cerebellopontine angle. Hemorrhagic cerebellar area is surgical operative wound.

neuroma; Fig. 26-10), the tumor occupying the cerebellopontine angle. The elongated component cells are arranged in irregular or twisted bundles with palisading of nuclei (see Fig. 12-10). Fascicular (Antoni type A) tissue arranged in an organoid formation has been referred to as a Verocay body. Reticular (Antoni type B) tissue forms a loose network of reticulin fibers about minute cystic spaces.

Neurofibroma. Neurofibroma is a diffuse or unencapsulated proliferation of nerve elements, sometimes single but more often multiple (Recklinghausen's neurofibromatosis). Patches of excessive melanin pigmentation of the skin (café au lait spots), pigmented moles, and soft fibromas of the skin (fibromata mollusca) are common stigmas accompanying Recklinghausen's disease (see Fig. 12-11). A neurofibroma cannot be enucleated from the parent nerve, since the nerve fibers run through the center of the tumor instead of around it. Neurofibromas may undergo malignant change.

Histologically, the tumors show an irregular reticular growth of Schwann cells, fibrous tissue, and nerve fibrils (shown by special stains). Proliferation of the tumor may occur within nerve sheaths, causing the involved nerves to become thick and tortuous (plexiform neurofibroma; Fig. 26-11).

Malignant schwannoma. Malignant schwannoma (neurogenic sarcoma) is composed of cells derived from the nerve sheath and may show some of the whorled interlacing bundles and nuclear palisading seen in neurilemomas. Nuclear hyperchromatism, cellularity, and rapid growth indicate the malignant character. The appearance may simulate fibrosarcoma or leiomyosarcoma. Insidious local infiltration occurs so that the tumor is likely to recur unless surgical resection is wide. Distant metastasis occurs mainly by the bloodstream.

Nerve cell tumors

Ganglioneuroma. Ganglioneuromas are the peripheral counterpart of the central neurocytoma. Grossly, they appear as fleshy masses, are often large, and usually are located along the thoracic and lumbar sympathetic trunk, bulging into the mediastinum or retroperitoneal region. They grow slowly and are benign. Microscopically, they show mature nerve cells in a profuse stroma of sheath cells, fibrous tissue, and varying amounts of neurofibrils and myelin (see Fig. 21-34). Ganglioneuroblastomas occur occasionally (p. 616).

Tumors of vascular and perivascular structures

Tumors of vascular and perivascular structures include hemangioma, hemangioendothelioma, sarcoma, and malignant lymphoma.

Hemangioma. Hemangioma is a vascular malformation that occurs most commonly over the surface of a cerebral hemisphere as a tangle of tortuous large and small vessels. Microscopically, it is similar to angiomas in other locations (p. 295).

Hemangioblastoma. Hemangioblastomas (hemangioendotheliomas) are most common in the cerebellum of adults. They appear as a small, firm, reddish "mural nodule" in the wall of a large, smooth cyst. Histologically, they are composed of many small blood vessels. A characteristic feature is the presence of intervascular swollen lipid-containing cells (foam cells or pseudoxanthoma cells). Similar tumors may occur elsewhere in the brain, in the spinal cord (sometimes with syringomyelia), or in the retina. Erythrocytosis has occasionally been associated, presumably caused by an erythropoietinlike substance secreted by the hemangioblastomas.

Association of the vascular tumors in the retina (von Hippel) with those in the central nervous system, particularly the cerebellum (Lindau), is referred to as *von Hippel–Lindau disease* (retinocerebellar angiomatosis). Other visceral lesions are commonly present also, e.g., polycystic lesions of the pancreas and liver and cysts and/or renal cell carcinoma of the kidney. Occasionally, pheochromocytoma is associated. A familial factor is demonstrable in about 20% of cases. The disease is transmitted as a modified mendelian dominant trait and is not sex linked.

Sarcoma. Malignant, rapidly growing sarcomatous lesions occur in the brain, growing

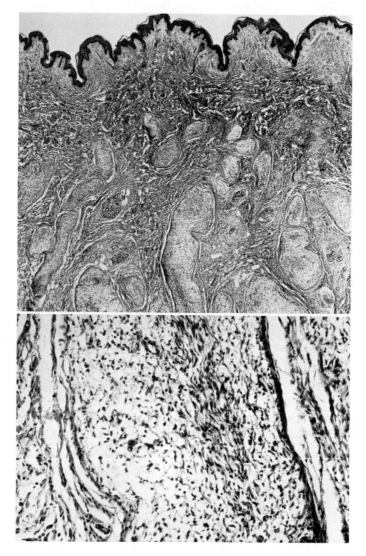

Fig. 26-11. Plexiform neurofibroma.

especially around blood vessels. These have been classified variously as fibrosarcomas, spindle cell sarcomas, and polymorphocellular sarcomas.

Malignant lymphoma. Malignant lymphomas occur infrequently in the epidural space and within the substance of the brain or cord. An example is the histiocytic type (reticulum cell sarcoma) that is believed to be derived from perivascular microglia or primitive reticulum cells.

Tumors of meninges

Meningiomas constitute about one fifth of all intracranial neoplasms, being second only to gliomas in frequency. They are essentially benign tumors that grow slowly and compress the brain by expansion. The most common

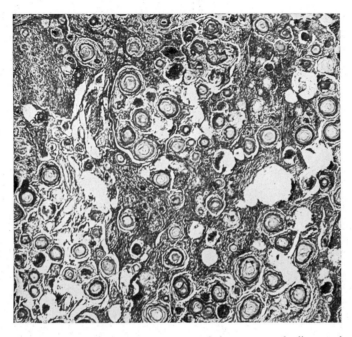

Fig. 26-12. Meningioma. Very numerous rounded psammoma bodies are shown.

sites are over the cerebral hemispheres, along the sagittal sinus, over the cribriform plate, and along the lesser wing of the sphenoid. They often erode the bone and sometimes stimulate bone growth into the tumor. Meningiomas also affect the spinal cord, where they are more common than gliomas. They are encapsulated, distinctly demarcated from brain or spinal cord, and almost always attached to the dura. The microscopic appearance varies greatly but is often highly cellular with a pronounced whorled arrangement. The central portion of the whorls undergoes degeneration and calcification, forming psammoma bodies (Fig. 26-12). Loose edematous meningiomas may be confused with astrocytomas, or the palisading of cells may suggest the appearance of a neurilemoma.

The exact origin of meningiomas is still debated, but it is commonly believed that they are of arachnoidal origin. In rare instances, a meningioma may not be localized but involves the brain surface over a wide area. Malignant fibrosarcomatous forms also occur. Fibrosarcomas of the dura resemble extracranial fibrosarcomas histologically. Pigmented meningiomas and melanomas of the meninges are rare. The latter are highly malignant.

Mixed tumors

Mixed tumors include *dermoid cysts* and *teratomas*. These tumors are thought to arise from congenital cell rests. Morphologically, they are similar to their counterparts elsewhere (p. 275). *Epidermoid tumors* (pearly tumors; cholesteatomas) are similar to dermoid cysts but lack hair, sebaceous glands, and other skin appendages.

Hypophyseal and pineal tumors

Hypophyseal tumors include the pituitary adenomas and craniopharyngiomas (pp. 577 and 581). *Pineal tumors* are described on p. 606.

Metastatic tumors

Metastatic tumors of the brain occur commonly from the lung and somewhat less commonly from a malignant melanoma, the large intestine, testis, breast, stomach, kidney, adrenal gland, and prostate gland. Skin tumors involving the orbit sometimes invade the brain.

Secondary tumors usually can be identified by their globular shape, sharp demarcation, and frequent multiplicity. Microscopically, they resemble the primary growth.

DEVELOPMENTAL AND CONGENITAL DISORDERS
Disorders related to faulty closure of bony structures

Related to faulty closure of the bony structures housing the medullary tube are numerous developmental disorders, which vary primarily in degree of involvement.

Rachischisis is a failure of formation of the dorsal arch throughout the length of the vertebral column, with exposure of the unclosed neural groove.

Myelocele is a spina bifida with protrusion of the spinal cord.

Meningocele is a leptomeningeal protrusion through a local defect in bone and dura with the leptomeninx underlying the skin. This may occur in the vertebral column or skull. *Meningomyelocele* is similar to meningocele, with the inclusion of spinal cord tissue in the protruding part. If the brain is the part involved, the condition is called *encephalocele*. *Syringomyelocele* is similar to meningomyelocele but with the addition of considerable distention of the central canal.

Spina bifida occulta is a congenital local dorsal arch defect (usually lumbar or sacral) in which the gap is filled with connective tissue to which the cord membranes are attached.

Malformations primarily involving brain tissue

Anencephaly is the condition wherein the forebrain and calvaria are absent. Often, there are significant pathologic changes elsewhere, such as atrophy of the adrenal glands. It probably is caused by defective organization in primordial tissues.

Porencephaly is an abnormal cavitation within the brain substance, the cavities usually communicating with the ventricles. The condition is looked on as a partial agenesia and is associated with maldevelopment elsewhere.

Heterotopias are persistent islands of tissue that, although normal for certain developmental stages, are abnormal when found in the mature brain.

Malformation of gyri is a common occurrence. Unusually large gyri are called *macrogyri* and unusually small ones *microgyri*.

Disturbances in brain volume are said to exist when brain weight in the adult varies beyond certain extremes. The average weight is around 1,350 g, and it is not uncommon to encounter brains weighing as little as 1,000 g or as much as 1,700 g. *Microcephaly* is the term applied to very small brains and *macrocephaly* to very large brains. Each condition is often associated with hydrocephalus.

Oxycephaly is a condition in which a tower-shaped skull is associated with premature synostosis of cranial sutures. Mental deficiency, papilledema, and eventually blindness result from disproportionate growth of the brain in the deformed skull.

Hydranencephaly exists when the forebrain is represented only by a thin membranous sac filled with water. The head size may be normal, and the fontanels close appropriately. In *hydromacrocephaly* the head is enlarged, with the fontanels and sutures widely open. The ventricular system is dilated, sometimes to a volume of several liters. Often, the chambers are confluent. Considerable brain tissue often persists in the outer shell. These cases represent the condition most often referred to as hydrocephalus.

Congenital hydrocephalus is the condition of an abnormal amount of intracranial cerebrospinal fluid present at, or shortly after, the time of birth. Several descriptive terms are applied to the condition, depending on gross variations. *External hydrocephalus* describes the condition wherein most of the fluid accumulates over the surface of the atrophic brain.

Internal hydrocephalus exists when the ventricular system is distended (Fig. 26-13). *Communicating hydrocephalus* exists when abnormally increased fluid is present although the connections between the ventricular system and the subarachnoid space are patent. *Noncommunicating hydrocephalus* occurs when there is an obstruction to the free flow between the ventricular system and the subarachnoid space.

Although hydrocephalus is commonly congenital in nature, it may occur any time after birth as a result of some acquired disturbance or disease.

Theoretically, the production of hydrocephalus may be brought about in three ways: (1) by overproduction of fluid, (2) by obstruction to its flow, and (3) by interference with its absorption into the venous system.

The production of cerebrospinal fluid fluctuates with venous pressure. An obstruction to venous return from the choroid plexus might cause excessive production of fluid. However, there is little evidence to incriminate excessive production of fluid as a cause of hydrocephalus. Exuberant growth or cysts of the choroid plexus are commonly found associated with infantile hydrocephalus but probably are not causative.

Obstruction to the flow of cerebrospinal fluid is noted commonly in the following locations: (1) the interventricular foramina (of Munro), (2) the cerebral aqueduct (of Sylvius), (3) the apertures of the fourth ventricle (of Magendie and Luschka), and (4) the subarachnoid space at the constricted tentorial aperture.

The etiology of the obstruction is often obscure, but causes include congenital atresia of the cerebral aqueduct, occluding tumors of the aqueduct in infants, and inflammation (e.g., ependymitis), particularly at the interventricular foramina and aqueduct of Sylvius. In some patients, *Toxoplasma* has been incriminated as the inciting organism. The infection is thought to be transmitted in utero, since the defect produced often can be allocated to early pregnancy by the stage of development of certain structures. This may be an important cause of congenital hydrocephalus (p. 210). Obstruc-

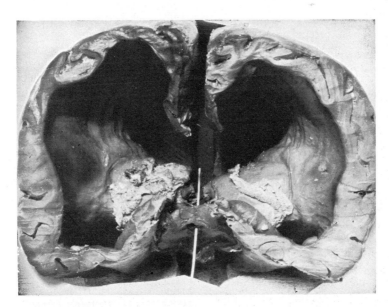

Fig. 26-13. Hydrocephalus. Note extreme dilatation of ventricles and thinness of cerebral substance.

tion with internal hydrocephalus may occur in children and adults as a result of tumors or inflammatory lesions (e.g., meningitis).

Interference with absorption of cerebrospinal fluid may occur from destruction of arachnoid granulations by meningitis. This mechanism of development of hydrocephalus also occurs in expanding central lesions of the brain, which, by compressing the brain against the skull, obliterate the subarachnoid space over the vertex.

Other congenital brain disorders

The following are examples of other congenital disorders resulting from various causes, such as some form of cerebral birth injury (cerebral palsy), developmental defect (tuberous sclerosis), chromosomal aberration (mongolism), and disturbance of lipid metabolism (amaurotic familial idiocy, a lipid storage disease).

Cerebral palsy (spastic diplegia; Little's disease) is characterized clinically by spasticity of the lower extremities, choreiform movements, and sometimes mental deficiency resulting from central neuronal degeneration. Grossly, the brain is usually small and shrunken, with patches of microgyri, and there may be gross defects in the cerebellum and pons. The cause is believed to be some form of cerebral birth injury, but it is not always possible to determine whether perinatal mechanical trauma, infection, anoxia, or metabolic abnormality is responsible. The syndrome is duplicated in infantile encephalomyelitides and in toxic reactions. Microscopically, the atrophied areas show gliosis.

Tuberous sclerosis is a heredofamilial disease that becomes manifest a few months to a few years after birth in mental deficiency, epileptiform seizures, cutaneous tumors similar to sebaceous adenomas, and often tumors of other organs. Grossly, the brain is small, firm, and dotted by areas of macrogyri that are pearly white and often nodular in form. Similar firm nodules may project into the ventricles. The nodules are composed of dense glial tissue and contain irregular giant cells and atypical glial elements. Hyperplasia of the sebaceous glands of the nose and cheeks (ade-

noma sebaceum), rhabdomyomas of the heart, and hamartomas of the kidneys are common accompaniments. The clinical syndrome characterized by mental changes and adenoma sebaceum of the skin in association ' with tuberous sclerosis of the brain is called *epiloia.*

Mongolism (Down's syndrome) is characterized by mongoloid features in an idiot child of white parents. It has been discovered that it is caused by the presence of an additional small acrocentric chromosome (p. 12). The head is usually small, the tongue is prominent, and the musculature is hypotonic. The brain is small, and there may be gross defects in the gyri. There is apparently a diminished number of cortical neurons, and the cortical architecture is distorted. Hypophyseal changes have been described (p. 580). The condition appears to cause some predisposition to leukemia. Associated congenital heart lesions (especially septal defects) may be present.

Amaurotic familial idiocy, a familial condition consisting of several forms, is a neuronal lipid storage disease. The infantile form is found mainly in Jewish people. Progressive muscle weakness develops in the early months of life, and mental development fails. There is a characteristic peculiar cherry-red spot in the retina, and later optic atrophy and blindness develop. The brain is atrophic and firm. The cerebellum may share in the atrophy. The characteristic histologic feature is distention of many of the nerve cells by a granular deposit of lipid (ganglioside) in the cytoplasm. The lipid deposit also involves cell processes. The degeneration of nerve cells and processes is followed by widespread gliosis. This infantile form is commonly known as *Tay-Sachs disease.*

In the juvenile form, which is more common in Gentiles, the cherry-red spot in the macula is absent, and the lipid in nerve cells stains well with the usual fat stains. A late infantile form and a very rare adult variety have also been described.

DEMYELINATING DISEASES

It was shown in a previous section that destruction or loss of myelin (demyelination) may occur secondary to injury to the cell body or axons in the central or peripheral nervous system, as in *wallerian degeneration* of the peripheral nerves (p. 733). However, there are a number of disorders of the nervous system in which demyelination may be primary. Typical examples of the *demyelinating (myelinoclastic) disorders* include the following.

Disseminated sclerosis (multiple sclerosis). Disseminated sclerosis (multiple sclerosis) is a relatively common disease of undetermined cause. The three main hypotheses regarding causation, all unproved, are that it is ischemic (resulting from thrombosis), that it is infective (possibly slow-virus infection), and that it is allergic (autoimmune disease). The onset usually is between the ages of 20 and 40 years.

The symptoms are varied, as would be expected from the irregular distribution of the lesions. Transient paresis, sensory disturbance, nystagmus, and retrobulbar neuritis are common features. A classic triad consists of nystagmus, intention tremor, and slurring speech. The disease clinically may have periods of remission and relapse, sometimes over a period of years. There are widespread scattered irregular lesions, predominantly in the white matter, that appear grossly as yellow-gray areas on the cut surface of the brain or cord. These stand out prominently as pale areas in Weigert preparations. They are most prominent in the long tracts of the cord, and lesions of the stem and cord figure conspicuously in the symptoms.

Microscopically, the lesion is a sharply outlined plaque of demyelination, and in degenerated areas of long standing, there may be gliosis. The early degeneration appears to spare the axis-cylinders, accounting for transient remissions. In the active process, fatty granule cells, lymphocytes, and plasma cells are present, form perivascular cuffs, and spill into the subarachnoid space. The older lesions are sclerotic and without myelin and inflammatory cells.

The optic nerve is often involved. If the optic neuritis dominates and is associated with an acute patchy encephalomyelitis, the condition is called *neuromyelitis optica* or *Devic's disease*. This condition is regarded by some authors as a separate clinical entity.

Schilder's disease. Schilder's disease *(encephalitis periaxialis diffusa* or *diffuse sclerosis)* is characterized by a subacute progressive course that leads to death within a year or so. Unlike multiple sclerosis, the disease is seen often in children and adolescents, although it may occur at any age. There is extensive demyelination in the cerebral white matter, usually in an asymmetrical manner, with one hemisphere being involved more than the other and the occipital lobes being predominantly affected in most instances. The lesions are sharply demarcated, and the arcuate fibers are often not involved. Microscopically, the destruction of myelin and the cellular response are similar to the changes seen in multiple sclerosis.

Postinfectious and postvaccinal encephalomyelitis. Encephalomyelitis characterized by perivascular demyelination and infiltration by lymphocytes and plasma cells may be seen after virus infections (e.g., measles, mumps, chickenpox) or after immunization with rabies or smallpox vaccine. Autoimmunity is believed to play a role in the development of the lesions, and the condition is referred to as ''allergic encephalomyelitis'' (pp. 89 and 166).

DYSMYELINATING DISORDERS (LEUKODYSTROPHIES)

As in demyelinating diseases, the myelin disturbance in the dysmyelinating disorders, or leukodystrophies, is primary. A major difference between the two types of disorders is that in the demyelinating diseases the myelin forms normally and then breaks down because of some factors, whereas in the dysmyelinating disorders the basic disturbance is defective myelin formation. In addition, the lesions in the leukodystrophies differ from those in the demyelinating diseases in that they are more likely to be bilateral and symmetrical, involve more of the nervous system, and occur in younger persons. The subcortical arcuate fibers in the affected regions usually are spared, as are the axons initially, although the latter may be destroyed later. Examples of the leukodystrophies are the following.

Krabbe's disease. Krabbe's disease *(globoid cell leukodystrophy)* is characterized by an accumulation of a PAS-positive material (galactocerebroside) that results from deficient activity of the enzyme galactocerebroside β-galactosidase. A striking feature is the presence of so-called *globoid cells,* which are large, often multinucleated, epithelioid cells found frequently in small clusters in the white matter, sometimes perivascularly. The abnormal material may be demonstrated in the globoid cells.

Metachromatic leukodystrophy. Metachromatic leukodystrophy *(sulfatide lipidosis)* is caused by a defect in the activity of the enzyme arylsulfatase A (cerebroside sulfatase), and this leads to an accumulation of excess galactosyl sulfatide (cerebroside sulfate) in the white matter. The abnormal material, which stains metachromatically, may be found in macrophages and extracellularly and sometimes in neurons. It also may be found in cells of the liver, gallbladder, and renal tubules, as well as in leukocytes of the peripheral blood and bone marrow. The Schwann cells and the cells of the nerve plexuses may also be affected.

NEUROMUSCULAR DISORDERS AND MYOPATHIES

Muscle disorders may result from disease of the central nervous system (motor neurons) and the peripheral nerves *(neuropathic muscle atrophy)* or from diseases not related to neurologic lesions (the *myopathies*). The latter include certain hereditary disorders (muscular dystrophies) and the myopathies associated with various systemic derangements (metabolic, endocrine, immunologic, etc.).

Neuromuscular disorders

Neuropathic muscle atrophy. A variety of diseases of the spinal cord (e.g., poliomyelitis) and peripheral nerves (trauma and the group of neuropathies), which are discussed elsewhere, may be accompanied by muscle weakness and atrophy.

Other neuromuscular disorders of hereditary nature or of unknown cause include those discussed in the following paragraphs.

Infantile spinal muscular atrophy. Infantile spinal muscular atrophy *(Werdnig-Hoffmann disease)* is an inherited disorder that has as its essential pathologic feature a paucity of cells in the anterior horn (in all levels of the spinal cord) and in the medulla. The clinical result is muscular hypotonia early in life. The term *amyotonia congenita* is sometimes used clinically for a weak hypotonic infant, but it is to be emphasized that amyotonia or hypotonia may be found in a variety of conditions. Werdnig-Hoffmann disease is often fatal in the first few years of life and must be distinguished from other conditions characterized by muscular hypotonia in infants and young children.

Friedreich's ataxia. Friedreich's ataxia is one of a group of hereditary diseases in which ataxia is prominent. Degenerative changes occur in tracts of the spinal cord, so that the cord appears smaller than normal. Myelin sheath degeneration, particularly in the spinocerebellar and posterior columns, is shown by light unstained areas in Weigert preparations. The degeneration apparently begins in the cells of Clark's column. Late in the disease, the pyramidal tracts may be involved. Gliosis follows the myelin degeneration. Degenerative changes may be seen in the cerebellum (e.g., loss of Purkinje cells), but they are not always present, and frequently the cerebellum is normal.

Amyotrophic lateral sclerosis. Amyotrophic lateral sclerosis appears in adults aged 40 or 50 years or over and runs a fairly rapid course to fatal termination. Clinically, there are weakness and atrophy of the skeletal muscles in the limbs, especially the hands and arms. The principal pathologic features are progressive degeneration of the pyramidal (corticospinal) tracts starting at the cerebral cortex and degenerative changes in the anterior horn cells and their analogous nuclei in the brainstem. Demyelination occurs as a result of the alterations in the motor nerve cells. The cause of amyotrophic lateral sclerosis is not known, but it is suspected that the disease may be one of the slow-virus infections. A variant of the disease is *progressive spinal muscular atrophy* in adults, in which anterior horn cell involvement is the predominant feature and the clinical course is more slowly progressive and more benign than in amyotrophic lateral sclerosis.

Hypertrophic interstitial neuropathy. Hypertrophic interstitial neuropathy is a familial inherited disease, but sporadic cases have been reported. It is characterized by a nodular proliferative condition of sheath cells and endoneurium along peripheral nerves, as well as demyelination and varying loss of axons. There may be an associated degeneration of posterior columns. Weakness and atrophy of skeletal muscles usually occur first in the lower extremities and then in the upper extremities.

Peroneal muscular atrophy. Peroneal muscular atrophy is a degeneration of the peroneal musculature with an associated neuropathy. There is atrophy of the calf muscles, with drop foot and clubfoot. The disease is hereditary and occurs in the first decade.

Myopathies

Several forms of muscle disease occur without involvement of the nervous system.

Muscular dystrophies. The muscular dystrophies are a group of inherited diseases characterized by degeneration and wasting of muscle fibers. The cause is unknown, but some intracellular enzyme or protein deficiency causing disturbance of metabolism of muscle cells is postulated. Microscopically, variation in size of muscle fibers is observed (i.e., atrophic fibers are admixed with large ones). In some fibers, striations are obscured, and others are homogenized. Adipose and fibrous tissues replace atrophic fibers. Elevation of serum enzyme levels, such as creatine phosphokinase (CPK), is evident.

There are several varieties of muscular dystrophy, involving different muscle groups and appearing at different ages. The most common form is the Duchenne type, or so-called pseudohypertrophic progressive muscular dystrophy, a sex-linked disorder that usually begins before the age of 5 years.

Other myopathies. Weakness of muscles occurs in several disorders of inflammatory or noninflammatory nature. Examples of such diseases are dermatomyositis, polymyositis, polyarteritis nodosa, endocrine disorders (hyperthyroidism, acromegaly, etc.), amyloidosis, sarcoidosis, and glycogen storage disease due to deficiency of muscle phosphorylase (McArdle's disease). Myasthenia gravis is referred to on p. 604.

Polymyositis is an inflammatory and degenerative disorder involving the striated muscles that is generally regarded as an autoimmune disease. When there is skin involvement, the disease is known as *dermatomyositis* (p. 685). There have been several reports of electron microscopic evidence of picornaviruslike particles in the muscle of patients with polymyositis and dermatomyositis. Recently, in a case of chronic myopathy (? polymyositis), not only were picornaviruslike crystals found in the muscle tissue, but the presence of coxsackievirus type A9 was verified by viral isolation. Further investigations may determine whether this virus is etiologically related to polymyositis.

DISEASES OF EXTRAPYRAMIDAL MOTOR SYSTEM

In diseases of the extrapyramidal motor system, the lesions are localized or predominant in extrapyramidal parts known to affect motor activity. These parts include the thalamus, basal nuclei (caudate, putamen, globus pallidus, claustrum, amygdaloid), and several lower stem nuclei (subthalamic body, nucleus ruber, substantia nigra). Clinically, there are disturbances in motor activity manifested by tremor, choreiform movement, torsion spasm, or rigidity without true motor paralysis. The symptoms vary with the topography of the lesion.

Progressive lenticular degeneration (Wilson's disease). Progressive lenticular degeneration is a genetic (autosomal recessive) defect in copper and ceruloplasmin metabolism that appears in adolescents or young adults, its varying course in untreated patients usually progressing to a fatal ending in a few months to 10 years. There is bilateral symmetric degeneration and cavitation of the putamen and, occasionally, the caudate nucleus. The involved tissue develops a spongy consistency.

Microscopically, there is a distinct glial proliferation with the production of giant astrocytes.

Associated with the disease in the basal nuclei is a cirrhosis of the liver. An increased copper content has been demonstrated in the liver and the brain and, in the latter, particularly in the putamen, caudate nucleus, and globus pallidus. In addition to the tremor and spasticity of skeletal muscles, often there is striking emotional disturbance. A characteristic feature is the appearance of greenish pigmentation along the corneal margin (Kayser-Fleischer ring). In some patients, accumulation of copper in the kidneys may impair tubular reabsorption, leading to aminoaciduria, glycosuria, phosphaturia, and uricosuria. Treatment with metal binding agents (e.g., penicillamine) may reduce tissue copper stores.

Acute chorea (Sydenham's chorea). Acute chorea usually appears between the ages of 5 and 15 years. It is commonly associated with rheumatic fever. There may be an associated rheumatic myocarditis. The cerebral lesions are difficult to localize, but such striatal involvements as areas of softening, focal degenerations, toxic changes in striatal cells, and inflammatory foci of mild degree have been described.

Clinically, the disease is characterized by rapid, involuntary, purposeless movements and considerable incoordination, especially of the upper extremity. Mentality is not affected. Recovery occurs usually within 2 or 3 months but occasionally later.

Chronic progressive chorea (Huntington's chorea). Chronic progressive chorea is a familial progressive disease appearing in persons past 30 years of age. Sporadic cases are said to occur also.

Profound mental changes are associated with the grimacing, gesticulation, and incoordination of the chorea. The corpus striatum is severely shrunken, with dissolution predominant among the smaller cells, and degeneration is found in the supragranular layers of the cerebral cortex. Secondary gliosis is present in lesions of long standing. The hereditary pattern of transmission of the disease is autosomal dominant. Certain investigators have observed that lymphocytes from patients with Huntington's chorea responded in vitro to the presence of brain tissue from patients with the disease by producing migration inhibition factor, a correlate of cellular immune response, and only rarely responded to brain tissue from patients without the disease. Lymphocytes from individuals without Huntington's chorea did not respond to the diseased brain tissue.

Paralysis agitans (Parkinson's disease; shaking palsy). Paralysis agitans is characterized clinically by coarse tremor (at rest) and muscle rigidity, which is most prominent in the upper extremity. Ordinarily, the condition is progressive, with the eventual appearance of the tremor in the lower extremity, jaw, and tongue and a significant alteration in gait.

Two distinct forms, idiopathic and secondary, are recognized. Idiopathic paralysis agitans, or Parkinson's disease, begins during or after the involutional period and progresses slowly. The secondary form (postencephalitic parkinsonism) is associated with epidemic encephalitis, a form of encephalitis that is rarely diagnosed today (p. 165). A secondary parkinsonism also may follow chronic manganese poisoning or severe carbon monoxide or nitrous oxide intoxication. The syndrome also may occur as a result of intake of drugs, such as reserpine, phenothiazines, or occasionally methyldopa. Some investigators believe that cerebral arteriosclerosis may play an etiologic role in some patients.

In Parkinson's disease, there are degenerative changes in the basal nuclei that rarely may be evident grossly as lacunar softenings. Often, the changes in the basal nuclei are evident only on quantitative study. Loss of nerve cells and nonspecific cellular changes (pigmentation, degeneration, swelling, and shrinkage) predominate. The substantia nigra and locus ceruleus are the principal sites of involvement in idiopathic paralysis agitans. In the postencephalitic form, the degeneration is more widespread. An abnormality of dopamine metabolism (a deficiency of dopa decarboxylase) has been recognized in parkinsonism. The administration of L-dopa alleviates the symptoms of the disorder.

DISEASES OF INTRACRANIAL VESSELS

The vascular system of the meninges includes three distinctive sets of vessels: the dural sinuses and their tributaries (emissary veins and superficial cerebral veins), the meningeal arteries, and the subarachnoid arteries. The dural sinuses and their tributaries are important in regard to both infections and hemorrhage, and the meningeal and subarachnoid arteries are important principally in relation to hemorrhage.

Sinus thrombosis. Sinus thrombosis is essentially a thrombophlebitis of a dural sinus. Cavernous sinus thrombosis is related to infections of the nose, upper lip, cheek, orbit, and sphenoid and posterior ethmoid paranasal sinuses. Superior sagittal sinus thrombosis occurs as a sequel to frontal sinusitis. Transverse sinus thrombosis is most often related to middle ear and mastoid infections. Superficial infections of the scalp and neck and retropharyngeal abscesses also can give rise to sinus thrombosis by conduction along appropriate emissary veins. There is usually an associated leptomeningitis, and sinus thrombophlebitis is thought to be important in the pathogenesis of some brain abscesses (p. 758).

Epidural hemorrhage. Epidural hemorrhage ordinarily refers to blood in the temporal region from traumatic rupture of the middle meningeal artery or its branches, but rarely it is caused by a tear of an emissary vein as it enters a dural sinus. This may be found in the posterior fossa from rupture of the mastoid emissary vein as it enters the transverse sinus. Epidural hemorrhage is limited in extravasation to individual bone areas because of the dural attachments at the suture lines. The clot forming between the dura and bone compresses the underlying brain tissue.

Subdural hemorrhage (subdural hematoma). Subdural hemorrhage occurs when bleeding from dural vessels extravasates in a subdural position, forming a hematoma. The hematoma may be acute or chronic, and the latter tends to become limited by granulation tissue, probably with fibroblasts of arachnoidal and dural origin. The bleeding point may be difficult to localize, but in recent traumatic cases it can often be traced to the junction of superficial cerebral veins with dural sinuses. Usually, there is a small amount of subarachnoid extravasation resulting from arachnoid tears.

The hematoma is most frequent over the frontal and parietal areas and is often bilateral. Although it is generally regarded as traumatic, spontaneous cases have occurred in blood dyscrasias, infections, and toxemias. The hematoma organizes at its periphery, usually retaining a fluid center. Its clinical effects result from the fact that it is a space-occupying mass.

Subarachnoid hemorrhage. Subarachnoid hemorrhage is from subarachnoid arteries, which lie superficially in the subarachnoid spaces of the base of the brain and deep in the sulci over the other surfaces, or from subarachnoid veins, which occupy a superficial position over the vertex (Fig. 26-14). Bleeding from the latter vessels occurs as a result of trauma, blood dyscrasias, or rupture of a sur-

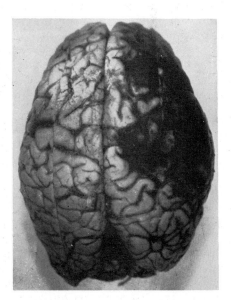

Fig. 26-14. Subarachnoid hemorrhage.

face angioma. Blood also may appear in the subarachnoid space by rupture from a hemorrhage in brain tissue or by conduction with cerebrospinal fluid from an intraventricular hemorrhage. However, subarachnoid bleeding most commonly is from a ruptured aneurysm. The aneurysms are usually basal in position at points of vessel branching. The most important aneurysms are congenital or mycotic and only rarely can be ascribed to arteriosclerosis and syphilis.

"Congenital" aneurysm. Congenital aneurysms (p. 293) are of fairly frequent occurrence. The angles of bifurcation of the arteries about the base of the brain are common sites (Fig. 26-15). They are caused by congenital weakness of the media at the point where the vessel branches. The aneurysm itself is not always congenital, although the defect in the vascular wall is a congenital or developmental abnormality. It may be associated with other developmental abnormalities, such as polycystic kidney. Small leakages may occur through the wall of the sac, giving rise to pigmentation and thickening of meninges in the neighborhood of the aneurysm. Rupture of the aneurysm results in a subarachnoid hemorrhage that is often rapidly fatal. The subarachnoid space about the region of the aneurysm (hence, usually at the base of the brain) is found filled by a recent blood clot. The clot may easily hide the aneurysm unless it is carefully removed. Occasionally, the hemorrhage extends into the ventricles. Aneurysms may be associated with cerebral infarction and sometimes with other complications, such as intracerebral hematoma and subarachnoid block with hydrocephalus.

Mycotic aneurysm. Mycotic aneurysms are produced by infected emboli lodging in cerebral vessels. Subacute bacterial endocarditis is the most common source of the embolus, and the middle cerebral artery is the most common site. Emboli bearing organisms of high virulence usually produce abscess or meningitis rather than mycotic aneurysm.

Birth injury. Birth injury may result from molding of the head during birth, which puts a strain on the falx of the dura and the tentorium over the cerebellum. A tear may result, sometimes with involvement of the dural sinuses or the great cerebral vein (of Galen), and some subarachnoid hemorrhage may be found also.

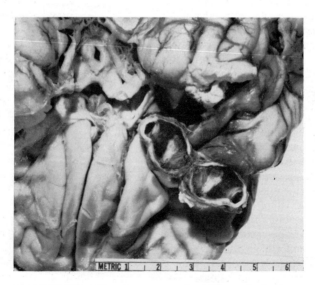

Fig. 26-15. Thrombosed aneurysm of middle cerebral artery.

INTRACEREBRAL VASCULAR DISEASES

Arteritis and vascular degeneration, with resulting thrombosis or hemorrhage, occur as a result of vascular damage from many poisons (carbon monoxide and arsenic) and in septic conditions (scarlet fever and pneumonia), blood dyscrasias (purpura and leukemia), polyarteritis nodosa, Buerger's disease, and syphilis. The brain tissue shows multiple small hemorrhages or softenings. Atherosclerosis and hypertension are the two important causes of intracerebral vascular disease.

Arteriosclerosis. Cerebral vessels are similar in structure to vessels elsewhere, although the small arteries contain a disproportionately large amount of connective tissue in their walls. With advancing age, muscle decreases, the internal elastic lamina undergoes reduplication, and there is a medial fibrosis. Arteriosclerosis of the larger vessels at the base of the brain is of the atherosclerotic type. Through weakening of the wall, aneurysms may form. Cerebral atherosclerosis may have no direct correlation with sclerotic changes elsewhere in the vascular system and has no constant relationship to hypertension. However, cerebral hyaline arteriolosclerosis is not uncommon with hypertension. Narrowing of the vascular lumina diminishes the blood supply and exerts a serious effect on brain tissue. Multiple perivascular zones of atrophy may be found in the brain as a result of atherosclerosis, in addition to larger softenings from thrombosis. Particularly susceptible to diminished blood supply are the striatum, hippocampus, dentate nucleus, and cerebral cortex.

Thrombosis. Thrombosis develops in cerebral vessels from the same causes as elsewhere. A sclerotic vessel usually is involved, and atherosclerosis is the most frequent underlying cause of cerebral infarction.

Embolism. Embolism of cerebral arteries originates mainly from thrombi in the left side of the heart (atrium or ventricle). Paradoxical embolism occurs from emboli breaking off in the right circulatory field and gaining access to the left side of the heart through an open foramen ovale or other right-to-left shunt. Air

and fat also act as emboli (p. 111). Massive infarction results most commonly from occlusion of branches of the middle cerebral artery, probably because this vessel is a direct continuation of the internal carotid artery. Consequently, the middle cerebral artery is in direct line for receiving emboli, as well as being subject to the wear and tear of direct pressure effects from the heart.

Infarction. Occlusion of a cerebral artery results in infarction of the region supplied by the vessel unless adequate collateral circulation is available. Even though abundant collaterals are present, they may be insufficient to maintain nutrition if an artery is blocked. Cerebral infarcts are characterized by softening. They may be ischemic or hemorrhagic. The clinical effects depend on the area of brain tissue involved.

The appearance of a cerebral infarct depends on its age. A recent ischemic infarct may be indistinguishable in a fresh brain, but after fixation it remains soft in comparison with surrounding tissue. If its age is greater than 2 or 3 days, it appears as a soft, semifluid area with a slightly yellowish color and an edematous, sometimes hemorrhagic, edge. Later, when the necrotic and liquefied material has been removed, the region is shrunken and depressed. If the infarcted area is large, it may have a cystlike center containing yellowish fluid *(apoplectic cyst)* encapsulated by glial tissue. A hemorrhagic infarct is initially an ischemic one in which considerable extravasation of blood occurs during its early stages.

Microscopically, a very recent infarct transiently contains neutrophilic leukocytes, but they soon disappear. Nerve cells, axis-cylinders, and neuroglial cells degenerate, and lipid of the myelin sheath is broken down and liquefied. The fatty and necrotic material undergoes phagocytosis and is removed by the ameboid microglial cells. These scavengers appear abundantly as rounded cells with a foamy or vacuolated cytoplasm (fatty granule cells or compound granular corpuscles). Healing occurs by proliferation of a granulation tissue composed of astrocytes, capillaries, and a few fibroblasts of the adventitia of adjacent vessels. Eventually, a dense neuroglial scar is formed. The damage is permanent, since there is no regeneration of the injured nerve cells and fibers.

Cerebral hemorrhage. Hemorrhages into the brain tissue itself may be either small petechial or perivascular hemorrhages or a massive hematoma. *Acute hemorrhagic leukoencephalitis* is an acute condition localized in the white matter of the cerebrum and characterized by focal perivascular hemorrhage, edema, demyelination, and necrosis. The cut surface of the white matter shows multiple hemorrhagic areas varying from minute points to several millimeters in diameter. The cause is unknown. Small petechial hemorrhages result from many types of trauma and may be found near gross cerebral lacerations. Petechial hemorrhages also may result from poisons such as carbon monoxide and arsphenamine, from cerebral fat embolism, or from purpuric or leukemic conditions (Fig. 26-16).

Massive intracerebral hemorrhage is caused by vascular disease with or without high blood pressure. It is a frequent result of hypertensive cardiovascular-renal disease. The vessels most commonly affected are the lenticulostriate branches of the middle cerebral artery, involving the basal ganglia and internal capsule. Less frequently, there is hemorrhage into the white matter of the cerebrum or into the pons or cerebellum. The actual mechanism of the hemorrhage is debatable, and it is usually impossible to find the point of vascular rupture. The brain bulges slightly on the side of the hemorrhage, where there is some flattening of the convolutions. Cutting through the brain tissue reveals the area of hemorrhage lacerating the brain substance. Rupture into a ventricle often occurs, and in such cases blood appears in the spinal fluid. Hemorrhage into cerebral tumor tissue may be grossly indistinguishable from the ordinary type of cerebral hemorrhage. Microscopic examination is necessary to confirm or rule out this possibility.

INTOXICATIONS AND VITAMIN DEFICIENCIES

Various degenerative lesions of the nervous system are caused by soluble toxins, chemical poisons, anesthesia, uremia, diabetic coma, hypoglycemia, and deficiency diseases.

The group caused by *soluble toxins* includes tetanus, botulism, and a heterogeneous group of undetermined cause referred to as "toxic" encephalopathy. *Tetanus* (p. 128) exerts its effect by its neurotropic toxin.

Chemical poisons, such as arsenic, lead, manganese, carbon monoxide, and alcohol, may give rise to degenerative changes in the nervous system. The mechanism is ascribed to actual toxic necrosis, implicating vascular structures primarily, or to relative or absolute anoxia. Pathologic alterations include edema, congestion, focal softenings, and hemorrhages. Actual inflammatory changes are rare. Because the changes are nonspecific, demonstration of the toxic substance is essential to diagnosis.

Streptomycin may cause degeneration and necrosis of neurons of the eighth cranial nerve nuclei, resulting in deafness and some vestibular dysfunction.

Anesthetic agents such as ether, chloroform, nitrous oxide, cyclopropane, and barbiturates have all been incriminated as occasional causes of death. Relative anoxia usually is described as the mechanism by which neuronal degeneration is induced. The cerebral changes produced by *anoxia* (e.g., in high altitude flying), circulatory arrest, carbon monoxide poisoning, hypoglycemia, and anesthetic agents are all very much alike, apparently influenced by both vascular and metabolic factors. Similar anoxic changes are found in fatalities after fever therapy. Ether and chloroform, as strong fat solvents, have been known to precipitate demyelination and are generally regarded as dangerous in any patient with a demyelinating disease. Microscopically, there may be found satellitosis, glial proliferation with the formation of glial nodes, and nonspecific changes in the nerve cell bodies, such as shrinkage and nuclear pyknosis.

Uremia may be accompanied by severe edema of the brain, with pressure marks and coning, and by cerebral anemia, believed to be caused by the swelling of the brain. The nerve cells are swollen, and sometimes there

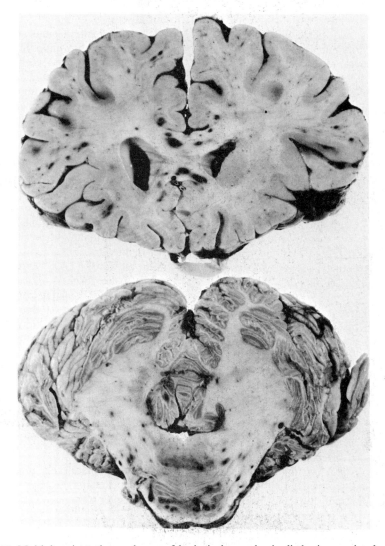

Fig. 26-16. Multiple minute hemorrhages of brain in hemorrhagic diathesis associated with leukemia.

is perivascular cuffing. The pathogenesis is obscure.

Diabetic coma is usually accompanied by little morphologic change. It usually is considered to result from relative anoxia rather than from toxemia. *Hypoglycemia* caused by insulin therapy or a tumor of pancreatic islet tissue may induce neurologic signs. Changes in the nervous system include chromatolytic, vacuolar, and pyknotic nerve cell alterations (nonspecific), formation of pseudogiant cells,

gemistocytosis, degeneration of axis-cylinders, and petechial hemorrhages.

Vitamin deficiency diseases, particularly pellagra, beriberi, pernicious anemia, rickets, and scurvy, may have associated nonspecific degenerative changes in the nervous system (p. 235). *Wernicke's encephalopathy,* associated with chronic alcoholism, is believed to be due to thiamine deficiency. The lesions, found in the mammillary bodies and in areas about the aqueduct and third and fourth ventricles, consist principally of degenerative changes and petechial hemorrhages. Deficiency of vitamin B$_{12}$, associated with pernicious anemia, results in *subacute combined degeneration of the spinal cord*. The lesions consist of patchy degeneration affecting the posterior and lateral columns of the cord, characterized by loss of myelin, oligodendroglia, and axons.

Burns, when extensive and severe, may result in cerebral edema, hyperemia, and small hemorrhages. Ganglion cells may show toxic changes, swelling, chromatolysis, and eccentric nuclei, and there may be small areas of demyelination. Degenerative changes in the brain, as well as in the peripheral nerves (neuropathy), occasionally occur as an unexplained remote effect of *visceral cancers,* e.g., bronchogenic carcinoma.

ENCEPHALITIS

Inflammatory diseases of the central nervous system may be caused by parasitic and fungal infections, syphilis, bacterial infections, rickettsial diseases, and viral diseases.

Parasitic and fungal infections. Parasitic and mycotic infections of the nervous system include those caused by *Toxoplasma, Trichina,* pork tapeworm (cysticercosis), malaria, and actinomycosis (Chapter 10). *Cryptococcus (Torula)* affects both the meninges and brain (p. 200). *Syphilis* frequently involves the central nervous system (p. 186).

Bacterial infection. Bacterial infection of the central nervous system may produce suppurative encephalitis or brain abscess. Staphylococci are the most common organisms, although streptococci, pneumococci, and others may be causative. Cultures at autopsy often yield mixed agents. The organism may be introduced by direct implantation (trauma or surgery), contiguous extension (e.g., from erosion of bone and dura over an otitis media), or metastatic extension (e.g., from bronchiectasis). A centrally located abscess sometimes has no identifiable primary focus, although it is assumed that all such abscesses are secondary to some other focus of infection, which is presumed to have disappeared while the brain abscess was developing. Lesions in which

brain abscess is commonly a complication include otitis media, sinus thrombophlebitis, bronchiectasis, empyema, lung abscess, bacterial endocarditis, and congenital heart disease with right-to-left shunts.

Brain abscesses occur most commonly in the temporal lobe and cerebellar hemispheres. If embolic, they are usually multiple. Grossly, the abscess is encapsulated and has a fluid, purulent center (Fig. 26-17). The developing abscess goes through the changes of focal necrosis, invasion by leukocytes, liquefaction and formation of pus, fatty granule cell reaction, peripheral fibrinous exudate, surrounding hyperemia and fibroblastic proliferation, and mild marginal gliosis. The fully formed abscess thus has four microscopic layers from within outward: (1) a central necrotic core (cavity of the abscess), (2) a vascular granulomatous border (reactive zone), (3) a zone of hyperemia and fibrosis, and (4) an external zone of gliosis (encephalitic zone).

Spontaneous resolution of a cerebral abscess probably does not occur. Rupture of an abscess results in disseminated suppurative encephalitis and purulent meningitis. Usually, encapsulation occurs in a variable time of a few days to a few weeks. Abscesses caused by aerobic bacteria tend to form better capsules than those caused by anaerobic bacteria or mixed infections.

Viral and rickettsial infections. Various viral and rickettsial infections produce encephalitis (Chapter 8).

MENINGITIS
Pachymeningitis

Inflammation of the dura may develop by spread from overlying bone. Hence, it may complicate osteomyelitis of the skull, compound fracture, etc. The dura tends to localize the lesion with the production of an *epidural abscess*. The overlying area of the scalp is swollen, congested, and edematous (so-called Pott's puffy tumor). Spinal epidural abscess may cause paraplegia. *Subdural abscess* may occur secondary to neighboring infections. This consists of a broad limited sheet of purulent material or organized exudate.

Peripachymeningitis is an inflammatory

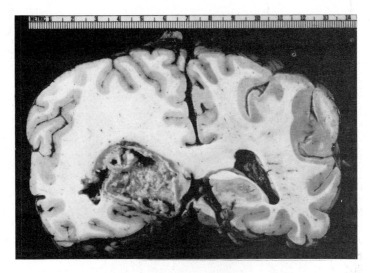

Fig. 26-17. Abscess of brain.

condition associated with Pott's disease of the spine (p. 710). *Pachymeningitis cervicalis hypertrophica* is a pronounced thickening of the dura in the cervical region that may be associated with syphilis.

Leptomeningitis

Inflammations of the leptomeninx may be purulent, caused by bacterial or actinomycotic infections, or nonpurulent, caused by tuberculous, syphilitic, lymphocytic, or *Cryptococcus* meningitis.

Purulent meningitis

Purulent meningitis may be caused by meningococci, pneumococci, streptococci, staphylococci, gonococci, *Haemophilus influenzae,* colon bacilli, and actinomyces. The most important of these is the meningococcus, which gives rise to the epidemic form of meningitis as well as to occasional sporadic cases.

In meningococcal meningitis, it has been suggested that the organism passes through the nasopharynx, where it leaves no trace, and then along the perineural sheath of the olfactory nerve and through the cribriform plate of the ethmoid to reach the meninges. However, the most likely route of meningeal infection is by the bloodstream. Acute fulminating forms of meningococcal infection are septicemic and systemic with hemorrhagic spots in the skin—hence, the term *spotted fever*. The purulent exudate is most abundant over the base of the brain, and extension commonly occurs to the spinal meninges. The infection usually spreads to the choroid plexus and the interior of the ventricles. Some degree of acute internal hydrocephalus results from an increased permeability of the choroid plexus, an outpouring of exudate into the ventricles, and interference with outflow caused by inflammatory swelling about the narrow ventricular openings. This condition, along with edema, congestion of blood vessels, and subarachnoid exudate, increases the intracranial pressure.

The other purulent meningitides resemble the meningococcal form both grossly and microscopically, necessitating identification of the organism for diagnosis. Streptococcal and pneumococcal exudates appear most abundantly over the vertex, whereas meningococcal exudate tends to aggregate at the base (Fig. 26-18). In meningitis caused by *Haemophilus influenzae,* the exudate is most abundant and diffuse. The microscopic appearance of an extensive purulent exudate in the leptomeninges is noted in Fig. 26-19.

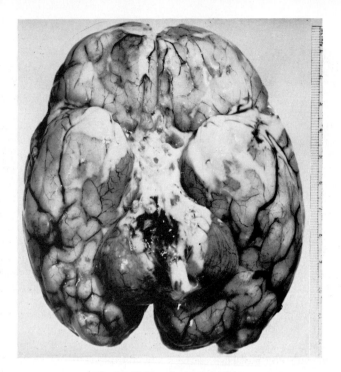

Fig. 26-18. Purulent meningitis.

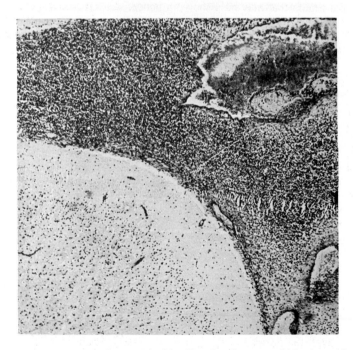

Fig. 26-19. Acute purulent meningitis. Note involvement of blood vessels.

Nonpurulent meningitis

A variety of infections may cause a meningitis with a nonpurulent type of exudate.

Tuberculous meningitis. Tuberculous meningitis is a nonpurulent meningitis that is secondary to a tuberculous lesion elsewhere and often only a part of a generalized miliary tuberculosis. In other cases, it is the most prominent active focus of tuberculosis in the body. It is almost invariably fatal. The brain is swollen, and a gelatinous, translucent, slightly greenish exudate may be evident in the subarachnoid space. If exudate is abundant, it usually involves the base of the brain and spreads through the sylvian cisterns. Tiny opaque yellowish flecks, which represent minute tubercles, are evident along the course of subarachnoid vessels or on the choroid plexus.

Microscopically, the inflammatory reaction and exudate are, in general, similar to tuberculosis elsewhere but tend to show more neutrophilic leukocytes. The predominant cells, however, are large mononuclear cells, lymphocytes, plasma cells, and epithelioid cells. Small areas of caseation and definite tubercles may be found. Giant cells are not numerous.

Since the inflammatory process often involves the superficial portions of the cortex, the condition is really a meningoencephalitis. Blood vessels passing through the exudate show adventitial inflammation and intimal thickening (tuberculous arteritis). Fibroblastic proliferation causes a meningeal thickening. Tubercles may be found involving the choroid plexus and ependyma.

The pathogenesis of tuberculous meningitis is a matter of dispute. The three main theories are (1) hematogenous infection of the cerebrospinal fluid, (2) hematogenous spread to the choroid plexus, with the development there of a tubercle that later infects the leptomeninges, and (3) hematogenous spread to the superficial cerebral cortex, with the development of a localized tubercle that later ruptures or spreads infection to the meninges.

Tuberculoma of the brain is a large solitary tuberculous lesion (Fig. 26-20). Its symptoms may cause confusion with a neoplasm. The microscopic structure is similar to that of tuberculous lesions elsewhere.

Lymphocytic choriomeningitis. Lymphocytic choriomeningitis is caused by a virus and

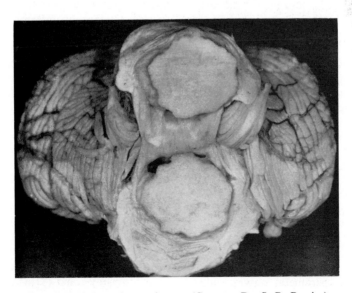

Fig. 26-20. Tuberculoma of pons. (Courtesy Dr. S. B. Pessin.)

has a transitory, nonfatal course. There is considerable lymphocytic infiltration of the subarachnoid spaces, with the appearance of large numbers of lymphocytes in the cerebrospinal fluid (p. 166).

Cryptococcus meningitis. *Cryptococcus* meningitis is a chronic meningeal irritation caused by a fungus, *Cryptococcus hominis* (p. 201).

Syphilitic meningitis. See p. 187.

INCREASED INTRACRANIAL PRESSURE

The relative rigidity of the cranial vault leads to increased intracranial tension from changes in volume of its contents. For this reason, space-occupying lesions, conditions limiting the flow of cerebrospinal fluid, and edema of the brain give rise to an elevated intracranial pressure. This brings about certain pathologic changes of great clinical importance.

The subarachnoid space often is obliterated, and the surface of the brain is dry. Underlying gyri are compressed and very flattened, and the sulci are obscured. The opposing walls of the ventricles may be in apposition. A distinctive characteristic is the appearance of pressure marks along the base of the brain. The cerebellar tonsils may be shoved over the brim of the foramen magnum, grooving the cerebellum (coning). In addition, the swollen temporal lobes may spread over the free margins of the tentorial aperture, with a consequent linear grooving on their medial surfaces. Compression of the upper part of the brainstem may be caused by the herniated portions of the temporal lobes. The result is interference with venous circulation of the pons, followed by passive congestion and pontine hemorrhages. *Papilledema* (choked disc), a swelling of the optic nerve head that may be seen ophthalmoscopically, is a possible effect of increased intracranial pressure.

DISEASES OF PERIPHERAL NERVES

The diseases of peripheral nerves, other than the neoplasms discussed previously, fall into the three ill-defined categories of neuralgia, neuropathy, and traumatic injury. The changes resulting from peripheral nerve trauma are those of wallerian degeneration and neuroma formation (pp. 732-733).

Neuralgia. The term *neuralgia* simply means pain, usually paroxysmal, along the course of one or more nerves. It does not refer to any particular disease. Such pain may be produced by known causes (e.g., compression or trauma of a nerve or its spinal roots, as in sciatic nerve involvement by a herniated intervertebral disc or tumor, and the various forms of neuropathy or neuritis of metabolic, nutritional, or infectious origin). However, the term is commonly applied to those conditions in which usually no definite cause or morphologic change in the nerves can be identified. Typical examples are trigeminal neuralgia (tic douloureux) and glossopharyngeal neuralgia. Although the cause of these neuralgias is usually not known, in some instances various inciting or precipitating factors may be recognized.

Neuropathy. The term *neuropathy* is used in referring to any degenerative or inflammatory changes in peripheral nerves. Sometimes, the term *neuritis* is used loosely for all disorders of peripheral nerves but should be restricted to the inflammatory lesions. When many nerves are involved, the condition is described as *polyneuropathy* or *polyneuritis;* if one nerve is involved, as *mononeuropathy* or *mononeuritis*. Various changes that may be found include hyperemia of the nerve sheath, transudation and swelling, cellular exudate, myelin degeneration, and swelling and fragmentation of axis-cylinders. Once continuity of fibers is broken, secondary wallerian degeneration occurs. From an etiologic standpoint, the neuropathies may be grouped under the following headings: (1) viral (herpes), (2) bacteriotoxic (scarlet fever and diphtheria), (3) deficiency or metabolic (beriberi and diabetes mellitus), (4) chemical (lead), (5) focal mechanical (tumor pressure), (6) focal infectious (leprosy), (7) hereditary (hypertrophic interstitial neuropathy), and (8) undetermined cause, possibly immunologic (Guillain-Barré syndrome). In each category there are more examples than those listed in the parentheses.

The so-called *infectious polyneuritis* or polyradiculitis *(Guillain-Barré syndrome)* is a polyneuropathy of sudden onset with widespread flaccid paralysis and increased protein in the spinal fluid without a corresponding increase in the number of cells. The etiology and pathogenesis have not been established, but one concept is that it is an allergic (autoimmune) phenomenon. It is often preceded by infections, particularly viral, and has been known to occur after vaccinations (e.g., swine flu vaccination). It may also be associated with pregnancy, malignant neoplasms (particularly lymphoproliferative lesions), and infectious mononucleosis. In some patients, however, there is no preceding or associated illness. Complement-dependent antimyelin antibodies have been demonstrated in the serum of patients with the Guillain-Barré syndrome, which supports the view that autoimmune mechanisms directed against myelin sheaths of the nerves may play a role in the pathogenesis.

REFERENCES

Abell, M. R., et al.: Hum. Pathol. **1**:503-551, 1970 (tumors of peripheral nervous system).

Adams, D. H., and Dickinson, J. P.: Lancet **1**:1196-1199, 1974 (etiology of multiple sclerosis).

Alpers, B. J., and Mancall, E. L.: Clinical neurology, ed. 6, Philadelphia, 1971, F. A. Davis Co.

Anderson, M. S.: Cancer **19**:585-590, 1966 (myxopapillary ependymoma).

Bannister, R.: Brain's clinical neurology, ed. 5, Oxford, 1978, Oxford University Press.

Barkley, D. S., et al.: Science **195**:314-316, 1977 (Huntington's disease—delayed hypersensitivity studies).

Blackwood, W., and Corsellis, J. A. N., editors: Greenfield's neuropathology, ed. 3, London, 1976, Edward Arnold (Publishers) Ltd.

Burger, P. C., and Vogel, F. S.: Am. J. Pathol. **92**:253-314, 1978 (cerebrovascular disease—a teaching monograph).

Burstein, S. D., et al.: Cancer **16**:289-305, 1963 (reticulum cell sarcoma of brain).

Crozier, R. E., and Ainley, A. B.: N. Engl. J. Med. **252**:83-88, 1955 (Guillain-Barré syndrome).

Crue, B. L.: Medulloblastoma, Springfield, Ill., 1958, Charles C Thomas, Publisher.

Harkin, J. C., and Reed, R. J.: Tumors of the peripheral nervous system. In Atlas of tumor pathology, Series 2, Fasc. 3, Washington, D.C., 1969, Armed Forces Institute of Pathology.

Kepes, J., and Kernohan, J. W.: Cancer **12**:364-370, 1959 (meningiomas).

Kernohan, J. W., and Sayre, C. P.: Tumors of the central nervous system. In Atlas of tumor pathology, Sect. 10, Fascs. 35 and 37, Washington, D.C., 1952, Armed Forces Institute of Pathology.

Koch, M. J., et al.: J.A.M.A. **228**:1555-1557, 1974 (multiple sclerosis).

Lampert, P. W.: Am. J. Pathol. **91**:175-208, 1978 (autoimmune and virus-induced demyelinating disease—a review).

Miles, J., and Bhandari, Y. S.: J. Neurol. Neurosurg. Psychiatry **33**:208-211, 1970 (cerebellar medulloblastomas in adults).

Minckler, J., editor: Pathology of the nervous system, vol. 1, New York, 1968, McGraw-Hill Book Co.

Minckler, J., editor: Pathology of the nervous system, vol. 2, New York, 1971, McGraw-Hill Book Co.

Minckler, J., editor: Pathology of the nervous system, vol. 3, New York, 1972, McGraw-Hill Book Co.

Pearce, G. W., and Walton, J. N.: J. Pathol. Bacteriol. **83**:535-550, 1962 (progressive muscular dystrophy).

Pearson, C. M.: N. Engl. J. Med. **292**:641-642, 1975 (myopathy with virallike structures).

Rubinstein, L. J.: Tumors of the central nervous system. In Atlas of Tumor Pathology, Series 2, Fasc. 6, Washington, D.C., 1972, Armed Forces Institute of Pathology.

Russell, D. S., and Rubinstein, L. J.: Pathology of tumours of the nervous system, ed. 4, Baltimore, 1977, The Williams & Wilkins Co.

Sakai, M., et al.: Arch. Neurol. **21**:526-544, 1969 (corpora amylacea).

Scotti, T. M.: Arch. Pathol. **63**:91-102, 1957 (plantar digital neuroma—Morton's toe).

Tang, T. T., et al.: N. Engl. J. Med. **292**:608-611, 1975 (chronic myopathy associated with coxsackievirus type A9).

Zacks, S. I.: Atlas of neuropathology, New York, 1971, Harper & Row, Publishers, Inc.

Zülch, K. J., and Wechsler, W.: Progr. Neurol. Surg. **2**:1-84, 1968 (pathology and classification of gliomas).

Index

Paragranuloma, Hodgkin's, 489
Parakeratosis, 681
  in contact dermatitis, 682
Paralysis
  agitans, 752
  familial periodic, hypokalemia in, 100
  immunologic, 77-78
Paraneoplastic syndromes, 251-252
  in liver cancer, 457
  in thymoma, 604
Paraphimosis, 377
Parathyroid glands, 598-602
  diseases of, 600-602
  structure and function of, 598-600
Parathyroid hormone, 598, 700
Paratyphoid fever, 545
Paresis, general, 188
Parkinson's disease, 752
  postencephalitic, 166
Parotid glands
  in mumps, 174, 518
  tumors of, 519-523
Parotitis, acute, 174, 518
Pasteurella
  pestis, 130
  tularensis, 131
Paul-Bunnell test in infectious mononucleosis, 481
Pearls, epithelial, in squamous cell carcinoma of skin, 690
Peliosis hepatis, 441
Pellagra, 235
Pemphigoid, bullous, 683
Pemphigus vulgaris, 93, 683
Penis, 377-378
Peptic ulcer, 530-535
Periarteritis nodosa, 287-288, 352
Pericardial lesions, 302-305
Pericarditis
  acute, 303
  adhesive, 304, 326
  chronic constrictive, 304-305
  in pneumonia, 409
  rheumatic, 307
  tuberculous, 145, 303-304
Pericytes, 298
Periodontal disease, 513
Periosteal fibrosarcoma, 712
Periostitis, syphilitic, 709
Peripachymeningitis, 758-759
Peripheral nerves
  in amyloid disease, 36
  in beriberi, 235
  in diabetes, 471
  diseases of, 762-763
  in leprosy, 148
  neurilemoma, 266, 267
  reaction to injury, 732
  regeneration of, 73
  sheath of Schwann, 731, 734
  tumors of, 742-743
Peritoneum, 571-573

Peritonitis, 571-572
  in appendicitis, 553
  biliary, 571-572
  coliform bacterial, 571
  gonococcal, 571
  periodic, 572
  pneumococcal, 571
  streptococcal, 571
  tuberculous, 145, 572
Perivascular cuffing in viral diseases, 162
Peroneal muscular atrophy, 751
Peroxisomes, 4
Pertussis, 128
Pesticides, toxic effects of, 230, 354
Petechiae, 102
  in scurvy, 236
Petrolatum, liquid, pneumonia from, 411-413
Petroleum products, toxic effects of, 227
Peutz-Jeghers syndrome, 561, 566, 697
Peyer's patches in typhoid fever, 544
Peyronie's disease, 377
Phagocytic cells, 476
  in bone, 700
Phagocytosis, 1, 61-63
  disorders of, 63
    infections in, 120
  by eosinophils, 59
  by giant cells, 62
  by macrophages, 58, 60, 62
  of nerve cells, 732
  by plasma cells, 59
  and resistance to infection, 120
Phagolysosome, 3, 62
Phagosome, 3, 62
Pharyngeal pouch syndrome, 603
Pharyngitis, 516
  acute febrile, 168
  streptococcal, 125
Pharyngoconjunctival fever, 168
Pharynx
  inflammations of, 516
  tumors of, 516-518
Phenacetin, nephritis from, 356, 358
Phenol poisoning, 221
Phenothiazines, adverse effects of, 227, 327
Phenotype, 8
Phenylketonuria, 16, 17
Pheochromocytoma, 326, 616-618
Phialophora infection, 204
Philadelphia chromosome, 14-15, 505
Phimosis, 377
Phlebitis, 293-294
Phleboliths, 111
Phlebothrombosis, 109, 294
Phlegmon, 67
Phocomelia, 228, 300
Phosphate stones, 362
Phosphatide lipidosis, 493
Phosphorus poisoning, 223
Photochromogens, 147
Phycomycosis, 198-199